Advanced Therapy in Surgical Oncology

Advanced Therapy in Surgical Oncology

Raphael E. Pollock, MD, PhD
Steven A. Curley, MD
Merrick I. Ross, MD
Nancy D. Perrier, MD

MD Anderson Cancer Center
University of Texas
Houston, Texas

2008
BC Decker Inc
Hamilton

BC Decker Inc
P.O. Box 620, L.C.D. 1
Hamilton, Ontario L8N 3K7
Tel: 905-522-7017; 800-568-7281
Fax: 905-522-7839; 888-311-4987
E-mail: info@bcdecker.com
www.bcdecker.com

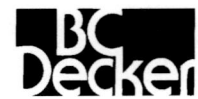

08 09 10 11 12 / WPC / 9 8 7 6 5 4 3 2 1

ISBN 978-1-55009-126-7
Printed in the United States of America by Walsworth Printing Company

Sales and Distribution

United States
BC Decker Inc
P.O. Box 785
Lewiston, NY 14092-0785
Tel: 905-522-7017; 800-568-7281
Fax: 905-522-7839; 888-311-4987
E-mail: info@bcdecker.com
www.bcdecker.com

Canada
McGraw-Hill Ryerson Education
Customer Care
300 Water St.
Whitby, Ontario   L1N 9B6
Tel: 1-800-565-5758
Fax: 1-800-463-5885

Foreign Rights
John Scott & Company
International Publishers' Agency
P.O. Box 878
Kimberton, PA 19442
Tel: 610-827-1640
Fax: 610-827-1671
E-mail: jsco@voicenet.com

Japan
United Publishers Services Limited
1-32-5 Higashi-Shinagawa
Shinagawa-Ku, Tokyo 140-0002
Tel: 03 5479 7251
Fax: 03 5479 7307

UK, Europe, Middle East
McGraw-Hill Education
Shoppenhangers Road
Maidenhead
Berkshire, England SL6 2QL
Tel: 44-0-1628-502500
Fax: 44-0-1628-635895
www.mcgraw-hill.co.uk

Singapore, Malaysia,Thailand, Philippines, Indonesia, Vietnam, Pacific Rim, Korea
McGraw-Hill Education
60 Tuas Basin Link
Singapore 638775
Tel: 65-6863-1580
Fax: 65-6862-3354

Australia, New Zealand
McGraw-Hill Australia
Pty LtdLevel 2, 82 Waterloo Road
North Ryde, NSW, 2113Australia

Customer Service Australia
Phone: +61 (2) 9900 1800
Fax: +61 (2) 9900 1980
Email: cservice_sydney@mcgraw-hill.com

Customer Service New Zealand
Phone (Free Phone): +64 (0) 800 449 312
Fax (Free Phone): +64 (0) 800 449 318
Email: cservice@mcgraw-hill.co.nz

Mexico and Central America
ETM SA de CV
Calle de Tula 59
Colonia Condesa
06140 Mexico DF, Mexico
Tel: 52-5-5553-6657
Fax: 52-5-5211-8468
E-mail: editoresdetextosmex@
prodigy.net.mx

Brazil
Tecmedd Importadora E Distribuidora
De Livros Ltda.
Avenida Maurílio Biagi, 2850
City Ribeirão, Ribeirão Preto –
SP – Brasil
CEP: 14021-000
Tel: 0800 992236
Fax: (16) 3993-9000
E-mail: tecmedd@tecmedd.com.br

India, Bangladesh, Pakistan, Sri Lanka
CBS Publishers & Distributors
4596/1A-11, Darya Ganj
New Delhi-2, India
Tel: 23271632
Fax: 23276712
E-mail: cbspubs@vsnl.com

PREFACE

Why a textbook in surgical oncology? What is so distinctive about this field that a comprehensive treatise is needed? To answer these questions it is important to first define the area of expertise encompassed by the discipline of surgical oncology. Next it is our obligation to convince you that this comprehensive textbook has value added by covering in depth all aspects of this dynamic field. Having accomplished these goals, we may then be able to identify those who might optimally benefit by consulting this new textbook.

Being a surgical oncologist is not synonymous with being a cancer surgeon. A cancer surgeon is a surgeon who operates on and removes solid tumors, whereas a surgical oncologist is an oncologist who uses surgery as his or her treating modality. This difference is important because it identifies the reality that surgical oncology is a cognitive rather than a technical and anatomically defined surgical specialty. As such, the surgical oncologist requires and receives additional training in the natural history of solid tumor disease as well as the multidisciplinary therapy of solid malignancy. Armed with this additional information, the surgical oncologist is in the optimal position to define the role of surgical intervention as defined against the larger timeline and continuum of tumor bearing that typifies the host-malignancy relationship.

In light of these distinctions, this textbook seeks to provide a broad-based cognitive presentation about the natural history of the major solid tumor systems that fall under the purview of the surgical oncologist. The role of non-surgical therapies is thoroughly discussed as are the many developments in the research laboratories that are becoming part of our standard therapeutic armamentarium now and in the relatively near future.

This textbook will be particularly useful to the surgical oncologist in practice or in training. Other oncology specialists who seek to learn more about the role of surgical oncology therapy in diseases of interest, as well as medical students, surgical residents, and surgical practitioners who have an abiding interest in the cancer patient will hopefully find this volume to be of value. We deeply appreciate your interest in this rapidly expanding surgical specialty, and hope that this textbook provides you with a useful entre to this important area of endeavor!

Raphael E. Pollock
Steven A. Curley
Merrick I. Ross
Nancy D. Perrier
July 2007

CONTRIBUTORS

Eddie K. Abdalla, MD
Department of Surgical Oncology
University of Texas
MD Anderson Cancer Center
Houston, Texas

Syed A. Ahmad, MD
Department of Surgery
University of Cincinnati
Cincinnati, Ohio

Daniel Albo, MD, PhD
Department of Surgery
Baylor College of Medicine
Houston, Texas

Waddah B. Al-Refaie, MD
Department of Surgical Oncology
University of Texas
MD Anderson Cancer Center
Houston, Texas

Frederick C. Ames, MD
Department of Surgical Oncology
University of Texas
MD Anderson Cancer Center
Houston, Texas

Keith D. Amos, MD
Department of Surgical Oncology
University of Texas
MD Anderson Cancer Center
Houston, Texas

Johanna R. Askegard-Giesmann, MD
Department of Surgery
Mayo Clinic
Rochester, Minnesota

Gildy V. Babiera, MD
Department of Surgical Oncology
University of Texas
MD Anderson Cancer Center
Houston, Texas

Matthew T. Ballo, MD
Department of Surgical Oncology
University of Texas
MD Anderson Cancer Center
Houston, Texas

Carlton C. Barnett Jr, MD Department of
Surgery
University of Texas Southwestern
    Medical Center
Dallas, Texas

Isabelle Bedrosian, MD
Department of Surgical Oncology
University of Texas
MD Anderson Cancer Center
Houston, Texas

David J. Bentrem, MD
Department of Surgery
Northwestern University
Chicago, Illinois

David H. Berger, MD
Department of Surgery
Baylor College of Medicine
Houston, Texas

Russell S. Berman, MD
Department of Surgery
New York University
New York, New York

Christina Bertocchi, MD
Department of Surgery
Drexel University College of Medicine
Pittsburgh, Pennsylvania

Therese Bevers, MD
Department of Gynecologic Oncology
University of Texas
MD Anderson Cancer Center
Houston, Texas

Shanda H. Blackmon, MD, MPH
Department of Thoracic and
    Cardiovascular Surgery
University of Texas
MD Anderson Cancer Center
Houston, Texas

Judy C. Boughey, MD
Department of Surgical Oncology
University of Texas
MD Anderson Cancer Center
Houston, Texas

Michael Bouvet, MD
Department of Surgery
VA San Diego Healthcare System
San Diego, California

Thomas Buchholz, MD
Department of Radiation Oncology
University of Texas
MD Anderson Cancer Center
Houston, Texas

Charles Catton, MD
Department of Radiation Oncology
University of Toronto
Toronto, Ontario, Canada

Abigail S. Caudle, MD
Department of Surgery
University of North Carolina
Chapel Hill, North Carolina

Anees B. Chagpar, MD, MSc
Department of Surgery
University of Louisville
Louisville, Kentucky

George J. Chang, MD
Department of Surgical Oncology
University of Texas
MD Anderson Cancer Center
Houston, Texas

Chusilp Charnsangavej, MD
Department of Radiology
University of Texas
MD Anderson Cancer Center
Houston, Texas

Herbert Chen, MD
Department of Surgery
University of Wisconsin
Madison, Wisconsin

Eugene A. Choi, MD
Department of Surgical Oncology
University of Texas
MD Anderson Cancer Center
Houston, Texas

Peter Chung, MD
Department of Radiation Oncology
University of Toronto
Toronto, Ontario, Canada

Gary L. Clayman, MD
Department of Head and Neck Surgery
University of Texas
MD Anderson Cancer Center
Houston, Texas

Janice N. Cormier, MD, MPH
Department of Surgical Oncology
University of Texas
MD Anderson Cancer Center
Houston, Texas

Charles S. Cox Jr, MD
Department of Pediatric Surgical
    Oncology
University of Texas
MD Anderson Cancer Center
Houston, Texas

Christopher H. Crane, MD
Department of Radiation Oncology
University of Texas
MD Anderson Cancer Center
Houston, Texas

Steven A. Curley, MD
Department of Surgical Oncology
University of Texas
MD Anderson Cancer Center
Houston, Texas

Alan PB Dackiw, MD, PhD
Department of Surgery
Johns Hopkins University School of
    Medicine
Baltimore, Maryland

Prajnan Das, MD, MS, MPH
Department of Radiation Oncology
University of Texas
MD Anderson Cancer Center
Houston, Texas

Shaheenah Dawood, MD
Department of Breast Medical Oncology
University of Texas
MD Anderson Cancer Center
Houston, Texas

Marc E. Delclos, MD
Department of Radiation Oncology
University of Texas
MD Anderson Cancer Center
Houston, Texas

Keith A. Delman, MD
Department of Surgery
Emory University
Atlanta, Georgia

Elijah Dixon, MD, MSc (Epi)
Department of Surgery
University of Calgary
Calgary, Alberta, Canada

Jay Douglas, MD
Department of Radiation Oncology
University of Washington
Seattle, Washington

Frederick R. Eilber, MD
Department of Surgical Oncology
University of California
Los Angeles, California

Fritz C. Eilber, MD
Department of Surgical Oncology
University of California
Los Angeles, California

Danielle D. Elliott, MD
Department of Pathology
University of Texas
MD Anderson Cancer Center
Houston, Texas

Cathy Eng, MD
Department of Surgical Oncology
University of Texas
MD Anderson Cancer Center
Houston, Texas

Nestor F. Esnaola, MD, MPH
Department of Surgery Medical
University of South Carolina
Charleston, South Carolina

Douglas B. Evans, MD
Department of Surgical Oncology
University of Texas
MD Anderson Cancer Center
Houston, Texas

David R. Farley, MD
Department of Surgery
Mayo Clinic
Rochester, Minnesota

Barry W. Feig, MD
Department of Surgery
University of Texas

MD Anderson Cancer Center
Houston, Texas

William E. Fisher, MD
Department of Surgery
Baylor College of Medicine
Houston, Texas

Jason B. Fleming, MD
Department of Surgery
University of Texas
Southwestern Medical Center
Dallas, Texas

Paul G. Gauger, MD
Department of Surgery
University of Michigan
Ann Arbor, Michigan

Jeff Gershenwald, MD
Department of Surgical Oncology
University of Texas
MD Anderson Cancer Center
Houston, Texas

Clive S. Grant, MD
Department of Surgery
Mayo Clinic
Rochester, Minnesota

Sanjay Gupta, MD
Department of Diagnostic Radiology
University of Texas
MD Anderson Cancer Center
Houston, Texas

Mouhammed Amir Habra, MD
Department of Surgery
Baylor College of Medicine
Houston, Texas

Frank Haluska, MD, PhD
Department of Hematology and
   Oncology
Tufts New England Medical Center
Boston, Massachusetts

Andrea A. Hayes-Jordan, MD
Department of Pediatric Surgical
   Oncology
University of Texas
MD Anderson Cancer Center
Houston, Texas

Luis J. Herrera, MD
Department of Thoracic and
   Cardiovascular Surgery
University of Texas
MD Anderson Cancer Center
Houston, Texas

Paulo Hoff, MD
Department of Surgical Oncology
University of Texas
MD Anderson Cancer Center
Houston, Texas

Wayne Hofstetter, MD
Department of Thoracic and
   Cardiovascular Surgery
University of Texas
MD Anderson Cancer Center
Houston, Texas

Jonathan C. Hundley, MD
Department of Surgery
University of Michigan
Ann Arbor, Michigan

Kelly K. Hunt, MD
Department of Surgical Oncology
University of Texas
MD Anderson Cancer Center
Houston, Texas

Rosa F. Hwang, MD
Department of Surgical Oncology
University of Texas
MD Anderson Cancer Center
Houston, Texas

Francesco Izzo, MD
Department of Surgical Oncology
G. Pascale National Cancer Institute
Naples, Italy

Jackie Jeruss, MD
Department of Surgery
Northwestern University
Chicago, Illinois

Kevin Kalinsky, MD
Department of Hematology and Oncology
Tufts New England Medical Center
Boston, Massachusetts

Andreas Karachristos, MD, PhD
Department of Surgery
Temple University School of Medicine
Philadelphia, Pennsylvania

Matthew H. Katz, MD
Department of Surgery
University of California
San Diego, California

Electron Kebebew, MD
Department of Surgery
University of California
San Francisco, California

Farid J. Kehdy, MD
Department of Surgery
University of Louisville
Louisville, Kentucky

Debra L. Kennamer, MD
Department of Anesthesiology and Pain
   Medicine
University of Texas
MD Anderson Cancer Center
Houston, Texas

Eric Kleinbaum, MD
Department of Sarcoma Medical
   Oncology
University of Texas
MD Anderson Cancer Center
Houston, Texas

Christopher Klem, MD
Department of Otolaryngology
Tripler Army Medical Center
Honolulu, Hawaii

Scott Kopetz, MD
Department of Gastrointestinal Medical
   Oncology

University of Texas
MD Anderson Cancer Center
Houston, Texas

Maria A. Kouvaraki, MD, PhD
Department of Surgical Oncology
University of Texas
MD Anderson Cancer Center
Houston, Texas

Steven J. Kronowitz, MD
Department of Plastic Surgery
University of Texas
MD Anderson Cancer Center
Houston, Texas

Henry M. Kuerer, MD, PhD
Department of Surgical Oncology
University of Texas
MD Anderson Cancer Center
Houston, Texas

Michael E. Kupferman, MD
Department of Head and Neck Surgery
University of Texas
MD Anderson Cancer Center
Houston, Texas

Ann S. La Casce, MD
Department of Medical Oncology
Harvard Medical School
Boston, Massachusetts

Kevin P. Lally, MD
Department of Pediatric Surgical
  Oncology
University of Texas
MD Anderson Cancer Center
Houston, Texas

Laura A. Lambert, MD
Department of Surgical Oncology
University of Texas
MD Anderson Cancer Center
Houston, Texas

Jeffrey E. Lee, MD
Department of Surgical Oncology
University of Texas
MD Anderson Cancer Center
Houston, Texas

Patrick P. Lin, MD
Department of Surgical Oncology
University of Texas
MD Anderson Cancer Center
Houston, Texas

Andrew M. Lowy, MD
Department of Surgery
University of Cincinnati
Cincinnati, Ohio

Anthony Lucci, MD
Department of Surgical Oncology
University of Texas
MD Anderson Cancer Center
Houston, Texas

Robert G. Maki, MD, PhD
Department of Medicine
Memorial Sloan-Kettering Cancer Center
New York, New York

Paul Mansfield, MD
Department of Surgical Oncology
University of Texas
MD Anderson Cancer Center
Houston, Texas

Robert C.G. Martin, MD
Department of Surgery
University of Louisville
Louisville, Kentucky

Kevin W. McEnery, MD
Department of Diagnostic Imaging
University of Texas
MD Anderson Cancer Center
Houston, Texas

Tamra McKenzie-Johnson, MD
Department of Surgical Oncology
University of Texas
MD Anderson Cancer Center
Houston, Texas

Kelly M. McMasters, MD, PhD
Department of Surgery
University of Louisville
Louisville, Kentucky

Funda Meric-Bernstam, MD
Department of Surgical Oncology
University of Texas
MD Anderson Cancer Center
Houston, Texas

Lavinia P. Middleton, MD
Department of Pathology
University of Texas
MD Anderson Cancer Center
Houston, Texas

George Miller, MD
Department of Surgery
Memorial Sloan-Kettering Cancer
  Center
New York, New York

Michael Miller, MD
Department of Plastic Surgery
University of Texas
MD Anderson Cancer Center
Houston, Texas

Bruce D. Minsky, MD
Department of Radiation Oncology
Memorial Sloan-Kettering Cancer Center
New York, New York

John T. Mullen, MD
Department of Surgical Oncology
University of Texas
MD Anderson Cancer Center
Houston, Texas

David W. Ollila, MD
Department of Surgery
University of North Carolina
Chapel Hill, North Carolina

Mark Onaitis, MD
Department of Surgery
Duke University Medical Center
Durham, North Carolina

Brian O'Sullivan, MD
Department of Radiation Oncology
University of Toronto
Toronto, Ontario, Canada

Alexander A. Parikh, MD
Department of Surgery
Temple University School of Medicine
Philadelphia, Pennsylvania

Janice L. Pasieka, MD
Department of Surgery
University of Calgary
Calgary, Alberta, Canada

Timothy M. Pawlik, MD, MPH
Department of Surgery
Johns Hopkins School of Medicine
Baltimore, Maryland

Nancy D. Perrier, MD
Department of Surgical Oncology
University of Texas
MD Anderson Cancer Center
Houston, Texas

Peter W.T. Pisters, MD
Department of Surgical Oncology
University of Texas
MD Anderson Cancer Center
Houston, Texas

Raphael E. Pollock, MD, PhD
Department of Surgical Oncology
University of Texas
MD Anderson Cancer Center
Houston, Texas

Chandrajit P. Raut, MD, MSc
Department of Surgery
|Harvard Medical School
Boston, Massachusetts

Emily Reiff, BS
Department of Surgery
University of California
San Francisco, California

Thereasa A. Rich, MS
Department of Surgical Oncology
University of Texas
MD Anderson Cancer Center
Houston, Texas

Steven E. Rodgers, MD, PhD
Department of Surgery
University of Miami
Miami, Florida

Miguel A. Rodriguez-Bigas, MD
Department of Surgical Oncology
University of Texas
MD Anderson Cancer Center
Houston, Texas

Mark S. Roh, MD
Department of Surgery
Drexel University College of Medicine
Pittsburgh, Pennsylvania

Kari M. Rosenkranz, MD
Department of General Surgery
Dartmouth-Hitchcock Medical Center
Lebanon, New Hampshire

Merrick I. Ross, MD
Department of Surgical Oncology
University of Texas
MD Anderson Cancer Center
Houston, Texas

Loren Rourke, MD
Department of Surgical Oncology
University of Texas
MD Anderson Cancer Center
Houston, Texas

Brian P. Rubin, MD, PhD
Department of Anatomic Pathology
University of Washington Medical Center
Seattle, Washington

Aysegul A. Sahin, MD
Department of Pathology
University of Texas
MD Anderson Cancer Center
Houston, Texas

Amod A. Sarnaik, MD
Department of Surgery
University of Cincinnati
Cincinnati, Ohio

Courtney L. Scaife, MD
Department of Surgery
University of Utah
Salt Lake City, Utah

Jonathan E. Schoeff, MD
Department of General Surgery
University of Cincinnati
Cincinnati, Ohio

Charles R. Scoggins, MD
Department of Surgery
University of Louisville
Louisville, Kentucky

Suzanne E. Shapiro, MS
Department of Surgical Oncology
University of Texas
MD Anderson Cancer Center
Houston, Texas

Thomas D. Shellenberger, DMD, MD
Department of Head and Neck Surgery
University of Texas
MD Anderson Cancer Center
Houston, Texas

Steven I. Sherman, MD
Department of Endocrine Neoplasia
University of Texas
MD Anderson Cancer Center
Houston, Texas

Timothy D. Sielaff, MD, PhD
Virginia Piper Cancer Institute
Minneapolis, Minnesota

Rebecca S. Sippel, MD
Department of Surgery
University of Wisconsin
Madison, Wisconsin

John M. Skibber, MD
Department of Surgical Oncology
University of Texas
MD Anderson Cancer Center
Houston, Texas

Eric A. Strom, MD
Department of Radiation Oncology
University of Texas
MD Anderson Cancer Center
Houston, Texas

Erich M. Sturgis, MD, MPH
Department of Head and Neck Surgery
University of Texas
MD Anderson Cancer Center
Houston, Texas

William Fraser Symmans, MD
Department of Pathology
University of Texas
MD Anderson Cancer Center
Houston, Texas

Mark S. Talamonti, MD
Department of Surgery
Northwestern University
Chicago, Illinois

Kenneth K. Tanabe, MD
Department of Surgery
Harvard Medical School
Boston, Massachusetts

William D. Tap, MD
Department of Surgical Oncology
University of California
Los Angeles, California

Richard L. Theriault, DO
Department of Breast Medical Oncology
University of Texas
MD Anderson Cancer Center
Houston, Texas

Geoffrey B. Thompson, MD
Department of Gastroenterologic and
    General Surgery
Mayo Clinic
Rochester, Minnesota

Jonathan C. Trent, MD, PhD
Department of Sarcoma Medical
    Oncology
University of Texas
MD Anderson Cancer Center
Houston, Texas

Todd M. Tuttle, MD
Department of Surgery
University of Minnesota
Minneapolis, Minnesota

Douglas Tyler, MD
Department of Surgery
Duke University Medical Center
Durham, North Carolina

Ara A. Vaporciyan, MD
Department of Thoracic and
    Cardiovascular Surgery
University of Texas
MD Anderson Cancer Center
Houston, Texas

Rena Vassilopoulou-Sellin, MD
Department of Endocrine Neoplasia
University of Texas
MD Anderson Cancer Center

Houston, Texas

Jean-Nicolas Vauthey, MD
Department of Surgical Oncology
University of Texas
MD Anderson Cancer Center
Houston, Texas

Huamin Wang, MD, PhD
Department of Pathology
University of Texas
MD Anderson Cancer Center
Houston, Texas

Thomas N. Wang, MD, PhD
Department of Surgery
Medical College of Georgia
Augusta, Georgia

Kevin T. Watkins, MD
Department of Surgery
Stony Brook University
Stony Brook, New York

Randal S. Weber, MD
Department of Head and Neck Surgery
University of Texas
MD Anderson Cancer Center
Houston, Texas

Bryan A. Whitson, MD
Department of Surgery
University of Minnesota
Minneapolis, Minnesota

Yan Xing, MD, MS
Department of Surgical Oncology
University of Texas
MD Anderson Cancer Center
Houston, Texas

James C. Yao, MD
Department of Gastrointestinal Medical
    Oncology
University of Texas
MD Anderson Cancer Center
Houston, Texas

Sam S. Yoon, MD
Department of Surgery
Harvard Medical School
Boston, Massachusetts

William F. Young Jr, MD, MSc
Department of Internal Medicine
Mayo Clinic College of Medicine
Rochester, Minnesota

Gunar K. Zagars, MD
Department of Radiation Oncology
University of Texas
MD Anderson Cancer Center
Houston, Texas

Jonathan S. Zager, MD
Department of Surgery
University of South Florida
Tampa, Florida

Daria Zorzi, MD
Department of Surgical Oncology
University of Texas
MD Anderson Cancer Center
Houston, Texas

CONTENTS

Section 3: Endocrine

Section 4: The Breast

Section 5: Sarcoma

Section 6: Pediatric Surgical Oncology

Section 7: Integument

CHAPTER 1

SURGICAL ONCOLOGY IN MULTIMODALITY CANCER CARE: HISTORY AND SCOPE

RAPHAEL E. POLLOCK, MD, PhD

The role of surgery in cancer care dates back to the ancient Egyptians and Greeks, who were the first to describe tumors and their therapy using written media. Up to the onset of general anesthesia in the midnineteenth century, oncology interventions with curative intent were primarily surgical, primarily heroic, and primarily unsuccessful. The era from 1850 to 1950 witnessed the development of standard surgical resection techniques as well as the emerging realization that surgical approaches were all too often debilitating to the patient, as well as fraught with failure to control the recurrence of malignancy, frequently at distant sites. In an attempt to mitigate these problems, the decade of 1950 to 1960 witnessed the emergence of radical surgical approaches, such as extended radical mastectomy for carcinoma of the breast and radical compartment resection for soft tissue tumors. However, this was also the era in which initial experiences with systemic treatments, such as chemotherapy, and regional approaches, such as external beam radiotherapy, first received appreciable attention. The time between 1960 and 1980 represented an era in which the first explorations of combined modality therapy were initiated. This was based on the reality that primary tumor local control was increasingly feasible because of earlier tumor detection coupled with the application of antibiotics and blood banking to improve surgical morbidity, the widespread acceptance of radiotherapy as a treatment modality, and the development and application of multidrug chemotherapy regimens. From 1980 to 2000, surgical techniques increasingly focused on organ preservation, quality of life, and the expanded use of chemotherapy and radiotherapy in the preoperative

setting, driven by a desire to downstage tumors prior to their resection, while simultaneously addressing subclinical regional and distant metastases, increasingly appreciated as the critical determinant of overall survival for most solid malignancies. Since the turn of the millennium, increasing attention has focused on the development of targeted molecular therapies in conjunction with the more traditional multimodality approaches developed over the previous decades.

The actual origin of each oncology discipline was from a parent medical specialty. The evolution of surgical oncology can be traced directly from surgery per se, coincident with the emergence of surgical subspecialty board certification mechanisms. This process has not yet been completed, as suggested by advocate and detractor concerns voiced in many segments of the surgical community regarding the prospect of board certification in this discipline. In contrast, radiation oncology originated within radiology and rapidly emerged as a freestanding board-certified specialty. Medical oncology likewise can find its origins within internal medicine, and fellowship training in medical oncology occurs after a residency in internal medicine. However, surgeons have also been historically involved in administering chemotherapy, and hormonal approaches began with the pioneering efforts of the urologist Charles Huggins, who won the Nobel Prize in 1965 for his work in prostate carcinoma.

It is difficult to specify what constitutes the definition of surgical oncology as a surgical or oncology discipline. Most would recognize that it is a cognitive rather than a technical surgical specialty. Unlike their general surgical counterparts, surgical oncologists focus primarily, if not

1

exclusively, on malignant disease, depending on practice milieu, and their approach is based on advanced training that includes extensive experience in the nonsurgical oncology disciplines, and also a refined understanding of the natural biology of malignant disease. Equipped with this broader background, a surgical oncologist has a keen appreciation of how surgical approaches interdigitate with the other cancer treatment modalities, and understands how surgery needs to be applied in a given malignant disease context. Whereas a cancer surgeon is a surgeon who uses surgical approaches to remove tumors, a surgical oncologist is an oncologist who uses surgery as his/her treatment modality. Although the differences may appear subtle, the cancer surgeon approaches the solid tumor problem within the context of a technical surgical specialty that is anatomically defined, whereas a surgical oncologist, although equipped with the same base technical skill set as a cancer surgeon, also evaluates the tumor problem from the perspective of the natural history of the disease, which in turn leads to the inclusion of other (nonsurgical) treatment modalities. This cognitive difference is critical in that it mandates that the surgical oncologist function as a coequal partner with the radiation oncology and medical oncology specialists to participate in the design of a treatment plan *prior* to the application of any therapeutic components.

At a time when radical surgery alone was the standard of care for most resectable solid tumors, the concept of multimodality care was already being instituted at the University of Texas M. D. Anderson Hospital and Tumor Institute by the founder and first president R. Lee Clark, MD. Beginning with the foundation of M. D. Anderson in 1941, Dr. Clark articulated a then revolutionary treatment approach to cancer:

> Dr. Clark believed that all known modalities should be re-evaluated in order to help the patient. Objective evaluation demanded that each specialist—the surgeon, the radiotherapist, and the internist—be of equal rank and be responsible for his particular modality … In neoplastic disease, group opinion is essential if the best results are to be achieved. This group approach was inaugurated early.[1]

From these early beginnings, the concept of multidisciplinary teams to care for the cancer patient have evolved into a large conglomeration of specialists, including a wide variety of physicians and allied health professionals (Table 1-1). It is important to recognize that family members are a critical component of the multidisciplinary cancer care team. The malignant process can rob patients of their autonomy and sense of self. Many patients relate that the day that they learned of their diagnosis was the day that their life irrevocably

Table 1-1 Members of Multidisciplinary Cancer Care Team

Primary care physician	Psycho-oncologist
Radiologist	Rehabilitation specialists
Pathologist	Oncology nurse
Surgical oncologist (all specialties)	Oncology pharmacist
Reconstructive surgeon	Family members
Anesthesiologist	ACP
Medical oncologist	Research nurse
(adult pediatrics)	Data manager
Radiation oncologist	

changed forever. Recruiting family members as a most critical support system can help restore a sense of hope for the future, and can also provide critical support to help the patient comply with and survive the treatment programs with their psychological sense of well-being as intact as possible.

For effective functioning as a multidisciplinary cancer care team, it is very important that team members support each other. An attitude regarding the team and its members typified by flexibility, collegiality, candor, tolerance for differences of opinion, and lack of ego are all important determinants of whether a team will ultimately be able to function effectively on behalf of the patient.

The structure in which the team interacts is usually in the format of a multidisciplinary planning conference. Team members commit to meeting on a regularly scheduled basis. The fundamental commitment to each other, and ultimately the shared patients, is that all relevant opinions will be solicited, discussed, and coalesced into a multimodality treatment plan for a given patient *before* rather than after any irreversible steps have been taken. The multidisciplinary conference provides a formalized structure in which patient care issues can be discussed. By enabling the collective examination of the evidence in support of a specific therapeutic approach, the underlying strength of the supporting data can be ascertained. This approach has the positive effect of diminishing the impact of modality-specific bias or reliance on anecdote, and leads to a better understanding of what each oncology discipline can contribute to the care of a specific patient, as well as the magnitude of temporal/biological/financial costs that will be incurred to accomplish these cancer management objectives.

The multidisciplinary conference also provides the aegis under which patients can be assessed for clinical trial protocol eligibility and can be accrued to prospective relational disease site databases. At the time of the conference, needed additional consultations can be scheduled with the full participation of all relevant practitioners. The organized and cohesive treatment plan can be presented and explained to the patient and their family, with expertise to answer specific questions being immediately available. The well-orchestrated conference builds on and helps further foster patient trust that a process is being put into play that will address their cancer issues. Most importantly, the conference creates an opportunity for dialogue, and sets in place an expectation that the dialogue will continue among the conferees moving forward, so that unanticipated problems necessitating departures from the plan can be addressed in real time. Patients come to believe in and understand this role of the multidisciplinary conference; it instills a sense of trust and hope for the future because the patient sees that "the experts are putting their heads together to help me with my problem."

As commitments are forged by team members such that cancer care becomes truly multimodal, the role of each conference participant is recast, such that they are functioning less as an independent practitioner and more as a team member contributing special expertise for the good of the whole. For example, the conference radiologist, in addition to interpreting any available radiological studies for a given patient, can also make recommendations or even select optimal imaging techniques for primary and possible metastasis tumor detection. The pathologist, in addition to the traditional roles of interpreting biopsy specimens obtained pre-, intra-, and postoperatively, can also facilitate use of newer molecular-based diagnostics and can advise about prognosis.

The surgical oncologist can offer advice about tumor biopsy methods; working with the conference pathologist, the most minimally invasive biopsy approach that will be diagnostic can be decided on, including decisions about whether radiological image guidance will be needed. The surgical oncologist can address issues of resectability and the likelihood of achieving negative margins, which in turn may impact on decisions to use chemotherapy and/or radiotherapy as preoperative neoadjuvants, especially when a tumor appears to be marginally resectable at presentation. The surgical oncologist can also offer insight about the role of surgery in the management of regional or distant disease, and whether such interventions should be undertaken concomitantly with the primary tumor resection or after the use of nonsurgical approaches.

The medical oncologist can provide a unique perspective about the utility of systemic approaches, such as chemotherapy or hormonal therapy, and whether it would be preferable to use these therapies as adjuvant treatments after surgery versus neoadjuvantly. Issues about concurrent versus sequential chemo- and radiotherapy delivery, and the timing of surgical interventions vis-à-vis neoadjuvant approaches, can be discussed.

Because of their historical role in caring for patients with disseminated disease, medical oncologists are also in a special position to discuss palliative care approaches and options with other conferees. The decision to offer a patient a palliative operation or a course of palliative radiotherapy cannot be made in a vacuum, and it is imperative that the availability of systemic approaches be fully discussed prior to such regional treatments being applied. For example, the advance knowledge that a palliative tumor resection is being contemplated and that a renally excreted chemotherapy agent is available for use after surgery may influence the decision about performing (or not performing) a kidney resection in continuity with a tumor versus using the drug *before* such an operation is performed.

The radiation oncologist can advise about the applicability of preoperative, intraoperative, and postoperative external beam approaches. The radiation oncologist can also help define the role of interstitial radiotherapy (brachytherapy), implantable radioemitters and the utility/availability of alternative energy sources such as electron beam, protons, etc. Discussing the entire regional approach prior to treatment is very important: Will the surgery alone necessitate resection of an organ that optimally should be preserved, and if so, can radiation prior to surgery downstage the tumor so that the threatened structure can be preserved? Will tumor-draining lymph nodes be removed or should they be treated prophylactically using radiation, and if so, before or after surgery? And what are the likely long-term radiation-induced effects on adjacent normal tissues? The impact of radiation on surgical decisions, such as flap selection (free versus rotational or local advancement), vascular grafting where issues such as creating an anastomosis in an irradiated field with possible long-term pseudoaneurysm formation relative to risk and likely location of a recurrence, or even biopsy scar orientation relative to a subsequent radiotherapy field and ultimate en bloc tumor resection, exemplify the complexity and necessity for multidisciplinary conferencing involving all specialists prior to any irrevocable decisions being made.

Many of these principles can be best illustrated in a patient vignette. Figure 1-1 depicts a patient referred to The University of Texas M. D. Anderson Cancer Center for consideration of hip disarticulation after initial treatment at another health care facility. The patient presented with a large, high-grade, deep (AJCC stage IIIB) synovial sarcoma of the left thigh. On presentation, the tumor was found to be growing through a previous biopsy site, which was now infected. MRI imaging (Figure 1-2) performed on presentation at M. D. Anderson demonstrated the large size of the tumor and

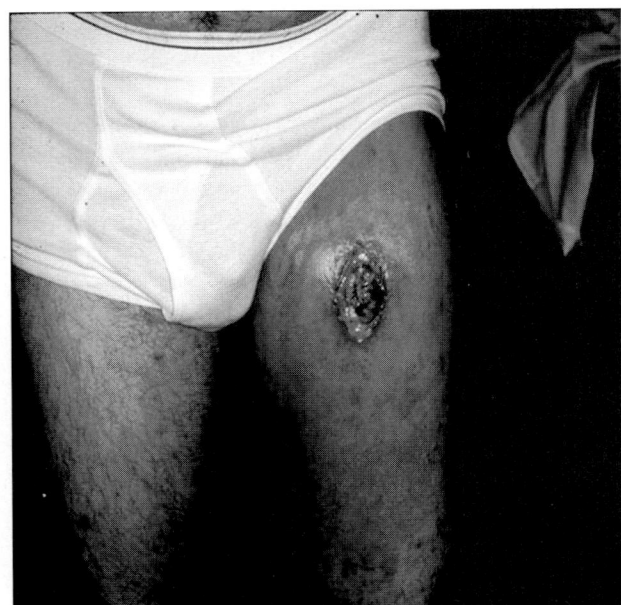

Figure 1-1 Clinical presentation of Stage IIIB soft tissue sarcoma of the thigh. Note the disrupted and infected biopsy wound, with tumor outgrowth.

also that the femoral neurovascular bundle was displaced medially and was not encased by tumor. The patient was discussed at the Sarcoma Multidisciplinary Conference. The pathology and radiology data were presented and discussed, revealing that the diagnosis was actually malignant fibrous histiocytoma (MFH) and not synovial sarcoma, but more importantly, that the tumor could be resected without resorting to amputation, in that the neurovascular structures were adjacent to (rather than surrounded by) tumor, and the femoral shaft was also not circumferentially engulfed by tumor. Pulmonary metastases were not detected on CT scan of the chest,

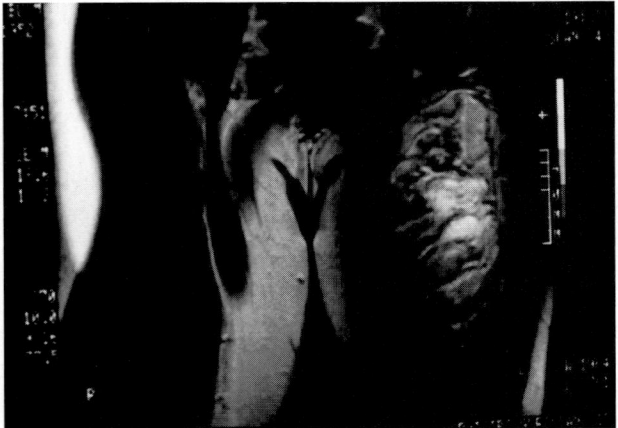

Figure 1-2 MRI scan demonstrating the massive size of this patient's sarcoma. Note the medial displacement of the neurovascular bundle.

and the roles of neoadjuvant versus adjuvant and preoperative versus postoperative radiotherapy were discussed. Surgical opinion was offered about tumor resectability, use of preoperative treatments in the face of an already disrupted and infected biopsy site, and the need for reconstructive surgery participation. Because of the high likelihood of subclinical dissemination to the lungs in stage IIIB MFH, and because preoperative primary tumor cytoreduction would facilitate limb salvage, a decision was reached to use preoperative chemotherapy and radiotherapy as part of an ongoing clinical trial after resolution of infection had been accomplished.

The tumor was stabilized by the preoperative nonsurgical treatments, and the patient remained

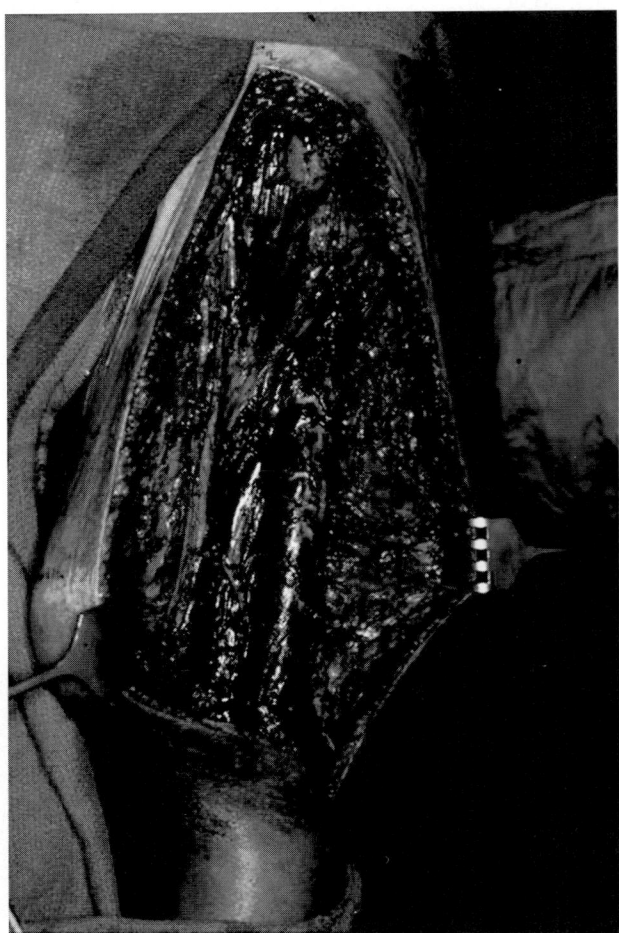

Figure 1-3 Intraoperative appearance of thigh after sarcoma resection. The neurovascular bundle is preserved, and the femur is also intact, although the periosteum has been resected. To promote wound healing in this irradiated tumor bed, while providing vascularized protection to the neurovascular bundle and femur, a dead space-obliterating ipsilateral rectus flap will be elevated and rotated into the tumor bed.

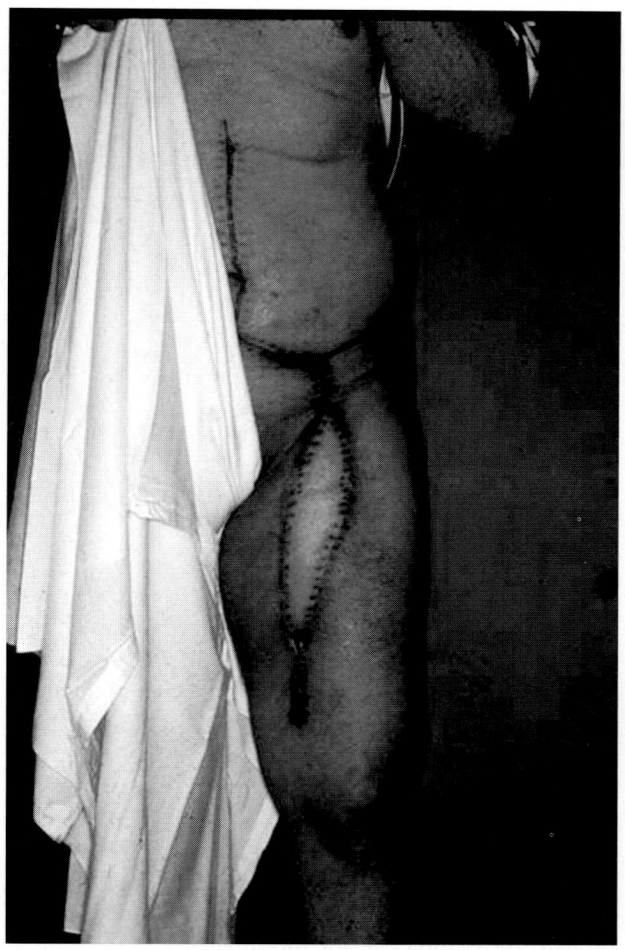

Figure 1-4 Patient appearance on return to clinic for postoperative follow-up. Full ambulatory capacity has been preserved.

metastasis free. A limb-sparing frozen section margin negative tumor resection was performed with preservation of the neurovascular bundle. A negative femur margin was obtained by including the femoral periosteum as the deep anteromedial margin of tumor resection (Figure 1-3). To protect the neurovascular bundle and femur from exposure in the event of wound breakdown, and to promote wound healing in an irradiated tumor bed by eliminating deadspace, an ipsilateral rectus abdominis myocutaneous flap was rotated into the tumor bed as per the plan originally developed by the reconstructive surgeons who also participate in the Sarcoma Multidisciplinary Conference at our institution (Figure 1-4). The final pathology report demonstrated negative margins of resection and 98% tumor necrosis. Adjuvant chemotherapy was completed, and the patient remains disease free more than a decade after resection.

As we move forward into the era of molecular staging, molecular-targeted therapy as both stand-alone as well as chemo- and radiosensitizer adjuncts, tissue-sparing proton beam therapy, tissue-engineered replacement body parts, robotic telesurgery, etc., the sophistication in planning and communication needed will become of even more paramount importance. Working together, the best is certainly yet to come!

References

1. Cumley RW, editor. The first twenty years of The University of Texas M. D. Anderson Hospital and Tumor Institute. Austin, TX: The University of Texas Press; 1964. p. 132.

CHAPTER 2

MOLECULAR UNDERPINNINGS

FUNDA MERIC-BERNSTAM, MD

Recent advances in cancer biology are revolutionizing cancer care. With discovery of biomarkers for cancer risk assessment, determination of prognosis, and prediction of response to specific therapies, these molecular markers are being increasingly incorporated into clinical practice. New targeted molecular therapies such as trastuzumab and imanitib have proven to be immensely useful in clinical applications, while many others are in development. The surgeon is often responsible not only for the initial diagnosis and management of solid tumors, but also for coordination of multidisciplinary care. It is essential that surgeons understand the principles of molecular oncology and be well-versed in the roles of molecular therapeutics and molecular markers so that they can incorporate these advances appropriately into clinical practice and coordinate delivery of state-of-the-art, personalized cancer care.

Molecular Basis of Carcinogenesis

CANCER INITIATION

There are three steps in tumorigenesis: initiation, promotion, and progression. Initiating events may lead a single cell to acquire a distinct growth advantage through gain of function of genes known as oncogenes, or loss of function of genes known as tumor suppressor genes. Recent evidence suggests that the genetic events leading to cancer initiation may be orchestrated by cancer stem cells—cancer cells that have the ability to self-renew.[1] With clonal progression, tumors that arise from a single cell accumulate additional mutations that confer increasingly aggressive behavior. Most tumors are thought to go through a progression from benign lesions to in situ tumors to invasive cancers (Figure 2-1).[2] Alterations in at least four or five genes are required for formation of a malignant tumor, while fewer changes are sufficient for a benign tumor.

Environmental factors can play a critical role in cancer initiation and progression. Any agent that can contribute to cancer formation is referred to as a "carcinogen." Carcinogens can be chemical (eg, vinyl chloride), physical (eg, radiation), or viral agents (hepatitis B).

CANCER GENES

In the past decade, more than 30 genes associated with autosomal dominant hereditary cancers have been identified (Table 2-1). Although hereditary cancer syndromes are rare, sporadic cancers have been found to have disruptions in the same cellular pathways altered in hereditary cancer syndromes, suggesting that these pathways are critical to the cell cycle and to normal cell growth and proliferation.

In the case of hereditary cancers, the individual carries a particular germline mutation in every cell. In most cases, a single mutation in a tumor suppressor gene is not thought to be sufficient for tumorigenesis. For example, hereditary retinoblastoma involves two mutations, one of which is germline, while nonhereditary retinoblastoma is due to two somatic mutations.[3] Therefore, both hereditary and nonhereditary forms of retinoblastoma involve the same number of mutations, an explanation of tumorigenesis known as the Knudson "two-hit" hypothesis. A "hit" may be a point mutation, a chromosomal deletion, or silencing of an existing gene.

In contrast, oncogenes are normal cellular genes that contribute to cancer development when they have a gain of function. These genes can be activated or overexpressed by translocation (eg, *abl*), promotor insertion (eg, c-*myc*), mutations (eg, *PI3K*), or amplification (eg, *HER2/neu*). Oncogenes may encode growth factors (eg, platelet-derived growth factor), growth factor receptors (eg, HER2/*neu*), intracellular signal transduction molecules (eg, Akt), nuclear transcription factors (eg, c-*myc*), or other molecules involved in regulation of cell growth and proliferation. Over 100 oncogenes have been identified.[4]

DEREGULATION OF THE CELL CYCLE

Mutations or alterations in the expression of cell-cycle proteins, growth factors, growth factor receptors (glo-

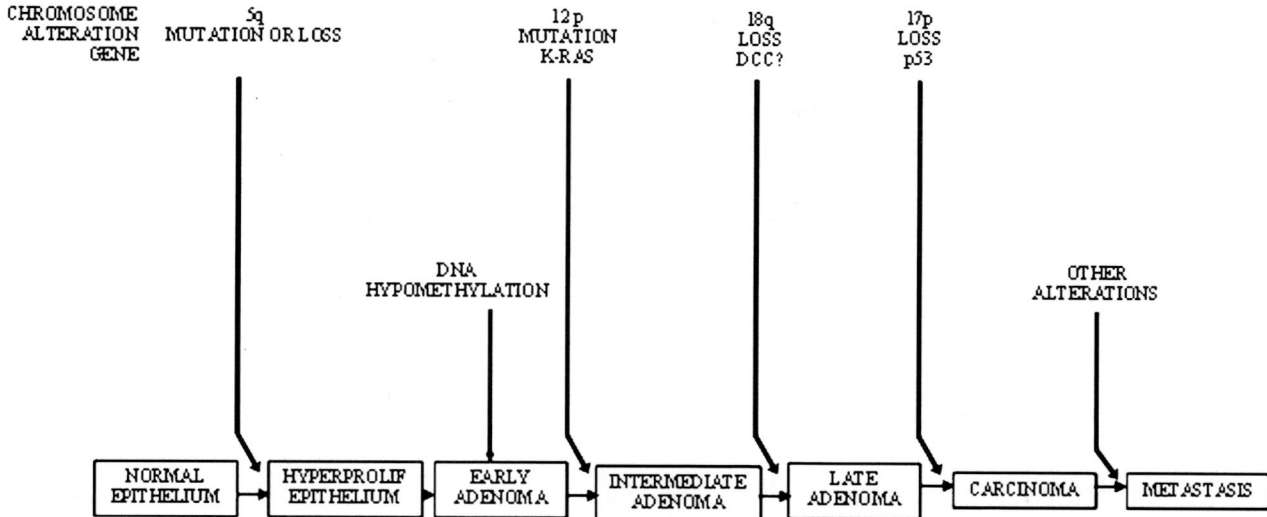

Figure 2-1 A genetic model for colorectal tumorigenesis. Tumorigenesis proceeds through a series of genetic alterations involving oncogenes and tumor suppressor genes. Individuals with familial adenomatous polyposis inherit a mutation on chromosome 5q, while in sporadic tumors the same region may be lost or mutated at a relatively early stage of tumorigenesis. A *ras* gene mutation (usually K-*ras*) occurs in one cell of a preexisting small adenoma, which, through clonal expansion, produces a larger and more dysplastic tumor. The chromosomes most frequently deleted include 5q, 17p, and 18q. Accumulation of these changes, rather than their order of appearance, seems most important. The tumor continues to progress once a carcinoma has formed, and the accumulated chromosomal alterations correlate with the ability of the carcinoma to metastasize and cause death. Source: Modified with permission from Fearon, et al.

Table 2-1 Selected Cancer Predisposition Genes

Syndrome	Component Tumors	Mode of Inheritance	Genes
Hereditary breast cancer and ovarian cancer syndrome	Breast cancer, ovarian cancer, prostate cancer, pancreatic cancer	Dominant	BRCA1, BRCA2
Li-Fraumeni syndrome	Soft tissue sarcoma, breast cancer, osteosarcoma, leukemia, brain tumors, adrenocortical carcinoma	Dominant	p53, CHEK2
Cowden syndrome	Breast cancer, thyroid cancer, endometrial and other cancers	Dominant	PTEN
Bannayan-Riley-Ruvalcaba syndrome	Breast cancer, meningioma, thyroid follicular cell tumors	Dominant	PTEN
Ataxia telangiectasia	Leukemia, lymphoma	Recessive	ATM
HNPCC	Colon cancer, endometrial cancer, ovarian cancer, renal pelvis cancers, ureteral cancers, pancreatic cancer, stomach and small bowel cancers, hepatobiliary cancers	Dominant	MLH1, MSH2, MSH6
Familial polyposis	Colon cancer	Dominant	APC
Hereditary gastric cancer	Stomach cancers	Dominant	CDH1
Juvenile polyposis	Gastrointestinal cancers, pancreatic cancer	Dominant	SMAD4/DPC4, BMPR1A
Peutz-Jeghers syndrome	Colon cancer, small-bowel cancer, breast cancer, ovarian cancer, pancreatic cancer	Dominant	STK11
Hereditary melanoma pancreatic cancer syndrome	Pancreatic cancer, melanoma	Dominant	CDKN2A/p16
Turcot syndrome	Colon cancer, basal cell carcinoma, ependymoma, medulloblastoma, glioblastoma	Dominant	APC, MLH1, PMS2
Familial gastrointestinal stromal tumor	Gastrointestinal stromal tumors	Dominant	KIT
Melanoma syndromes	Malignant melanoma	Dominant	CDKN2 (p16), CDK4, DMM
von Hippel-Lindau syndrome	Hemangioblastomas of retina and central nervous system, renal cell cancer, pheochromocytomas	Dominant	VHL
MEN1, Multiple Endocrine Neoplasia 1	Pancreatic islet cell tumors, pituitary adenomas, parathyroid adenomas	Dominant	MEN1
MEN2, Multiple Endocrine Neoplasia 2	Medullary thyroid cancer, pheochromocytoma, parathyroid hyperplasia	Dominant	RET

merular filtration rate), intracellular signal transduction proteins, and nuclear transcription factors can all lead to disturbances in cell cycle control, allowing unregulated cell growth and proliferation. The cell cycle is divided into four phases. During the synthetic or S phase, the cell generates a single copy of its genetic material, while in the mitotic or M phase, cellular components are partitioned between the two identical daughter cells.[5] The G_1 and G_2 phases represent gap phases during which the cells prepare themselves for completion of the S and M phases, respectively. When cells cease proliferation, they exit the cell cycle and enter the quiescent state referred to as G_0. The proliferative advantage of tumor cells is associated with their ability to bypass quiescence.[5]

DEREGULATION OF APOPTOSIS

The growth of a tumor mass is dependent not only on an increase of proliferation of tumor cells, but also on a decrease in their rate of apoptosis, or programmed cell death (Figure 2-2). Apoptosis is a genetically regulated program to dispose of cells. The initiator caspases (8, 9, 10) cleave the downstream executioner caspases (3, 6, 7), which carry out apoptosis.[6] Two principal molecular pathways signal apoptosis by cleaving the initiator caspases: the mitochondrial (intrinsic) pathway and the death receptor (extrinsic) pathway. In the mitochondrial pathway, death results from the release of cytochrome c from the mitochondria. The mitochondrial pathway can be stimulated by many factors, including deoxyribonucleic acid (DNA) damage, reactive oxygen species, or withdrawal of survival factors. The permeability of the mitochondrial membrane, regulated by Bcl-2 proteins, determines whether the apoptotic pathway will proceed.[6]

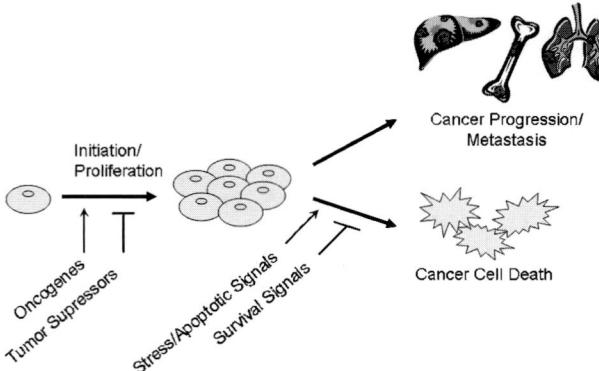

Figure 2-2 The balance of apoptosis and survival signaling. Cancer cells acquire a growth advantage through gain of oncogenes or loss of tumor suppressor genes. Cancer growth and progression is dependent not only on an increase of proliferation of tumor cells, but also on a decrease in apoptosis, as determined by the balance of apoptotic and survival signals.

The Bcl-2 family of regulatory proteins includes proapoptotic proteins (eg, Bax, Bad, Bak) and antiapoptotic proteins (eg, Bcl-2, Bcl-xL).

In the death receptor pathway, cell-surface death receptors Fas, tumor necrosis factor receptor 1 (TNFR1), and Death Receptor 5 (DR5), bind their ligands FasL, tumor necrosis factor (TNF), and TNF-related apoptosis-inducing ligand (TRAIL), respectively.[6] When the receptors are bound by their ligands, they form a death-inducing signaling complex (DISC), and procaspase-8 and procaspase-10 are cleaved, yielding active initiator caspases.[7] The death receptor pathway may be regulated at the cell surface by the expression of "decoy" receptors, which are closely related to the death receptors but lack a functional death domain. Thus they bind death ligands but do not transmit a death signal.[6] Another regulatory group is the fas-associated death domain protein (FADD)-like interleukin-1 protease-inhibitory proteins (FLIPs). FLIPs have homology to caspase-8; they bind DISC and inhibit activation of caspase-8. Furthermore, inhibitors of apoptosis proteins, such as X-linked inhibitor of appoptosis (XIAP) and survivin, block caspase-3 activation and have the ability to regulate both the death receptor and the mitochondrial pathway. In human cancers, aberrations in the apoptotic program include increased expression of decoy receptors; increased expression of antiapoptotic proteins Bcl-2, survivin, and c-FLIP; mutations or downregulation of proapoptotic molecules; and activation of survival signaling pathways.[6,7]

Molecular Determinants of Cancer Progression

CANCER INVASION

A critical step in cancer progression is the ability to invade the surrounding normal tissue. Tumors in which the malignant cells appear to lie exclusively above the basement membrane are referred to as "in situ" cancer, while tumors in which the malignant cells are demonstrated to breach the basement membrane, penetrating into surrounding stroma, are termed "invasive" cancer. The ability to invade involves changes in adhesion, motility, and proteolysis of the extracellular matrix (ECM). Serine, cysteine, and aspartic proteinases and matrix metalloproteinases (MMPs) have all been implicated in cancer invasion. Urokinase plasminogen activators (uPA) and tissue plasminogen activators (tPA) are serine proteases that convert plasminogen into plasmin. Plasmin, in return, can degrade several ECM components and may activate MMPs.[8] uPA level has been correlated with tissue invasion and metastasis and cancer progression.

ANGIOGENESIS

Another critical step for tumor progression is angiogenesis, the establishment of new blood vessels from a preexisting vascular bed. Tumors develop an angiogenic phenotype as a result of accumulated genetic alterations and in response to local selection pressures such as hypoxia. Many of the common oncogenes and tumor suppressor genes play a role in inducing angiogenesis.[9] Angiogenesis is mediated by factors produced by various cells, including tumor cells, endothelial cells, stromal cells, and inflammatory cells. Of the angiogenic stimulators, the best studied is the vascular endothelial growth factor (VEGF). VEGF has various functions, including increasing vascular permeability, inducing endothelial cell proliferation and tube formation, and inducing endothelial cell synthesis of proteolytic enzymes such as uPA.[8–10] Furthermore, VEGF may mediate blood flow by its effects on the vasodilator nitric oxide,[10] and act as an endothelial survival factor, thus protecting the integrity of the vasculature.[11] The proliferation of new lymphatic vessels, termed lymphangiogenesis, is also thought to be controlled by the VEGF family.

Tumor angiogenesis is regulated by several factors in a coordinated fashion. In addition to upregulation of proangiogenic molecules, suppression of naturally occurring inhibitors also can encourage angiogenesis. Angiogenesis is a prerequisite not only for primary tumor growth but also for metastasis. In the primary tumor, as determined by microvessel density and expression of VEGF, angiogenesis has been demonstrated to be an independent predictor of distant metastatic disease and survival in several cancers,[9,12] emphasizing its importance in cancer biology.

METASTASIS

Metastases arise from the spread of cancer cells from the primary site and the formation of new tumors in distant sites. The metastatic process consists of a series of steps that need to be completed successfully. The primary cancer needs to develop access to the circulation and needs to survive in the circulation. Next, the circulating cells arrest in a new organ and extravasate into the new tissue. Then the cells need to grow in the new tissue and establish vascularization. Only a small subset of circulating cancer cells initiate micrometastases, while an even smaller portion go on to grow into macrometastasis.

Many models of cancer metastasis have been proposed. One model suggests that the ability of a primary tumor to metastasize is determined by the genes that are expressed by an individual tumor. This model suggests that the ability to metastasize may be predictable by analysis of the tumor's gene expression profile. Indeed, several studies have identified a gene expression profile or a "molecular signature" that is associated with metastasis.[13] A second model proposes that dissemination of metastatic cells occurs early, and is independent of the primary tumor characteristics. The third model is based on the multistep tumorigenesis theory and suggests that tumor cells progressively accumulate genetic mutations that confer the ability to metastasize; thus, not all cells within the tumor can metastasize, only a clone arising within the tumor can metastasize. The fourth model suggests that only a self-renewing subpopulation of stem cells within the primary tumor have the ability to form new tumors and metastasize. All of these models of metastasis are in evolution, awaiting molecular marker-based assays to delineate the relative contribution of each molecular mechanism to human metastasis.

Molecular Therapeutics

Over the past decade, increasing understanding of cancer biology has led to the idea of personalized medicine and the emerging field of molecular therapeutics. The basic principle of molecular therapeutics is to exploit the molecular differences between normal and cancer cells, and to develop therapies that "target" a biologically important molecule (eg, HER2/*neu*) or a biologically important process (eg, angiogenesis). The ideal molecular target would be expressed exclusively in the cancer cells, be the driving force of proliferation of the cancer cells, and be critical to cancer cell survival but not to the survival of normal cells. A large number of molecular targets are currently being explored, both preclinically and in clinical trials. The major groups of targeted therapies include inhibitors of glomerular filtration rate, inhibitors of intracellular signal transduction, cell-cycle inhibitors, apoptosis-based therapies, and antiangiogenic compounds.

Cell signaling molecules, especially protein kinases, have come to the forefront as attractive therapeutic targets with the success of imitanib mesylate, which targets bcr-abl in chronic myelogenous leukemia and c-kit in gastrointestinal stromal tumors, and trastuzumab, which targets HER2/*neu* in breast cancer. Protein kinases are enzymes that covalently attach phosphates to the side chain of serine, threonine, or tyrosine residues of specific proteins. Studies of the human genome have revealed over 500 protein kinases.[14] Several protein kinases have oncogenic properties, and many other protein kinases have been shown to be activated aberrantly in cancer cells. Therefore, these protein kinases are being pursued aggressively in molecular therapeutics. Potential targets can be addressed via different strategies, such as transcriptional downregulation, targeting of messenger ribonucleic acid (mRNA) with small inhibitory ribonucleic acid (RNA) or antisense strategies, targeting of protein with monoclonal antibodies or direct inhibition of protein activity with small molecule inhibitors, and induction of immunity against the protein. Most of the compounds in development are monoclonal antibodies such as trastuzumab or small-molecule kinase inhibitors such as imatinib. Some of the kinase inhibitors in clinical development include inhibitors of epidermal growth factor receptor, Src, Ras, Raf, mitogen-activated protein extracellular regulated kinase, mammalian target of rapamycin, cyclin-dependent kinase, protein kinase C, and 3-phosphoinositide-dependent protein kinase 1. Other targeted therapies being evaluated in clinical trials include farnesyltransferase inhibitors, inhibitors of cellular chaperone heat shock protein90 (hsp90), proteosome inhibitors, as well as therapies targeting the apoptotic pathway, such as TRAIL-based therapies and bcl-2 inhibition/downregulation strategies. Although few targeted molecular therapies have been successfully incorporated into our clinical armamentarium to date, it is clear that these agents will eventually play a critical role in achieving our goal of delivering personalized cancer therapy.

Molecular Markers of Cancer Risk

Molecular markers of cancer risk consist of markers of environmental risk (carcinogen exposure and carcinogen damage) and markers of inherited risk. Recently, it has become possible to offer genetic testing for several cancer-predisposing genes to individuals considered to be at inherited risk on the basis of their family and personal history. With genetic testing, patients presenting with a cancer can be assessed for their risk of metachronous tumors, while disease-free individuals with a family history can be better stratified by cancer risk. For example, patients who have a family history suggestive of hereditary breast/ovarian cancer syndrome should be offered genetic counseling. Statistical models have been demonstrated to be accurate counseling tools to predict the probability of carrying a deleterious mutation in BRCA1 and BRCA2, and can assist in decision making regarding the utility of genetic testing.[15]

Carriers of deleterious mutations can be offered more intensive surveillance, chemoprevention, or prophylactic surgery such as bilateral mastectomy and bilateral salpingo-oopherectomy (BSO). Prophylactic surgery is also considered for other hereditary cancer syndromes such as familial adenomatous polyposis (total colectomy or proctocolectomy), hereditary nonpolyposis colon cancer (total colectomy, hysterectomy, and BSO), hereditary gastric cancer (total gastrectomy), and multiple endocrine neoplasia type B (total thyroidectomy). The decision regarding the role of prophylactic surgery is influenced by patient age, projected life-time cancer risk, effectiveness of cancer surveillance, expected survival with the cancer type, and the physical and psychological morbidity of the risk-reducing surgery. Although "knowledge is power," the psychological implications of genetic testing and the limitations of testing both need to be considered in patient care planning.

Most of the familial aggregation of tumors is not accounted for by mutations in the known high-penetrance genes. For example, only 30% of the estimated proportion of familial risk for colorectal cancers (CRCs), 30% of that for breast cancers, and 10% of that for melanomas can be explained by mutations in known heritable cancer genes.[16] The rest may be attributable to other yet unidentified high-penetrance genes or to a large number of alleles that each confer a small genotypic risk (eg, 1.5- to 2-fold risk), combined additively or multiplicatively to confer a range of susceptibilities in the population.[17] Recent efforts have focused on single nucleotide polymorphisms (SNPs), which are variations in the DNA sequence when a single nucleotide (A, T, C, or G) is altered in the genome sequence. For a variation to be considered an SNP, it must occur in at least 1% of the population. As many as three million SNPs have been identified. While mutations that inactivate critical genes can have obvious clinical consequences, SNPs in genes such as carcinogen metabolizers or DNA repair genes may produce subtle alterations, with an increased sensitivity to environmental exposure, and subsequent cancer development. Although in the past decade several studies have evaluated the association between SNPs and cancer, few loci have been unequivocally identified. For example, of 50 studies examining the risk of CRC conferred by variations in 13 genes, 16 significant associations were found, but only three were reported in more than one study: APC –I1307K, HRAS1-VNTR, and MTHFR-Ala677Val.[17] With the recent availability of SNP microarrays and other approaches to high-throughput SNP profiling, genomewide risk associations will be increasingly feasible in the next few years, potentially leading to clinically useful risk assessment tools.

Diagnostic Markers

Because cancer outcome is determined by stage at presentation, much work is being done to improve early diagnosis. Areas of research include evaluation of better anatomic imaging approaches, as well as attempts to identify molecular differences between normal cells and tumor cells that can be exploited for functional imaging (such as protein emission tomography scanning) or with imaging using novel molecular targeting approaches (eg, nanoparticles). Serum and plasma markers are under especially active investigation because they may allow early diagnosis of a cancer or may be used to follow a cancer's response to therapy or monitor for recurrence.

Unfortunately, many of the tumor markers used so far have low sensitivities and specificities. Tumor markers can be elevated in benign conditions. Further, tumor markers may not be elevated in all patients with cancer, especially in the early stages, when a serum marker would be most useful for diagnosis. Therefore, when using a tumor marker to monitor recurrence, it is important to be certain that the tumor marker was elevated prior to primary therapy. The best example of a clinically useful serum marker at this time is prostate-specific antigen (PSA). PSA levels have been shown to be useful in monitoring the effectiveness of prostate cancer treatment and for recurrence after therapy.

High-throughput technologies such as matrix-assisted laser-desorption-ionization time-of-flight (MALDI-TOF) mass spectroscopy and liquid chromatography-ion-spray tandem mass spectroscopy (LC-MS/MS) have revolutionized the field of proteomics and are now being used to compare serum protein profiles between patients with cancer and individuals without cancer. Investigators have recently begun to compare the proteomic profiles of patients with prostate cancer and ovarian cancer to those of controls, identifying unique proteins in the sera of cancer patients.[18,19] Identification of unique serum proteins as well as unique proteomic profiles for most cancer types is being actively pursued as a means of developing potential diagnostic biomarkers. The proteomic field is still in its infancy and is confounded by artifacts of sample collection, storage and processing, and mass spectrometry instruments, as well as bioinformatics analysis. If, however, attempts to identify early serum or plasma markers are successful, it would dramatically enhance cancer detection and the delivery of cancer care.

Prognostic Markers

SELECTION OF PROGNOSTIC FACTORS

Standard prognostic factors include clinical and pathological staging, especially tumor size, nodal status, and the presence or absence of distant metastases. The term "prognostic marker" is usually used to describe molecular markers that predict disease-free survival, disease-free survival, disease-specific survival (DSS), or overall survival (OS). The goal is to identify prognostic markers that can give information on prognosis independent of other clinical characteristics, and therefore can provide information in addition to what can be projected on the basis of clinical presentation. Such markers would allow us to further classify patients as being at higher or lower risk within clinical subgroups, and therefore to identify patients who may benefit most from adjuvant therapy. A potential application of these markers would be to distinguish patients at high risk for recurrence, who are candidates for adjuvant systemic therapy, from patients at low risk of recurrence, who could be spared the toxicity of this therapy.

Thousands of papers have been published looking at potential prognostic markers for several cancer types. Most of these studies have evaluated the expression of a single gene through studies that are retrospective, have small sample sizes and differing endpoints, and have used different methods of marker detection. In most cases, these molecular markers have not been validated in well-designed, Level of Evidence I studies, and have therefore not been incorporated into clinical practice.

Most hospitals have the ability to store tissue in paraffin, while many fewer have the ability to store frozen biopsies or surgical specimens. Thus markers that can be assessed from tissue in paraffin have a competitive advantage in being much more widely applicable. For example, uPA/PAI 1 overexpression appears to be a very strong prognostic for breast cancer.[20] The expression of this marker is usually determined by enzyme-linked immunosorbent assay, requiring fresh or frozen tissue; this likely limits the widespread use of this marker in the US and many other countries.

HIGH-THROUGHPUT GENE EXPRESSION PROFILING

An exciting new approach to prognostic markers relies not on the evaluation of a few genes, but rather the expression of several dozen or several thousand genes. The most widely studied technology relies on DNA segments (complementary DNA or oligonucleotides) representing different genes that are arrayed on glass slides (chips) or membranes, to which cRNA derived from the patient's tissue (usually tumor) is hybridized. This technology allows determination of the levels of expression of thousands of mRNA segments in comparison to either a reference RNA or the average signal from the microarray. Using microarray technology, investigators from the Netherlands Cancer Institute identified a 70-gene prognostic signature that appears to distinguish breast cancer patients with a poor prognosis from patients with a good prognosis.[21,22] The utility of this prognostic profile is being validated in a prospective clinical trial. Gene expression profiles that are associated with prognosis have also been described in CRC, gastric cancer, and other cancer types.[23–25]

Despite major technological advances in array technology, a number of factors still limit its widespread use, including the need for fresh/frozen tissue; differences in array technology, array platforms, and methods of analysis; and challenges in implementation of large validation studies including study design, patient selection, and specimen availability and processing. In addition to being a potential prognostic tool itself, gene expression profiling also has the potential to identify novel prognostic markers, which can then be assessed individually with more widely accessible techniques, such as immunohistochemistry (IHC), or can be further pursued as therapeutic targets.

Another powerful approach that has been introduced recently is the ability to perform quantitative reverse transcriptase polymerase chain reaction (RT-PCR) on multiple genes using paraffin-embedded tissue. Paik and colleagues recently demonstrated that a RT-PCR assay of 21 genes, used in a prospectively defined algorithm, predicted distant recurrence and OS in tamoxifen-treated patients with node-negative and estrogen receptor–positive breast cancer.[26] This assay (Oncotype DX assay, Genomic Health) is the first of many molecular diagnostic tests and services likely to reach the market over the next few decades.

High-throughput technologies also can be utilized to evaluate tumors at the genomic level. Such approaches currently include comparative genomic hybridization and SNP arrays. Moreover, high-throughput approaches to mutational analysis are being pursued.

Some investigators have argued that as the functional unit, proteins may be preferable for evaluation of gene expression. Indeed, gene expression can be regulated posttranscriptionally at the level of protein translation and stability, and protein function can be modulated by posttranslational changes such as glycosylation and phosphorylation. In addition to standard IHC-based approaches, high-throughput proteomic approaches such as reverse-phase arrays are being expored.[27]

CIRCULATING TUMOR CELLS AND MICROMETASTASES

For most solid tumors, our current staging strategy is based on determination of nodal involvement on the basis of histologic evaluation and distant metastases on the basis of appropriate imaging studies. Over the past decade there has been considerable debate as to whether utilization of

molecular technologies can help identify patients with low volume, subclinical nodal and distant disease burden, and whether this would be of prognostic significance.

The routine utilization of sentinel node technology for staging breast cancer and melanoma has made these diseases especially appropriate to test this hypothesis, by allowing scrutiny of relatively few lymph nodes rather than dozens of nodes. In both breast cancer and melanoma models, use of multimarker RT-PCR has been able to detect expression of at least one marker in a significant number of patients with IHC-negative nodes.[28,29] In retrospective studies in melanoma, molecular upstaging has been found to be a significant independent prognostic factor for recurrence and OS.[28] The prognostic value of molecular staging of sentinel nodes for breast cancer is being evaluated in a multi-institutional prospective study.[29]

There is compelling evidence for the prognostic value of micrometastasis in the bone marrow. In a recent pooled analysis of bone marrow micrometastasis in breast cancer, micrometastases were reported to be found in 31% of the 4,703 patients with stage I, II, or III cancer.[30] Patients with larger tumors, higher-grade tumors, positive nodes, and/or hormone receptor–positive tumors were more likely to have bone marrow micrometastasis. On multivariate analysis, bone marrow micrometastasis was an independent predictor of poor outcome. Ongoing work is evaluating the role of routine assessment of bone marrow status and the best way to incorporate this information into our clinical practice.

It has been suggested that circulating cancer cells can be an effective tool in selecting patients who are at high risk of relapse. The use of RT-PCR to detect circulating cancer cells as a prognostic marker is under active investigation by many groups, but is especially challenging because of its high sensitivity and its great potential for contamination and false-positive results. In one study, semiquantitative RT-PCR for three melanoma markers—tyrosinase, p97, and MelanA/MAET1—was used to detect circulating melanoma cells; the investigators concluded that detection of circulating melanoma cells has no additional prognostic value.[31] In another recent study, however, melanoma patients with stage II or III disease who had a positive RT-PCR for tyrosinase mRNA in their peripheral blood had a significantly lower DSS rate.[32] Therefore, the clinical value of this approach remains controversial.

There is, however, rapidly accumulating data supporting the use of the number of circulating tumor cells (CTCs) as a prognostic factor. In a prospective multicenter trial, the number of CTCs ($\geq$ 5 CTCs per 7.5 mL whole blood versus < 5 CTCs) before treatment of metastatic breast cancer was an independent predictor of progression-free and OS rates.[33] Serial monitoring of CTCs during or after therapy also has been proposed to be prognostic.[34,35]

Predictive Markers

The trend in systemic therapy is toward personalized medicine. Until recently it has been presumed that all cancers of a certain cell origin are the same, and all patients are offered the same systemic therapy. Not all patients respond to these therapies, however, emphasizing the biological variability within tumors. Therefore, the intent is to determine the underlying biology of each tumor in order to tailor therapy accordingly. "Predictive markers" are markers that can prospectively identify or enrich for patients who will benefit from a certain therapy.

There is increasing interest in identifying predictive markers for chemotherapy so that patients can be given the regimens that they are most likely to benefit from; those who are not likely to benefit from existing conventional therapies can be spared the toxicity of the therapy and be offered investigational therapies. The approaches utilized include high-throughput techniques such as transcriptional profiling. Preliminary work suggests that transcriptional profiling may be utilized successfully to identify molecular signatures that correlate with response to chemotherapy in general or to certain agents specifically.[36,37]

There is special interest in identifying predictive markers for targeted therapies. Existing predictive markers include estrogen receptor and HER2/*neu* for breast cancer, and c-kit for gastrointestinal stromal tumors, which can identify/enrich for patients who can potentially benefit from antiestrogen therapies (eg, tamoxifen), anti-HER2/*neu* therapies (eg, trastuzumab), and imatinib, respectively. If indeed a drug acts through a target, one would expect that the target should be expressed in the tumor. However, expression of the target alone may not be an adequate marker of response, as has been observed in clinical trials with inhibitors of EGFR. Instead, markers predictive of response should be able to select patients whose tumor growth is dependent on the target. Clinical trials conducted in unselected populations may lead to the elimination of therapies that could be efficacious in a selected subpopulation. For example, studies have demonstrated that although most patients with non–small-cell lung cancer have no response to gefitinib, a subgroup of patients have activating mutations of EGFR that render their tumors clinically responsive.[38,39] Identification of predictive markers will ultimately rely on a detailed understanding of the biologic rationale, as well as the careful molecular scrutiny of responders and nonresponders early in clinical trials.

Pharmacodynamic Markers of Response

Traditionally patients are given two to three cycles (weeks or months) of systemic therapy and then subjected to imaging to determine whether their tumors are responding. Pharmacodynamic markers of response can determine early in the treatment course whether the disease is responding at a molecular level. One set of markers, which determine whether the desired target is being inhibited, are often referred to as "markers of biological activity."

When targeted agents are brought to clinical trials, there is often uncertainty regarding the optimal dose. Traditional approaches of drug dose selection based on maximally tolerated dose may not be applicable—a dose leading to inhibition of the target should be sufficient. Markers that demonstrate target function, such as downstream signaling, are sought. For example, if kinase A phosphorylates protein B, phosphorylated B could be a marker of target function that could identify the effectiveness of an inhibitor of kinase A. A decline in downstream signaling would demonstrate whether the target was inhibited, and thus whether biologically relevant drug doses were achieved. If downstream signaling were not inhibited, this may suggest that dosing was inadequate, that genetic variations in speed of clearance/metabolism play a role, that compensatory feedback loops were activated and overcame the effect of target inhibition, that the individual has a mutation in the target, or that the drug is simply ineffective in inhibiting the target in vivo.

It is important to note that target inhibition may be necessary but not sufficient for response. Thus, markers of target inhibition may not be adequate markers of response. Other surrogate markers of response may include markers of proliferation (eg, Ki-67), markers of apoptosis, or other specific mechanism-dependent endpoints. Serial biopsies of the tumor could be utilized to assess these biomarkers. Another area of immense research activity is the development of molecular imaging strategies. The effects of molecular therapies on functional endpoints such as glucose uptake and cell proliferation are all being evaluated with significant early promise, while novel tracers to image-specific targets are also in development.

Towards the Future

An important goal in molecular oncology is to prevent a larger portion of cancers from developing, and once cancer develops, to detect it earlier, when higher cure rates can be achieved with surgery alone. A potential algorithm for incorporating molecular markers and molecular-targeted therapies into our clinical practice is shown in Figure 2-3. It is very likely that, in the near future, once a cancer diagnosis is made, molecular characterization of the tumor in addition to clinical staging will facilitate a more accurate prognostic assessment. This will allow for identification of patients at low risk of systemic recurrence, sparing them the toxicity of systemic therapy. Patients at higher risk will be able to undergo systemic therapy with traditional as well as novel agents that they are more likely to respond to, and less likely to experience adverse events with, as determined by predictive biomarker profiling. Thus, our rapidly improving understanding of cancer biology, as well as evolving technologies, will be incorporated into our clinical practice to result in personalized medicine that can achieve greater efficacy and an improved quality of life.

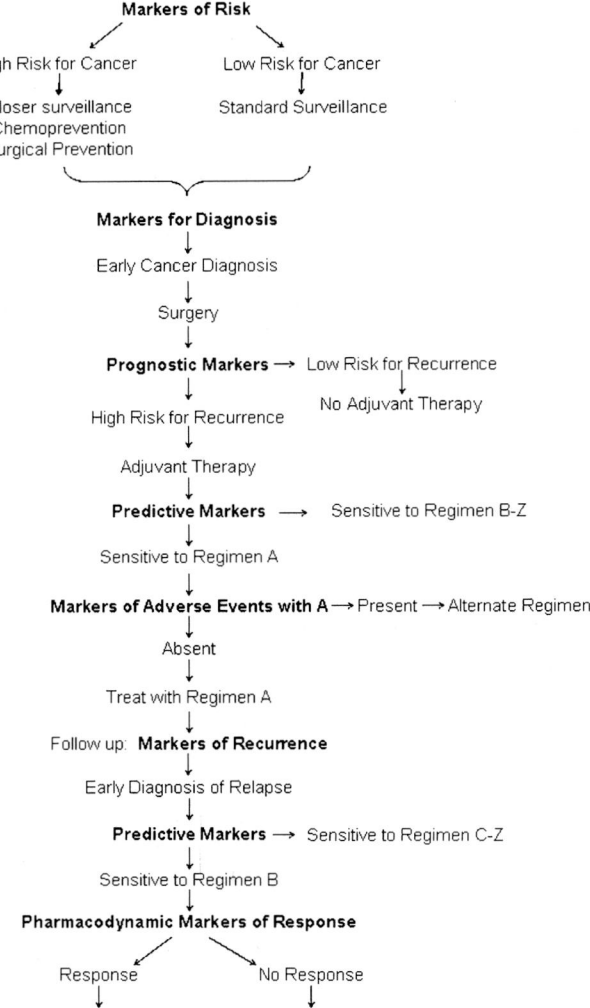

Figure 2-3 An algorithm for incorporating molecular markers and molecular-targeted therapies into clinical practice. Markers of risk can be utilized to select patients at higher risk of cancer development, and these patients can be offered closer observation or more aggressive preventive options. In the future, new diagnostic markers may assist in earlier diagnosis. Once a diagnosis is made, molecular characterization of the tumor can allow a more accurate prognostic assessment. Patients at low risk of systemic recurrence can be spared the toxicity of systemic therapy. Patients at higher risk will be able to undergo systemic therapy with agents that they are more likely to respond to, and less likely to experience adverse events with, as determined by predictive biomarker profiling. In patients with evaluable tumors (in the recurrent or metastatic setting, or in the neoadjuvant setting) pharmacodynamic markers of response can be used to further evaluate the success of selected therapies.

References

1. Bjerkvig R, Tysnes BB, Aboody KS, et al. The origin of the cancer stem cell: current controversies and new insights. Nat Rev Cancer 2005;5:899–904.

2. Fearon ER, Vogelstein B. A genetic model for colorectal tumorigenesis. Cell 1990;61:759–67.

3. Knudson AG. Two genetic hits (more or less) to cancer. Nat Rev Cancer 2001;1:157–62.

4. Blume-Jensen P, Hunter T. Oncogenic kinase signalling. Nature 2001;411:355–65.

5. Malumbres M, Barbacid M. To cycle or not to cycle: a critical decision in cancer. Nat Rev Cancer 2001;1:222–31.

6. Corn PG, El-Deiry WS. Derangement of growth and differentiation control in oncogenesis. Bioessays 2002;24:83–90.

7. Igney FH, Krammer PH. Death and anti-death: tumour resistance to apoptosis. Nat Rev Cancer 2002;2:277–88.

8. Liekens S, De Clercq E, Neyts J. Angiogenesis: regulators and clinical applications. Biochem Pharmacol 2001;61:253–70.

9. Fox SB, Gasparini G, Harris AL. Angiogenesis: pathological, prognostic, and growth-factor pathways and their link to trial design and anticancer drugs. Lancet Oncol 2001;2:278–89.

10. Reinmuth N, Parikh AA, Ahmad SA, et al. Biology of angiogenesis in tumors of the gastrointestinal tract. Microsc Res Tech 2003;60:199–207.

11. Nor JE, Christensen J, Mooney DJ, et al. Vascular endothelial growth factor (VEGF)-mediated angiogenesis is associated with enhanced endothelial cell survival and induction of Bcl-2 expression. Am J Pathol 1999;154:375–84.

12. Weidner N, Semple JP, Welch WR, et al. Tumor angiogenesis and metastasis—correlation in invasive breast carcinoma. N Engl J Med 1991;324:1–8.

13. Ramaswamy S, Ross KN, Lander ES, et al. A molecular signature of metastasis in primary solid tumors. Nat Genet 2003;33:49–54.

14. Dancey J, Sausville EA. Issues and progress with protein kinase inhibitors for cancer treatment. Nat Rev Drug Discov 2003;2:296–313.

15. Berry DA, Iversen ES Jr, Gudbjartsson DF, et al. BRCAPRO validation, sensitivity of genetic testing of BRCA1/BRCA2, and prevalence of other breast cancer susceptibility genes. J Clin Oncol 2002;20:2701–12.

16. Hemminki K, Bermejo JL. Relationships between familial risks of cancer and the effects of heritable genes and their SNP variants. Mutat Res 2005;592:6–17.

17. Houlston RS, Peto J. The search for low-penetrance cancer susceptibility alleles. Oncogene 2004;23:6471–6.

18. Paweletz CP, Liotta LA, Petricoin EF 3rd. New technologies for biomarker analysis of prostate cancer progression: laser capture microdissection and tissue proteomics. Urology 2001;57:160–3.

19. Petricoin EF, Ardekani AM, Hitt BA, et al. Use of proteomic patterns in serum to identify ovarian cancer. Lancet 2002;359:572–7.

20. Look MP, van Putten WL, Duffy MJ, et al. Pooled analysis of prognostic impact of urokinase-type plasminogen activator and its inhibitor PAI-1 in 8377 breast cancer patients. J Natl Cancer Inst 2002;94:116–28.

21. van 't Veer LJ, Dai H, van de Vijver MJ, et al. Gene expression profiling predicts clinical outcome of breast cancer. Nature 2002;415:530–6.

22. van de Vijver MJ, He YD, van't Veer LJ, et al. A gene-expression signature as a predictor of survival in breast cancer. N Engl J Med 2002;347:1999–2009.

23. Barrier A, Lemoine A, Boelle PY, et al. Colon cancer prognosis prediction by gene expression profiling. Oncogene 2005;24:6155–64.

24. Arango D, Laiho P, Kokko A, et al. Gene-expression profiling predicts recurrence in Dukes' C colorectal cancer. Gastroenterology 2005;129:874–84.

25. Chen CN, Lin JJ, Chen JJ, et al. Gene expression profile predicts patient survival of gastric cancer after surgical resection. J Clin Oncol 2005;23:7286–95.

26. Paik S, Shak S, Tang G, et al. A multigene assay to predict recurrence of tamoxifen-treated, node-negative breast cancer. N Engl J Med 2004;351:2817–26.

27. Petricoin EF, Zoon KC, Kohn EC, et al. Clinical proteomics: translating benchside promise into bedside reality. Nat Rev Drug Discov 2002;1:683–95.

28. Takeuchi H, Morton DL, Kuo C, et al. Prognostic significance of molecular upstaging of paraffin-embedded sentinel lymph nodes in melanoma patients. J Clin Oncol 2004;22:2671–80.

29. Mikhitarian K, Martin RH, Mitas M, et al. Molecular analysis improves sensitivity of breast sentinel lymph node biopsy: results of a multi-institutional prospective cohort study. Surgery 2005;138:474–81.

30. Braun S, Vogl FD, Naume B, et al. A pooled analysis of bone marrow micrometastasis in breast cancer. N Engl J Med 2005;353:793–802.

31. Palmieri G, Ascierto PA, Perrone F, et al. Prognostic value of circulating melanoma cells detected by reverse transcriptase-polymerase chain reaction. J Clin Oncol 2003;21:767–73.

32. Voit C, Kron M, Rademaker J, et al. Molecular staging in stage II and III melanoma patients and its effect on long-term survival. J Clin Oncol 2005;23:1218–27.

33. Cristofanilli M, Budd GT, Ellis MJ, et al. Circulating tumor cells, disease progression, and survival in metastatic breast cancer. N Engl J Med 2004;351:781–91.

34. Cristofanilli M, Hayes DF, Budd GT, et al. Circulating tumor cells: a novel prognostic factor for newly diagnosed metastatic breast cancer. J Clin Oncol 2005;23:1420–30.

35. Koyanagi K, O'Day SJ, Gonzalez R, et al. Serial monitoring of circulating melanoma cells during neoadjuvant bio-chemotherapy for stage III melanoma: outcome prediction in a multicenter trial. J Clin Oncol 2005;23:8057–64.

36. Ayers M, Symmans WF, Stec J, et al. Gene expression profiles predict complete pathologic response to neoadjuvant paclitaxel and fluorouracil, doxorubicin, and cyclophosphamide chemotherapy in breast cancer. J Clin Oncol 2004;22:2284–93.

37. Chang JC, Wooten EC, Tsimelzon A, et al. Gene expression profiling for the prediction of therapeutic response to docetaxel in patients with breast cancer. Lancet 2003;362:362–9.

38. Lynch TJ, Bell DW, Sordella R, et al. Activating mutations in the epidermal growth factor receptor underlying responsiveness of non–small-cell lung cancer to gefitinib. N Engl J Med 2004;350:2129–39.

39. Paez JG, Janne PA, Lee JC, et al. EGFR mutations in lung cancer: correlation with clinical response to gefitinib therapy. Science 2004;304:1497–500.

CHAPTER 3

SURGICAL TREATMENT OF SQUAMOUS CANCER OF THE ESOPHAGUS

LUIS J. HERRERA, MD

ARA A. VAPORCIYAN, MD

Squamous cell carcinoma (SCC) of the esophagus is the most common histological type of esophageal cancer worldwide.[1,2] The incidence of esophageal SCC has significant geographical variation, and in certain high-risk regions, esophageal cancer represents one of the leading causes of death.[3] In the US, SCC of the esophagus has been eclipsed as the most common histology by the steep increase in the incidence of esophageal adenocarcinoma; however, squamous cell histology still represents approximately 45% of esophageal carcinomas with an estimated 6,500 new cases in 2005.[1,4] Most of the surgical experience with esophageal SCC comes from China and Japan, where this histologic type represents more than 80% of esophageal cancers. Due to its overall poor prognosis, multimodality treatment options are often preferred in an attempt to improve survival and local tumor control.

Surgery remains the main component of treatment for SCC of the esophagus. However, variability exists regarding the surgical approach to esophageal cancer. Despite decades of surgical treatment, significant controversy remains regarding the optimal approach for surgical resection, the extent of resection, and degree of lymphadenectomy. In addition, surgical treatment of this disease often presents significant challenges due to tumor location and aggressive locoregional involvement. In this chapter we review the current concepts in the surgical management of esophageal SCC.

Etiology and Epidemiology

In the US, the most common risk factors for esophageal SCC are chronic tobacco use and alcohol consumption.[5]

Chronic esophageal irritation associated with achalasia and esophageal injury due to lye ingestion has also been associated with the development of cancer. Other important risk factors commonly associated with the development of esophageal cancer include environmental and dietary factors such as consumption of hot beverages, vitamin deficiencies, and heavy exposure to nitrates. These factors tend to play a more prominent role in Asian cultures.[6]

In 2005 it is estimated that approximately 14,520 Americans will be diagnosed with esophageal cancer, and 13,570 will die of this malignancy. Of the new cases, 11,220 will occur in men and 3,300 will occur in women.[4] In the US, the incidence of SCC is gradually declining, while the incidence of adenocarcinoma has risen precipitously (Figure 3-1).[2,7] Squamous histology is more commonly seen in African-American males, where its incidence has remained relatively stable, and is also more common in patients with significant smoking and drinking habits.[8] However, esophageal SCC continues to be the most common histologic type worldwide. In certain regions such as Iran, Turkey, China, and India, esophageal SCC is one of the leading causes of death, with incidences surpassing 100 cases per 100,000, compared to an incidence of 7.7 cases per 100,000 men and 2 cases per 100,000 women in the US.[3,9]

Diagnosis

The presentation of SCC of the esophagus commonly includes dysphagia to a varying degree. Other common signs and symptoms include weight loss, regurgitation,

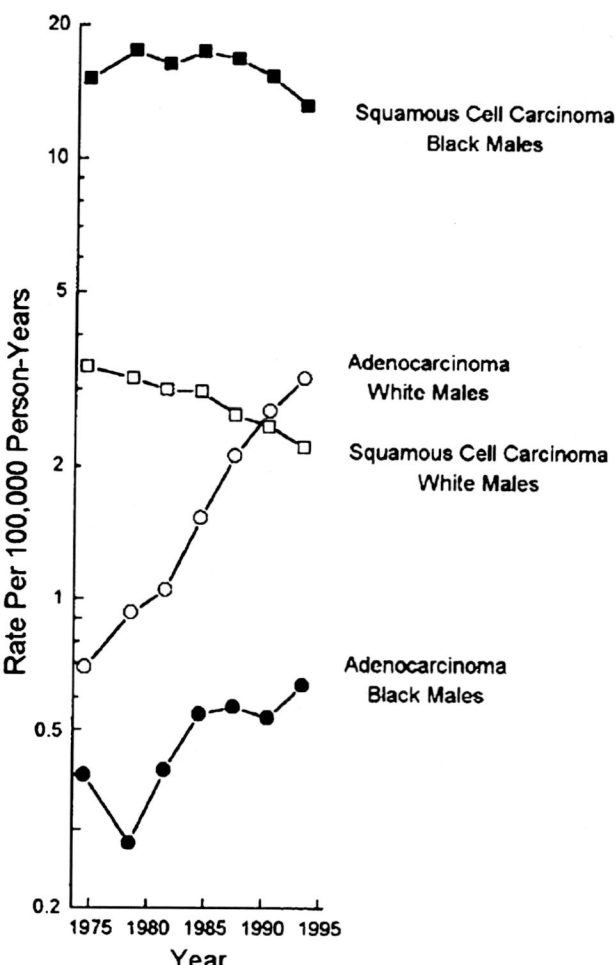

Figure 3-1 Trends in age-adjusted incidence for esophageal carcinoma by race and cell type.[2]

Staging

An essential component for planning any treatment for esophageal SCC is accurate staging evaluation. The current staging for esophageal carcinoma is based on the classification by the American Joint Committee on Cancer and is listed in Table 3-1.[10] Esophageal SCC with celiac node involvement is frequently staged M1b due to the predominant upper- and middle-third presentation of this histology. This classification may not always represent distant disease. Akiyama and colleagues performed a detailed description of lymph node involvement in esophageal cancer according to tumor location and depth of invasion.[11] In cervical esophageal tumors with positive lymph node metastasis, the location of the lymph node metastasis was intrabdominal in 31% of cases. Similarly, distal-third tumors had cervical lymph node metastasis in 9.8%. Once the tumor invades the submucosa, lymph node metastases are present in 30% of cases.[12]

The staging evaluation of esophageal cancer begins with the EUS, which can evaluate the T and N status accurately. As mentioned earlier, EUS has become the primary modality for evaluation of the extent of locoregional disease, in particular the T staging. EUS can correctly establish the level of invasion (T stage) in 89% of patients and the nodal status (N stage) in 73% of patients.[13]

CT scan of the chest and upper abdomen is also useful for staging with the ability to detect distant metastases, and with lesser accuracy, the extent of locoregional disease. The accuracy of CT scan for nodal staging in esophageal cancer is 67% (55% sensitivity and 83% specificity).[14] PET scanning has become a useful adjunct in the staging of esophageal cancer with more sensitivity for the detection of metastatic and regional lymph node disease. PET can complement CT scans in the detection of metastatic disease. In a series of 100 esophageal cancer cases, 16% of patients were found to have PET-positive metastatic disease that was not detected with CT scans.[15] In addition, PET scanning may have an important role in assessing the response to neoadjuvant therapy. Swisher and colleagues at the University of Texas M. D. Anderson Cancer Center evaluated the utility of PET scanning after induction chemoradiotherapy (CRT) for restaging, for prediction of response, and for prognosis. Pathologic response was found to correlate with the post-CRT PET standardized uptake value (SUV) and a post-CRT SUV higher than 4 was found to be the only preoperative factor to correlate with decreased survival (2-year survival rate of 33% versus 60%; $p = .01$).[16]

Given the more common involvement of the mid and upper esophagus in SCC of the esophagus, broncho-

respiratory symptoms, chest pain, and gastrointestinal bleeding. Advanced disease at presentation is common, with 28% of patients demonstrating distant metastatic disease at the time of diagnosis.[8] Evaluation of dysphagia usually involves a contrast esophagogram, which will identify a classic intraluminal mass with narrowing and proximal dilatation. Endoscopy is the definitive diagnostic tool for esophageal SCC, especially when accompanied by esophageal endoscopic ultrasound (EUS). The combination of these two procedures improves diagnosis and staging with assessment of the Tumor (T) and Nodal (N) stage, the location of the tumor (proximal, mid, distal esophagus), and histologic confirmation. In addition, an important factor to be evaluated during endoscopy is the suitability of the stomach as an esophageal replacement.

Advanced esophageal SCC can also be diagnosed using computed tomography (CT) and positron emission tomography (PET); however, these tests are more commonly involved in the staging of esophageal cancer.

Table 3-1 TNM Staging for Esophageal Cancer: American Joint Committee on Cancer Staging System[10]

Primary tumor stage (T)	
Tx	Primary tumor cannot be assessed
T0	No evidence of primary tumor
T1*	Tumor invades the lamina propria or submucosa
T2	Tumor invades the muscularis propria
T3	Tumor invades through muscularis propria into periesophageal tissue
T4	Invasion into adjacent structure (trachea, pericardium, spine, aorta)
Nodal involvement (N)	
Nx	Regional lymph nodes cannot be assessed
N0	No regional lymph node metastases
N1	Regional lymph node metastasis
Distant metastasis (M)	
Mx	Distant metastasis cannot be assessed
M0	No evidence of distant metastasis
M1	Distant metastases
M1a	Celiac lymph node metastasis in lower-third esophageal cancers
	Cervical lymph node metastasis in upper-third esophageal cancer
	Extrathoracic lymph node involvement in middle-third lesions
M1b	Other distant metastasis

C = clinical staging; P = pathological staging; Y refers to restaging after induction treatment.
*T1 patients are sometimes subclassified into T1a (intramucosal tumor not extending into submucosa) and T1b (tumor invading submucosa).

scopic evaluation of the airway to assess for tracheobronchial invasion is an essential part of staging SCC, in particular if EUS demonstrates a T3 lesion. More invasive staging modalities such as thoracoscopic and laparoscopic staging have been used. In addition to identification of pleural and peritoneal metastasis, biopsy of nodal stations can increase nodal staging accuracy to 93%; however, the cost and utility of this approach is generally warranted only in the patient with higher likelihood of having metastatic disease based on preoperative imaging.[17]

Preoperative Evaluation

Patients presenting with SCC of the esophagus are frequently elderly and often have significant medical comorbidities. In addition, many patients present with malnutrition and heavy exposure to alcohol and tobacco. It is necessary to identify patients with limited cardiopulmonary reserve who would not tolerate extensive operations due to a high likelihood of complications.

Standard evaluation includes a complete history and physical examination with a careful assessment of any comorbidities identified. The physiologic studies most commonly obtained include pulmonary function studies and stress evaluation of the heart. The presence of other comorbidities leads to additional preoperative testing in order to exclude patients with an excessive risk of operative morbidity or mortality.

Another essential component in the preoperative evaluation is the nutritional assessment of the esophageal SCC patient. Changes in diet secondary to the progressive dysphagia often result in patients that are malnourished even without significant weight loss. Aggressive preoperative nutritional support is frequently warranted. Placement of enteral access is frequently necessary in patients with dysphagia and planned induction chemotherapy or CRT. In extreme cases, CRT or surgical treatment may need to be delayed to allow correction of severe malnutrition. Nasoenteric or jejunostomy tubes are preferred over gastric tubes, which may damage the stomach and jeopardize its use as an esophageal replacement.

Surgical Options for Squamous Cell Cancer of the Esophagus

The surgical approach to esophageal SCC depends on the location of the tumor, the tumor stage, and the surgeon's level of experience. There is significant controversy regarding the extent of resection, the level of regional lymph node dissection, and the method of reconstruction. Regardless of the approach, the essential requirements of any operation are the same: to achieve a complete surgical resection and, if possible, restore enteral continuity.

The definition of complete surgical resection is the center of most of the controversy regarding the surgical management of this disease. At the least, it should include proximal, distal, and radial margins that are microscopically free of disease and regional nodal assessment. The accepted proximal and distal margins are 5 cm when possible. Most of the controversy surrounds the radial margin. Hence, the surgical approach to this disease has significant variability and is often influenced by surgeon's preference, training, and treatment philosophy.

Method of Resection

We have broadly categorized the methods of resection by the location of the esophagogastric anastomosis. While lower third tumors can be resected using any of these methods, upper-third and some middle-third tumors may only be approached using cervical anastomotic techniques.

CERVICAL ANASTOMOSIS

Transhiatal Esophagectomy

Transhiatal resection of the esophagus preceded the development of the transthoracic approach to esophagectomy, mainly due to anesthetic limitations at the time. First performed by Turner in 1936, the transhiatal procedure then became disfavored once intrathoracic surgery was possible, due to the superior visualization obtained with a transthoracic approach.[18] In 1978 Orringer and Sloan reintroduced transhiatal esophagectomy as an option for elective palliation of esophageal cancer and dysphagia with reduced perioperative morbidity rates.[19] Since then, the transhiatal approach has gained significant popularity, but controversy still exists regarding its adequacy as a cancer operation for carcinoma of the esophagus. Although a complete celiac lymph node dissection is performed, only a limited mediastinal lymph node dissection is possible. Many authors suggest this limitation does not adversely impact disease-free or overall survival. Moreover, the transhiatal approach avoids the morbidity associated with an additional thoracotomy incision. In a recent review by Orringer of 1,085 patients undergoing transhiatal esophagectomy, the hospital mortality rate was 4%, and significant postoperative complications occurred in 20% of patients. The anastomotic leak rate was 13% and recurrent laryngeal nerve injury occurred in less than 7%, with permanent hoarseness in less than 1% of patients.[20] In a more recent review of modifications in anastomotic technique, clinically significant cervical anastomotic leaks occurred in only 2.7% of patients.[21] Other specific but rare complications after transhiatal esophagectomy include bleeding from direct injury of the azygos vein, bleeding form the esophageal bed, and injury of the tracheobronchial tree during blunt mobilization.

Three-Field Esophagectomy (McKeown Modification)

As first described in 1976, the patient was placed in the left lateral decubitus position with the right arm prepped into the field. The abdominal procedure was performed first, followed by a right thoracotomy and then a right cervical approach to the esophagus.[22]

The procedure has subsequently been modified and now begins with a right thoracotomy to mobilize the esophagus. The thoracotomy is closed and the patient is repositioned supine, exposing the left neck for access to the cervical esophagus. This surgical approach is most useful for tumors located in the middle third of the esophagus, particularly when avoiding a thoracic anastomosis is desired. In addition, a total esophagectomy is performed, which maximizes the proximal resection margin. Compared to a transhiatal esophagectomy, the addition of the thoracotomy increases the morbidity but allows safe dissection of tumors adjacent to the tracheobronchial tree and a complete mediastinal lymph node dissection. The lymph node dissection commonly includes the celiac and mediastinal fields, but a cervical lymphadenectomy can be performed to achieve a complete three-field lymph node dissection.

INTRATHORACIC ANASTOMOSIS

Transthoracic Esophagectomy (Ivor-Lewis)

The first successful esophagectomies via a transthoracic approach were described by Lewis and by Tanner in 1946 and 1947, respectively, and this approach is still used extensively today.[23,24] Initially associated with significant morbidity and high mortality rates, modern series report a reduced mortality rate of approximately 3% to 6%, and a morbidity rate of 26% to 34%.[25,26] This operation offers excellent exposure for resection of lower and some middle-third esophageal tumors, and allows regional lymph node dissection in the abdomen and in the chest.

Apart from the added morbidity and postoperative pain associated with the use of a thoracotomy, the main disadvantage of this approach has been the intrathoracic location of the anastomosis. Historically the consequences of an intrathoracic anastomotic leak were more life threatening than a cervical anastomotic leak; however, improvement in perioperative care and a more aggressive approach to patients with intrathoracic leaks have resulted in decreased mortality rates. Intrathoracic anastomotic leak-associated mortality rates of 20 to 33% have been reported.[27,28] However, in a recent review of the experience at the M. D. Anderson Cancer Center, the mortality rate associated with an intrathoracic anastomotic leak was no different to that of patients without a leak (3.3% versus 2.5%, $p = .55$). During a 34-year experience at this institution, the leak-associated mortality rate was markedly reduced from 43% to 3.3% ($p = .016$). This was partly attributed to an increased proportion of successful reoperations attempting to repair the leak, combined with a liberal use of reinforcing muscle flaps.[29]

Left Thoracoabdominal Approach

The left thoracoabdominal approach to resection is more suitable for distal-third esophageal carcinoma; therefore, it less commonly applied to esophageal SCC. However, when distal lesions are encountered, it remains a viable option for resection. Although similar to an Ivor-Lewis operation, the advantages of this approach include the ability to perform a resection under direct visualization via a single incision without the need to reposition the patient, while allowing performance of a two-field lymph node dissection. The disadvantage of this approach is the limited access to the middle and upper third of the esophagus due to the constraints of the aortic arch in the left chest.

CONDUITS

The stomach is the most commonly utilized esophageal substitute due to the simplicity of preparation, reliable blood supply, and adequate length. However, in certain cases, the stomach will not be appropriate and alternative conduits are required. The colon is the second most frequently utilized conduit. Some authors favor colonic interposition because of better functional outcomes, less esophageal reflux, and a lower incidence of regurgitation. However, the blood supply of the colon is limited due to atherosclerotic disease in many older patients. Preoperative angiography is required to assure patency of the marginal artery of Drummond prior to using the colon as an esophageal substitute.

In certain situations, neither the stomach nor colon can be used. For short segment distal-esophageal defects, a pedicled Roux short jejunal segment or a free jejunal graft allows for a functional conduit. In more challenging cases where a long segment esophageal substitute is needed, our preferred approach for reconstruction has been a supercharged pedicled long segment of jejunum. The distal end of the vascular arcade is revascularized with a microvascular anastomosis in the cervical area.[30]

Surgical Controversies

EXTENT OF RESECTION

Transhiatal versus Transthoracic Resection

Several retrospective studies comparing results of transhiatal and transthoracic esophagectomies have reported increased postoperative complication rates after transthoracic resection.[31,32] Three prospective evaluations of transhiatal versus transthoracic esophagectomies have been performed[33,34,36] (Table 3-2). The patient numbers were small, but revealed no significant difference in morbidity or mortality rates, and in one study there was comparable 3-year survival rates in stage III patients.[34] In a more recent prospective randomized trial comparing transhiatal resection with transthoracic en bloc esophagectomy, it was noted that perioperative mortality was not different between the two groups, but the transthoracic resection group had a higher incidence of pulmonary complications. There was not a statistically significant difference in survival; however, after 3 years there appeared to be a trend towards improved survival with transthoracic resection[36] (Figure 3-2).

Total en bloc Esophagectomy

This operation is usually combined with a three-field esophagectomy but with a wider resection of the esophagus. It involves en bloc resection of the posterior pericardium, both pleural envelopes, azygos vein, thoracic duct, and a thorough regional lymph node dissection. Proponents argue that this allows complete resection of the esophagus with a radial margin of normal mediastinal periesophageal tissues. A modification of the en bloc procedure preserves the azygos vein, but still includes a posterior mediastinectomy including the thoracic duct.[37] Retrospective studies have reported improved survival rates using en bloc esophagectomy

Table 3-2 Summary of Recent Trials Evaluating Outcomes after Transhiatal Esophagectomy versus Transthoracic Resection for Esophageal Carcinoma

Study	Patients	Operation	In-Hospital Mortality	Anastomotic Leak	Pulmonary Complication	Survival
Hulscher et al. 2002[36]	220 PRT AdenoCA	THE 106	2 (2%)	15 (14%)	29 (27%)	5-yr 29%
		TTE 114	5 (4%)	18 (16%)	65 (57%)	5-yr 39%
Horstmann et al. 1995[35]	87 RS	THE 46	7 (15%)	23 (50%)	16 (35%)	3-yr 21%
		TTE 41	4 (10%)	10 (24%)	12 (29%)	3-yr 17%
Goldminc et al. 1993[34]	67 pts PRT	THE 32	2 (6%)	2 (6%)	6 (19%)	No difference
		TTE 35	3 (8.5%)	3 (9%)	7 (20%)	
Chu et al. 1997[33]	39 PRT	THE 20	3 (15%)	NR	14 (70%)	Median 16 mo
		TTE 19	0 (0%)		11 (56%)	Median 13.5 mo

NR = not reported; PRT = prespective randomized trial; RS = retrospective series; THE = transhiatal esophagectomy; TTE = transthoracic esophagectomy.

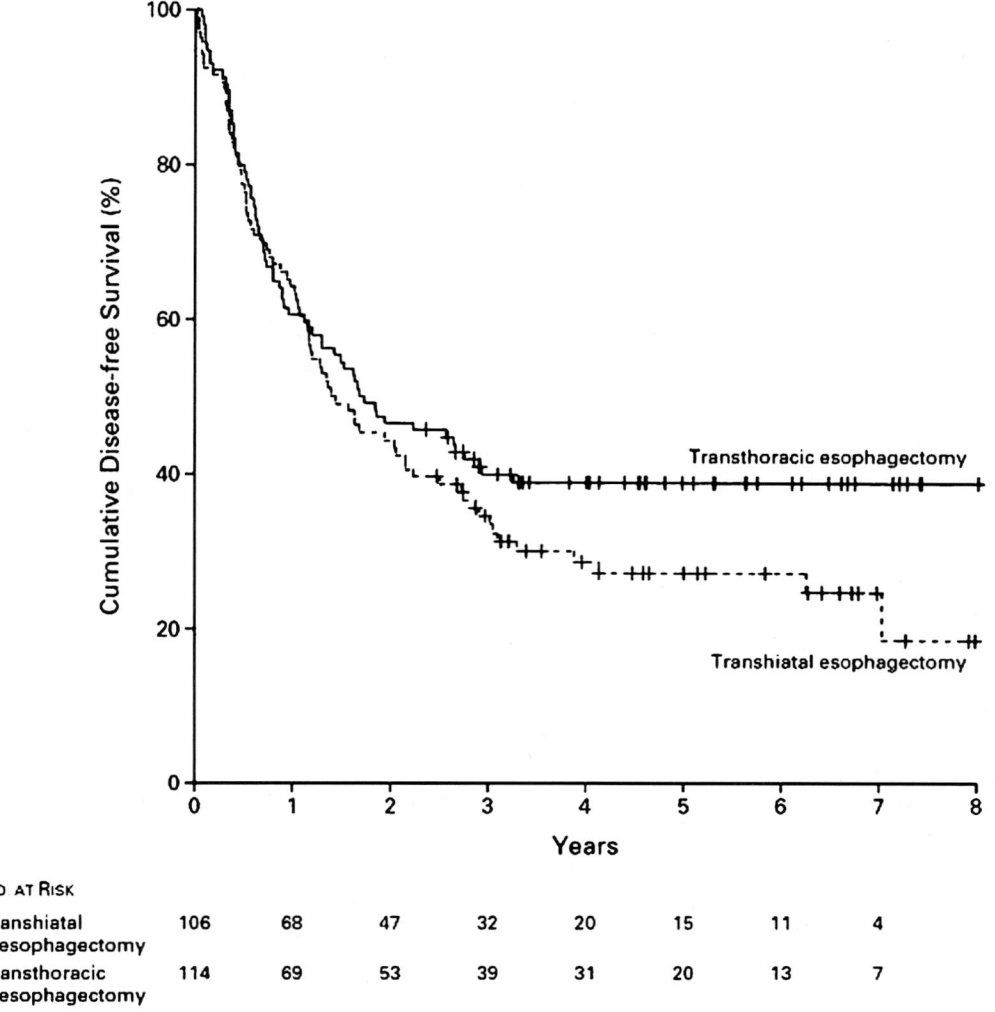

No at Risk								
Transhiatal esophagectomy	106	68	47	32	20	15	11	4
Transthoracic esophagectomy	114	69	53	39	31	20	13	7

Figure 3-2 Kaplan–Meier curves showing disease-free survival among patients randomly assigned to transhiatal esophagectomy or transthoracic esophagectomy with extended en bloc lymphadenectomy.[36]

when compared to standard transthoracic esophagectomy. No prospective data are available comparing these two techniques.[37,38] In the series reported by Altorki and colleagues, the in-hospital mortality rate following en bloc esophagectomy was 4.8%, with 40% having postoperative complications. The overall and disease-free 5-year survival rate with en bloc esophagectomy was 46% and 40%, respectively.[37]

Three-Field Lymphadenectomy

The variable nodal drainage pattern of the esophagus has provoked some surgeons to perform extended lymphadenectomy that includes the upper mediastinum, along both recurrent laryngeal nerves, the brachiocephalic trunk, and bilateral cervical nodes [39]. Three-field lymph node dissections was first popularized by the Japanese in the 1980s due to a reported 30 to 40% incidence of

isolated cervical lymph node metastasis after resection.[39,40] Some series in the US have reported comparable incidences of metastasis in the cervical lymph nodes with 40% of patients with squamous cancer demonstrating cervical lymph node involvement. In 13% of patients the cervical nodes were the only site of involvement.[41,42] In the East, especially in Japan, extensive lymph node dissection is advocated as standard procedure for esophageal SCC, including resection of abdominal, lower and upper mediastinal, and occasionally the cervical lymph nodes.[39] This aggressive approach has been applied to SCC of the lower thoracic esophagus, where a three-field dissection improved survival in patients with upper- or middle-mediastinal lymph node metastasis when compared to a two-field dissection (30% versus 5.6%, $p = .005$). However, the overall 5-year survival rate for the group of 156 patients was not different between those having a two-field (45%) versus a three-field lymph node dissection (51.7%), $p = .406$.[43] In another series of patients undergoing three-field lymphadenectomy from Japan, Nakagawa and colleagues reported on 174 patients, with an overall 5-year survival of 55%, and a 43% overall recurrence rate.[44] Locoregional recurrence occurred in 17.5% of patients. Of patients with cervical lymph node metastasis, 63% had a locoregional recurrence despite this aggressive lymphadenectomy. Despite a very low mortality rate of 1.3%, the complication rate was 75%, with recurrent laryngeal nerve injury being the most frequent at 58%.[44]

Cervical Esophageal Tumors

Esophageal squamous cell carcinomas arising in the cervical esophagus represent 7 to 10% of all esophageal tumors. Cervical esophageal cancers can be challenging tumors to address surgically due to the proximity to the cricopharyngeus muscle. In addition, early lymph node metastasis can involve paratracheal and deep cervical lymph node stations.[45]

It is crucial to determine the extent of the cancer and its distance from the cricopharyngeus muscle. Every effort is made to preserve the upper-esophageal sphincter because resection increases both the technical complexity of the procedure and the incidence of aspiration. Inability to achieve a clear proximal margin of at least 1 cm from the cricopharyngeus requires pharyngo-laryngo-esophagectomy, first described by Ong and Lee in 1960.[46] Concomitant laryngectomy at the time of esophagectomy was required in up to 94% of cervical esophageal tumors.[47] The hypopharynx, esophagus, and larynx are resected en bloc, with creation of a terminal tracheostomy. A bilateral cervical lymphadenectomy is performed. Esophageal reconstruction depends on the level of the distal margin. If the disease is localized to the upper-cervical esophagus, a free jejunal interposition graft with microvascular anastomosis provides a good conduit. Additional reconstructive options include a pectoralis or deltopectoral myocutaneous flaps. A partial sternectomy or manubrium resection can facilitate exposure. If the distal extent of the tumor does not allow a clear margin at the cervical level, then a complete esophagectomy via a transhiatal or transthoracic approach can be performed, using the stomach, colon, or a supercharged pedicled jejunal transfer as reconstruction options.

The impact of these aggressive procedures in quality of life has led many to use external beam radiotherapy as the primary method of treatment for these tumors. However, the results with definitive radiation for upper-third tumors have been inferior to surgery; local recurrence rates of up to 80% have been reported following irradiation.[48] As an alternative, definitive chemoradiation therapy is effective for the treatment of cervical esophageal carcinomas, with the main advantage being avoidance of the morbidity and loss of function associated with laryngectomy. In a series of 34 patients with cervical esophageal carcinoma treated with chemotherapy based on 5-Flurouracil and cisplatin with concurrent external beam radiation therapy with a mean dose of 61.2 Gy, the local control rate was 88% with a projected 5-year survival rate of 55%.[49] Salvage surgical therapy for patients who demonstrate persistent or recurrent disease may be feasible; however, is often associated with increased morbidity and mortality rates.

Summary

Squamous cell carcinoma of the esophagus, although currently less frequent than adenocarcinoma in the US, is still a commonly encountered malignancy for esophageal surgeons. The frequent upper-esophageal location of the tumor, propensity for airway involvement, and the physiologic status of the patient can make the surgical treatment of this disease quite challenging. However, despite improvement in multimodality therapy, surgery remains the mainstay of treatment of this disease. The surgical approach to esophageal SCC depends on the location of the tumor, the tumor stage, and the surgeon's preference. Given that most tumors are located in the middle and upper esophagus, three-field esophagectomy is often a favored approach. Superior results with cervical lymphadenectomy in Japan and China have not been consistently reproduced in the US and are not routinely performed.

References

1. Blot WJ, Devesa SS, Kneller RW, Fraumeni FF Jr. Rising incidence of adenocarcinoma of the esophagus and gastric cardia. JAMA 1991;265:1287–9.

2. Devesa SS, Blot WJ. Fraumeni FF Jr. Changing patterns of esophageal and gastric adenocarcinoma in the United States. Cancer 1998;83:2049–53.

3. Kirby TJ, Rice TW. The epidemiology of esophageal carcinoma. The changing face of a disease. Chest Surg Clin North America 1994;4:217–25.

4. American Cancer Society: Cancer Facts and Figures 2005. Atlanta, GA: American Cancer Society, 2005.

5. Ribeiro U Jr, Posner MC, Safatle-Ribeiro AV, Reynolds JC. Risk factors for squamous cell carcinoma of the oesophagus. Br J Surg 1996;83:1174–85.

6. Gamliel Z. Incidence, epidemiology and etiology of esophageal cancer. Chest Surg Clin N Am 2000;10:441–50.

7. Blot WJ, McLaughlin JK. The changing epidemiology of esophageal cancer. Semin Oncol 1999;26:2–8.

8. U.S. Cancer Statistics Working Group. *United States Cancer Statistics: 1999–2002 Incidence and Mortality Web-based Report Version.* Atlanta: Department of Health and Human Services, Centers for Disease Control and Prevention, *and* National Cancer Institute; 2005. Available at: www.cdc.gov/cancer/npcr/uscs.

9. Surveillance, Epidemiology, End Results (SEER) Program (www.seer.cancer.gov) SEER*Stat Database: Incidence—SEER 9 Regs Public-Use, Nov 2004 Sub (1973–2002), National Cancer Institute, DCCPS, Surveillance Research Program, Cancer Statistics Branch, released April 2005, based on the November 2004 submission.

10. Esophagus. In: American Joint Committee on Cancer: AJCC Cancer Staging Manual. 6th ed. New York, NY: Springer, 2002. p. 91–8.

11. Akiyama H, Tsurumaru M, Kawamura T, Ono Y. Principles of surgical treatment for carcinoma of the esophagus: analysis of lymph node involvement. Ann Surg 1981;194:438–46.

12. Lu YK, Li YM, Gu YZ. Cancer of esophagus and esophagogastric junction: analysis of results of 1,025 resections after 5 to 20 years. Ann Thorac Surg 1987;43:176–81.

13. Meining A, Dittler HJ, Wolf A, et al. You get what you expect? A critical appraisal of imaging methodology in endosonographic cancer staging. Gut 2002;50:599–603.

14. LoCicero J 3rd. Will multimodality therapy solve the enigma of long-term survival for squamous cell carcinoma of the esophagus? Semin Surg oncol 1993;9:14–8.

15. Luketich JD, Schauer PR, Meltzer CC, et al. Role of positron emission tomography in staging esophageal cancer. Ann Thorac Surg 1997;64:765–9.

16. Swisher SG, Erasmus J, Maish M, et al. 2-Fluoro-2-deoxy-D-glucose positron emission tomography imaging is predictive of pathologic response and survival after preoperative chemoradiation in patients with esophageal carcinoma. Cancer 2004;101:1776–85.

17. Krasna MJ. Advances in staging of esophageal carcinoma. Chest 1998;113:107S–111S.

18. Turner GC. Carcinoma of the esophagus. The question of its treatment by surgery Lancet 1936;1:130.

19. Orringer MB, Sloan H. Esophagectomy without thoracotomy. J Thorac Cardiovasc Surg 1978;76:643–54.

20. Orringer MB, Marshall B, Iannettoni MD. Transhiatal esophagectomy: clinical experience and refinements. Ann Surg 1999;230:392–400.

21. Orringer MB, Marshall B, Iannettoni MD. Eliminating the cervical esophagogastric anastomotic leak with a side-to-side stapled anastomosis. J Thorac Cardiovasc Surg 2000;119:277–88.

22. McKeown KC. Total three-stage oesophagectomy for cancer of the oesophagus. Br J Surg 1976;63:259–62.

23. Lewis I. The surgical treatment of carcinoma of the esophagus with special reference to a new operation for growths of the middle third. Br J Surg 1946;34:18.

24. Tanner NC. The present position of carcinoma of the esophagus. Post Grad Med 1947;23:109.

25. Ellis FH Jr, Heatley GJ, Krasna MJ, et al. Esophagogastrectomy for carcinoma of the esophagus and cardia: a comparison of findings and results after standard resection in three consecutive eight-year intervals with improved staging criteria. J Thorac Cardiovasc Surg 1997;113:836–46.

26. Kelsen DP, Ginsberg R, Pajak TF, et al. Chemotherapy followed by surgery compared with surgery alone for localized esophageal cancer. N Engl J Med 1998;339:1979–84.

27. Agrawal S, Deshmukh SP, Patil PK, et al. Intrathoracic anastomosis after oesophageal resection for cancer. J Surg Oncol 1996;63:52–6.

28. Ellis FH Jr, Heatley GJ, Krasna MJ, et al. Esophagogastrectomy for carcinoma of the esophagus and cardia: a comparison of findings and results after standard resection in three consecutive eight-year intervals with improved staging criteria. J Thorac Cardiovasc Surg 1997;113:836–46.

29. Martin LW, Swisher SG, Hofstetter W, et al. Intrathoracic leaks following esophagectomy are no longer associated with increased mortality. Ann Surg 2005;242:392–9.

30. Ascioti AJ, Hofstetter WL, Miller MJ, et al. Long-segment, supercharged, pedicled jejunal flap for total esophageal reconstruction. J Thorac Cardiovasc Surg 2005;130:1391–8.

31. Pac M, Basoglu A, Kocak H, et al. Transhiatal versus transthoracic esophagectomy for esophageal cancer. J Thorac Cardiovasc Surg 1993;106:205–9.

32. Putnam JB Jr, Suell DM, McMurtrey MJ, et al. Comparison of three techniques of esophagectomy within a residency training program. Ann Thorac Surg 1994;57:319–25.

33. Chu KM, Law SY, Fok M, Wong J. A prospective randomized comparison of transhiatal and transthoracic resection for lower-third esophageal carcinoma. Am J Surg 1997;174:320–4.

34. Goldminc M, Maddern G, Le Prise E, et al. Oesophagectomy by a transhiatal approach or thoracotomy: a prospective randomized trial. Br J Surg 1993;80:367–70.

35. Horstmann O, Verreet PR, Becker H, et al. Transhiatal oesophagectomy compared with transthoracic resection and systematic lymphadenectomy for the treatment of oesophageal cancer. Eur J Surg 1995;161:557–67.

36. Hulscher JB, van Sandick JW, de Boer AG, et al. Extended transthoracic resection compared with limited transhiatal

resection for adenocarcinoma of the esophagus. N Engl J Med 2002;347:1662–9.

37. Altorki N, Skinner D. Should en bloc esophagectomy be the standard of care for esophageal carcinoma? Ann Surg 2001; 234:581–7.

38. Skinner DB, Little AG, Ferguson MK, et al. Selection of operation for esophageal cancer based on staging. Ann Surg 1986;204:391–401.

39. Isono K, Sato H, Nakayama K. Results of a nationwide study on the three-field lymph node dissection of esophageal cancer. Oncology 1991;48:411–20.

40. Kato H, Tachimori Y, Watanabe H, et al. Lymph node metastasis in thoracic esophageal carcinoma. J Surg Oncol 1991;48:106–11.

41. Altorki NK, Skinner DB. Occult cervical nodal metastasis in esophageal cancer: preliminary results of three-field lymphadenectomy. J Thorac Cardiovasc Surg 1997;113: 540–4.

42. Altorki N, Kent M, Ferrara C, Port J. Three-field lymph node dissection for squamous cell and adenocarcinoma of the esophagus. Ann Surg 2002;236:177–83.

43. Igaki H, Tachimori Y, Kato H. Improved survival for patients with upper and/or middle mediastinal lymph node metastasis of squamous cell carcinoma of the lower thoracic esophagus treated with 3-field dissection. Ann Surg 2004;239:483–90.

44. Nakagawa S, Kanda T, Kosugi S, et al. Recurrence pattern of squamous cell carcinoma of the thoracic esophagus after extended radical esophagectomy with three-field lymphadenectomy. J Am Coll Surg 2004;198:205–11.

45. Ando N, Ozawa S, Kitagawa Y, et al. Improvement in the results of surgical treatment of advanced squamous esophageal carcinoma during 15 consecutive years. Ann Surg 2000;232:225–32.

46. Ong GB, Lee TC. Pharyngogastric anastomosis after oesophago-pharyngectomy for carcinoma of the hypopharynx and cervical oesophagus. Br J Surg 1960;48:193–200.

47. Kron IL, Joob AW, Levine PA, Cantrell RW. Blunt esophagectomy and gastric interposition for tumors of the cervical esophagus and hypopharynx. Am Surg 1986;52: 140–1.

48. Collin CF, Spiro RH. Carcinoma of the cervical esophagus: changing therapeutic trends. Am J Surg 1984;148:460–6.

49. Burmeister BH, Dickie G, Smithers BM, et al. Thirty-four patients with carcinoma of the cervical esophagus treated with chemoradiation therapy. Arch Otolaryngol Head Neck Surg 2000;126:205–8.

CHAPTER 4

MANAGEMENT OPTIONS FOR BARRETT'S ESOPHAGUS WITH DYSPLASIA

WAYNE HOFSTETTER, MD

Introduction

An estimated 10% of the U.S. population suffers from significant gastroesophageal reflux disease, an affliction that in some patients leads to insidious epithelial changes known as intestinal metaplasia of the specialized type, more commonly known as Barrett's esophagus (BE) (Figure 4-1). On the basis of population studies and autopsy findings, researchers have projected that BE exists in 1% of the U.S. population,[1] and we now know that anywhere from 0.3 to 1%/year of these patients will have progression from BE to an invasive cancer.[2–3] The natural history of the development of an esophageal adenocarcinoma arising in a segment of BE has been shown to progress through a metaplasia-dysplasia-cancer sequence; therefore, a diagnosis of BE with high-grade dysplasia (BE/HGD) has serious implications for the patient.[4] Patients with Barrett's esophagus have a significantly higher risk of esophageal carcinogenesis than those of the general population, usually estimated as 30 to 40 times higher.[5]

Paramount to a discussion of treatment options for BE with dysplasia is establishing the subclassifications of the diagnosis. The dysplasia associated with BE is classified as either low grade or high grade, according to the amount of atypia, heterogeneity, and nuclear disorganization seen under light microscopy; this is correlative to the risk of developing adenocarcinoma of the esophagus. [6] Low-grade dysplasia (LGD) confers a

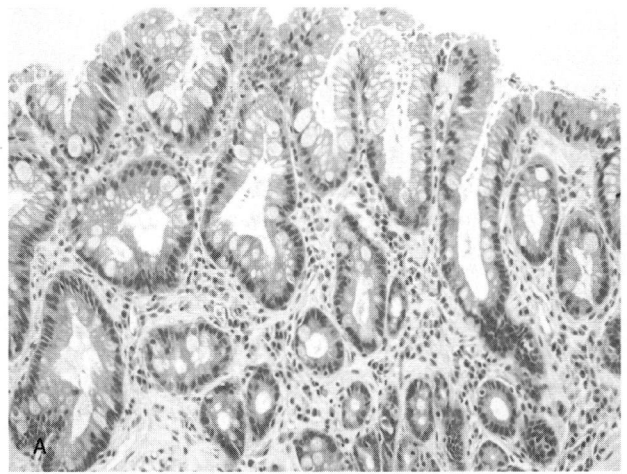 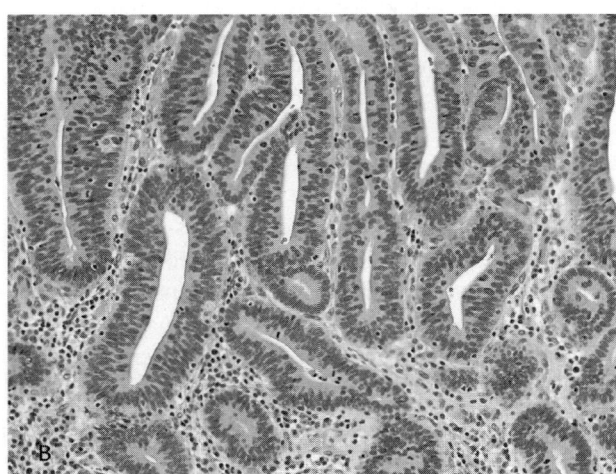

Figure 4-1 Barrett's Esophagus. *A*, Specialized intestinal metaplasia without dysplasia. Columnar epithelium with goblet cells are apparent and the nuclei are homogeneous, normochromic, and in linear array. *B*, High grade dysplasia—nuclear heterogeneity, disarray, and polymitotic figures. Photos courtesy of Tsung T. Wu, MD.

negligibly higher risk of progression to cancer than does nondysplastic BE, but these patients may have progression to cancer, with or without a recognized sequenced evolution to HGD, so this diagnosis does warrant serious attention. Patients who have BE/HGD carry the highest risk of developing esophageal adenocarcinoma. It is also important to note that frequently the diagnosis of HGD is made simultaneously with a diagnosis of invasive cancer and many clinicians consider the diagnosis of HGD to be a marker for a synchronous invasive carcinoma. At this time, treatment options for patients with BE/LGD are observation on adequate acid suppression, consideration of a reflux reducing procedure (fundoplication), or mucosal ablation. None of these procedures have yet been shown to be superior to the others in avoiding eventual progression; therefore, they are currently considered to be equivalent, although this debate will go on.[7] For the purposes of this chapter, we will focus on BE/HGD because of the significant cancer risk to these patients and because the treatment recommendations remain somewhat controversial.

Criteria such as length (long segment versus short segment), presence of ulceration, and focality (focal versus diffuse) are felt to be indicators of malignant potential. Long-segment BE, defined as more than 3 cm long, carries the highest risk of progression to BE/HGD, and the risk increases proportional to the length of the segment and the age of the patient.[8] However, recent reports of the malignant potential of short-segment BE (less than 3 cm in length) suggest that patients with this diagnosis also have a significant risk for invasive cancer and should be followed just as closely and frequently as patients with long-segment BE.[9] Likewise, characteristics of unifocal or multifocal/diffuse dysplastic disease can be used as predictors of progression. A finding of long-segment BE with multifocal or diffuse HGD was typically correlated with the highest risk of progression to cancer, but patients with a focal area of HGD may have a similar risk for carcinogenesis as well. Whereas these "minor criteria" are debated and may be of limited value as prognostic indicators, they are important when choosing among available treatment modalities. As we evaluate BE patients, this information is gathered and heavily influences the treatment recommendations.

Many researchers have attempted to quantify the risk of existing or eventual progression to cancer in patients with a diagnosis of BE/HGD (ie, the natural history of HGD). Reports from retrospective and prospective surveillance studies have reported that between 16 and 60% of patients with HGD will develop adenocarcinoma within 5 to 7 years[10–11] (this is the risk of developing a new, "incident" cancer, found subsequent to any existing "prevalent" cancer being ruled out). This indicates that a diagnosis of HGD does not always lead to a diagnosis of invasive cancer and that some patients may not have disease progression. Importantly, careful surveillance of HGD patients in these studies revealed that most who had progression to cancer were identified at an early and potentially curable stage, emphasizing the importance of recurrent screening to detect early-stage disease and initiate treatment.

On the other hand, the issue of HGD as a marker for an existing cancer has been reviewed from the standpoint of patients who have been resected. Invasive cancer is routinely found in approximately 40% (range, 30–75%) of patients who undergo resection for a diagnosis limited to BE/HGD.[12–15] This has been seen in centers where careful surveillance was performed but did not reveal the invasive cancer before resection. Furthermore, these reports indicate that several of the undetected cancers were at a more advanced state, already involving the submucosa and regional lymph nodes in some patients. Therefore, it is appropriate to say that HGD represents an intraepithelial cancer, which has the ability to progress to invasion, and in a significant number of patients it also may be an indicator that an invasive cancer already exists. At this time, we do not possess the necessary tools to ensure that we are capturing all patients who undergo surveillance with early-stage disease.

Diagnostic Studies

Once the diagnosis is made, it is mandatory to confirm it with a second endoscopy with separate biopsies, and we strongly advocate confirmation by a second pathologist.[16] This is especially important in a situation where a patient may have been referred with a diagnosis that was made on a first endoscopy and reviewed by a single pathologist who may or may not have significant experience in esophageal dysplasia. Confirmation is mandatory. Patients who present with a new diagnosis of HGD and have never been on proton pump inhibitors should be allowed to go on medication and be rescheduled for confirmatory biopsies in several weeks. It is not infrequent that what appeared to be HGD under the microscope is actually BE with little or no dysplasia complicated by overlying inflammation, a finding which frequently confounds the diagnosis of HGD. If the second set of biopsies shows metaplasia without HGD, then the patient should be placed on close follow-up with surveillance biopsies in 3 months. An interesting finding of a randomized trial of acid reduction plus photodynamic therapy versus acid reduction alone showed that a significant number (39%) of patients regressed from HGD with medical therapy (proton pump inhibitors) alone.[17] It is very likely that the nuclear disorganization and atypia seen on the initial biopsies of these patients was at least in part due to acute inflammatory changes. An often-quoted study performed in a Veterans Affairs hospital showed that only 16% of patients with HGD who were managed by surveillance endoscopy and biopsy alone had progression to invasive carcinoma.[10] The study has been criticized as having a rate of progression to cancer that is one-third of the rate seen in many of the other cohort studies and for having only one pathologist confirm the diagnosis of HGD.

We recommend that all patients with BE/HGD undergo endoscopy with high-frequency endoscopic ultrasonography (EGD/EUS). The ultrasound modality of the study can visualize the layers of the esophagus and is therefore a good, but imperfect, indicator of the depth of penetration of an invasive process. Of specific interest is any visible nodular or ulcerated area; a finding frequently correlated to a diagnosis of invasion. A fairly accurate T stage can be obtained from EGD/EUS using high-frequency ultrasound, and these findings may change the treatment recommendations for a particular patient. During the EGD, biopsies should be taken in 4 quadrants every 1 to 2 cm to search for invasive cancer. However, it is important to realize that some prevalent cancers may still go undetected because BE with HGD can be a diffuse process and random biopsies can result in a false-negative result owing to sampling errors. The Seattle Barrett's Program has advocated 4-quadrant biopsies at 1 cm intervals with jumbo forceps in patients with HGD to increase the detection rate of invasive carcinoma. In their hands, this resulted in the diagnosis of significantly more prevalent cancers than biopsies done every 2 cm.[18]

Treatment

When the diagnosis of BE with HGD is confirmed, several treatment options are available to patients and physicians, allowing individualization to patient needs and comorbidities. Currently, the four main categories of therapies are the following:

1) Observation with serial endoscopies (surveillance)
2) Mucosal ablation
   a) Photodynamic therapy (PDT)
   b) Argon plasma coagulation (APC)
   c) Neodymium-doped yttrium aluminium garnet (Nd:YAG) laser ablation
3) Endoscopic Resection
   a) Endoscopic mucosal resection (EMR)
   b) Endoscopic submucosal dissection (ESD)
4) Esophagectomy
   a) Vagal-sparing
   b) Minimally invasive
   c) Traditional transhiatal or transthoracic

Surveillance as a treatment strategy for BE/HGD is appropriate in a selected group of patients. Recent advances suggest that we may soon gain the ability to predict which patients with BE will have progression to invasive cancer and which patients might remain stable for many years, or even have disease regression. In one sophisticated center, esophageal biopsies were analyzed by flow cytometry for nuclear tetraploidy and aneuploidy.[19] The group of patients found to be at the highest risk for adenocarcinoma consisted of those who had HGD and a significant amount of aneuploidy. Certainly prospective identification of this cohort would warrant early intervention rather than surveillance. However, researchers at other centers have not been able to duplicate these findings.[20] Furthermore, some centers that have used surveillance as a treatment modality have not had a similar experience regarding ability to diagnose most patients with invasive cancer at an early stage. In a retrospective experience by Reed and colleagues, of 13 patients who underwent observation, 7 later presented with an invasive cancer, 4 of which were advanced (stage II-IV).[12] Furthermore, as mentioned previously, one must carefully note that cancers detected within the early phase of any surveillance protocol (usually the first year) are eliminated from the "progression" subset and considered prevalent rather than incident cancers and are not accounted for in the final analysis. This assumes that the cancers were adequately detected at an early stage at the outset of the HGD diagnosis. Most notable in the reported surveillance studies is a short duration of follow-up of usually less than 5 years, which is too short a time to allow accurate assessment of the natural history of HGD. Given available technology and a lack of patient compliance with vigorous biopsy protocols, treating physicians are often left without the ability to assess accurately which patients have an occult cancer, which will remain stable, or which will progress to an unresectable carcinoma. Therefore, we advocate a surveillance strategy only for patients who have no evidence of carcinoma on multiple endoscopies and are not candidates for any type of more aggressive therapy. This is essentially a strategy of competing risks: the risk of observation versus that of intervention. Patients at extreme age with significant comorbidities or who are at high risk of complications related to resection or even anesthetic for endoscopic therapies may be compelled to avoid invasive treatments. Patients who are healthy enough to receive therapy should be seen and reviewed in a multidisciplinary setting involving a gastroenterologist, a surgeon, and a pathologist. BE/HGD in this setting is appropriately treated with resection, mucosal ablation, or EMR. Factored into this decision are the minor criteria of length of the affected segment of esophagus, the presence of a visible lesion, and patient data on age and comorbidities.

Mucosal Ablation

Several methods of limited esophageal mucosal ablation have been used over the years. The most popular current modalities are the thermal ablative methods such as APC, intravenous photosensitizing/light-induced cell necrosis (PDT), or laser ablation. In theory, ablation of the metaplastic cellular epithelium of the esophagus allows multipotent progenitor cells in normal squamous cell epithelium at the boundaries of the metaplastic area to proliferate and re-epithelialize the iatrogenically injured area, replacing the treated segment of the esophagus with normal epithelium, a process that is essentially equivalent to skin burn wound healing. However, the efficacy of thermal ablation techniques is limited by several obstacles, including the following: (1) the limited ability to predict the actual depth of destruction; (2) predicting and attaining the necessary depth of penetration; (3) the lack of a histologic specimen; (4) "pseudoregression," or the overgrowth of squamous epithelium hiding metaplastic epithelium (shown to occur in 37% of PDT patients in an abstract presented before the American Society for Gastrointestinal Endoscopy in 2004 by Ohana and colleagues); and (5) significant morbidity, including esophageal stricture and skin photosensitivity. There is also the issue of the necessity to perform multiple procedures at a significant cost for repeated treatments. Because patients generally are asked to wait several months between treatments, a complete course can take 6 months to more than a year to complete, during the course of which frequent endoscopic procedures and extensive biopsies are required. Moreover, the patient must remain on intensive endoscopic surveillance for life. However, if one can successfully and reliably ablate the diseased area while preserving a patent and functional esophagus, this could be an improvement over resection, with the attendant higher morbidity and mortality rates associated with a major surgical procedure. It is important to note that the appropriateness of nonoperative management of this disease is still controversial because of the lack of long-term data for many of the modalities. We advocate that any patient treatment for HGD with any modality other than the currently recommended standard (resection) be done in a protocol setting whenever possible.

Photodynamic Therapy

Given the disappointing results of a recent randomized trial using PDT versus medical therapy,[17] in which 13% of patients treated with PDT had progression to invasive carcinoma in a short follow-up period (24 months) after treatment, PDT is not recommended as a sole modality for younger, healthier patients with HGD. Results from that trial predicted that, after 3 years, 50% of patients can expect to have a recurrence of intestinal metaplasia with HGD. Half the treated patients required 3 treatments with a 3-month waiting period and a 30-day period of photosensitivity between treatments. About 36% had post-treatment esophageal strictures, and a third of these patients required more than 10 dilations. On the positive side, however, 39% of patients on observation and acid suppression alone showed regression (at least in the short term), and some patients were free of dysplasia after ablation therapy even after 43 months. Unfortunately, survival after progression to cancer was not an end point to the study; therefore, we were not informed of the eventual outcome of these patients. Results of the aforementioned and other ablation studies suggest that it may be feasible in patients who have recurrence or progression to be identified at an early stage of disease by aggressive follow-up, and therefore, be good candidates for further curative therapy. While this may be the case in the future, there is very limited evidence-based medical information to suggest this now. Therefore, we do not advocate mucosal ablation as the sole modality for HGD; however, it may be reasonable to consider PDT and observation for patients with BE/HGD who are not candidates for more invasive therapy.

Endoscopic Mucosal Resection

Another endoscopic therapy that is gaining popularity in the local treatment of dysplastic BE is EMR. Patients with either short- or long-segment BE have been treated with EMR, but this modality is best suited to patients with a short segment or patchy areas of intestinal metaplasia with or without dysplasia. Patients with extended segments of intestinal metaplasia, although potentially treatable with EMR, may have higher recurrence rates and need more repetitive procedures. The procedure can be performed through a single or double working channel endoscope, and experience with this treatment has shown exceptionally low morbidity rates. Some of the advantages of EMR over other endoscopic treatments for BE include (1) the ability to provide a specimen for pathologic review; this is especially important in a patient with surgical options; (2) patients can be serially treated over less time than is possible with PDT; and (3) EMR can be either diagnostic or therapeutic. For example, in one published series, researchers reported that the larger tissue samples obtained by EMR compared with EUS and random biopsies resulted in a change in the diagnosis in 40% of patients.[21] In half of these cases, invasive carcinoma was discovered; in the other half, the diagnosis was downgraded from invasive carcinoma to HGD, from HGD to BE without dysplasia, or even from cancer to benign epithelium. Patients who are confirmed to have HGD on EMR and are reasonably healthy should consider the choice of undergoing major surgical resection, completing the EMR as a definitive resection, or adding mucosal ablation to a definitive EMR. Existing data using this technique in patients with HGD suggest a complete local response is possible in most patients.[22] On an intention-to-treat basis, approximately 70% were free of HGD after initial treatment; however, a caveat to interpreting this data is that all of the current studies are hampered by a very short follow-up period after EMR (in the range of 9–34 months).

EMR is clinically best suited for patients with short-segment BE/HGD (Figure 4-2). In these cases, the whole area can be resected, submitted to pathology, and subsequently, the treated area of the esophagus is monitored closely by endoscopy. Therefore, at this time, the patients we consider for therapeutic EMR are those who (1) do not have a surgical option either because of comorbidity or informed decision, (2) are elderly patients with a higher risk of undergoing an esophagectomy and whose diagnostic EGD/EMR shows a resectable (long or short) segment of HGD, or (3) have very localized intestinal metaplasia and HGD that can be easily resected and followed up endoscopically. The

clinician should be aware that this treatment modality may result in a lower overall cure rate compared with resection (although the effects on long-term survival are still not adequately studied) and that intensive follow-up is still necessary after EMR. Furthermore, current EMR techniques using suction-ligation or strip techniques frequently result in an incomplete resection and positive margins. Because of this, combination therapy (EMR and PDT) has been utilized in clinical trials[22] and has shown excellent local remission rates (the ablated area remains free of disease); however, recurrences of HGD or early cancers within the diseased esophagus are very common (30%). Long-term follow-up data are again lacking.

To combat the limitation of a partial endoscopic resection, a deeper endoscopic resection has been advocated and practiced in Japan, Germany, and some U.S. centers. Transluminal endoscopic submucosal dissection (ESD) results in an "en bloc" resection of mucosa and submucosa all the way to the level of the muscularis propria, and this virtually eliminates the worry of the piecemeal resection seen in EMR-suction-ligation or EMR-strip biopsy techniques. Unfortunately, this promising technique has had trouble with high perforation and stricture rates and is currently still being investigated. It is not approved by the U.S. Food and Drug Administration for esophageal procedures at this time.

Surgery

The current rationale for recommending surgery for patients with severely dysplastic esophageal epithelium stems completely from our inability to separate accurately the patients who have BE/HGD with a high

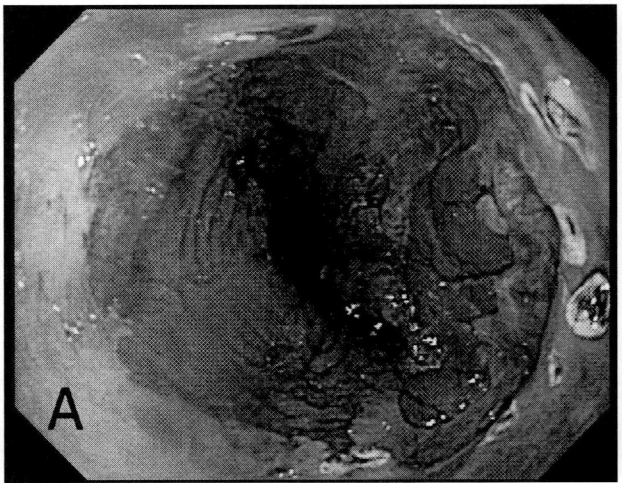 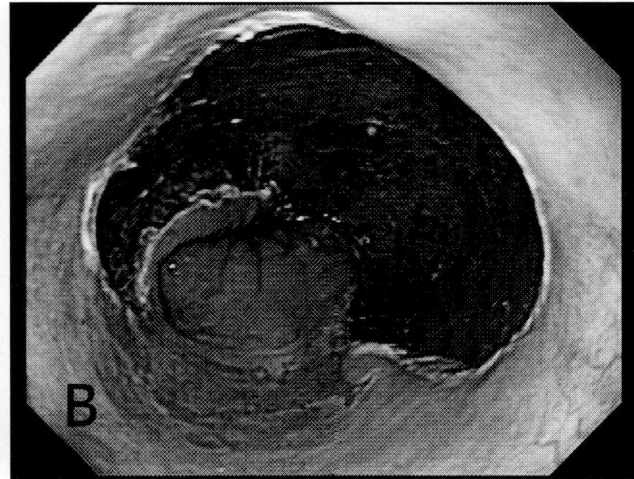

Figure 4-2 Endoscopic Mucosal Resection. *A*, Pre-endoscopic mucosal resection (EMR) chromoendoscopic (methylene blue) view of distal esophagus showing short segment of salmon-colored mucosa consistent with Barrett's esophagus and a suspicious nodular area from 2 o'clock to 5 o'clock. *B*, Post-EMR view of resected area. Photos courtesy of Norio Fukami, MD.

probability of malignant progression (or even an occult cancer) from those who do not. We are too well aware of the current limitations in curing patients with esophageal adenocarcinoma with nodal disease; therefore, our goal is to intervene before the disease reaches this stage. Esophageal cancer spreads through lymphatic channels, which lie mostly within the submucosa of the esophagus. As evidence, adenocarcinoma arising within the mucosa of the gastroesophageal junction can invade into the submucosal layer and can spread a considerable distance upward along the esophagus or downward into the submucosa of the stomach, "creeping behind the walls," so to speak. Similarly, deeper invasion of carcinoma is an independent risk factor for lymph node involvement. The critical anatomic juncture separating patients with early esophageal cancer that can be easily cured from patients who are at higher risk of regional or distant recurrence (and are cured very infrequently) is invasion across the muscularis mucosa. This occurs long before a patient is symptomatic and can also occur in patients who are under active endoscopic surveillance. In studies on patients with early esophageal cancer undergoing resection where detailed and systematic lymph node dissection has been performed, between 30 and 50% of patients with adenocarcinoma who present with superficial to intermediate submucosal invasion have lymph node metastases.[23] In a subset of patients with only lymphovascular invasion within the mucosa and no clear evidence of submucosal invasion, up to 10% can be found to have lymph node involvement. Rarely, even patients thought to have only HGD have presented with lymph node involvement. Presumably, these patients had unrecognized areas of invasive carcinoma that led to lymphatic spread, but this underscores the importance of sampling error even with surgical pathology. It is specifically the subset of patients with BE/HGD and the early undetected cancer that may benefit most from resection of the esophagus.

The recent literature reviewing single-institution experience with operative intervention for HGD echoes the findings of studies from nearly a decade ago, further emphasizing the slow progress made in the field of early detection. The data show that more than 40% of the patients who undergo resection after a diagnosis of BE/HGD actually have invasive carcinoma within the pathologic specimen despite the findings on preoperative endoscopy and careful biopsies.[13,23] This has been shown to occur even in situations of previous BE surveillance. More important, in one recently published review, 18 of 49 BE/HGD patients who underwent resection were found to have invasive cancer on pathologic examination, and 11 of these 18 had an invasion of the submucosa or deeper. Approximately 10% (5 of 49)

had lymph node involvement.[12] Although these figures are higher than those seen in other published data, this is indicative of what can result in a program with a significant esophageal experience where surveillance biopsies are being performed in a routine manner.

Surgical resection is the standard treatment for BE with carcinoma in situ. However, the overall difficulty and morbidity of this operation precludes its application to patients with significant comorbidities or advanced age. This cohort accounts for a fairly large percentage of patients presenting with this disease and this leaves a treatment void that is filled by the previously discussed treatment modalities, including endoscopic therapies or acid suppression and observation. As physicians have gained experience and some success with less invasive therapies, the indications for performing a resection in a higher-risk patient population have come under scrutiny and forms the crux of the controversy regarding endoscopic therapy versus resection. Clearly, this is a personal choice made by an informed patient/physician team. One must weigh the relative risk of morbidity or mortality for any given procedure versus the presumed potential for carcinogenesis.

Overall, the results for resection are excellent. The 5-year overall survival rate is generally reported as 80 to 90% in multiple series of HGD patients.[13] Local control for HGD approaches 100% and regional/distant control depends on the existence of deeper invasion and on lymph node involvement if an invasive cancer is discovered. As the invasion reaches into the submucosal layer, survival drops precipitously at 5 years, emphasizing the need to detect disease at a very early stage. Operative mortality rates are low (approximately 2%) for this group of patients, who are at significantly lower risk than patients undergoing surgery for more advanced cancers. Quality of life is considered to be comparable with "normal" after recovery from esophagectomy, and for the most part, morbidity is overstated in most medical literature (though this should not be trivialized either).

Surgical Options

There are several options for surgical resection, and studies have shown no significant superiority of one method over the others. Some surgeons have moved toward nerve-sparing or minimally invasive techniques in an effort to reduce the potential short- and long-term morbidities of the procedure. A minimally invasive esophagectomy can be done with some efficiency in centers with experienced surgeons and may offer advantages in shorter recovery time.[24] Vagal-sparing esophagectomy (Figure 4-3) is reported to result in lower morbidity rates for dumping and issues with maintaining

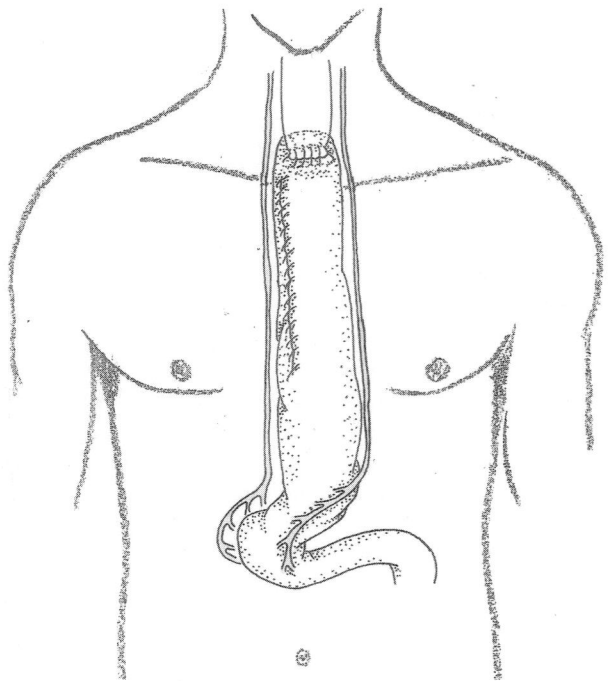

Figure 4-3 Vagal-Sparing Esophagectomy. Schematic shows retained vagal trunks and antral innervation after vagal-sparing gastric pull-up procedure. Illustration courtesy of Shanda Blackmon, MD.

weight postoperatively than a resection involving a vagotomy.[25] Either of these procedures would be suitable in a patient with HGD or even very early invasive carcinoma, a caveat being that if a patient is discovered to have a visible esophageal lesion at the time of resection, a frozen section would be appropriate, and if it shows evidence of invasion into the muscularis mucosa or deeper, the patient should undergo a lymph node dissection for a more complete resection and proper staging. Therefore, in any surgical approach where there is an incomplete or no nodal dissection routinely performed, a frozen section analysis should be performed on any visible nodules or ulcerated areas as well as at the margins. Standard techniques of resection (subtotal and total esophagectomy, with or without thoracotomy) are used worldwide with equally excellent results when performed by experienced groups.

Conclusion

To summarize, early detection and treatment prior to development of an unresectable or locoregionally advanced cancer is the goal for therapy for BE/HGD. Promising new endoscopic techniques such as chromoendoscopy and optical coherence tomography may facilitate the detection of HGD and early cancers, and

these could potentially enable a more effective method of selection among various therapies. Molecular techniques are also evolving that could assess the carcinogenesis of a patient who has developed BE. Currently, however, some type of invasive therapy for patients with HGD is advocated if they are medically able to undergo such treatment. EMR is an underutilized diagnostic modality that may also be a therapeutic option for patients with a manageable segment of metaplasia. Overall, we recommend that a young, fit patient, with many years of risk ahead of him or her and a confirmed diagnosis of BE/HGD should undergo surgery; an elderly patient should undergo mucosal ablation or EMR, (short-segment BE is amenable to EMR, whereas very long segments may require PDT or both EMR and PDT); and patients with significant comorbid conditions should undergo surveillance to rule out the existence of an occult cancer and then be enrolled in an active surveillance program.

References

1. Spechler SJ, Lee E, Ahnen D, et al. Long-term outcome of medical and surgical therapies for gastroesophageal reflux disease: follow-up of a randomized controlled trial. JAMA 2001;285:2331–8.

2. O'Connor JB, Falk GW, Richter JE. The incidence of adenocarcinoma and dysplasia in Barrett's esophagus: report on the Cleveland Clinic Barrett's Esophagus Registry. Am J Gastroenterol 1999;94:2037–42.

3. Ronkainen J, Aro P, Storskrubb T, et al. Prevalence of Barrett's esophagus in the general population: an endoscopic study. Gastroenterology 2005;129:1825–31.

4. Pera M, Manterola C, Vidal O, Grande L. Epidemiology of esophageal adenocarcinoma. J Surg Oncol 2005;92:151–9.

5. Bresalier R. Barrett's metaplasia: defining the problem. Semin Oncol 2005;32:S21–4.

6. Chandrasoma P. Controversies of the cardiac mucosa and Barrett's oesophagus. Histopathology 2005;46:361–73.

7. Sampliner RE. A population prevalence of Barrett's esophagus—finally. Gastroenterology 2005;129:2101–3.

8. Gopal DV, Lieberman DA, Magaret N, et al. Risk factors for dysplasia in patients with Barrett's esophagus (BE): results from a multicenter consortium. Dig Dis Sci 2003;48:1537–41.

9. Kamberoglou DK, Savva SC, Kalapothakos PN, et al. Prevalence and risk factors associated with specialized intestinal metaplasia at the esophagogastric junction. Hepatogastroenterology 2002;49:995–8.

10. Schnell TG, Sontag SJ, Chejfec G, et al. Long-term nonsurgical management of Barrett's esophagus with high-grade dysplasia. Gastroenterology 2001;120:1607–19.

11. Reid BJ, Levine DS, Longton G, et al. Predictors of progression to cancer in Barrett's esophagus: baseline histology and flow cytometry identify low- and high-risk patient subsets. Am J Gastroenterol 2000;95:1669–76.

12. Reed MF, Tolis G, Edil BH, et al. Surgical treatment of esophageal high-grade dysplasia. Ann Thorac Surg 2005;79: 1110–5.

13. Peters JH, Clark GW, Ireland AP, et al. Outcome of adenocarcinoma arising in Barrett's esophagus in endoscopically surveyed and nonsurveyed patients. J Thorac Cardiovasc Surg 1994;108:813–21.

14. Thomas T, Richards CJ, De Caestecker JS, Robinson RJ. High-grade dysplasia in Barrett's oesophagus: natural history and review of clinical practice. Aliment Pharmacol Ther 2005;21:747–55.

15. Tharavej C, Hagen JA, Peters JH, et al. Predictive factors of coexisting cancer in Barrett's high-grade dysplasia. Surg Endosc 2006;20:439–43.

16. Sharma P, McQuaid K, Dent J, et al. A critical review of the diagnosis and management of Barrett's esophagus: the AGA Chicago workshop. Gastroenterology 2004;127:310–30.

17. Overholt BF, Lightdale CJ, Wang KK, et al. Photodynamic therapy with porfimer sodium for ablation of high-grade dysplasia in Barrett's esophagus: international, partially blinded, randomized phase III trial. Gastrointest Endosc 2005;62:488–98.

18. Reid BJ, Blount PL, Feng Z, et al. Optimizing endoscopic biopsy detection of early cancers in Barrett's high-grade dysplasia. Am J Gastroenterol 2000;95:3089–96.

19. Rabinovitch PS, Longton G, Blount PL, et al. Predictors of progression in Barrett's esophagus III: baseline flow cytometric variables. Am J Gastroenterol 2001;96:3071–83.

20. Koppert LB, Wlinhoven BPL, van Dekken H, et al. The molecular biology of esophageal adenocarcinoma. J Surg Oncol 2005;92:169–90.

21. Nijhawan PK, Wang KK. Endoscopic mucosal resection for lesions with endoscopic features suggestive of malignancy and high-grade dysplasia within Barrett's esophagus. Gastrointest Endosc 2000;52:328–32.

22. May A, Gossner L, Pech O, et al. Local endoscopic therapy for intraepithelial high-grade neoplasia and early adenocarcinoma in Barrett's oesophagus: acute-phase and intermediate results of a new treatment approach. Eur J Gastroenterol Hepatol 2002;14:1085–91.

23. Nigro JJ, Hagen JA, DeMeester TR, et al. Occult esophageal adenocarcinoma: extent of disease and implications for effective therapy. Ann Surg 1999;230:433–8.

24. Luketich JD, Alvelo-Rivera M, Buenaventura PO, et al. Minimally invasive esophagectomy outcomes in 222 patients. Ann Surg 2003;238:179–88.

25. Banki F, Mason RJ, DeMeester SR, et al. Vagal-sparing esophagectomy: a more physiologic alternative. Ann Surg 2002;236:324–35.

CHAPTER 5

COMBINED MODALITY THERAPY FOR SQUAMOUS CELL CANCER OF THE ESOPHAGUS

BRUCE D. MINSKY, MD

Combined modality therapy (CMT) has been used in a variety of approaches in the treatment of squamous cell cancer of the esophagus. These include preoperative, postoperative, and primary nonoperative treatment. Most contemporary trials of CMT in esophagus cancer include patients with both squamous cell and adenocarcinomas. This trend will continue as the incidence of adenocarcinoma compared with squamous cell cancers increases.[1] However, the impact of histology on outcome is unclear. At the present time the data are conflicting with some series reporting different results by histology whereas other series report no difference. Fortunately, the US Intergroup randomized trials are stratified by histology. Until these data are available, the impact of histology cannot be adequately assessed and it is reasonable to treat both histologies in a similar fashion.

This chapter will primarily review the use of primary CMT for squamous cell carcinomas. Trials examining radiation alone or CMT in the adjuvant setting will not be discussed.

Combined Modality Therapy

STANDARD APPROACHES

Although there are 6 randomized trials comparing radiation therapy alone with CMT, the only trial designed to deliver adequate doses of systemic chemotherapy with concurrent radiation therapy was the Radiotion Therapy Oncology Group (RTOG) 85-01 trial (Figure 5-1).[2–4] This Intergroup trial primarily included patients with squamous cell carcinoma. Patients received four cycles of 5-fluorouracil (FU)/Cisplatin. Radiation

therapy (50 Gy) was given concurrently beginning day 1 of chemotherapy. The control arm was radiation therapy alone, albeit a higher dose (64 Gy) than the CMT arm.

Patients who received CMT had a significant improvement in median survival (14 months versus 9 months), and 5-year survival (27% versus 0%, $p < .0001$).[3] With a minimum follow-up of 5 years, the 8-year survival was 22%.[4] Histology did not significantly influence the results with 21% of patients with squamous cell carcinomas (N = 107) alive at 5 years compared with 13% of patients with adenocarcinoma (N = 23), p = NS. Although African-Americans had larger primary tumors and all were squamous cell cancers, there was no difference in survival compared with whites.[5] The incidence of local failure as the first site of failure (defined as local persistence or recurrence) was also decreased in the combined modality arm (47% versus 65%). The protocol was closed early due to the positive results; however, following this early closure, an additional 69 eligible patients were treated with the same CMT regimen. In this nonrandomized combined modality group, the 5-year survival was 14% and local failure was 52%.

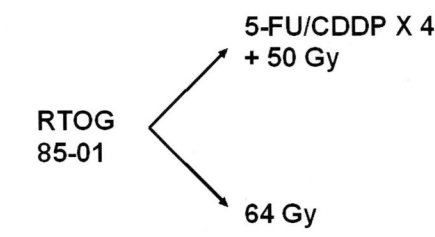

Figure 5-1 RTOG 85-01.

Combined modality therapy is associated with a higher incidence of toxicity. In the 1997 report of the RTOG 85-01 trial, patients who received CMT had a higher incidence of acute grade 3 toxicity (44% versus 25%) and acute grade 4 toxicity (20% versus 3%) compared with radiation therapy alone. Including the one treatment-related death (2%), the incidence of total acute grade 3+ toxicity was 66%.[3] The 1999 report examined late toxicity. The incidence of late grade 3+ toxicity was similar in the CMT arm compared with the radiation alone arm (29% versus 23%).[4] However, grade 4+ toxicity remained higher (10% versus 2%, respectively). Interestingly, the nonrandomized CMT group experienced a similar incidence of late grade 3+ toxicity (28%), however, lower incidence of grade 4 toxicity (4%) and there were no treatment-related deaths.

Based on the positive results from the RTOG 85-01 trial, the conventional nonsurgical treatment for esophageal carcinoma is CMT. Because the local failure rate in RTOG 85-01 CMT arm was 45%, new approaches such as intensification of CMT and escalation of the radiation dose were developed in an attempt to help improve these results.

INTENSIFICATION OF COMBINED MODALITY THERAPY

Neoadjuvant Chemotherapy

A limited number of Phase I/II trials have tested the use of neoadjuvant chemotherapy prior to CMT using non–5-FU-containing regimens such as paclitaxel/cisplatin[6,7] or CPT-11/cisplatin.[8] The majority of patients in these trials had adenocarcinoma and, although optional, most underwent surgery. Bains and colleagues reported that of 38 patients who presented with dysphagia, 92% had relief following the completion of 2 cycles (weeks 1 and 4) of neoadjuvant paclitaxel and cisplatin.[6] Similar results have been reported by Ilson and colleagues in 19 patients who received 2 cycles neoadjuvant CPT-11 plus cisplatin weeks 1, 2, 4, 5 prior to the start of CMT.[8] Treatment was well tolerated with no grade 3+ nonhematological toxicity, and only 5% of patients required a feeding tube. Of the 16 patients who presented with dysphagia, 81% had dysphagia relief following the completion of neoadjuvant chemotherapy.

Another potential advantage of neoadjuvant chemotherapy is the early identification of those patients who may or may not respond to the regimen being delivered. Ott and colleagues found that the response to a fluorodeoxyglucose/positron emission tomography (FDG-PET) scan 2 weeks after the start of cisplatin/5-FU/leucovorin followed by surgery in 35 patients with adenocarcinoma of the gastroesophageal junction or stomach was able to predict patients who responded, based on the surgical specimens, to chemotherapy.[9] Although investigational, if the nonresponders can be identified early, changing the chemotherapeutic regimen may be helpful.

In summary, although the early trials primarily using 5-FU/cisplatin-based neoadjuvant regimens did not suggest a benefit, more recent trials using paclitaxel and CPT-11-based regimens reveal more favorable response rates and rapid improvement of dysphagia.

Intensification of the Radiation Dose

Another approach to the dose intensification of CMT is increasing the radiation dose either by brachytherapy and/or external beam.

Brachytherapy

Intraluminal brachytherapy allows the escalation of the dose to the primary tumor while protecting the surrounding dose limiting structures such as the lung, heart, and spinal cord.[10] Brachytherapy has been used both as a primary therapy (usually as a palliative modality)[11] as well as a boost following external beam radiation therapy or CMT.[12] Although there are technical and radiobiological differences between high- and low-dose rates, there are no clear therapeutic advantages.

Series which escalate the close by combining brachytherapy with either external beam or CMT report similar results to series which do not use brachytherapy. Calais and colleagues reported a local failure rate of 43% and a 5-year actuarial survival of 18%.[13] Even with the more favorable subset of patients with clinical T1-2 disease, Yorozu and colleagues reported a local failure rate of 44% and a 5-year survival of 26%.[14]

In the RTOG 92-07 trial, 75 patients (92% with squamous cell cancers) of the thoracic esophagus received the RTOG 85-01 combined modality regimen (5-FU/Cisplatin/50 Gy) followed by a boost during cycle 3 of chemotherapy with either low- rate or high-dose rate intraluminal brachytherapy.[15] Although the complete response rate was 73%, with a median follow-up of only 11 months, local failure as the first site of failure was 27%. Acute toxicity included 58% grade 3, 26% grade 4, and 8% treatment-related deaths. The cumulative incidence of fistula was 18%/year and the crude incidence was 14%. Of the 6 treatment-related fistulas, 3 were fatal. Given the significant toxicity, this treatment approach should be used with caution.

Based on this experience, the American Brachytherapy Society has developed guidelines for esophageal brachytherapy.[16] For patients treated in the curative setting, brachytherapy should be limited to tumors ≤ 10 cm with no evidence of distant metastasis. Contraindications include tracheal or bronchial involvement, cervical esophagus location, or stenosis that cannot be bypassed. The applicator should have an external diameter of 6 to 10 cm. If CMT is used (defined as 5-FU-based chemotherapy plus 45 to 50 Gy), the recommended doses of brachytherapy are 10 Gy in 2 weekly fractions of 5 Gy each for high-dose rate and 20 Gy in a single fraction at 4 to 10 Gy/hr for low-dose rate. The doses should be prescribed to 1 cm from the source. Lastly, brachytherapy should be delivered after the completion of external beam and not concurrently with chemotherapy.

In patients treated in the curative setting, the addition of brachytherapy does not appear to improve the results compared with radiation therapy or CMT alone. Therefore, the additional benefit of adding intraluminal brachytherapy to radiation or CMT, although reasonable, remains unclear.

External-Beam

Conventional Fractionation

Some investigators have advocated CMT using higher external beam doses. Data from retrospective series suggest improved local regional control with higher radiation doses.[17] Calais and colleagues[18] and the INT 0122 trial[19] reported that doses of 64.8 to 65 Gy are tolerable. Based on the tolerability of 64.8 Gy in the INT 0122 trial, this higher dose of radiation was used in the experimental arm of the Intergroup esophageal trial INT 0123 (RTOG 94-05). INT 0123 was the follow-up trial to RTOG 85-01. In this trial, patients with either squamous cell (85%) or adenocarcinomas (15%) who were selected for a nonsurgical approach were randomized to a slightly modified RTOG 85-01-combined modality regimen with 50.4 Gy versus the same chemotherapy with 64.8 Gy (Figure 5-2).

The modifications to the original RTOG 85-01 CMT arm included 1) using 1.8 Gy fractions to 50.4 Gy rather than 2 Gy fractions to 50 Gy, 2) treating with 5 cm proximal and distal margins for 50.4 Gy rather than

treating the whole esophagus for the first 30 Gy, followed by a cone down with 5 cm margins to 50 Gy, 3) cycle 3 of 5-FU/cisplatin did not begin until 4 weeks following the completion of radiation therapy rather than 3 weeks, and 4) cycles 3 and 4 of chemotherapy are delivered every 4 weeks rather than every 3 weeks.

The INT 0123 was closed to accrual in 1999 when an interim analysis revealed that it was unlikely that the high-dose arm would achieve a superior survival compared to the standard-dose arm. For the 218 eligible patients, there was no significant difference in median survival (13.0 months versus 18.1 months) or 2-year survival (31% versus 40%) in the high-dose versus standard-dose arm.[20] Although 11 treatment-related deaths occurred in the high-dose arm compared with two in the standard-dose arm, 7 of the 11 occurred in patients who had received ≤ 50.4 Gy.

In order to help determine if the unexplained increase in treatment-related deaths in the high-dose arm was the factor responsible for the inferior survival rate, a separate survival analysis was performed that included only patients who received the assigned dose of radiation. Despite this biased analysis, there was still no survival advantage with the high-dose arm.

Although the crude incidence of local failure and/or persistence of local disease (50% versus 55%) and distant failure (9% versus 16%) were lower in the high-dose versus the standard-dose arm, this did not reach statistical significance. At 2 years, the cumulative incidence of local failure was 56% for the high-dose arm versus 52% for the standard-dose arm ($p = .71$). Therefore, based on the INT 123 trial, the standard dose of external beam radiation remains 50.4 Gy.

The modifications to the original RTOG 85-01 CMT arm outlined above did not adversely affect the local control or survival rate of the control arm of INT 0123. Therefore, the radiation doses and field design used in the control arm of INT 0123 should be used.

Altered Fractionation

In addition to increasing the total dose, radiation can be intensified by accelerated or hyperfractionation. Wang and colleagues randomized 101 patients with squamous cell cancer to continuous accelerated hyperfractionated radiation (66 Gy) versus late-course accelerated hyperfractionated radiation (68.4 Gy).[21] Compared with patients who received late-course accelerated hyperfractionated radiation, those treated with continuous accelerated hyperfractionated radiation had a significantly higher incidence of grade 3+ esophagitis (61% versus 10%, p < .001), but no benefit in local control or survival. Zhao and colleagues treated 201 patients with squamous cell cancer using 41.4 Gy followed by late-

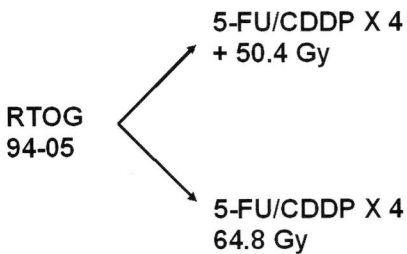

Figure 5-2 RTOG 94-05.

course accelerated hyperfractionation to 68.4 Gy.[22] The results were similar to RTOG 85-01 (38% local failure and 26% 5-year survival. Although these approaches are reasonable, most series report an increase in acute toxicity without any clear therapeutic benefit. These regimens remain investigational.

Split course radiation is inferior to continuous course. In a randomized trial from France, 95 patients with squamous cell cancers who received continuous course had a significantly higher local control rate (57% versus 29%), 2-year event-free survival (33% versus 23%), and a borderline significant 2-year survival rate (37% versus 23%).[23]

Novel Radiation Approaches

Based on the more favorable dose distribution of protons, Sugahara and colleagues treated 46 patients (45 with squamous cell) with a combination of protons or combined protons/photons to a median dose of 82 Gy or 76 Gy, respectively.[24] Although 23 of 46 patients had T1 disease, the local failure was still 35% and 5-year survival was only 13%.

Nutting and colleagues compared two-phase conformal radiotherapy with intensity-modulated radiation therapy (IMRT) in 5 patients who received 55 Gy plus concurrent chemotherapy.[25] Treatment plans using both techniques were performed and were compared using dose-volume histograms and normal tissue complication probabilities. The IMRT field using 9 equispaced field provided no improvement over conformal radiation because the larger number of fields in the IMRT plan distributed a low dose over the entire lung. In contrast, IMRT using 4 fields equal to the conformal fields offered an improvement in lung sparing.

Radiation Field Design and Treatment Techniques

Radiation field design for esophageal cancer requires careful techniques.[26] There are a number of sensitive organs which, depending on the location of the primary tumor, will be in the radiation field. These include but are not limited to skin, spinal cord, lung, heart, intestine, stomach, kidney, and liver. Minimizing the dose to these structures while delivering an adequate dose to the primary tumor and local/regional lymph nodes requires patient immobilization and computed tomography (CT)-based treatment planning for organ identification, lung correction, and development of dose-volume histograms.

Although CT can identify adjacent organs and structures, it may be limited in defining the extent of the primary tumor. To assess the consistency of target volume delineation, Tai and colleagues sent sample cases with CT scans to 48 radiation oncologists throughout Canada and asked them to complete questionnaires regarding treatment techniques as well as outline the boost target volumes.[27] There was substantial inconsistency in defining the planning target volume, both in the transverse and longitudinal dimensions. Therefore, in addition to a CT scan, it is helpful to obtain a barium swallow at the time of radiation therapy simulation. The integration of other imaging modalities in radiation treatment planning, such as esophageal ultrasound[28] and PET scan,[29,30] are under active investigation. Comparing PET, ultrasound, and CT for treatment planning, Konski and colleagues reported that PET underestimated the tumor length compared with CT and ultrasound identified more nodes versus PET and CT.[28]

In a separate study Tai and colleagues reported that the results of 12 Canadian radiation oncologists drew cervical esophagus target volumes based on the RTOG 94-05 protocol design both before and after a one-on-one training session.[31] A pre- and post-training session survey revealed less variability in the longitudinal positions of the target volumes, thereby illustrating the importance of specialized training.

Recent studies have examined the effectiveness of PET in the staging of esophageal cancer.[29] Following standard staging for esophageal cancer, which included CT and endoscopy, undetected metastatic disease was detected by PET in 15% of patients in the series by Flamen and colleagues[32] and 20% in the series by Downey and colleagues.[33] Given the potential for CT to understage metastatic disease, PET should be part of the standard work-up for patients receiving CMT.

As with surgery, the success of radiotion treatment is also related, in part, to patient volume. The 1996–1999 US Patterns of Care study of 414 patients (49% with squamous cell cancers) treated with a component of radiation therapy at 59 institutions reported that, by multivariate analysis, there was a significant improvement in survival in those patients treated at centers where ≥ 500 versus < 500 new cancer patients were seen each year.[34]

NEW CHEMOTHERAPEUTIC AGENTS

Because 75 to 80% of patients die of metastatic disease, advances in systemic therapies are necessary. The most widely used regimen combined with radiation has been 5-FU and cisplatin. There are new chemotherapeutic agents in both in current practice and development. Most are being developed as preoperative regimens and are combined with radiation doses of 45 to 50.4 Gy. These include both cytotoxic and targeted small molecules. Paclitaxel-[6,7,35] and docetaxel-based[36] CMT regimens have shown encouraging results. The RTOG randomized phase II trial E-0113 compared paclitaxel plus cisplatin, with/or without 5-FU. Other agents such as Irinotecan,[8,37,38] herceptin,[39] oxaliplatin,[40] are being used as platforms for new regimens. Trials are ongoing testing the combination of radiation, irinotecan/cisplatin plus bevacizumab or cetuximab. Whether these investigational approaches offer improved results compared to conventional 5-FU/cisplatin-based CMT regimens is not known. The development of the ideal regimens and schedules remains an active area of clinical investigation.

PREDICTORS OF RESPONSE TO COMBINED MODALITY THERAPY

Berger and colleagues reported that of patients receiving preoperative CMT (only 17% had squamous cell cancers), complete response was associated with a significant improvement in survival.[41] Therefore, it would be helpful to predict those tumors that have a higher likelihood of responding to CMT. Unfortunately, most studies have limited numbers of patients and the results are conflicting. Markers such as $Bcl-X_L$,[42] $p53$,[43] membrane phospholipids,[44] CDC25B,[45] $Ki-67$, EGFR, cyclin D1, VEGF, MVD, thymidylate synthase, dihydropyrimidine dehydrogenase, and glutathione s-transferase,[46] lymphocytic infiltration,[47] and $c-erbB-2$[48] have been correlated with response and/or outcome. With the further discovery and understanding of various tumor suppressor genes, in the future, molecular markers may be helpful in selecting treatment.

Kalha and colleagues found that post-treatment ultrasound did not accurately predict the pathologic response after CMT.[49] However, Weider and colleagues reported that changes in metabolic activity measured by PET 14 days after starting CMT in patients with squamous cell cancers correlated with tumor response and patient survival.[50]

IS SURGERY NECESSARY AFTER COMBINED MODALITY THERAPY?

Two trials examine whether surgery is necessary after CMT. In the FFCD 9102 trial, 445 patients with clinically resectable T3-4N0-1M0 squamous cell or adenocarcinoma of the esophagus received CMT; however, the randomization was limited to patients who responded to initial CMT. Patients initially received 2 cycles of 5-FU, cisplatin, and concurrent radiation (either 46 Gy at 2 Gy/day or split course 15 Gy weeks 1 and 3).[51] The 259 patients who had at least a partial response were then randomized to surgery versus additional CMT, which included 3 cycles of 5-FU, cisplatin, and concurrent radiation (either 20 Gy at 2 Gy/day or split course 15

Gy). There was no significant difference in 2-year survival (34% versus 40%, $p = .56$) or median survival (18 months versus 19 months) in patients who underwent surgery versus additional CMT. The data suggest that patients who initially respond to CMT should complete CMT rather than stop and undergo surgery. Using the Spitzer index, there was no difference in global quality of life (QOL); however, a significantly greater decrease in QOL was observed in the postoperative period in the surgery arm (7.52 versus 8.45, $p < .01$, respectively).[52]

The German Oesophageal Cancer Study Group compared preoperative CMT followed by surgery versus CMT alone.[53] In this trial, 172 eligible patients $\leq$ 70 years old with uT3-4N0-1M0 squamous cell cancers of the esophagus were randomized to preoperative therapy (3 cycles of 5-FU, leucovorin, etoposide, and cisplatin, followed by concurrent etoposide, cisplatin, plus 40 Gy) followed by surgery versus CMT alone (the same chemotherapy but the radiation dose was increased to 60 to 65 Gy +/- brachytherapy). Despite a decrease in local failure for those who were randomized to preoperative therapy followed by surgery versus CMT alone (36% versus 58%, $p = .003$), there was no significant difference in 3-year survival (31% versus 24%).

PALLIATION OF DYSPHAGIA

Dysphagia is a common problem in patients with esophageal cancer. Not only is it the most frequently presenting symptom, but it can remain a problem up to the time of the patient's death. Coia and colleagues reported that within 2 weeks following the start of CMT, 45% had improvement in dysphagia, and by the completion of the 6th week, 83% had improvement.[54] Overall, 88% had an improvement in dysphagia with a median time to maximum improvement of 4 weeks. Histology and stage had no impact of the rate of palliation. Intraluminal brachytherapy is also an effective albeit more limited method of achieving palliation of dysphagia in 40 to 90% of patients.[55,56]

ACUTE AND LONG-TERM TOXICITY OF RADIATION THERAPY

There are limited toxicity data in patients who received conventional doses of radiation therapy. Patients will experience lethargy and esophagitis commencing 2 to 3 weeks after the start of radiation; these symptoms usually resolve 1 to 2 weeks following the completion of therapy.

The most carefully documented acute toxicity data in patients receiving CMT were reported in the RTOG 85-01[2,3] and 94-05 trials and were previously discussed.[20] The effect of radiation on pulmonary function was examined by Gergel and colleagues.[57] Patients received 39.6 Gy with anterior/posterior fields followed by obliques to a total dose of 50.4 Gy plus concurrent oxaliplatin and 5-FU. Pulmonary function tests performed both preradiation and a median of 16 days postradiation revealed significant declines in DLCO and total lung capacity.

RADIATION TREATMENT IN THE SETTING OF A TRACHEOESOPHAGEAL FISTULA

The presence of a malignant tracheoesophageal fistula is an unfavorable prognostic feature. Although the experience is very limited, data from the Mayo Clinic suggest that radiation does not necessarily increase the severity of a malignant tracheoesophageal fistula and it may be administered safely. A total of 10 patients with a malignant tracheoesophageal fistula received 30 to 66 Gy external beam radiation, the median survival was 5 months and none experienced an enlarging or more debilitating fistula following radiation.[58]

References

1. Pohl H, Welch HG. The role of overdiagnosis and reclassification in the marked increase of esophageal adenocarcinoma incidence. J Natl Cancer Inst 2005;97:142–6.

2. Herskovic A, Martz LK, Al-Sarraf M, et al. Combined chemotherapy and radiotherapy compared with radiotherapy alone in patients with cancer of the esophagus. New Engl J Med 1992;326:1593–8.

3. Al-Sarraf M, Martz K, Herskovic A, et al. Progress report of combined chemoradiotherapy versus radiotherapy alone in patients with esophageal cancer: An intergroup study. J Clin Oncol 1997;15:277–84.

4. Cooper JS, Guo MD, Herskovic A, et al. Chemoradiotherapy of locally advanced esophageal cancer. Long-term follow-up of a prospective randomized trial (RTOG 85-01). JAMA 1999;281:1623–7.

5. Streeter OE, Martz KL, Gaspar LE, et al. Does race influence survival for esophageal cancer patients treated on the radiation and chemotherapy arm of RTOG # 85-01? Int J Radiat Oncol Biol Phys 1999;44:1047–52.

6. Bains MS, Stojadinovic A, Minsky B, et al. A phase II trial of preoperative combined-modality therapy for localized esophageal carcinoma: initial results. J Thorac Cardiovasc Surg 2002;124:270–7.

7. Goldberg M, Lampert C, Colarusso P, et al. Survival following intensive preoperative combined modality therapy with paclitaxel, cisplatin, 5-fluorouracil, and radiation in resectable esophageal carcinoma: a phase I report. Proc ASCO 2002;21:154a.

8. Ilson DH, Bains M, Kelsen DP, et al. Phase I trial of escalating-dose irinotecan given weekly with cisplatin and concurrent radiotherapy in locally advanced esophageal cancer. J Clin Oncol 2003;21:2926–32.

9. Ott K, Fink U, Becker K, et al. Prediction of response to preoperative chemotherapy in gastric carcinoma by metabolic imaging: results of a prospective trial. J Clin Oncol 2003;21:4604–10.

10. Armstrong JG. High dose rate remote afterloading brachytherapy for lung and esophageal cancer. Sem Radiat Oncol 1993;4:270–7.

11. Maingon P, d'Hombres A, Truc G, et al. High dose rate brachytherapy for superficial cancer of the esophagus. Int J Radiat Oncol Biol Phys 2000;46:71–6.

12. Okawa T, Dokiya T, Nishio M, et al. Multi-institutional randomized trial of external radiotherapy with and without intraluminal brachytherapy for esophageal cancer in Japan. Int J Radiat Oncol Biol Phys 1999;45:623–8.

13. Calais G, Dorval E, Louisot P, et al. Radiotherapy with high dose rate brachytherapy boost and concomitant chemotherapy for stages IIB and III esophageal carcinoma: results of a pilot study. Int J Radiat Oncol Biol Phys 1997;38:769–75.

14. Yorozu A, Dokiya T, Oki Y, et al. Curative radiotherapy with high-dose-rate brachytherapy boost for localized esophageal carcinoma: dose-effect relationship of brachytherapy with the balloon type applicator system. Radiother Oncol 1999;51:133–9.

15. Gaspar LE, Qian C, Kocha WI, et al. A phase I/II study of external beam radiation, brachytherapy and concurrent chemotherapy in localized cancer of the esophagus (RTOG 92-07): preliminary toxicity report. Int J Radiat Oncol Biol Phys 1997;37:593–9.

16. Gaspar LE, Nag S, Herskovic A, et al. American Brachytherapy Society (ABS) consensus guidelines for brachytherapy of esophageal cancer. Int J Radiat Oncol Biol Phys 1997;38:127–32.

17. Zhang Z, Liao Z, Jin J, et al. Dose response relationship in locoregional control for patients with stage II-III esophageal cancer treated with concurrent chemotherapy and radiotherapy. Int J Radiat Oncol Biol Phys 2005;61:656–64.

18. Calais G, Jadaud E, Chapet S, et al. High dose radiotherapy (RT) and concomitant chemotherapy for nonresectable esophageal cancer. Results of a phase II study. Proc ASCO 1994;13:197.

19. Minsky BD, Neuberg D, Kelsen DP, et al. Final report of intergroup trial 0122 (ECOG PE-289, RTOG 90-12): Phase II trial of neoadjuvant chemotherapy plus concurrent chemotherapy and high-dose radiation for squamous cell carcinoma of the esophagus. Int J Radiat Oncol Biol Phys 1999;43:517–23.

20. Minsky BD, Pajak T, Ginsberg RJ, et al. INT 0123 (RTOG 94-05) phase III trial of combined modality therapy for

esophageal cancer: high dose (64.8 Gy) versus standard dose (50.4 Gy) radiation therapy. J Clin Oncol 2002;20: 1167–74.

21. Wang Y, Shi XH, He SQ, et al. Comparison between continuous accelerated hyperfractionated and late-course accelerated hyperfractionated radiotherapy for esophageal carcinoma. Int J Radiat Oncol Biol Phys 2002;54:131–6.

22. Zaho KL, Shi XH, Jiang GL, et al. Late course accelerated hyperfractionated radiotherapy for localized esophageal carcinoma. Int J Radiat Oncol Biol Phys 2004;60:123–9.

23. Jacob JH, Seitz JF, Langlois C, et al. Definitive concurrent chemo-radiation therapy (CRT) in squamous cell carcinoma of the esophagus (SCCE): preliminary results of a French randomized trial comparing standard versus split course irradiation (FNCLCC-FFCD 9305). Proc ASCO 1999;18:270a.

24. Sugahara S, Tokuuye K, Okumura T, et al. Clinical results of proton beam therapy for cancer of the esophagus. Int J Radiat Oncol Biol Phys 2005;61:76–84.

25. Nutting CM, Bedford JL, Cosgrove VP, et al. A comparison of conformal and intensity-modulated techniques for oesphageal radiotherapy. Radiother Oncol 2001;61:157–63.

26. Phillips TL, Minsky BD, Dicker AP. Cancer of the Esophagus, in Leibel SA, Phillips TL. (eds): Textbook of Radiation Oncology, 1st ed. Philadelphia: W.B. Saunders; 1998. p. 601–23.

27. Tai P, van Dyk J, Yu E. Variability of target volume delineation in cervical esophageal cancer. Int J Radiat Oncol Biol Phys 1998;42:277–88.

28. Konski A, Doss M, Milestone B. The integration of 18-fluoro-deoxy-glucose positron emission tomography and endoscopic ultrasound in the treatment-planning process for esophageal carcinoma. Int J Radiat Oncol Biol Phys 2005;61:1123–8.

29. Larson SM, Schoder H, Yeung H. Positron emission tomography/computerized tomography functional imaging of esophageal and colorectal cancer. Cancer J 2004;10:243–50.

30. van Westreenen HL, Heeren PA, Jager PL. Pitfalls of positive findings in staging esophageal cancer with F-18-fluorodeoxyglucose positron emission tomography. Ann Surg Oncol 2003;10:1100–5.

31. Tai P, van Dyk J, Battista J. Improving the consistency in cervical esophageal target volume definition by special training. Int J Radiat Oncol Biol Phys 2002;53:766–44.

32. Flamen P, van Cutsem E, Lerut T. Positron emission tomography for assessment of the response to induction radiochemotherapy in locally advanced oesphageal cancer. Ann Oncol 2002;13:361–8.

33. Downey RJ, Akhurst T, Ilson D. Whole body 18FDG-PET and the response of esophageal cancer to induction therapy: results of a prospective trial. J Clin Oncol 2003; 21:428–32.

34. Suntharalingam M, Moughhan J, Coia LR. Outcome results of the 1996–1999 patterns of care survey of the national practice for patients receiving radiation therapy for carcinoma of the esophagus. J Clin Oncol 2005;23:2325–31.

35. Nutting CM, Bedford JL, Cosgrove VP. A comparison of conformal and intensity-modulated techniques for oesphageal radiotherapy. Radiother Oncol 2001;61:157–63.

36. Font A, Garcia-Alfonso P, Arellano A. Preoperative combined multimodal therapy with docetaxel plus 5-fluorouracil and concurrent hyperfractionated radiotherapy for locally advanced esophageal cancer. Proc ASCO 2002;21:128b.

37. Ilson DH, Minsky B, Kelsen D. Irinotecan cisplatin and radiation in esophageal cancer. Oncology 2002;16s:11–5.

38. D'Adamo DR, Bains M, Minsky B. A phase I trial of paclitaxel, cisplatin, irinotecan, and concurrent radiation therapy in locally advanced esophageal cancer. Proc ASCO 2003;22:349.

39. Safran H, DiPetrillo T, Nadeem A. Neoadjuvant herceptin, paclitaxel, cisplatin, and radiation for adenocarcinoma of esophagus: a phase I study. Proc ASCO 2002;21:141a.

40. Khushalani KI, Leichman CG, Proulx G. Oxaliplatin in combination with protracted-infusion fluorouracil and radiation: report of a clinical trial for patients with esophageal cancer., J Clin Oncol, 2002;20:2844–50.

41. Berger AC, Farma J, Scott WJ. Complete response to neoadjuvant chemoradiotherapy in esophageal carcinoma is associated with significantly improved survival. J Clin Oncol 2005;23:4330–7.

42. Sarbia M, Stahl M, Fink U. Expression of apoptosis-regulating proteins and outcome of esophageal cancer patients treated by combined therapy modalities. Clin Cancer Res 1998;4:2991–7.

43. Pomp J, Davelaar J, Blom J. Radiotherapy for oesophagus carcinoma: the impact of p53 on treatment outcome., Radiother Oncol, 1998;46:179–84.

44. Merchant TE, Minsky BD, Lauwers GY. Esophageal cancer phospholipids correlated with histopathologic findings: a 31P NMR study., NMR Biomed, 1999;12:184–8.

45. Kishi K, Doki Y, Miyata H. Prediction of the response to chemoradiation and prognosis in oesophageal squamous cancer. Br J Surg 2002;89:597–603. (Abstract).

46. Hironaka S, Hasebe T, Kamijo T. Biopsy specimen microvessel density is a useful prognostic marker in patients with T2-4M0 esophageal cancer treated with chemoradiotherapy. Clin Cancer Res 2002;8:124–30.

47. Morita M, Kuwano H, Araki K. Prognostic significance of lymphocytic infiltration following preoperative chemoradiotherapy and hyperthermia for esophageal cancer. Int J Radiat Oncol Biol Phys 2001;49:1259–66.

48. Akamatsu M, Matsumoto T, Oka K. c-erbB-2 oncoprotein expression related to chemoradioresistance in esophageal

squamous cell carcinoma. Int J Radiat Oncol Biol Phys 2003;57:1323–7.

49. Kalha I, Kaw M, Fukami N. The accuracy of endoscopic ultrasound for restaging esophageal carcinoma after chemoradiation therapy. Cancer 2004;101:940–7.

50. Wieder HA, Brucher BLDM, Zimmermann F. Time course of tumor metabolic activity during chemoradiotherapy of esophageal squamous cell carcinoma and response to treatment. J Clin Oncol 2004;22:900–8.

51. Bedenne L, Michel P, Bouche O. Randomized phase III trial in locally advanced esophageal cancer: radiochemotherapy followed by surgery versus radiochemotherapy alone (FFCD 9102), Proc ASCO, 2002;21:130a.

52. Bonnetain F, Bedenne L, Michel P. Definitive results of a comparative longitudinal quality of life study using the Spitzer index in the randomized multicentric phase III trial FFCD 9102 (surgery vs. radiochemotherapy in patients with locally advanced esophageal cancer). Proc ASCO 2003; 22:250.

53. Stahl M, Stuschke M, Lehmann N. Chemoradiation with and without surgery in patients with locally advanced squamous cell carcinoma of the esophagus. J Clin Oncol 2005;23:2310–7.

54. Coia LR, Soffen EM, Schultheiss TE. Swallowing function in patients with esophageal cancer treated with concurrent radiation and chemotherapy. Cancer 1993;71: 281–6.

55. Sur RK, Singh DP, Sharma SC. Radiation therapy of esophageal cancer: role of high dose rate brachytherapy. Int J Radiat Oncol Biol Phys 1992;22:1043–6.

56. Sur RK, Donde B, Levin VC. Fractionated high dose rate intraluminal brachytherapy in palliation of advanced esophageal cancer. Int J Radiat Oncol Biol Phys 1998;40: 447–53.

57. Gergel TJ, Leichman LL, Nava HR. Effect of concurrent radiation therapy and chemotherapy on pulmonary function in patients with esophageal cancer: dose-volume histogram analysis. Cancer J 2002;8:451–60.

58. Gschossmann JM, Bonner JA, Foote RL. Malignant tracheoesophageal fistula in patients with esophageal cancer. Cancer 1993;72:1513–21.

CHAPTER 6

SURGICAL TREATMENT OF GASTROESOPHAGEAL JUNCTION ADENOCARCINOMA

DAVID J. BENTREM, MD

MARK S. TALAMONTI, MD

Although the overall incidence of gastric cancer has remained stable in the West, there is a well documented shift from distal lesions to more proximal lesions involving the gastroesophageal junction (GEJ) and cardia.[1] These tumors are defined as being within 5 cm proximal or distal to the anatomic cardia. Siewert and colleagues have classified these lesions as follows: type I: distal esophagus, arising from specialized intestinal metaplasia and may infiltrate the GEJ from above; type II: "true carcinoma of the cardia arising from cardiac epithelium; and type III: subcardial carcinoma that may infiltrate the GEJ from below.[2] Surgery remains the mainstay for the curative treatment of these lesions. However, despite adequate surgery, survival rates remain poor. The use of adjuvant chemotherapy and radiotherapy has been examined in multiple previous clinical trials without convincing evidence of efficacy. Novel agents and methods of delivery are being investigated, and recent trials will affect the treatment of GEJ carcinomas in the US.

Diagnosis/Clinical Staging

Although subtle symptoms such as epigastric discomfort and indigestion may develop with early stage tumors, the patient often ignores these findings, and presentation is usually delayed. It is not uncommon for patients with vague epigastric symptoms to be treated with a presumptive diagnosis of benign "gastritis" for several months prior to further evaluation. Lesions involving the distal esophagus will present predominantly with dys-

phagia, whereas lesions in the gastric cardia commonly manifest with pain and evidence of bleeding. As lesions progress, weight loss will become apparent (Table 6-1).[3] Physical examination will reveal the degree of weight loss and the presence of any widespread nodal disease, such as metastases to supraclavicular lymph nodes.

Routine hematologic studies may disclose an iron deficiency anemia, and occult blood may be identified in the stool. The carcinoembryonic antigen (CEA) level may be elevated in advanced disease but is insensitive as a means to detect or screen for early disease. A double-contrast barium swallow is a useful test for evaluating dysphagia, yet is less effective in screening for lower GEJ/cardia lesions.[4] Endoscopy allows for direct visualization and biopsy of the tumor (Figure 6-1). In addition to establishing the diagnosis of cancer, endoscopic visualization of the esophagus, stomach, and duodenum can provide direct and useful surgical information about the extent of disease. The size, location, and morphology of the tumor, including the proximal and distal extent of disease, will be useful in planning the extent of surgical resection.

Barium study and upper endoscopy define luminal involvement of the tumor, but do not determine radial extension of the tumor. A computed tomography (CT) scan (Figure 6-2) and endoscopic ultrasound (EUS) are useful for defining locoregional disease. CT scan can evaluate for distant metastases, particularly in the liver and lung, as well as celiac lymph nodes possibly involved by metastatic disease. Unless the stomach is adequately distended during examination, CT is limited in its ability to characterize the degree of gastric wall involvement of

Table 6-1

Clinical Variable	N	Median Disease-Free Survival (Months)	5-year Disease-Free Survival (Months)
Gender			
Female	36	31.2	36.4
Male	74	37.2	40.6
Race			
Caucasian and other	85	37.8	41.7
African-American	25	30.1	32.7
Age			
<65 years	46	34.5	41.2
65-74 years	41	37.0	42.2
>75 years	23	30.2	30.1
Symptoms			
Pain			
Yes	41	31.8	37.0
No	69	36.7	40.1
Weight loss			
Yes	38	21.1*	25.0*
No	72	37.9	41.4
Dysphagia			
Yes	26	30.6	34.2
No	84	36.9	42.3
GI Bleeding			
Yes	23	37.0	40.4
No	87	30.4	35.6
Obstruction			
Yes	21	29.1	27.9
No	89	36.6	41.5
Abdominal Mass			
Yes	5	22.2*	27.0*
No	105	36.1	41.2

Outcome based on symptoms at presentation. Adapted from Talamonti MS.[3]
*$p < .05$ on univariate analysis.

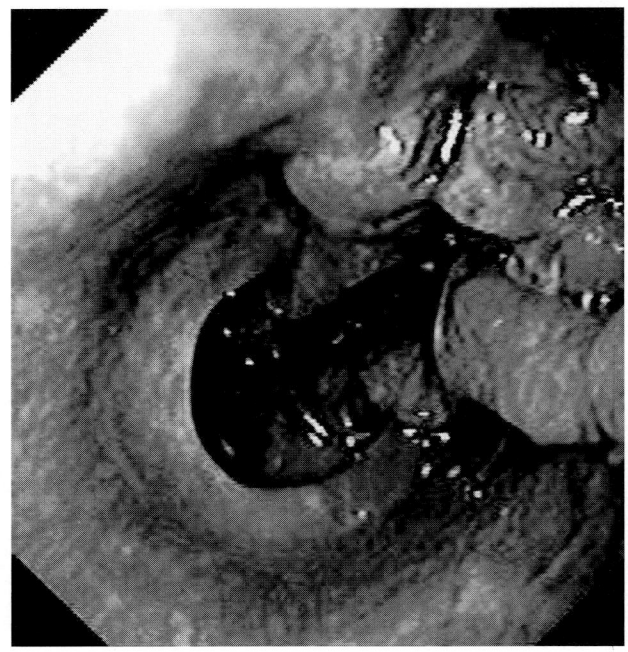

Figure 6-1 Endoscopic image of gastroesophageal junction malignancy.

improves to greater than 75%.[5,7,8] The addition of fine-needle aspiration (FNA) cytology of regional lymph nodes should also improve N-stage determination.[7] FNA cytology of perigastric and regional lymph nodes provides a more reliable and objective assessment of regional node metastases. Advances in EUS technology may have added

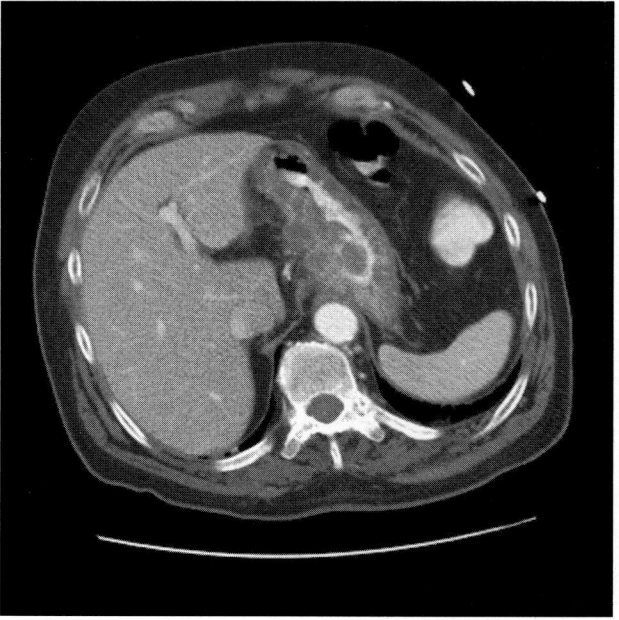

Figure 6-2 Computed tomography scan demonstrating gastric wall thickening associated with malignancy.

the tumor. The gastric wall near the GEJ and cardia is particularly difficult to evaluate because the axial images may obliquely transverse the curved gastric wall. EUS is more effective in determining the depth of invasion (T stage). It is often used to define high-risk patients (serosal or nodal involvement), eligible for enrollment into neoadjuvant protocols. Endoscopic ultrasound is not as effective at determining individual T stage,[5] yet the accuracy of detecting intramural versus transmural invasion is 75 to 85%.[5–8]

CT scans, and to a lesser degree EUS, are less accurate in detecting paraesophageal lymph node involvement by morphology alone. The size of the lymph node may not reflect tumor involvement. Small lymph nodes may harbor microscopic tumor cells, whereas enlarged nodes may be chronically inflamed. The accuracy of CT scan is approximately 50% for detecting regional nodal involvement.[9] EUS is not much improved when determining individual N stage,[5] yet when distinguishing between node negative versus node positive disease, the accuracy advantages in planning operative strategies. We have found that for cancers of the gastroesophageal junction and proximal stomach, EUS characterization can help determine the surgical choice between total gastrectomy with esophagojejunal reconstruction versus esophagogastrectomy via either an Ivor-Lewis approach or transhiatal technique. Preoperative lymph node mapping with EUS-FNA may also aid in planning precise regional lymphadenectomy. We continue to use the combination of EUS-FNA and CT scan to plan the type of gastric resection and reconstruction, particularly when defining the proximal extent of disease for adenocarcinomas of the cardia, GEJ, and distal esophagus.

Whole-body positron emission tomography (PET) is a useful modality being used increasingly to evaluate for distant metastatic lesions not identified or indeterminate by CT scan.[10,11] PET scanning utilizes preferential uptake of 5-fluorodeoxyglucose (FDG) by malignant cells to identify lesions < 1cm in size. Luketich and colleagues found that PET scans could identify unsuspected distant metastases in up to 20% of patients with esophageal carcinoma and an otherwise negative metastatic survey.[10] Because of this ability and the need for accurate preoperative assessment in patients entering clinical trials, PET scan is usually done after the preliminary survey with CT and EUS.

Operative Staging

Laparoscopy is a valuable adjunct in evaluating small volume metastases on the surface of the liver or peritoneum. Laparoscopy also provides information regarding serosal invasion by the primary tumor and involvement of perigastric or portal lymph nodes. For lesions with esophageal extension, some groups will also use the thoracoscope to further stage the lesion prior to selection of a treatment strategy.[12] Two series confirm the value of laparoscopy in the management of these lesions. Lowy and colleagues from M. D. Anderson reported on 71 patients who underwent preoperative CT and laparoscopy.[13] Unsuspected peritoneal or hepatic metastases were found by laparoscopy in 20 patients (28%). The median survival for these patients was 5 months. Similarly, Burke and colleagues from Memorial Sloan-Kettering found unsuspected disease in 37% of patients.[14] Patients who underwent laparoscopy alone did not require any subsequent palliative operations. Peritoneal cytology can be performed at the time of laparoscopy, and, if positive, is the most significant predictor of outcome for patients undergoing an R0 resection (Figure 6-3).[15] In one study of 371 patients undergoing an R0 resection for gastric cancer, 6.5% had positive cytology from peritoneal washings.[15] Median

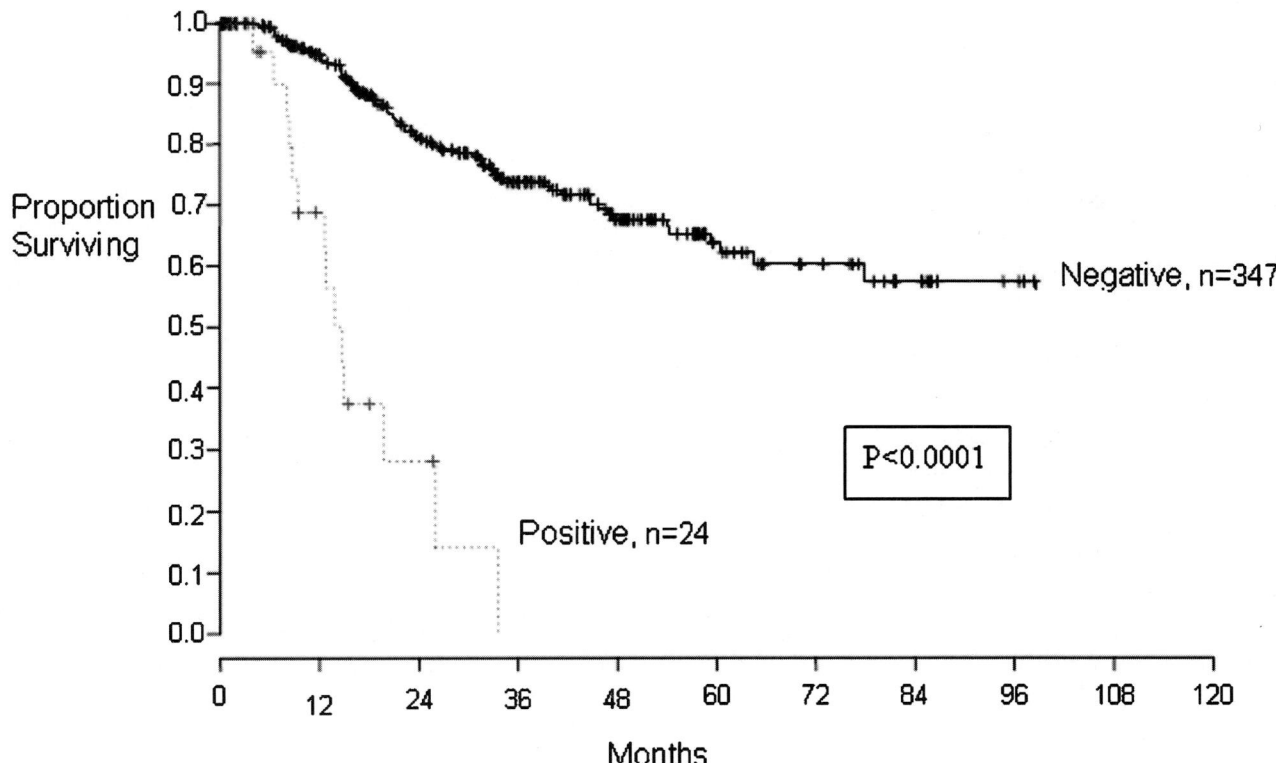

Figure 6-3 Disease-specific survival for patients with positive peritoneal washings.

survival of patients with positive cytology was less than 15 months.

Treatment

Surgical therapy remains the mainstay for patients with localized lesions who are fit for major resection. In the absence of metastatic disease, resection of all gross disease with negative microscopic margins offers the only chance for long-term survival.[16,17] Appropriate surgical resection depends upon the location and extent of the primary tumor. Surgical strategy should provide the optimal cancer operation with minimal morbidity. For patients with GEJ or proximal gastric lesions, the surgeon will have to make a choice between performing a transabdominal total gastrectomy with esophagojejunal anastomosis versus a combined transthoracic and transabdominal resection of the distal esophagus and proximal stomach with intrathoracic esophagogastric anastomosis (traditional Ivor-Lewis procedure) or transhiatal esophagectomy with cervical esophagogastric anastomosis. In general, if the tumor is limited to the proximal portion of the stomach with minimal extension past the GEJ, a total gastrectomy with intra-abdominal esophagojejunal anastomosis is our procedure of choice. This operation assures a completely negative histologic distal margin. We recognize that a longer (> 5 cm) negative distal margin will not enhance survival for patients with proximal lesions, but this procedure may minimize postgastrectomy complications compared to proximal subtotal gastrectomy. Functionally, total gastrectomy with Roux-en-Y reconstruction has the advantage of avoiding alkaline reflux gastritis associated with proximal subtotal gastrectomy. This operation also facilitates complete perigastric lymph node removal relative to a proximal subtotal gastrectomy.

TRANSHIATAL VERSUS TRANSTHORACIC ESOPHAGECTOMY

For lesions involving the GEJ and distal esophagus, esophagectomy is required in order to obtain an adequate esophageal margin (Figure 6-4). Most surgeons experienced with both techniques do not see a clear advantage of one method, and certainly no randomized trial clearly identifies a preferred approach. Hulscher and colleagues assigned 220 patients with adenocarcinoma of the mid-to-distal esophagus or gastric cardia involving the distal esophagus either to transhiatal esophagectomy or to transthoracic esophagectomy with extended en bloc lymphadenectomy.[18] Perioperative morbidity was higher after transthoracic esophagectomy, but there was no significant difference in in-hospital mortality.

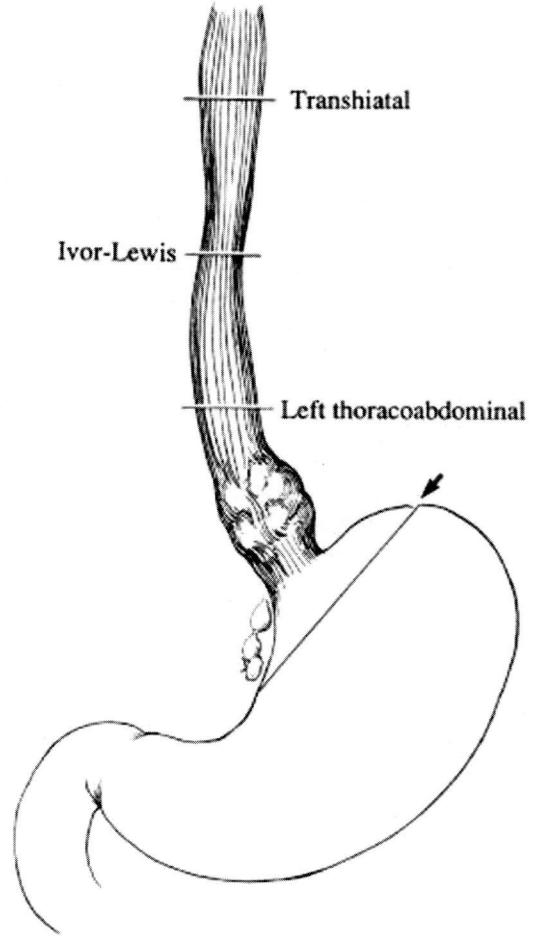

Figure 6-4 Regardless of the incisional approach used, the operative procedure required to resect lesions of the gastroesophageal junction with esophageal extension is a partial esophagogastrectomy. A portion of the proximal stomach is resected (arrow) and, different lengths of proximal esophagus may be resected as indicated. (Reproduced with permission from Heitmiller RF.[52] Cancer of the esophagus. In: Bayless TM, ed. Current therapy in gastroenterology and liver disease. 4th ed. St. Louis: Mosby-Year Book, 1994:81.

Furthermore, there was no significant difference in overall survival (OS) or disease-free survival (DFS) for patients who underwent transhiatal esophagectomy versus those who underwent transthoracic esophagectomy.

There are several maneuvers common to both approaches. For all patients, the colon is prepared by preoperative cathartics and oral antibiotics in case the need arises for a secondary conduit. An upper midline incision is made from xiphoid to umbilicus. The xiphoid process may be resected to enhance exposure of the esophageal hiatus. If occult liver or peritoneal metastases or any nodal involvement outside the field of dissection are encountered, we do not proceed with the resection. The left lobe of the liver is gently retracted medially. The greater omentum is dissected free from the transverse colon. The suitability of the stomach as a conduit is assessed. If using the stomach for reconstruction upon entry into the lesser sac through the greater omentum, dissection up the greater curve is maintained at least 2 cm away from the right gastroepiploic artery. Division of the omentum is carried out between clamps with extreme care to preserve the right gastroepiploic arcade. Excessive traction may result in injury to the gastroepiploic vein as it inserts into the middle colic vein leading to venous congestion in the newly formed conduit. We routinely perform a drainage procedure (either pyloromyotomy or pyloroplasty) to aid in emptying of the gastric conduit. This latter step remains controversial regarding its effects on dumping syndromes versus the prevention of delayed gastric emptying.

In the lesser sac, dissection is carried along the anterior surface of the pancreas and includes the lymph nodes along the splenic, common hepatic and left gastric arteries, in addition to the perigastric lymph nodes. A splenectomy is not performed due to increased morbidity unless there is direct extension of tumor into the spleen.[19] After the stomach is elevated superiorly and the gastropancreatic attachments are divided, the fold containing the left gastric artery and coronary vein is exposed. These vessels can be either suture ligated or ligated with an endostapler near its origin from the celiac axis.

Esophagectomy with thoracotomy involves dissection of the thoracic esophagus under direct vision. This is combined with a laparotomy if a right thoracotomy is performed, or if a left thoracotomy is made, the diaphragm can be incised and/or the incision can be carried across the costal margin into the abdomen (thoracoabdominal). Once the stomach is mobilized and the hiatus dissected as described above, the abdomen is closed and the patient is turned to the left lateral decubitus position. A bean bag is generally used to aid in stabilizing the patient on the table. A right posterolateral thoracotomy is made through the fifth intercostal space. The serratus anterior muscle is preserved. The pleural cavity is entered, and the inferior pulmonary ligament is divided. The deflated lung is retracted superomedially to expose the posterior mediastinal pleura over the esophagus. The intrathoracic esophagus is dissected from the surrounding tissues. The azygous vein is divided, the mediastinal lymph nodes are dissected (two-field lymphadenectomy), and the mobilized stomach is brought up into the chest. A high intrathoracic anastomosis using either a hand sewn or stapled technique is performed after resection of the lower esophagus and proximal

stomach. Two chest tubes are placed, and we secure the posterior tube in place using absorbable suture in proximity with the anastomosis. Anastomotic leak rates continue to be as high as 20%.[20] Thoracic anastomosis poses a more difficult problem and can lead to mediastinitis and sepsis; however, a recent series by Martin and colleagues found that the morbidity associated with an intrathoracic anastomotic leak was not as significant in terms of associated mortality as previously believed.[21]

The transhiatal approach for resection of the esophagus and proximal stomach is performed through a laparotomy with mobilization of the stomach as described above with the addition of an extensive Kocher maneuver to insure adequate conduit length and a tension-free anastomosis. The distal esophagus is dissected extensively and under direct visualization through the enlarged hiatus. A Penrose drain is placed around the lower esophagus and used for traction. Utilizing lighted retractors and malleable retractors, visualization is usually possible up to the level of the aortic arch. With the Penrose drain providing downward traction, a dissection plane is then created posterior to the esophagus, with fingertips against the esophagus progressing cephalad. Improved instrumentation, such as the LigaSure device (Valleylab, Boulder Colorado), limits the amount of blunt dissection and mobilization necessary to free the circumference of the thoracic esophagus.

A second incision is made along the anteromedial border of the left sternocleidomastoid (SCM) muscle. The SCM and carotid sheath are reflected laterally and the trachea is reflected medially to expose the underlying esophagus. A Penrose drain again is used to encircle the cervical esophagus and provide traction. Using blunt finger dissection, the posterior cervical esophagus is dissected free of the prevertebral fascia and ultimately joins the dissection plane from below. The cervical esophagus is transected with a linear stapler and the specimen is delivered through the posterior mediastinum into the abdomen. The proximal stomach is divided with multiple firings of a linear stapler. Great care is taken to achieve a gastric margin of several centimeters. The esophagus and GEJ are retracted to the right and the linear stapler is fired through the cardia and fundus well away from the tumor. This achieves the negative gastric margin while simultaneously creating the gastric conduit. The gastric conduit is then placed up through the mediastinum into the neck. Similar to the intrathoracic procedure, either a hand-sewn or stapled anastomosis is performed between the gastric conduit and the cervical esophagus. A Jackson-Pratt drain is placed in a dependent portion of the cervical wound. Prior to wound closure, the mediastinum is evaluated for hemostasis. There is an increased risk of hemorrhage from either the azygous vein or the esophageal branches of the thoracic aorta; however, tumors of the distal esophagus and GEJ can be dissected under direct vision with adequate exposure via the enlarged hiatus. Anastomotic leaks in the neck can usually be treated with opening of the cervical wound and observation with minimal additional morbidity.

En bloc esophagectomy is a more radical approach to carcinomas of the esophagus and GEJ.[22,23] In this operation the intrathoracic esophagus is resected along with the paraesophageal tissues including the adjacent pericardium, pleura, thoracic duct, and a portion of the right crus in an en bloc fashion. Extensive lymphadenectomy is performed to include intrathoracic nodal basins in addition to those of the upper abdomen taken as part of D2 dissection (left gastric, celiac, common hepatic, splenic, perigastric, and paraesophageal lymph nodes). A cervical incision is used to complete the anastomosis. Such extensive surgery not only takes more operative time but also increases postoperative morbidity. Arguments against the radical lymphadenectomy procedures are that after obtaining negative margins, it is the biologic nature and staging of the tumor rather than the extent of the operation that influences survival in esophageal cancer; thus, a more extensive operation is unlikely to improve overall patient survival.

TOTAL VERSUS PROXIMAL GASTRECTOMY

The goals of the total gastrectomy are (1) clear proximal and distal margins and (2) removal of draining lymph node basins, including those along the right and left gastric arteries, splenic, and common hepatic arteries as well as the perigastric lymph nodes. The gastrocolic omentum is mobilized free from the transverse colon and its mesentery. The standard dissection is continued back to the inferior border of the pancreas and the pancreatic capsule is dissected upward. Branches to the right gastroepiploic vessels are divided. The right gastric artery is identified and ligated. The nodal tissue is then dissected free along the common hepatic artery. The proximal duodenum is divided with a linear stapler. After division of the left gastric artery, the stomach is elevated and the dissection is carried up to the GEJ. A noncrushing clamp or a purse-string applier is placed on the mobilized esophagus and the resection is completed. We perform an end-to-side esophagojejunostomy with a circular stapler and favor a Roux-en-Y reconstruction with a direct esophagoenterostomy rather

than a jejunal pouch. We utilize an adequate D2 lymphadenectomy to accurately stage these patients with the goal of evaluating a minimum of 15 lymph nodes.[24]

Proximal gastrectomy can be performed for GEJ/cardia lesions without esophageal extension. In this operation, the stomach and distal esophagus are mobilized as described above. A Satinsky clamp or purse-string applier is placed at the site of the esophageal transection, and the esophagus is then divided. The proximal stomach is divided with multiple firings of the linear stapler to fashion a gastric tube or conduit as is done with the intrathoracic (Ivor-Lewis) anastomosis. Either a hand-sewn or stapled anastomosis is performed. Harrison and colleagues reported on 98 patients with proximal gastric cancer who underwent either a total or proximal gastrectomy.[25] There was no significant difference in length of stay, hospital mortality, or long-term survival. Functional or quality of life measures were not assessed.

Minimally invasive surgical (MIS) techniques using laparoscopy and/or thoracoscopy can be employed. For patients at high risk for complications with thoracotomy due to poor lung function, the esophagus and mediastinal lymph nodes can be mobilized with the thoracoscope. This avoids thoracotomy and the resultant potential compromise in postoperative respiratory function.

For any of the procedures above, the absolute goal is to obtain negative histologic margins of resection.[16,17] Once negative margins are obtained, we feel the biologic behavior of the tumor and not the magnitude of the resection determines survival.[26]

MULTIMODALITY THERAPY: PREOPERATIVE VERSUS POSTOPERATIVE

Unfortunately, cancer recurrence is common even after a curative resection.[27] Multimodality therapy has been used with the goal of extending OS for high-risk patients. Risk stratification prior to definitive therapy is an important challenge in the management of patients with GEJ cancer, with the goal of selecting high-risk patients for whom more aggressive multimodality therapy might be appropriate. Chemotherapy given concurrently with radiation therapy (RT) represents the most common way these two modalities are combined in the treatment of gastroesophageal cancers. Many phase II studies using preoperative chemotherapy or chemoradiotherapy, predominately containing patients with esophageal cancer, have reported improved survival compared with historical controls. Some large series have shown no improvement in survival compared with surgery alone.[28,29]

However, Walsh and colleagues performed a randomized, controlled trial of induction chemoradiotherapy (CRT) with cisplatin and 5-fluorourcil (5-FU) and external beam RT (40 Gy) followed by surgery versus resection alone.[30] The pathologic complete response rate was 25% following CRT, and the 3-year survival rate in the CRT group was 32% compared to 6% in the surgery alone group. This study provided support for the currently held view that preoperative multimodality treatment is justified for patients with advanced T stage and/or N stage adenocarcinoma of the distal esophagus.

For more distal lesions without esophageal involvement, the Intergroup trial 0116 demonstrated a survival advantage for patients treated with surgery and adjuvant chemoradiotherapy. MacDonald and colleagues reported on 556 patients with gastric adenocarcinoma (20% of patients having proximal or GEJ lesions) who were randomized after curative resection to observation or postoperative therapy with 5-FU, leucovorin, and 4500 cGy of fractionated radiotherapy.[31] The median survival was 36 months in the adjuvant chemoradiotherapy group versus 27 months in the surgery alone group ($p = .05$). This study, combined with the relative success of preoperative combined modality therapy for more proximal lesions, has led to the development of similar treatment regimens for GEJ lesions.

Neoadjuvant chemotherapy with or without radiation therapy is being investigated as a strategy to improve outcome in patients with locally advanced gastric cancer.

Ajani and colleagues reported a multi-institutional, nonrandomized study of preoperative chemoradiotherapy (5-FU/LV and cisplatin with 45 Gy of RT) in patients with potentially resectable gastric cancer.[32] Seventy-six percent of patients had proximal gastric lesions. The median survival was 33.7 months with a pathologic complete response rate of 30%. The MAGIC trial is a randomized, controlled trial nearing completion from the Royal Marsden Hospital using preoperative chemotherapy (epirubicin, cisplatin, and continuous-infusion 5-FU) in operable gastric and lower esophageal cancer with encouraging preliminary results and may define a future control arm for preoperative systemic therapy.[33]

Current active agents for pre- or postoperative therapy are cisplatin, 5-FU, epirubicin, and paclitaxel. The addition of targeted biologic agents such as vascular endothelial growth factor (VEGF) receptor or epidermal growth factor receptor (EGFR) inhibitors is also under investigation. One possible limitation of neoadjuvant therapy is treating nontarget populations (patients who might not benefit from additional therapy). Improvements in imaging and the combination of preoperative staging modalities should help risk-stratify patients to identify those at high risk of recurrence and most likely to benefit from neoadjuvant therapy.

RESPONSE

Traditionally, radiographic studies have been used to define response, but there are limitations in using morphologic criteria to assess response for solid tumors.[34] It can be difficult to distinguish between tumor and residual fibrosis. Histopathologic response scores have been used to define the percentage of viable tumor relative to therapy-induced fibrosis.[35] Many investigators advocate the value of histologic response for a variety of gastrointestinal solid tumors types, although a meaningful threshold has not been found consistently. For distal locoregional esophageal cancer, Chirieac and colleagues identified a 50% or greater histologic response to neoadjuvant chemoradiation for esophageal cancer as a significant factor in improved DFS and OS for patients who underwent chemoradiation follow by esophagectomy.[36,37] PET scan response after neoadjuvant therapy is a promising area under investigation.[38,39] Downey and colleagues[40] correlated a greater than 60% decrease in standardized uptake value (SUV) on PET scans after neoadjuvant therapy with improved 2-year DFS and OS rates. Swisher and colleagues found that a postneoadjuvant treatment PET scan SUV of greater than 4 was an independent predictor of decreased OS (HR = 3.5).[41]

For gastric cancer, Lowy and colleagues identified histologic response (90% or greater) as the only independent predictor of an improved outcome after neoadjuvant chemotherapy.[42] After neoadjuvant chemoradiotherapy, Ajani and colleagues also identified a significant histologic response after chemoradiotherapy as a predictor of survival for patients with gastric cancer on univariate analysis.[32]

Palliation

Greater than 25% of patients with GEJ adenocarcinoma are not candidates for curative surgery because of advanced disease or medical comorbidities. The aim of palliative therapies is to reestablish swallowing in order to stabilize the patient's body weight and nutritional status. Dilation can be employed. The complication rate is low (less than 10%); however, the duration of therapeutic benefit is short, usually lasting only 2 to 4 weeks.[43] Full dose radiotherapy is an excellent non-invasive option for improving the patient's capacity to swallow. Success rates, measured as prolonged maintenance of esophageal patency and relief of dysphagia, range from 50 to 70%.[44] Higher success rates for relief of dysphagia have been seen with endoscopic stent placement. Expandable metal stents are being used with success rates of 80 to 90%.[45]

Outcomes

In experienced centers, the 30-day perioperative mortality after resection of GEJ cancers is less than 5% (Table 6-2). In a literature review of 1,201 papers on the surgical treatment of esophageal carcinoma by Muller and colleagues, the overall hospital mortality rate was 13%.[46] The overall complication rate was 36% for the 46,692 patients included in their review. The overall incidence of clinically apparent anastomotic leaks was 12% and did not vary based on whether it was stapled or hand sewn. Finally, the incidence of postoperative pneumonia was similar whether the procedure was transthoracic (26%) or extrathoracic (21%), yet patients who underwent a transthoracic procedure had a higher incidence of postoperative atelectasis than those who did not (23% versus 10%). Rizk and colleagues[20] documented an anastomotic leak rate of 21% in a recent series of 510 patients from Memorial Sloan-Kettering, and these "technical complications" not only correlated with increased length of stay and in-hospital mortality, but also with significantly decreased OS. Several reports have used state administrative databases to identify improved outcome based on volume when performing excision of the esophagus. Begg and colleagues reported mortality rates after esophagectomy at low volume centers of 17.3% versus 3.4% at high volume centers.[47]

In the Statewide Planning and Research Cooperative System analysis of 207 hospitals and over 1,100 surgeons, Hannan and colleagues reported on 3,711 gastrectomies with an overall mortality rate of 6.2%, presumably including both total and partial gastrectomies in the assessment.[48] The observed mortality rates decreased significantly from 11.2% in the lowest-volume quartile of hospitals to 2.9% in the highest-volume quartile, and similarly, a drop from 8.8% mortality to 6.2% mortality for low- and high-volume surgeons, respectively. Using the Medicare claims data base, Birkmeyer and colleagues found the adjusted mortality rates decreased from 11.4% in the lowest-volume hospitals to 8.6% in the highest-volume hospitals.[49]

Recurrence/Surveillance

To define effective monitoring for cancer recurrence, there must be a thorough understanding of the pattern of disease failure. Adenocarcinoma of the GEJ can recur with local extension into adjacent structures and can develop lymphatic, peritoneal, or distant metastases. Locoregional failures occur commonly within the region of the gastric bed and nearby lymph nodes. Autopsy studies demonstrate locoregional failure ultimately in 50 to 70% of patients.[50] Similarly, peritoneal seeding or distant metastases are seen in 20 to 40% of patients at reoperation, and ultimately as a component of failure in 40 to 70% of patients.[50] The most common sites of visceral metastasis are the liver and lungs. Predictably, patients at greatest risk for locoregional failure are those with primary tumors penetrating through the serosa of the stomach or with extensive lymph node involvement. D'Angelica and colleagues reported on 367 patients with gastric adenocarcinoma after an R0 (margins negative) resection.[51] Among the documented recurrences, 79% were detected within 2 years of operation. Proximal lesions had a higher risk of both locoregional and distant recurrence compared with more distal gastric lesions. The median time to death from the time of recurrence was 6 months.

No rigid recommendations can currently be made for periodic imaging. Patients at high risk for both local recurrence and distant failure may be monitored selectively with frequent testing if considered eligible for investigational trials at the time that recurrent disease is detected.

Conclusions

The incidence of adenocarcinoma of the GEJ continues to rise, likely related to the increasing incidence of Barrett's esophagus and chronic gastroesophageal reflux disease. The treatment of adenocarcinomas of the GEJ is related to stage, and it is therefore essential to accurately stage the patient prior to treatment, particularly in the

Table 6-2

Study	N	Adjusted Perioperative Mortality	
Begg, 1998[47]	503	≤ 5 esophageal cases/10yr 17.3%	≥ 11 esophageal cases/10yr 3.4%*
Birkmeyer, 2002[49]	6337	< 2 esophageal cases/yr 20.3%	> 19 esophageal case/yr 8.4%*
Birkmeyer, 2002[49]	31,944	< 5 gastric cases/yr 11.4%	> 21 gastric cases/yr 8.6%*
Hannan, 2002[48]	3,711	< 16 gastric cases/4yr 11.2%	> 63 gastric cases/4yr 2.9%*

Outcome volume relationship measured by perioperative mortality after esophagectomy or gastrectomy.
*Statistically significant.

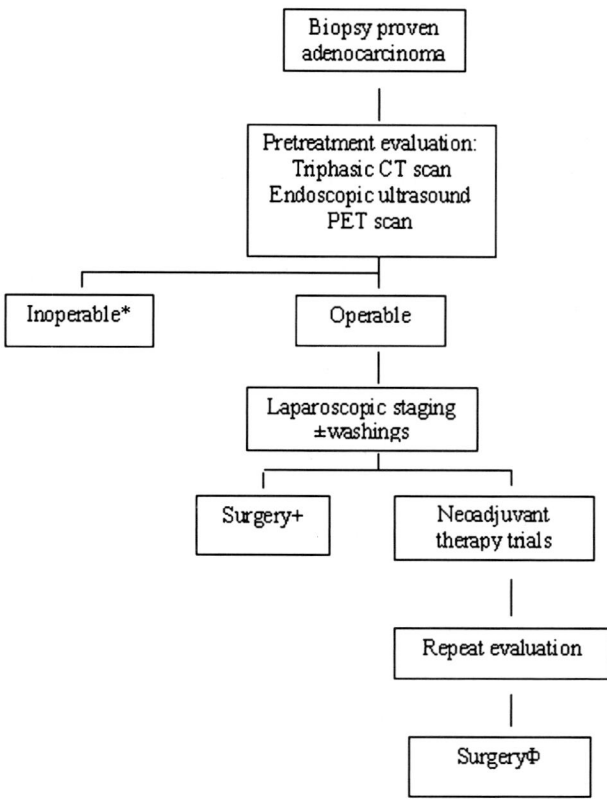

Figure 6-5 Treatment algorithm for tumors of the gastroesophageal junction.

setting of neoadjuvant protocols (Figure 6-5). The extent of resection depends on the exact location and size of the tumor, which then determines the level of anastomosis for esophagoplasty. With the evaluation of potentially better chemotherapeutic agents and the advent of molecularly directed therapy, there is increasing hope for improving the outcome of patients with adenocarcinoma of the GEJ.

References

1. Blot WJ, Devesa SS, Kneller RW, Fraumeni JF Jr. Rising incidence of adenocarcinoma of the esophagus and gastric cardia. Jama 1991;265:1287–9.

2. Rudiger Siewert J, Feith M, Werner M, Stein HJ. Adenocarcinoma of the esophagogastric junction: results of surgical therapy based on anatomical/topographic classification in 1,002 consecutive patients. Ann Surg 2000;232:353–61.

3. Talamonti MS, Kim SP, Yao KA, et al. Surgical outcomes of patients with gastric carcinoma: the importance of primary tumor location and microvessel invasion. Surgery 2003; 134:720–7; discussion 727–9.

4. Chernin MM, Amberg JR, Kogan FJ, et al. Efficacy of radiologic studies in the detection of Barrett's esophagus. AJR Am J Roentgenol 1986;147:257–60.

5. Bentrem DJ, Gerdes H, Tang L, et al. Clinical correlation of endoscopic ultrasound with pathologic stage and outcome in patients undergoing curative resection for gastric cancer. Ann Surg Oncol 2005. [In press].

6. Fok M, Cheng SW, Wong J. Endosonography in patient selection for surgical treatment of esophageal carcinoma. World J Surg 1992;16:1098–103; discussion 103.

7. Dittler HJ, Siewert JR. Role of endoscopic ultrasonography in esophageal carcinoma. Endoscopy 1993;25:156–61.

8. Dittler HJ, Siewert JR. Role of endoscopic ultrasonography in gastric carcinoma. Endoscopy 1993;25:162–6.

9. Reeders JW, Bartelsman JF. Radiological diagnosis and preoperative staging of oesophageal malignancies. Endoscopy 1993;25:10–27.

10. Luketich JD, Schauer PR, Meltzer CC, et al. Role of positron emission tomography in staging esophageal cancer. Ann Thorac Surg 1997;64:765–9.

11. Meltzer CC, Luketich JD, Friedman D, et al. Whole-body FDG positron emission tomographic imaging for staging esophageal cancer comparison with computed tomography. Clin Nucl Med 2000;25:882–7.

12. Sugarbaker DJ, DeCamp MM, Liptay MJ. Surgical procedures to resect and replace the esophagus. In: Zinner MJ, Schwartz SI, Ellis H, editors. Maingot's abdominal operations, Vol I. Stamford: Appleton & Lange, 1997. p. 885–95.

13. Lowy AM, Mansfield PF, Leach SD, Ajani J. Laparoscopic staging for gastric cancer. Surgery 1996;119:611–4.

14. Burke EC, Karpeh MS, Conlon KC, Brennan MF. Laparoscopy in the management of gastric adenocarcinoma. Ann Surg 1997;225:262–7.

15. Bentrem D, Wilton A, Mazumdar M, et al. The value of peritoneal cytology as a preoperative predictor in patients with gastric carcinoma undergoing a curative resection. Ann Surg Oncol 2005;12:347–53.

16. Brennan MF. Benefit of aggressive multimodality treatment for gastric cancer. Ann Surg Oncol 1995;2:286–7.

17. Brennan MF, Karpeh MS Jr. Surgery for gastric cancer: the American view. Semin Oncol 1996;23:352–9.

18. Hulscher JB, van Sandick JW, de Boer AG, et al. Extended transthoracic resection compared with limited transhiatal resection for adenocarcinoma of the esophagus. N Engl J Med 2002;347:1662–9.

19. Brady MS, Rogatko A, Dent LL, Shiu MH. Effect of splenectomy on morbidity and survival following curative gastrectomy for carcinoma. Arch Surg 1991;126:359–64.

20. Rizk NP, Bach PB, Schrag D, et al. The impact of complications on outcomes after resection for esophageal and gastroesophageal junction carcinoma. J Am Coll Surg 2004;198:42–50.

21. Martin LW, Swisher S, Hofstetter W, et al. Intrathoracic leaks following esophagectomy are no longer associated with increased mortality. American Surgical Association 2005;125th annual mtg:16.

22. Skinner DB. En bloc resection for neoplasms of the esophagus and cardia. J Thorac Cardiovasc Surg 1983;85:59–71.

23. Skinner DB, Dowlatshahi KD, DeMeester TR. Potentially curable cancer of the esophagus. Cancer 1982;50(11 Suppl):2571–5.

24. Karpeh MS, Leon L, Klimstra D, Brennan MF. Lymph node staging in gastric cancer: is location more important than Number? An analysis of 1,038 patients. Ann Surg 2000;232:362–71.

25. Harrison LE, Karpeh MS, Brennan MF. Proximal gastric cancers resected via a transabdominal-only approach. Results and comparisons to distal adenocarcinoma of the stomach. Ann Surg 1997;225:678–83; discussion 683–5.

26. Orringer MB. Transhiatal esophagectomy without thoracotomy for carcinoma of the thoracic esophagus. Ann Surg 1984;200:282–8.

27. Hochwald SN, Kim S, Klimstra DS, et al. Analysis of 154 actual five-year survivors of gastric cancer. J Gastrointest Surg 2000;4:520–5.

28. Parker EF, Reed CE, Marks RD, et al. Chemotherapy, radiation therapy, and resection for carcinoma of the esophagus. Long-term results. J Thorac Cardiovasc Surg 1989;98:1037–42, discussion 1042–4.

29. Kelsen DP, Ginsberg R, Pajak TF, et al. Chemotherapy followed by surgery compared with surgery alone for localized esophageal cancer. N Engl J Med 1998;339:1979–84.

30. Walsh TN, Noonan N, Hollywood D, et al. A comparison of multimodal therapy and surgery for esophageal adenocarcinoma. N Engl J Med 1996;335:462–7.

31. MacDonald JS, Smalley SR, Benedetti J, et al. Chemoradiotherapy after surgery compared with surgery alone for adenocarcinoma of the stomach or gastroesophageal junction. N Engl J Med 2001;345:725–30.

32. Ajani JA, Mansfield PF, Janjan N, et al. Multi-institutional trial of preoperative chemoradiotherapy in patients with potentially resectable gastric carcinoma. J Clin Oncol 2004;22:2774–80.

33. Allum W, Cunningham D, Weeden S. Perioperative chemotherapy in operable gastric and lower oesophageal cancer: a randomized, controlled trial (the MAGIC trial). Proc Am Soc Clin Oncol 2003;22:249.

34. Miller AB, Hoogstraten B, Staquet M, Winkler A. Reporting results of cancer treatment. Cancer 1981;47:207–14.

35. Salzer-Kuntschik M, Delling G, Beron G, Sigmund R. Morphological grades of regression in osteosarcoma after polychemotherapy—study COSS 80. J Cancer Res Clin Oncol 1983;106 Suppl:21–4.

36. Chirieac LR, Swisher SG, Ajani JA, et al. Posttherapy pathologic stage predicts survival in patients with esophageal carcinoma receiving preoperative chemoradiation. Cancer 2005;103:1347–55.

37. Swisher SG, Hofstetter W, Wu TT, et al. Proposed revision of the esophageal cancer staging system to accommodate pathologic response (pP) following preoperative chemoradiation (CRT). Ann Surg 2005;241:810–7; discussion 817–20.

38. Weber WA, Ott K, Becker K, et al. Prediction of response to preoperative chemotherapy in adenocarcinomas of the esophagogastric junction by metabolic imaging. J Clin Oncol 2001;19:3058–65.

39. Cerfolio RJ, Bryant AS, Ohja B, et al. The accuracy of endoscopic ultrasonography with fine-needle aspiration, integrated positron emission tomography with computed tomography, and computed tomography in restaging patients with esophageal cancer after neoadjuvant chemoradiotherapy. J Thorac Cardiovasc Surg 2005;129:1232–41.

40. Downey RJ, Akhurst T, Ilson D, et al. Whole body 18FDG-PET and the response of esophageal cancer to induction therapy: results of a prospective trial. J Clin Oncol 2003;21:428–32.

41. Swisher SG, Maish M, Erasmus JJ, et al. Utility of PET, CT, and EUS to identify pathologic responders in esophageal cancer. Ann Thorac Surg 2004;78:1152–60; discussion 1152–60.

42. Lowy AM, Mansfield PF, Leach SD, et al. Response to neoadjuvant chemotherapy best predicts survival after curative resection of gastric cancer. Ann Surg 1999;229:303–8.

43. Lundell L, Leth R, Lind T, et al. Palliative endoscopic dilatation in carcinoma of the esophagus and esophagogastric junction. Acta Chir Scand 1989;155:179–84.

44. Caspers RJ, Welvaart K, Verkes RJ, et al. The effect of radiotherapy on dysphagia and survival in patients with esophageal cancer. Radiother Oncol 1988;12:15–23.

45. Reed CE. Endoscopic palliation of esophageal carcinoma. Chest Surg Clin N Am 1994;4:155–72.

46. Muller JM, Erasmi H, Stelzner M, et al. Surgical therapy of oesophageal carcinoma. Br J Surg 1990;77:845–57.

47. Begg CB, Cramer LD, Hoskins WJ, Brennan MF. Impact of hospital volume on operative mortality for major cancer surgery. Jama 1998;280:1747–51.

48. Hannan EL, Radzyner M, Rubin D, et al. The influence of hospital and surgeon volume on in-hospital mortality for colectomy, gastrectomy, and lung lobectomy in patients with cancer. Surgery 2002;131:6–15.

49. Birkmeyer JD, Siewers AE, Finlayson EV, et al. Hospital volume and surgical mortality in the United States. N Engl J Med 2002;346:1128–37.

50. Alexander RH, Kelsen DG, Tepper JC. Cancer of the stomach. In DeVita VT, Hellman S, Rosenberg SA, editors. Cancer: principles and practice of oncology. Philadelphia: JB Lippincott Co.; 1997. p. 1021.

51. D'Angelica M, Gonen M, Brennan MF, et al. Patterns of initial recurrence in completely resected gastric adenocarcinoma. Ann Surg 2004;240:808–16.

52. Heitmiller RF. Cancer of the esophagus. In: Bayless TM, editor. Current therapy in gastroenterology and liver disease, 4th ed. St. Louis: Mosby-Year Book, 1994. p. 81.

Chapter 7

Stomach

Carlton C. Barnett Jr, MD

Jason B. Fleming, MD

Statistics from 2005 identified 21,860 new cases of gastric cancer last year in the US, and 11,550 mortalities from gastric cancer in that same time period.[1] These results produce an actuarial 5-year survival rate of approximately of 20% for patients diagnosed with gastric cancer <http://seer.cancer.gov>. There is currently no unified screening strategy for gastric cancer in the US. Symptoms of gastric cancer are often vague and nonspecific, which leads to a delay in diagnosis and presentation of most patients in this country at an advanced stage with a generally poor outcome. Also contributing to a low survival rate is the fact that locoregional failure after surgical treatment of gastric carcinoma is frequent (40 to 65%) and nearly always results in cancer-related death.[2,3] Recently, however, the Intergroup trial (INT 0116) demonstrated improved outcomes for patients who receive an R0 (negative margin) surgical resection and postoperative chemotherapy (bolus 5-FU) and radiation (45Gy delivered 2 cm beyond all involved nodal basins).[4] Specific data on the surgical aspects of the patients in this trial identified apparent shortcomings in the surgical management of gastric carcinoma in the US. Specifically, more than half (54%) of enrolled patients received an inadequate (D0) lymphadenectomy according to published standards.[5] Importantly, computerized models developed to predict the site and extent of lymphadenectomy accurately predict which of the patient groups in the trial would have a poor outcome as a result of inadequate surgery.[6] We believe data from this and other well-performed clinical trials demonstrate the critical importance of a well-performed surgical resection in the cancer-related outcome of gastric cancer patients. In this chapter we present our application of the surgical data in the care of patients with gastric adenocarcinoma.

Initial Work-up

When patients are diagnosed with gastric adenocarcinoma, it is important to perform a timely and accurate staging work-up with consultation by a multidisciplinary Gastrointestinal (GI) Oncology program. This group necessarily includes medical, surgical, and radiation oncologists as well as pathologists, gastroenterologists, diagnostic radiologists, and nursing coordinators. In this way each patient receives an individual recommendation for their case based upon review of all the diagnostic and staging information and an evidence-based treatment pathway.

Diagnostic studies usually begin with a diagnostic upper endoscopy, which provides a gross estimation of tumor size and the presence of risk factors, such as bleeding from the cancer, that might influence immediate treatment decisions. Importantly, endoscopic biopsy yields a tissue diagnosis and important information on histologic variants (eg signet ring). Endoscopic ultrasound (EUS), while not absolutely necessary, is helpful in evaluating patients with locally advanced disease. In patients with advanced tumors defined as uT3-uT4, ie, tumors infiltrating the serosa or neighboring structures, the diagnostic concordance of EUS was 91.1%.[7] Moreover, occult lesions identified in the liver or lymph nodes can be biopsied in some instances confirming metastatic disease.[8] Endoscopic ultrasound is somewhat limited in terms of biopsies of nodal metastasis as the primary tumor must often be traversed to get to suspicious appearing nodes causing contamination.[9] Patients should also receive a chest X-ray and thin cut axial imaging via an intravenous contrast-enhanced computed tomography scan. Lesions suspicious for metastasis can be further evaluated with PET scanning.[10–12] We obtain an upper GI contrast study in patients with lesions in the upper third of the stomach for anatomic location of the tumor relative to the gastroesophageal (GE) junction. Additionally, lack of distensability of the stomach as it fills with contrast can be detected and suggests tumor infiltration usually undetected by routine endoscopy (Figure 7-1). In addition to the above imaging modalities, patients

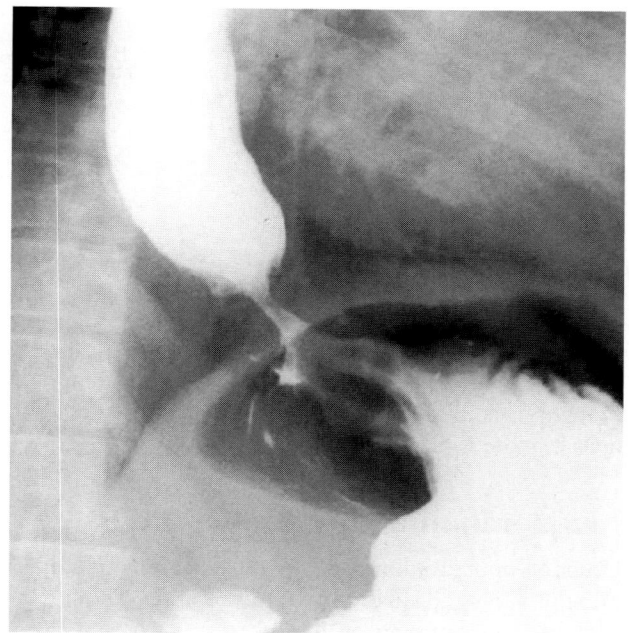

Figure 7-1 Contrasted esophagogram shows poor distensability at the gastroesophageal junction indicative of significant proximal extension of a gastric cancer.

should also have a complete blood count, chemistry panel, serum albumin, prealbumin and carcinoembryonic antigen level drawn. The nutritional parameters are helpful in stratifying patients for potential treatment pathways. After all the initial data have been obtained and reviewed, patients can generally be placed in one of two groups (Figure 7-2); group 1 are stage IV patients

based on the presence of obvious metastatic disease; group 2 has evidence of locoregional disease only. Group 2 can be further divided into three groups: (A) candidates for curative therapy (R0) resection; (B) patients with good performance status with locoregional disease that will prevent resection for cure (R1/R2 resection); (C) patients who are unresectable for cure (R1/R2) and are unfit for any operative intervention. This chapter will focus on the surgical management of patients with resectable locoregional disease.

Laparoscopic Staging

Even the best axial imaging modalities have limited value when staging gastric cancer.[12] The primary advantage of laparoscopic exploration is the prevention of a nontherapeutic laparotomy.[13] Patients found to have even occult peritoneal metastases have a limited life expectancy (less than one year),[14] and recovery from full laparotomy can unduly delay palliative chemoradiation treatments in symptomatic patients. Laparoscopy offers an additional low morbidity study, which allows for more accurate staging. Previous studies have shown that patients with negative laparoscopy have greater than a 90% chance of undergoing and R0 resection and that staging laparoscopy alters the management of gastric cancer in approximately 30% of cases (Table 7-1).[15–17] Although others have found that positive cytology sent at the time of laparoscopy strongly correlates with outcome,[14,18,19] we have found that careful visual inspection via multiple laparoscopic ports identifies intra-abdominal metastatic disease in 30 to 40% of cases and is superior to cytology

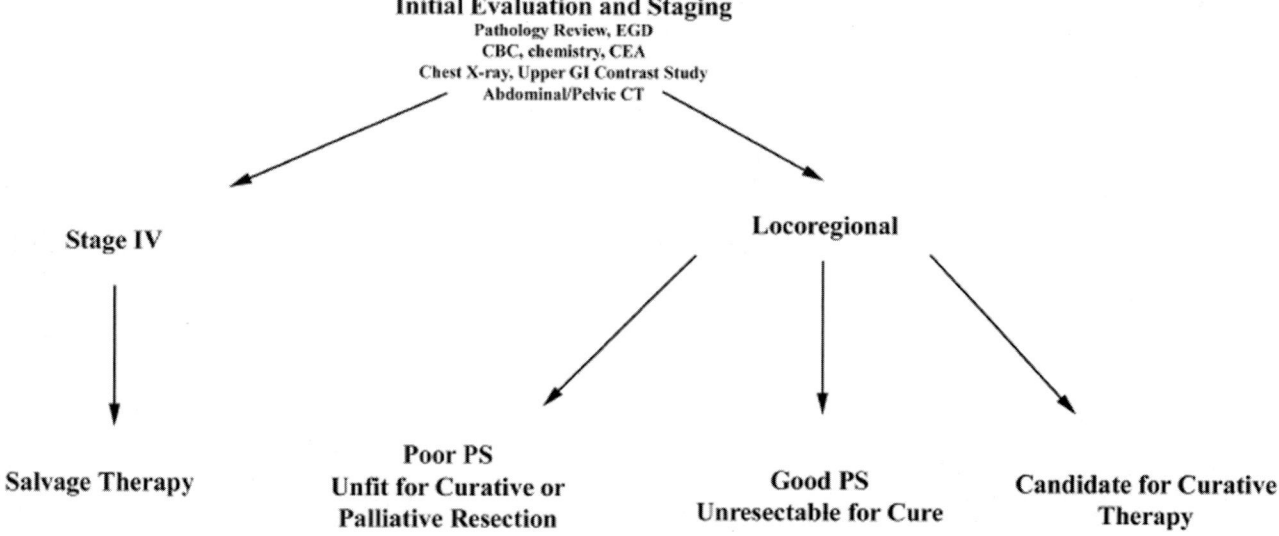

Figure 7-2 Initial work-up and pathways of care employed for patients with gastric adenocarcinoma. CBC = complete blood count; CEA = serum carcinoembryonic antigen; CT = computed tomography; EGD = esophagogastroduodenoscopy; PS = performance status.

Table 7-1 Laparoscopy for Staging

Author	Dates	Tumor Location	Number of Patients	Laparoscopy Changed stage or plan(%)	Hepatic Metastases (%)	Peritoneal Metastases (%)
Feussner[39]	*	Stomach	111	41	9	
Burke[19]	90-95	Stomach	110	29	3	
Davies[40]	93-96	Stomach	105	**	7	
Stell[16]	88-91	Stomach	103***	31	21	
Lowy[15]	91-95	Stomach	69	23	4	
Summary			498	Range 23-41% Mean 31%	Range 3-21% Mean 9%	Range 10-24% Mean 19%

alone in staging patients with gastric and esophageal carcinomas.[13] Our technique is as follows: after the induction of general anesthesia, a 10 to 12 mm Hasson trocar is placed in the standard fashion at the umbilicus. The abdomen is then insufflated with CO_2 to a pressure of 15 mmHg. Using a 30-degree scope, all peritoneal surfaces are carefully examined. Care should be taken to prevent bleeding into the peritoneal cavity because this can make visualization somewhat more difficult. At this point 1 L of warmed saline can be introduced through the Hasson trocar and the camera can be driven "under water"[20] for improved visualization of the diaphragm over segments 7 and 8 of the liver, the undersurface of the left lobe of the liver, and within the lesser sac. Additional ports are placed as needed to allow for careful inspection of all peritoneal surfaces. The liver is also elevated and the lesser omentum/gastrohepatic ligament is divided to allow complete visualization of the lesser sac (Figure 7-3). Following this the patient is placed in Trendelenberg position to allow visualization of the pouch of Douglas and the root of the mesentery. Starting in Trendelenberg position, the omentum can be manipulated to allow it to be completely examined.[13] At this point, if all laparoscopic findings are negative, we will proceed to open laparotomy. In our experience, careful laparoscopy will "up-stage" a significant number of patients (30 to 40%) and avoid unnecessary lapar-

otomy.[13] If staging laparoscopy is negative, the patient is brought back to the flat supine position and prepared for open exploration.

Exploration and Operative Exposure

Either an upper midline or bilateral subcostal abdominal incision allows adequate access to the upper abdominal contents. Our decision on the opening incision is based on the patient's body habitus and predicted operative needs. For example, a patient with a narrow-angled costal margin at the xiphoid or a proximal gastric tumor would likely receive a midline incision, while a patient potentially requiring dissection of splenic hilar nodes or multivisceral resection would received a bilateral subcostal incision. We generally preserve the ligamentum teres as a vascularized pedicle from its origin to its insertion on the umbilicus because this is potentially useful later to cover the stump of the left gastric artery. After the falciform ligament is taken down over the dome of the liver, a self-retaining table attached retractor can be placed. The authors find that either a Thompson-Farley (Thompson Surgical Instruments Inc., Traverse City, MI) or Omni-Tract (Omni-Tract Surgical, St. Paul, MN) retractor works well.

At this point, the greater omentum is removed from the colon in a right to left fashion. We do not pursue

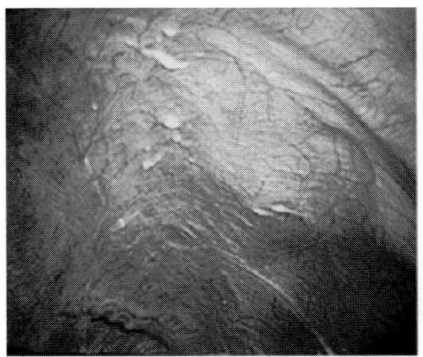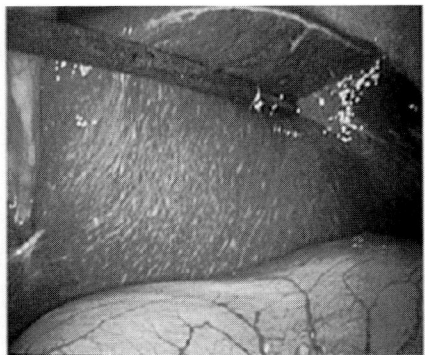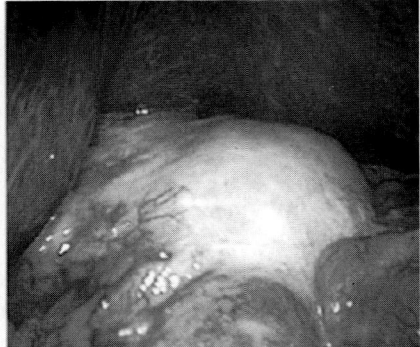

Figure 7-3 Images from exploratory laparoscopy revealing diaphragmatic studding of metastatic tumor nodules (A), elevation of the left lobe of the liver for exposure (B), locally advanced disease (C).

complete removal of the omental bursa as is suggested by others[21] because this is non-lymph node-bearing tissue, and if microscopic tumor implants exist on this surface, they are undoubtedly present throughout the peritoneal cavity, and likely also present within the liver. Additionally, dissecting the omentum free from the transverse colon contributes to blood loss, which in our opinion negatively influences the outcome of surgery, particularly if the patient receives an autologous transfusion.[22] As demonstrated by others, we have found that using an ultrasonic shear device greatly assists our speed and reduces blood loss during this portion of the operation.[23,24] Use of this device also facilitates the continuance of the dissection of the greater omentum to the level of the short gastric vessels so that the omentum and greater curve of the stomach are efficiently mobilized with a single maneuver.

Extent of Gastric Resection

Gastric adenocarcinoma cells infiltrate beneath normal-appearing mucosa, increasing the risk of unsuspected R1 (margin positive) resections. To achieve a R0 gastric resection, we perform a total or subtotal gastrectomy based upon the anatomic position and characteristics of the primary tumor. The proximal margin must be at least 6 cm from tumor to the cut edge because this distance has been shown to have the least chance of a positive margin. Therefore, if the tumor is within 6 to 8 cm of the GE junction we perform a total gastrectomy. Tumors that penetrate the serosa are more likely to infiltrate to the proximal margin, and a total gastrectomy is also performed in these patients.[25] Our preference, however, is to perform a subtotal gastrectomy. Total gastrectomy is technically a more demanding procedure and is more often associated with splenectomy, which has an adverse effect on postoperative complications and on susceptibility to infections.[26–28] It has been shown in randomized studies that patients undergoing a subtotal gastrectomy with negative resection margins have the same long-term survival rate as those receiving a total gastrectomy, and the subtotal gastrectomy patients have a reduced incidence of nutritional problems.[29,30]

To determine the extent of gastric resection, the left triangular ligament of the liver is divided and the left lobe of the liver is retracted medially to expose the upper stomach and GE junction. If a total gastrectomy is necessary, the short gastric vessels are ligated with ultrasonic shears: for a subtotal gastrectomy the short gastric vessels to the proximal stomach remnant are left intact to ensure adequate blood supply to a potentially small gastric remnant. If a total gastrectomy is planned, the esophagus can be divided between two firings of a noncutting linear stapling device; alternatively, a Satinsky clamp can be placed across the intra-abdominal esophagus 1 to 2 cm above the planned line of transection. The esophagus is then divided with a number 10 blade. If a subtotal gastrectomy is planned, a linear cutting stapling device is used with the necessary number of firings to divide the stomach. A full thickness tissue specimen in the proximal transection margin should be sent at this point for frozen section examination to determine microscopically clear margins; based on data regarding distance and the risk of a positive margin, we specifically mark and ask the surgical pathologist to examine the cut edge that is closest to the primary tumor. The distal transection is performed with a cutting or noncutting linear stapler 3 cm distal to the pylorus to avoid retained antral tissue in the duodenal stump and to prevent a positive distal margin that may occur when tumor cells invade distally into the pyloric channel. The authors generally divide the distal (duodenal) margin first and the proximal margin after the lymphadenectomy and distal gastric mobilization is complete and the jejunojejunostomy of the Roux-en-Y limb is completed. The surgeon should, however, be ready to adjust the procedure based on tumor location.

Extent of Lymphadenectomy

The difficulty in determining the extent of lymphadenectomy lies in the fact that the presence of micrometastatic nodal disease cannot be determined at the time of operation. Based on results from the MRC[28] and Dutch[31] trials, the extent of lymphadenectomy to be employed during gastrectomy has been debated. Centers of excellence can demonstrate a significant survival advantage in patients who receive a D2 resection, but the risk of bleeding and splenectomy is higher when a D2 dissection is attempted.[32,33] Taken together, this data supports an approach designed to remove all microscopically positive lymph nodes without placing the patient at unnecessary surgical risk.

With adequate preparation the surgeon can predict the extent of lymphadenectomy needed based on available patient data. This can be accomplished using the Maruyama Index of Unresected Disease (Maruyama Program).[34] The pertinent lymph node stations have been well-defined by the Japanese Research Society for Gastric Cancer[35] (Figure 7-4 A and B) and the lymphatic drainage from the stomach is predictable based on the location of the primary cancer (Figure 7-5). We believe that a rational anatomic approach can be applied without difficult algorithms. In general, stations 1 to 6 consist of perigastric lymph node stations and should be dissected en bloc with the stomach during mobilization and taken

A

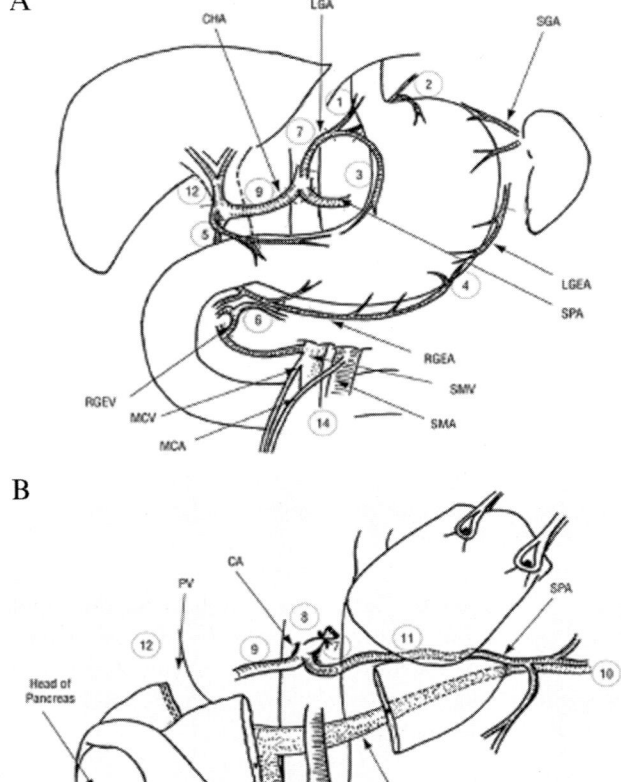

B

Figure 7-4 The location of gastric lymph node stations, as defined by the Japanese Research Society for Gastric Cancer. Reproduced with permission Khatri et al.[21]

artery is then transected using either an endovascular stapler or divided using a 3-0 prolene suture with a pledgett. The pledgett may prove quite useful in the case of significant atherosclerosis of the aorta. Nodes along the splenic artery and in the splenic hilum (station 10 and 11) can be evaluated after mobilization of the greater curve of the stomach; however, we do not routinely remove these nodes because the risk of pancreatic or splenic injury is increased. We do not routinely remove nodal stations 13 to 16 because these are extraregional stations and disease in these extraregional node stations makes an R0 resection unlikely.

Locally Advanced Disease

Patients in randomized trials examining D2 lymphadenectomy experienced a significant increase in postoperative morbidity and mortality if the spleen or pancreas was resected.[28,32] Additionally, patients with T4 disease by ultrasound have only a 37% chance of achieving R0 resection.[14] Consequently, our preference is to identify T4 patients before open exploration and offer these patients the option of preoperative chemoradiation (as part of an investigational protocol) in the hope of decreasing tumor volume and increasing the chance for an R0 resection. In patients with axial radiography that delineates T4 disease, we rely upon endoscopic ultrasound and laparoscopy before and after chemoradiation. This allows us to identify occult stage IV disease. Therefore, we only perform hepatic, pancreatic, or splenic resections en bloc with the stomach in an effort to achieve an R0 resection in carefully selected patients with direct tumor extension.

Reconstruction

It is our preference to perform a simple Roux-en-Y reconstruction using a defunctionalized jejunal limb of at least 50 cm. We do not create a pouch (eg, Hunt-Rodino-Lawrence) with the jejunal limb because randomized trials have not demonstrated a difference in morbidity or nutritional parameters when compared to standard Roux-en-Y methods.[36] In fashioning the limb we pay particular attention to division of the mesenteric arcade and prefer to use mosquito clamps to individually clamp the vessels in the jejunal mesentery using fine sutures to ligate these vessels. This is done to avoid ischemia, which increases the risk of leak at the esophagojejunostomy and poor motility attributed to the use of a Roux limb. After the Roux limb has been fashioned to the appropriate length for a tension free anastomosis, we perform the obligate jejuno-jenostomy first to prevent undue tension or manipulation of the

according to tumor location (eg, station 1 to 4 for proximal and 3 to 6 for distal tumors). This will achieve a D1 resection for patients with either proximal or distal tumors. The primary drainage pathway for the antrum, body, and even the cardia of the stomach is to the celiac nodal basin (stations 7 to 9). Incision of the hepatogastric ligament and mobilization of the greater curvature of the stomach exposes the named arteries from which the appropriate nodal tissue can be dissected using the ultrasonic shears. Nodal tissue is then dissected from the hepatic artery (station 9) toward the previously identified left gastric artery and included with celiac (station 7) and left gastric nodes (station 8). With appropriate dissection of lymph node-bearing tissue, the proximal hepatic and splenic artery should be visible, as well as the left gastric artery coursing from posterior toward the anteriorly retracted stomach. With this exposure the left gastric

LN Station	Upper Third	Middle Third	Lower Third	Entire Stomach
1. R Cardiac	N1	N1	N2	N1
2. L Cardiac		N2	N3	
3. Lesser Curvature		N1	N1	
4. Greater Curvature				
5. Suprapyloric	N2			
6. Infrapyloric				
7. LGA		N2	N2	N2
8. CHA				
9. CA				
10. Splenic Hilum				
11. SPA			N3	
12. Hepatoduodenal	N3	N3		N3
13. Retro-pancreatic				
14. Transverse Mesocolon				
15. MCA				
16. Para-aortic	N4	N4	N4	N4

Figure 7-5 Pertinent lymph node stations for D1 and D2 dissection depending on location of primary tumor. Reproduced with permission from Khatri et al.[21]

esophago- or gastrojejunostomy. At this point, if a total gastrectomy has been performed, we prefer a hand-sewn single-layer esophagojejunostomy performed in a similar method to that described by Blumgart for difficult bile duct anastomosis.[37] Whether stapled or sewn, the esophagojejunostomy must be performed as an end-to-side anastomosis because the leak rate is 2% versus 20% when constructed in an end-to-end configuration. If a subtotal gastrectomy is performed, we fashion a two-layer end to side gastrojejunostomy.

At the completion of the primary anastomosis we place a jejunostomy feeding tube in the jejunum distal to the jejuno-jejunostomy using a Witzel tunnel technique. A closed suction drain is placed if an esophagojejunostomy is constructed or if there is concern about injury to the pancreas. A nasogastric tube placed by the anesthesiologist is secured in place just proximal to our anastomosis.

Postoperative Care

With appropriate attention to intraoperative detail, the postoperative course should be uncomplicated; however, the morbidity and mortality of this procedure is surprisingly high.[38] Patients begin to receive continuous jejunostomy tube feeds at 10 cc per hour on postoperative day 2. These are advanced by 10 cc per hour every 24-hour period until patients are receiving 30 cc per hour. We do not increase the feeds beyond this level until the patients have flatus. For patients who undergo a total gastrectomy, we leave the nasogastric tube and drain in place for 5 days. At that time, if they have flatus we obtain an oral contrast radiographic swallow study. The surgeon should be present to review this "real-time" study to ensure there

is no leak. If the anastomosis is intact, the operating surgeon removes the nasogastric tube. In patients who have undergone a subtotal gastrectomy, the nasogastric tube is removed once the patients have flatus. After the removal of the nasogastric tube, the patient is given clear liquids to drink for approximately 24 hours prior to being started on six small "postgastrectomy" meals per day. If the patients are able to tolerate oral intake, we convert the jejunostomy tube feeds to nocturnal feeds. It has been our practice to have the patient take "two cans" of tube feeds per night. This eliminates confusion regarding setting up pumps and provides approximately one-quarter of the patient's caloric and fluid needs per day. Tube feeds are continued in this fashion for approximately 2 weeks after the patient is discharged home. If the patient is doing well, then the jejunostomy tube can be safely pulled at 4 weeks post discharge. In patients who have marginal or poor oral intake postoperatively, the jejunostomy tube is a useful bridge to allow them to complete adjuvant chemoradiation without complications. There is wide variance in postoperative management, but this strategy has been safe and effective in our institution. We do not see large advantages to feeding patients early because this has not in our opinion been associated with early discharge; one readmission and subsequent prolonged hospitalization for a premature discharge will negate the perceived cost saving for a multitude of patients.

References

1. Jemal A, Murray T, Ward E, et al. Cancer Statistics, 2005. CA Cancer J Clin 2005;55:10–30.

2. Gunderson LL, Sosin H. Adenocarcinoma of the stomach: areas of failure in a re-operation series (second or symptomatic look) clinicopathologic correlation and implications for adjuvant therapy. Int J Radiat Oncol Biol Phys 1982;8:1–11.

3. Gunderson LL, Martin JK, O'Connell MJ, et al. Local control and survival in locally advanced gastrointestinal cancer. Int J Radiat Oncol Biol Phys 1986;12:661–5.

4. Macdonald JS, Smalley SR, Benedetti J, et al. Chemoradiotherapy after surgery compared with surgery alone for adenocarcinoma of the stomach or gastroesophageal junction. N Engl J Med 2001;345:725–30.

5. Hundahl SA. Surgical quality in trials of adjuvant cancer therapy. J Surg Oncol 2002;80:177–80.

6. Hundahl SA, Macdonald JS, Benedetti J, Fitzsimmons T. Surgical treatment variation in a prospective, randomized trial of chemoradiotherapy in gastric cancer: the effect of undertreatment. Ann Surg Oncol 2002;9:278–86.

7. Mancino G, Bozzetti F, Schicchi A, et al. Preoperative endoscopic ultrasonography in patients with gastric cancer. Tumori 2000;86:139–41.

8. Prasad P, Schmulewitz N, Patel A, et al. Detection of occult liver metastases during EUS for staging of malignancies. Gastrointest Endosc 2004;59:49–53.

9. Eloubeidi M, Wallace M, Reed C, et al. The utility of EUS and EUS-guided fine needle aspiration in detecting celiac lymph node metastasis in patients with esophageal cancer: a single-center experience. Gastrointest Endosc 2001;54:714–9.

10. Tian J, Chen L, Wei B, et al. The value of vesicant 18F-fluorodeoxyglucose positron emission tomography (18F-FDG PET) in gastric malignancies. Nucl Med Commun 2004;25:825–31.

11. Weber WA, Ott K. Imaging of esophageal and gastric cancer. Semin Oncol 2004;31:530–41.

12. Abdalla EK, Pisters PWT. Staging and preoperative evaluation of upper gastrointestinal malignancies. Semin Oncol 2004;31:513–29.

13. Wilkiemeyer MB, Bieligk SC, Ashfaq R, et al. Laparoscopy alone is superior to peritoneal cytology in staging gastric and esophageal carcinoma. Surg Endosc 2004;18:852–6.

14. Bentrem D, Wilton A, Mazumdar M, et al. The value of peritoneal cytology as a preoperative predictor in patients with gastric carcinoma undergoing a curative resection. Ann Surg Oncol 2005;12:347–53.

15. Lowy AM, Mansfield PF, Leach SD, Ajani J. Laparoscopic staging for gastric cancer. Surgery 1996;119:611–4.

16. Stell DA, Carter CR, Stewart I, Anderson JR. Prospective comparison of laparoscopy, ultrasonography and computed tomography in the staging of gastric cancer. Br J Surg 1996;83:1260–2.

17. Fleming J. Laparoscopy in the evaluation of patients with upper gastrointestinal malignancies. In: Jones DB, Wu JS, Soper NJ, editors. Laparoscopic surgery: principles and techniques. New York: Marcel-Dekker; 2004.

18. D'Ugo DM, Pende V, Persiani R, et al. Laparoscopic staging of gastric cancer: an overview. J Am Coll Surg 2003;196:965–74.

19. Burke EC, Karpeh MS Jr, Conlon KC, Brennan MF. Peritoneal lavage cytology in gastric cancer: an independent predictor of outcome. Ann Surg Oncol 1998;5:411–5.

20. Abdalla EK, Barnett CC, Pisters PWT, et al. Subaquatic laparoscopy for staging of intraabdominal malignancy. J Am Coll Surg 2003;196:155–8.

21. Khatri VP, Douglass HO Jr. D2.5 dissection for gastric carcinoma. Arch Surg 2004;139:662–9.

22. Heiss MM, Allgayer H, Gruetzner KU. Prognostic influence of blood transfusion on minimal residual disease in resected gastric cancer patients. Anticancer Res 1997;17:2657–61.

23. Tsimoyiannis EC, Jabarin M, Tsimoyiannis JC, et al. Ultrasonically activated shears in extended lymphadenectomy for gastric cancer. World J Surg 2002;26:158–61.

24. Lee WJ, Chen TC, Lai IR, et al. Randomized clinical trial of Ligasure versus conventional surgery for extended gastric cancer resection. Br J Surg 2003;90:1493–6.

25. Bozzetti F, Bonfanti G, Bufalino R, et al. Adequacy of margins of resection in gastrectomy for cancer. Ann Surg 1982;196:685–90.

26. Brady MS, Rogatko A, Dent LL, Shiu MH. Effect of splenectomy on morbidity and survival following curative gastrectomy for carcinoma. Arch Surg 1991;126:359–64.

27. Bozzetti F, Marubini E, Bonfanti G, et al. Total versus subtotal gastrectomy: surgical morbidity and mortality rates in a multicenter Italian randomized trial. The Italian Gastrointestinal Tumor Study Group. Ann Surg 1997;226:613–20.

28. Cuschieri A, Weeden S, Fielding J, et al. Patient survival after D1 and D2 resections for gastric cancer: long-term results of the MRC randomized surgical trial. Surgical Cooperative Group. Br J Cancer 1999;79:1522–30.

29. Bozzetti F, Marubini E, Bonfanti G, et al. Subtotal versus total gastrectomy for gastric cancer: five-year survival rates in a multicenter randomized Italian trial. Italian Gastrointestinal Tumor Study Group. Ann Surg 1999;230:170–8.

30. Gouzi J, Huguier M, Fagniez P, et al. Total versus subtotal gastrectomy for adenocarcinoma of the gastric antrum. A French prospective controlled study. Ann Surg 1989;209:162–6.

31. Bonenkamp JJ, Hermans J, Sasako M, et al. Extended lymph-node dissection for gastric cancer. N Engl J Med 1999;340:908–14.

32. Bonenkamp JJ, Songun I, Hermans J, et al. Randomised comparison of morbidity after D1 and D2 dissection for gastric cancer in 996 Dutch patients. Lancet 1995;345:745–8.

33. Cuschieri A, Fayers P, Fielding J, et al. Postoperative morbidity and mortality after D1 and D2 resections for gastric cancer: preliminary results of the MRC randomised controlled surgical trial. The Surgical Cooperative Group. Lancet 1996;347:995–9.

34. Guadagni S, de Manzoni G, Catarci M, et al. Evaluation of the Maruyama computer program accuracy for preoperative estimation of lymph node metastases from gastric cancer. World J Surg 2000;24:1550–8.

35. Maruyama K, Gunven P, Okabayashi K, et al. Lymph node metastases of gastric cancer. General pattern in 1931 patients. Ann Surg 1989;210:596–602.

36. Bozzetti F, Bonfanti G, Castellani R, et al. Comparing reconstruction with Roux-en-Y to a pouch following total gastrectomy. J Am Coll Surg 1996;183:243–8.

37. Blumgart LH, Kelley CJ. Hepaticojejunostomy in benign and malignant high bile duct stricture: approaches to the left hepatic ducts. Br J Surg 1984;71:257–61.

38. Rizk NP, Bach PB, Schrag D, et al. The impact of complications on outcomes after resection for esophageal and gastroesophageal junction carcinoma. J Am Coll Surg 2004;198:42–50.

39. Feussner H, Omote K, Fink U, et al. Pretherapeutic laparoscopic staging in advanced gastric carcinoma. Endoscopy 1999;31:342–7.

40. Davies J, Chalmers AG, Sue-Ling HM, et al. Spiral computed tomography and operative staging of gastric carcinoma: a comparison with histopathological staging. Gut 1997;41:314–9.

CHAPTER 8

MANAGEMENT OF GASTRIC LYMPHOMAS/MALT

GEORGE MILLER, MD

RUSSELL S. BERMAN, MD

Introduction

The oncologic management of the patient with gastric lymphoma has been dramatically influenced by improved understanding of the pathogenesis and disease biology of this malignancy. Just about every aspect of the approach to gastric lymphoma has changed over the past two decades, from the histologic classification of what constitutes gastric lymphoma to the therapeutic interventions to treat it. Therefore, whereas it is the goal of this chapter to provide clinical guidelines for gastric lymphoma management, it is critical to briefly discuss the advances, at the biologic and molecular levels, that have resulted in the evolving concepts in gastric lymphoma therapy.

HISTORICAL PERSPECTIVES

Gastric lymphoma is the most common type of extranodal non-Hodgkin's lymphoma (NHL) and accounts for approximately 8% of all diagnosed NHL. Approximately 3,000 new cases of gastric lymphoma are diagnosed annually in the United States. The definition of gastric lymphoma has been revised over the past 25 years, with a resulting coincident rise in the diagnosis of this disease entity. Therefore, while the incidence of gastric adenocarcinoma has been decreasing, the incidence of gastric lymphoma has experienced a steady increase.

Until two decades ago, gastric lymphomas were classified by their endoscopic appearance, a system first proposed in 1950.[1] The vast majority of lymphomas diagnosed were large, advanced tumors with regional nodal involvement. On the occasion that a gastric lymphoma was found incidentally in a biopsy specimen, an incorrect diagnosis of carcinoma was not uncommon.

Furthermore, gastric resection was the only accepted treatment for this disease.

In the early 1980s, three independent and critical discoveries were reported that marked the onset of a major change in the classification, diagnosis, and treatment of gastric lymphoma.[2] First, Isaacson and Wright found that gastric lymphomas most often arise from mucosa associated lymphoid tissue (MALT).[3] MALT is of similar histology to the Peyer's patches found in other areas of the alimentary tract, but is not found in the normal human stomach. Second, Marshall and Warren implicated the bacteria *Heliobacter pylori* as an agent involved in the pathogenesis of chronic gastritis.[4] *H. pylori* would soon be found to be a primary causative agent in the development of MALT. Finally, Murayama and colleagues described a case series of early gastric lymphomas with limited infiltration of the gastric mucosa or submucosa.[5]

Pathogenesis

Primary gastric lymphomas are almost exclusively extranodal marginal B-cell lymphomas. T-cell lymphomas are rare, accounting for only 1% of all gastric lymphomas. Gastric B-cell lymphomas are further subcategorized by the World Health Organization classification as being either low grade (indolent) or high grade (aggressive). Nearly 98% of low-grade gastric lymphomas arise in the histologic setting of MALT and are often referred to as low-grade MALT lymphomas. Normal stomach mucosa does not contain any lymphatic tissue because gastric acid and a thick layer of viscous mucous usually protect the gastric mucosa from stimulation by bacteria and antigens that can trigger lymphoid infiltration. However, colonization of the stomach by *H. pylori*, an organism that can neutralize the gastric pH by secreting urase, can lead to the accumulation of gastric lymphoid tissue containing B-cell follicles. *H. pylori* infection has been documented in up to 98% of patients with gastric lymphoma.[6] In addition, epidemiological studies have shown a 6-fold increased risk of developing gastric MALT lymphoma in individuals infected with *H. pylori*.[7] These observations have been further bolstered by animal studies that showed that *Heliobacter* infection directly resulted in gastric lymphoma formation in mice.[8] It is thought that the persistent antigenic stimulation by *H. pylori*, as well as the local immune response in the form of T cells specific for *H. pylori*, results in the expansion of a monoclonal B-cell clone. The growth of a pathologic B-cell clone can progressively replace the mixed lymphoid population in MALT and give rise to lymphoma. Interestingly, the presence of a B-cell clone that would become the predominant cell in the transformation of a MALT lymphoma has been demonstrated in patients with *H. pylori* gastritis several years before the development of lymphoma.[9] Less frequently, *Heliobacter heilmannii*, a close relative of *H. pylori*, can infect the gastric mucosa and also result in the acquisition of MALT and the development of lymphoma.

In the Unites States, gastric lymphoma is estimated to occur in between 1:30,000 and 1:80,000 *H. pylori*-infected individuals. A central question to be answered is why the minority of infected patients go on to develop malignancy. It is likely that additional microbial, environmental, or host genetic factors are necessary for lymphomagenesis. Investigators have discovered a number of genetic alterations in the malignant B-cell clones of gastric lymphoma patients that appear to contribute to neoplastic progression. The most common mutation is the t(11;18)(q21;q21) translocation, which is present in 30 to 40% of gastric lymphoma cases. This translocation results in a survival advantage for the transformed B-cell clone by producing the chimeric fusion product *AP12-MALT1*, which in turn can activate NFκB, a transcription factor for several survival-related genes.[10] A second nonrandom translocation t(1;14)(p22;q32) is hypothesized to confer an increased capacity for autonomous growth.[11] Trisomy 3, a genetic mutation seen in many types of lymphomas, has been variably reported in up to 60% of gastric MALT lymphoma cases.[12] However, its precise significance is uncertain. Studies of *TP53*, a tumor suppressor gene involved in regulating apoptosis, have shown a loss of heterozygosity in approximately 7% of low-grade and 29% of high-grade (large-cell) lymphomas.[13] In addition, mutations in *TP53* were discovered in 19% and 33% of low-grade and high-grade MALT lymphomas, respectively. It is thought that partial inactivation of *TP53* is involved in the development of low-grade lymphoma, whereas complete inactivation of *TP53* may be associated with transformation to high-grade lymphoma. Similarly, inactivation of the *p16* gene, a cyclin-dependent kinase inhibitor and negative regulator of the cell cycle, is thought to be a critical event in the progression from low-grade to high-grade lymphoma.[14] Mutations in the gene encoding Fas/CD95, a receptor involved in apoptosis and the deletion of autoreactive lymphocytes, have also been detected in 60% of MALT lymphoma patients in a small series of patients.[15] Additionally, point mutations in the regulatory region of the c-*MYC* oncogene have been discovered in nearly 20% of early gastric MALT lymphomas.[16] Microsatellite instability has also been reported to be a common genetic feature in MALT and is found in approximately 50% of cases.[17] The precise role of each genetic alteration in the pathogenesis of gastric lymphoma is still speculative and is being investigated.

Histology

Most gastric lymphomas are localized in the antrum or body of the stomach, but the disease is multifocal in approximately one-third of cases. Histologically, neoplastic cells infiltrate the marginal zone around reactive lymphoid follicles and invade the gastric glands forming characteristic lymphoepithelial lesions. Tumor cells can eventually expand and invade the deeper layers of the stomach wall. There is a continuous histologic spectrum of lesions that can be seen during the progression from *H. pylori* gastritis to low-grade MALT lymphoma, and the diagnosis of early lymphoma can be challenging even for experienced pathologists. However, Isaacson and Spencer[18] described two specific criteria that must be present on histologic sampling to establish the diagnosis of a low-grade gastric MALT lymphoma. The first histologic requirement is that the gastric glands are replaced by uniform infiltrates of cells that appear similar to follicle center centrocytes, monocytoid B cells, or small lymphocytes. The second histologic criteria is lymphoid destruction of the gastric glands (Figure 8-1A). Low-grade MALT lymphoma, which fulfills the above criteria, accounts for approximately 40% of gastric lymphomas. The remainder (60%) are classified as high-grade lymphomas. Histologically, transformation to high-grade lymphoma is seen with increased numbers of large blast cells that form sheets or clusters and ultimately efface all residual low-grade tumor (Figure 8-1B). One-third of high-grade gastric lymphomas are found with an associated low-grade MALT element, raising the possibility that high-grade lymphomas develop from initial low-grade lesions.

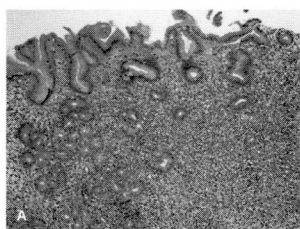 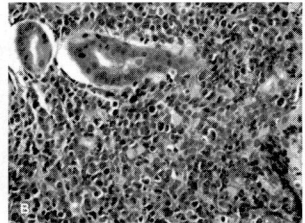

Figure 8-1 *A*, Low-grade gastric MALT lymphoma. *B*, High-grade gastric lymphoma. Histology courtesy of Ibrahim Sherif, MD, PhD. Department of Pathology, New York University School of Medicine.

Clinical Features, Diagnosis, and Staging

There exists considerable epidemiologic variation in the prevalence of gastric lymphoma by geographic region. The highest incidence of gastric lymphoma appears to be in northeastern Italy, where 13.2 people per 100,000 population per year are affected. By contrast, in the United Kingdom, the incidence is approximately 1 person per 100,000 population per year.[19] It has been suggested that the geographic variation may reflect the rates of *H. pylori* in each region.

The median age of patients affected with gastric lymphoma is 60 to 65 years, with males being affected more frequently than females, in some studies, at approximately a 2:1 ratio. Other reports have demonstrated no gender predominance. Although gastric lymphoma usually arises in patients 50 years or older, the disease has been reported in patients in their second decade of life. In younger patients, gastric lymphoma is often seen in patients infected with human immunodeficiency virus (HIV).[20] Other risk factors include immunosupression after organ transplantation, inflammatory bowel disease, and celiac disease.

Abdominal or epigastric pain is the most common presenting symptom in patients with gastric lymphoma and is the primary complaint in more than 50% of patients. Symptoms of dyspepsia or early satiety are also commonly noted, whereas constitutional "B" symptoms are rare except in cases of advanced disease. Physical exam is normal in approximately 60% of patients with gastric lymphoma. Nevertheless, physical findings may include epigastric tenderness (20–35%) or a palpable mass (17–25%). Fever, jaundice, hepatosplenomegaly, and lymphadenopathy are uncommon and are frequently signs of advanced disease presentation. In early disease, signs and symptoms may mimic other abdominal pathologies, including gall bladder or biliary tract disease, gastritis or peptic ulcer disease, pancreatic pathology, and

other forms of gastric cancer. Laboratory tests are usually noncontributory. On rare occasions, however, patients may present with an elevated β_2-microglobulin (4%) or lactic dehydrogenase (LDH) (1%).

After a comprehensive history is obtained and physical examination performed, the work-up of patients suspected of harboring gastric lymphoma should proceed with gastroduodenal endoscopy. Ulcers are found on endoscopy in nearly 50% of gastric lymphoma patients. An additional 20 to 30% have areas of patchy mucosal erythema or superficial erosions. Multiple biopsies should be obtained from each area of the stomach as well as from all suspicious sites. If the diagnosis of gastric lymphoma remains ambiguous after histological analysis, polymerase chain reaction (PCR) assays may be employed to confirm the presence of B-cell monoclonality in the gastric tissue. However, one should be cautioned that in up to 30% of cases of biopsy-proven gastric lymphoma, B-cell monoclonality cannot be identified on PCR analysis.[21] False positives are also possible (10–15%). In addition to confirming the diagnosis of lymphoma, the presence or absence of *H. pylori* infection should be established by histology, PCR, the urea breath test, or through serological studies. Finally, an important adjunct in the work-up of these patients is to determine whether the tumor harbors the t(11;18)(q21;q21) mutation. This assessment can be made using either PCR or fluorescence in situ hybridization (FISH) techniques and is available in many institutions. The implications of the t(11;18)(q21;q21) mutation in the treatment of gastric lymphoma are considerable, as will be detailed below.

The optimal staging system for gastric lymphoma remains controversial. The Lugano staging system, the Musshoff modification of the Ann Arbor system, and tumor-nodes-metastasis (TNM) staging system have been variably used and all are satisfactory (Table 8-1). Regardless of the system employed, staging should begin with an endoscopic ultrasound (EUS) evaluation. EUS is the best modality available to assess the vertical extent of disease and has been shown to have an 89% sensitivity, 97% specificity, and 95% overall accuracy in determining the depth of gastric lymphoma invasion. EUS also has a sensitivity of 44% and a specificity of 100% in detecting perigastric lymphadenopathy.[22] Before the widespread availability of EUS, computed tomography (CT) was the standard imaging modality to assess the extent of gastric wall invasion. The hallmark of gastric lymphoma on CT scan is gastric wall thickening. However, lymphoma may be difficult to distinguish definitively from adenocarcinoma on CT scan. In addition, approximately 50% of patients with low-grade gastric lymphoma do not have appreciable abnormalities in their gastric wall on CT

Table 8-1 Staging Systems for Gastric Lymphoma

Lugano Staging System for GI Lymphomas		Modified Ann Arbor Classification	TNM Staging System
Stage I	Tumor confined to GI Tract: Single primary site or multiple, noncontiguous site	IE$_1$	T1 N0 M0 (Mucosa, Submucosa)
		IE$_2$	T2 N0 M0 (Muscularis propria)
		IE$_2$	T3 N0 M0 (Serosa)
Stage II	Tumor extending into abdomen from primary GI site		
	− II$_1$ = Local, paragastric or paraintestinal nodal involvement	IIE$_1$	T1-3 N1 M0 (Perigastric lymph nodes)
	− III$_2$ = Distant, mesenteric, para-aortic, paracaval, pelvic, inguinal nodal involvement	IIE$_2$	T1-3 N2 M0 (More distant regional lymph nodes)
Stage II$_E$	Penetration of serosa to involve adjacent organs or tissues	IE$_2$	T4 N0 M0 (Invasion of adjacent structures)
Stage IV	Disseminated extranodal involvement, or, concomitant supradiaphragmatic nodal involvement	IIIE	T1-4 N3 M0 (Lymph nodes on both sides of the diaphragm)
		IVE	T1-4 N0-3 M1 (Distant metastases, eg, bone marrow or additional extranodal sites)

GI = gastrointestinal; TNM = tumor nodes metastasis.

scan.[23] Nevertheless, CT scanning can be useful in detecting lymphadenopathy (seen in approximately 50% of patients) and distant disease. The combination of EUS and CT scanning of the chest, abdomen, and pelvis usually obviates the need for more invasive procedures such as a staging laparotomy. The staging work-up should also include bone marrow examination and upper airway examination, including indirect laryngoscopy, to determine the presence or absence of Waldeyer's ring involvement by tumor.

Treatment

H. PYLORI ERADICATION

For most of the twentieth century, surgical gastrectomy was the only effective therapeutic option for patients with gastric lymphoma, resulting in approximately 90% cure rates for patients with localized disease. The long-term morbidity for patients who underwent gastrectomy, however, was not insignificant. More recently, specifically over the past 20 years, chemotherapy and radiation therapy, either alone or in combination, were shown to have efficacies rivaling gastrectomy with less morbidity. However, in 1993, based on the association between *H. pylori* infection and gastric lymphoma, Wotherspoon and colleagues treated patients harboring low-grade gastric MALT lymphomas with therapy directed against *H. pylori* and achieved complete remission in 5 of 6 patients.[24] Table 8-2 lists the outcome of selected studies in which gastric lymphoma was treated with *H. pylori* eradication. Stolte and colleagues reported on the largest

series of low-grade gastric MALT lymphomas treated with *H. pylori* eradication therapy alone. Complete remission was achieved in 81% of patients, with only 10% being unresponsive to treatment.[2] The reported medication regimen used for *H. pylori* eradication has varied widely, but most drug combinations have comparable efficacies. There are currently 8 regimens approved by the U.S. Food and Drug Administration (FDA) to treat *H. pylori* infection (Table 8-3).

Randomized clinical trials comparing *H. pylori* eradication therapy with traditional treatment modalities

Table 8-2 Outcomes of Selected Studies Treating Gastric Lymphoma with *H. pylori* Eradication Therapy

First Author	Year	Number of Patients	Complete Remission (%)
Wotherspoon	1993	6	83
Savio	1996	12	92
Montalban	1997	9	89
Pinotti	1997	49	67
Nobre-Leitao	1998	17	100
Steinbach	1999	28	50
Kato	1999	19	84
Nakamura	1999	37	35
Suzuki	1999	16	88
Oda	1999	30	50
Yamashita	1999	25	64
Suekane	1999	22	68
Dragosics	2000	19	84
Ruskoné-Formestaux	2001	34	56
Stolte	2002	120	81
Fischbach	2004	90	62

Table 8-3 FDA-Approved Treatment Regimes for *H. pylori* Eradication

	Regimen	Dose	Frequency	Duration	Eradication Rates
1	Omeprazole	20 mg	BID	10 days	
	Clarithromycin	500 mg	BID	10 days	85–90%
	Amoxicillin*	1 g	BID	10 days	
2	Lansoprazole	30 mg	BID	10 days	
	Clarithromycin	500 mg	BID	10 days	85–90%
	Amoxicillin*	1 g	BID	10 days	
3	Lansoprazole	30 mg	BID	10 days	
	Clarithromycin	500 mg	TID	10 days	85–90%
	Amoxicillin*	1 g	BID	10 days	
4	Bismuth subsalicylate	525 mg	QID	14 days	
	Metronidazole	500 mg	QID	14 days	84–95%
	Tetracycline	500 mg	QID	14 days	
	H2 receptor antagonist	As directed	As directed	28 days	
5	Lansoprazole	30 mg	TID	14 days	50–90%
	Amoxicillin*	1 g	TID	14 days	
6	Omeprazole	40 mg	Daily	14 days	
	Clarithromycin	500 mg	TID	14 days	50–80%
	Omeprazole	20 mg	Daily	additional 14 days	
7	Ranitidine bismuth citrate (RBC)	400 mg	BID	28 days	not available
	Clarithromycin	500 mg	BID	14 days	
8	RBC	400 mg	BID	28 days	not available
	Clarithromycin	500 mg	TID	14 days	

*Amoxicillin may be substituted with metronidazole, 500 mg BID, in penicillin-allergic patients.
QD = once daily; BID = twice daily; TID = three times daily; QID = four times daily.

are lacking. Nevertheless, because of the ease of its administration and its lack of debilitating side effects, *H. pylori* eradication therapy has been rapidly accepted as the standard first-line therapy for most patients with gastric MALT lymphoma. However, a number of factors have been identified that can predict the success of treatment and may account for the variability in reported remission rates (see Table 8-2). First, all patients to be treated with agents aimed at eradicating *H. pylori* should first be confirmed to be *H. pylori* positive. Approximately 2 to 10% of patients with gastric lymphoma are *H. pylori* negative and would not benefit from eradication therapy. Next, the presence of t(11:18) mutation, present in 30 to 40% of gastric lymphoma patients, is the most consistent predictor of nonresponse to *H. pylori* eradication therapy. In a recent study, none of the 22 patients who exhibited the t(11:18) translocation responded to *H. pylori* eradication treatment.[25] In another study, only 2 of 44 t(11:18)-positive patients responded to *H. pylori* eradication therapy, whereas 46 of 67 translocation-negative patients responded.[26] The presence of another mutation commonly found in gastric lymphomas patients, Trisomy 3, has also recently been shown to predict unresponsiveness to *H. pylori* eradication therapy.[12]

Although *H. pylori* negativity and t(11:18) positivity are the strongest predictors of failure of *H. pylori*

eradication therapy, a number of other clinicopathologic variables affect outcome of treatment directed against *H. pylori*. The vertical extent of gastric wall invasion, as determined by EUS, is predictive of response to antibiotic therapy. For example, Ruskoné-Fourmestraux and colleagues showed that the response rate to *H. pylori* eradication therapy was 78% in cases when disease was limited to the mucosa, but decreased to 43%, 20%, and 25% when the lymphoma invaded the submucosa, muscularis propria, and serosa, respectively.[27] The presence of nodal involvement is also an independent predictor of poor response to *H. pylori* treatment. In one study, none of the 10 patients who developed perigastric or distant lymphadenopathy responded to *H. pylori* eradication, whereas a larger trial demonstrated a 76% complete remission rate in patients who were free of perigastric lymph node involvement on EUS. Those with suspicious perigastric nodes had a 33% remission rate.[28] The presence or absence of nodal disease and the depth of gastric wall invasion have each been shown to be independent predictors of response to *H. pylori* eradication therapy on multivariate analysis. Similarly, the presence of systemic disease is associated with high failure rates.

High histologic grade was originally considered a contraindication to *H. pylori* eradication therapy. However, a number of recent reports have shown that both high-grade and low-grade gastric lymphomas underwent similar rates of remission in response to antibiotic treatment. In 1 series, 7 of 8 patients with high-grade, stage I or II disease exhibited complete histological remission after treatment with antibiotic therapy directed against *H. pylori*.[29] The appropriateness of *H. pylori* eradication therapy as first-line treatment for high-grade disease is further bolstered by the fact that the t(11:18) mutation, which is associated with nonresponse to antibiotic treatment, is seen primarily in patients with low-grade disease.

Based on the above discussion, the patient optimally suited for a trial of *H. pylori* eradication therapy is one with a low-grade, *H. pylori*-positive, t(11:18)-negative gastric lymphoma, with disease limited to the mucosa and with the absence of nodal or systemic disease. Although *H. pylori*-negative and t(11:18)-positive status and the presence of systemic disease are contraindica-

tions to a course of *H. pylori* eradication therapy, the presence of invasion beyond the gastric mucosa or involvement of perigastric lymph nodes may still warrant a trial of antibiotic treatment, given the minimal side effects of any of the anti-*H. pylori* treatment protocols. Furthermore, the relatively indolent nature of gastric lymphoma makes disease progression during the course of *H. pylori* treatment unlikely (Figure 8-2).

Surveillance Following *H. pylori* Eradication Therapy

Randomized clinical trials delineating the optimal surveillance following a course of *H. pylori* eradication therapy do not presently exist. Therefore, recommendations for follow-up can be based only on reasonable practice patterns, and not on an evidence-based approach. All patients should have repeat endoscopic

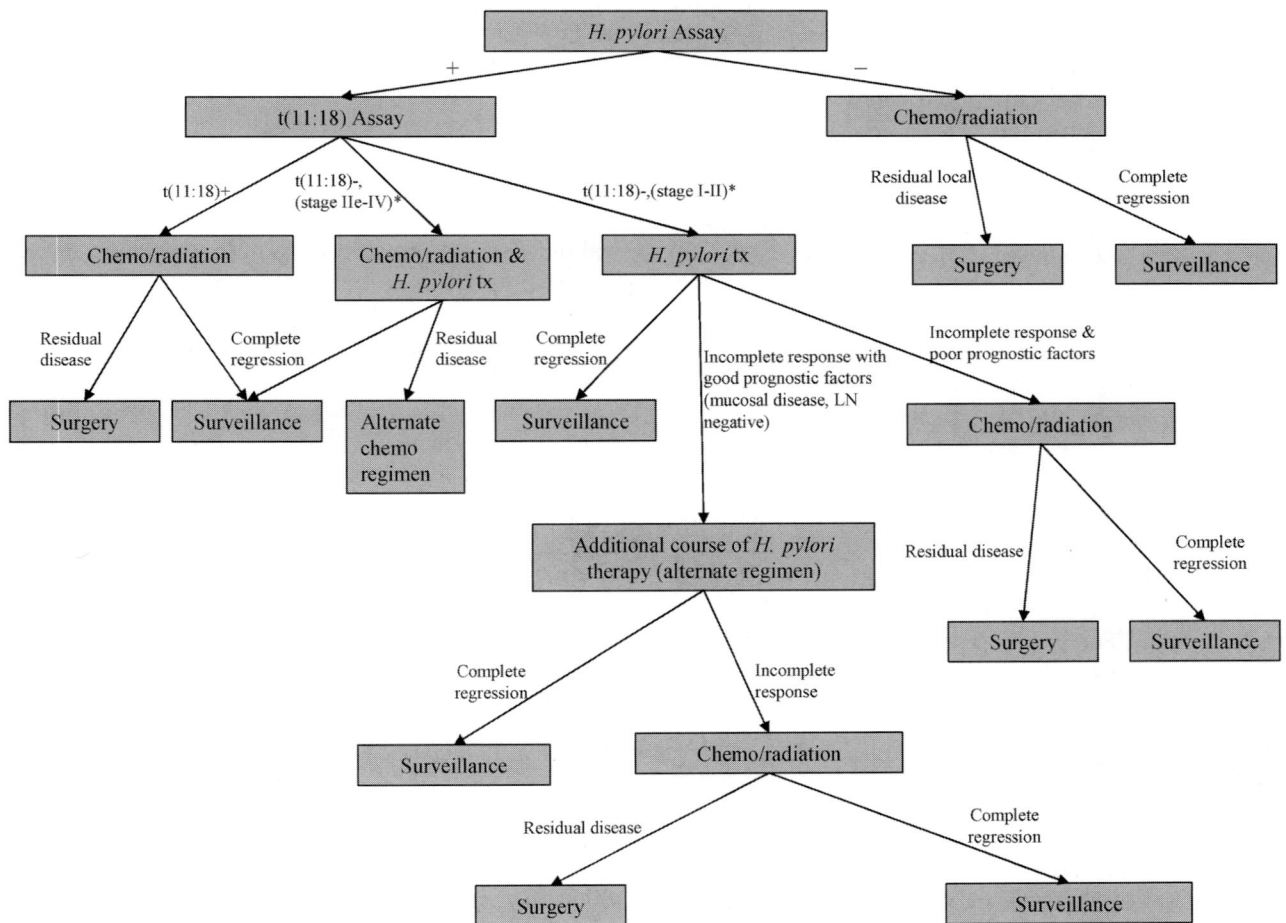

*Refers to Lugano Staging System

Figure 8-2 Authors' proposed treatment algorithm for gastric lymphoma.

biopsies approximately 6 weeks after completing antibiotic-based therapy. After repeat biopsies, patients would then fall into 1 of 3 categories based on pathological evaluation: complete responders, partial responders, and nonresponders. Complete responders should then undergo repeat endoscopic biopsy every 6 months for the next 2 years, and then yearly thereafter. Other groups have recommended endoscopy and biopsy every 3 to 6 months.[30] Because of the lack of long-term follow-up data and the unknown durability of *H. pylori* eradication therapy, we presently continue surveillance indefinitely. Isolated reports exist of complete responders who recurred several years after the conclusion of antibiotic-based treatment.[27] Furthermore, PCR analysis has shown the persistence of a monoclonal B-cell population in the stomach in more than 70% of complete histologic responders.[31] The clinical significance of this residual monoclonal B-cell population and its potential to induce recurrent disease is uncertain. A further mandate for long-term surveillance in patients considered to have been cured of gastric lymphoma stems from the fact that gastric lymphoma patients are at higher risk of the later development of gastric adenocarcinoma. This may be a result of both malignancies sharing a common pathogenesis in *H. pylori* infection.[32]

For patients who exhibit partial response to *H. pylori* eradication therapy, repeat endoscopic biopsies every 2 to 3 months may represent a cautious approach until complete regression is achieved. The median time interval to disease regression after *H. pylori* eradication therapy is approximately 5 months, but can range from 1 to 18 months. If complete lymphoma eradication is not achieved by 18 months, then further therapeutic approaches, including chemotherapy or radiation therapy, should then be employed. Other institutions have recommended that for patients with high success rates (disease limited to gastric wall, no nodes, no evidence of t(11;18) translocation), persistent lymphoma after 12 months is an indication to proceed with radiation or chemotherapy. For low-success patient groups, with only partial response to *H. pylori* eradication therapy, Yoon and colleagues proceed with other therapies much earlier.[30]

For patients who do not exhibit any response to initial antimicrobial treatment, an alternative anti-*H. pylori* regimen may be employed (see Table 8-3). This option is particularly appropriate for patients whose tumors display favorable prognostic features, such as disease limited to the mucosa and absence of lymph node involvement. Lack of response to initial antimicrobial therapy is frequently a result of the resistance of a particular *H. pylori* strain to metronidazole. However,

continued unresponsiveness to antimicrobial therapy after the addition of a second regimen or evidence of distant disease mandates treatment with chemotherapy and/or radiotherapy (see Figure 8-2).

Chemotherapy, Radiotherapy, and Surgery

For patients who fail to respond to *H. pylori* eradication therapy or who are not candidates for antimicrobial treatment by the criteria outlined above, the optimal therapeutic option is uncertain given the paucity of randomized controlled trials investigating the relative merits of surgery, radiation, and chemotherapy. However, level II and III data suggest that similar outcomes can be achieved with any of the above treatment options. Given the potential morbidity of gastrectomy, patients are generally managed with radiation and/or chemotherapy, with surgery reserved for nonresponders or for patients with complications such as hemorrhage, perforation, or unremitting obstruction. This recommendation is supported by the German Multicenter Study Group, which reported a prospective, nonrandomized study of patients ($n = 185$) with stage I and II gastric lymphoma comparing surgical to nonsurgical treatment.[33] In the surgery group, patients underwent gastrectomy followed by radiation with or without chemotherapy. In the nonsurgical group, nearly all patients received chemotherapy and radiation. The event-free survival rate and the 5-year survival rate ($> 80\%$ for both groups) were not significantly different between treatment groups, suggesting that gastrectomy was not required to achieve therapeutic aims. It must be stressed, however, that this was a nonrandomized study. Similarly, Aviles and colleagues randomized 241 patients with stage I or II gastric lymphoma to receive surgery, chemotherapy, or radiotherapy. With a median follow-up of 7.5 years, the overall survival rates (75–87%) were not significantly different among the various treatment arms.[34] A number of other retrospective analyses have shown similar results.[35,36]

Although the available data suggest that chemotherapy and radiation therapy have comparable efficacies against gastric lymphoma, the optimal scenarios for the employment of each therapeutic modality have not been studied adequately . Similarly, the relative benefits of single-agent chemotherapy versus multiagent chemotherapy or combined radiation and chemotherapy versus either modality alone is still uncertain. Single alkylating agent chemotherapy with either cyclophosphamide or chlorambucil has shown reasonable efficacy in nonrandomized trials with overall 5-year survival rates of approximately 75%.[37] More recently, many centers have employed the COP (cyclophosphamide, vincristine, and prednisone), CHOP (cyclophosphamide, doxorubicin, vincristine, and prednisone), or the MCP (mitoxantrone, chlorambucil, and prednisone) regimens with comparable efficacy.[33,38] These regimens have been variably employed either alone or in combination with radiation therapy. Rituximab, a monoclonal antibody directed against CD20, the B-cell surface antigen, has also recently been shown to be effective in patients not suitable for or unresponsive to *H. pylori* eradication therapy.[39] Rituximab has been used alone or in combination with CHOP. All of the aforementioned chemotherapeutic regimens are well tolerated by most patients with grade III or IV toxicities encountered infrequently.

Whereas chemotherapy is necessary in the treatment armamentarium for patients with distant disease, for individuals with lymphoma confined to the stomach, radiation therapy alone may be employed with good results. In a report from Memorial Sloan-Kettering Cancer Center, 17 patients with stage I or II gastric MALT lymphoma, without evidence of *H. pylori* infection or refractory to *H. pylori* eradication therapy, were treated for 4 weeks with low-dose radiation therapy to the stomach and the adjacent lymph nodes (median total dose 30 Gy). One hundred percent of patients achieved a biopsy-proven complete response, and all were disease free at a median follow-up of 27 months.[40] Acute toxicities such as gastric perforation and bleeding as a result of radiation therapy are rarely seen.

Although surgery was, at one time, the standard therapeutic modality for gastric lymphoma, its current role is limited. Surgery should be considered in cases of persistent local disease in the stomach after treatment with chemotherapy or radiotherapy. In addition, surgery is indicated in the uncommon patient with gastric perforation or in cases of unremitting bleeding or gastric outlet obstruction recalcitrant to conservative measures. Furthermore, in unusual cases, an individual patient's comorbidity profile and risk/benefit analysis may suggest a greater tolerance for surgery rather than for radiation or chemotherapeutic options. When surgery is necessary, complete gastrectomy is prudent because gastric lymphoma is frequently multicentric.

Future Directions

Research is necessary on both the molecular and clinical levels to enhance our understanding of the pathogenesis of gastric lymphoma and to optimize the treatment of patients with this disease. Regarding lymphoma acquisition and pathogenesis, current research is focused on elucidating the necessary microbial, host, and environmental factors that determine why a select minority of patients harboring *H. pylori* progress to gastric lymphoma. In addition, basic investigations studying the interplay of the proteins expressed by the mutated genes in gastric lymphoma patients will facilitate our understanding of disease progression and can lead to novel therapeutic interventions. For example, the discovery of NFκB activation as a common pathway in many of the genetic mutations linked to gastric lymphomagenesis suggests this may be an appropriate therapeutic target using proteasome inhibition.[41] On a clinical level, evaluation of the long-term durability of *H. pylori* eradication therapy in achieving lasting lymphoma remission is critical for its continued use as an effective first-line therapy. Furthermore, large multicenter randomized controlled trials are needed to determine the most appropriate of the currently available therapeutic options for patients at each disease stage who either fail or are not candidates for *H. pylori* eradication therapy.

References

1. Palmer E. The sarcoma of the stomach. Am J Dig Dis 1950; 17:186–95.

2. Stolte M, Bayerdorffer E, Morgner A, et al. *Helicobacter* and gastric MALT lymphoma. Gut 2002;50:19–24.

3. Isaacson P, Wright DH. Malignant lymphoma of mucosa-associated lymphoid tissue. A distinctive type of B-cell lymphoma. Cancer 1983;52:1410–6.

4. Marshall BJ, Warren JR. Unidentified curved bacilli in the stomach of patients with gastritis and peptic ulceration. Lancet 1984;1:1311–5.

5. Murayama H, Kikuchi M, Eimoto T, et al. Early lymphoma coexisting with reactive lymphoid hyperplasia of the stomach. Acta Pathol Jpn 1984;34:679–86.

6. Eidt S, Stolte M, Fischer R. *Helicobacter pylori* gastritis and primary gastric non-Hodgkin's lymphomas. J Clin Pathol 1994;47:436–9.

7. Parsonnet J, Hansen S, Rodriguez L, et al. *Helicobacter pylori* infection and gastric lymphoma. N Engl J Med 1994; 330:1267–71.

8. O'Rourke JL, Dixon MF, Jack A, et al. Gastric B-cell mucosa-associated lymphoid tissue (MALT) lymphoma in an animal model of 'Helicobacter heilmannii' infection. J Pathol 2004;203:896–903.

9. Zucca E, Bertoni F, Roggero E, et al. Molecular analysis of the progression from *Helicobacter pylori*-associated chronic

gastritis to mucosa-associated lymphoid-tissue lymphoma of the stomach. N Engl J Med 1998;338:804–10.

10. Auer IA, Gascoyne RD, Connors JM, et al. t(11;18)(q21;q21) is the most common translocation in MALT lymphomas. Ann Oncol 1997;8:979–85.

11. Willis TG, Jadayel DM, Du MQ, et al. Bcl10 is involved in t(1;14)(p22;q32) of MALT B cell lymphoma and mutated in multiple tumor types. Cell 1999;96:35–45.

12. Taji S, Nomura K, Matsumoto Y, et al. Trisomy 3 may predict a poor response of gastric MALT lymphoma to *Helicobacter pylori* eradication therapy. World J Gastroenterol 2005;11:89–93.

13. Du M, Peng H, Singh N, et al. The accumulation of p53 abnormalities is associated with progression of mucosa-associated lymphoid tissue lymphoma. Blood 1995;86:4587–93.

14. Neumeister P, Hoefler G, Beham-Schmid C, et al. Deletion analysis of the p16 tumor suppressor gene in gastrointestinal mucosa-associated lymphoid tissue lymphomas. Gastroenterology 1997;112:1871–5.

15. Gronbaek K, Straten PT, Ralfkiaer E, et al. Somatic Fas mutations in non-Hodgkin's lymphoma: association with extranodal disease and autoimmunity. Blood 1998;92:3018–24.

16. Peng H, Diss T, Isaacson PG, Pan L. c-myc gene abnormalities in mucosa-associated lymphoid tissue (MALT) lymphomas. J Pathol 1997;181:381–6.

17. Niv E, Bomstein Y, Bernheim J, Lishner M. Microsatellite instability in gastric MALT lymphoma. Mod Pathol 2004;17:1407–13.

18. Isaacson PG, Spencer J. Malignant lymphoma of mucosa-associated lymphoid tissue. Histopathology 1987;11:445–62.

19. Doglioni C, Wotherspoon AC, Moschini A, et al. High incidence of primary gastric lymphoma in northeastern Italy. Lancet 1992;339:834–5.

20. Powitz F, Bogner JR, Sandor P, et al. Gastrointestinal lymphomas in patients with AIDS. Z Gastroenterol 1997;35:179–85.

21. Zucca E, Roggero E, Pileri S. B-cell lymphoma of MALT type: a review with special emphasis on diagnostic and management problems of low-grade gastric tumours. Br J Haematol 1998;100:3–14.

22. Caletti G, Ferrari A, Brocchi E, Barbara L. Accuracy of endoscopic ultrasonography in the diagnosis and staging of gastric cancer and lymphoma. Surgery 1993;113:14–27.

23. Choi D, Lim HK, Lee SJ, et al. Gastric mucosa-associated lymphoid tissue lymphoma: helical CT findings and pathologic correlation. Am J Roentgenol 2002;178:1117–22.

24. Wotherspoon AC, Doglioni C, Diss TC, et al. Regression of primary low-grade B-cell gastric lymphoma of mucosa-associated lymphoid tissue type after eradication of *Helicobacter pylori*. Lancet 1993;342:575–7.

25. Inagaki H, Nakamura T, Li C, et al. Gastric MALT lymphomas are divided into three groups based on responsiveness to *Helicobacter pylori* eradication and detection of API2-MALT1 fusion. Am J Surg Pathol 2004;28:1560–7.

26. Liu H, Ye H, Ruskoné-Fourmestraux A, et al. (11;18) is a marker for all stage gastric MALT lymphomas that will not respond to *H.* pylori, eradication. Gastroenterology 2002;122:1286–94.

27. Ruskoné-Fourmestraux A, Lavergne A, Aegerter PH, et al. Predictive factors for regression of gastric MALT lymphoma after anti-*Helicobacter pylori* treatment. Gut 2001;48:297–303.

28. Levy M, Copie-Bergman C, Traulle C, et al. Conservative treatment of primary gastric low-grade B-cell lymphoma of mucosa-associated lymphoid tissue: predictive factors of response and outcome. Am J Gastroenterol 2002;97:292–7.

29. Morgner A, Miehlke S, Fischbach W, et al. Complete remission of primary high-grade B-cell gastric lymphoma after cure of *Helicobacter pylori* infection. J Clin Oncol 2001;19:2041–8.

30. Yoon S, Coit D, Portlock C, et al. The diminishing role of surgery in the treatment of gastric lymphoma. Ann Surg 2004;240:28–37.

31. Neubauer A, Thiede C, Morgner A, et al. Cure of *Helicobacter pylori* infection and duration of remission of low-grade gastric mucosa-associated lymphoid tissue lymphoma. J Natl Cancer Inst 1997;89:1350–5.

32. Copie-Bergman C, Locher C, Levy M, et al. Metachronous gastric MALT lymphoma and early gastric cancer: is residual lymphoma a risk factor for the development of gastric carcinoma? Ann Oncol 2005;16:1232–36.

33. Koch P, del Valle F, Berdel WE, et al. Primary gastrointestinal non-Hodgkin's lymphoma: II. Combined surgical and conservative or conservative management only in localized gastric lymphoma—results of the prospective German Multicenter Study GIT NHL 01/92. J Clin Oncol 2001;19:3874–83.

34. Aviles A, Nambo MJ, Neri N, et al. Mucosa-associated lymphoid tissue (MALT) lymphoma of the stomach: results of a controlled clinical trial. Med Oncol 2005;22:57–62.

35. Ferreri AJ, Cordio S, Paro S, et al. Therapeutic management of stage I-II high-grade primary gastric lymphomas. Oncology 1999;56:274–82.

36. Brincker H, D'Amore F. A retrospective analysis of treatment outcome in 106 cases of localized gastric non-

Hodgkin lymphomas. Danish Lymphoma Study Group, LYFO. Leuk Lymphoma 1995;18:281–8.

37. Hammel P, Haioun C, Chaumette MT, et al. Efficacy of single-agent chemotherapy in low-grade B-cell mucosa-associated lymphoid tissue lymphoma with prominent gastric expression. J Clin Oncol 1995;13:2524–9.

38. Wohrer S, Drach J, Hejna M, et al. Treatment of extranodal marginal zone B-cell lymphoma of mucosa-associated lymphoid tissue (MALT lymphoma) with mitoxantrone, chlorambucil and prednisone (MCP). Ann Oncol 2003;14:1758–61.

39. Martinelli G, Laszlo D, Ferreri AJ, et al. Clinical activity of rituximab in gastric marginal zone non-Hodgkin's lymphoma resistant to or not eligible for anti-*Helicobacter pylori* therapy. J Clin Oncol 2005;23:1979–83.

40. Schechter NR, Portlock CS, Yahalom J. Treatment of mucosa-associated lymphoid tissue lymphoma of the stomach with radiation alone. J Clin Oncol 1998;16:1916–21.

41. Kahl BS. Update: gastric MALT lymphoma. Curr Opin Oncol 2003;15:347–52.

CHAPTER 9

MANAGEMENT OF GASTRIC CARCINOID TUMORS

JONATHAN E. SCHOEFF, MD

ANDREW M. LOWY, MD

SYED A. AHMAD, MD

Introduction

The term carcinoid has long been used to describe a group of tumors derived from a neuroendocrine lineage. Over time, the descriptions of many tumors have fallen within the classification of carcinoid. However, it is now clear that these tumors may differ greatly from one another in both their cellular make-up and pathobiological behavior. The cell of origin for most carcinoid tumors is the enterochromaffin cell (EC) or "Kulchitsky cell" first described by Kulchitsky in 1897.[1] The term "Karzinoide" (carcinoma-like) was originally coined by Oberndorfer in 1907 to describe a novel gastrointestinal tumor that behaved in a much more indolent fashion than had previously been described for adenocarcinoma of a similar anatomic location.[2]

Carcinoid tumors can be classified as gastroenteropancreatic neuroendocrine tumors (GEP-NETs) based on morphology, histology, and clinical characteristics.[3] GEP-NETs have come to be recognized as a heterogeneous group consisting of carcinoids, neuroendocrine tumors of the pancreas, melanoma, pheochromocytoma, and medullary thyroid cancer.[4] It has become evident that even amongst gastrointestinal carcinoids, the behavior, sex predilection, association with endocrine symptomatology, and even production of specific proteins differ greatly (Table 9-1).

Over the past 30 years, the incidence and location of carcinoid tumors have changed. Previously, the incidence of gastrointestinal carcinoids predominated, and amongst those, appendiceal was the most common.[5] More recently, Modlin and colleagues[6] demonstrated an increase in the incidence of extra-abdominal carcinoid tumors, and a concomitant decrease in gastrointestinal carcinoids. This series also demonstrated an increase in the incidence of gastric carcinoid, now representing 8.7% of all cases, which is the focus of this review.

Biology of Gastric Carcinoids

The gastric carcinoid has for many years remained enigmatic to researchers and clinicians. These tumors have generated much interest given their unique relationship to the hormone gastrin, the increasing incidence over the last 50 years, and association with several genetic disorders.[7] Based on immunohistochemical markers, distribution, and tumor biology, it is apparent that not all gastric carcinoids are similar and that several subtypes exist.

The EC cell, which is the progenitor for all other carcinoid tumors, does not appear to be the cell of origin for gastric carcinoid tumors. The role of the EC cell in gastric mucosa is secretion of somatostatin, which acts directly on the enterochromafin-like cell (ECL) to inhibit histamine production. It is the enterochromafin-like cell that appears to be the cell of origin for all gastric carcinoids. The ECL is the most abundant neuroendocrine (NE) cell and is exclusive to the fundus, comprising 35% of the human fundic endocrine cell mass. This cell type stains positive for chromogranin A (CgA) and can also be identified by vesicular monoamine transporter staining (VMAT$_2$).[8] ECL plays a pivotal role in normal gastric function and appears to be a central regulator of gastric acid secretion via production of histamine.

The relationship of gastrin to the ECL in the progression from hyperplasia to neoplasia is a major focus of current research. Multiple studies have demon-

Table 9-1 Clinical, Histological, Immunohistochemical Classification of NE Tumors

Classification of Neuroendocrine (NE) Tumors of GI Tract

	Origin								
	Stomach				Proximal Small Bowel	Appendix	Ileum	Colon	Rectum
	Type I	Type II	Type III	Type IV					
Gross appearance	small, multifocal, polypoid .5–1 cm often in body/fundus	small, multifocal typically <1.5 cm	larger, solitary tumor w/ 33% > 2 cm at dx	solitary tumor often advanced at time of dx > 4 cm	commonly solitary	solitary, solid tumor	solitary, solid tumor advanced at time of dx > 2 cm	very rare lesion, often solitary > 2 cm	small < 1 cm, mobile, submucosal tumor
Sex	F>>M	M=F	M>F	M>F	M»F	F	M»F	M=F	M=F
Clinically	no sx or vague gastric symptoms	no sx or vague gastric symptoms	atypical carcinoid syndrome	atypical carcinoid syndrome	no hormonal syndrome associated	malignant carcinoid syndrome rare	malignant carcinoid syndrome common		
Histology	well differentiated confined to mucosa and submucosa	well differentiated confined to mucosa and submucosa	well differentiated with submucosal invasion	poorly differentiated with submucosal invasion	well differentiated	solid, "island-like" pattern	solid, "island-like" pattern	poorly differentiated	
Cell Type	ECL	ECL	Mixed cellular type including EC and X	ECL or uncommonly EC	EC	EC	EC	EC	EC
Markers									
Chromogranin A	++	+	+	−	+	+	+	+	+
NSE	+	+	+	+	+	+	+	+	+
Synaptophysin	−	−	−	−	−	−	−	+	+
Xenin	−	−	−	−	+	−	−	+	−
Bioactive products									
Histamine	+	+	±	±	−	−	−	−	−
Seratonin	−	−	±	±	±	++	+++	+	+
Substance P	−	−	−	−	−	+	+	−	−
Associated disorders	CAG	MEN-1 (ZE)	sporadic	sporadic	sporadic	sporadic	sporadic	sporadic	sporadic
Metastasis	−	−	+	++	−	−	+++	++	+

ECL = enterochromaffin-like cell; EC = enterochromaffin cell; NSE = neuron-specific enolase; CAG = chronic atrophic gastritis; MEN-1 (ZE) = multiple endocrine neoplasia type 1, Zollinger-Ellison.

strated that increasing levels of plasma gastrin initiate and maintain the neoplastic changes seen in these cells.[9,10] A hypergastrinemic state caused by selective histamine (H2) antagonists and proton pump inhibitors (PPIs) in an animal model has been associated with ECL neoplasia.[11] This relationship has been further defined by the ability of somatostatin to inhibit ECL neoplasia in a similar animal model. Given the unique relationship between gastric carcinoids and hypergastrinemic states, some propose that these tumors represent a distinct pathobiological entity from carcinoid tumors found elsewhere in the gastrointestinal tract.[12]

Classification of Gastric Carcinoids

During the last two decades, advances in immunohisto-chemical techniques and genetic markers have provided more accurate reclassification of carcinoid tumors. In 1980, the World Health Organization (WHO) used the term carcinoid to identify all NETs except pancreas, thyroid, paraganglionoma, small cell lung cancer, and Merkel cell carcinoma of the skin.[3] It has now become clear that these tumors, although sharing common features, differ greatly in their pathobiology. The most recent WHO classification describes three classes and still maintains an association with the old terminology.[13] The term carcinoid is still maintained and associated with the first class, termed "well-differentiated neuroendocrine tumor." This class of tumor follows a relatively benign course and includes appendiceal and nonsporadic gastric carcinoids. The second class, designated "well-differentiated neuroendocrine carcinoma," is used synonymously with malignant carcinoid tumor, or those tumors with low-grade malignant potential and the potential for metastases. The third class is the "poorly differentiated neuroendocrine carcinomas," which are high-grade malignancies that metastasize early and include small cell carcinoma of the lung and the controversial type IV gastric carcinoid tumor[8] described later in this text.

Over the years, the gastric carcinoids have become classified into three widely accepted subtypes. The first two types are associated with other disease processes and/or syndromes and are related to hypergastrinemia. The type I gastric carcinoid is associated with chronic atrophic gastritis (CAG), most commonly type A (CAG-A); however, it may also be associated with CAG-B. The incidence is increased with the duration of CAG diagnosis. Type 2 lesions are associated with the Zollinger-Ellison syndrome (ZES) and are most commonly seen in patients with the multiple endocrine neoplasia type 1 syndrome (MEN-1). Type 3 lesions are

sporadic and do not have any association with hypergastrinemia.

Considerable focus has been placed on the histological evaluation of these tumors. This analysis is important in proper identification and classification of carcinoid tumors and may prove valuable in prognostication of these lesions based on recent reports in the literature.[14,15] Neoplasia is defined by nodules > 5 mm in size or by invasion of submucosal planes. Rindi and colleagues[15] describe histopathological predictors of malignancy as being histological grades 2 and 3, size > 3 cm, 9 or more mitoses per high-power field, or > 300 Ki67-positive cells per 10 high-power fields. Based on histological findings alone, these factors identified 26 of 33 (79%) malignant carcinoids (metastatic or deeply invasive). Benign tumors were size generally < 1 cm and/or were growth restricted to the mucosa. In the same series, these histological findings identified 46 of 69 (67%) tumors with benign behavior.

Type I and II Gastric Carcinoid Tumors

TYPE I GASTRIC CARCINOID TUMORS

Type I gastric carcinoids are the most common carcinoid tumors of the stomach, comprising 68 to 83%[16] of all cases and occurring most often during the fifth decade of life. They occur more frequently in females than males, with a ratio of 2 to 3:1.[17] Grossly, these lesions appear as small (< 1 cm), multicentric lesions localized to the fundus.[18] The vast majority are associated with chronic atrophic gastritis (CAG), the etiology of which is either autoimmune pathology or *Helicobacter pylori* infection. CAG-A is associated with autoimmune disorders in which antiparietal and anti-intrinsic factor antibodies result in an achlohydric state and pernicious anemia. The resultant parietal cell destruction interrupts the normal feedback inhibition of acid on G-cell secretion of gastrin. The subsequent hypergastrinemic state has a trophic effect on ECL, ultimately leading to neoplasia. A similar phenomenon is seen with iatrogenic achlorhydria in animal models using PPIs. Approximately 2 to 9% of patients with CAG-A will develop type I gastric carcinoid tumors.[19] CAG-B is associated with *H. pylori* infection and is typically asymptomatic. CAG-B is less commonly linked to the development of gastric carcinoid tumors and is more likely related to the development of gastric adenocarcinoma. Patients with type I gastric carcinoids are at an increased risk of developing gastric adenocarcinoma.

Biologically, type I gastric carcinoids behave less aggressively than sporadic (type III) gastric carcinoids. Typically, they are well differentiated, limited to the mucosa or submucosa, and rarely demonstrate angioinvasion. Larger size tumors (1–2 cm) may occasionally exhibit malignant behavior. Lymph node metastases can be seen in 3 to 8% of these lesions with distant metastases occurring in only 2%.[17] Patients with type I carcinoid typically present with vague gastrointestinal complaints, including abdominal pain, seen in approximately 69 to 78%[9,20] of patients. Approximately 57 to 72% of patients will present with signs and symptoms of anemia.[20]

TYPE II GASTRIC CARCINOID

Type II gastric carcinoids are significantly less common than type I, comprising 8% of all gastric carcinoids.[18] There is no sex predilection in this subset of patients, and the mean age at diagnosis is somewhat younger, usually appearing around 45 to 50 years of age. Grossly, they are often multiple (in 90% of cases) and small, with 80% of type II lesions being less than 2 cm.[8]

The majority of type II gastric carcinoids associated with ZES occurs in the setting of the MEN-1 syndrome (MEN-1-ZES). In 1 study, 13 to 37% of patients with MEN-1-ZES developed type II lesions. In contrast, less than 2% of patients with sporadic ZES developed type II carcinoids.[21] This finding strongly suggests an interaction of a genetic component with the underlying hypergastrinemia in the pathogenesis of this subtype of gastric carcinoid. The MEN-1 syndrome is now recognized to be associated with loss of heterozygosity (LOH) of the gene product on 11q13, the Menin gene, which normally acts as a tumor suppressor gene. Seventy-five percent of type II gastric carcinoid tumors demonstrate LOH at 11q13.[22] It has been hypothesized that, when mutated, the Menin product becomes dysfunctional and its inhibitory effects on ECL hyperplasia in the setting of hypergastrinemia are lost.

Biologically, type II carcinoids behave somewhat more aggressively than type I, but are still considerably less aggressive than type III. In one study, 90% of lesions were limited to the mucosa or submucosa, and lymph node and distant metastases were seen in 30% and 12% of cases, respectively.[23] While a small percentage of patients present with vague gastrointestinal symptoms, most present with symptoms and signs of peptic ulcer disease. Upwards of 90% of patients with type II lesions either had upper gastrointestinal bleeding or a history of peptic ulcer disease diagnosed on endoscopy.[17]

DIAGNOSIS AND TREATMENT OF TYPE I AND II GASTRIC CARCINOID TUMORS

The diagnostic work-up for type I and II lesions is quite similar. While these lesions vary as to the etiology of

hypergastrinemia, they exhibit similar behavior. A high index of suspicion for gastric carcinoid should be maintained in any patient with a known personal or family history of autoimmune gastritis or the MEN syndromes. Surveillance is now recommended and supported by several large reports in the literature.[24,25] Upper endoscopy with biopsy is the most valuable diagnostic tool in this subset of patients.[24,25] A standardized sampling technique has been described by Bordi and colleagues[25] and involves selective biopsies of the greater and lesser curvatures of the stomach. In a series of 149 patients, Bordi and colleagues noted a 3.4% incidence of dysplastic lesions and a 1.2% incidence of carcinoid tumors in otherwise unremarkable mucosa endoscopically, with an equal distribution between the greater and lesser curvatures of the stomach.[25] Based on these data, this sampling strategy is now recommended and employed as a screening modality in these high-risk populations.

In those patients who present with symptoms consistent with the carcinoid or atypical carcinoid syndrome, both urinary and serum levels of biochemical markers should be obtained. While urinary 5-hydroxyindoleacetic acid (5-HIAA) is the standard for diagnosing most GI carcinoids, type I and II gastric carcinoids have not been shown to cause elevated 5-HIAA urinary levels consistently. In 36 patients with known gastric carcinoid tumors, urinary 5-HIAA was elevated in only 17%.[9] The gold standard for diagnosis of gastric carcinoids is plasma chromogranin.[26] Significantly elevated levels of chromogranin A and B have been reported in both type I and II tumors[20].

Endoscopy is usually performed to obtain tissue and a diagnosis. Radiological imaging studies such as computed tomography (CT) scans and chest radiographs are performed to evaluate for metastatic disease. More recently, somatostatin receptor scintigraphy (SRS) with ^{111}In-labeled octreotide has become the standard for radiographic evaluation. Relatively high sensitivity and specificity rates for identification of primary gastric carcinoids on the order of 75 to 95%[27–29] and 95%, respectively,[27] have been reported. Finally, positron emission tomography (PET) is under investigation in the work-up of these patients. In 1 study, patients undergoing 11C-labeled 5-HTP (hydroxytryptophan) PET (11C-5-HTP-PET) were more likely to have their primary lesions as well as metastatic disease diagnosed compared with contrast-enhanced CT. PET scans may also prove to be more effective in identifying primary lesion(s) than SRS.[30]

Type I and II gastric carcinoids are managed in the same way. We have developed a treatment algorithm at our institution based on the current literature (Figure 9-

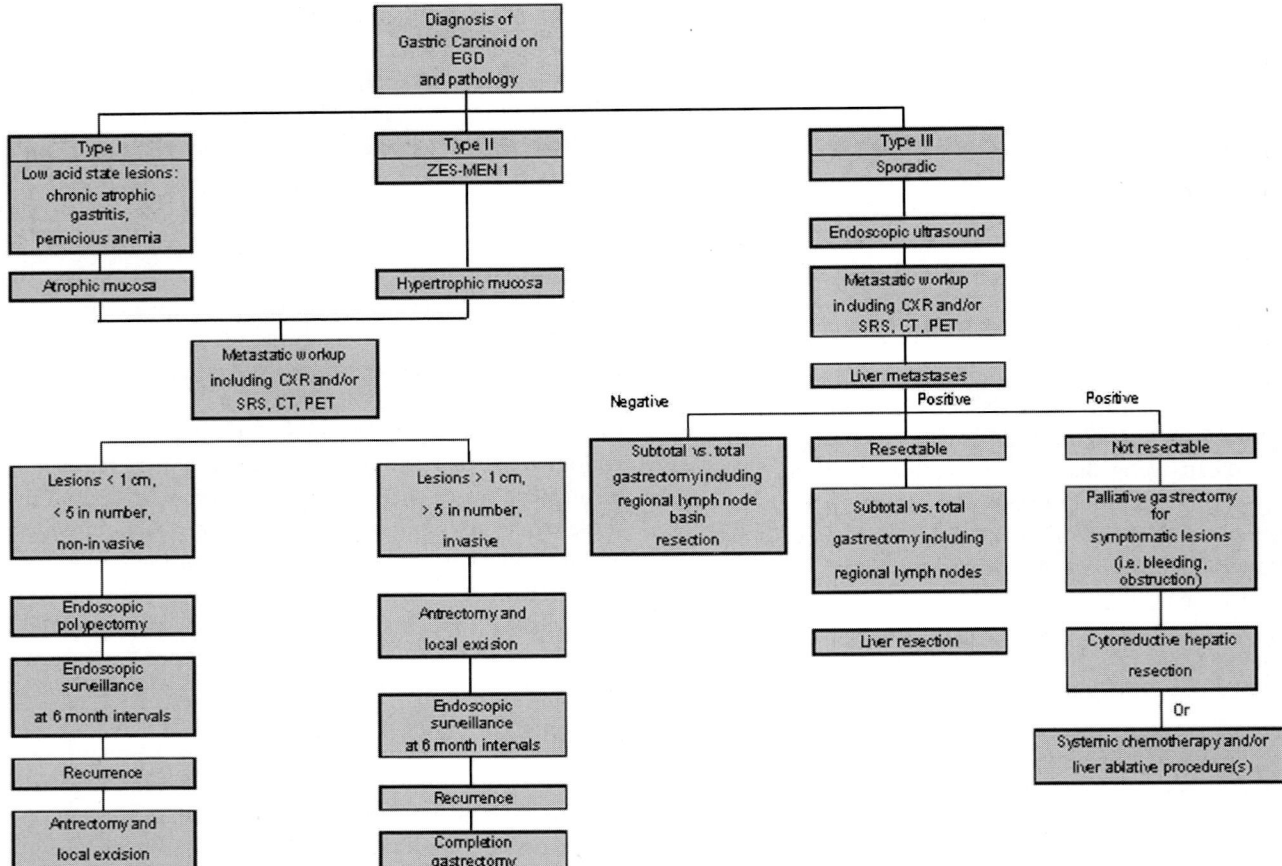

Figure 9-1 Algorithm for management of gastric carcinoids.

1), which we employ for the management of gastric carcinoid tumors. In the past, type I and II tumors were managed with total gastrectomy and regional lymph node dissection. More conservative practices have been employed recently to include antrectomy in lieu of total gastrectomy based on the association of hypergastrinemia to the progression of ECL neoplasia. However, given the prognosis of type I and II lesions, several authors believe that the standard of care should shift to an even more conservative approach using endoscopic resection and surveillance.[12,17] This novel endoscopic approach is supported in the literature. For multiple tumors (up to 5), less than 1 cm in greatest dimension, with no evidence of metastatic disease on imaging studies, endoscopic polypectomy and surveillance endoscopy every 6 months shows equivalent survival to operative intervention without the associated morbidity and mortality of operation. If the tumor recurs, antrectomy and local excision are recommended at that time. The rationale for this approach is that in removing the antrum, which serves as the sole source of gastrin, the hypergastrinemic state is resolved. Local excision of

tumor burden is then often sufficient given the removal of the neoplastic stimulus. This approach is certainly less effective in the presence of a gastrin-secreting tumor, in which case every effort should be made to remove the source of hypergastrinemia. In some case reports, the conservative approach using endoscopic polypectomy has been successful in managing tumors > 1 cm in patients who are poor operative candidates.[31] It is obvious that a consensus approach still remains to be reached, given the many different therapeutic strategies that have been described and employed; however, based on the current literature we consider the standard of care to be endoscopic polypectomy for lesions less than 1 cm in greatest diameter, when the total tumor number is less than 5.

As with lesions less than 1 cm, considerable controversy exists regarding the management of gastric carcinoids measuring 1 to 2 cm. While gastrectomy is an option, antrectomy alone with greater than 5 tumors has been shown to result in regression of tumors in the remaining stomach in long-term follow-up.[32] Based on the most recent literature, there is little, if any, role for endoscopic management of these tumors. For tumors > 2 cm, the standard of care is resection of the tumor with wide margins, including antrectomy, given the widely recognized increased incidence of metastatic disease.[33] Depending on the location and number of lesions, it may be more feasible to perform a subtotal or total gastrectomy. Several authors argue for subtotal versus total gastrectomy for all lesions > 2 cm, regardless of association with hypergastrinemic states.[34] Based on the current literature, we routinely perform an antrectomy with local tumor excision and recommend this approach for these larger lesions. In the case of patients with type I and II lesions > 1 cm initially, who present with recurrent disease, a completion gastrectomy is the next step in surgical management.

Type III Gastric Carcinoid Tumors

Type III tumors represent almost a quarter of all gastric carcinoids. Approximately 80% of all type III lesions are diagnosed in males.[18] The mean age of diagnosis is similar to that of the type II lesion, between 45 and 50 years of age. Grossly, these lesions are usually solitary, arise in normal gastric mucosa, and are considerably larger than type I and II tumors at the time of diagnosis, with a median diameter of 2 cm.[8] These lesions often exhibit a mixed cellular population that may include EC cells, although other gastric neuroendocrine cells have been identified.[35] These tumors may contain serotonin-, somatostatin-, or gastrin-positive cells. Unlike the type I and II lesions, sporadic gastric carcinoid tumors are not associated with any genetic syndrome(s).

These tumors, in contrast to their more benign counterparts, demonstrate rapid local invasion and dissemination, with approximately 15% of lesions presenting with regional nodal metastases at the time of diagnosis.[8,18] Several larger series have demonstrated that size greater than 2 cm at initial presentation portends a higher risk for metastatic disease. Up to 50%[8,18] will be found to have distant metastatic disease on initial presentation. This subtype of tumor is clearly associated with significantly higher mortality and relatively early demise following diagnosis.

DIAGNOSIS AND TREATMENT OF TYPE III GASTRIC CARCINOID TUMORS

The diagnosis of type III carcinoids is often delayed given the lack of specific symptomatology associated with the disease. The spectrum of presentation ranges from vague left upper quadrant abdominal pain to the typical or atypical carcinoid syndrome. Upwards of 80% of patients with type III tumors will present with severe abdominal pain warranting endoscopy, at which time the diagnosis is often made.[17] Althouhg many physicians associate the "malignant carcinoid syndrome" with these tumors, it is actually uncommon. Less than 10% of patients with sporadic gastric carcinoid tumors will present with symptoms of carcinoid syndrome.[36] The syndrome results from a failure of the liver to metabolize secreted hormones from carcinoid tumors and is seen with metastatic disease in the liver where the hormones are secreted directly into the systemic circulation. It was once thought that the constellation of symptoms was due to the synthesis of serotonin and the precursor 5-hydroxytryptophan (5-HTP). It is now clear that multiple bioactive substances are secreted by these tumors and it is likely that they all play varied roles in the syndrome. The most common manifestations are vasomotor and cardiac symptoms including flushing and tachycardia. These symptoms are seen in approximately 90% of patients with the syndrome. Gastrointestinal hypermotility, as well as bronchospasm, sweating, and hypotension are seen in approximately 75% of patients.[37] Any combination of these symptoms may be present in patients with metastatic carcinoid tumors.

In the case of gastric carcinoids, the classic carcinoid syndrome is even less common. Given the diversity of cell types found in type III lesions, it is possible to see the typical syndrome; however, the "atypical carcinoid syndrome" is more common. This syndrome is characterized by profound cutaneous flushing (purplish in appearance), severe itching, bronchospasm, and lacrimation, which are attributed to overactive histamine production.[38] These symptoms are often provoked by ingestion of certain foods, in particular cheese and wine.[8,18]

The work-up for type III lesions is similar to that of type I and II in several ways. As with type I and II subtypes, urinary 5-HIAA is not considered a reliable marker.[8] Marked elevation of serum levels of chromogranin A and B are demonstrated with these lesions. Also, tele-methylimidazoleacetic acid (t-MeImAA), a urinary metabolite of histamine, is usually elevated in type III lesions. Contrast-enhanced CT or SRS often reveals a solitary lesion, and there is an increased incidence of metastatic disease on initial presentation. Orlefors and colleagues have demonstrated a significant increase in radiographical diagnosis of type III tumors and metastatic disease using whole-body 11C-5-HTP-PET when compared with CT and SRS. In 58% of patients studied, PET identified more lesions than CT or SRS. Many authors recommend the use of SRS for preoperative planning and identification of metastatic disease; however, as new data emerges regarding PET, this modality may supersede CT and SRS.[39] It is important to obtain tissue for histological diagnosis as well as serum biochemical markers to confirm diagnosis.

The treatment algorithm for type III clinically localized lesions is much less controversial. Given the aggressive behavior of this tumor, these lesions are treated similarly to gastric adenocarcinoma. Based on anatomic location, subtotal versus total gastrectomy and en bloc lymph node resection is the standard of care. The presence of hepatic metastases does not preclude surgical intervention with curative intent; however, it is desirable if the presence of hepatic metastases can be identified prior to operative intervention.

Given the significant incidence of metastatic disease associated with the type III tumor, several treatment strategies for liver metastases have been developed and will be covered in detail in other chapters. Surgical treatment of metastatic disease is an option that has been employed by multiple centers. In patients without significant liver disease that might preclude resection, and in patients who are otherwise appropriate operative candidates, surgical resection may decrease symptoms (in patients presenting with the atypical or typical carcinoid syndromes) and improve survival. There have been several case reports documenting this strategy; however, to date there have been no large randomized trials to evaluate this approach. In 3 separate small trials, the 4- to 5-year survival following hepatic resection was between 70 and 85%.[40–42] In another small trial, Yao and colleagues reported the best outcomes in patients with fewer than 5 liver lesions and a previous resection of the primary tumor.[41]

In patients with unresectable metastatic disease, traditional systemic chemotherapeutic options have yielded poor results. Multiple single and combination drug regimens have been studied, including streptozotocin, 5-fluorouracil, doxorubicin, and cyclophosphamide, which have shown modest partial response rates of 20 to 40%. Etoposide, either alone or in combination with cisplatin, has also been utilized to treat metastatic disease. In a prospective series, Moertel and colleagues demonstrated a 7% response rate. However, in another series of patients with poorly differentiated NETs, an overall response rate of 67% was noted.[43] More recently, radiolabeled somatostatin analogues, including ^{111}In-DTPA-D-Phe1-octreotide and 90-yttrium-DOTA-D-Phe1-Tyr3-octreotide, have been used with some success in the treatment of disseminated disease.[44,45]

Prognosis

The data that exist regarding the prognosis of these tumors are based on the general classification of gastric carcinoids as a homogenous group. The more recent separation of gastric carcinoid into subtypes, unfortunately, is often not reflected in the larger epidemiological studies that have been reported. Five-year survival rates of gastric carcinoids in general are 63%.[7] Additionally, those gastric carcinoids confined locally without metastatic disease demonstrate a 69% 5-year survival.[8] These values likely reflect a bias toward the type III lesions, given the well-recognized benign natural history of type I and II lesions. In one study, Rappel and colleagues report an age-corrected 5-year survival rate of 100% in 88 patients with type I lesions.[46] Rappel's work represents the largest analysis of carcinoid tumor subsets to date. Regardless of subtype, there is a reported 21.2% 5-year survival for gastric carcinoids with distant disease at the time of diagnosis. Amongst all gastric carcinoid tumors, predictors of metastatic disease include tumors > 2 cm, tumors demonstrating angioinvasion, or invasive tumors infiltrating the muscularis propria.

In addition to what is already known regarding the three types of gastric carcinoid tumors, there are several authors who now describe a type IV gastric carcinoid lesion.[8,13] Whether or not this is truly a carcinoid tumor of similar biological origin to the other subtypes versus a poorly differentiated neuroendocrine tumor (similar to small cell lung malignancy) remains to be determined. In a small series of 12 patients with type IV tumors,[47] 75% occurred in men, and hypergastrinemia was seen in 33% of all patients. Atrophic gastritis was frequently associated with these lesions, and 25% of these patients demonstrated ECL hyperplasia. At the time of diagnosis, these tumors are usually solitary and have a mean diameter greater than 4 cm. In another small series, metastatic disease was present in all patients at the time of diagnosis.[48] Relative to the 3 recognized subtypes of gastric carcinoid, this type is considerably more aggressive and, therefore, should not be treated surgically unless there is no evidence of metastatic disease or surgery is required for palliative purposes. In the article by Rindi and colleagues, the mean survival of patients with these lesions was only 7 months.[47] Agreement remains to be reached regarding the origin and classification of this fourth type of gastric neuroendocrine tumor.

References

1. Oberndorfer S. Karzinoide: tumoren des dünndarms. Frankf Z Pathol 1907;1:425–429.

2. Modlin IM, Shapiro MD, Kidd M. Siegfried Oberndorfer: origins and perspectives of carcinoid tumors. Hum Pathol 2004;35:1440–51.

3. Kloppel G, Perren A, Heitz PU. The gastroenteropancreatic neuroendocrine cell system and its tumors: the WHO classification. Ann N Y Acad Sci 2004;1014:13–27.

4. Kulke MH, Mayer RJ. Carcinoid tumors. N Engl J Med 1999;340:858–68. Barakat MT, Meeran K, Bloom SR. Neuroendocrine tumours. Endocr Relat Cancer 2004;11: 1–18.

5. Godwin JD II. Carcinoid tumors. An analysis of 2,837 cases. Cancer 1975;36:560–9.

6. Modlin IM, Lye KD, Kidd M. A 5-decade analysis of 13,715 carcinoid tumors. Cancer 2003;97:934–59.

7. Modlin IM, Lye KD, Kidd M. A 50-year analysis of 562 gastric carcinoids: small tumor or larger problem? Am J Gastroenterol 2004;99:23–32.

8. Modlin IM, Lye KD, Kidd M. Carcinoid tumors of the stomach. Surg Oncol 2003;12:153–72.

9. Gough DB, Thompson GB, Crotty TB, et al. Diverse clinical and pathologic features of gastric carcinoid and the relevance of hypergastrinemia. World J Surg 1994;18:473–80.

10. Hakanson R, Tielemans Y, Chen D, et al. Time-dependent changes in enterochromaffin-like cell kinetics in stomach of hypergastrinemic rats. Gastroenterology 1993;105:15–21.

11. Bilchik AJ, Nilsson O, Modlin IM, et al. H2-receptor blockade induces peptide YY and enteroglucagon-secreting gastric carcinoids in mastomys. Surgery 1989;106:1119–27.

12. Modlin IM, Gilligan CJ, Lawton GP, et al. Gastric carcinoids. The Yale experience. Arch Surg 1995;130:250–6.

13. Solcia E, Klöppel G, Sobin LH, et al. Histological typing of endocrine tumours. 2nd ed. In: Sobin LH, editor. World Health Organization international histological classification of tumours. Berlin: Springer; 2000.

14. Solcia E, Bordi C, Creutzfeldt W, et al. Histopathological classification of nonantral gastric endocrine growths in man. Digestion 1988;41:185–200.

15. Rindi G, Azzoni C, La Rosa S, et al. ECL cell tumor and poorly differentiated endocrine carcinoma of the stomach: prognostic evaluation by pathological analysis. Gastroenterology 1999;116:532–42.

16. Bordi C, D'Adda T, Azzoni C, Ferraro G. Pathogenesis of ECL cell tumors in humans. Yale J Biol Med 1998;71:273–84.

17. Gilligan CJ, Lawton GP, Tang LH, et al. Gastric carcinoid tumors: the biology and therapy of an enigmatic and controversial lesion. Am J Gastroenterol 1995;90:338–52.

18. Modlin IM, Kidd M, Lye KD. Biology and management of gastric carcinoid tumours: a review. Eur J Surg 2002;168: 669–83.

19. Borch K, Renvall H, Liedberg G. Gastric endocrine cell hyperplasia and carcinoid tumors in pernicious anemia. Gastroenterology 1985;88:638–48.

20. Granberg D, Wilander E, Stridsberg M, et al. Clinical symptoms, hormone profiles, treatment, and prognosis in patients with gastric carcinoids. Gut 1998;43:223–8.

21. Jensen RT. Management of the Zollinger-Ellison syndrome in patients with multiple endocrine neoplasia type 1. J Intern Med 1998;243:477–88.

22. Debelenko LV, Emmert-Buck MR, Zhuang Z, et al. The multiple endocrine neoplasia type I gene locus is involved in the pathogenesis of type II gastric carcinoids. Gastroenterology 1997;113:773–81.

23. Rindi G, Luinetti O, Cornaggia M, et al. Three subtypes of gastric argyrophil carcinoid and the gastric neuroendocrine carcinoma: a clinicopathologic study. Gastroenterology 1993;104:994–1006.

24. Sjoblom SM, Sipponen P, Miettinen M, et al. Gastroscopic screening for gastric carcinoids and carcinoma in pernicious anemia. Endoscopy 1988;20:52–6.

25. Bordi C, Azzoni C, Ferraro G, et al. Sampling strategies for analysis of enterochromaffin-like cell changes in Zollinger-Ellison syndrome. Am J Clin Pathol 2000;114: 419–25.

26. Modlin IM, Tang LH. The gastric enterochromaffin-like cell: an enigmatic cellular link. Gastroenterology 1996;111: 783–810.

27. Gibril F, Reynolds JC, Lubensky IA, et al. Ability of somatostatin receptor scintigraphy to identify patients with gastric carcinoids: a prospective study. J Nucl Med 2000;41: 1646–56.

28. Kolby L, Wangberg B, Ahlman H, et al. Somatostatin receptor subtypes, octreotide scintigraphy, and clinical response to octreotide treatment in patients with neuroendocrine tumors. World J Surg 1998;22:679–83.

29. Wangberg B, Nilsson O, Johanson VV, et al. Somatostatin receptors in the diagnosis and therapy of neuroendocrine tumor. Oncologist 1997;2:50–8.

30. Sundin A, Eriksson B, Bergstrom M, et al. PET in the diagnosis of neuroendocrine tumors. Ann N Y Acad Sci 2004;1014:246–57.

31. Gonzalez Ramirez A, Lopez Roses L, Santos Blanco E, et al. Multiple gastric carcinoid tumors: endoscopic management. J Clin Gastroenterol 1996;23:75–7.

32. Hirschowitz BI, Griffith J, Pellegrin D, Cummings OW. Rapid regression of enterochromaffin-like cell gastric carcinoids in pernicious anemia after antrectomy. Gastroenterology 1992;102(4 Pt 1):1409–18.

33. Thirlby RC. Management of patients with gastric carcinoid tumors. Gastroenterology 1995;108:296–7.

34. Shi W, Buchanan KD, Johnston CF, et al. The octreotide suppression test and [^{111}In-DTPA-D-Phe1]-octreotide scintigraphy in neuroendocrine tumours correlate with responsiveness to somatostatin analogue treatment. Clin Endocrinol (Oxf) 1998;48:303–9.

35. Arnold R, Koppel G, Rothmund. Carcinoid tumors. International symposium on pathology, clinical aspects and therapy. Digestion 1994;55Suppl 3:1–113.

36. Lips CJ, Lentjes EG, Hoppener JW. The spectrum of carcinoid tumours and carcinoid syndromes. Ann Clin Biochem 2003;40(Pt 6):612–27.

37. Oates JA. The carcinoid syndrome. N Engl J Med 1986;315: 702–4.

38. Vinik AI. Carcinoid tumors. In: De Groot LJ, Jameson JL, editors. Endocrinology, 4th ed. Philadelphia: WB Saunders; 2001. p. 2533–46.

39. Orlefors H, Sundin A, Garske U, et al. Whole-body (11)C-5-hydroxytryptophan positron emission tomography as a universal imaging technique for neuroendocrine tumors: comparison with somatostatin receptor scintigraphy and computed tomography. J Clin Endocrinol Metab 2005;90: 3392–400.

40. Chamberlain RS, Canes D, Brown KT, et al. Hepatic neuroendocrine metastases: does intervention alter outcomes? J Am Coll Surg 2000;190:432–45.

41. Yao KA, Talamonti MS, Nemcek A, et al. Indications and results of liver resection and hepatic chemoembolization for metastatic gastrointestinal neuroendocrine tumors. Surgery 2001;130:677–85.

42. Jaeck D, Oussoultzoglou E, Bachellier P, et al. Hepatic metastases of gastroenteropancreatic neuroendocrine tumors: safe hepatic surgery. World J Surg 2001;25:689–92.

43. Moertel CG, Kvols LK, O'Connell MJ, Rubin J. Treatment of neuroendocrine carcinomas with combined etoposide and cisplatin. Evidence of major therapeutic activity in the anaplastic variants of these neoplasms. Cancer 1991;68: 227–32.

44. Barakat MT, Meeran K, Bloom SR. Neuroendocrine tumours. Endocr Relat Cancer 2004;11:1–18.

45. Wangberg B, Nilsson O, Johanson VV, et al. Somatostatin receptors in the diagnosis and therapy of neuroendocrine tumor. Oncologist 1997;2:50–8, .

46. Rappel S, Altendorf-Hofmann A, Stolte M. Prognosis of gastric carcinoid tumours. Digestion 1995;56:455–62.

47. Rindi G, Bordi C, Rappel S, et al. Gastric carcinoids and neuroendocrine carcinomas: pathogenesis, pathology, and behavior. World J Surg 1996;20:168–72.

48. Ahlman H, Kolby L, Lundell L, et al. Clinical management of gastric carcinoid tumors. Digestion 1994;55 Suppl 3:77–85.

CHAPTER 10

THE CURRENT STATUS OF ADJUVANT AND NEOADJUVANT THERAPY FOR GASTRIC CANCER

AMOD A. SARNAIK, MD

ANDREW M. LOWY, MD

Gastric carcinoma comprises 2% of all cancers in the US, while worldwide it ranks second in incidence and remains a leading cause of death. The survival of gastric cancer patients in the US has not significantly changed over the past 30 years. More than half of patients in the US present with Stage III or Stage IV disease and have 5-year survival rates of 10 to15% and 0 to 5%, respectively. In Western series, even those patients with Stage I and II disease have relatively poor 5-year survival rates of 50% or less.[1] These discouraging results have led researchers to investigate adjuvant and neoadjuvant therapy as a means to improve outcome. In this chapter the results of adjuvant and neoadjuvant studies for both locally advanced and resectable gastric cancer are discussed.

Role of Surgery

Surgical resection remains the only curative therapy for gastric cancer. Although the precise definition may vary, a potentially curative (R0) resection should involve removal of the primary tumor and at least the perigastric (D1) lymph nodes, with resection margins grossly and microscopically free of tumor cells. In several comprehensive reports, R0 resection is associated with increased 5-year survival (mean 35 to 60%) versus noncurative resection (mean 3 to 20%). The overall R0 resection rate in the US averages 40 to 50% for all patients presenting with gastric cancer. Reported median survival for patients following R0 resection ranges from 18 to 24 months, whereas patients with residual disease after resection survive an average of 6 to 12 months.[1] Therefore, any therapy that increases the R0 resection rate would be expected to increase the overall survival of patients with gastric cancer.

Patterns of Failure

The development of rational strategies of adjuvant and neoadjuvant therapy requires thorough understanding of the patterns of relapse. Patterns of recurrence following gastrectomy have been evaluated by autopsy studies, second-look laparotomy, and clinical evaluation using physical exam and diagnostic imaging. Gastric cancer may spread by several routes including lymphatic and hematogenous metastasis, intraperitoneal dissemination, and direct invasion. In a large number of cases, it spreads along several routes simultaneously, creating a mixed pattern of recurrence. Gunderson and Sosin, in their retrospective study of second-look laparotomies, found that 80% of patients had evidence of cancer at reoperation or other follow-up.[2] Of these, local recurrence and/or regional lymph node metastasis occurred as the only site of failure in 54% and as a component of failure in 88%. Distant metastasis alone was uncommon, but was found as a component in over 25% of the failure group. In this study and in others, local-regional relapse is usually defined as tumor in the gastric remnant, perigastric lymph nodes and gastric bed. Intra-abdominal failure usually includes liver, peritoneal, or distant lymph node involvement. In a clinical study, Landry and colleagues noted that 52% of patients developed distant metastatic disease following curative resection.[3] Several other studies have shown varied rates and location of recurrence and these results are summarized in Table 10-1. As shown, local-regional failure is present in about 47 to 78% while metastases to the liver, bone, lung, or other organs are present in 22 to 53%. R0 resection is associated with a lower overall recurrence rate and a smaller percentage of local-regional failures versus distant failures.[3,4,5]

The differences noted between the above studies probably relate to the variability in the average stage of disease, pathological grade and surgical treatment, in addition to the varying definitions of local-regional, intra-abdominal, and distant recurrence. Furthermore, autopsy studies are mostly an expression of late-stage disease and, consequently, distant metastases are more common.[6]

In summary, patients with gastric cancer tend to have high rates of both local and distant relapse after resection. Following R0 resection, distant failures tend to become even more important. Therefore, in designing adjuvant and neoadjuvant therapies, one needs to address local as well as distant spread of gastric cancer.

Role of Lymphadenectomy

The extent of lymphadenectomy has been a source of major controversy in the surgical management of gastric cancer and will be more extensively discussed in an additional chapter in this publication. While not fully resolved, after several large prospective randomized trials, it can be safely stated that at least a D1 lymph node dissection should be performed for all patients with clinically localized gastric cancer. Unfortunately, several studies have revealed that at least in the US, less than a D1 dissection is perhaps the most commonly performed procedure. Using data from Intergroup 0116, the largest

adjuvant gastric cancer study ever performed in the US, Estes and colleagues examined the extent of lymphadenectomy in 453 patients. According to Japanese rules, the extent of lymphadenectomy was D0 in 54.2%, D1 in 38.1%, D2 in 6.2%, and D3 in 1.5%.[7] These statistics make interpretation of adjuvant and neoadjuvant studies difficult in that it can be argued that the effects of adjuvant treatments may simply be compensating for poor surgical therapy.

Adjuvant Chemotherapy

In 1950, Owen Wangensteen, discouraged by the failure of extended lymph node dissection and second-look operations to improve the survival of patients with gastric cancer, pleaded with the medical community for "a more powerful tool than surgery" for patients with this malignancy. Numerous trials have now been conducted investigating the potential benefit of adjuvant systemic chemotherapy following surgical resection. These studies have involved a host of different chemotherapeutic agents, dosing regimens, timing of therapy, and follow-up. A vast majority of these trials have failed to demonstrate a clear and reproducible benefit for adjuvant chemotherapy versus surgery alone. Despite this, several meta-analyses on postoperative adjuvant trials have suggested a modest benefit for patients receiving postoperative chemotherapy with hazard ratios in the range of 0.72 to 0.84.[8–11] The most pivotal trials are discussed below and outlined in Table 10-2.

Grau and colleagues randomized gastric cancer patients to either high-dose mitomycin C or no therapy following surgical resection.[12] A total of 134 patients were followed for a median time of 9 years. A statistically significant survival advantage was demonstrated for the mitomycin C group. However, other studies have failed

Table 10-1 Patterns of Recurrence Following Surgical Resection of Gastric Cancer

	Method	Number of patients	Loco-regional	Peritoneal	Liver	Extra-abd/distant mets
Duarte, 1981	Autopsy	77	85%	38%	42%	39% lung, 30% mediastinal LN
Gunderson, 1982	2nd Look laparotomy	86	69%	42%	-	23%
Wisbeck, 1986	Autopsy	16 (R0 resection)	94%	50%	44%	37%
Meyer, 1987	Autopsy, 2nd look	130	47%	34%	12%	7%
Koga, 1987		255	28%	50%	-	22% (lung, liver, bone)
Landry, 1990	Clinical, autopsy	88	56%	-	-	76%
Esaki, 1990	Autopsy	173	-	58%	51%	-
Wanebo, 1993	Clinical, autopsy	1089	40%	-	-	60%

LN = lymph node.

Table 10-2 Randomized Trials of Adjuvant Chemotherapy or Chemoradiation for Gastric Cancer

Author	n	Treatment Arms	Results
GI Tumor Study Group, 1982	142	Post-op 5-FU, methyl CCNU vs surg alone	Median survival > 48 mo (treatment) vs 33 mo (surg alone) $p < 0.03$
Higgens et al., 1983	312	Post-op 5-FU, methyl CCNU vs surg alone	No survival benefit or improved rate of recurrence
Engstrom et al., 1985	180	Post-op 5-FU, methyl CCNU vs surg alone	No survival benefit or improved rate of recurrence
Estape et al., 1990	70	Post-op mitomycin C vs surg alone	10 yr survival rate 52% (treatment) vs 16% (surg alone) $p < 0.001$
Krook et al., 1991	125	Post-op 5-FU, doxorubicin vs surg alone	No survival benefit
Grau et al., 1993	134	Post-op mitomycin C vs surg alone	10 yr survival rate 39% (treatment) vs 26% (surg alone) $p < 0.02$
Lise et al., 1995	314	Post-op FAM2 vs surg alone	No survival benefit, but treatment improved time to relapse $p = 0.02$
MacDonald et al., 1995	193	Post-op FAM vs surg alone	No survival benefit
MacDonald et al., 2001	556	Post-op 5-FU, leucovorin, radiation vs surg alone	Median survival 36 mo (treatment) vs 27 mo (surg alone) $p = 0.005$

5-FU = 5-Flurouracil.

to reproduce a survival advantage for mitomycin C-treated patients as part of a polychemotherapy regimen. MacDonald and colleagues followed 193 patients randomized to surgery and 5-Flurouracil (FU), adriamycin, and mitomycin C versus surgery alone for a median time of 9.5 years without a discernible improvement in survival.[13] Lise and colleagues observed an increase in time to recurrence but no overall survival advantage with a similar adjuvant treatment regimen in 314 patients.[14] The Gastrointestinal Tumor Study Group evaluated the effect of postoperative methyl-CCNU and 5-FU versus surgery alone in a well-designed prospective randomized trial.[15] At a median follow-up of 48 months, median survival for the surgery alone group was 33 months, while the postoperative chemotherapy group had not yet reached its median survival. However, other trials including a similarly structured Eastern Cooperative Oncology Group trial and the Veterans Administration Surgical Oncology Group trial failed to reproduce this survival advantage.[16] Even in Japan, where adjuvant therapy has been standard since the 1970s, few trials have demonstrated a significant survival benefit.

Rationale for Neoadjuvant Therapy

Largely because of the disappointing results obtained with adjuvant chemotherapy, many investigators have explored the potential of neoadjuvant therapy. There are several lines of evidence, both theoretical and established data, to support a neoadjuvant approach. These include the ability to downstage a tumor preoperatively, potentially increase curative resection rates, and to utilize more conservative operative approaches. Neoadjuvant therapy allows the identification of responders to a particular chemotherapeutic regimen and consequently the selection of more effective agents or the discontinuation of therapy in "nonresponders." Patients with rapidly progressive disease may be identified and spared the morbidity of nontherapeutic surgery. Furthermore, a neoadjuvant approach provides for simultaneous early treatment of both the primary tumor as well as subclinical metastases before the primary tumor is removed. Perhaps the most salient argument for preoperative therapy is patient compliance. Due to the complex nature of gastric surgery, many patients experience prolonged postoperative recovery, often with significant weight loss and fatigue. Gastric surgery often results in significant delays in initiation of postoperative adjuvant therapy. Neoadjuvant therapy had been associated with higher rates of compliance in the treatment of other gastrointestinal malignancies such as pancreatic and rectal cancer. Finally, a reduction in tumor burden preoperatively could decrease the overall catabolic state of the patient, improve nutritional status, and therefore improve the patient's condition for surgery.

Potential adverse effects of preoperative chemotherapy include a delay in definitive local control with surgery, potentially leading to tumor progression; allowing time for the development of resistant tumor clones; and exposing the patient to potential toxicities that further delay operative resection or render the patient unable to tolerate surgery. Consequently, preoperative identification of patients most likely to benefit from therapy remains critical when planning neoadjuvant therapy.

The Appropriate Patient for Neoadjuvant Therapy

Modern chemotherapeutic regimens have substantial and significant toxicities; therefore, preoperative identification of the subset of patients who would benefit from neoadjuvant therapy is important in designing treatment protocols. To identify patients who are high risk for recurrent disease, the American Joint Committee on Cancer staging system for gastric cancers accounts for tumor penetration (T), nodal involvement (N), and the presence of metastatic disease (M). Patients considered at high risk for recurrence are generally T2–4, N (any), M0. Patients with T2N0 lesions are most controversial because some studies report excellent survival with surgery alone, while others such as the recent American College of Surgeons study found recurrence rates of 50%.[1] Patients with early stage disease (T1N0M0) have excellent cure rates (> 90% 5-year survival) following R0 resection. These patients, rare in western series, are best spared the potential morbidity of preoperative chemotherapy.

Preoperative Staging

Traditionally, definitive staging was obtained at the time of operation in conjunction with postoperative pathologic analysis. However, in order to select appropriate patients for neoadjuvant therapy, accurate preoperative staging is essential. Preoperative staging is also critical to evaluate the effectiveness of neoadjuvant therapy and for proper comparisons between different treatment regimens.

Computed tomography (CT) scanning had traditionally been the most frequently used modality for the staging of gastric cancer. With multidetector CT scanners in routine use, the sensitivity for the detection of visceral metastatic disease, particularly hepatic metastases, is in excess of 80% for lesions over 1 cm in size.[17] Although CT scanning is sensitive in the detection of visceral metastatic disease, its sensitivity in the detection of peritoneal metastases remains poor. Furthermore, its accuracy in determining the T status in gastric cancers has been reported to be less than 50%, and for N status, about 50 to 70%. Experience with magnetic resonance imaging is limited, but most reports fail to show any superiority over CT scanning in predicting tumor stage.

Endoscopic ultrasound (EUS) has become the imaging modality of choice in the local-regional staging of gastric cancer. EUS is unique in its ability to discern individual layers of the gastric wall that correlate with histological analysis and results in accurate determination of tumor depth. Several authors report the accuracy of EUS in predicting the T stage of gastric cancer to be 80 to 92%.[18] Most of the difficulty remains in determining T2 (subserosal invasion) versus T3 (serosal invasion). Since the advent of EUS-guided lymph node biopsy, the diagnostic accuracy of regional lymph node status has improved with the ability to confirm histologically the presence or absence of metastatic disease.

Laparoscopy and laparoscopic ultrasound are techniques that help bridge the gap between EUS and CT scanning. Laparoscopy can help determine the T stage by direct inspection of the primary lesion and by laparoscopic ultrasound examination of the stomach. As with EUS, it is possible to evaluate suspicious lymph nodes with biopsy. Finally, laparoscopy is most valuable in the diagnostic of subcentimeter peritoneal and liver surface metastases not visualized by CT scan. Compared to preoperative ultrasound and CT, laparoscopy has been shown to be more sensitive in detecting peritoneal metastases and may prevent nontherapeutic laparotomy in patients with metastatic disease undetected by preoperative ultrasound and CT.[19]

Neoadjuvant Therapy Trails

Unresectable/Locally Advanced Gastric Cancer

A potential role for neoadjuvant therapy in patients with gastric cancer was first suggested by reports in the 1970s and 1980s. These trials suggested that preoperative therapy induced a significant response and enabled operative resection in some patients initially deemed unresectable (Table 10-3). One of the earliest studies of neoadjuvant chemotherapy was reported in 1985 by Bonatsos and colleagues.[20] Five patients with unresectable gastric carcinoma were treated with two cycles of 5-FU, adriamycin, and mitomycin C (FAM). All five patients had symptomatic improvement, and the therapy was generally well tolerated. In 3 of the 4 responders, R0 resection was later possible, and 1 patient remained disease-free after 2 years. Verschueren et al. reported 17 patients with unresectable disease in 1988.[21] Four cycles of 5-FU and methotrexate were administered, and 13 of the patients underwent a second-look laparotomy. Seven of the 13 (54%) were deemed resectable, and the median survival for the entire group was 14 months. Although

Table 10-3 Neoadjuvant Chemotherapy Trials for Unresectable Locally Advanced Gastric Cancer

Author	n	Regimen	Complete and Partial Clinical Response Rate	Resection Rate (R0 and R1)	Median survival
Verschuren et al., 1988	17	5FU/MTX	-	54%	16 mo
Wilke et al., 1989	34	EAP	70%	-	18 mo
Plukker et al., 1991	20	5FU/MTX	-	40%	22 mo
Lerner et al., 1992	36	EAP	33%	-	7.5 mo
Rougier et al., 1994	30	5 FU/CP	75%	77%	16 mo
Fink et al., 1995	30	EAP	60%	80%	17 mo*
Kang et al., 1996	53	EFP±postop	-	79%	43 mo
	54	surg±postop	-		30 mo

*24 months in patients with neoadjuvant therapy followed by R0 resection.
5-FU = 5-Fluorouracil; CP = cisplatin; EAP = etoposide, adriamycin, and cisplatin; EFP = etoposide, 5-FU, and cisplatin therapy; MTX = methotrexate.

both these studies were limited in terms of patient numbers and duration of follow-up, they did establish that neoadjuvant therapy was feasible and potentially beneficial in otherwise unresectable patients.

The first large phase II trial of neoadjuvant chemotherapy was reported by Wilke and colleagues in 1989.[22] Thirty-four patients with surgically proven locally advanced, unresectable gastric cancer were treated with an aggressive regimen of etoposide, adriamycin, and cisplatin (EAP). Patients received between 2 and 4 cycles of chemotherapy. Response and toxicity data were available for 33 patients. A complete clinical and radiographic response was noted in 7 of 33 patients (21%), and an additional 16 patients (49%) achieved a partial response. Twenty patients underwent a second-look laparotomy, and 5 complete clinical responses were pathologically confirmed. Fifteen patients underwent R0 resection, and an additional 3 had only microscopically positive margins (R1 resection). A total of 20 patients were rendered disease-free after the combination of chemotherapy, surgery, and consolidation chemotherapy, and 40% remained without evidence of disease at a median follow-up of 20 months. The median survival for all patients was 18 months, and the median survival for the 20 patients who completed the entire treatment regimen was 24 months. The primary toxicity of the EAP regimen was leukopenia and thrombocytopenia, but there was no increase in perioperative or operative morbidity compared to historical controls undergoing surgery alone. This trial suggested that preoperative chemotherapy could induce a response in a significant number of patients, could down-stage patients previously deemed unresectable to a resectable status, and that the combination of preoperative chemotherapy, surgical resection, and consolidation chemotherapy could result in reasonable survival rates.

Unfortunately, a subsequent report by Lerner and colleagues in 1992 failed to reproduce the high response rate reported by Wilke and colleagues.[23] In a phase II trial of 36 patients with surgically unresectable disease treated with a similar neoadjuvant EAP chemotherapy protocol, the overall response rate was 33%, with only 8% experiencing a complete clinical response. Five patients underwent subsequent surgical resection, and only 1 was rendered free of gross disease. In addition, hospitalization was required in 22% of the treatment courses, and 4 patients (11%) died of treatment-related toxicity. The authors concluded that the EAP regimen did not provide a significant advantage over other less toxic regimens.

Although the toxicity of the EAP regimen caused many centers to abandon its use, an additional trial was reported in 1995 by Fink and colleagues.[24] In this prospective phase II trial, neoadjuvant EAP was administered to 30 patients with locally advanced gastric carcinoma diagnosed by staging laparoscopy or EUS. A total of three to four cycles of preoperative chemotherapy were scheduled, and 27 patients received at least two cycles. A complete clinical response was observed in 8 of these 27 patients (30%), and 9 additional patients had evidence of major clinical response. R0 resection was performed in 24 patients (80%), with no deaths or significant perioperative morbidity. When surgical specimens were compared with preoperative clinical staging, down-staging occurred in 50% of the cases. Overall median survival time was 17 months, and the 2-year actuarial survival rate was 30%. For patients having undergone neoadjuvant therapy and subsequent curative resection, the median survival and 2-year survival rates were 24 months and 36%, respectively. Tumor recurrence after curative resection was observed in 17 of 23 patients after a median time of 7 months. Local or regional failure occurred in 11 patients, and distant metastatic disease occurred in 5 patients. Leukopenia and thrombocytopenia were cited as the most common side effects, and hospital admissions secondary to chemotherapy-related toxicity was necessary in 13 of 30 patients.

There were no Grade III or IV nonhematological complications or treatment-related deaths.

Other groups have used less toxic preoperative chemotherapeutic agents in patients with locally advanced disease felt not to be amenable to curative resection. Plukker and colleagues administered 4 cycles of 5-FU and methotrexate to 20 patients with stage IIIB or IV disease.[25] Seventeen patients (85%) completed all four cycles of therapy, and 14 underwent operative resection. Eight patients (40%) demonstrated a response allowing for curative resection, and an additional 6 patients showed evidence of tumor down-staging. For the entire group, only 2 patients (10%) remained alive and disease-free at 54 months. Therefore, although the 5-FU/methotrexate regimen was completed with acceptable toxicity in this study, the regimen did not significantly improve long-term survival.

A study was reported in 1994 by Rougier and colleagues utilizing preoperative 5-FU and cisplatin in 30 patients with locally advanced gastric cancers.[26] A total of two to three cycles were given, and an overall clinical response rate of 56% was noted in 27 patients; however, there were no complete pathologic responses. Surgical resection was performed in 28 of the 30 patients. A 60% curative resection rate was obtained, with an additional 22% of patients having microscopic residual disease. Overall median survival was 16 months with 5 patients alive at 4 years. Although overall toxicity was acceptable, there was one treatment-related death.

Newman and colleagues in 2002 studied the preoperative use of CPT-11/cisplatin in 22 patients with locally advanced gastric cancer.[27] Of the 19 patients who underwent operation, 17 (89%) underwent curative resections. While there were no complete pathologic responses, there appeared to be significant tumor down-staging, as postoperative pathologic staging yielded 16% T3 lesions compared to preoperative clinical staging of 85% T3 lesions. Postoperatively, the patients were administered intraperitoneal chemotherapy in an attempt to reduce peritoneal recurrence. The patients were followed for a median time of 15 months, and median survival had not been reached.

A small phase III trial was reported by Kang and colleagues comparing neoadjuvant chemotherapy followed by surgery versus surgery alone for patients with locally advanced gastric cancer, as documented by preoperative imaging studies.[28] Fifty-three patients received etoposide, 5-FU, and cisplatin therapy (EFP) for two or three cycles prior to surgery, and another 54 patients underwent surgery alone. Some patients received 3 to 6 additional cycles of chemotherapy after surgery according to the surgical stage. Of 101 evaluable patients, the overall curative resection rate was significantly higher in the neoadjuvant group (79% versus 61%), and the postoperative stage was significantly lower. Although there was an observed trend towards improved overall survival in the neoadjuvant group (3.6 years) versus surgery alone (2.5 years), this difference did not reach statistical significance, perhaps because of the relative small number of patients. There were no differences noted in operative morbidity or mortality.

In summary, several phase II trials have demonstrated that preoperative chemotherapy was feasible despite potential toxicities, and that median survival was higher than that of historical controls undergoing surgery alone.

Table 10-4 Neoadjuvant Trials for Potentially Resectable Gastric Cancer

Author	n	Regimen	Clinical Response	Pathologic Complete Response	Curative Resection (R0)	Median Survival
Ajani, 1991	25	EFP pre & postop	24%	-	72%	15 mo*
Leichman, 1992	38	Preop: 5 FU/leu/CP	-	8%	76%	17+ mo
Ajani, 1993	48	EAP pre & postop	31%	0%	77%	15.5 mo
Swartz, 1993	29	Preop: FAMTX Postop: IP Flu/CP, IV FU	-	-	56%	-
Kelsen, 1996	56	Preop: FAMTX Postop: IP FU/CP, IV FU	-	-	61%	15.3 mo**
Ajani, 1999	30	Preop: 5-FU, CP, IFNβ-2b	34%	7%	83%	30 mo
Lowy, 2001	24	Preop: EBXRT+FU IORT	74%	11%	-	-
Allum, 2003	250	Preop: ECF chemo	-	79%	-	-
	253	Surg alone	-	69%	-	-
Ajani, 2004	34	Preop: EBXRT+FU/leu/CP	48%	30%	70%	33.7 mo

* Median survival for resected patients not reached at 25 mo,
**31 months in patients undergoing curative resections.
FU = Fluorouracil; CP = cisplatin; EBXRT = external beam radiation therapy; ECF = epirubicin, cisplatin, and 5-FU; EFP = etoposide, 5-FU, and cisplatin therapy; FAMTX = 5-FU, doxorubicin, and methotrexate; IFN = interferon; IORT = intraoperative radiation therapy; IV = intravenous.

Current investigations center on the development of more active regimens incorporating new agents, including novel biologic agents.

Potentially Resectable Disease

Based on the encouraging results from trials of locally advanced disease, neoadjuvant strategies have been applied to patients with potentially resectable gastric cancer (Table 10-4). Ajani and colleagues reported a trial evaluating the use of preoperative EFP in 25 consecutive patients with potentially resectable disease as determined by CT scan.[29] Patients were administered two courses of preoperative chemotherapy, and those who responded received an additional three cycles of EFP postoperatively. Six patients (24%) were noted to have a major clinical response. Eighteen patients (72%) underwent a potentially curative resection, and three resected specimens contained only microscopic foci of tumor. No complete pathologic responses were identified, and minor responses were more common than major responses. The most common site of recurrence following surgery was the peritoneal cavity. At a median follow-up of 25 months, the median survival for the entire group was 15 months, while the median survival for resected patients was not reached.

In an attempt to achieve a 5 to 10% complete pathologic response rate, a follow-up trial was performed at the M. D. Anderson and Dana Farber Cancer Centers studying a similar regimen in 48 patients with potentially resectable gastric cancer.[30] Three cycles of preoperative EAP were given with responders receiving an additional two postoperative cycles. Six patients (12%) were judged to have a complete clinical response to preoperative therapy while 9 (19%) had a partial response. Among the 41 patients taken to surgery, 37 underwent a potentially curative resection (90% of the operated patients, 77% of the total). No complete pathologic responses were identified, and substantial toxicity was encountered, requiring dose reduction in 77% of the patients and hospitalization in 40%. At a median follow-up of 16 months, actuarial median survival was 15.5 months. The authors concluded that although the EAP regimen was modestly active and could achieve a complete clinical response in a small number of patients, substantial toxicities were present that may limit therapeutic efficacy.

Ajani and colleagues in 1999 studied the use of five preoperative cycles of 5-FU, cisplatin, and interferon alfa-2b without any planned postoperative chemotherapy.[31] Of 30 patients enrolled, 14 received all five cycles. Twenty-nine patients (97%) underwent attempted resection, 25 patients (83%) had an R0 resection, 2 patients

(7%) had a complete pathologic response. The median duration of follow-up was 30 months, and the median survival time was 30 months. The authors concluded that it is feasible to administer prolonged preoperative chemotherapy in patients with potentially resectable gastric cancer, and that larger studies need to be pursued to determine if this treatment enhances curative resection rates and prolongs survival.

Other centers have reported the use of preoperative chemotherapy combined with postoperative intraperitoneal 5-FU and cisplatin. In a study from the Memorial Sloan-Kettering Cancer Center, 23 of 29 patients with high risk T3-4 M0 tumors staged by endoscopic ultrasound received three cycles of preoperative 5-FU, doxorubicin, and methotrexate (FAMTX) followed by surgical resection.[32] Sixteen of these patients were resectable, and 13 of 23 underwent curative resection. Postoperatively, intraperitoneal 5-FU and cisplatin in combination with continuous systemic 5-FU infusion was delivered. One-third of patients ultimately undergoing resection showed evidence of pathologic downstaging in response to neoadjuvant therapy when compared to preoperative EUS staging. At a follow-up time of 6 months, 39% remained disease-free. In a follow-up article, Kelsen and colleagues reported the use of the FAMTX regimen in a total of 56 patients with high risk T3-4, N (any), M0 cancers staged by endoscopic ultrasound (mostly stage IIIA or B).[33] The same FAMTX regimen was continued and delivered for three courses before surgery. Postoperative intraperitoneal cisplatin and fluorouracil with concurrent intravenous (IV) fluorouracil were administered to patients following resection. The dose-limiting toxicity was primarily myelosuppression, with 60% of the patients experiencing at least one episode of neutropenic fever. Eight-nine percent of patients underwent surgical exploration and 61% underwent curative resection. Comparison of pathologic tumor stage with EUS-predicted tumor stage showed down-staging in 51% of patients. There was no observed increase in operative morbidity or mortality rates when comparing patients undergoing a similar operative procedure without neoadjuvant chemotherapy. The median survival was 15.3 months with a median follow-up of 29 months. For patients who underwent curative resection, the median survival duration was 31 months, suggesting that preoperative chemotherapy could increase the curative resection rate and perhaps overall survival.

Leichman and colleagues reported a series of 59 patients with gastric cancer, over 40% harboring stage III or IV disease.[34] Patients were initially treated with continuous infusion of 5-FU for 3 weeks with weekly

IV leucovorin and cisplatin on days 1 and 29. After two cycles of chemotherapy, the patients underwent operation. For patients who underwent curative resection, postoperative intraperitoneal chemotherapy with floxuridine and cisplatin was given. Preoperative chemotherapy resulted in a 45% response rate as assessed by CT. An R0 resection was accomplished in 40 patients (71%). The median follow-up was 43 months, and the median survival for patients undergoing curative resection was 52 months.

Lowy and colleagues studied prognostic factors associated with survival in three separate M. D. Anderson phase II trials utilizing neoadjuvant chemotherapy in potentially resectable gastric cancer patients.[35] On multivariate analysis, response to neoadjuvant chemotherapy correlated with increased survival as responders exhibited an actuarial 5-year survival rate of 83% versus 31% for nonresponders ($p < 0.05$). Compared to T stage, tumor grade, nodal positivity or number of positive nodes, response to chemotherapy was the single most important predictor of overall survival.

These studies suggest that in patients with resectable disease, neoadjuvant chemotherapy can result in clinical and pathologic responses in a significant percentage of patients. Curative resection rates are promising and overall survival may be improved over historical controls.

In 2003, Allum and colleagues reported preliminary results from a phase III study known as the MAGIC trial.[36] In this study, 503 patients with locally advanced adenocarcinoma of the distal esophagus, gastroesophageal junction, or the stomach were randomized to undergo three preoperative and three postoperative doses of epirubicin, cisplatin, and 5-FU or surgery alone. Of the patients randomized to the neoadjuvant arm, 88% completed their preoperative therapy and 40% finished their postoperative therapy. Curative resection was achieved in 79% of the patients who received neoadjuvant therapy versus 69% in the surgery alone group ($p = 0.02$). Neoadjuvant therapy resulted in significant pathologic down-staging because 54% of the patients in the neoadjuvant arm had T1 or T2 pathology versus 36% in the surgery alone arm ($p = 0.01$). Initial survival data demonstrated a hazard ratio of 0.70 ($p = 0.002$) for disease-free survival in favor of the chemotherapy arm. The hazard ratio for overall survival was 0.80, which approached, but did not reach statistical significance ($p = 0.06$). Longer follow-up data from the MAGIC trial are not yet mature, but these promising initial results support the efficacy of neoadjuvant therapy and further investigations of this kind.

Chemoradiation

Given the high rates of local and regional relapse that occur even following curative resection, it is logical to investigate the use of radiation therapy as an adjuvant in the treatment of gastric cancer. An important gastric adjuvant study, the Intergroup 0116 trial, examined the use of surgery plus adjuvant chemoradiation (5-FU, leucovorin [LV] and 4,500 cGy of external beam radiation [EBXRT]) versus surgery alone.[37] Patients received postoperative 5-FU/LV for one cycle followed by chemoradiation with 5-FU/LV given on days 1 to 4 and during the last three days of radiation, followed by 2 additional months of 5-FU/LV. A total of 556 patients have now been followed for a median time of greater than 6 years. The 3-year survival rates were 50% for the chemoradiation group versus 41% for the surgery alone group ($p = 0.005$). The 3-year relapse-free survival rates were 48% for the chemoradiation group versus 31% for the surgery alone group ($p = 0.001$). Of note, 41% of patients in the chemoradiation group exhibited significant toxicity that included hematologic, gastrointestinal, influenza-like, and infectious side effects. Cessation of therapy due to toxicity occurred in 17% of the enrolled patients, and a treatment-related mortality rate of 1% was observed. The predominant difference in recurrence patterns between the treatment arms was a decrease in local failure rate in the chemoradiation arm. Subset analyses revealed no significant treatment interactions between sex, T-stage, N-stage, location, or D-level, thus chemoradiation was beneficial across these subsets. However, only a small number of patients with Stage II disease were enrolled in the study. The D-level (extent of regional lymphadenectomy) was prognostic for survival, but a mere 10% of patients underwent D2 dissections. As previously discussed, the high proportion of patients who underwent substandard lymphadenectomy has been the major point of criticism for this study. Nevertheless, Intergroup 0116 has set standards for future regimens to be judged against and it has raised important issues regarding the quality of surgery that must be addressed in future study designs. Since the design of Intergroup 0116, there have been significant advances in drug development and radiation technique. The use of novel chemoradiation combination regimens awaits larger, prospective randomized trials.

A pilot study from M. D. Anderson investigated the role of preoperative chemoradiation, surgery, and intraoperative radiation therapy in patients with potentially resectable gastric carcinoma.[38] Twenty-four patients entered the trial and received concurrent continuous infusion 5-FU and 45 Gy of external beam radiation followed by surgical resection and intraoperative radiation (10 Gy). Twenty-three patients completed the preoperative protocol and 19 of these (83%) underwent an R0 resection. Of the resected patients, 2 (11%) had a complete pathologic response and 12 (63%) had a partial pathologic response. Surgical complications were comparable to gastrectomy alone. This study was notable for the high rate of compliance with the radiotherapy regimen and the fact that infusional 5-FU was utilized as opposed to bolus, which was used in Intergroup 0116.

Ajani and colleagues recently reported results from a multi-institutional trial combining the use of neoadjuvant chemotherapy and chemoradiation in patients with potentially resectable gastric carcinoma.[39] Thirty-three patients completed induction chemotherapy comprising fluorouracil, leucovorin, cisplatin, and then chemoradiation comprising fluorouracil and 45 Gy of EBXRT prior to operative resection. Twenty-eight patients (85%) underwent surgery. An R0 resection was achieved in 23 patients (70%). A complete pathologic response was observed in 10 patients (30%), and a partial pathologic response was observed in an additional 8 patients (24%). The median survival time was 33.7 months, and patients having a complete or partial pathologic response had a significantly longer survival of 63.9 months. One patient died during induction chemotherapy, and one patient died following surgery. The long-term survival data of this study are particularly impressive considering 94% of patients had an EUS-determined stage of T3, and 65% had an EUS-determined stage of N1. A recently closed Phase II study by the Radiation Therapy Oncology Group (RTOG) utilized a similar design, examining the efficacy of sequential neoadjuvant chemotherapy and chemoradiation using 5-FU, cisplatin and paclitaxel. The results of this study are not yet available but will provide additional information about the potential utility of this aggressive strategy.

Future Directions and Conclusions

Based on the results of Intergroup 0116, fit patients with resected gastric cancer that is Stage II or greater in the US should be considered for adjuvant 5-FU-based chemoradiation. For patients with early stage disease, or those in whom a D2 lymphadenectomy was performed with no or minimal lymph node disease on pathology, the results of Intergroup 0116 must be interpreted with caution. These subgroups comprised a very small percentage of the study population; thus, decisions regarding adjuvant treatment are even more difficult. Neoadjuvant treatment incorporating sequential chemotherapy and chemoradiation is promising but remains investigational for patients with resectable disease. Several phase II trials have demonstrated that preoperative chemotherapy can result in a significant clinical response rate and perhaps increase the curative resection rate for patients with locally advanced disease. For patients with locally advanced unresectable disease, it is clear that the only hope of surgical cure is associated with a response to neoadjuvant treatment. Identifying more active regimens is the source of ongoing studies. These largely involve the incorporation of newer agents such as the taxanes and oxaliplatin, in combination with biologics such as epidermal growth factor receptor inhibitors and anti-angiogenesis agents.

In designing new trials, several points are worth considering. First, accurate preoperative staging is crucial to evaluate resectability and subsequent response of the cancer to preoperative therapy. Traditional methods such as CT scanning, endoscopy, and upper gastrointestinal studies alone are inadequate; more modern techniques such as endoscopic ultrasonography and laparoscopy with laparoscopic ultrasound should be employed in combination with CT scanning when staging these tumors. The role of positron emission tomography scan in initial staging and in response to neoadjuvant treatment deserves inclusion as an endpoint in future neoadjuvant trial design. Second, definitions of locally advanced, potentially resectable, and unresectable tumors must be clearly defined in order to make valid comparisons of response to various preoperative regimens. Finally, surgical quality control remains a variable that has been difficult to control, but which clearly holds implications for the evaluation of both clinical trial results. Standardization of resection techniques, though difficult, must be attempted in order to compare adjuvant and neoadjuvant trials conducted in the US, Europe, and Asia.

References

1. Wanebo H, Kennedy B, Chmeil J, et al. Cancer of the stomach: a patient care study by the American College of Surgeons. Ann Surg 1993;218:583–92.

2. Gunderson L, Sosin H. Adenocarcinoma of the stomach: areas of failure in a re-operation series (second or symptomatic look) clinicopathologic correlation and implications for adjuvant therapy. Int J Radiat Oncol Biol Phys 1982;8:1–11.

3. Landry J, Tepper J, Wood W, et al. Patterns of failure following curative resection of gastric carcinoma. Int J Radiat Oncol Biol Phys 1990;19:1357–62.

4. Meyer H, Pichlmayr R. Patterns of recurrence in relation to therapeutic strategy in gastric cancer. Scand J Gastroenterol 1987;22(Suppl 133):45–8.

5. Koga S, Takebayashi M, Kaibara N, et al. Pathological characteristics of gastric cancer that develop hematogenous recurrence, with special reference to the site of recurrence. J Surg Oncol 1987;36:239–42.

6. Viadana E, Bross D, Pickren J. The metastatic spread of cancers of the digestive system in man. Oncology 1978;35: 114–26.

7. Estes NC, MacDonald JS, Touijer K, et al. Inadequate documentation and resection for gastric cancer in the United States: a preliminary report. Am Surg 1998;64:680–5.

8. Janunger KG, Hafstrom L, Glimelius B. Chemotherapy in gastric cancer: a review and updated meta-analysis. Eur J Surg 2002;168:597–608.

9. Earle CC, Maroun JA. Adjuvant chemotherapy after curative resection for gastric cancer in non-Asian patients: revisiting a meta-analysis of randomised trials. Eur J Cancer 1999;35:1059–64.

10. Mari E, Floriani I, Tinazzi A, et al. Efficacy of adjuvant chemotherapy after curative resection for gastric cancer: a meta-analysis of published randomised trials. A study of the GISCAD (Gruppo Italiano per lo Studio dei Carcinomi dell'Apparato Digerente). Ann Oncol 2000;11: 837–43.

11. Panzini I, Gianni L, Fattori PP, et al. Adjuvant chemotherapy in gastric cancer: a meta-analysis of randomized trials and a comparison with previous meta-analyses. Tumori 2002;88:21–7.

12. Grau J, Estape J, Alcobenda F, et al. Mitomycin C as an adjuvant treatment to resected gastric cancer: a randomized trial on 134 patients. Eur J Cancer 1993;29A: 340–2.

13. MacDonald J, Fleming T, Peterson R, et al. Adjuvant chemotherapy with 5-FU, adriamycin, and mitomycin C (FAM) versus surgery alone for patients with locally advanced gastric adenocarcinoma: a southwest oncology group study. Ann Surg Oncol 1995;2:488–94.

14. Lise M, Nitti D, Marchet A, et al. Prognostic factors in resectable gastric cancer: results of EORTC study no. 40813 on FAM adjuvant chemotherapy. Ann Surg Oncol 1995;2: 495–501.

15. The Gastrointestinal Tumor Study Group. Controlled trial of adjuvant chemotherapy following curative resection for gastric cancer. Cancer 1982;49:1116–22.

16. Leach S, Lowy A, Mansfield P, et al. Adjuvant therapy for resectable gastric adenocarcinoma: preoperative and post-operative chemotherapy trials. J Infusional Chemo 1995;5: 104–11.

17. Halvorsen R, Yee J, McCormick V. Diagnosis and staging of gastric cancer. Sem Oncol 1996;23:325–35.

18. Pollack B, Chak A, Sivak M. Endoscopic ultrasonography. Sem Oncol 1996;23:336–46.

19. Lowy A, Mansfield P, Leach S, et al. Laparoscopic staging for gastric cancer. Surgery 1996;119:611–4.

20. Bonatsos C, Aust J, Meisner D, et al. Preoperative chemotherapy for patients with locally advanced gastric carcinoma. Proc ASCO 1985;4:83.

21. Verschueren R, Willemse P, Sleijfer D, et al. Combined chemotherapeutic-surgical approach of locally advanced gastric cancer. Proc ASCO 1988;7:93.

22. Wilke H, Preusser P, Fink U, et al. Preoperative chemotherapy in locally advanced and nonresectable gastric cancer: A phase II study with etoposide, doxorubicin, and cisplatin. J Clin Oncol 1989;7:1318–26.

23. Lerner A, Gonin R, Steele G, et al. Etoposide, doxorubicin and cisplatin chemotherapy for advanced gastric adenocarcinoma: Results of a phase II trial. J Clin Oncol 1992;10: 536–40.

24. Fink U, Schumacher C, Stein H, et al. Preoperative chemotherapy for stage III–IV gastric carcinoma: feasibility, response and outcome after complete resection. Br J Surg 1995;82:1248–52.

25. Plukker J, Mulder N, Sleijfer D, et al. Chemotherapy and surgery for locally advanced cancer of the cardia and fundus: phase II study with methotrexate and 5-fluorouracil. Br J Surg 1991;78:955–8.

26. Rougier P, Lasser P, Ducreux M, et al. Preoperative chemotherapy of locally advanced gastric cancer. Ann Oncol 1994;5:S59–68.

27. Newman E, Marcus S, Potmesil M, et al. Neoadjuvant chemotherapy with CPT-11 and cisplatin downstages locally advanced gastric cancer. J Gastrointest Surg 2002; 6:212–23.

28. Kang Y, Choi D, Im Y, et al. A phase III randomized comparison of neoadjuvant chemotherapy followed by surgery versus surgery for locally advanced stomach cancer. Proc ASCO 1996;15:215.

29. Ajani J, Ota D, Jessup J, et al. Resectable gastric carcinoma. Cancer 1991;68:1501–6.

30. Ajani J, Mayer R, Ota D, et al. Preoperative and postoperative combination chemotherapy for potentially resectable gastric carcinoma. J NCI 1993;85:1839–44.

31. Ajani J, Mansfield P, Lynch P, et al. Enhanced staging and all chemotherapy preoperatively in patients with potentially resectable gastric carcinoma. J Clin Oncol 1999;17: 2403–11.

32. Schwartz G, Kelsen D, Christman K, et al. A phase II study of neoadjuvant FAMTX and postoperative intraperitoneal cisplatin in high risk patients with gastric cancer. Proc ASCO 1993;12:195.

33. Kelsen D, Karpeh M, Schwartz G, et al. Neoadjuvant therapy of high-risk gastric cancer: a phase II trial of preoperative FAMTX and postoperative intraperitoneal

fluorouracil-cisplatin plus intravenous fluorouracil. J Clin Oncol 1996;14:1818–28.

34. Leichman L, Silberman H, Leichman C, et al. Preoperative systemic chemotherapy followed by adjuvant postoperative intraperitoneal therapy for gastric cancer: a University of Southern California pilot program J Clin Oncol 1992;10: 1933–42.

35. Lowy A, Mansfield P, Leach S, et al. Response to neoadjuvant chemotherapy best predicts survival after curative resection of gastric cancer. Ann Surg 1999;229: 303–8.

36. Allum W, Cunningham D, Weeder S. Perioperative chemotherapy in operable gastric and lower oesophageal cancer: a randomized controlled trial (the MAGIC trial, ISRCTN 93793971). Proc Am Soc Clin Oncol 2003; 22:249.

37. MacDonald J, Smalley S, Benedetti J, et al. Chemoradiotherapy after surgery compared with surgery alone for adenocarcinoma of the stomach or gastroesophageal junction. N Engl J Med 2001;345:725–30.

38. Lowy A, Feig B, Janjan N, et al. A pilot study of preoperative chemoradiotherapy for resectable gastric cancer. Ann Surg Oncol 2001;8:519–24.

39. Ajani J, Mansfield N, Janjan N, et al. Multi-institutional trial of preoperative chemoradiotherapy in patients with potentially resectable gastric carcinoma. J Clin Oncol 2004; 22:2774–80.

CHAPTER 11

SURGICAL TREATMENT OF HEPATOCELLULAR CARCINOMA

STEVEN E. RODGERS, MD, PhD

TIMOTHY M. PAWLIK, MD, MPH

EUGENE A. CHOI, MD

EDDIE K. ABDALLA, MD

Hepatocellular carcinoma (HCC) is a major health problem affecting more than half a million people worldwide each year. It is the fifth most common malignant neoplasm among men and the eighth most common among women.[1] Surgical resection, whether by partial hepatectomy or transplantation, is the only potentially curative treatment for HCC. Unfortunately, surgical therapy can be applied in only a small minority (10 to 25%) of patients who present with this disease. The frequent association of HCC with severe underlying liver disease further complicates treatment and limits therapeutic options in most patients. Finally, HCC is difficult to study because of the tremendous biologic variability in its behavior. Tumor doubling times can vary from as little as 9 weeks to as many as 20 months; thus, measures of outcome are difficult to compare. This chapter discusses the risk factors, staging, and surgical strategies that may be used to treat HCC and highlights a selective but aggressive approach to hepatic resection of HCC.

Risk Factors

HEPATITIS

Worldwide, infection with hepatitis viruses is the most common etiologic factor in the development of HCC. In Europe and the US, the incidence of HCC is less than 10 per 100,000 people. However, in parts of Asia and Africa, the incidence has been reported to be as high as 35 to 50 per 100,000 people. The higher rate in these regions is due in large part to a much higher prevalence of chronic hepatitis B virus (HBV) infection. Although HCC is still relatively rare in the US, its incidence has risen steadily over the last three decades. The increase is likely related to an increase in the prevalence of chronic hepatitis C virus (HCV) infection in the American population. Both HBV and HCV infections are associated with the development of HCC, and although the carcinogenic mechanisms of these viruses are poorly understood, they appear to differ. HBV is a double-stranded DNA virus that integrates into the host deoxyribonucleic acid (DNA), causing alterations in cell signaling pathways, apoptosis, and cell cycle control. These alterations lead to an increased risk of carcinogenesis. In contrast, HCV is a single-strand ribonucleic acid (RNA) virus that does not integrate into the host genome. Instead, it induces fibrosis and subsequent cirrhosis, and it is believed to lead to HCC through chronic inflammatory stimulation.

Hepatitis viral status has been suggested as a prognostic indicator of patient survival after surgical resection. However, recent studies have called into question this relationship between chronic hepatitis virus infection and prognosis. Among patients who undergo resection for HCC, those who are seronegative for the hepatitis viruses and those infected with HBV have larger tumors at diagnosis and thus a higher incidence of vascular invasion than patients infected with HCV. Patients with chronic HCV infection have a higher incidence of underlying hepatic fibrosis and cirrhosis, smaller tumors (probably as a result of screening), and a lower incidence of vascular invasion. Thus, likely because of a balance between prognostic factors (large tumor size and vascular invasion for HBV and fibrosis for HCV), the overall prognosis is not necessarily related to hepatitis status, per se.[2] For this reason, seropositivity alone is not used as a selection criterion when determining which patients are candidates for surgical treatment.

OTHER RISK FACTORS

In the US and Europe, chronic alcohol use leading to cirrhosis is a significant risk factor for the development of HCC. Unlike HBV and HCV infection, the prevalence of alcoholic cirrhosis has remained relatively stable in the US population over the last 20 years. Likewise, the prevalence of HCC attributable to alcoholic cirrhosis has remained essentially unchanged during this period.[3,4] Carcinogenesis in alcoholic liver disease appears to be due to cirrhosis and chronic inflammation.

Many patients who present with HCC and cirrhosis do not have a history of hepatitis virus infection or alcohol abuse. In the absence of a known cause of HCC, these patients have been described to have "cryptogenic" liver disease. Recent data suggest that many of these patients may have nonalcoholic steatohepatitis (NASH), or nonalcoholic fatty liver disease (NAFLD), a spectrum of hepatic parenchymal disorders resembling alcohol-related liver disease.[5] The characteristic histologic features of NASH/NAFLD disappear as the condition progresses to cirrhosis; therefore, the diagnosis is difficult to make when patients present with HCC. However, diabetes and obesity, both risk factors for NASH/NAFLD, are disproportionately common in patients with HCC due to cryptogenic liver disease. Understanding of this type of liver disease is expanding rapidly since the link between obesity, fibrosis/cirrhosis, and HCC was postulated only recently.[6,7] Significant interest has emerged in this relatively new, potentially preventable cause of chronic liver disease and HCC.

In sub-Saharan Africa and parts of Asia, some human populations are routinely exposed to aflatoxins through the consumption of foods harboring mold, particularly *Aspergillus* species. These aflatoxins are potent hepatocarcinogens. Either alone, or in synergy with the effects of chronic HBV infection, aflatoxin exposure is associated with a higher-than-normal risk of HCC. Other factors that may be associated with the development of HCC include oral contraceptive use, cigarette smoking, and hereditary conditions such as hemochromatosis and Wilson's disease.

Staging Systems for HCC

Accurate staging of HCC is important because it not only provides prognostic data but also may aid in selecting patients for specific treatment regimens. Studies have reported divergent outcomes and predictors of survival after treatment of HCC,[8–11] and a variety of staging systems and treatment schemes that rely on clinical parameters have been devised. These include the Okuda staging system, the Barcelona Clinic Liver Cancer (BCLC) classification system, and the Cancer of the Liver Italian Program (CLIP) staging system. The most internationally recognized staging system, however, is the American Joint Committee on Cancer/Union Internationale Contre le Cancer (AJCC/UICC) tumor, node, metastasis (TNM) classification scheme. This system combines clinical and pathologic data to provide the most accurate staging and prognostic scoring system for resectable HCC. Because all these systems are mentioned frequently in the literature, a brief discussion of each follows.

OKUDA STAGING SYSTEM

In 1985, Okuda and colleagues proposed an HCC staging system based on both serum liver function tests and tumor extension.[12] In the Okuda staging system, patients are divided into three stages of disease based on tumor extent (< 50% vs. > 50% liver replacement), ascites status (absence vs. presence), bilirubin level (< 3 mg/dl vs. > 3 mg/dl), and serum albumin level (< 3 g/dl vs. > 3 g/dl) (Table 1). While this was the first classification system to consider both tumor factors and liver function, the staging system was devised based on an analysis predominantly of patients with advanced-stage HCC. The Okuda staging system does not include factors that affect prognosis in patients with early stage, resectable HCC; therefore, its utility is limited to assessing the prognosis of patients with advanced, unresectable disease.

Table 1 Okuda Staging System for Hepatocellular Carcinoma

		Points
Tumor Size	> 50%	1
	< 50%	0
Ascites	Yes	1
	No	0
Albumin	< 3 g/dL	1
	> 3 g/dL	0
Bilirubin	> 3 mg/dL	1
	< 3 mg/dL	0
Stage	I	0
	II	1 or 2
	III	3 or 4

Adapted from Okuda et al.[12]

CANCER OF THE LIVER ITALIAN PROGRAM CLASSIFICATION

In 1998, the CLIP staging system was developed in an attempt to provide more accurate prognostic information.[13] The CLIP system was derived from findings in a retrospective study but has subsequently been validated prospectively.[14] The score is based on the Child-Pugh classification of liver function (see "Evaluating Liver Function" below), tumor morphology (both size and number of nodules), serum alpha fetoprotein (AFP) level, and presence or absence of portal vein thrombosis (Table 2). The CLIP score stratifies patients according to prognosis better than the Okuda staging system. Patients with CLIP scores of 0, 1, 2, 3, and 4 have median survival times of 36, 22, 9, 7, and 3 months, respectively.

Despite its ability to help predict a patient's prognosis, the CLIP score does have several limitations. In the initial cohort of 435 patients used to derive the CLIP classification, only 12 (2.8%) underwent a surgical procedure, while 182 (41.8%) had no locoregional treatment, suggesting that most patients had advanced HCC.[13] Because the system is based on findings in patients with advanced disease, it is not as applicable to patients who present with early stage disease who are eligible for surgical resection.

BARCELONA CLINIC LIVER CANCER CLASSIFICATION

The BCLC classification system was developed as a "staging system" for HCC, but it has been criticized as being a treatment algorithm rather than a true staging system. In fact, it was created by correlating outcome with treatment for HCC.[15,16] This system first divides patients into two groups; those with earlier-stage/good-performance-status disease (BCLC stages A to C) are candidates for treatment, and those who have advanced disease (BCLC Stage D) are designated for palliative or symptomatic treatment only. BCLC stages A to C include patients who have Okuda stage 1 or 2 disease, with a performance status of 0 to 2 and a Child-Pugh classification of A or B. These groups are further stratified for treatment based on tumor status.

Unfortunately, this algorithmic approach allocates only patients with solitary lesions and normal portal pressure for resection. Patients with more than one lesion are excluded from resection. Additionally, many patients who meet the Milan criteria for liver transplantation (see "Liver Transplantation" in this chapter) are assigned to receive radiofrequency ablation (RFA) or ablation with alcohol by the BCLC algorithm. Patients with "intermediate-stage" disease are considered to be candidates for chemoembolization or randomized trials. Patients with slightly more advanced-stage disease, particularly those with extrahepatic disease, are designated to receive experimental agents or be entered into randomized trials.

The main criticism of this algorithm is that it excludes many patients from potentially curative treatments. For example, Ng and colleagues reported a 5-year survival rate of 39% among patients with large or multinodular HCC who had undergone surgical resection; these patients would have been relegated to undergo only trial-based or palliative therapy by the BCLC algorithm.[17] Similarly, Pawlik and colleagues reported that hepatic resection in carefully selected patients with HCCs measuring 10 cm or more yielded a 5-year survival rate of 25%.[18] Again, these patients would have been excluded from surgical resection by the BCLC system. These data emphasize that the use of morphologic criteria to exclude patients from consideration for surgery, as proposed by the BCLC system, is inappropriate. Treatments are evolving quickly, and this algorithm is rapidly becoming outdated. Additionally, the BCLC algorithm remains biased toward palliative therapies and largely undermines the multidisciplinary assessment and treatment of patients.

AMERICAN JOINT COMMITTEE ON CANCER/UNION INTERNATIONALE CONTRE LE CANCER STAGING SYSTEM

The AJCC/UICC TNM staging system for HCC was introduced in 1988. Although widely adopted, initial versions of the AJCC/UICC system failed to stratify patients effectively according to prognosis and were very complex.[19,20] In 2002, Vauthey and colleagues analyzed the outcomes of 557 patients who underwent surgical resection for HCC and identified vascular invasion, tumor number,

Table 2 Cancer of the Liver Italian Program (CLIP) Staging System*

		Points
Child-Pugh Class	A	0
	B	1
	C	2
Tumor Morphology	Uninodular; Extension ≤ 50%	0
	Multinodular; Extension ≤ 50%	1
	Massive or Extension > 50%	2
AFP (ng/ml)	< 400	0
	≥ 400	1
Portal Vein Thrombosis	No	0
	Yes	1

Each patient is assigned a score (from 0 to 6) by adding points from the four categories listed. Adapted from Cancer of the Liver Italian Program (CLIP) Investigators.[13]
AFP = alpha fetoprotein.

tumor size, and the presence of cirrhosis/fibrosis as independent predictors of survival.[21] Based on these analyses, a new simplified staging system was proposed and adopted in the latest AJCC/UICC guidelines (Table 3).[21, 22] This system has subsequently been validated in several cohorts of European and Asian patients.[23–25]

In the current (sixth) edition of the AJCC/UICC staging system, patients with a single tumor of any size and no vascular invasion are designated T1. Patients with evidence of microvascular invasion and those with multiple tumors less than 5 cm are designated T2. Patients with major vascular invasion and those with multiple tumors, any one of which is greater than 5 cm, are designated T3. In the absence of lymph node metastasis (N0) and distant metastasis (M0), T1, T2, and T3 tumors correspond respectively to stage I, stage II, and stage IIIA disease. The presence of lymph node metastasis (N1) places patients in the stage IIIB category, and the presence of distant metastasis (M1) places patients in the stage IV category.

Another important feature of the new AJCC/UICC TNM staging system is its provision for a separate reporting of hepatic fibrosis. Although not yet a formal part of the staging, fibrosis is noted because fibrosis status affects survival within every T classification.[21] In the case of stage I disease, 5-year survival is 64% for patients without underlying fibrosis (F0) versus 49% for patients with moderate-to-severe fibrosis (F1). In the case of stage II disease, 5-year survival is 46% for F0 patients, but only 30% for F1 patients; for stage IIIA disease, 5-year survival is 17% for F0 patients, and 9% for F1 patients. Thus, the new AJCC/UICC criteria provide a more precise means of evaluating the effect of fibrosis and cirrhosis on prognosis. Compared to other HCC staging systems, the AJCC/UICC system better stratifies patients into prognostic groups, especially those with early disease (Table 4).[23–25] The AJCC/UICC system has recently been validated in a large cohort of patients treated by liver transplantation.[26]

Preoperative Considerations

EVALUATING LIVER FUNCTION

The most commonly employed system for evaluating liver function in patients with cirrhosis is the Child-Pugh

Table 3 American Joint Committee on Cancer/Union Internationale Contre le Cancer (AJCC/UICC) TNM Staging System

Primary Tumor (T)

TX Primary tumor cannot be assessed
T0 No evidence of primary tumor
T1 Single tumor without vascular invasion
T2 Single tumor with vascular invasion or multiple tumors (none > 5 cm)
T3 Multiple tumors (any > 5 cm or tumor involving major branch of portal or hepatic vein)

Regional Lymph Nodes (N)

NX Regional lymph nodes cannot be assessed
N0 No regional lymph node metastasis
N1 Regional lymph node metastasis

Distant Metastasis (M)

MX Distant metastasis cannot be assessed
M0 No distant metastasis
M1 Distant metastasis

Fibrosis Score (F) *

F0 Ishak Grade 0-4 fibrosis (none to moderate)
F1 Ishak Grade 5-6 fibrosis (severe fibrosis/cirrhosis)

Stage Grouping

Stage I	T1	N0	M0
Stage II	T2	N0	M0
Stage IIIA	T3	N0	M0
Stage IIIB	any T	N1	M0
Stage IV	any T	any N	M1

F score is not formally included in assessment of stage, but the staging manual recommends notation of F score because the F score stratifies prognosis for each stage grouping. Adapted from the AJCC Manual for Staging of Cancer.[22]
TNM = tumor, node, metastasis.

Table 4 Comparison of 5-Year Survival Rates Based on Staging Classifications from Three Hepatocellular Carcinoma Staging Systems

Staging System	Stage	5-Year Survival (%)
AJCC/UICC[21]	I, F0	64
	I, F1	49
	II, F0	46
	II, F1	30
	IIIA, F0	17
	IIIA, F1	9
	IIIB	0
	IV	0
CLIP[76]	0	67
	1	17
	2	0
	3	0
	4	0
	5	0
	6	0
Okuda[76]	1	35
	2	0
	3	0

AJCC/UICC = American Joint Committee on Cancer/Union Internationale Contre le Cancer; CLIP = Cancer of the Liver Italian Program.

classification scheme. The Child-Pugh score is derived from three laboratory parameters (bilirubin level, albumin level, and prothrombin time) and two clinical factors (presence or absence of ascites and encephalopathy). The Child-Pugh score is useful in assessing global liver function; however, it alone is not adequate to guide surgical management of HCC. Other measures that can be used to evaluate hepatic metabolic function include indocyanine green (ICG) retention rate, galactose elimination, and aminopyrine clearance. Most of the experience with ICG retention rate comes from Japan because this test is not widely used in the West. Although retention rates at 15 minutes after intravenous injection ICG (0.5 mg/kg) have been correlated with outcomes for *minor* resections in some series, the ICG test may be impractical for use in surgical planning for *major* hepatectomy because it provides an overall measurement of function and does not differentiate between the function of liver to be resected and that of the anticipated liver remnant. Prior to major hepatic resection, we promote a systematic evaluation of the volume of the anticipated liver remnant in the context of the level of underlying liver disease (see "Liver Volume Measurement" in this chapter). Finally, some centers routinely measure portal pressures as an indicator of liver function. In most patients, portal pressure can be assessed indirectly. Patients considered for surgical resection must have no evidence of esophageal varices,

splenomegaly, or thrombocytopenia (platelet counts > 100,000). Noninvasive (duplex) or invasive portal pressure measurement may be used when necessary.

LIVER VOLUME MEASUREMENT

Liver volume and severity of underlying liver disease are linked to liver function. In fact, by determining the residual liver volume corrected for the degree of liver disease, the surgeon can make reasonable estimates of postresection hepatic function. Several studies have been performed to determine the safe limits of resection based on the liver volume remaining after resection and the degree of underlying liver disease.[27–30] For patients with normal livers, a remnant as small as 20% of the standardized total liver volume (TLV) is the safe limit of resection.[28] A study of patients undergoing hepatic resection at The University of Texas M. D. Anderson Cancer Center showed that the rates of complications, extended hospital stays, and intensive care unit admissions, as well as the incidence of liver failure, were low when the future liver remnant (FLR) exceeded 20% of the TLV in patients with normal liver (compared to patients with FLR < 20% standardized TLV).[28] This result was validated in a series of 127 consecutive extended hepatectomies with only one mortality.[31] In patients with cirrhosis or severe fibrosis, the safe limit of resection is approximately 60% of the TLV, but may be significantly less in some patients.[29,30] These guidelines have also been proposed for use in the selection of patients for portal vein embolization (PVE) (see "Portal Vein Embolization" in this chapter).

The method of liver volume measurement is very important. In an attempt to estimate the function of the FLR, it is not the actual volume that is predictive but, rather, the FLR volume standardized to the patient's size. Larger patients need a larger volume of liver than smaller patients; similarly, patients with diseased livers require a larger volume than patients with normal livers. As in liver transplantation, the liver volume can be standardized to the patient size using body weight or body surface area (BSA) because of the close correlation between TLV and these parameters.

At the M. D. Anderson Cancer Center, we have standardized our approach to FLR volume estimation by utilizing highly accurate three-dimensional (3-D) computed tomography (CT) volumetry. Measuring the total liver to obtain an index of reference is not useful because the size of the diseased liver is not consistent among patients who have tumors, who have preexisting areas of hepatic hypertrophy or atrophy, or who have large or small livers due to cirrhosis, biliary dilatation, or infiltration of tumor into the liver. Instead, the nondiseased FLR is measured by 3-D CT volumetry and then standardized to a calculated TLV, based on a formula derived from the close association between TLV and BSA[32]:

$$TLV\ (cm^3) = -794.41 + 1267.28 \times BSA\ (m^2)$$

Thus, the standardized FLR volume calculation utilizes the *measured* FLR volume from 3-D CT volumetry as the numerator and the *calculated* TLV as the denominator:

Standardized FLR (%) = measured FLR volume/ calculated TLV

The standardized FLR volume has been correlated with surgical outcome in several studies.[27,28,33] When the FLR is adequate based on the guidelines above, patients can undergo resection immediately. When the volume is inadequate, they are considered for preoperative PVE.

PORTAL VEIN EMBOLIZATION

A major advance in preparing patients with small FLRs for extensive liver surgery is preoperative PVE.[34,35] In fact, in most comprehensive hepatobiliary centers, preoperative PVE is now considered the standard of care before major hepatectomy in selected patients.[36] PVE redirects portal flow to the intended FLR to initiate hypertrophy of the nonembolized segments. This strategy has been shown to improve the functional reserve and volume of the FLR before surgery. At the M. D. Anderson Cancer Center and several other centers worldwide, PVE has been adopted for routine use in selected patients to reduce postoperative morbidity and enable safe, potentially curative hepatectomy for patients not previously considered candidates for resection because the anticipated FLR was marginal.[27-29,37]

The indications for PVE as outlined above relate to the relative size of the FLR and to the degree of underlying liver disease. PVE is indicated in patients with normal liver when the standardized FLR volume is < 20% of the TLV[28] and in patients with cirrhosis or severe underlying liver disease when the FLR volume is < 40% of the TLV.[38,29]

Several approaches to PVE have been described. The preferred approach respects and does not transgress the FLR and, thus, punctures the liver to be resected by a percutaneous "ipsilateral" approach. Under sonographic guidance, a portal vein branch on the side of the liver to be resected is cannulated. Then, using fluoroscopy, catheters are inserted, and through these catheters the portal branches are occluded using small particles for outflow occlusion and coils for inflow occlusion. With a complication rate of 5 to 8%, PVE is safe and has been shown to increase the size of the FLR 8 to 16%, depending on the extent of underlying liver disease

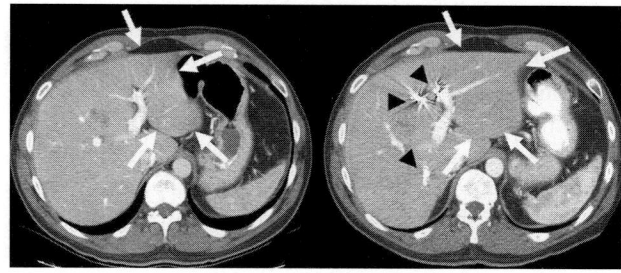

Figure 1 Portal phase computed tomograms revealing the left lateral bisegment before (left panel) and 1 month after (right panel) portal vein embolization extended to segment IV. Segments II and III (outlined by white arrows) increased in volume from 18% to 27% of the standardized total liver volume. Embolization coils are marked with black arrows.

(Figure 1).[38,39] Both normal and diseased livers will undergo hypertrophy, although normal livers enlarge at a faster rate than diseased livers. Also, systemic factors, such as diabetes, can slow hepatic hypertrophy.

In the last few years, the indications for, approaches to, and benefits of PVE prior to major hepatectomy in patients with cirrhosis and before extended hepatectomy in patients without cirrhosis have been refined. PVE is known to be highly important in increasing the safety and feasibility and decreasing the morbidity and mortality of these procedures.[35,36] Using a systematic approach to FLR volume measurement, morbidity for extended hepatectomy can be as low as 31%.[31] A recent randomized trial proved the benefit of right PVE before right hepatectomy in cirrhotic patients.[38] Thus, volumetry and PVE have secured important places in the evaluation and preparation of patients for major hepatectomy for HCC. PVE may be combined with other treatments, such as transarterial chemoembolization (discussed below).

Operative Considerations

Modern hepatic surgery centers take an aggressive but careful approach to the treatment of HCC, and perioperative morbidity and mortality rates following hepatic resection for HCC have decreased markedly as a result. Better patient selection, careful preparation for surgery, and changes in intraoperative technique—specifically with respect to operative blood loss, transfusion requirements, and the duration of operation—all contribute to improved outcomes. Factors that may affect these variables include the routine use of intraoperative ultrasound (IOUS), techniques of hepatic parenchymal dissection, and methods of hepatic vascular control.

INTRAOPERATIVE ULTRASOUND

IOUS is generally considered critical for performing a safe and complete liver resection. This technique permits evaluation of the anatomic relationships between the tumor and intrahepatic structures—most importantly, the major blood vessels. Additionally, IOUS allows for the detection and characterization of lesions not evident on preoperative imaging and may detect subcentimeter lesions that are not yet palpable. IOUS has been shown to alter the planned procedure in 19 to 49% of cases in some series,[40,41] although improved detection rates for small lesions by modern cross-sectional imaging has decreased the rate of new-lesion detection at IOUS. IOUS will always remain a critical surgical tool, both in determining the intrahepatic anatomy and in establishing the proper transection plane. Particularly in patients with cirrhosis, for whom conservation of nonmalignant parenchyma is critical to outcome, IOUS enables removal of the tumor and its portal supply, while preserving the maximum amount of remaining parenchyma and vasculature.

DISSECTION TECHNIQUES

In recent years, numerous dissection tools and techniques for liver surgery have emerged, including use of the Cavitron Ultrasonic Surgical Aspirator (CUSA, Valleylab, Boulder CO), the argon beam coagulator, the TissueLink floating-ball radiofrequency (RF) dissector (TissueLink Medical, Dover, NH), and various vascular stapling devices.[42] Although retrospective studies have reported that several of these new techniques decrease blood loss relative to older methods,[43,44] a prospective randomized trial comparing CUSA with the more conventional clamp crush dissection method in 132 patients undergoing liver resection showed no difference in blood loss or operative time.[45] A two-surgeon technique using the CUSA and TissueLink dissector was reported recently.[46] This method facilitates simultaneous dissection with the CUSA by one surgeon and tissue coagulation with the TissueLink dissector by the second surgeon. This combination allows for rapid, safe identification of intrahepatic structures and efficient parenchymal transection.[46] Others use vascular staplers for rapid, low-blood-loss major resection.[42] Many techniques can be used to transect the liver parenchyma, depending on what instruments are available, but surgeon experience is among the most important factors determining outcome from hepatic resection, regardless of the technique. Common to all techniques of safe parenchymal transection is clear identification of intrahepatic structures using

a combination of IOUS and dissection, ensuring precise ligation and division of hepatic venous, portal venous, and biliary branches.

VASCULAR CLAMPING TECHNIQUES

At the beginning of the twentieth century, J.H. Pringle demonstrated that inflow vascular occlusion could reduce liver bleeding. Since that time, low-blood-loss hepatic surgery has become standard, particularly because it was found that morbidity is reduced when transfusion can be avoided.[47,48] Although some liver resections may be safely and routinely performed without vascular clamping, resection with minimal blood loss remains an important concern in hepatic surgery. Vascular clamping techniques include inflow occlusion, segmental vascular occlusion, and total hepatic vascular exclusion (HVE). Each technique has a place in liver surgery, and each has a different systemic and hepatic effect. Some techniques, particularly total HVE, can be associated with hemodynamic changes that some patients can not tolerate.[49]

Hepatic pedicle clamping (Pringle's maneuver) is the simplest, most widely used technique to reduce blood loss during liver surgery. It interrupts the arterial and portal venous inflow to the liver but has no direct effect on backflow bleeding from branches of the hepatic veins. Following pedicle clamping, the decrease in cardiac preload causes a 10% drop in cardiac output. At the same time, the reflex elicited by clamping increases the systemic vascular resistance to generate a 10% increase in mean arterial pressure. Thus, pedicle clamping is extremely well-tolerated in almost all patients. Continuous interruption of hepatic inflow to a normal liver under normothermic conditions is safe for up to 60 minutes. In cirrhotic patients, however, the intermittent clamping technique is preferred. The intermittent method involves alternating periods of clamping (15 to 20 minutes) with periods of restored flow (5 minutes). This method is much better tolerated than continuous clamping in patients with cirrhosis, as indicated by decreased alteration of serum liver function tests and improved hemodynamic stability.[50] In normal livers, intermittent clamping can enable total clamp times of > 120 minutes. To reduce backflow bleeding, central venous pressure should be maintained below 6 mmHg. Additionally, to further reduce backflow bleeding, the infrahepatic inferior vena cava (IVC) may be clamped without causing major hemodynamic compromise.

Hemihepatic or segmental vascular clamping selectively interrupts the arterial and portal venous inflow to the hemiliver or segment to be excised and provides clear demarcation of the limits of resection. This technique avoids ischemia to the remnant liver, splanchnic venous congestion, and systemic hemodynamic consequences. This procedure may be performed together with occlusion of the ipsilateral hepatic vein. Segmental vascular clamping is particularly useful in patients with small HCC tumors and underlying liver disease because ischemic injury to the remaining liver parenchyma is minimized. Also, the portal territory of the tumor is better delineated than with other techniques, allowing true segment-oriented hepatic resection.[49]

HVE consists of both total hepatic inflow and outflow vascular occlusion. Outflow vascular occlusion is achieved by mobilizing the liver completely from the IVC below the hepatic veins and occluding the IVC above and below the liver (with ligation of the right adrenal vein). This method of totally isolating the liver from the systemic circulation is occasionally employed during resection of tumors adjacent to or involving the major hepatic veins or the IVC. HVE may also be considered when significant backflow bleeding occurs because of persistently elevated central venous pressure. In most cases, HVE offers little advantage over inflow occlusion alone, and it is poorly tolerated in 10 to 15% of patients.[51,52] In patients with cirrhosis, HVE has little or no role because of poor liver and patient tolerance.

The vascular occlusion technique chosen will depend on the reason for resection, the tumor location, the presence or absence of associated underlying liver disease, the patient's cardiovascular status, and the surgeon's experience.

SURGICAL MARGINS OF RESECTION

A surgical margin of resection (tumor-free margin) at least 1 cm in size has traditionally been the goal during resection of HCC. The importance of margin width, however, is controversial. Although early studies reported a longer recurrence-free survival time for patients with a margin width ≥ 1 cm than for those with narrower margins,[53,54] modern series have shown no correlation between prognosis and surgical margin width.[55,56] In a recent study of 288 patients who underwent surgical resection for HCC at the University of Hong Kong, recurrence-free and overall survival times did not differ between patients who had histologically negative narrow surgical margins (< 1 cm) and patients who had wide surgical margins (≥ 1 cm).[57]

HCC spreads through the liver along portal venous tracts and frequently recurs within adjacent areas of the liver despite the use of wide surgical margins.[58] For this reason, portal-oriented resection may provide lower rates of recurrence and longer survival times than nonanatomic wedge resection. Thus, margin negative resections performed using an anatomic portal-oriented approach should be the surgeon's primary goal when resecting

HCC, and wide surgical margins (≥ 1 cm) should be attempted whenever feasible.

Liver Transplantation

Orthotopic liver transplantation (OLT) has evolved as a treatment for patients with early HCC and severe underlying liver disease. During the 1980s, attempts at OLT for unresectable HCC produced disappointing results, with 5-year survival rarely achieved and recurrence rates as high as 75%.[59,60] Recognition that patients with small tumors had better survival rates than other patients after undergoing transplantation led to a reassessment of this treatment modality for HCC. A new set of criteria for the selection of transplantation candidates was proposed by Bismuth and colleagues[61] in 1993 and later amended by Mazzaferro and colleagues.[62] The new criteria, now known as the Milan criteria, are based on the small series reported by Mazzaferro and colleagues (48 patients), in which no patient had a tumor with vascular invasion and only a 4-year survival rate was reported. According to these criteria, patients eligible for OLT include those with a solitary liver tumor not exceeding 5 cm in maximum diameter or up to three tumors not exceeding 3 cm in diameter. Following adoption of these criteria by the international transplant community, the 5-year overall survival rate in a multicenter series of patients undergoing OLT for HCC in the US rose to 61%.[63] In Europe, 5-year survival rates as high as 70% and disease-free survival rates of nearly 60% have been reported for carefully selected patients.[64] The lower survival rates reported in the multicenter series may reflect the fact that patients are selected for transplantation based solely on tumor morphology (size and number), without accounting for the presence of microscopic vascular invasion. Vascular invasion is one of the strongest prognostic indicators for treatment outcome in HCC, and patients with unrecognized microscopic vascular invasion have shorter disease-free and overall survival times following OLT.

In a univariate analysis of risk factors in 344 patients who underwent OLT at the University of Pittsburgh, the presence of microscopic or major vascular invasion in the explant specimen was associated with a significantly shorter median overall survival time (7.8 years for microscopic and 1.7 years for macroscopic invasion, respectively) than that of patients who had no evidence of vascular invasion (9.1 years).[65] Although microscopic vascular invasion cannot be identified until after the tumor is removed, preoperative evidence of major vascular invasion is an absolute contraindication to OLT. Given the recent improvements in overall and disease-free survival times after OLT for HCC, this treatment has become increasingly popular for patients with small tumors and nonpreserved liver function. However, the use of OLT is limited by the strict selection criteria and by a shortage of organs.

BRIDGE TREATMENT TO TRANSPLANTATION

Long waiting periods and the frequency with which HCC patients "drop out" of the waiting list for OLT because of tumor progression have led to the exploration of bridge treatments to control tumor growth during the wait-time for organs for OLT. The preferred bridge therapies are nonsurgical, including in-situ tumor ablation and transarterial chemoembolization (which are described in the following sections in this chapter). Partial hepatic resection has been proposed as a potential bridge treatment because it offers the opportunity for surgical staging and examination of the pathologic specimen.[66,67] However, concern regarding the technical difficulty of the subsequent OLT and possible decreased overall survival in the case of postresection OLT may limit its utility; thus, this issue is still being hotly debated.[68]

In-situ Tumor Ablation

Despite a trend toward earlier diagnosis, the majority of patients who present with HCC are not candidates for surgical resection. Many of these patients are considered unresectable not because of the tumor burden but because they have severe underlying liver disease. For this group of patients, direct ablation of the liver tumors has been proposed. A subset of these patients includes those who are awaiting liver transplantation but need local tumor control in the interim period. Numerous ablative techniques have been described for both curative and palliative treatment of HCC, including cryosurgery, percutaneous ethanol injection, and RFA.

CRYOSURGERY

Cryosurgery involves subjecting the tumor and surrounding liver parenchyma to two or more freeze-thaw cycles with freezing (-40° to -50°C) performed using a thick, solid probe inserted into the tumor during surgery. Although this method of tumor destruction can be effective, it can result in cracking of the hepatic tissue and bleeding from the probe tract and can be associated with significant systemic effects, including multiple organ failure and death. This method has therefore been largely abandoned.

PERCUTANEOUS ETHANOL INJECTION

Percutaneous ethanol injection involves the injection of absolute ethanol into tumors, typically under ultrasound guidance. The ethanol causes cellular dehydration and vascular thrombosis, leading to tumor necrosis. Morbidity and mortality rates associated with this treatment are very low, and destruction of target lesions ≤ 2 cm in diameter is usually complete. Several studies have documented acceptable survival rates after this treatment for extremely small tumors in well-selected patients, but the rate of recurrent disease in the liver is high. In two-thirds of patients, recurrence is seen in distant segments of the liver within 3 years.[69] Even higher recurrence rates are observed in patients with larger (> 2 cm) tumors. Although this technique can be repeated as recurrent lesions appear and thus may provide a bridge to transplantation, it has not been widely adopted as a preferred method of ablating larger lesions.

RFA

For many patients who are not candidates for surgical resection or who are awaiting transplantation, RFA provides a safe alternative method for local control of HCC. RFA causes tumor destruction by using RF energy to heat the tumor tissue. The probe used to deliver the RF energy may be inserted into the tumor by open, laparoscopic, or percutaneous approaches. Ultrasound guidance (or CT guidance for the percutaneous approach) is typically used for placement of the RFA probe. For maximal benefit, a 360°, 1-cm margin of liver parenchyma is destroyed around the target lesion. The size of tumor that can be treated is limited by the size of the ablation zone created by the RFA probe. Tumors ≤ 3 cm in size may be ablated with a single treatment, but larger lesions require multiple passes of the probe in order to create overlapping ablation zones. Recurrence rates after RFA are much higher for tumors > 3 cm, but good results have been shown for smaller tumors.[70]

Recently, interest has increased in the use of RFA as an alternative treatment for HCC in patients who are candidates for surgical resection because RFA preserves a maximal volume of hepatic parenchyma. Several non-randomized trials have been reported comparing overall survival and recurrence-free survival in patients treated with either RFA or surgical resection.[71–73] Results of these studies are presented in Table 5. They demonstrate significantly higher 3-year recurrence-free and overall survival rates for the resection patients than for patients who underwent RFA. Given these data, surgical resection remains the preferred treatment modality whenever possible. However, RFA has secured an important role in patients with HCC rendered unresectable by underlying cirrhosis. RFA is also a widely used bridge to transplantation.

RFA has also been used in conjunction with surgical resection. By combining the two techniques, patients

Table 5 Non-randomized Comparative Trials of RFA versus Surgical Resection for Hepatocellular Carcinoma

Author, year	No. of Tumors	Tumor Size	No. of Patients	Treatment	3-year DFS	3-year OS
Montorsi, 2005[71]	1	< 5 cm	58	RFA	31%	61%
			40	Resection	59%	73%
Hong, 2005[73]	1	≤ 4 cm	55	RFA	40%	73%
			93	Resection	55%	84%
Vivarelli, 2004[72]	1–4	43 pts ≤ 3 cm	79*	RFA	20%	33%
		115 pts > 3 cm	79	Resection	50%	65%

*Patients with tumors ≤ 3 cm and > 3 cm were evenly distributed between RFA and resection groups.
DFS = disease-free survival; OS = overall survival; RFA = radiofrequency ablation.

who might otherwise be considered to have unresectable disease can undergo potentially curative treatment. This strategy allows resection of the portion of the liver containing the majority of lesions. RFA is then performed on any small lesions that remain in the liver remnant, preserving an adequate volume of functional liver parenchyma. Adding RFA to hepatic resection is well tolerated and adds minimal complexity or morbidity to the operation.[74]

One factor that may limit the effectiveness of RFA is the heat-sink effect seen when the lesion to be ablated is in close proximity to large blood vessels. Blood flow within these vessels or within the tumor itself reduces the thermal effect of the RFA probe, reducing the ablation zone. The Pringle maneuver may be used to decrease blood flow around the target lesion, resulting in larger ablation zones. An open surgical technique, however, is required to employ the Pringle maneuver. RFA can be used to treat lesions abutting the IVC or the major hepatic veins without damaging the vessel wall, but recurrence at the vessel wall is common. Tumors near the hilar plate, however, must be avoided when using RFA. The large bile ducts in this area do not tolerate heat, and biliary strictures, fistulae, or bilomas can result.

The choice of whether to perform RFA percutaneously, laparoscopically, or as part of an open surgical procedure depends on several factors: the severity of comorbid conditions and underlying liver disease; the number, size, and location of the lesions to be ablated; the presence of adhesions from prior surgical procedures; and the need to perform other treatments at the same time. Patients with only a few small lesions that are remote from the main bile ducts and intrahepatic vessels are often good candidates for the percutaneous approach. Those who are not candidates for general anesthesia because of comorbidities may have the percutaneous approach as their only option. An operative (open or laparoscopic) approach to RFA is needed when the lesions are near the dome of the liver, adjacent to the diaphragm, or in close proximity to other organs. An open surgical RFA approach may also be preferred in patients with larger tumors (> 4 cm) or multiple tumors. The open technique allows for more accurate placement of the RFA probe, ensuring adequate overlap of multiple ablation zones. Laparoscopically guided RFA can be performed in patients who have just a few small lesions located centrally within the liver. Laparoscopic ultrasound allows for precise localization of the target lesions. A laparoscopic approach may be difficult in patients who have extensive intra-abdominal adhesions from prior operations.

Chemoembolization

Many patients who present with HCC are considered to have unresectable disease because they have large, multifocal tumors, though they may have relatively well-preserved liver function. These patients are poor candidates for percutaneous ethanol injection or RFA because of the size or number of lesions. Attempts to provide local control and palliation in these patients have led to the development of chemoembolization.

Chemoembolization, or transarterial chemoembolization (TACE), is a technique that combines intra-arterial chemotherapy and embolization of selected vessels feeding tumors within the liver. Chemotherapeutic agents, such as doxorubicin or cisplatin (or a combination), are combined with an iodized oil (lipiodol) and delivered transarterially to intrahepatic branches of the hepatic artery. The infusion is typically followed by delivery of an embolic agent, such as gelatin sponge (Gelfoam), polyvinyl alcohol, or starch microspheres. The procedure results in extensive tumor necrosis in more than half the patients treated. Randomized controlled trials from Hong Kong[75] and Barcelona[76] have shown significant improvements in overall survival in patients treated with TACE compared with those treated with best supportive care or with transarterial embolization (TAE) alone. These studies reported 3-year survival rates of 26%[75] and 29%[76] among patients who underwent TACE, compared to 3% and 11%, respectively, for those receiving symptomatic treatment alone

Table 6 Randomized Controlled Trials of Arterial Embolization for Hepatocellular Carcinoma

Author, year	No. of Patients		Treatment	Overall Survival		
				1-year	2-year	3-year
Llovet, 2002[76]	112	40	TACE	82%	63%	29%
		37	TAE	75%	50%	29%
		35	Best supportive	63%	27%	17%
Lo, 2002[75]	80	40	TACE	57%	31%	26%
		40	Best supportive	32%	11%	3%

TACE = transarterial chemoembolization; TAE = transarterial (bland) embolization.

(Table 6). The different outcomes in the two studies reflect the criteria used to select patients for embolization in each trial—patients in the Hong Kong trial had more advanced disease than those in the Barcelona trial. Both studies show a survival advantage was conferred by TACE, despite the differences in selection criteria. Although the Barcelona study demonstrates equivalent 3-year survival rates for patients receiving TACE and TAE, fewer deaths in the TACE group were secondary to tumor progression. This finding led to the conclusion that TACE was superior to TAE. Among patients with unresectable HCC, fewer than 30% are candidates for TACE, which requires relatively well-preserved hepatic function, adequate renal function, and no evidence of extrahepatic metastatic disease. Patients with advanced HCC and poor hepatic function are susceptible to liver failure after TACE. Main portal vein occlusion is another relative contraindication to TACE, although patients with segmental portal vein or hepatic vein occlusion can be treated selectively (and were included in the Hong Kong trial).[75] TACE is used occasionally as a bridge to OLT or sequentially to complement RFA, and has been used in conjunction with PVE before major resection.

Summary

Selecting a treatment for HCC requires a patient-oriented, multidisciplinary approach. The interplay of HCC and underlying liver disease complicates treatment of this worldwide health problem in most patients. Treatment is guided by overall patient condition, degree of underlying liver disease, liver function, and tumor stage. The available treatments, including resection, transplantation, percutaneous ablation, and chemoembolization are complementary across the spectrum of disease.

Resection can be used to treat small, large, and multifocal tumors in a broad spectrum of patients when careful preoperative planning and preparation with PVE are used appropriately. Surgical resection can also be combined with techniques of in-situ ablation. Resection is limited by the degree of underlying liver disease and can be used only in patients with adequate liver function

and relatively normal portal pressure. Transplantation can simultaneously treat underlying liver disease, remove the entire "field of cancerization" for future tumors, and resect early stage HCC. This modality is limited by organ availability, the need for systemic immunosuppression (which could stimulate the proliferation of recurrent HCC) and its failure to effectively treat patients with intermediate- and advanced-stage cancer.

Percutaneous ablation by alcohol or RF energy can be used effectively in patients with a few small tumors and in those for whom laparotomy or major resection are contraindicated because of systemic disease, poor performance status, or marginal liver function. Most ablation treatments are restricted by tumor proximity to intra- and extrahepatic structures. TACE is an option for patients with multiple and bilateral tumors, can be used in patients with marked cirrhosis, and like ablation, can be used repeatedly in the same patient. TACE is generally reserved for patients with relatively good liver function, but it cannot be used when portal thrombosis is extensive. Systemic therapy has a very limited role in HCC, although some combination therapies may enable down-staging and subsequent resection of tumors in highly selected patients with good liver function.

Although many combinations and sequences of treatments can potentially be used in the treatment of HCC, the great majority of patients are not candidates for aggressive treatment and ultimately succumb to their disease. Parallel advances in surgical techniques, patient preparation for surgery, and the development of new treatment strategies will be necessary to improve outcomes for this intriguing and complex disease.

References

1. Bosch FX, Ribes J, Diaz M, Cleries R. Primary liver cancer: worldwide incidence and trends. Gastroenterology 2004; 127(5 Suppl 1):S5–16.

2. Pawlik TM, Poon RT, Abdalla EK, et al. Hepatitis serology predicts tumor and liver-disease characteristics but not prognosis after resection of hepatocellular carcinoma. J Gastrointest Surg 2004;8(7):794–804; discussion 804–5.

3. El-Serag HB, Mason AC. Risk factors for the rising rates of primary liver cancer in the United States. Arch Intern Med 2000;160(21):3227–30.

4. Davila JA, Morgan RO, Shaib Y, et al. Hepatitis C infection and the increasing incidence of hepatocellular carcinoma: a population-based study. Gastroenterology 2004;127(5):1372–80.

5. Regimbeau JM, Colombat M, Mognol P, et al. Obesity and diabetes as a risk factor for hepatocellular carcinoma. Liver Transpl 2004;10(2 Suppl 1):S69–73.

6. Ratziu V, Bonyhay L, Di Martino V, et al. Survival, liver failure, and hepatocellular carcinoma in obesity-related cryptogenic cirrhosis. Hepatology 2002;35(6):1485–93.

7. Bugianesi E, Leone N, Vanni E, et al. Expanding the natural history of nonalcoholic steatohepatitis: from cryptogenic cirrhosis to hepatocellular carcinoma. Gastroenterology 2002;123(1):134–40.

8. Vauthey JN, Marsh RW, Davis GL. Treatment of unresectable hepatocellular carcinoma. N Engl J Med 1995;333(13):877; author reply 878.

9. Fong Y, Sun RL, Jarnagin W, Blumgart LH. An analysis of 412 cases of hepatocellular carcinoma at a Western center. Ann Surg 1999;229(6):790–9; discussion 799–800.

10. Ikai I, Yamamoto Y, Yamamoto N, et al. Results of hepatic resection for hepatocellular carcinoma invading major portal and/or hepatic veins. Surg Oncol Clin N Am 2003; 12(1):65–75, ix.

11. Kosuge T, Makuuchi M, Takayama T, et al. Long-term results after resection of hepatocellular carcinoma: experience of 480 cases. Hepatogastroenterology 1993;40(4):328–32.

12. Okuda K, Ohtsuki T, Obata H, et al. Natural history of hepatocellular carcinoma and prognosis in relation to treatment. Study of 850 patients. Cancer 1985;56(4):918–28.

13. Cancer of the Liver Italian Program (CLIP) Investigators. A new prognostic system for hepatocellular carcinoma: a retrospective study of 435 patients. Hepatology 1998;28(3):751–5.

14. Cancer of the Liver Italian Program (CLIP) Investigators. Prospective validation of the CLIP score: a new prognostic system for patients with cirrhosis and hepatocellular carcinoma. Hepatology 2000;31(4):840–5.

15. Llovet JM, Bru C, Bruix J. Prognosis of hepatocellular carcinoma: the BCLC staging classification. Semin Liver Dis 1999;19(3):329–38.

16. Llovet JM, Fuster J, Bruix J. The Barcelona approach: diagnosis, staging, and treatment of hepatocellular carcinoma. Liver Transpl 2004;10(2 Suppl 1):S115–20.

17. Ng KK, Vauthey JN, Pawlik TM, et al. Is hepatic resection for large or multinodular hepatocellular carcinoma justified? Results from a multi-institutional database. Ann Surg Oncol 2005;12(5):364–73.

18. Pawlik TM, Poon RT, Abdalla EK, et al. Critical appraisal of the clinical and pathologic predictors of survival after resection of large hepatocellular carcinoma. Arch Surg 2005;140(5):450–7; discussion 457–8.

19. Staudacher C, Chiappa A, Biella F, et al. Validation of the modified TNM-Izumi classification for hepatocellular carcinoma. Tumori 2000;86(1):8–11.

20. Izumi R, Shimizu K, Ii T, et al. Prognostic factors of hepatocellular carcinoma in patients undergoing hepatic resection. Gastroenterology 1994;106(3):720–7.

21. Vauthey JN, Lauwers GY, Esnaola NF, et al. Simplified staging for hepatocellular carcinoma. J Clin Oncol 2002; 20(6):1527–36.

22. American Joint Committee on Cancer. AJCC Staging Manual. 6th ed. New York: Springer-Verlag, 2002.

23. Wu CC, Cheng SB, Ho WM, et al. Liver resection for hepatocellular carcinoma in patients with cirrhosis. Br J Surg 2005;92(3):348–55.

24. Ramacciato G, Mercantini P, Cautero N, et al. Prognostic evaluation of the new American Joint Committee on Cancer/International Union against cancer staging system for hepatocellular carcinoma: analysis of 112 cirrhotic patients resected for hepatocellular carcinoma. Ann Surg Oncol 2005;12(4):289–97.

25. Poon RT, Fan ST. Evaluation of the new AJCC/UICC staging system for hepatocellular carcinoma after hepatic resection in Chinese patients. Surg Oncol Clin N Am 2003; 12(1):35–50, viii.

26. Vauthey JN, Ribero D, Abdalla EK, et al. Outcome of liver transplantation with hepatocellular carcinoma: validation of a uniform staging after surgical treatment. J Am Coll Surg 2007 (in press).

27. Vauthey JN, Chaoui A, Do KA, et al. Standardized measurement of the future liver remnant prior to extended liver resection: methodology and clinical associations. Surgery 2000;127(5):512–9.

28. Abdalla EK, Barnett CC, Doherty D, et al. Extended hepatectomy in patients with hepatobiliary malignancies with and without preoperative portal vein embolization. Arch Surg 2002;137(6):675–80; discussion 680–1.

29. Kubota K, Makuuchi M, Kusaka K, et al. Measurement of liver volume and hepatic functional reserve as a guide to decision-making in resectional surgery for hepatic tumors. Hepatology 1997;26(5):1176–81.

30. Shirabe K, Shimada M, Gion T, et al. Postoperative liver failure after major hepatic resection for hepatocellular carcinoma in the modern era with special reference to remnant liver volume. J Am Coll Surg 1999;188(3):304–9.

31. Vauthey JN, Pawlik TM, Abdalla EK, et al. Is extended hepatectomy for hepatobiliary malignancy justified? Ann Surg 2004;239(5):722–30; discussion 730–2.

32. Vauthey JN, Abdalla EK, Doherty DA, et al. Body surface area and body weight predict total liver volume in Western adults. Liver Transpl 2002;8(3):233–40.

33. Hemming AW, Reed AI, Howard RJ, et al. Preoperative portal vein embolization for extended hepatectomy. Ann Surg 2003;237(5):686–91; discussion 691–3.

34. Makuuchi M, Thai BL, Takayasu K, et al. Preoperative portal embolization to increase safety of major hepatectomy for hilar bile duct carcinoma: a preliminary report. Surgery 1990;107(5):521–7.

35. Abdalla EK, Hicks ME, Vauthey JN. Portal vein embolization: rationale, technique and future prospects. Br J Surg 2001;88(2):165–75.

36. Madoff DC, Abdalla EK, Vauthey JN. Portal vein embolization in preparation for major hepatic resection: evolution of a new standard of care. J Vasc Interv Radiol 2005;16(6):779–90.

37. Nagino M, Kamiya J, Kanai M, et al. Right trisegment portal vein embolization for biliary tract carcinoma: technique and clinical utility. Surgery 2000;127(2):155–60.

38. Farges O, Belghiti J, Kianmanesh R, et al. Portal vein embolization before right hepatectomy: prospective clinical trial. Ann Surg 2003;237(2):208–17.

39. Madoff DC, Hicks ME, Abdalla EK, et al. Portal vein embolization with polyvinyl alcohol particles and coils in preparation for major liver resection for hepatobiliary malignancy: safety and effectiveness—study in 26 patients. Radiology 2003;227(1):251–60.

40. Rifkin MD, Rosato FE, Branch HM, et al. Intraoperative ultrasound of the liver. An important adjunctive tool for decision making in the operating room. Ann Surg 1987; 205(5):466–72.

41. Parker GA, Lawrence W Jr, Horsley JS 3rd, et al. Intraoperative ultrasound of the liver affects operative decision making. Ann Surg 1989;209(5):569–76; discussion 576–7.

42. Smith DL, Arens JF, Barnett CC Jr, et al. A prospective evaluation of ultrasound-directed transparenchymal vascular control with linear cutting staplers in major hepatic resections. Am J Surg 2005;190(1):23–9.

43. Hodgson WJ, Morgan J, Byrne D, DelGuercio LR. Hepatic resections for primary and metastatic tumors using the ultrasonic surgical dissector. Am J Surg 1992;163(2):246–50.

44. Rees M, Plant G, Wells J, Bygrave S. One hundred and fifty hepatic resections: evolution of technique towards blood-less surgery. Br J Surg 1996;83(11):1526–9.

45. Takayama T, Makuuchi M, Kubota K, et al. Randomized comparison of ultrasonic vs clamp transection of the liver. Arch Surg 2001;136(8):922–8.

46. Aloia TA, Zorzi D, Abdalla EK, Vauthey JN. Two-surgeon technique for hepatic parenchymal transection of the noncirrhotic liver using saline-linked cautery and ultrasonic dissection. Ann Surg 2005;242(2):172–7.

47. Makuuchi M, Takayama T, Gunven P, et al. Restrictive versus liberal blood transfusion policy for hepatectomies in cirrhotic patients. World J Surg 1989;13(5):644–8.

48. Shimada M, Matsumata T, Akazawa K, et al. Estimation of Risk of Major Complications after Hepatic Resection. American Journal of Surgery 1994;167(4):399–403.

49. Abdalla EK, Vauthey JN, Couinaud C. The caudate lobe of the liver: implications of embryology and anatomy for surgery. Surg Oncol Clin N Am 2002;11(4):835–48.

50. Belghiti J, Noun R, Malafosse R, et al. Continuous versus intermittent portal triad clamping for liver resection—a controlled study. Annals of Surgery 1999;229(3):369–375.

51. Delva E, Barberousse JP, Nordlinger B, et al. Hemodynamic and biochemical monitoring during major liver resection with use of hepatic vascular exclusion. Surgery 1984;95(3): 309–18.

52. Belghiti J, Noun R, Zante E, et al. Portal triad clamping or hepatic vascular exclusion for major liver resection. A controlled study. Ann Surg 1996;224(2):155–61.

53. Nonami T, Harada A, Kurokawa T, et al. Hepatic resection for hepatocellular carcinoma. Am J Surg 1997;173(4):288–91.

54. Chau GY, Lui WY, Tsay SH, et al. Prognostic significance of surgical margin in hepatocellular carcinoma resection: an analysis of 165 Childs' A patients. J Surg Oncol 1997; 66(2):122–6.

55. Fuster J, Garcia-Valdecasas JC, Grande L, et al. Hepatocellular carcinoma and cirrhosis. Results of surgical treatment in a European series. Ann Surg 1996;223(3):297–302.

56. Yoshida Y, Kanematsu T, Matsumata T, et al. Surgical margin and recurrence after resection of hepatocellular carcinoma in patients with cirrhosis. Further evaluation of limited hepatic resection. Ann Surg 1989;209(3):297–301.

57. Poon RT, Fan ST, Ng IO, Wong J. Significance of resection margin in hepatectomy for hepatocellular carcinoma: a critical reappraisal. Ann Surg 2000;231(4):544–51.

58. Regimbeau JM, Abdalla EK, Vauthey JN, et al. Risk factors for early death due to recurrence after liver resection for hepatocellular carcinoma: results of a multicenter study. J Surg Oncol 2004;85(1):36–41.

59. Penn I. Hepatic transplantation for primary and metastatic cancers of the liver. Surgery 1991;110(4):726–34; discussion 734–5.

60. Iwatsuki S, Gordon RD, Shaw BW Jr, Starzl TE. Role of liver transplantation in cancer therapy. Ann Surg 1985; 202(4):401–7.

61. Bismuth H, Chiche L, Adam R, et al. Liver resection versus transplantation for hepatocellular carcinoma in cirrhotic patients. Ann Surg 1993;218(2):145–51.

62. Mazzaferro V, Regalia E, Doci R, et al. Liver transplantation for the treatment of small hepatocellular carcinomas in patients with cirrhosis. N Engl J Med 1996;334(11):693–9.

63. Yoo HY, Patt CH, Geschwind JF, Thuluvath PJ. The outcome of liver transplantation in patients with hepatocellular carcinoma in the United States between 1988 and 2001: 5-year survival has improved significantly with time. J Clin Oncol 2003;21(23):4329–35.

64. Llovet JM, Schwartz M, Mazzaferro V. Resection and liver transplantation for hepatocellular carcinoma. Semin Liver Dis 2005;25(2):181–200.

65. Iwatsuki S, Dvorchik I, Marsh JW, et al. Liver transplantation for hepatocellular carcinoma: a proposal of a prognostic scoring system. J Am Coll Surg 2000;191(4): 389–94.

66. Poon RT, Fan ST, Lo CM, et al. Long-term survival and pattern of recurrence after resection of small hepatocellular carcinoma in patients with preserved liver function: implications for a strategy of salvage transplantation. Ann Surg 2002;235(3):373–82.

67. Belghiti J, Cortes A, Abdalla EK, et al. Resection prior to liver transplantation for hepatocellular carcinoma. Ann Surg 2003;238(6):885–92; discussion 892–3.

68. Adam R, Azoulay D, Castaing D, et al. Liver resection as a bridge to transplantation for hepatocellular carcinoma on cirrhosis: a reasonable strategy? Ann Surg 2003;238(4):508–18; discussion 518–9.

69. Ebara M, Ohto M, Sugiura N, et al. Percutaneous ethanol injection for the treatment of small hepatocellular carcinoma. Study of 95 patients. J Gastroenterol Hepatol 1990; 5(6):616–26.

70. Curley SA. Radiofrequency ablation of malignant liver tumors. Ann Surg Oncol 2003;10(4):338–47.

71. Montorsi M, Santambrogio R, Bianchi P, et al. Survival and recurrences after hepatic resection or radiofrequency for hepatocellular carcinoma in cirrhotic patients: a multivariate analysis. J Gastrointest Surg 2005;9(1):62–7; discussion 67–8.

72. Vivarelli M, Guglielmi A, Ruzzenente A, et al. Surgical resection versus percutaneous radiofrequency ablation in the treatment of hepatocellular carcinoma on cirrhotic liver. Ann Surg 2004;240(1):102–7.

73. Hong SN, Lee SY, Choi MS, et al. Comparing the outcomes of radiofrequency ablation and surgery in patients with a single small hepatocellular carcinoma and well-preserved hepatic function. J Clin Gastroenterol 2005;39(3):247–52.

74. Pawlik TM, Izzo F, Cohen DS, et al. Combined resection and radiofrequency ablation for advanced hepatic malignancies: results in 172 patients. Ann Surg Oncol 2003; 10(9):1059–69.

75. Lo CM, Ngan H, Tso WK, et al. Randomized controlled trial of transarterial lipiodol chemoembolization for unresectable hepatocellular carcinoma. Hepatology 2002; 35(5):1164–71.

76. Llovet JM, Real MI, Montana X, et al. Arterial embolisation or chemoembolisation versus symptomatic treatment in patients with unresectable hepatocellular carcinoma: a randomised controlled trial. Lancet 2002;359(9319):1734–9.

77. Levy I, Sherman M. Staging of hepatocellular carcinoma: assessment of the CLIP, Okuda, and Child-Pugh staging systems in a cohort of 257 patients in Toronto. Gut 2002; 50(6):881–5.

CHAPTER 12

SURGICAL TREATMENT OF COLORECTAL CANCER LIVER METASTASES

STEVEN A. CURLEY, MD

The liver, second only to lymph nodes as the most common site of metastasis from other solid tumors, is a common site of colorectal cancer (CRC) metastasis. A subset of patients with metastatic CRC have liver-only disease, or liver and resectable extrahepatic disease, and are candidates for surgical treatment. Resection of liver metastases can be performed with minimal mortality rates in these patients, and this procedure can provide long-term survival benefit in a significant proportion. Beliefs regarding which patients with hepatic metastases are candidates for resection or other surgical treatment need to be reevaluated through critical examination of extant data, and also by considering the impact of improved diagnostic imaging techniques, new cytotoxic and targeted molecular therapies, and improved patient selection and treatment criteria.

Candidates for Hepatic Resection

Data from the Registry of Hepatic Metastases reported in 1986 by Hughes and colleagues were instrumental in helping to define which patients may be good candidates for surgical resection of liver metastases.[1] The Registry included data on consecutive patients from 24 institutions who had undergone hepatic resection for CRC metastases. This retrospective review of 859 patients showed that hepatic resection was associated with a 5-year overall survival (OS) rate of approximately 33% and a disease-free survival (DFS) rate of approximately 25%. Patterns of recurrence were examined in a subgroup of 607 patients who underwent curative resection of isolated hepatic metastases, and indicated that adverse prognostic factors included extrahepatic disease, resec-

tion margin < 1.0 cm, a short disease-free interval (< 12 months), stage of primary tumor (II versus III), and number of metastases (> 3 or 4). Other large data sets from the US and Europe that have been reported have demonstrated similar 5-year survival rates with resection (Table 1): 28% among 1,568 patients as reported by Nordlinger and colleagues of the Association Francaise de Chirurgie (1996)[2]; 36% among 1,001 patients (median survival [MS], 42 months) as reported by Fong and colleagues (1999)[3]; and 33% among 597 patients (MS, 32 months) as reported by Scheele and co-workers (2001).[4]

There are, however, issues with the Hepatic Tumor Registry data (to some extent, shared with the other large data sets) regarding dogmatic acceptance of the identified prognostic factors to select candidates for surgical resection. These issues center on the fact that the data from all of these studies were collected retrospectively over an extended period of time. The Hepatic Tumor Registry data were collected from chart reviews from patients from 24 US institutions treated between 1948 and 1985.[1] In the years these patients were treated with liver resection, preoperative and intraoperative staging were not performed to current standards, with very few patients

Table 1 Survival Following Resection of Colorectal Cancer Liver Metastases; Results from Large Retrospective Series

Study	Number of patients	5-year overall survival rate	Median survival
Hughes et al 1986[1]	859	33%	-
Nordlinger et al 1996[2]	1,569	28%	-
Fong et al 1999[3]	1,001	36%	42 months
Scheele et al 2001[4]	597	33%	32 months

undergoing state-of-the-art computed tomography (CT) or magnetic resonance imaging (MRI). Few, if any, of the patients underwent intraoperative ultrasound imaging, which even in the era of modern CT and MRI detects additional hepatic metastases in up to 23% of patients.[5,6] In addition, the patient population was highly selected, with most (607 of 859) having a solitary liver metastasis.

Despite the authors' conclusion that candidates with more than 3 or 4 metastases were not candidates for resection, close scrutiny of the data indicated a 5-year actuarial survival rate of 18% among patients with > 3 metastases.[1] Systemic chemotherapy for patients with metastatic liver disease is improving, with newer agents providing better survival rates than the traditional 5-fluorouracil (5-FU)-based regimens.[7–11] Although the role of regional chemotherapy remains relatively undefined, it is clear that benefit can be achieved via this route in some cases. Novel biologic and molecular targeted agents are being evaluated that in combination with cytotoxic agents have further improved response rates.[12–15] These considerations have led surgical investigators to question the standard indications and contraindications for resection of colorectal cancer liver metastases. We must redefine and expand the role of surgery as part of the multimodality approach to treat patients with hepatic metastases, including patients who previously have not been considered candidates for surgical treatment.

Surgical Treatment of Patients with Multiple Metastases

Recent studies have demonstrated that resection in patients with four or more hepatic metastases from CRC can yield long-term survival in some patients. For example, Minagawa and colleagues reported that while survival was improved in patients with a solitary metastasis compared to those with multiple metastases, those undergoing complete resection of multiple liver lesions, including some patients with up to 20, still achieved 10-year survival rates in excess of 20%.[16] This study is the only report of a 10-year survival rate after resection of ≥ 4 CRC liver metastases. Several series reported since 2000, including Minagawa's, report 5-year survival rates that range from 21 to 37% after resection of multiple CRC liver metastases.[16–20] These modern day studies indicate that the total tumor volume, rather than the absolute number of metastases, is an important prognostic variable.[18] Furthermore, with thoughtful patient selection and planning of the volume of liver to be resected, mortality rates of $< 2\%$ should be expected in patients with multiple metastases. Aggressive resections of five or more hepatic segments is possible in some patients, particularly using modern volumetric liver

imaging studies to determine which patients would benefit from preoperative portal vein embolization (see the Chapter 11 on "Surgical Treatment of Hepatocellular Carcinoma" for indications and techniques for preoperative portal vein embolization).

Our group has examined our prospective database at The University of Texas M. D. Anderson Cancer Center that includes more than 1,300 patients undergoing resection of CRC liver metastases since 1995. Among 159 patients with 4 to 12 liver metastases that were treated with surgery (resection or resection and radiofrequency ablation), there was a 5-year actuarial DFS rate of 22% and a 5-year OS rate of 51%.[21] The median overall survival in these 159 patients was 62.1 months. The favorable long-term survival data in our study relates to the fact these patients were carefully selected. Every patient had no radiographic or intraoperative evidence of extrahepatic disease at the time of surgical treatment of their hepatic metastases, most received neoadjuvant chemotherapy (89.9%), the majority (72.7%) had reduction in tumor volume following preoperative chemotherapy, and all patients underwent thorough intraoperative ultrasonography to detect additional small lesions not evident on preoperative imaging studies. The number of tumors treated did not affect long-term survival probability. On multivariate analysis of predictive factors, only response to neoadjuvant chemotherapy remained an independent predictor of OS. Our data suggest that tumor biology (response to cytotoxic therapy) rather than morphologic criteria (tumor number, size) determines long-term prognosis.

A study from France confirms the significance of response to neoadjuvant chemotherapy in patients with more than four colorectal cancer liver metastases undergoing surgical treatment. A group of 131 consecutive patients who underwent surgical treatment of four or more colorectal cancer liver metastases after neoadjuvant chemotherapy was recently reported.[22] Of these 131 patients, 58 (44%) had a decrease in tumor volume with neoadjuvant chemotherapy, 39 (30%) had stable disease on chemotherapy, and 34 (26%) had tumor progression on chemotherapy. The 5-year survival rate for patients who responded to chemotherapy or had stable disease was 37% and 30%, respectively, compared to a 5-year survival rate in patients who progressed on chemotherapy of only 8% ($p < .0001$). DFS was also significantly lower in the patients who progressed on chemotherapy compared to the other two groups. This French study corroborates the findings from our study at the University of Texas M. D. Anderson Cancer Center, indicating that tumor biology, including response to chemotherapy, is more significant as a predictor of long-term outcome than the number of tumors.

Resection Margins

The retrospective Hepatic Tumor Registry data suggested that a tumor-free resection margin of < 1 cm was associated with a reduced probability of long-term survival.[1] Subsequently, several authors suggested that an inability to obtain at least a 1 cm tumor-free margin was either an absolute[23] or relative[24] contraindication to surgery for CRC liver metastases. However, until recently there has not been a rigorous evaluation of the effect of < 1 cm margins on either local recurrence or long-term survival in such patients.

A critical evaluation on the effect of surgical margin status on survival and local recurrence was recently reported.[25] A multicenter evaluation of 557 patients who underwent only hepatic resection for colorectal metastases found that the margin status was positive in 45 patients (8.1%), negative by 1 to 4 mm in 129 (23.1%), negative by 5 to 9 mm in 85 (15.3%), and was ≥ 1 cm in 298 (53.5%). The median survival for patients with a positive margin was 49.6 months, while the median survival in patients with negative margins had not yet been reached. A positive margin was associated with a significantly higher risk for a local recurrence, while there was no difference in local recurrence rates or in long-term survival rates comparing margins of 1 to 4 mm, 5 to 9 mm, or ≥ 1-cm. The 5-year survival rate for patients with margins 1 to 4 mm was 62.3%, 5 to 9 mm was 71.1%, and ≥ 1 cm was 63.0% ($p = 0.63$). In contrast, the 5-year survival rate in patients with positive margins was 17.1% ($p = .01$ versus all patients with negative margins; 63.8% 5-year survival rate). Thus, aggregate data suggest that a surgical margin of at least 1 mm appears to be acceptable and is not associated with a significantly higher risk of local recurrence or reduced probability of long-term survival. Surgeons should clearly use intraoperative ultrasonography and meticulous surgical technique to assure a tumor-free margin, even if it is minimal. It is not surprising that even a limited-margin complete resection can be associated with long-term survival given that colorectal liver metastases histopathologically are well circumscribed, are associated with satellitosis in only 16% of cases, extension through Glisson's capsule is uncommon (14.5%), and same-segment micrometastases are rare (2%).[25]

Stage of Primary CRC and Interval to Diagnosis of Metastases

The large retrospective studies on survival of patients undergoing resection for CRC liver metastases suggested that patients with node-positive (stage III) primary tumors, short interval between diagnosis of the primary cancer and development of liver metastases (synchronous or < 12 months), or both had a reduced probability of long-term survival.[1–4] Importantly, these studies predated the availability of modern cytotoxic chemotherapy agents, including oxaliplatin and irinotecan, and targeted biologic agents, including bevacizumab (antibody against vascular endothelial growth factor receptor) and cetuximab (antibody against epidermal growth factor receptor), which have significantly improved the outcome of patients with advanced CRC compared to the previously available agents 5-FU and leucovorin.[7–11] Recent surgical studies have failed to demonstrate any predictive significance for stage of the primary tumor or interval between the diagnosis of primary tumor and liver metastases.[21,22,25–28] These recent studies include a significant number of patients who have received neoadjuvant and/or adjuvant chemotherapy in addition to surgical treatment of their CRC liver metastases. The availability of current combination drug therapy regimens that include active cytotoxic and biologic agents may explain in part why stage of the primary tumor and interval between diagnosis of primary and metastatic disease are not significant prognostic variables in reports from the last 5 years.

Unfortunately, at this time there are no large prospective, randomized trials that have provided definitive proof for improved DFS or OS rates in patients receiving neoadjuvant or adjuvant chemotherapy and surgical treatment of their CRC liver metastases. Currently, the National Surgical Adjuvant Breast and Bowel Project is conducting a phase III trial (C-09) that compares two different adjuvant chemotherapy treatments following surgical treatment of CRC liver metastases (Figure 1). All patients in this two-arm study receive adjuvant chemotherapy; there is no surgery alone arm. The CLOCC (Chemotherapy plus Local ablation versus Chemotherapy) Intergroup trial in Europe and the US is designed to evaluate the role of local tumor ablation therapy in addition to systemic chemotherapy to determine if there is a benefit for thermal tumor ablation treatment plus chemotherapy compared to chemotherapy alone. This trial does not include an ablation alone arm, so again there will be no comparison of surgical treatments alone versus surgical treatments and chemotherapy. There are no ongoing trials that will compare surgical treatment of CRC liver metastases versus surgical treatment combined with chemotherapy. Because modern studies have demonstrated that there is no negative prognostic value for stage of the primary CRC or interval between diagnosis of primary and metastatic disease, patients should not be excluded from receiving aggressive surgical treatment of their liver metastases based on stage of primary tumor or whether the metastases were diagnosed synchronously or metachronously.

C-09 SCHEMA

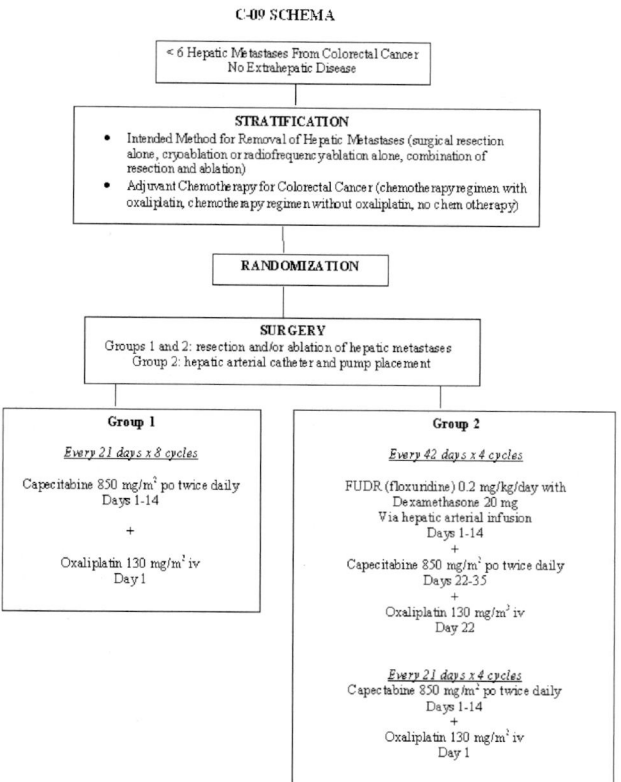

Figure 1 Randomization and treatment schema for the National Surgical Adjuvant Breast and Bowel Project (NSABP) phase III trial C-09.

Unresectable Liver Metastases or Extrahepatic Disease

The retrospective surgical series regarding outcome of patients undergoing resection for CRC liver metastases are based on highly selected subsets of patients. The majority of patients who develop CRC liver metastases will never be considered for surgical therapy because they present with extensive liver replacement by tumor liver lesions that are unresectable based on intrahepatic location, the pattern of metastases involves too many hepatic segments precluding resection that will leave an adequate volume of perfused liver (even with portal vein embolization), or the presence of extrahepatic metastatic disease to lymph nodes, lungs, the peritoneal cavity, or some other extrahepatic site. Based on the report by the Registry of Hepatic Metastases, the presence of extrahepatic disease came to be considered as an absolute contraindication to resection of liver metastases.[1] The presence of extrahepatic disease has clearly been demonstrated to be a negative prognostic factor in retrospective studies of CRC liver metastases treated with surgery alone.[1-4] This surgical dogma has been challenged in the modern era of multimodality management for CRC metastatic to the liver. A study by Adam and colleagues reported on a single institution experience of 1,439 consecutive patients presenting with CRC liver metastases.[29] At initial presentation, 1,104 (77%) of these patients were deemed to have unresectable disease and were treated by chemotherapy, while 335 (23%) were resectable and underwent surgical treatment. There were two very interesting findings from this study. First, among the 1,104 nonresectable patients, 138 (13%) had significant reduction in their tumor volume with chemotherapy and became candidates for a potentially curative surgical procedure. These 138 patients were treated with either resection alone or resection combined with thermal ablation. The overall 5- and 10-year survival rates in these 138 patients was 33% and 23%, respectively, with DFS rates at the same intervals of 22% and 17%, respectively. The second important finding was that an extrahepatic tumor was present at the time of surgical treatment in 52 of these 138 patients (38%). All of these patients underwent surgical treatment of their liver metastases along with resection of lung, lymph node, peritoneal, or other metastatic disease. When it was possible to treat all metastatic disease surgically, there was no significant decrease in the long-term survival probability compared to patients who underwent treatment of liver metastases alone.

Other groups have confirmed the finding that the presence of extrahepatic disease should not be an absolute contraindication to aggressive surgical therapy for CRC liver metastases.[16,30] When it is possible to treat hepatic and extrahepatic CRC metastases completely, particularly when combined with aggressive multimodality chemotherapeutic management, 5-year survival rates of 30% or higher may be achieved. Thus, patients who initially present with extrahepatic metastatic disease or with liver metastases thought to be unresectable when evaluated by an experienced hepatobiliary surgeon should receive state-of-the-art systemic chemotherapy. This is followed by complete surgical extirpation of all malignant disease when safe and feasible in those patients with significant reduction in their metastatic disease. The operative mortality rate (0.7%) and morbidity rate (28%) after aggressive surgical treatment of patients initially presenting with unresectable CRC liver metastases, with or without resectable extrahepatic disease, indicates that these operations can be performed safely with complication rates not higher than those in patients undergoing primary surgical treatment of resectable CRC liver metastases.[1-4,16-29]

Resection and Thermal Ablation of Liver Metastases

We recently reported the results of a prospective study of outcomes following surgical treatment of CRC liver metastases using hepatic resection only, radiofrequency ablation (RFA) plus resection for multiple tumors, or RFA only when patients had tumor in an in unresectable site in the liver. The study group consisted of 348 consecutive patients with colorectal liver metastases and no extrahepatic disease treated for cure with hepatic resection with or without RFA, as well as 70 patients found at laparotomy to have liver-only disease (patients were not candidates for curative treatment based on involvement of too many liver segments) (Figure 2). Of the 190 (45%) undergoing resection alone, 122 (64%) had a hemihepatectomy or more (91 with hemihepatectomy, 31 with extended resection) and 46 (24%) had an associated procedure (consisting of resection in 26, placement of an intra-arterial hepatic artery infusion pump in 13, or another intra-abdominal procedure in 7 [ileostomy or colostomy reversal]). Among the 101 (24%) patients undergoing resection and ablation, 56 (55%) had hemihepatectomy or more (37 with hemihepatectomy and 19 with extended resection), and 27 (27%) had an associated procedure (consisting of hepatic arterial infusion-pump placement in 19 and bowel resection in 8). An example of a case in which a combined approach of resection and ablation was used is illustrated in Figure 3. Among the 57 (14%) patients undergoing RFA alone, there was a median of 2 tumors (1 to 8) treated per patient, and tumors in all 8 hepatic segments were ablated; 8 patients (14%) had hepatic

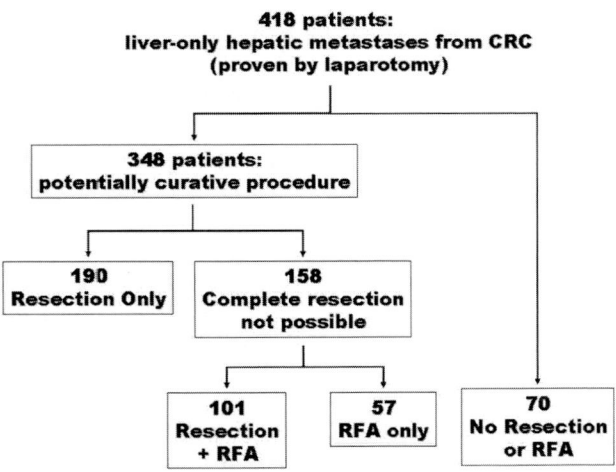

Figure 2 Treatment of 418 consecutive patients with liver-only colorectal cancer metastases at the University of Texas M. D. Anderson Cancer Center. CRC = colorectal cancer; RFA = radiofrequency ablation.

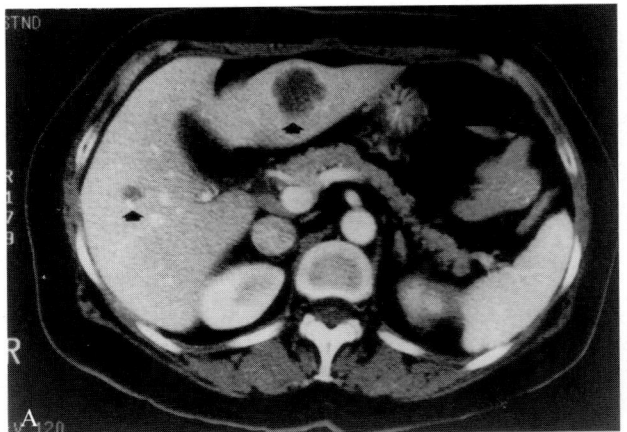

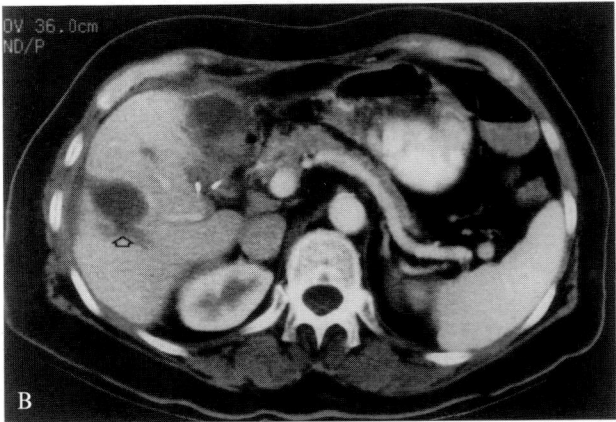

Figure 3 Example of case treated with resection and radiofrequency ablation. The patient had a large tumor in the left lateral segment. Also visible is one of four smaller tumors in the right lobe. The large tumor was resected, as was one of the smaller tumors near the dome. The other tumors were ablated, with ablation including a surrounding zone of the parenchyma to ensure a negative margin.

intra-arterial pumps placed. A total of 70 patients (17%) did not undergo resection or ablation after laparotomy revealed multiple hepatic metastases on ultrasound that were not detected on initial imaging studies; hepatic artery infusion pumps were placed in the majority of these patients for delivery of regional chemotherapy.

There were no significant differences among the resection-only, resection plus RFA, and RFA-only groups with regard to patient risk factors (gender, race, age > 65 years), primary tumor characteristics affecting prognosis (T stage, N stage, colon versus rectal cancer, DFS ≤ 12 months), liver tumor risk factors (carcinoembryonic antigen [CEA] > 200 ng/mL, tumor > 5 cm, number of tumors), or perioperative risk factors (hepatectomy versus segmental or wedge resection, surgical margin, blood loss). Rates of major complications were higher in the resection-only group (14%) and the resection plus RFA group (16%) than in the RFA-only group (4%).

There was a trend toward a higher 90-day mortality rate in the resection plus RFA group (7%) compared with the resection-only group (1%,) and the RFA-only group (0%); two patients in the resection plus RFA group died due to postoperative myocardial infarction.

The 5-year OS rate among the 348 patients treated with curative intent was 44%. Survival with resection alone (58% at 5 years) was significantly greater than with either resection plus ablation (28%) or RFA alone (19%, $p < .001$), with no significant difference between the approaches including RFA. The overall 4-year survival rates after resection, RFA + resection, and RFA-only were 65%, 36%, and 22%, respectively ($p < .0001$); however, 4-year survival rates with resection plus RFA and RFA-only were still substantial and significantly improved over that achieved with chemotherapy alone (5%) in the 70 patients not treated with resection or RFA ($p = .0017$). The recurrence-free survival rate was also significantly better in the resection-only group compared to the other two surgical groups ($p < .0001$).[28]

Multivariate analysis showed that presence of > 3 metastases was associated with significantly greater risk of death than presence of a solitary metastasis (hazard ratio [HR] 2.05; 95% confidence interval [CI], 1.11 to 3.78; $p = .021$); however, patients with > 3 metastases still had 5-year survival rates in excess of 50%. Both resection plus RFA (HR, 2.14; 95% CI, 1.28 to 3.59; $p = .004$) and RFA-only (HR, 2.79; 95% CI, 1.68 to 4.62; $p < .0001$) treatments were associated with a significantly increased risk of death compared with resection alone on multivariate analysis. Overall, although outcomes are improved with resection alone in patients with disease that was amenable to such treatment, the findings with regard to the approaches of resection plus RFA and RFA alone showed that both reasonable survival and low local-recurrence rates could be achieved (Table 2). Most notably, the 5-year survival rate of 58% seen in patients with disease that was treated successfully with resection

Table 2 Summary of Outcomes with Resection plus Radiofrequency Ablation (RFA) and RFA alone

	Resection + RFA	RFA alone
Recurrence rate	27%	44%
Liver	27%	9%
True local (incomplete ablation)	5%	9%
Recurrence-free survival		
1-year	46%	41%
4-year	18%	2%
Overall survival		
1-year	80%	92%
4-year	36%	22%

Adapted from Abdalla EK, et al.[28]

Table 3 Survival Following Resection of Colorectal Cancer Liver Metastases: Reports Since 2000

Study	Number of patients	5-year overall survival rate	Median survival
Choti et al 2002[26]	133	58%	-
Fernandez et al 2004[27]	100	58%	NR
Abdalla et al 2004[28]	190	58%	68 months
Pawlik et al 2005[25]	557	58%	74 months

NR = not reached.

alone is identical to the 5-year survival rates reported in three other recent studies (Table 3).[25–27] Importantly, with modern surgical and anesthesia management in patients undergoing major liver resection for colorectal metastases, 90-day operative mortality rates are $< 2\%$ and morbidity rates are below 30%.[25–28] Our prospective evaluations of new resection techniques reveal that these operations are safe, even when extended hepatectomy is required, and are associated with transfusion rates of 5% or less.[31–33]

Concerns with Neoadjuvant Therapy

Systemic chemotherapy may convert some patients with unresectable CRC liver metastases to a resectable status, and response to neoadjuvant chemotherapy in patients with resectable disease is an important prognostic indicator of improved probability of long-term survival.[21,29,34,35] The use of neoadjuvant chemotherapy in patients with resectable CRC liver metastases must be carefully considered in multidisciplinary treatment planning involving medical oncologists and hepatobiliary surgical oncologists. Concerns about the anti-angiogenic activity of bevacizumab impairing hepatic regeneration after resection coupled with the long circulating half-life of this drug has led to the recommendation to wait 6 to 8 weeks after the last dose of this drug before preceding with liver resection.[36] Neoadjuvant chemotherapy regimens that are based on oxaliplatin or irinotecan can produce specific types of liver injury. Oxaliplatin-based chemotherapy was reported to cause sinusoidal obstruction, veno-occlusive lesions in the microvasculature of nontumoral liver, and perisinusoidal fibrosis in over half of the patients receiving neoadjuvant therapy.[37] Both irinotecan and oxaliplatin treatment have been found to produce nonalcoholic steatohepatitis (NASH), and the severity of NASH is greater in patients who are also obese.[38] Hepatic steatosis or steatohepatitis was identified as an independent variable predicting increased perioperative morbidity and mortality rates in a retrospective study of 135 patients undergoing resection of CRC liver metastases.[39] Data suggest that steatosis impairs hepatic regeneration after resection and the rates of liver insufficiency and hyperbilirubinemia are higher in patients with hepatic steatosis compared to patients with normal liver. Another recent study found that patients with steatosis who underwent a major liver resection had a nonsignificant trend toward higher mortality compared to patients with a nonsteatotic liver.[40] The same study indicated there was a significantly higher complication rate in patients with steatosis compared to patients with a normal liver, with the most notable increase in complications being related to wound problems (seromas, infections, and hernias) and to liver-related problems (cholangitis, biliary obstruction, liver failure or insufficiency, ascites, perihepatic fluid collection, and perihepatic abscess).

A multi-institution review of 406 patients who underwent resection of CRC liver metastases using a standardized system to score the severity of NASH and nonalcoholic fatty liver disease (NAFLD) has been recently completed.[41,42] Preoperative chemotherapy was administered to 248 (61%), while 158 (39%) patients received no neoadjuvant treatment. Patients received a variety of chemotherapy regimens based on 5-FU alone, or 5- FU and irinotecan or 5- FU and oxaliplatin. Patients who received oxaliplatin were found to have sinusoidal dilatation at a much higher frequency compared to patients who did not receive chemotherapy ($p < .001$). In contrast, patients who received irinotecan had an approximately 20% incidence of NASH, which was significantly greater than the 4% rate seen in patients who received no chemotherapy ($p < .001$). The most striking finding of this study was that only NASH was associated with an increased 90-day mortality rate (14.7%) after liver resection while patients with other types of liver injury or normal liver had a postoperative mortality rate of only 1.6% ($p < .001$). Clearly, very careful consideration must be given to the type and duration of neoadjuvant chemotherapy to be delivered to patients, particularly in patients who are also obese. In patients who have preoperative imaging or intraoperative evidence of either NAFLD or NASH, consideration should be given to obtaining a core liver biopsy to assess the severity of steatohepatitis. The presence of severe NASH should lead the surgeon to question the safety of a major liver resection and lower the threshold to consider preoperative portal vein embolization in an attempt to reduce postoperative morbidity and liver failure rates.

Conclusion

The gold standard in the treatment of CRC liver metastases remains complete resection. Complete resection can be performed safely with low morbidity and mortality as well as low local recurrence rates, even with minimal tumor-free margins. Local hepatic tumor ablation techniques do have a role in treatment of patients with unresectable disease. Ablation, with or without resection, appears to provide long-term survival benefit in some patients who, on the basis of having multiple metastases or tumor involving key vascular structures, would otherwise not be considered candidates for surgery. However, it needs to be emphasized that no data currently exist to suggest that either RFA or RFA combined with resection provides survival comparable to complete resection, and that long-term survival rates in patients treated with thermal ablation techniques are still being established. Aggressive surgical management combined with neoadjuvant and adjuvant chemotherapy regiments has yielded 5-year survival rates that exceed 50%. All patients with CRC liver metastases should be evaluated by a multidisciplinary team consisting of hepatobiliary surgical oncologists, medical oncologists, pathologists, and diagnostic imaging specialists to optimize the management of this fascinating group with stage IV disease.

References

1. Hughes KS, Simon R, Songhorabodi S, et al. Resection of the liver for colorectal carcinoma metastases: a multi-institutional study of patterns of recurrence. Surgery 1986; 100:278–84.

2. Nordlinger B, Guiguet M, Vaillant JC, et al. Surgical resection of colorectal carcinoma metastases to the liver. A prognostic scoring system to improve case selection, based on 1,568 patients. Association Francaise de Chirurgie. Cancer 1996;77:1254–62.

3. Fong Y, Fortner J, Sun RL, et al. Clinical score for predicting recurrence after hepatic resection for metastatic colorectal cancer: analysis of 1,001 consecutive cases. Ann Surg 1999;230:309–18; discussion 318–21.

4. Scheele J, Altendorf-Hofmann A, Grube T, et al. Resection of colorectal liver metastases. What prognostic factors determine patient selection? [article in German]. Chirurg 2001;72:547–60.

5. Scaife CL, Ng CS, Ellis LM, et al. Accuracy of preoperative imaging of hepatic tumors with helical computed tomography. Ann Surg Oncol 2006;13:1–5.

6. Conlon R, Jacobs M, Dasgupta D, Lodge JP. The value of intraoperative ultrasound during hepatic resection compared with improved preoperative magnetic resonance imaging. Eur J Ultrasound 2003;16:211–6.

7. Levi F, Zidani R, Brienza S, et al. A multicenter evaluation of intensified, ambulatory, chronomodulated chemotherapy with oxaliplatin, 5-fluorouracil, and leucovorin as initial treatment of patients with metastatic colorectal

carcinoma. International Organization for Cancer Chronotherapy. Cancer 1999;85:2532–40.

8. Douillard JY, Cunningham D, Roth AD, et al. Irinotecan combined with fluorouracil compared with fluorouracil alone as first-line treatment for metastatic colorectal cancer: a multicentre randomised trial. [erratum appears in Lancet 2000 Apr 15;355(9212):1372]. Lancet 2000;355: 1041–7.

9. Giacchetti S, Perpoint B, Zidani R, et al. Phase III multicenter randomized trial of oxaliplatin added to chronomodulated fluorouracil-leucovorin as first-line treatment of metastatic colorectal cancer. J Clin Oncol 2000;18:136–47.

10. de Gramont A, Figer A, Seymour M, et al. Leucovorin and fluorouracil with or without oxaliplatin as first-line treatment in advanced colorectal cancer. J Clin Oncol 2000;18:2938–47.

11. Goldberg RM, Sargent DJ, Morton RF, et al. A randomized controlled trial of fluorouracil plus leucovorin, irinotecan, and oxaliplatin combinations in patients with previously untreated metastatic colorectal cancer. [see comment]. J Clin Oncol 2004;22:23–30.

12. Varadhachary GR, Hoff PM. Front-line therapy for advanced colorectal cancer: emphasis on chemotherapy. Sem Oncol 2005;32:S40–42.

13. Goldberg RM. Advances in the treatment of metastatic colorectal cancer. Oncologist 2005;10:40–8.

14. Chong G, Cunningham D. The role of cetuximab in the therapy of previously treated advanced colorectal cancer. Sem Oncol 2005;32:S55–8.

15. Marshall J. The role of bevacizumab as first-line-therapy for colon cancer. Sem Oncol 2005;32:S43–7.

16. Minagawa M, Makuuchi M, Torzilli G, et al. Extension of the frontiers of surgical indications in the treatment of liver metastases from colorectal cancer: long-term results. Ann Surg 2000;231:487–99.

17. Bolton JS, Fuhrman GM. Survival after resection of multiple bilobar hepatic metastases from colorectal carcinoma. Ann Surg 2000;231:743–51.

18. Ercolani G, Grazi GL, Ravaioli M, et al. Liver resection for multiple colorectal metastases: influence of parenchymal involvement and total tumor volume, vs number or location, on long-term survival. Arch Surg 2002;137:1187–92.

19. Weber SM, Jarnagin WR, DeMatteo RP, et al. Survival after resection of multiple hepatic colorectal metastases. Ann Surg Oncol 2000;7:643–50.

20. Kokudo N, Imamura H, Sugawara Y, et al. Surgery for multiple hepatic colorectal metastases. J Hepatobiliary Pancreat Surg 2004;11:84–91.

21. Pawlik TM, Abdalla EK, Ellis LM, et al. Debunking dogma: surgery for four or more colorectal liver metastases is justified. J Gastrointest Surg 2006;10:240–8.

22. Adam R, Pascal G, Castaing D, et al. Tumor progression while on chemotherapy: a contraindication to liver resection for multiple colorectal metastases? Ann Surg 2004;240:1052–61; discussion 1061–4.

23. Cady B, Jenkins RL, Steele GD Jr, et al. Surgical margin in hepatic resection for colorectal metastasis: a critical and improvable determinant of outcome. Ann Surg 1998;227: 566–71.

24. Shirabe K, Takenaka K, Gion T, et al. Analysis of prognostic risk factors in hepatic resection for metastatic colorectal carcinoma with special reference to the surgical margin. Br J Surg 1997;84:1077–80.

25. Pawlik TM, Scoggins CR, Zorzi D, et al. Effect of surgical margin status on survival and site of recurrence after hepatic resection for colorectal metastases. Ann Surg 2005; 241:715–22.

26. Choti MA, Sitzmann JV, Tiburi MF, et al. Trends in long-term survival following liver resection for hepatic colorectal metastases. Ann Surg 2002;235:759–66.

27. Fernandez FG, Drebin JA, Linehan DC, et al. Five-year survival after resection of hepatic metastases from colorectal cancer in patients screened by positron emission tomography with F-18 fluorodeoxyglucose (FDG-PET). Ann Surg 2004;240:438–7; discussion 447–50.

28. Abdalla EK, Vauthey JN, Ellis LM, et al. Recurrence and outcomes following hepatic resection, radiofrequency ablation, and combined resection/ablation for colorectal liver metastases. Ann Surg 2004;239:818–25; discussion 825–7.

29. Adam R, Delvart V, Pascal G, et al. Rescue surgery for unresectable colorectal liver metastases downstaged by chemotherapy: a model to predict long-term survival. Ann Surg 2004;240:644–57; discussion 657–8.

30. Elias D, Ouellet JF, Bellon N, et al. Extrahepatic disease does not contraindicate hepatectomy for colorectal liver metastases. Br J Surg 2003;90:567–74.

31. Smith DL, Arens JF, Barnett CC Jr, et al. A prospective evaluation of ultrasound-directed transparenchymal vascular control with linear cutting staplers in major hepatic resections. Am J Surg 2005;190:23–9.

32. Aloia TA, Zorzi D, Abdalla EK, Vauthey JN. Two-surgeon technique for hepatic parenchymal transection of the noncirrhotic liver using saline-linked cautery and ultrasonic dissection. Ann Surg 2005;242:172–7.

33. Vauthey JN, Pawlik TM, Abdalla EK, et al. Is extended hepatectomy for hepatobiliary malignancy justified? Ann Surg 2004;239:722–30; discussion 730–2.

34. Tanaka K, Adam R, Shimada H, et al. Role of neoadjuvant chemotherapy in the treatment of multiple colorectal metastases to the liver. Br J Surg 2003;90:963–9.

35. Allen PJ, Kemeny N, Jarnagin W, et al. Importance of response to neoadjuvant chemotherapy in patients under-

going resection of synchronous colorectal liver metastases. J Gastrointest Surg 2003;7:109–15; discussion 116–7.

36. Ellis LM, Curley SA, Grothey A. Surgical resection after downsizing of colorectal liver metastasis in the era of bevacizumab. J Clin Oncol 2005;23:4853–5.

37. Rubbia-Brandt L, Audard V, Sartoretti P, et al. Severe hepatic sinusoidal obstruction associated with oxaliplatin-based chemotherapy in patients with metastatic colorectal cancer. Ann Oncol 2004;15:460–6.

38. Fernandez FG, Ritter J, Goodwin JW, et al. Effect of steatohepatitis associated with irinotecan or oxaliplatin pretreatment on resectability of hepatic colorectal metastases. J Am Coll Surg 2005;200:845–53.

39. Behrns KE, Tsiotos GG, DeSouza NF, et al. Hepatic steatosis as a potential risk factor for major hepatic resection. J Gastrointest Surg 1998;2:292–8.

40. Kooby DA, Fong Y, Suriawinata A, et al. Impact of steatosis on perioperative outcome following hepatic resection. J Gastrointest Surg 2003;7:1034–44.

41. Kleiner DE, Brunt EM, Van Natta M, et al. Design and validation of a histological scoring system for nonalcoholic fatty liver disease. Hepatology 2005;41:1313–21.

42. Vauthey JN, Pawlik TM, Ribero D, et al. Chemotherapy regimen predicts steatohepatitis and an increase in ninety-day mortality after surgery for hepatic colorectal metastases. J Clin Oncol 2006;24:2065–72.

CHAPTER 13

Surgical Treatment of Neuroendocrine Liver Metastases

Todd M. Tuttle, MD

Timothy D. Sielaff, MD, PhD

Bryan A. Whitson, MD

Gastrointestinal (GI) neuroendocrine tumors (NETs) are rare malignancies with an incidence of 1 to 2 per 100,000 people.[1] A substantial proportion of these patients will have either synchronous or metachronous liver metastases. Metastatic disease is often confined to the liver, but usually involves both lobes. As a result, most patients with NET liver metastases are not candidates for complete surgical resection. Because NET liver metastases may cause local symptoms (pain) and systemic effects from hormone secretion (5-hydroxytryptamine, gastrin, insulin, and vasoactive intestinal peptide [VIP]), treatment strategies must not only address tumor control, but also overall quality of life.

Although a small fraction of NETs originate in the liver, most metastasize to the liver from other sites. The majority of NETs arise sporadically, but a few occur in the setting of multiple endocrine neoplasia syndrome type 1 (MEN-1). GI NETs are generally classified as either carcinoid or islet cell tumors. Midgut carcinoids originate in the distal duodenum, jejunum, ileum, appendix, ascending colon, and liver. These tumors secrete high levels of serotonin, are usually responsible for carcinoid syndrome, and represent the majority of carcinoid liver metastases. Small bowel carcinoid tumors are multifocal in 25% of patients and may be associated with other malignancies, such as adenocarcinoma of the large bowel. Islet cell tumors include gastrinomas, glucagonomas, insulinomas, VIPomas, nonfunctioning tumors, and polypeptide-secreting tumors.

The long-term survival of patients with untreated liver metastases from NETs is significantly longer as compared with patients with colorectal cancer (CRC) liver metastases. Moertel reported a 30% 5-year survival rate for patients with untreated liver metastases from NETs.[2] With advances in medical therapy of hormonal symptoms (somatostatin analogues, proton-pump inhibitors), survival of patients with metastatic NETs is usually dependent upon control of liver metastases. However, nonsurgical therapies alone have had limited success in improving overall survival.

Radiographic Evaluation of NET Liver Metastases

Axial imaging studies and whole body scintigraphy can be used in combination to stage patients at the time of initial presentation of NET and before initiating liver-directed therapy for metastatic disease. As the fidelity of the imaging tests improves, the ability to stage patients accurately and predict response to therapy will improve as well.

Many patients with NET develop symptoms associated with liver metastases. Conventional computed tomography (CT) is an important tool, but studies not performed with a dedicated liver protocol (in which arterial phase contrast images are obtained) can underestimate the extent of disease. As many as 75% of neuroendocrine liver metastases are hypervascular.[3]

Thirty percent of metastatic lesions are identified best in the arterial phase, and 6% of these may be seen exclusively in the arterial phase.[4]

Somatostatin receptor scintigraphy (SRS) is performed with the injection of indium-111 labeled octreotide (Pentetreotide; OctreoScan—Maloinckrodt Medical, The Netherlands) exploiting the expression of somatostatin subtype II receptors in the majority of NET.[5] SRS appears to be highly accurate, and when compared to conventional CT scanning alone, it is associated with an upstaging of a significant number of patients. In a study directly comparing CT, magnetic resonance imaging (MRI), and SRS, Dromain and colleagues reported 66 consecutive patients who had NETs with and without liver metastases.[6] MRI detected significantly more liver metastases than CT and SRS; CT detected more liver metastases than SRS alone. The relative sensitivities of SRS, CT, and MRI were 49.3%, 78.5%, and 95.2%, respectively. The imaging characteristics of the metastases were hypervascular in 77% of patients and hypovascular in 23% of patients. A miliary (diffuse) pattern was seen in 22% of patients. Of the patients who had a negative SRS, 17.5% were found to be positive on CT and MRI. These authors conclude that MRI is an essential tool in the evaluation of patients with NET liver metastasis, but that SRS plays a complimentary role in detecting extrahepatic disease. They also found that somatostatin analogue therapy did not have a negative impact on the performance of SRS. New techniques such as 5-hydroxy-L-tryptophan positron emission tomography may prove to be useful in the future. While a routine contrast-enhanced CT is sufficient for the general evaluation of patients with NET, a liver protocol MRI is recommended for the evaluation of a patient as a prelude to liver-directed therapy. SRS should also be performed in these patients to evaluate for the presence and extent of extrahepatic disease.

Laboratory Evaluation of NET Liver Metastases

Serotonin and 5-hydroxy indole acetic acid (5-HIAA) have been used to diagnose and follow patients with carcinoid tumors for many years. Serotonin levels can be measured in platelets, serum, and the urine; the serotonin breakdown product, 5-HIAA, can be measured in the urine. Midgut tumors tend to have the highest levels of urinary 5-HIAA and serum/platelet serotonin. Patients with gastric and pancreatic carcinoid tumors tend to have higher levels of urinary serotonin.

Elevated 5-HIAA levels are associated with the presence of liver metastases and a risk of death.[7] 5-HIAA levels have been shown to fluctuate with the efficacy of therapy, and these fluctuations are thought to reflect reduced tumor proliferation. However, 5-HIAA levels do not necessary correlate with symptomatology.[8]

While urinary 5-HIAA levels have been a standard in the clinical management of patients with neuroendocrine malignancies, plasma chromogranin A (a molecule important to the generation and sorting of intracellular granules) levels are increasingly employed. Serum chromogranin A levels are useful in detecting NETs, though levels may also be elevated in patients with adenocarcinomas as well.[9] Serum chromogranin A levels are elevated in over 90% of patients with metastatic NET and are the best test for following patients with metastatic and symptomatic NETs as it correlates with tumor burden.[10] The preferential use of serum chromogranin A is recommended for the surveillance of patients undergoing liver-directed therapy for NETs.

Nonsurgical Therapy

The primary aims of medical therapy for NET liver metastases are palliation of symptoms and tumor control or regression. Somatostatin analogs, such as octreotide, inhibit release and action of multiple GI hormones and improve symptoms from hyperfunctioning NET metastases. Treatment with octreotide relieves symptoms from carcinoid syndrome in approximately 75% of patients, may control tumor growth, and in a small proportion of patients cause regression in liver metastases.[11] Adverse reactions to octreotide are predominantly GI in origin and include nausea, loose stools, cholelithiasis, and abdominal discomfort. Many patients become partially resistant to long-term octreotide therapy.

Single-agent chemotherapy has been ineffective in controlling tumor growth of metastatic NETs. The results of streptozocin alone or in combination with 5-fluoruracil (5-FU) or anthracyclines have been disappointing. Octreotide plus interferon-alpha may improve tumor response rates, but overall survival is not significantly improved.[12] Other treatment strategies include therapeutic meta-iodobenzylguanidine (MIBG) and radiolabeled-somatostatin analogues.

In patients with unresectable liver metastases, selective hepatic artery ligation or embolization can produce objective tumor response rates and transient reduction in hormone secretion. Antitumor responses and reduction in tumor markers may be enhanced with hepatic arterial chemoembolization. Chemoembolization typically involves a cocktail of chemotherapeutic drugs (streptozocin, 5-FU, doxorubicin, cisplatin, etc.) with saline and iodine containing oil that is then injected into the branches of the hepatic artery distal to the origin of the gastroduodenal artery. Embolization is subsequently performed with gelatin foam or microspheres injected into the arterial branches supplying the tumors. Kim and colleagues reported an overall partial response rate of 37% after chemoembolization for 30 patients with liver metastases from carcinoid or islet cell tumors.[13] Contraindications to chemoembolization include complete portal vein occlusion, hepatic failure, or prior biliary anastomosis. Presently, chemotherapy and embolization should be reserved for patients with unresectable or recurrent NET metastases. Minor side effects after chemoembolization are common and typically include abdominal pain, fever, elevated liver transaminases, nausea, and vomiting. Major complications are rare, but bleeding ulcers, infection, and hepatic and renal failure have been reported.

Surgical Therapy

PERIOPERATIVE CONSIDERATIONS

Special perioperative risks must be considered for patients with NET liver metastases. Induction of general anesthesia may induce life-threatening carcinoid crisis manifested by hypotension and bronchospasm. Thus, preoperative and perioperative octreotide treatment is required for patients with carcinoid liver metastases. Existing cardiac valvular disease from metastatic carcinoid tumors may be associated with increased central venous pressure, which can lead to massive bleeding during hepatic parenchymal dissection. Sarmiento and Que report that 28% of patients with carcinoid liver metastases had coexisting valvulopathy.[14] Thus, these patients should be evaluated with electrocardiogram, chest radiograph, and echocardiograms before liver resection. If severe valvular disease is detected, then valve repair should be performed prior to hepatic

resection. Cholecystectomy should be completed at the time of liver resection because many patients will require future octreotide therapy, which may induce cholelithiasis or chemoembolization, which may cause gallbladder necrosis or chemical cholecystitis. Intraoperative hepatic ultrasonography is mandatory to identify and treat all liver metastases.

RESECTION OF LIVER METASTASES

Liver resection is the key element of multimodality therapy for NET liver metastases. Table 1 lists the modern series that include at least 15 nonrepetitive patients undergoing liver resection for NET.[15–21] The 5-year survival rate is approximately 60 to 70% after liver resection. These results compare favorably to historical data, which estimate 30% 5-year survival for untreated patients.[2] Effective symptomatic relief is achieved in approximately 90% of patients after liver resection. Complete surgical resection is not likely in patients with 75% or more of their liver replaced with tumor. Even though these tumors are usually bilateral and require major hepatic resections, operative mortality and morbidity rates are acceptable and similar to those reported for resection of colorectal liver metastases.

In the largest reported series of liver resection for NETs, Sarmiento and colleagues described the outcome of 170 patients treated at the Mayo Clinic from 1977 to 1998.[16] Small-bowel carcinoid was the most common primary tumor. Hepatic metastases were bilateral in 76% of patients. Complete resection (R0) was possible in 75 patients (44%). Partial or complete relief of symptoms from excess hormone secretion was achieved in 96% of patients; the median time to symptom recurrence was 45.5 months. Tumor recurrence rates were 84% at 5 years and 94% at 10 years. Complete tumor resection was associated with significantly lower recurrence rates. The survival rate was 61% at 5 years and 35% at 10 years; median survival was 81 months.

Retrospective studies have demonstrated that patients who undergo liver resection have improved survival as compared with those patients with unresected

Table 1 Results of Liver Resection for NET Liver Metastases

Author	Year	N	Operative Mortality (%)	Complete Resection (%)	Survival
Chamberlain[15]	2000	34	6	44%	5 yr: 76%
Sarmiento[16]	2003	170	1.2	44%	5 yr: 61%
Chen[17]	1998	15	0	100%	5 yr: 73%
Grazi[18]	2000	19	0	84%	4 yr: 93%
Norton[19]	2003	16	0	100%	5 yr: 82%
Nave[20]	2001	31	0	32%	5 yr: 47%
Dousset[21]	1996	17	5.9	71%	5 yr: 46%

Table 2 Factors Limiting Survival Analyses for NET Liver Metastases

1. Rare tumors
2. Prolonged survival in untreated patients
3. Variable natural history
4. Retrospective studies spanning several decades
5. Heterogenous tumors
   a) Functional versus. nonfunctional
   b) Hereditary versus spontaneous
   c) Carcinoid versus islet cell tumors
6. No universally accepted staging system
7. Difficulty in subtyping tumors with immunohistochemistry

tumors.[15,17] In a retrospective analysis of 38 patients, Chen and colleagues from Johns Hopkins reported a 5-year survival rate of 73% after liver resection for NET metastases versus 29% for patients who did not undergo resection.[17] However, such survival analyses of NET livermetastases are significantly limited by multiple factors listed in Table 2. Nevertheless, the available data strongly suggest that liver resection prolongs overall survival and improves quality of life, but rarely produces a "cure."

Many patients with NET liver metastases have intact primary tumors in the stomach, small intestine, or pancreas. We recommend synchronous resection of the primary tumor, liver metastases, and extrahepatic metastases if all disease can be safely removed (Figure 1). Norton and colleagues described the outcomes of 16 patients with liver plus extrahepatic disease treated with aggressive surgery at the University of California San Francisco.[19] Liver-directed surgery included 5 right or left hepatectomies, 1 extended right hepatectomy, 10 wedge resections, and 2 radiofrequency ablation (RFA) procedures. All liver disease was completely treated as determined by intraoperative ultrasound. Small bowel resection, gastrectomy, pancreatectomy, and low anterior resection were performed to treat extrahepatic disease. Despite extensive surgery, postoperative complications occurred in only 19% patients with no operative deaths. All 8 patients with carcinoid syndrome had amelioration of symptoms and lowering of serum tumor markers. Two of the five patients with gastrinoma had complete amelioration of symptoms and lowering of serum tumor markers. The actuarial 5-year survival rate from this series was 82%.

PROGNOSTIC FACTORS

Because most surgical series are relatively small, identifying prognostic factors after liver resection for NET is difficult. The most consistent prognostic factor is completeness of resection. Nave and colleagues reported that the 5-year survival rate was significantly improved if all disease was completely resected (complete resection: 86%; incomplete resection: 26%).[20] Tumor type (carcinoid versus islet cell) does not appear to be a significant prognostic factor.[16] Likewise, gender, patient age, and preoperative hormonal symptoms probably do not influence survival after liver resection. Existing data do not support the use of adjuvant chemotherapy for asymptomatic patients after liver resection for all gross disease.

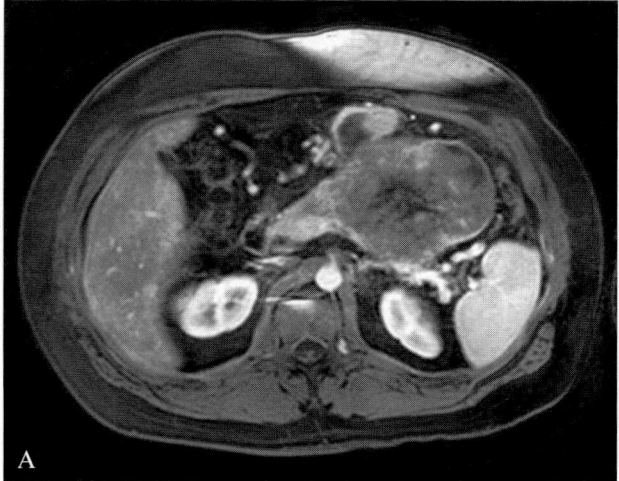
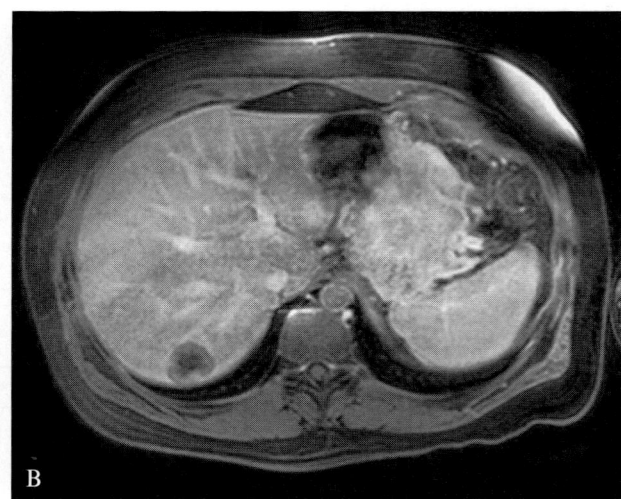

Figure 1 Magnetic resonance imaging demonstrates a 10 cm pancreatic neuroendocrine tumor (A) with liver metastases (B). Concurrent distal pancreatectomy, splenectomy, and liver resection were performed with no postoperative complications. The patient was discharged from the hospital 6 days after surgery.

RFA

RFA is an effective ablative treatment that has been used primarily to treat unresectable hepatocellular carcinoma and CRC liver metastases. Because most NET liver metastases are multiple and bilateral, RFA may be used either alone or combined with chemoembolization or resection. The three main approaches to RFA are open, laparoscopic, and percutaneous. Open RFA is especially useful to treat central or deep-seated lesions while other metastases are resected. Berber and colleagues reported the outcomes of 34 patients with NET liver metastases (including 7 patients with metastatic medullary thyroid cancer) treated with laparoscopic RFA.[22] Laparoscopic RFA was safe with no perioperative mortality, 5% morbidity rate, and average hospital stay of 1.1 days. Preoperative symptoms were ameliorated in 95% of patients, with significant or complete symptom control in 80% of patients for a mean of 10.1 months. Percutaneous RFA is preferred for patients who have significant comorbidities and are poor candidates for general anesthesia or have hostile abdomens (for instance, after hepatic resection). However, percutaneous RFA is limited by the inability to perform intraoperative hepatic ultrasound, resulting in failure to recognize small tumors not visualized on preoperative imaging and by the lack of peritoneal staging.

PALLIATIVE LIVER RESECTION

For patients with unresectable metastases, some authors have recommended cytoreductive surgery (R2) if 90% or more of gross disease can be treated.[14] The rationale for incomplete surgical treatment is that NET liver metastases are typically slow growing tumors, and cytoreductive surgery may provide effective palliation and prolong survival. Moreover, because a "cure" is rarely achieved in patients with NET liver metastases, complete resection may be regarded as a more thorough cytoreduction. McEntee and colleagues reported that 50% of patients with symptomatic endocrinopathies treated with palliative surgery experienced complete symptom relief after surgery; however, the mean duration of complete relief was only 6 months.[23]

Presently, no solid data exist to guide surgeons in determining how much tumor volume (95% versus 90% versus 80%, etc.) should be resected in an effort to improve the symptoms and prolong the survival of patients with unresectable tumors. Furthermore, because symptom-free survival is significantly less after incomplete resection, the rationale for performing radical non-R0 resections is unclear. If preoperative imaging indicates that complete resection is not possible, we prefer to utilize minimally invasive treatments such as laparo-scopic RFA and chemoembolization for symptom control. These therapies do not "burn bridges" and frequently can be repeated as necessary.

SURVEILLANCE AFTER LIVER-DIRECTED THERAPY

The goal of a postoperative surveillance program after liver resection is to identify recurrent tumor with the premise that early intervention improves outcome. The most common site of recurrent disease after liver resection for NETs is within the remnant liver. Repeat liver resection or RFA may prolong overall and symptom-free survival for selected patients with isolated liver recurrence. With the objective of identifying recurrent tumor amenable to either resection or RFA, we obtain abdominal CT scans every 4 months for 2 years and then every 6 months thereafter. Chromogranin A or other specific serum hormone levels (eg, gastrin) are obtained at the same intervals.

Liver Transplantation for NET

The initial liberal application of liver transplantation for metastatic NET in the early 1990s is now tempered by a variety of factors, including a relative scarcity of organs, increasing waiting lists, and guarded results in metastatic cancers. Synchronous radical resections of primary tumors at the time of liver transplantation, including Whipple resections, distal pancreatectomy, and ileocolectomy have been reported. In a multicenter study from France, the mortality of upper abdominal exenteration in the immediate postop period was 57%; all patients who underwent pancreatic-duodenal replacement died of complications of the procedure.[24]

In patients with control of the primary disease, the symptom-free survival following liver transplantation ranges widely in the literature from 5 to over 100 months.[25] Most of these patients will experience tumor recurrence after transplantation; the 5-year disease-free survival rate in the literature is less than 25%. The overall 5-year survival rate for patients with metastatic carcinoid tumors in the largest series was 69%, though the median disease-free survival was 48 months.[25]

Clearly, a very small minority of patients with metastatic NET will be candidates for liver transplantation. Patients who have severe, and otherwise refractory, symptoms caused by isolated liver metastases would be the best candidates for the effective use of this limited resource, even if palliation is the ultimate goal. Strong relative contraindications would be older patients and patients with extensive primary disease who require synchronous upper abdominal exenteration or who have other significant extrahepatic disease.

CONCLUSIONS AND RECOMMENDATIONS

Liver resection can provide safe, effective, and long-lasting symptomatic relief of metastatic NETs. Although prospective randomized trials are not available, liver resection appears to improve survival as compared with other nonoperative therapies. If the primary tumor has not been resected, the authors recommend synchronous liver and primary tumor resection. Likewise, extrahepatic metastases, including enlarged portal lymph nodes, should also be resected at the time of liver resection if an R0 resection can be achieved. Liver resection, even when combined with other surgical procedures, has a low mortality rate and can be performed with acceptable morbidity at specialized centers. RFA complements liver resection for patients with multiple tumors, bilobar disease, or central lesions. Although some authors have recommended cytoreductive surgery (R2 resection) for patients with unresectable tumors, we prefer laparoscopic RFA and chemoembolization in an effort to ameliorate symptoms and prolong survival. Although complete resection is the cornerstone of multimodality treatment for NET liver metastases, nearly all patients develop recurrent disease. Hepatic artery chemoembolization is recommended for patients with extensive NET liver metastasis not amenable to resection or RFA. The initial enthusiasm for liver transplantation has diminished and its role in the management of NET liver metastases is not clear.

References

1. Modlin IM, Sandor A. An analysis of 8305 cases of carcinoid tumors. Cancer 1997;79:813–29.

2. Moertel CG. Karnofsky memorial lecture. An odyssey in the land of small tumors. J Clin Oncol 1987;5:1502–22.

3. Dromain C, de Baere T, Baudin E, et al. MR imaging of hepatic metastases caused by neuroendocrine tumors: comparing four techniques. AJR Am J Roentgenol 2003; 180:121–8.

4. Paulson EK, McDermott VG, Keogan MT, et al. Carcinoid metastases to the liver: role of triple-phase helical CT. Radiology 1998;206:143–50.

5. Hofland LJ, Lamberts SW, van Hagen PM, et al. Crucial role for somatostatin receptor subtype 2 in determining the uptake of [111In-DTPA-D-Phe1]octreotide in somatostatin receptor-positive organs. J Nucl Med 2003;44: 1315–21.

6. Dromain C, de Baere T, Lumbroso J, et al. Detection of liver metastases from endocrine tumors: a prospective comparison of somatostatin receptor scintigraphy, computed tomography, and magnetic resonance imaging. J Clin Oncol 2005;23:70–8.

7. Onaitis MW, Kirshbom PM, Hayward TZ, et al. Gastrointestinal carcinoids: characterization by site of origin and hormone production. Ann Surg 2000;232:549–56.

8. Faiss S, Pape UF, Bohmig M, et al. Prospective, randomized, multicenter trial on the antiproliferative effect of lanreotide, interferon alfa, and their combination for therapy of metastatic neuroendocrine gastroenteropancreatic tumors—the International Lanreotide and Interferon Alfa Study Group. J Clin Oncol 2003;21:2689–96.

9. Syversen U, Ramstad H, Gamme K, et al. Clinical significance of elevated serum chromogranin A levels. Scand J Gastroenterol 2004;39:969–73.

10. Ardill JE, Erikkson B. The importance of the measurement of circulating markers in patients with neuroendocrine tumours of the pancreas and gut. Endocr Relat Cancer 2003;10:459–62.

11. di Bartolomeo M, Bajetta E, Buzzoni R, et al. Clinical efficacy of octreotide in the treatment of metastatic neuroendocrine tumors. A study by the Italian Trials in Medical Oncology Group. Cancer 1996;77:402–8.

12. Kolby L, Persson G, Franzen S, Ahren B. Randomized clinical trial of the effect of interferon alpha on survival in patients with disseminated midgut carcinoid tumours. Br J Surg 2003;90:687–93.

13. Kim YH, Ajani JA, Carrasco CH, et al. Selective hepatic arterial chemoembolization for liver metastases in patients with carcinoid tumor or islet cell carcinoma. Cancer Invest 1999;17:474–8.

14. Sarmiento JM, Que FG. Hepatic surgery for metastases from neuroendocrine tumors. Surg Oncol Clin N Am 2003; 12:231–42.

15. Chamberlain RS, Canes D, Brown KT, et al. Hepatic neuroendocrine metastases: does intervention alter outcomes? J Am Coll Surg 2000;190:432–45.

16. Sarmiento JM, Heywood G, Rubin J, et al. Surgical treatment of neuroendocrine metastases to the liver: a plea for resection to increase survival. J Am Coll Surg 2003;197: 29–37.

17. Chen H, Hardacre JM, Uzar A, et al. Isolated liver metastases from neuroendocrine tumors: does resection prolong survival? J Am Coll Surg 1998;187:88–92.

18. Grazi GL, Cescon M, Pierangeli F, et al. Highly aggressive policy of hepatic resections for neuroendocrine liver metastases. Hepatogastroenterology 2000;47:481–6.

19. Norton JA, Warren RS, Kelly MG, et al. Aggressive surgery for metastatic liver neuroendocrine tumors. Surgery 2003; 134:1057–63.

20. Nave H, Mossinger E, Feist H, et al. Surgery as primary treatment in patients with liver metastases from carcinoid tumors: a retrospective, unicentric study over 13 years. Surgery 2001;129:170–5.

21. Dousset B, Saint-Marc O, Pitre J, et al. Metastatic endocrine tumors: medical treatment, surgical resection, or liver transplantation. World J Surg 1996;20:908–14.

22. Berber E, Flesher N, Siperstein AE. Laparoscopic radio-frequency ablation of neuroendocrine liver metastases. World J Surg 2002;26:985–90.

23. McEntee GP, Nagorney DM, Kvols LK, et al. Cytoreductive hepatic surgery for neuroendocrine tumors. Surgery 1990; 108:1091–6.

24. Le Treut YP, Delpero JR, Dousset B, et al. Results of liver transplantation in the treatment of metastatic neuroendocrine tumors. A 31-case French multicentric report. Ann Surg 1997;225:355–64.

25. Routley D, Ramage JK, McPeake J, et al. Orthotopic liver transplantation in the treatment of metastatic neuroendocrine tumors of the liver. Liver Transpl Surg 1995;1: 118–21.

CHAPTER 14

SURGICAL MANAGEMENT OF NONCOLORECTAL, NONNEUROENDOCRINE LIVER METASTASES

DANIEL ALBO, MD, PhD

THOMAS WANG, MD, PhD

Liver metastases from noncolorectal, nonneuroendocrine (NCNN) tumors, even if they appear to be limited to a single organ, are generally considered to be a disseminated disease that requires systemic rather than local therapy. However, it has been reported that in 5 to 12% of patients with NCNN, liver metastases can be confined to the liver. Most of these patients are treated palliatively, with a median survival after the detection of liver metastases of only 2 to 14 months.

Modern systemic treatments can, however, achieve approximately 60% response rates, and in some cases, can control tumor progression, albeit temporarily. For most of these patients, the clinical course consists of a succession of more or less prolonged remissions, followed by repeated relapses. Remission consolidation strategies are needed for patients with NCNN liver metastases who respond to chemotherapy.

It is in this context that several groups have started to consider surgical options in the management of this selected group of patients. Liver surgery offers the only chance for cure in patients with a variety of primary and metastatic liver tumors. Furthermore, there is an increasing role for surgical cytoreduction in multimodality treatments for cancer. In this chapter we summarized the available data and different therapeutic options on the surgical management of liver metastases in patients with metastatic NCNN tumors.

Surgical Management of NCNN Liver Metastases: Rationale

The rationale for hepatic metastasectomy in patients with NCNN liver metastases recently outlined by Bathe and colleagues[1] is summarized below.

METASTASES FROM NCNN TUMORS ARE FREQUENTLY ISOLATED TO THE LIVER

Autopsy studies have provided a better understanding of the natural history of NCNN cancer. Lee and colleagues summarized the findings of seven autopsy series of patients with breast carcinoma.[2] The liver was the third most common site of metastases (50 to 71%), behind only the lung (55 to 77%) and bone (49 to 74%). Even at autopsy, the incidence of metastasis confined to the liver at autopsy is 5 to 12%. While accurate data are unavailable, it is likely that an even greater proportion of patients have metastases isolated to liver in the antemortem period. Similar findings have been reported for other types of NCNN liver metastases.[3–5]

METASTATIC DEPOSITS IN THE LIVER MAY GIVE RISE TO FURTHER DISSEMINATION TO OTHER ORGANS

Viadana and colleagues attempted to define the way in which cancer spreads using autopsy studies of patients with a variety of metastatic NCNN tumors.[4,5] They reasoned that dissemination of cancer could occur by two processes. The first is a one-step process in which cancer cells are spread directly from the primary tumor to metastatic sites throughout the body. The second is a "cascade" phenomenon in which metastases originating from the primary gives rise to other metastases. They showed that the organs most frequently involved with metastases were the lung, liver, and bone. With the exception of central nervous system metastases, metastases to other organs were strikingly unusual in the absence of seeding in the lungs, liver, or bone. Mathematical analysis supported the hypothesis that these major sites of involvement were sources of further dissemination to other sites. Others have also shown that metastatic tumor spread is a step-wise process whereby metastases act as the source of further dissemination.[6] Thus, removal of an isolated metastasis from the liver may, to some degree, prevent further dissemination to other organs.

CURE OF METASTATIC NCNN LIVER METASTASES IS UNUSUAL USING CHEMOTHERAPY ALONE

The most common treatment strategy for NCNN liver metastases is chemotherapy and/or hormonal therapy. Unfortunately, despite considerable toxicity, significant improvements in long-term outcomes are rarely achieved.

Cure of metastatic breast cancer with systemic chemotherapy is rarely possible. The long-term prognosis of patients with metastatic breast cancer has recently been reported in a group of patients treated at the University of Texas M. D. Anderson Cancer Center with front-line treatment protocols containing doxorubicin and an alkylating agent.[7] Of 1,581 patients, only 263 (16.6%) achieved complete responses and just 49 (3.1%) remained in complete remission for more than 5 years. Of the latter, 26 of 1,581 continued in complete remission after a median follow-up of 191 months.

These data showed that it is rarely possible to cure patients with metastatic breast cancer with systemic chemotherapy, demonstrating the limitations of standard therapy and emphasizing the need for alternative therapeutic approaches. Response rates and outcomes are similarly poor for other types of NCNN liver metastases patients, including renal, noncolorectal gastrointestinal (GI) and sarcoma malignancies.[8–10]

LIVER METASTASES ARE PARTICULARLY RESISTANT TO MOST HORMONAL AND CHEMOTHERAPEUTIC AGENTS

Hormonal treatments are rarely effective against liver metastases, which tend to be hormone receptor-negative.[11] Thus, chemotherapy is frequently used as a first-line treatment of visceral metastatic disease. Liver metastases are generally considered to be less responsive to chemotherapy than metastases in other sites, and patients with liver lesions have a shorter duration of survival than patients with metastatic disease at other sites.[11,12]

METASTASECTOMY IS ASSOCIATED WITH GOOD LONG-TERM RESULTS IN SELECTED PATIENTS

Various advances in perioperative care and in technique have resulted in significant improvements in outcome following hepatic resections.[13] Operative mortality rates of less than 5% following hepatic resection are consistently reported in most recent series.[14–16] Similarly, low morbidity rates of approximately 10 to 15% have been reported in most modern series. Liver failure is extremely uncommon following limited resections in patients with normal underlying liver function. Improved appreciation for the segmental anatomy of the liver and better techniques for obtaining vascular control are among the factors that have led to improved postoperative outcome. It is likely that a further improvement in postoperative morbidity and mortality rates has resulted from the fact that fewer surgeons are doing more of these procedures, leading to a greater concentration of experience.

NEW MODELS OF THE DEVELOPMENT OF LIVER METASTASES SUGGEST THAT ACHIEVEMENT OF A "COMPLETE RESPONSE" IS MOST CRITICAL FOR LONG-TERM CONTROL OF DISEASE

The continuous growth model is the conventional paradigm of the development of metastases in breast cancer. The model assumes continuous tumor growth of micrometastases until recurrence is clinically detectable. Growth and therapeutic responses are described by Gompertzian growth kinetics. Unfortunately, this continuous growth model is inconsistent with many clinical observations. In particular, the model does not explain how patients followed closely for long periods of time without evidence of disease suddenly return for evaluation with large recurrences. These recurrences are often too big to have been missed by the previous examination, suggesting a sudden acceleration of growth for some reason that is unexplained by the conventional model.

Recently, Retsky and colleagues detailed an alternative model to describe the development of liver metastasis: the tumor dormancy model.[17] The underlying hypothesis is that micrometastases present in the preclinical phase grow at various rates depending on tumor and/or host factors. Micrometastases may escape dormancy by at least two mechanisms: (a) the removal of an angiogenesis inhibitor, or (b) the transformation of a subpopulation of tumor cells to an angiogenic phenotype. In the conventional view, metastatic breast cancer is commonly believed to be incurable, and long-term survivals are attributed to the indolent nature of their disease, which is related to tumor growth kinetics. In contrast, the new tumor dormancy model predicts that the achievement of a complete response results in the depletion of tumor cells of the angiogenic phenotype, resulting in the resumption of the same conditions that occur for early stage breast cancer. The data described by Demicheli and colleagues support this contention.[18] Thus, according to the model, achievement of a complete response is critical to long-term control of disease and this can be achieved surgically in selected cases.

Surgical Management of NCNN Liver Metastases: Options

RESECTION OF NCNN LIVER METASTASES: THE CONCEPT OF "ADJUVANT SURGERY"

Liver resection for colorectal and neuroendocrine liver metastases has gained wide acceptance. Since 1980, single institution series exceeding 100 patients have reported actuarial 5-year survival rates of up to 46%.[13,14,16,19–21] Liver resection for symptomatic neuroendocrine metastases may offer significant long-term palliation or even cure in some cases.[22] With modern advances in preoperative and intraoperative imaging (eg, intraoperative ultrasound), anesthetic management, critical care support, and operative technique, major liver resections are now possible with mortality rates of less than 5% and low morbidity rates.[13,14,16,19–21]

Results of surgical therapy for metastatic colorectal and neuroendocrine tumors have been extensively reported in the literature, but data supporting surgical therapy for NCNN liver metastases are more limited. As improvements in hepatic surgery progress, proper patient selection to include metastatic disease to the liver from other primaries must be investigated. NCNN

liver metastases usually indicate the presence of disseminated cancer with an extremely poor prognosis. Median survival after the detection of liver metastasis rarely reaches 14 months despite chemotherapy.[23] Most of these patients receive palliative therapy only. The relative rarity of NCNN metastases confined to the liver explains the paucity of data supporting surgery as a treatment option for these patients. Isolated metastases to the liver are detected in only 5 to 12% of patients with metastatic NCNN tumors.[2,3] Unlike colorectal cancer (CRC) liver metastases, which can be considered as a stage of localized regional disease reaching the liver by the portal route, apparently "isolated" (unique or multiple) NCNN liver metastases are only the visible part of true distant dissemination and reflect an initial selection of patients with metastatic disease. Most of these patients begin with systemic chemotherapy and wait some months without a detectable sign of extrahepatic disease before being referred to the surgeon. In this small group of selected patients, it became clear that surgery capable of removing all detectable neoplastic disease could profoundly modify the host defenses in favor of the host. In this manner, hepatectomy for NCNN liver metastases should have a place in the therapeutic arsenal. Over the last decade, a growing body of evidence in the world literature has accumulated to support adjuvant surgery in NCNN liver metastases. Some of the available data are summarized in Table 1.[24–31]

Although long-term survival following resection of NCNN liver metastases confined to the liver is a realistic goal, recurrences in the liver and other visceral foci continue to be a problem. Resection should therefore be considered part of a cytoreductive strategy, which potentiates systemic treatment with an agent active against visceral sites of disease. Hepatic metastasectomy can only afford improvements in survival in patients with NCNN liver metastases if their disease is stabilized with chemotherapy and/or endocrine therapy. Surgical resection of NCNN liver metastases should improve local disease control and allow deferral of chemotherapy when possible. Therefore, liver-directed surgical therapies should be considered a local adjuvant treatment of the liver when the patient has already responded to systemic treatment. This type of treatment strategy has been termed "adjuvant surgery."[23]

Several North American centers have recently reported their experience with liver resections for patients with isolated NCNN liver metastases (see Table 1). In one of the largest published series, Weitz and colleagues reported their results on 141 patients who underwent hepatic resection for liver metastases from NCNN carcinoma.[24] The thirty-day postoperative mortality rate was 0%. Overall, 33% of the patients developed

Table 1 Summary of results from recent series of resective therapy for NCNN liver metastases.

Series	Origin	Patient number	Operative mortality (%)	Median survival (months)	1-year survival (%)	3-year survival (%)	5-year survival (%)	Favorable Prognostic Factors
Harrison et al., 1997	New York, USA	96	0	32	80	45	37	DFI>36m, R0 resection, Non-GI origin
Hemming et al., 2000	Toronto, Canada	37	0	46	85	55	45	Non-GI origin, R0 resection
Cordera et al., 2005	Minnesota, USA	64	1.5		81	43	30	DFI>24m
Weitz et al., 2005	New York, USA	141	0				36	DFI>24m, R0 resection, Reproductive tract tumors
Elias et al., 1998	Villejuif, France	127	2			60	40	Non-GI and non-melanoma origin, R0 resection
Ercolani et al., 2005	Bologna, Italy	142	0			49.5	34.3	Non-GI origin, R0 resection
Lang et al., 1999	Hannover, Germany	127	5.8	32			25	R0 resection
Laurent et al., 2001	Bordeaux, France	39	0		81	40	35	DFI>24m

DFI: Disease-free interval; R0: Margin-negative; GI: Gastrointestinal.

postoperative complications. The median follow-up was 26 months; the median follow-up for survivors was 35 months. There were 24 actual 5-year survivors. The actuarial 3-year relapse-free survival rate was 30% with a median of 17 months. The actuarial 3-year cancer-specific survival rate was 57% with a median of 42 months. Primary tumor type and length of disease-free interval from the primary tumor were significant independent prognostic factors for relapse-free and cancer-specific survival. Margin status was significant for cancer-specific survival and showed a strong trend for relapse-free survival. The authors concluded that hepatic resection for metastases from NCNN carcinoma is safe, can offer long-term survival in selected patients, and should be considered if all gross disease can be removed, especially in patients with metastases from reproductive tract tumors or a disease-free interval greater than 2 years.

Several European centers have also recently reported their outcomes following liver resections for NCNN liver metastases (see Table 1). In one of the largest series reported, Elias and colleagues reported their outcomes following hepatic resections in 147 patients with NCNN liver metastases.[30] The perioperative mortality rate was 2%. The crude 5-year survival rate was 36%, and survival rate without progressive disease was 28%. No difference was observed in survival when synchronous and metachronous liver metastases (LM) were compared, or when patients with more or fewer than three LM were compared. Five-year survival rates were 20% for 35 breast cancers, 46% for 20 testicular tumors, 18% for 13 sarcomas, and slightly less than 20% for 11 gastric carcinomas, 10 melanomas, and 7 tumors of the gallbladder, according to the primary. Survival exceeded 20% for 6 gynecologic tumors, but was disappointing for head and neck cancers when the primary was unknown or when the tumor was truly undifferentiated.

Several potential prognostic factors after hepatectomy for NCNN liver metastases have been evaluated in recent series. The primary tumor type bears a direct relationship with outcomes.[24,27–30] The best outcomes have been reported for reproductive tract malignancies. Good outcomes have also been reported for selected sarcomas, urinary tract, and breast malignancies. Outcomes after hepatectomies for metastatic melanoma, noncolorectal GI malignancies, squamous cell carcinomas of the head and neck, and tumors of unknown primary have been very poor. Achieving a negative margin during hepatectomy (R0 resection) has also been consistently found to be an important independent prognostic factor.[24,26–30] Finally, consideration of tumor biology is also important, as reflected by the fact that metastases that develop after a short interval from the primary tumor treatment (less than 24 to 36 months) carry a poorer prognosis.[24,25,27,31]

From the available data in the literature, and as suggested by Elias and colleagues, certain guidelines are emerging regarding the indications for liver resection and the use of adjuvant chemotherapy in patients with NCNN liver metastases:

1. Liver resections should be reserved for NCNN liver metastases patients that have disease confined to the liver. A thorough preoperative workup is necessary for adequate patient selection.
2. Margin-negative (R0) resection should be the goal of therapy. Outcomes following incomplete (R1/R2) are poor. Achievement of a "complete response" is most critical for long-term control of disease.
3. The number of liver metastases and their synchronous or metachronous emergence rela-

tive to the primary tumor are not prognostic factors of outcome after liver resection. Although shorter intervals ($<$ 36 months) between the primary tumor and the development of liver metastases results in worse outcomes, it does not necessarily contraindicate liver resection.

4. The histology of the primary tumor bears a direct relationship to outcomes after hepatectomy for NCNN liver metastases. Hepatectomies for gynecological, urological, breast, and sarcoma malignancies carry a prognosis that is similar to that of patients with colorectal primaries. Hepatectomies are therefore indicated for these patients. Conversely, hepatectomies for noncolorectal GI malignancies (esophagus, stomach, pancreas, and biliary neoplasms), head and neck tumors, melanomas, and unknown primary tumors have a very poor prognosis. Liver resection in these patients needs to be individualized.

5. A multidisciplinary approach should be used in the management of these patients. Even when the disease appears to be confined to the liver, it is likely that subclinical micrometastases are already present elsewhere. Chemotherapy, hormonal therapy, and/or biological cancer therapies should play a central role in the therapeutic armamentarium for these patients. Surgery should be viewed as the "adjuvant" therapy for patients with NCNN liver metastases.

6. Chemotherapy, hormonal therapy, and/or biological cancer therapies can be administered before or after surgical resection. A possible advantage of preoperative chemotherapy is the ability to determine responsiveness to the agents used prior to resection. Disadvantages of preoperative chemotherapy include potential hepatotoxicity with changes in both the metastases and the liver parenchyma, leading to potential increase in operative blood loss and perioperative risk as well as to a more difficult visualization of the metastases by preoperative and intraoperative imaging (eg, computed tomography, ultrasound). In order to exploit the advantages and minimize the disadvantages of preoperative chemotherapy, oncologists should refer these patients to the liver surgeon early, after two or three courses of chemotherapy. Prolonged preoperative treatments should be avoided. Chemotherapy, hormonal therapy, and/or biological cancer therapy treatments can be completed postoperatively after recovery from surgery.

RADIOFREQUENCY ABLATION

Radiofrequency ablation (RFA) is a modality for local tumor destruction with minimal local and systemic complications.[32,33] RFA is a localized thermal treatment technique designed to produce tumor destruction by heating tumor tissue to temperatures that exceed 60°C. New multiple array needles recently developed have replaced single array needles and have made RFA relevant (Figure 1). The insulated needle electrode shaft is placed into the tumor with the array retracted. Using real-time ultrasound guidance, the array is then deployed from the needle tip into the tumor. These deployed multiple array hooks create a series of electrodes across which the radiofrequency (RF) current can be passed. The multiple array electrodes are a technologic innovation that permits ablation of much larger zones of tissue compared to simple needle electrodes. An RF needle electrode can be advanced into the unresectable liver tumor via either a percutaneous, laparoscopic, or open (laparotomy) route. Tumors less than 2.5 cm in their greatest diameter can be ablated with the placement of a needle electrode with an array diameter of 3.5 cm when the electrode is positioned in the center of the tumor. For larger tumors, multiple placements and deployments of the electrode array may be necessary to completely destroy the tumor. Treatment is planned such that the zones of coagulative necrosis overlap to ensure complete destruction of the tumor (Figure 2).

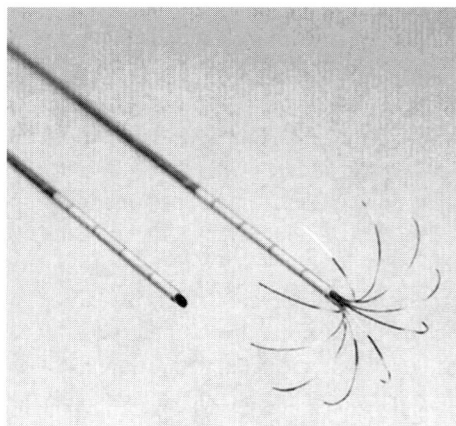

Figure 1 Insulated shaft 15-gauge RF needle electrodes showing the multiple array retracted into the needle sheath (left) and fully deployed from the needle tip (right). The 10 individual tines of the multiple arrays are clearly seen with the array deployed to the full 4 cm diameter.

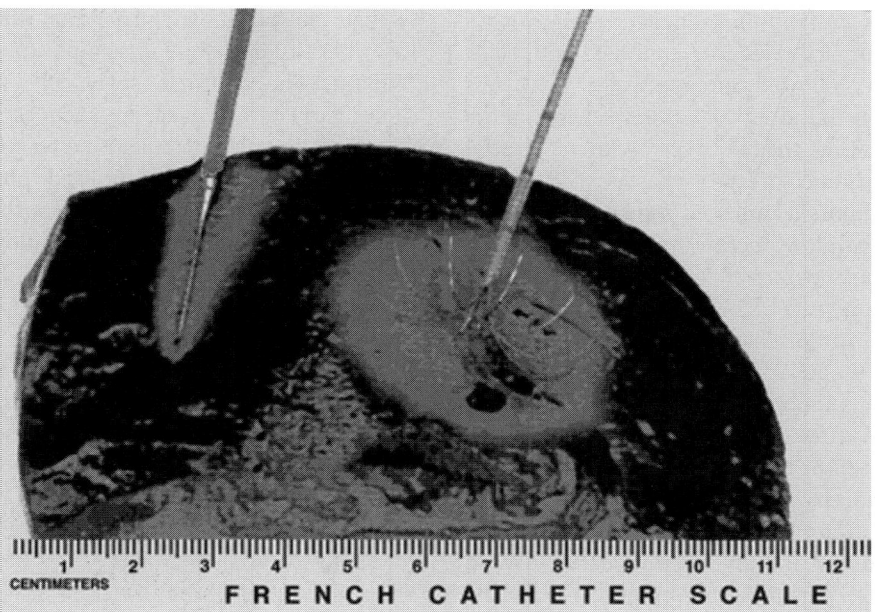

Figure 2 Differences in the size and extent of zones of coagulative necrosis in bovine liver treated with RFA using a simple needle electrode (left) compared to a multiple array LeVeen needle electrode (right).

The selection of patients to be treated with RFA should be based on rational principles and goals. Any local therapy for malignant hepatic tumors, be it surgical resection, RFA, or some other tumor ablative technique, is generally performed with curative intent, but a significant proportion of patients will subsequently develop clinically detectable hepatic or extrahepatic recurrence from their coexistent micrometastatic disease. Thus, RFA is performed mostly in patients with no preoperative or intraoperative evidence of extrahepatic disease, and only for tumor histologies with a reasonable probability of disease metastatic only to the liver. Occasionally, patients with tumor types usually associated with disseminated, systemic metastatic disease (eg, NCNN malignancies) may be considered for RFA if they have been treated with at least 6 months of effective systemic chemotherapy and have only liver metastasis or low-volume extrahepatic disease otherwise well controlled with chemotherapy and/or hormonal therapy. This latter group of patients is a small, highly selected subset from which a few patients could derive long-term survival benefit from aggressive liver-directed surgical therapy.

Several investigators have reviewed their series of RFA for primary and secondary hepatic tumors with subset analysis of NCNN tumor RFA outcomes.[34–36] Bleicher and colleagues reviewed their RFA experience at the John Wayne Cancer Center to identify variables affecting local recurrence.[34] 447 unresectable liver tumors were ablated in 153 patients between 1997 and 2001. The majority of tumors were colorectal and hepatocellular carcinoma, making up 52% of the histologies. Neuroendocrine tumors made up 8.5% of the histologies. The NCNN group included breast (11.1%), melanoma (8.5%), sarcoma (3.9%), ovarian cancer (3.9%), noncolorectal GI cancers (3.2%), lung cancer (1.3%), and others (6.5%). The authors found that colorectal carcinomas and hepatocellular histologies exhibited a univariate increase in recurrence, whereas breast and carcinoid tumors recurred significantly less frequently. Because size was not different among tumor types, the investigators felt that this may be a function of the differences in the parenchymal milieu, the tumor itself, or efficiency of ablation of particular tissue types. Because the neuroendocrine tumors, including the carcinoid tumor histology, were not separated from the NCNN tumors, we are unable to determine the actual recurrence of the NCNN group after RFA. The authors concluded that size has the highest correlation with local recurrence, but multiple tumors and pathology may also predict local recurrence risk. Large, complex lesions can be safely serially ablated, but because of morbidity and recurrence, RFA should not replace resection as the primary treatment of resectable liver tumors.

Similar to the John Wayne Cancer Center series, Pawlik and colleagues from the University of Texas M. D. Anderson Cancer Center demonstrated that RFA of hepatic metastases can result in improved patient outcome.[36] The authors successfully demonstrated the safety and efficacy of hepatic resection combined with RFA. In their study, patients with multifocal hepatic malignancies were treated with surgical resection combined with RFA. All patients were followed prospectively to assess complications. Seven hundred and thirty-seven tumors in 172 patients were treated (124 with colorectal metastases; 48 with noncolorectal metastases). RFA was used to treat 350 tumors. Combined modality treatment was well tolerated with low operative times and minimal blood loss. The postoperative complication rate was 19.8% with a mortality rate of 2.3%. At a median follow-up of 21.3 months, tumors had recurred in 98 patients (56.9%). Failure at the RFA site was uncommon (2.3%). A combined total number of tumors treated with resection and RFA >10 was associated with a faster time to recurrence ($p = .02$). The median actuarial survival time was 45.5 months. Patients with noncolorectal metastases had an improved survival ($p = .03$), whereas RF ablating a lesion > 3 cm adversely impacted survival (HR = 1.85, $p = .04$). Again, we are unable to draw any conclusions concerning the effect of RFA combined with resection of the NCNN tumor metastases group because the patients having a neuroendocrine histology were included as part of the noncolorectal metastases group.

Finally, Berber and colleagues from the Cleveland Clinic investigated the application of RFA for NCNN liver tumors utilizing a laparoscopic approach in all of their patients.[37] This recent study is the only one of its kind dealing specifically with RFA of NCNN hepatic metastases. Between January 1996 and March 2005, 53 patients with NCNN tumors underwent laparoscopic RFA. The histologic cell types included sarcoma (n = 18), breast cancer (n = 10), esophageal cancer (n = 4), melanoma (n = 4), lung cancer (n = 3), ovarian cancer (n = 2), pancreatic cancer (n = 2), unknown primary cancer (n = 2), cholangiocarcinoma (n = 2), rectal squamous cancer (n = 2), renal cancer (n = 2), papillary thyroid cancer (n = 1), and hemangioendothelioma (n = 1). The 53 patients underwent ablation of 192 lesions, with 8 patients undergoing repeat treatment. The hospital stay averaged 1 day and there was no 30-day mortality. Complications included one postoperative hemorrhage, one liver abscess, and one wound infection. Tumors recurred locally for 17% of the lesions over a mean follow-up period of 24 months. The overall median survival was 33 months for the whole series, more than 51 months for breast cancer, and 25 months for sarcoma. The 5-year actuarial survival for all the patients was reported to be greater than 40%. The authors concluded that laparoscopic RFA can safely and effectively treat NCNN hepatic metastases. Their results convincingly support the efficacy of cytoreduction of NCNN by laparoscopic RFA when other treatment methods have failed. However, one area of concern of this investigation

is that the authors mention that the majority of the sarcomas studied were gastrointestinal stromal tumors (GISTs). The treatment of GISTs may benefit from molecularly targeted agents such as imatinib mesylate (Gleevec), thereby affecting a better prognosis regardless of the surgical treatment utilized. How many of these patients were initially treated with Gleevec is not mentioned. A considerable pathological response to Gleevec in the "sarcoma" group would significantly skew the survival data towards an improved outcome in the largest subset of this study.

Livraghi and colleagues have recently reported their experience in the use of RFA for the treatment of liver metastases in patients with breast cancer.[38] Twenty-four consecutive patients with 64 metastases measuring 1.0 to 6.6 cm in diameter (mean, 1.9 cm) underwent ultrasonography-guided percutaneous RFA with 18-gauge, internally cooled electrodes. Treatment was performed with the patient under conscious sedation and analgesia or general anesthesia. A single lesion was treated in 16 patients, and multiple lesions were treated in 8 patients. Follow-up with serial computed tomography ranged from 4 to 44 months (mean, 10 months; median, 19 months). Complete necrosis was achieved in 59 (92%) of 64 lesions. Among the 59 lesions, complete necrosis required a single treatment session in 58 lesions (91%) and two treatment sessions in one lesion (2%). In 14 (58%) of 24 patients, new metastases developed during follow-up. Ten (71%) of these 14 patients developed new liver metastases. Currently, 10 (63%) of 16 patients whose lesions were initially confined to the liver are free of disease. One patient died of progressive brain metastases. No major complications occurred. Two minor complications were observed. On the basis of these results, the authors concluded that RF ablation appears to be a safe, relatively simple, and effective treatment for liver metastases from breast cancer. The absence of major complications and the high rate of local control achieved in this series suggest that RFA may be a valid alternative to surgery in a select population of patients with metastatic breast cancer. They also noted that even if the proportion of patients with liver-only metastases from breast cancer is relatively lower than that from other primary tumors, the high overall prevalence of breast cancer suggests that a large number of patients may be eligible for RFA treatment (Figure 3).

CRYOABLATION

Cryosurgery is based on the cyclic application of extremely low temperatures (-196°C) to the tumor through a probe, which is positioned in the tumor, cooled with either circulating liquid nitrogen or argon.[39–45] Tumor cell destruction occurs by ice crystal formation during

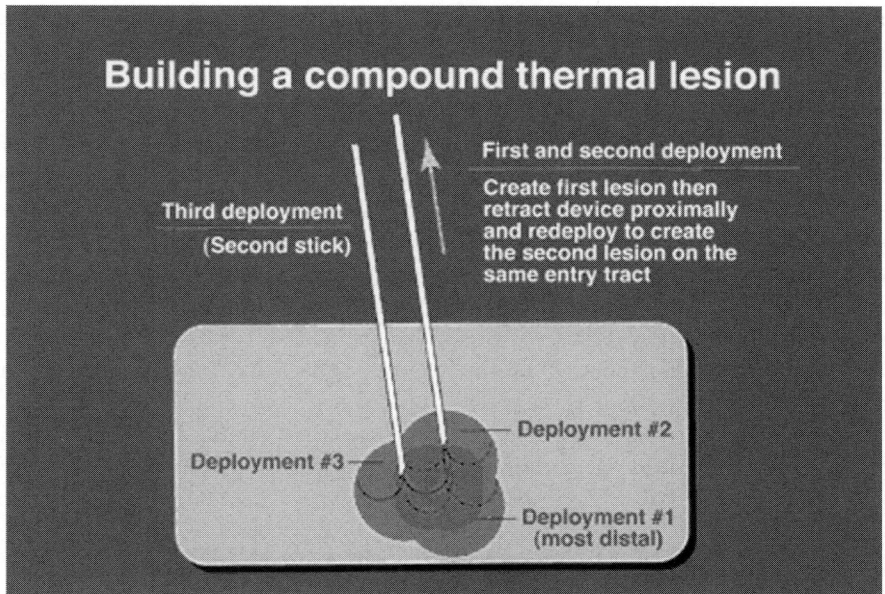

Figure 3 A schematic diagram indicating sequential placement of an RF needle electrode with deployment of the multiple array at each site to produce overlapping zones of coagulative necrosis to treat a liver tumor >2.5 cm in diameter. Three-dimensional planning must be performed for liver tumors too large to be treated with a single deployment of the needle electrode. Ultrasonography is used to guide needle placement and array deployment to assure that the entire tumor (brown area) and a surrounding zone of normal hepatic parenchyma (orange areas) are ablated. The array should be deployed first at the most posterior interface of tumor and normal liver because the RF-ablated tissue becomes hyperechogenic with ultrasonographic shadowing. Thus, it would be difficult to place accurately the multiple array deep, or posterior, to a previously ablated zone of tissue.

the repeated freezing and thawing process, resulting in cellular dehydration, protein denaturation, and microcirculatory failure. Cryosurgical treatment of hepatic malignancies may be used when conventional surgical resection is restricted by anatomical limitations or as an adjunct to resection, in the treatment of hepatic malignancies. Cryosurgery can be performed by open and minimally invasive percutaneous approaches.

More recently, the advent of other ablative techniques with potentially higher efficacy and lower morbidity (eg, RFA) has decreased the enthusiasm for the use of cryoablation in the management of hepatic malignancies.[32,42,46] In particular, cryoablation requires more expensive and cumbersome equipment, is associated with higher morbidity and mortality rates, and has higher recurrence rates than RFA. Malignant cells are more resistant to lethal damage from freezing compared to normal cells, but are more sensitive to hyperthermic damage than normal cells.[47] Two nonrandomized studies have compared RFA with cryosurgery. The first report to appear was that of Pearson and colleagues, who compared cryosurgery and RF using an open laparotomy approach.[33] In this series, 40.7% of the patients, including 1 postoperative death, had complications following cryosurgery compared with 3.3% and no

deaths following RF. Local recurrences were identified in 13.6% of the patients following cryosurgery and in 2.2% following RF. As a result, this group prefers RF to cryosurgery for treating primary and metastatic hepatic tumors.

Bilchik and colleagues used cryosurgery and RF, either alone or as complementary treatments to each other, using various approaches, including laparotomy, laparoscopy, or percutaneous approaches.[42] They found significantly higher rates of blood loss, thrombocytopenia, and pleural effusion following cryosurgery. Although mortality rates following either treatment were similar (3.0% for cryosurgery and 2.5% for RF), the overall local recurrence rate was higher for the cryosurgery group (15% following cryosurgery alone compared with 10% following RF alone). In a study by Adam and colleagues comparing percutaneous cryoablation to percutaneous RFA for unresectable hepatic malignancies including NCNN liver metastases, higher morbidity and mortality rates were observed in the cryosurgery group compared to the RF group (3.5% versus 0% and 29% versus 24%, respectively).[45] The two methods proved to be equally efficient for initial treatment success; however, local recurrences were higher following percutaneous cryosurgical treatment. Overall, the local recurrence following percutaneous cryosurgical treatment was 60% of patients and 53% of tumors compared with 16% of patients and 18% of tumors following percutaneous RFA. Moreover, the differences in the rates of local recurrence were amplified following treatment for metastatic hepatic malignancies (71% and 19% for tumors and 78% and 18% for patients following cryosurgical and RFA, respectively). Furthermore, by multivariate analysis, treatment by cryotherapy had an independent influence on local recurrence.

Cryosurgical ablation of hepatic metastases from colon carcinoma has become a useful adjunct in the management of patients whose tumors are not amenable to surgical resection. Various investigators have evaluated the efficacy of cryoablation in treating noncolorectal hepatic metastases. However, similar to RFA, few of these studies have focused primarily on the effect of cryoablation of NCNN tumor metastases but include neuroendocrine tumors in their evaluation of this treatment modality. Bilchik and colleagues from the John Wayne Cancer Center evaluated cryoablation of noncolorectal hepatic metastases from breast cancer, ovarian cancer, and thyroid cancer.[48] Although this study also included patients with neuroendocrine tumors and primary hepatic tumors in this noncolorectal group, median survival was 32 months following curative surgery (range 16 to 45 months) and 25 months following palliative surgery (range 2 to 42 months). The authors concluded that cryosurgical ablation of noncolorectal hepatic metastases is safe, provides excellent palliation of symptoms, and in selected patients can be performed with curative intent.

Goering and colleagues. reviewed their treatment outcomes using cryosurgical ablation and conventional resection techniques for noncolorectal liver metastases.[49] Forty-two patients undergoing 48 hepatic tumor ablative procedures from February 1991 through May 2001 at a single institution were retrospectively reviewed. Overall survival and local hepatic tumor recurrence-free survival were analyzed for different surgical procedures and primary tumor types. Overall survival rates at 1, 3, and 5 years were 82%, 55%, and 39%, respectively (median survival 45 months). Local hepatic tumor recurrence-free survival rates for resection only (n = 25) and cryosurgery with or without resection (n = 23) at 3 years are 24% and 19%, respectively. The survival rates at 5 years are 40% and 37%, for resection-only and cryosurgery with or without resection, respectively. The authors concluded that cryoablation of hepatic tumor for metastatic noncolorectal primary tumors results in survival and local hepatic tumor recurrence rates similar to resection alone. The combination of cryosurgery and resection extended the cohort of patients with surgically treatable

disease. Although this study also included patients with neuroendocrine tumors in this noncolorectal group, the investigators did do subset analysis and stratify survival data according to the three major tumor classes: neuroendocrine, genitourinary, and soft-tissue sarcoma hepatic metastases. Three-year survival data for neuroendocrine, genitourinary, and soft tissue tumors were 91%, 52%, and 34%, respectively, which is comparable to resection and superior to no treatment. The authors concluded that hepatic cryoablation for metastases could be justified for renal, adrenal, Wilm's, and testicular liver tumors by providing a survival advantage when compared to nonoperative management. The authors also believe that careful selection of patients with hepatic metastases from sarcomas, breast, ovarian, and melanoma may yield improved long-term survival after hepatic cryoablation.

Conclusions

Discussions today about the possible role for surgery in the management of NCNN liver metastases appear to be at a similar state than they were two decades ago about the role of surgery in the management of CRC liver metastases. As our understanding of the tumor biology of metastatic NCNN cancer evolves, so do the indications for possible surgical intervention in the management of liver metastasis in the subset of patients with metastatic NCNN cancer that present with either liver-only disease or with additional low-volume extrahepatic disease well controlled with chemotherapy and/or hormonal therapy. As our technical, anesthetic, critical care, imaging, and interventional radiology capabilities evolve, so do the surgical indications for the surgical management in these subset of patients with metastatic NCNN tumors.

Most recent series of surgical resection in patients with metastatic NCNN tumors confined to the liver show survival rates comparable to that of similar series in patients with metastatic CRC. The results of surgical resection in this subset of patients are far superior to even the most aggressive chemotherapy protocols. Furthermore, surgery and chemotherapy appear to be complementary in the management of these patients, a concept recently referred to as "adjuvant surgery." In this model, surgery achieves good locoregional control of the typically chemoresistant liver metastasis, and systemic chemotherapy helps reduce the incidence of extrahepatic recurrences. Long-term survival, and possibly even cure, appears possible in a this highly selected group of patients.

Cryosurgical and RFA techniques are safe and effective methods to control unresectable hepatic malignancies. However, despite successful initial tumor devascularization, many tumors recur, in local, hepatic, or extra-hepatic sites. In retrospective studies, RFA seems to result in lower morbidity and mortality rates and a lower rate of local recurrence than cryosurgical ablation, particularly in those with metastatic malignancies. These retrospective results open the way to a prospective randomized trial comparing the two treatments to state definitively the suggested superiority of RF. It is further expected that the more recent advancements in the area of RF probes, which allow the creation of up to a 7 cm destruction area, will further lower the rate of local recurrence by helping to reduce the requirement for overlapping ablations during the treatment of larger tumors. Nevertheless, the overall risk of recurrence after ablative treatment of hepatic malignancies stresses the need to consider liver resection whenever possible because it is a more definitive tumor treatment, and to restrict the indications of in situ tumor destruction to patients with unresectable disease. We believe it is premature to compare liver resection with in situ tumor destruction in patients with resectable disease, particularly for those with metastases. Long-term follow-up data are necessary to fully evaluate the role of these ablative techniques in the management of patients with metastatic hepatic malignancies.

References

1. Bathe OF, Kaklamanos IG, Moffat FL, et al. Metastasectomy as a cytoreductive strategy for treatment of isolated pulmonary and hepatic metastases from breast cancer. Surg Oncol 1999;8(1):35–42.

2. Lee YT, Terry R. Surgical treatment of carcinoma of the breast. I. Pathological finding and pattern of relapse. J Surg Oncol 1983;23(1):11–5.

3. Tongaonkar HB, Kulkarni JN, Kamat MR. Solitary metastases from renal cell carcinoma: a review. J Surg Oncol 1992;49(1):45–8.

4. Viadana E, Bross ID, Pickren JW. The relationship of histology to the spread of cancer. J Surg Oncol 1975;7(3): 177–86.

5. Viadana E, Au KL. Patterns of metastases in adenocarcinomas of man. An autopsy study of 4,728 cases. J Med 1975;6(1):1–14.

6. Bross ID, Viadana E, Pickren J. Do generalized metastases occur directly from the primary? J Chronic Dis 1975;28(3): 149–59.

7. Greenberg PA, Hortobagyi GN, Smith TL, et al. Long-term follow-up of patients with complete remission following combination chemotherapy for metastatic breast cancer. J Clin Oncol 1996;14(8):2197–205.

8. Neves RJ, Zincke H, Taylor WF. Metastatic renal cell cancer and radical nephrectomy: identification of prognostic factors and patient survival. J Urol 1988;139(6):1173–6.

9. Ochiai T, Sasako M, Mizuno S, et al. Hepatic resection for metastatic tumours from gastric cancer: analysis of prognostic factors. Br J Surg 1994;81(8):1175–8.

10. Ng EH, Pollock RE, Romsdahl MM. Prognostic implications of patterns of failure for gastrointestinal leiomyosarcomas. Cancer 1992;69(6):1334–41.

11. Fumoleau P. Treatment of patients with liver metastases. Anticancer Drugs 1996;7 Suppl 2:21–3.

12. Gregory WM, Smith P, Richards MA, et al. Chemotherapy of advanced breast cancer: outcome and prognostic factors. Br J Cancer 1993;68(5):988–95.

13. Curley SA, Cusack JC Jr, Tanabe KK, et al. Advances in the treatment of liver tumors. Curr Probl Surg 2002;39(5):449–571.

14. Fuhrman GM, Curley SA, Hohn DC, Roh MS. Improved survival after resection of colorectal liver metastases. Ann Surg Oncol 1995;2(6):537–41.

15. Fong Y, Fortner J, Sun RL, et al. Clinical score for predicting recurrence after hepatic resection for metastatic colorectal cancer: analysis of 1001 consecutive cases. Ann Surg 1999;230(3):309–18; discussion 18–21.

16. Scheele J, Altendorf-Hofmann A, Stangl R, Schmidt K. [Surgical resection of colorectal liver metastases: Gold standard for solitary and radically resectable lesions]. Swiss Surg 1996;Suppl 4:4–17.

17. Retsky M, Demicheli R, Hrushesky W, et al. Recent translational research: computational studies of breast cancer. Breast Cancer Res 2005;7(1):37–40.

18. Demicheli R, Retsky MW, Swartzendruber DE, Bonadonna G. Proposal for a new model of breast cancer metastatic development. Ann Oncol 1997;8(11):1075–80.

19. Fong Y, Cohen AM, Fortner JG, et al. Liver resection for colorectal metastases. J Clin Oncol 1997;15(3):938–46.

20. Adam R, Vinet E. Regional treatment of metastasis: surgery of colorectal liver metastases. Ann Oncol 2004;15 Suppl 4: iv103–6.

21. Minagawa M, Makuuchi M, Torzilli G, et al. Extension of the frontiers of surgical indications in the treatment of liver metastases from colorectal cancer: long-term results. Ann Surg 2000;231(4):487–99.

22. Sarmiento JM, Que FG. Hepatic surgery for metastases from neuroendocrine tumors. Surg Oncol Clin N Am 2003; 12(1):231–42.

23. Pocard M, Pouillart P, Asselain B, et al. Hepatic resection for breast cancer metastases: results and prognosis (65 cases). Ann Chir 2001;126(5):413–20.

24. Weitz J, Blumgart LH, Fong Y, et al. Partial hepatectomy for metastases from noncolorectal, nonneuroendocrine carcinoma. Ann Surg 2005;241(2):269–76.

25. Laurent C, Rullier E, Feyler A, et al. Resection of noncolorectal and nonneuroendocrine liver metastases: late metastases are the only chance of cure. World J Surg 2001;25(12):1532–6.

26. Lang H, Nussbaum KT, Weimann A, Raab R. Liver resection for non-colorectal, non-neuroendocrine hepatic metastases. Chirurg 1999;70(4):439–46.

27. Hemming AW, Sielaff TD, Gallinger S, et al. Hepatic resection of noncolorectal nonneuroendocrine metastases. Liver Transpl 2000;6(1):97–101.

28. Harrison LE, Brennan MF, Newman E, et al. Hepatic resection for noncolorectal, nonneuroendocrine metastases: a fifteen-year experience with ninety-six patients. Surgery 1997;121(6):625–32.

29. Ercolani G, Grazi GL, Ravaioli M, et al. The role of liver resections for noncolorectal, nonneuroendocrine metastases: experience with 142 observed cases. Ann Surg Oncol 2005;12(6):459–66.

30. Elias D, Cavalcanti de Albuquerque A, Eggenspieler P, et al. Resection of liver metastases from a noncolorectal primary: indications and results based on 147 monocentric patients. J Am Coll Surg 1998;187(5):487–93.

31. Cordera F, Rea DJ, Rodriguez-Davalos M, et al. Hepatic resection for noncolorectal, nonneuroendocrine metastases. J Gastrointest Surg 2005;9(9):1361–70.

32. Curley SA. Radiofrequency ablation of malignant liver tumors. Oncologist 2001;6(1):14–23.

33. Pearson AS, Izzo F, Fleming RY, et al. Intraoperative radiofrequency ablation or cryoablation for hepatic malignancies. Am J Surg 1999;178(6):592–9.

34. Bleicher RJ, Allegra DP, Nora DT, et al. Radiofrequency ablation in 447 complex unresectable liver tumors: lessons learned. Ann Surg Oncol 2003;10(1):52–8.

35. Curley SA, Izzo F, Delrio P, et al. Radiofrequency ablation of unresectable primary and metastatic hepatic malignancies: results in 123 patients. Ann Surg 1999;230(1):1–8.

36. Pawlik TM, Izzo F, Cohen DS, et al. Combined resection and radiofrequency ablation for advanced hepatic malignancies: results in 172 patients. Ann Surg Oncol 2003; 10(9):1059–69.

37. Berber E, Ari E, Herceg N, Siperstein A. Laparoscopic radiofrequency thermal ablation for unusual hepatic tumors: operative indications and outcomes. Surg Endosc 2005;19(12):1613–7.

38. Livraghi T, Goldberg SN, Solbiati L, et al. Percutaneous radio-frequency ablation of liver metastases from breast cancer: initial experience in 24 patients. Radiology 2001; 220(1):145–9.

39. Ravikumar TS. The role of cryotherapy in the management of patients with liver tumors. Adv Surg 1996;30:281–91.

40. Seifert JK, Heintz A, Junginger T. Cryotherapy for primary and secondary liver tumours. Zentralbl Chir 2002;127(4): 275–81.

41. Sheen AJ, Poston GJ, Sherlock DJ. Cryotherapeutic ablation of liver tumours. Br J Surg 2002;89(11):1396–401.

42. Bilchik AJ, Wood TF, Allegra D, et al. Cryosurgical ablation and radiofrequency ablation for unresectable hepatic malignant neoplasms: a proposed algorithm. Arch Surg 2000;135(6):657–62; discussion 62–4.

43. Wallace JR, Christians KK, Pitt HA, Quebbeman EJ. Cryotherapy extends the indications for treatment of colorectal liver metastases. Surgery 1999;126(4):766–72; discussion 72–4.

44. Finlay IG, Seifert JK, Stewart GJ, Morris DL. Resection with cryotherapy of colorectal hepatic metastases has the same survival as hepatic resection alone. Eur J Surg Oncol 2000; 26(3):199–202.

45. Adam R, Hagopian EJ, Linhares M, et al. A comparison of percutaneous cryosurgery and percutaneous radiofrequency for unresectable hepatic malignancies. Arch Surg 2002;137(12):1332–9; discussion 40.

46. Barnett CC Jr. Curley SA. Ablative techniques for hepatocellular carcinoma. Semin Oncol 2001;28(5):487–96.

47. Hoffmann NE, Bischof JC. The cryobiology of cryosurgical injury. Urology 2002;60(2 Suppl 1):40–9.

48. Bilchik AJ, Sarantou T, Wardlaw JC, Ramming KP. Cryosurgery causes a profound reduction in tumor markers in hepatoma and noncolorectal hepatic metastases. Am Surg 1997;63(9):796–800.

49. Goering JD, Mahvi DM, Niederhuber JE, et al. Cryoablation and liver resection for noncolorectal liver metastases. Am J Surg 2002;183(4):384–9.

CHAPTER 15

BENIGN LIVER TUMORS

SAM S. YOON, MD

KENNETH K. TANABE, MD

Introduction

The management of benign liver tumors is a frequent clinical demand for the practicing surgical oncologist. Benign liver tumors are common in the general population, being present in about 9% of individuals.[1] Although most individuals never have any symptoms related to these tumors, these lesions are now regularly discovered owing to the increased use of radiologic imaging such as ultrasound (US) and computed tomography (CT). The majority of the benign liver tumors are innocuous, but it is important to be aware of their imaging characteristics, natural history, management, and potential complications. Benign tumors must often be differentiated from malignant tumors, especially when they are discovered in the evaluation of patients with underlying cancer. In patients with gastrointestinal symptoms and a liver lesion, one must determine if such symptoms are secondary to the liver tumor or more common gastrointestinal disorders. Thus the clinician responsible for managing such patients must have knowledge of the (1) imaging modalities required to adequately evaluate undiagnosed liver lesions, (2) radiologic features that differentiate one type of tumor from another, and (3) scenarios in which definitive biopsy is necessary. Once a benign liver tumor is diagnosed, knowledge of its natural history and the risk of complications are necessary to determine whether intervention or follow-up is required. Finally, the surgeon who evaluates patients with these tumors requires knowledge of the optimal techniques of resection and outcomes following resection.

Classification

Benign liver lesions can be classified into cystic and solid lesions. The former includes simple cysts, polycystic liver disease, biliary cystadenoma, parasitic cysts (eg, hydatid disease), and traumatic lesions (eg, hematoma or biloma). The most common solid tumors are hepatic hemangioma, focal nodular hyperplasia, and liver cell adenoma.

Benign tumors of the liver can also be classified by their cell of origin (Table 1). This chapter will focus on four benign liver tumors: hepatic hemangioma, focal nodular hyperplasia, liver cell adenoma, and biliary cystadenoma. Regenerative nodules usually occur in the setting of cirrhosis or chronic liver disease and must be differentiated from hepatocellular carcinoma. Hepatic cysts are common, usually easily identified on magnetic resonance imaging (MRI), and almost never are symptomatic. Bile duct hamartomas are small, gray-white nodules commonly found under the liver capsule at the time of laparotomy, and they often require biopsy to differentiate them from small metastatic lesions.

Initial Patient Evaluation

The majority of benign liver tumors are asymptomatic and are found incidentally. For patients who present with gastrointestinal symptoms, the clinical history is important for diagnosing other conditions, such as cholelithiasis or peptic ulcer disease, that may be the source of the symptoms. It is also important to obtain information

Table 1 Benign Tumors of the Liver

Cell of origin	Tumor
Hepatocyte	Focal nodular hyperplasia
	Liver cell adenoma
	Regenerative nodule
Cholangio-epithelial	Biliary adenoma or cystadenoma
	Simple cysts
Mesenchymal	Hemangioma
	Bile duct hamartoma

regarding a history of hepatitis, cirrhosis, alcohol use, and oral contraceptive or estrogen use. On physical examination, liver tumors are usually not palpable unless quite large, but the examiner should determine if any abdominal or flank tenderness exists in the location of the liver tumor. Serum liver function tests are generally normal. In certain cases, measurement of alpha fetoprotein (AFP), carcinoembryonic antigen (CEA), and carbohydrate antigen (CA) 19-9 may help differentiate benign from malignant tumors. Benign liver tumors rarely have elevations in these tumor markers, whereas patients with hepatocellular carcinoma, colorectal cancer liver metastases, and cholangiocarcinoma will often have elevations in one or more of these serum markers.

Radiologic Evaluation and Diagnosis

Radiologic evaluation plays an increasingly important role in diagnosing unknown liver tumors. The primary modalities used are ultrasound (US), computed tomography (CT), and magnetic resonance imaging (MRI). Often, two or all three of these modalities are used to reach a diagnosis. Other tests that may be required in certain circumstances include sulfur colloid scans (eg, liver-spleen scan), positive emission tomography (PET), and angiography. In some cases, noninvasive imaging is inadequate in establishing a diagnosis.

Ultrasound is very useful in differentiating between solid and cystic neoplasms of the liver, but is less useful in differentiating between types of solid tumors. The fluid content within cysts results in minimal signal, and thus cysts appear as hypoechoic masses with through-transmission. Whereas certain solid tumors of the liver have specific ultrasound characteristics, the appearance of any solid lesion on ultrasound is not specific enough to yield a definitive diagnosis.[2] Color flow Doppler can be used in conjunction with ultrasound to assess the relationship of the tumor to major blood vessels as well as assess blood flow within tumors.

CT scans to evaluate liver lesions should be obtained in three phases of intravascular contrast: arterial phase, portal venous phase, and delayed. Some hypervascular tumors can be identified on precontrast or arterial images and may be undetectable if only portal venous phase images are obtained. Arterial phase images can also detect small hypervascular lesions as hyperdense areas compared with adjacent normal liver. The portal venous phase images are most helpful for detecting lesions such as metastases that appear hypodense compared with normal liver parenchyma, because they receive their blood supply principally from the hepatic artery, whereas the normal liver receives its blood supply principally from the portal vein.

MRI is usually the most useful modality in differentiating between various types of liver tumors. MRI and CT are relatively equivalent in detecting lesions, but MRI often provides better differentiation in determining the type of tumor. On T1-weighted images, the liver is dark gray, whereas fluid (water density) is dark, and on T2-weighted images, the liver is gray and fluid is bright. Almost all liver masses are hypodense on T1-weighted images, and 90% are hyperdense on T2-weighted images.[3] Intravenous contrast is usually administered for liver MRI in the form of gadolinium, and certain benign liver lesions have a characteristic enhancement pattern.

Table 2 lists the characteristic CT and MRI features of the three most common benign, solid liver tumors. MRI is especially good for diagnosing hemangiomas, with reported accuracies ranging from 84 to 95%.[4] Hepatic hemangiomas are hypodense on T1-weighted images and become intensely bright on T2-weighted images in what is known as the light bulb sign (Figure 1). Following gadolinium administration, there is a characteristic initial peripheral nodular enhancement followed by centripetal filling of the lesion from the periphery toward the center (Figure 1B). This centripetal filling occurs more commonly in intermediate-sized lesions between 1.5 and 5 cm.[5]

In the past, several other tests have been used to diagnose hepatic hemangiomas but now uncommonly are required. Labeled red blood cell scintigraphy using planar and SPECT mode demonstrates pooling on

Table 2 CT and MRI Features of Benign Liver Tumors

Imaging Modality	Hemangioma	Focal Nodular Hyperplasia	Hepatic Adenoma
CT Noncontrast	Hypodense	Hypo- or isodense central scar	Hypodense
Contrast	Initial patchy peripheral enhancement followed by centripetal filling	Enhances early; isodense late	Enhances early, hypodense late
MRI			
T1	Hypodense	Isodense; hypodense central scar	Hyperdense
T2	Hyperdense (light bulb)	Iso- or hyperdense; hyperdense central scar	Hyperdense
Gadolinium	Initial patchy peripheral enhancement followed by centripetal filling	Enhances early with hypodense scar Isodense late with hyperdense scar	Enhances early; isodense late

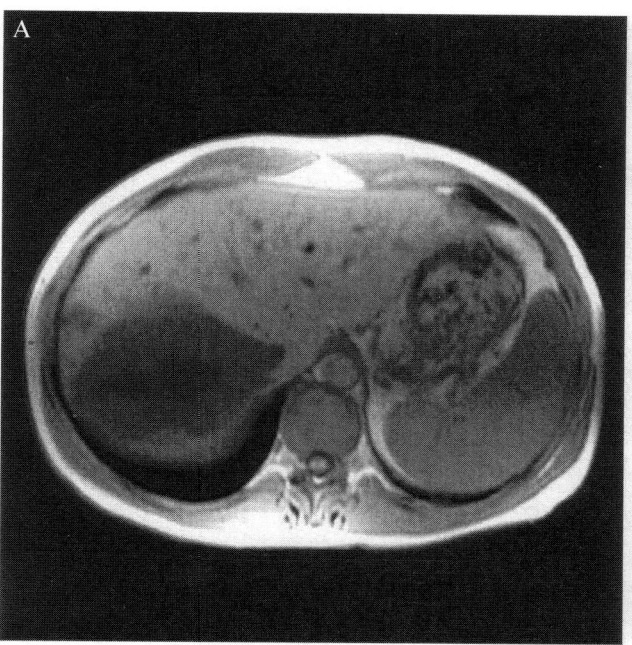 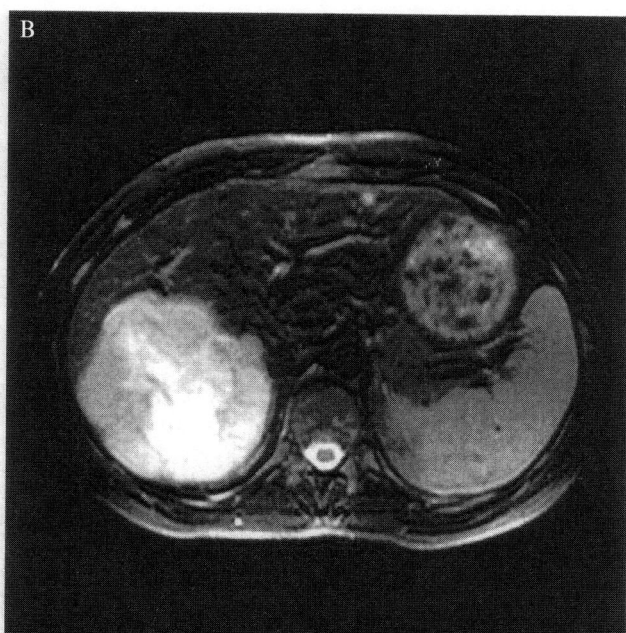

Figure 1 T1- (A) and T2-weighted (B) images of a hepatic hemangioma.

delayed images at 30 to 60 minutes and is highly specific in diagnosing hemangiomas.[6] Angiography is also highly accurate in establishing the diagnosis of hemangioma, and demonstrates one or more large feeding vessels followed by diffuse pooling of contrast in what has been described as a "cotton-wool" pattern.[7]

The diagnoses of focal nodular hyperplasia (FNH) and liver cell adenoma are often more difficult than that for hemangiomas, given they can have variable appearances on CT scan or MRI (see Table 2). Thus the diagnosis of these tumors may require additional studies. Focal nodular hyperplasia has a central scar evident on imaging studies about 60% of the time. On MRI, T1-weighted images usually show an isodense lesion with a hypodense scar if present, whereas T2-weighted images usually show a hyperdense lesion with a hyperdense scar. Gadolinium contrast results in early enhancement with a hypodense scar followed later by an isodense lesion with a hyperdense scar. FNH on sulfur colloid scanning with technetium 99m-labeled sulfur colloid has normal or increased uptake, whereas most other lesions have decreased uptake.[2] Finally, angiography reveals a hypervascular lesion with a characteristic spoke-wheel pattern. The diagnostic imaging of liver cell adenoma is often indeterminate. On MRI, these lesions appear hyperdense on both T1- and T2-weighted images. After gadolinium, they enhance early and are isodense late. Liver cell adenoma can often resemble a well-differentiated hepatocellular carcinoma on imaging studies.

Biliary cystadenomas appear as multiloculated masses in which the wall enhances with administration of contrast. Solid components, including papillary projections into the cyst lumen, identified on either contrast-enhanced CT or MRI raise the suspicion for malignant transformation. Fine septal calcifications may be identified on CT. Biliary duct dilatation is uncommon.

Benign liver tumors such as hemangiomas, FNH, liver cell adenomas, and biliary cystadenoma generally do not demonstrated increased ^{18}F-fluorodeoxyglucose (FDG) uptake on FDG-positron emission tomography (PET) scans. Thus, PET studies can be used to differentiate these benign tumors from malignant tumors such as colorectal cancer or other solid tumor liver metastases and hepatocellular carcinomas, which generally have increased FDG uptake.[8]

The use of percutaneous biopsy for undiagnosed liver lesions requires careful clinical judgment. Biopsies should be reserved for clinical situations in which the diagnosis will make a difference in management. Thus, for symptomatic lesions that will require resection, biopsy is not necessary. For patients with a history of malignancy and with an undiagnosed liver lesion that may be a metastasis versus a benign tumor, biopsy may be useful. The diagnosis of metastasis can often be made by comparing biopsy material from the liver tumor with that of the primary tumor. However, biopsy of many benign lesions often yields equivocal results. For hepatic hemangiomas, percutaneous biopsies are often nondiagnostic[9] and carry the risk of hemorrhage.[10] FNH on biopsy appears similar to liver cirrhosis with regenerating nodules and connective tissue septa,[11] and so biopsies can be nondiagnostic or incorrect. Biopsies are rarely helpful when used to diagnose a liver cell adenoma, as the inability to distinguish this entity accurately from a well-differentiated hepatocellular carcinoma is well known. Similarly, biopsy of biliary cystadenoma is rarely helpful given these lesions are mostly cystic. In one series, 19 of 30 preoperative percutaneous biopsies for what later proved to be benign liver tumors were incorrect or indeterminate.[12]

Hemangioma

GENERAL

Hepatic hemangiomas are the most common solid benign tumor of the liver, with an incidence in autopsy series of up to 7.3%.[13] They are found more commonly in women than men of any age, with a median age of presentation between 50 and 60 years. These lesions are considered to be congenital vascular malformations and enlarge by ectasia rather than neoplastic growth. They can be single or multiple and range in size from less than 1 cm in diameter to giant lesions that replace much of the liver. Macroscopically, hemangiomas are dark, reddish-purple lesions that can have a smooth or lobulated surface (Figure 2A). Hepatic hemangiomas can often be distinguished from other common liver tumors by their compressibility and changes in consistency in relation to central venous pressure. A Valsalva maneuver delivered by the anesthesiologist during an open laparotomy may produce an increase in consistency. Histologic analysis of these tumors reveals large blood-filled spaces lined by endothelial cells and separated by thin fibrous septa (Figure 2B).

CLINICAL PRESENTATION, NATURAL HISTORY, AND COMPLICATIONS

The vast majority of hepatic hemangiomas are small (< 5 cm) and asymptomatic, and even large hemangiomas rarely cause symptoms. These tumors are usually discovered during abdominal imaging to investigate unrelated conditions or at the time of laparotomy. In those with symptoms, the most common symptom is abdominal pain or discomfort. The pathogenesis of abdominal pain or discomfort secondary to these tumors is unclear. Intratumoral thrombosis can lead to inflammation that may cause discomfort for 1 to 3 weeks, and intratumoral bleeding or enlargement can stretch Glisson's capsule, causing pain. Large tumors can cause a mass effect on the stomach or duodenum, resulting in early satiety, nausea, or vomiting. The gastrointestinal symptoms that lead to the discovery of hepatic hemangiomas are often not due to the tumor. Farges and colleagues reported that 24% of patients had persistent symptoms following resection of hepatic

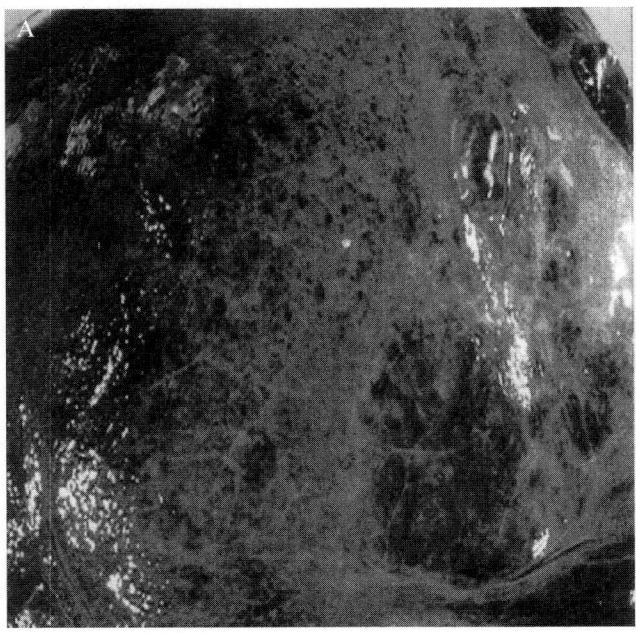 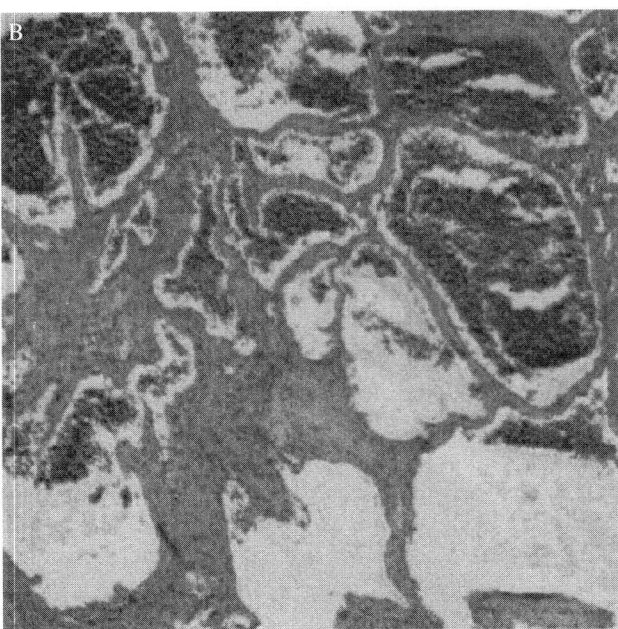

Figure 2 Gross (A) and microscopic (B) photos of a hepatic hemangioma.

hemangiomas, suggesting these patients had other etiologies for their pain.[14]

The natural history of hepatic hemangiomas is such that they rarely cause symptoms or problems over the life span of affected individuals.[15] In a study of 163 patients with a mean follow-up of nearly 8 years, only 9 tumors increased in size, whereas 7 tumors decreased in size.[14] Five patients had significant complications, and 8 patients required resection. In our own series of 63 patients, only 2 lesions increased in size by over 1 cm.[9] Numerous other series have confirmed that the vast majority of hepatic hemangiomas may be safely followed with a very low risk of complications.

Other rare clinical presentations include spontaneous rupture with intraperitoneal hemorrhage and Kasabach-Merritt syndrome. There have been only 30 cases of spontaneous rupture of a giant cavernous hemangioma reported in the literature.[16] In such cases, patients with active bleeding may benefit from angiography and embolization to stabilize this life-threatening complication prior to definitive surgical resection. Kasabach-Merritt syndrome is a clinical diagnosis characterized by thrombocytopenia and consumptive coagulopathy, which results from platelet trapping in large hemangiomas followed by activation of platelets and the coagulation cascade.[17] In our own series, we had 2 patients with this rare syndrome, and both patients had resolution of their thrombocytopenia and coagulopathy after resection of their hemangiomas.[9] Budd-Chiari syndrome characterized by thrombotic or nonthrombotic obstruction to hepatic venous outflow can also occur.[14] Malignant transformation of hepatic hemangiomas has not been reported.

MANAGEMENT

Once the diagnosis of hepatic hemangioma is established, treatment depends on the degree of symptoms, certainty of diagnosis, and the presence of complications. For asymptomatic patients, a follow-up MRI in 6 months may be obtained to ensure that the tumor is not significantly growing and to reassure anxious patients. Subsequent to this, follow-up imaging can be performed only as needed. For patients with gastrointestinal symptoms, abdominal ultrasound and upper endoscopy may be necessary to rule out gallstone disease or peptic ulcer disease as the etiology for symptoms. A period of watchful waiting for 2 to 3 months may be appropriate for patients without severe symptoms to determine if these symptoms may resolve on their own. Patients with persistent or worsening symptoms that cannot be attributed to other causes may be considered for surgical resection. There is no definitive link between hepatic hemangiomas and oral contraceptive use or exogenous estrogen. In general, we do not recommend stopping the use of these agents. For women of childbearing age, we also do not discourage pregnancy, given the risk of rapid growth or rupture is very small. For symptomatic women or women with giant hepatic hemangiomas, one can consider stopping oral contraceptives to determine the effect on symptoms or rate of growth.

In addition to severe or persistent symptoms, another indication for resection is the inability to exclude malignancy. Shimizu and colleagues reviewed 32 patients who were thought preoperatively to have a possible liver malignancy but subsequently proved to have benign diagnoses.[18] They identified three criteria that suggested benign lesions: size less than 4 cm, discrepancy in radiologic diagnoses, and stability in size. Patients in our hemangioma series who underwent surgery to exclude malignancy were more commonly male, asymptomatic, had a history of cancer, and had smaller lesions compared with patients who underwent surgery for other indications.[9] Although the majority of patients with hepatic hemangiomas can have a diagnosis established nonoperatively, there exist a minority of patients who cannot be definitively diagnosed and in which the clinical scenario warrants resection. Rarely, surgical resection of hepatic hemangiomas is necessary when significant complications arise. Such complications include tumor rupture with intraperitoneal hemorrhage, Kasabach-Merritt syndrome, and Budd-Chiari syndrome.

Resection of hepatic hemangiomas can be performed using a variety of techniques, including enucleation, formal hepatic resection, and laparoscopic techniques.[7,9,19–27] Morbidity rates are low and mortality is rare (Table 3). Formal hepatic resection is often necessary for small, deep tumors suspected of being malignant. Such tumors cannot be visualized well intraoperatively, and a margin of normal tissue should be obtained. For tumors known to be hemangioma, we feel enucleation is the procedure of choice. One study reported fewer intra-abdominal complications with enucleation compared with hepatic resection,[1] whereas other studies used only hepatic resection.[7,26]

We perform enucleation similar to the technique described by Baer and colleagues.[20] There are several advantages of enucleation over hepatic resection, including preservation of a maximal amount of functional liver, eliminating the need for outflow control of the hepatic veins, and limiting blood loss. For a large hemangioma, especially those located in the central liver, one can obtain a preoperative CT angiogram (Figure 3A and B). These studies are used to identify the main feeding arteries to the hemangioma and delineate the relationship to surrounding vessels, which are often obscured on standard imaging because of compression. Prior to enucleation, the liver is mobilized from its ligamentous

Table 3 Summary of Surgical Series of Liver Hemangioma Resection

Author	Year	Number pts	Avg/Median Size (cm)	Surgery						Morbidity		Mortality
				Enuc	Segment	Lobe	N (%) Extend	Nonanat	Laparosc	Major	Minor	
Schwartz[19]	1987	16	10	2 (13)	7 (44)	5 (31)	2 (13)	0	0	NR	NR	0
Baer[20]	1992	10	14.5	10 (100)	0	0	0	0	0	1	NR	0
Belli[7]	1992	24	11	0	17 (71)	4 (17)	0	3 (13)	0	0	2	0
Lise[21]	1992	25	8.5	3 (12)	4 (16)	6 (24)	0	12 (48)	0	2	NR	0
Petri[25]	1993	51	5.6	29 (51)	0	2 (4)	1 (2)	19 (37)	0	5	8	0
Brouwers[26]	1997	24	11	0	4 (17)	13 (54)	4 (17)	3 (13)	0	5	NR	0
Weimann[27]	1997	69	8.3	26 (38)	18 (26)	11 (16)	0	14 (20)	0	5	8	0
Gedaly[1]	1999	28	6.5	23 (82)	1 (4)	2 (7)	2 (7)	0	0	6	6	0
Ozden[22]	2000	39	10	33 (85)	3 (8)	3 (8)	0	0	0	5	NR	1
Reddy[23]	2001	34	6.9	0	22 (65)	11 (32)	1 (3)	0	0	NR	NR	0
Popescu[24]	2001	57	9	38 (67)	11 (19)	4 (7)	0	3 (5)	1 (2)	6	NR	0
Yoon[9]	2003	52	11	31 (60)	8 (15)	5 (10)	1 (2)	6 (12)	1 (2)	10	12	0

Enuc = enucleation; Segment = segmentectomy or sectorectomy; Lobe = lobectomy; Extend = extended lobectomy;
Nonanat = nonanatomic resection; Laparosc = laparoscopically assisted resection; NR = not reported.

attachments. Blood loss can be minimized by maintaining a low central venous pressure, elevating the liver anteriorly following mobilization, and using an intermittent Pringle maneuver. A crush clamp or other parenchymal dissection technique is used to identify the normal parenchyma/fibrous capsule interface, and dissection proceeds along this plane. Early ligation of the major inflow vessels during enucleation allows manual decompression of a large hemangioma and often dramatically facilitates their manipulation.

Surgical resection remains the definitive treatment of symptomatic hemangioma, but other less effective options include transarterial embolization,[28] radiotherapy,[29] and hepatic artery ligation.[30] For large, symptomatic hemangiomas that are not resectable and that are causing hepatic dysfunction, liver transplantation has been performed.[31]

Focal Nodular Hyperplasia

GENERAL

FNH is the second most common benign solid tumor of the liver, and one autopsy study identified these lesions

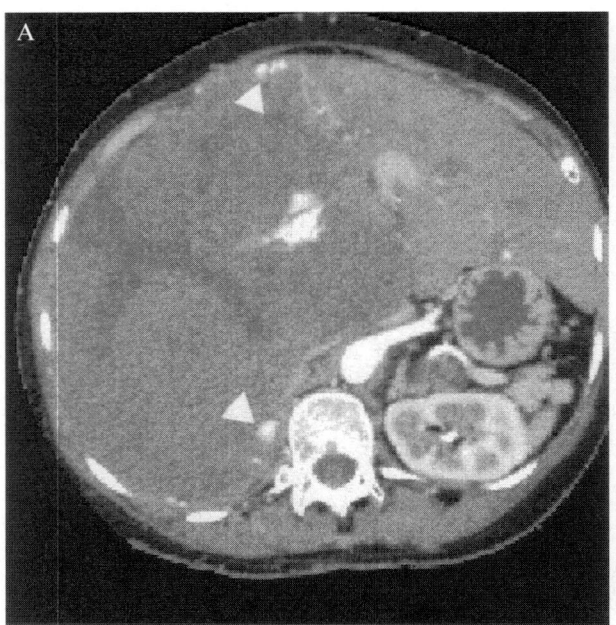
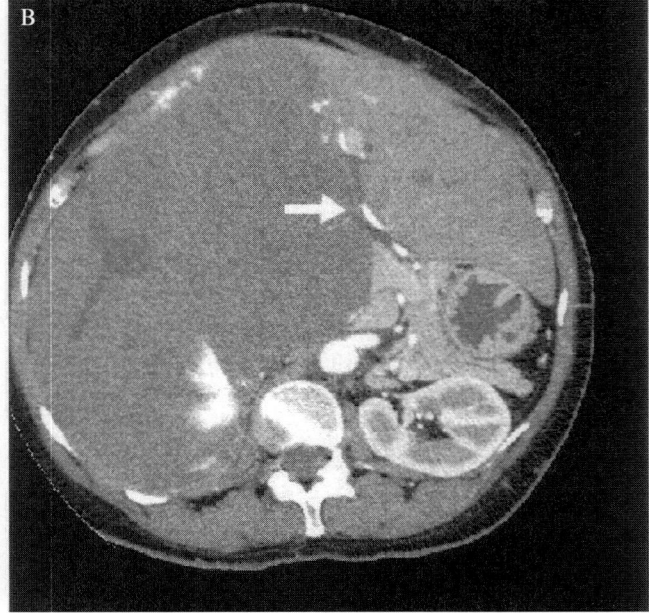

Figure 3 CT angiogram of a hepatic hemangioma. *A,* Arrowheads demonstrate peripheral nodular enhancement and *B,* arrow demonstrates feeding arterial vessel.

in 0.31% of adult livers.[32] These tumors are thought to be secondary to injury or developmental vascular malformations, and are usually found as solitary tumors. They are found much more commonly in women of childbearing age, and oral contraceptives may act to accelerate the growth of these tumors, although this association is less clear than with liver cell adenoma. The majority of FNH tumors are small (< 5 cm), but these tumors can grow to significant sizes. Grossly these lesions are usually well-defined, nodular, or dimpled masses, and their color varies from tan to yellow-brown (Figure 4A). Many of these tumors have a central scar that can contain an abnormally large artery that branches into smaller vessels radiating through the fibrous septa to the periphery of the lesion, producing the characteristic spoke-wheel appearance during angiography. Histologically, FNH tumors resemble cirrhotic liver parenchyma and are composed of cords of benign hepatocytes subdivided by thin fibrous septae radiating from a central scar (Figure 4B).

CLINICAL PRESENTATION, NATURAL HISTORY, AND COMPLICATIONS

Like hepatic hemangiomas, FNH tumors are usually discovered during abdominal imaging to investigate unrelated conditions or at the time of laparotomy. The majority of tumors are asymptomatic. In those patients with symptoms, the most common symptom is abdominal pain or discomfort.[27] Larger tumors can cause a mass effect, resulting in early satiety, nausea, or vomiting.

The natural history is such that it is extremely rare for these lesions to cause symptoms or problems. Hugh and colleagues summarized observation series totaling 115

FNH patients and found only 14 patients who had persistent symptoms or increased tumor size, and only 9 patients required intervention at some point.[15] Significant complications associated with FNH such as spontaneous rupture with intraperitoneal hemorrhage rarely occur, and malignant transformation has not been reported.

MANAGEMENT

The management of FNH resembles that of hepatic hemangiomas. For asymptomatic patients, a follow-up MRI in 6 months may be obtained to ensure stability in size, and further follow-up beyond that time can be performed as needed. For patients with symptoms, a thorough investigation should be performed to rule out other causes. The authors usually recommend stopping oral contraceptive use and using alternative methods of birth control in symptomatic patients or patients with extremely large tumors, although it is recognized that not all physicians are strict regarding this recommendation. For patients with significant or persistent symptoms that cannot be attributed to other conditions, surgical resection should be considered. For less severe symptoms, patients can be followed for 2 to 3 months to determine if such symptoms persist or worsen. Lesions that cannot be definitively diagnosed may require short-term follow-up (2–3 months) or surgical resection, depending on the clinical scenario.

For surgical resection, superficial FNH tumors can usually be excised in a wedge resection along with a small amount of normal hepatic parenchyma. Large or deep lesions may require a formal anatomic resection. These tumors are not compressible and do no have an easily

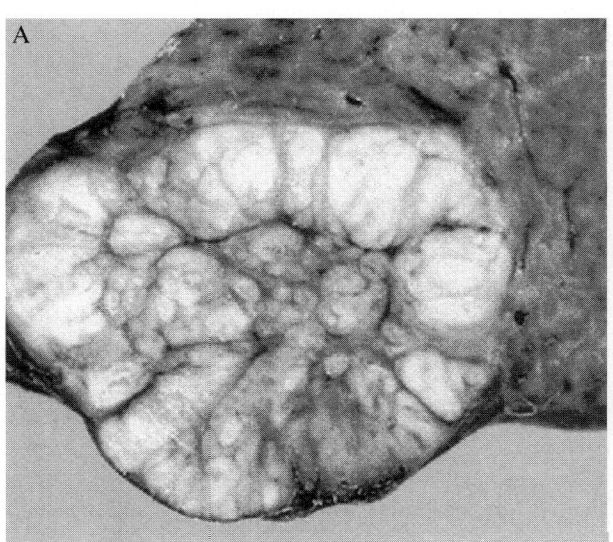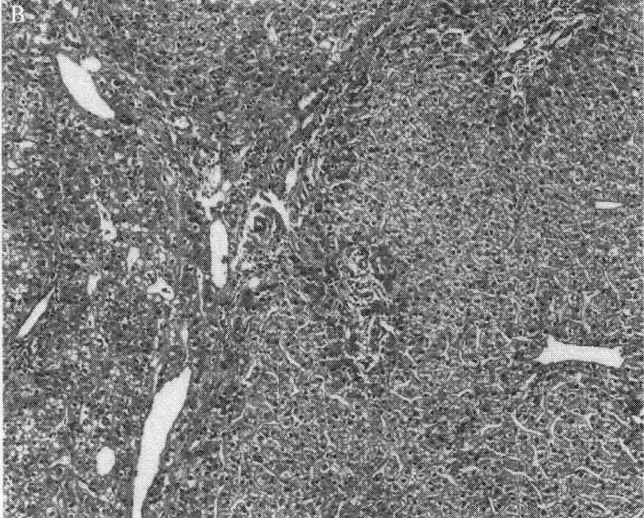

Figure 4 Gross (A) and microscopic (B) photos of focal nodular hyperplasia.

defined tumor/normal parenchyma interface, so enucleation is less commonly performed than for hemangiomas.[12] In one series of 61 patients who underwent resection of FNH, 13 (21%) underwent enucleation, 16 (26%) nonanatomic resection, 16 (26%) segmental resection, 15 (25%) hepatectomy or extended hepatectomy, and 1 (2%) liver transplantation.[27] The complication rate was 28% and there were no peri- or postoperative deaths.

Liver Cell Adenoma

GENERAL

Liver cell adenoma is the third most common benign solid tumor of the liver. Similar to FNH, these lesions are found much more commonly in women of childbearing age. These tumors are composed of a benign proliferation of hepatocytes. The true incidence of hepatic adenomas from autopsy series is unknown; however, it is clear that the incidence increased following the introduction of oral contraceptives.[33] There is a much stronger association of liver cell adenoma with oral contraceptive use than occurs with FNH. Adenomas occur 30 to 40 times more commonly in women with a history of long-term oral contraceptive use. These tumors are usually solitary, round, and range in size from less than 1 cm in diameter to greater than 30 cm. On gross examination, a liver cell adenoma is typically soft with a smooth surface and fleshy appearance, with a yellow-to-brown color, and may contain areas of necrosis or hemorrhage within (Figure 5A). They often have prominent vessels around the periphery and within the tumor, and these tumors lack a true capsule. Under the microscope, liver cell adenomas demonstrate sheets of benign-appearing hepatocytes without portal tracts or hepatic veins (Figure 5B).

CLINICAL PRESENTATION, NATURAL HISTORY, AND COMPLICATIONS

Liver cell adenomas are more often symptomatic than hemangiomas or FNH, and their natural history does not always follow an innocent course. There are published reports of spontaneous hemorrhage, rupture, and hepatocellular carcinoma arising within liver cell adenomas.[34] In the past, many patients with liver cell adenomas presented with symptoms; however, the proportion of patients with symptoms appears to be declining as more are identified incidentally during an abdominal imaging study.

Abdominal mass or pain is the most common presenting symptom in patients with liver cell adenomas. Most commonly, nonspecific abdominal pain leads to imaging tests that initially discover the adenoma. It seems unlikely in most of these instances that the adenoma was the source of abdominal pain, and usually these adenomas are better classified as incidentally identified. Pain actually referable to a liver cell adenoma is most commonly in the right upper quadrant or epigatrium, and may radiate to the right flank or back.

A minority of patients will present with the more dramatic and potentially life-threatening clinical symptoms arising from rupture and acute hemorrhage.[35] There is a common but unproven notion that pregnancy exerts significant effects on liver cell adenomas, largely because of one study in which 5 of 6 women who were pregnant or within 6 weeks of pregnancy presented with rupture compared with less than 30% of other women diagnosed with hepatic adenomas.[33]

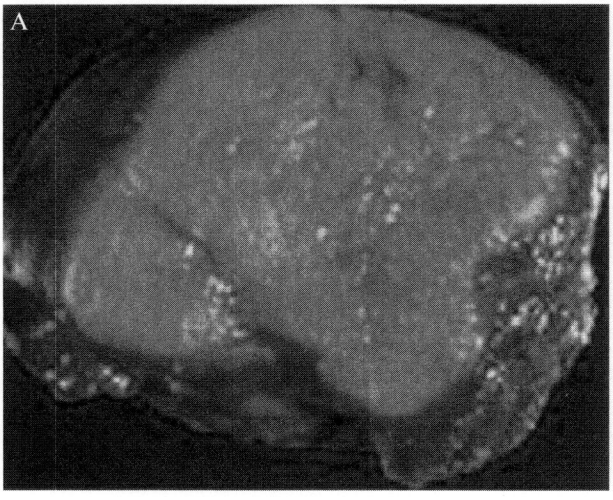
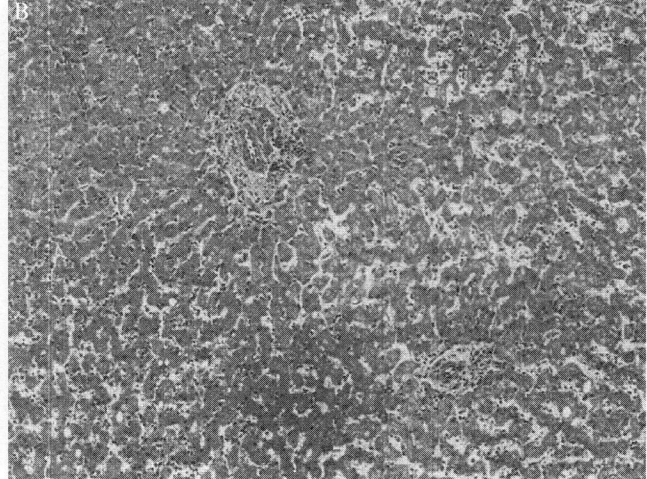

Figure 5 Gross (A) and microscopic (B) photos of a liver cell adenoma.

Case reports of hepatocellular carcinoma arising within a liver cell adenoma raise the notion that malignant transformation is possible.[34] Fortunately, based on the relative infrequency of these reports and the small numbers of patients involved, it appears that the risk of malignant transformation is quite low.

MANAGEMENT

Nearly all patients with liver cell adenomas should be considered for surgical resection. Patients who present with asymptomatic (incidentally identified) liver cell adenomas who are taking oral contraceptives or steroids may be cautiously observed following discontinuation of these medications. Regression of liver cell adenomas in response to this maneuver has been reported.[36] It is the authors' practice to obtain scans every 3 months following discontinuation of oral contraceptives, followed by less frequent scans once regression is achieved. Resection is recommended if no regression is observed within 6 months, or if the tumor increases in size during observation. The principal reason to resect lesions that do not regress is the potential for spontaneous hemorrhage, as opposed to the very small risk of malignant transformation. In patients whose lesions regress following discontinuation of oral contraceptives or steroids, subsequent development of hepatocellular carcinoma has been reported,[37] but based on the infrequency of such reports, this is felt to be a very low risk. In patients with asymptomatic liver cell adenomas who are not taking oral contraceptives, the risks of resection should be weighed against the possibility of rupture and hemorrhage. The risk of the latter is difficult to calculate, but generally increases with lesion size. The rapidly falling mortality rates associated with liver surgery argue for resection of such lesions in general, although lesion location, patient comorbidity, and surgeon experience must be factored into the decision. Patients who present with rupture and bleeding should undergo urgent operation to resect the adenoma. Hepatic angiography and embolization to reduce or control bleeding transiently prior to surgery is used rarely in emersent situations. Patients who present with pain should undergo resection when feasible.

Surgical removal of liver cell adenomas generally requires dividing liver parenchyma along traditional surgical dissection planes, although nonanatomical resections may be used when more convenient and safe. Unlike hemangiomas, there is rarely a suitable dissection plane to allow enucleation of liver cell adenomas. In addition, the differential diagnosis commonly includes malignant lesions, which further argues against attempts at enucleation. Standard surgical techniques for liver resection are generally employed, including use of low central venous pressure, complete liver mobilization, and vascular inflow occlusion. Subtotal resection may be considered in patients whose tumors are symptomatic and involve all hepatic veins, or both left and right main portal trunks. In patients with lesions that are unresectable because of involvement of bilateral hepatic vascular structures and in which continued lesion growth has become life threatening, liver transplantation is a reasonable option. The minimal experience with radiation, radiofrequency ablation, cryoablation, and arterial embolization argues for selective use of these approaches only in patients whose tumors are not suitable for resection based on tumor size, location, or patient comorbidities.

Biliary Cystadenoma

GENERAL

Biliary cystadenoma is the only cystic lesion included in this chapter; it is an entity that should not be forgotten when formulating differential diagnoses. These lesions are generally large, located in the right lobe, and more prevalent in middle-aged women.[38] These lesions contain mucinous fluid, although the presence of blood may indicate transformation to a biliary cystadenocarcinoma. These tumors are relatively rare, and the notion that they are congenital in nature is unconfirmed. Biliary cystadenomas are lined by benign biliary epithelium; malignant transformation of this epithelium may occur. The presence of benign biliary epithelium in most biliary cystadenocarcinomas suggests that most arise from malignant transformation of intially benign cystadenomas.

CLINICAL PRESENTATION, NATURAL HISTORY, AND COMPLICATIONS

Biliary cystadenomas are typically asymptomatic and identified incidentally during abdominal imaging. As is observed with other types of benign liver tumors, nonspecific abdominal pain may lead to imaging tests that initially discover the liver lesion. Biliary cystadenomas are slow growing. Hemorrhage, rupture, biliary obstruction, and cholangitis are inordinately rare.[13] When multilocular in appearance, biliary cystadenomas are more readily distinguished from liver cysts; however, unilocular biliary cystadenomas are nearly impossible to distinguish from simple congenital hepatic cysts. The differential diagnosis of complex cystic lesions also includes hemorrhage into simple cysts, parasitic cysts (eg, hydatid disease), and cystic metastases. Metastatic liver tumors that undergo cystic change can usually be diagnosed correctly based on the clinical context and radiographic appearance.

MANAGEMENT

In patients with a large, asymptomatic, simple liver cyst, serial imaging on an annual basis may be recommended. Lesion growth or changes in the internal structure of the lesion suggest the possibility of biliary cystadenocarcinoma, for which surgical exploration and resection is indicated. Needle biopsy is of little value. For patients in whom the differential diagnosis includes a simple cyst and a biliary cystadenoma, laparoscopic excision of a cyst wall segment for pathologic evaluation is the most direct and least invasive method to establish a diagnosis. Simple cysts may be left open to the peritoneum, and biliary cystadenomas should be excised because of the potential for malignant transformation. Enucleation or removal by liver resection may be used to remove biliary cystadenomas, recognizing that incomplete enucleation or resection will almost certainly lead to recurrence. For patients with complex cystic lesions in whom a diagnosis of biliary cystadenoma is entertained, needle biopsy is not generally recommended because of the low diagnostic accuracy. Rather, surgical exploration is indicated, with complete enucleation or removal by liver resection. Outcomes following resection of biliary cystadenomas are generally quite good, whereas patients with cystadenocarcinomas must be followed long term to assess for recurrent or metastatic disease.[39]

Summary

Benign liver tumors often present a significant challenge in diagnosis and treatment. For lesions causing significant symptoms or complications, definitive diagnosis is not necessary and one may proceed to definitive surgical resection. For asymptomatic tumors, MRI usually is the diagnostic imaging study of choice, and can be complemented by additional studies such as CT scans and ultrasound. Percutaneous biopsy may be warranted in patients to rule out a primary or secondary malignant tumor, but biopsy is often incorrect or nondiagnostic for benign liver lesions. Asymptomatic or minimally symptomatic hemangiomas, FNH, and cystadenomas may be safely followed, given the risk of significant complications is low. Cystadenomas may progress to cystadenocarcinomas, so these lesions require continued follow-up. Liver cell adenomas in general should be resected, given their risk of hemorrhage, but a period of observation off oral contraceptives can be considered to allow for regression. Numerous surgical series have demonstrated that benign liver tumors can be resected with low morbidity and almost no mortality. Uncommonly, benign liver tumors grow to very large sizes and cause significant problems such that alternative management strategies including liver transplantation are necessary.

References

1. Gedaly R, Pomposelli JJ, Pomfret EA, et al. Cavernous hemangioma of the liver: anatomic resection vs. enucleation. Arch Surg 1999;134:407–11.

2. DeMatteo RP, Fong Y. Imaging of hepatobiliary neoplasms. Surg Oncol Clin N Am 1999;8:59–89.

3. Wittenberg J, Stark DD, Forman BH, et al. Differentiation of hepatic metastases from hepatic hemangiomas and cysts by using MR imaging. AJR Am J Roentgenol 1988;151:79–84.

4. Mitchell P, Hodgson TJ, Seaman S, et al. Stereotactic radiosurgery and the risk of haemorrhage from cavernous malformations. Br J Neurosurg 2000;14:96–100.

5. Semelka RC, Brown ED, Ascher SM, et al. Hepatic hemangiomas: a multi-institutional study of appearance on T2-weighted and serial gadolinium-enhanced gradient-echo MR images. Radiology 1994;192:401–6.

6. Middleton ML. Scintigraphic evaluation of hepatic mass lesions: emphasis on hemangioma detection. Semin Nucl Med 1996;26:4–15.

7. Belli L, De Carlis L, Beati C, et al. Surgical treatment of symptomatic giant hemangiomas of the liver. Surg Gynecol Obstet 1992;174:474–8.

8. Delbeke D, Martin WH, Sandler MP, et al. Evaluation of benign vs malignant hepatic lesions with positron emission tomography. Arch Surg 1998;133:510–6.

9. Yoon SS, Charny CK, Fong Y, et al. Diagnosis, management, and outcomes of 115 patients with hepatic hemangioma. J Am Coll Surg 2003;197:392–402.

10. Terriff BA, Gibney RG, Scudamore CH. Fatality from fine-needle aspiration biopsy of a hepatic hemangioma. AJR Am J Roentgenol 1990;154:203–4.

11. Foster JH. Benign liver tumours. In: Blumgart LH, editor. Surgery of the liver and biliary tract. 2nd ed. Edinburgh: Churchill Livingstone; 1994. p. 1325–39.

12. Charny CK, Jarnagin WR, Schwartz LH, et al. Management of 155 patients with benign liver tumours. Br J Surg 2001; 88:808–13.

13. Ishak KG, Rabin L. Benign tumors of the liver. Med Clin North Am 1975;59:995–1013.

14. Farges O, Daradkeh S, Bismuth H. Cavernous hemangiomas of the liver: are there any indications for resection? World J Surg 1995;19:19–24.

15. Hugh TJ, Poston GJ. Benign liver tumors. In: Blumgart LH, Fong Y, editors. Surgery of the liver and biliary tract. 3rd ed London: W. B. Saunders; 2000. p. 1397–422.

16. Cappellani A, Zanghi A, Di Vita M, et al. Spontaneous rupture of a giant hemangioma of the liver. Ann Ital Chir 2000;71:379–83.

17. Gilon E, Ramot B, Sheba C. Multiple hemangiomata associated with thrombocytopenia: remarks on the patho-

genesis of the thrombocytopenia in this syndrome. Blood 1959;14:74–9.

18. Shimizu S, Takayama T, Kosuge T, et al. Benign tumors of the liver resected because of a diagnosis of malignancy. Surg Gynecol Obstet 1992;174:403–7.

19. Schwartz SI, Husser WC. Cavernous hemangioma of the liver. A single institution report of 16 resections. Ann Surg 1987;205:456–65.

20. Baer HU, Dennison AR, Mouton W, et al. Enucleation of giant hemangiomas of the liver. Technical and pathologic aspects of a neglected procedure. Ann Surg 1992;216:673–6.

21. Lise M, Feltrin G, Da Pian PP, et al. Giant cavernous hemangiomas: diagnosis and surgical strategies. World J Surg 1992;16:516–20.

22. Ozden I, Emre A, Alper A, et al. Long-term results of surgery for liver hemangiomas. Arch Surg 2000;135:978–81.

23. Reddy KR, Kligerman S, Levi J, et al. Benign and solid tumors of the liver: relationship to sex, age, size of tumors, and outcome. Am Surg 2001;67:173–8.

24. Popescu I, Ciurea S, Brasoveanu V, et al. Liver hemangioma revisited: current surgical indications, technical aspects, results. Hepatogastroenterology 2001;48:770–6.

25. Petri A, Karacsonyi S, Nagy KK. Surgical treatment of cavernous haemangiomas of the liver. Langenbecks Arch Chir 1993;378:322–4.

26. Brouwers MA, Peeters PM, de Jong KP, et al. Surgical treatment of giant haemangioma of the liver. Br J Surg 1997;84:314–6.

27. Weimann A, Ringe B, Klempnauer J, et al. Benign liver tumors: differential diagnosis and indications for surgery. World J Surg 1997;21:983–91.

28. Deutsch GS, Yeh KA, Bates WB 3rd, Tannehill WB. Embolization for management of hepatic hemangiomas. Am Surg 2001;67:159–64.

29. Gaspar L, Mascarenhas F, da Costa MS, et al. Radiation therapy in the unresectable cavernous hemangioma of the liver. Radiother Oncol 1993;29:45–50.

30. Nishida O, Satoh N, Alam AS, Uchino J. The effect of hepatic artery ligation for irresectable cavernous hemangioma of the liver. Am Surg 1988;54:483–6.

31. Russo MW, Johnson MW, Fair JH, Brown RS Jr. Orthotopic liver transplantation for giant hepatic hemangioma. Am J Gastroenterol 1997;92:1940–1.

32. Wanless IR, Albrecht S, Bilbao J, et al. Multiple focal nodular hyperplasia of the liver associated with vascular malformations of various organs and neoplasia of the brain: a new syndrome. Mod Pathol 1989;2:456–62.

33. Rooks JB, Ory HW, Ishak KG, et al. Epidemiology of hepatocellular adenoma. The role of oral contraceptive use. JAMA 1979;242:644–8.

34. Janes CH, McGill DB, Ludwig J, Krom RA. Liver cell adenoma at the age of 3 years and transplantation 19 years later after development of carcinoma: a case report. Hepatology 1993;17:583–5.

35. Kerlin P, Davis GL, McGill DB, et al. Hepatic adenoma and focal nodular hyperplasia: clinical, pathologic, and radiologic features. Gastroenterology 1983;84(5 Pt 1):994–1002.

36. Edmondson HA, Reynolds TB, Henderson B, Benton B. Regression of liver cell adenomas associated with oral contraceptives. Ann Intern Med 1977;86:180–2.

37. Tesluk H, Lawrie J. Hepatocellular adenoma. Its transformation to carcinoma in a user of oral contraceptives. Arch Pathol Lab Med 1981;105:296–9.

38. Wheeler DA, Edmondson HA. Cystadenoma with mesenchymal stroma (CMS) in the liver and bile ducts. A clinicopathologic study of 17 cases, 4 with malignant change. Cancer 1985;56:1434–45.

39. Akwari OE, Tucker A, Seigler HF, Itani KM. Hepatobiliary cystadenoma with mesenchymal stroma. Ann Surg 1990;211:18–27.

CHAPTER 16

LAPAROSCOPIC SURGERY FOR HEPATOBILIARY AND PANCREATIC NEOPLASMS

KEVIN T. WATKINS, MD

New instrumentation and more experience with laparoscopic surgery have made resection of hepatic and pancreatic tumors possible in carefully selected patients. It is crucial that surgeons have thorough training in both open and laparoscopic resection techniques. In laparoscopic surgery for malignant disease, there are areas that are now well-accepted practice and those that are controversial.

There are three areas where laparoscopic surgery can be applied in managing solid organ tumors: staging, resection, and palliation. Out of these three, the area most widely studied to date is staging to assess resectability of tumors,[1] Staging laparoscopy is a minimally invasive technique that can offer the operating surgeon invaluable information prior to embarking on a major resection or neoadjuvant treatment plans. Improvements in abdominal imaging have increased the sensitivity of identifying local tumor progression or the presence of distant disease. Staging laparoscopy can identify small volume peritoneal deposits that cannot be identified on standard imaging studies. Intraoperative laparoscopic ultrasound offers a more detailed evaluation of local tumor infiltration and can screen the hepatic parenchyma for small metastatic deposits. Significantly smaller deposits of metastatic disease can be identified and suspicious tissue can be biopsied for confirmation of the diagnosis. Presence of metastatic disease then obviates the need for a laparotomy if the plan was for a standard resection. Nontherapeutic laparotomies in this patient population lead to significant morbidity and should be avoided if at all possible.

Staging Laparoscopy for Pancreatic or Liver Malignancies

For pancreatic adenocarcinoma patients, as many as one-third of the cancers of the pancreatic head are found to have metastatic disease at time of surgery, and metastatic disease may be present in up to two-thirds of patients with cancer of the body and tail of the pancreas. The vast majority of these patients with metastatic disease will require no surgical palliation and should be spared laparotomy when possible.[2]

Staging laparoscopy can be performed to different degrees, but the basic principles are similar. Trocar placement is designed to allow these incisions to be incorporated into an incision for definitive resection. The entire peritoneal surface is inspected and any suspicious lesions are biopsied and sent for frozen section pathologic evaluation. Spoon or cup biopsy forceps can be used to obtain biopsies. Typically, hemostasis at biopsy sites can be achieved with standard cautery. The lymph nodes along the hepatic artery are inspected and the lesser sac is entered and inspected. Laparoscopic ultrasound is used to assess the liver and lymph node basins. Liver metastases can either be biopsied with a laparoscopic wedge resection or by the use of ultrasound-guided core biopsy. Typically, core biopsy is performed in a similar fashion to radiofrequency ablation as discussed below. The ultrasound can also be used to identify the tumor in the pancreas or liver and assess for local resectability. Care must be taken when evaluating tumors for vascular involvement. Obvious tumor encasement of vessels can be used to identify lesions that would be unresectable. Tumor encroachment on the vessels should be evaluated more thoroughly at laparotomy and cannot necessarily be used as documentation of unresectability for pancreatic cancer.

Once adequate laparoscopic inspection has been performed, the procedure can be converted to a standard open resection as planned. Conversely, if the patient is to enter a neoadjuvant treatment protocol, a feeding jejunostomy tube can be placed at the time of laparoscopy for nutritional supplementation through therapy.

Laparoscopic Radiofrequency Ablation

For small hepatocellular carcinomas (HCC), laparoscopy can play a significant role in management. Long-term survival is possible with radiofrequency ablation (RFA) of HCC and can be performed by a variety of techniques.[3] Since the majority of patients with HCC have concomitant liver disease, laparotomy is associated with a significant risk for wound and other postoperative complications. Although more technically challenging, laparoscopy can offer the same benefits of open RFA with less morbidity. In many cases RFA can be performed percutaneously; however, not all tumor locations are amenable to this approach. Laparoscopy gives the added benefit of being able to perform intraoperative ultrasound on the entire liver to survey for other potential lesions, as well as stage for distant spread of disease.

To perform laparoscopic RFA, camera port insertion should be performed to center on the location of the liver tumor. For lesions in the lateral portion of the right lobe or very posterior lesions, consideration should be made to place the patient in the left lateral decubitus position. Care must be taken in patients with portal hypertension when positioning the trocars. For initial entry, a Hasson trocar technique is recommended since placement of a Veress needle into a dilated venous branch can cause devastating results. Typically, nonbladed trocars are used for all other port placements. The camera port is placed approximately 4 to 6 cm below the location of a subcostal incision and is positioned to center on the tumor. A 12 mm port is then positioned for laparoscopic ultrasound probe insertion. In general, for right-sided lesions this is placed to the left side of the camera in the position of a subcostal incision. The opposite placement is used for left-sided lesions. For very anterior lesions, these two trocars will typically suffice. For more posterior or superior tumors, it is common to place a 5 mm trocar to use an instrument to help guide the needle RFA placement. This trocar is placed approximately 12 to 15 cm from the ultrasound port on the opposite side within the location of a subcostal incision.

After localization of the tumor with ultrasound and deciding the direction the RFA needle will take to reach the tumor, the RFA needle is introduced through the abdominal wall. A coaxial sheath is first placed to allow for exchange of needles if it is necessary to perform a core biopsy prior to ablation. This sheath can be placed through an intercostal space if necessary; in this case, respiration should be held during placement of the sheath to help prevent the possibility of pneumothorax. Laparoscopic ultrasonography is used to guide needle placement and to observe deployment of the radiofrequency array in the same fashion used for open ablation. After the ablation is performed, it is necessary to inspect the site of needle entry into the liver with decreased insufflation pressures. This is important since insufflation pressure may tamponade bleeding, which then becomes evident with lower intraperitoneal pressures. All trocar sites should be closed with fascial sutures to reduce leak of ascitic fluid; typically, this can be performed using a Carter-Thompson type suture passer.

Laparoscopic Liver Resection

Laparoscopic resection of solid organ tumors is in its infancy but is gaining in popularity. There are a myriad of techniques employed to perform liver resections laparoscopically. Standard surgical procedures in patients with cirrhosis carry significant morbidity and mortality. A laparoscopic approach in cirrhotic patients can significantly diminish postoperative wound complications, including leak of ascitic fluid, if all trocar fascial wounds are closed, including those from 5 mm trocars.

With advances in open hepatic resection techniques, mortality rates have significantly decreased. In performing hepatic resections laparoscopically, one of the principle disadvantages has been the inability to visualize consistently during parenchymal transection, because even mild hemorrhage from the liver edge can obscure a laparoscopic field. It is also difficult to perform parenchymal transection rapidly with standard laparoscopic techniques in order to diminish warm ischemia time when employing inflow occlusion. Many surgeons have, therefore, shifted to performing laparoscopically assisted liver resections utilizing a hand access port of some variety. This makes performing parenchymal transection more expeditious and allows better use of vascular inflow occlusion. Advances in instrumentation, such as ultrasonic shears and saline-enhanced electrocautery, have allowed for reduction in blood loss during laparoscopic parenchymal transection.

The most concerning potential risk specific to laparoscopic hepatic surgery is that of air embolism into an open branch of the hepatic veins. This could be especially important if the laparoscopic resection is performed utilizing hypovolemic (low central venous pressure) anesthetic techniques. Many surgeons compensate for this potential risk by lowering insufflation pressures when dissecting and transecting liver near the hepatic venous branches. It is also important to remember that the insufflation pressure during the laparoscopic procedure could tamponade hemorrhage from the cut surface of the liver. The effect of insufflation tamponade has allowed for parenchymal transection without vascular inflow occlusion. This can limit blood loss during transection, but it is particularly important that the cut surface be inspected with minimal insufflation at the end of the procedure to ensure there is not ongoing hemorrhage.

Laparoscopic hepatic resections can be performed in a variety of ways. This technique should generally be reserved for patients who require minor resections or resections for benign disease. Limited resections can also be performed to obtain tissue for diagnostic purposes. Resection can be performed with or without hand assistance. The decision on the use of a hand port should be based on several factors: size of the resected specimen, use of inflow occlusion, region of the liver to be resected, and the individual surgeon's comfort level. The hand assistance port can aid with retraction of a large specimen and permits tactile sensation and evaluation. Patient selection is one of the most important factors. Not all patients should undergo attempts at laparoscopic resection. The most approachable tumors for laparoscopic resection are those that present anterior and inferior on the liver. Lateral tumors can be resected laparoscopically with the patient in the decubitus position, but are technically more challenging and require meticulous port selection to obtain the proper angles to approach the tumor (Figure 1). Port selection is of paramount importance in being able to perform these laparoscopic resections. The position of the camera port will change depending on which segment the lesion occupies. Camera port positions that are too low on the abdomen make visualization difficult as the resection proceeds. The initial camera port position should be placed approximately 6 to 8 cm below the costal margin and should be positioned such that a direct line of view can be obtained over the transection line. For right-sided lesions, this would be toward the patient's left side of the tumor, with the converse being true for left-sided lesions.

The initial laparoscopic approach to tumors requires intraoperative localization of the tumor and surrounding vascular structures. Ultrasound is used to identify the known lesions and also to scan for other additional small liver tumors. The ligamentous attachments of the liver are preserved during resection to keep the liver

suspended. This and patient positioning generally obviates the need for a retractor to constantly support the liver. After the target lesion is identified, the resection is mapped out over the surface of the liver. Ultrasound can be used to inspect for vasculature along the lines of parenchymal transection. The TissueLink™ EndoSH (TissueLink Medical, Inc., Dover, NH) hook (Figure 2) is used to precoagulate and dissect the liver parenchyma. It can seal most vascular and biliary branches encountered. Larger segmental vascular branches are dissected free from the surrounding hepatic parenchyma and clipped or divided using an endoscopic vascular stapler. Alternatively, ultrasound can be used to detect and guide positioning of the stapler when parenchymal transection approaches larger vascular structures. This offers less chance of tearing the vessels when dissecting them free from the parenchyma since it is difficult to control tension in the line of dissection. Other coaptive devices (Ultrasonic shears, Ligasure™ [Valleylab, Boulder, CO]) can be used for parenchymal transection; however, they require the jaws of the instrument to be introduced blindly into the liver tissue, which may cause more ongoing slow hemorrhage that obscures visualization.

Specimen retrieval is performed in several different ways. The surgical specimen should be retrieved in a pouch to prevent the specimen from contacting the wound tract. For small resections, a single port site incision can be extended (Figure 3a). Larger specimens can be retrieved through a separate site, such as a small transverse suprapubic incision (Figure 3b). If hand access is being employed, the specimen can be removed through this port.

With minimally invasive techniques, liver resection can be performed with short hospital stays and low morbidity. When the potential for liver dysfunction is low, with small volume parenchymal resections, hospital stays can be less than 24 hours. In our series of 17 patients, the mean hospital stay was 29 hours, with 11 patients being discharged in less than 23 hours.[4] Long-term follow-up to determine if the laparoscopic approach to resection of malignant liver tumors has equivalent oncologic outcome compared with open resection does not yet exist. As long as the same basic principles of resection are maintained, the outcomes should be equivalent. It is important to perform adequate resections to assure a negative resection margin (see Figure 1d).

Laparoscopic Pancreatectomy

Since the mid-1990s, laparoscopic pancreatic resections have been reported in the literature.[5] The majority of

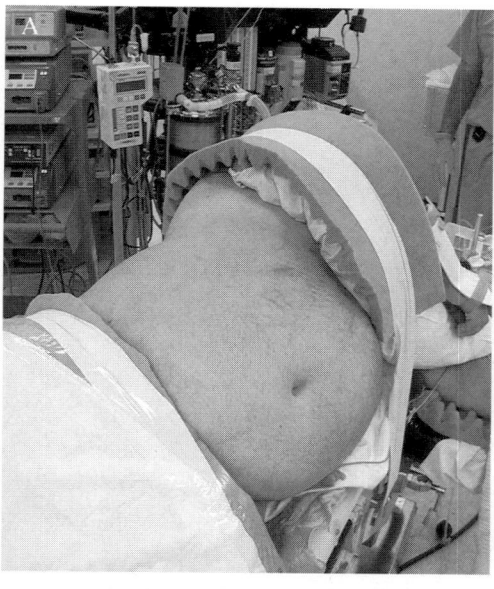 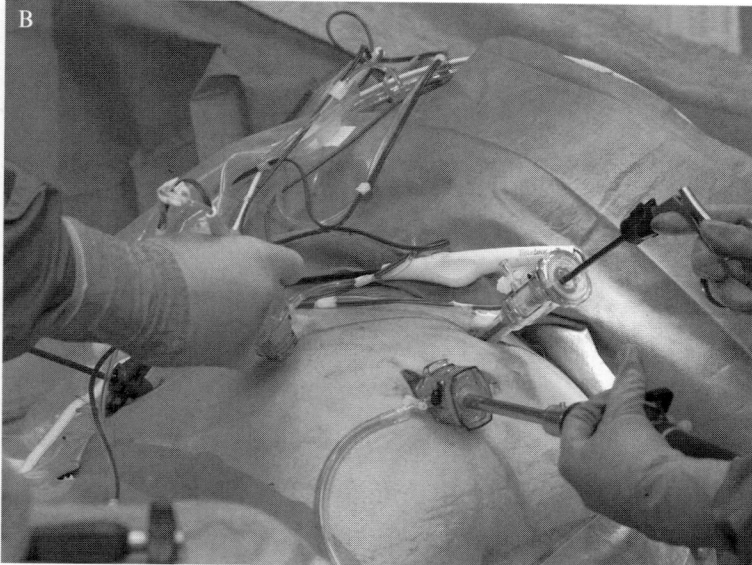

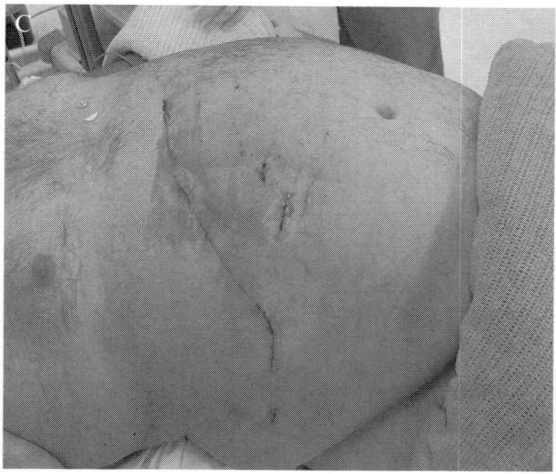 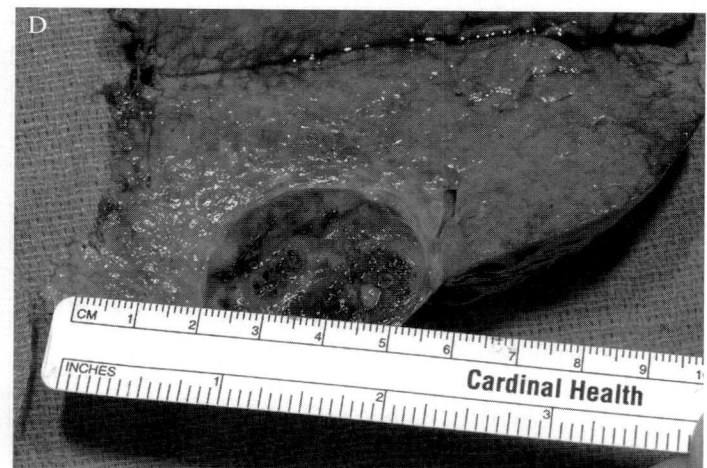

Figure 1 Lateral positioning for laparoscopic liver resection of a Segment 6 hepatocellular carcinoma. (a) Patient position, (b) Trocar position, (c) Final incisions, (d) Specimen and margin.

these resections involve three basic entities: chronic pancreatitis, neuroendocrine tumors, and cystic or benign neoplasms. The majority of the literature has focused on neuroendocrine tumors. Resection of these pancreatic lesions is often possible through a laparoscopic approach.

Neuroendocrine Tumors

The use of laparoscopy to localize and resect functional endocrine tumors of the pancreas is relatively well established.[6] The use of laparoscopic ultrasound is invaluable in localizing tumors that are not seen on preoperative imaging studies. Additionally, ultrasound can help plan resection by identifying the proximity of

tumor to structures such as the pancreatic duct, splenic vein, and common hepatic artery. Enucleation and distal pancreatic resections have been performed laparoscopically for islet cell tumors. Care must be taken when performing enucleation of lesions in the head of the pancreas as nearby structures, particularly the pancreatic duct and bile duct, must be clearly delineated with ultrasound. The ability to perform splenic preservation with distal pancreatic resections of neuroendocrine tumors is very much dependent on tumor size and location. If possible, splenic preservation should be attempted, but not at the risk of substantial bleeding, which could lead to conversion to an open procedure.

For functional neuroendocrine pancreatic tumors, preoperative tumor localization is usually possible with

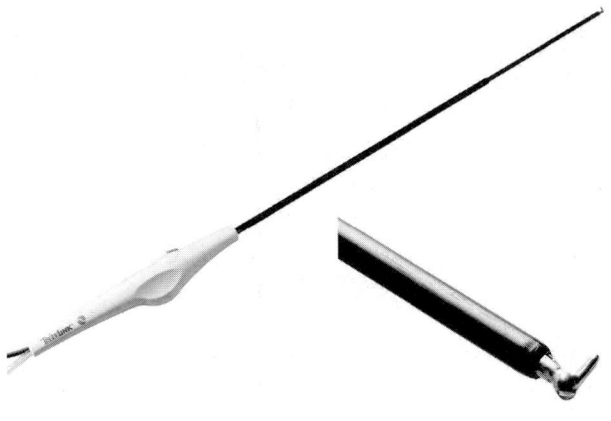

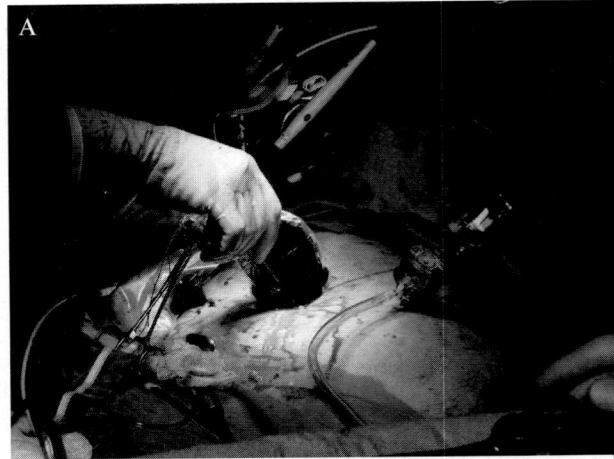

Figure 2 TissueLink™ EndoSH saline-enhanced electrocautery. Continuous saline flow yields topical radiofrequency cautery effects.

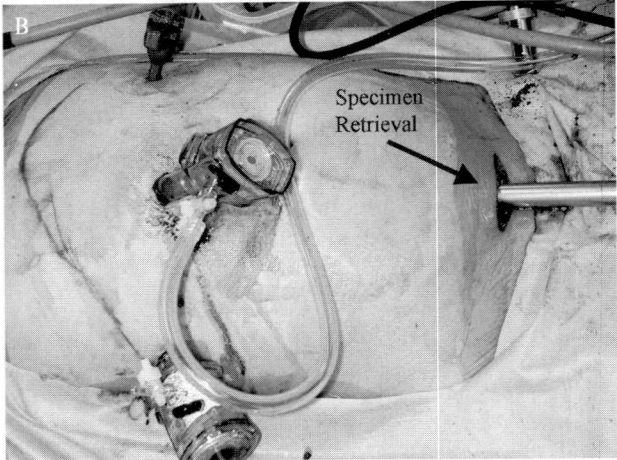

Figure 3 Specimen delivery for laparoscopic liver resection. (a) Extension of trocar site, (b) Suprapubic incision.

the combination of computed tomography (CT) scan and endoscopic ultrasound. In instances where CT scan does not identify the lesion and endoscopic ultrasound is not available, then intraoperative laparoscopic ultrasound can be used to localize the lesion. It is preferable to localize the lesion preoperatively to plan a laparoscopic resection strategy. Since laparoscopic enucleation of lesions of the pancreas carries a fistula rate of nearly 33%,[6] it is best to perform limited distal pancreatectomies for lesions in the tail. Lesions in the head and body of the pancreas can be enucleated once identification of the main pancreatic duct is clear. Lesions in the body that abut the main pancreatic duct and lesions in the head of the pancreas near the main pancreatic and bile ducts are best approached through open laparotomy.

Preoperative tumor localization helps in planning port positions. For lesions of the pancreatic body and tail, camera port position should be placed to the left of the midline, while the camera port should be placed to the right of midline for lesions of the pancreatic head. The preferred patient orientation for enucleation would be in the split-leg position. Placing the patient in a decubitus position can be employed when performing a distal resection with splenectomy, but does not generally aid in enucleations or spleen-preserving resections. The operating surgeon is positioned between the legs of the patient. The operating surgeon works through a 12 mm right-hand port and a 5 mm left-hand port. For work to the patient's left of the portal vein, the assistant stands on the left side of the table and holds the camera and assists with a right-hand lateral 5 mm port. Lesions in the head are approached with the assistant on the patient's right

side holding the camera with the right hand and using a lateral 5 mm left-handed port. The procedure is begun by widely exposing the pancreas in the region where the tumor is located. For lesions in the pancreatic head, this generally requires mobilizing the duodenal sweep by performing a Kocher maneuver in addition to opening the gastrocolic ligament. For tumors in the body and tail, the exposure is obtained by dividing the gastrocolic ligament and mobilizing any posterior adhesions of the stomach to the anterior surface of the pancreas. Enucleations can be performed with a variety of devices, including simple cautery, ultrasonic tissue dissection devices, and saline-enhanced cautery instruments. Hemostasis in the pancreas can be obtained with most of these devices or with the use of fibrin sealants or other hemostatic agents. The tumor should be removed in a laparoscopic pouch and examined to ensure complete resection. When adequate hemostasis has been obtained, the area should be drained with a closed suction device because of the high fistula rates reported following laparoscopic approaches to enucleate pancreatic tumors.

Laparoscopic Distal Pancreatectomy

For resection of tumors of the tail or body of the pancreas, laparoscopy has the potential to decrease postoperative morbidity. The published series to date have shown short-term outcome data similar to open laparotomy resection.[7,8] There is appropriate concern regarding an increased pancreatic fistula rate in laparoscopic resections.

Figure 4a shows our standard port positions for laparoscopic spleen-sparing distal pancreatectomy. For resections where splenectomy is planned for malignant lesions, a hand access port would typically be employed to remove the intact specimen and also to aid with tactile sensation and retraction (Figure 4b).

The procedure begins by dividing the gastrocolic ligament to gain access to the lesser sac. All posterior adhesions of the stomach to the pancreas are divided. Intraoperative ultrasound is employed to map the location of the lesion in the pancreas as well as to scan for possible nodal or hepatic metastases. Ultrasound can also be used to help choose a point of transection of the pancreas to ensure an adequate margin away from the malignant lesion. On occasion, especially in cystic pancreatic lesions, other pancreatic lesions may be identified with ultrasound.

Once the point of transection of the pancreas is identified, the pancreas is dissected free from attachments to the retroperitoneum in that location. By dissecting posterior to the pancreas, the splenic vein and artery can be identified. Not infrequently, it is difficult to identify the artery from an inferior pancreatic dissection; in these circumstances the splenic artery can be identified coursing along the superior border of the pancreas. It is important to visualize and control these vessels when performing splenic vessel preservation. The pancreas is divided at the point of transection by precoagulating with a saline-enhanced electrocautery (TissueLink™ EndoSH), and then dividing sharply with endoscopic scissors. The saline-enhanced electrocautery is the only treatment applied to the cut surface of the pancreas.[9] There have been no occurrences of pancreatic fistula using this technique.[10] Other methods of dividing the pancreas include the use of stapling devices or ultrasonic shears; the cut surface of the pancreas can be oversewn with sutures to close the pancreatic duct.

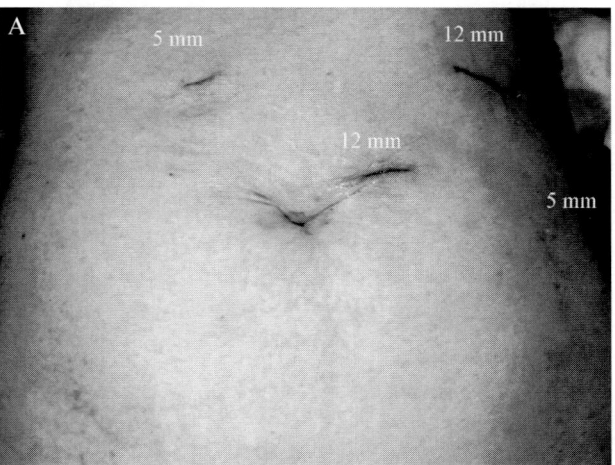

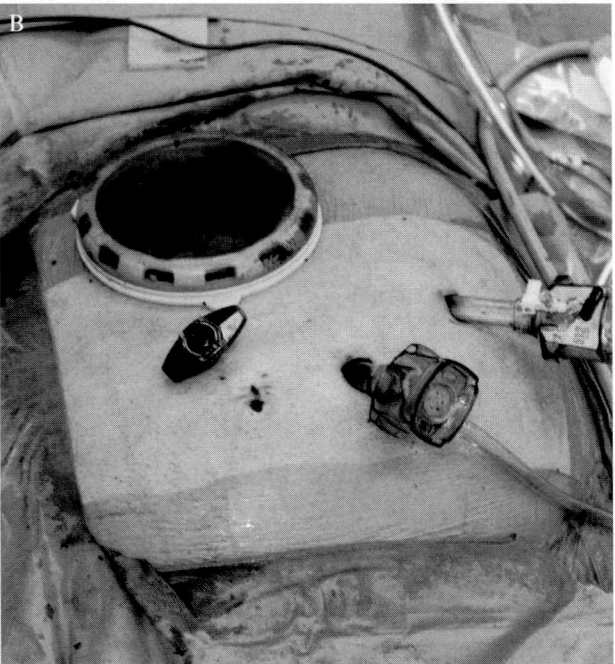

Figure 4 Trocar positions for laparoscopic distal pancreatectomy. (a) Splenic preserving, (b) Hand access in patient undergoing en bloc resection.

When performing distal pancreatectomy with splenectomy, the splenic artery and vein are divided at this point in the operation. The splenic artery is first ligated with a suture and then divided distal to the ligature with a vascular linear cutting stapler. The vein is divided using a vascular linear cutting stapler. When splenic artery identification is difficult, the vein can be divided first, which generally provides identification and access to divide the artery. After dividing the splenic artery and vein, the pancreas is mobilized from the retroperitoneum in a medial to lateral rotation. If a hand access port is utilized, the procedure is performed with the patient in a supine position. When using only standard laparoscopic ports, the procedure is performed with the patient in a decubitus position. Once the pancreas is dissected free from the retroperitoneum, the short gastric blood vessels and retroperitoneal attachments of the spleen are divided. The spleen is then dissected lateral to medial until the specimen can be delivered. When splenectomy is performed for benign conditions, the spleen can be morcelized prior to specimen extraction.

If splenic vessel preservation is planned, access to the splenic artery and vein should first be gained prior to attempting to dissect the pancreas free from the vessels. This allows for rapid vascular control with stapled ligation and division if vascular injury is encountered, which may save conversion to an open procedure. Many techniques can be employed to dissect the pancreas away from the splenic vessels. This is a tedious procedure that requires patience to complete successfully. Our preferred approach is to utilize the TissueLink EndoSH (see Figure 2) to dissect out the small branches to and from the pancreas from the splenic artery or vein, respectively, and coagulate them and then divide them sharply with scissors. These branches can also be divided with other coaptive devices, such as ultrasonic shears. Vascular clips can also be used, but generally get in the way of dissection and can be pulled off with retraction of the pancreas, leading to trouble-some hemorrhage.

If dissection of the distal pancreas from the splenic vessels is not possible, splenic preservation can be performed utilizing the short gastric vessels.[7] It is important to preserve the short gastric vessels because the blood supply to the spleen will be based on these vessels if the splenic artery and vein are ligated and divided. The splenic artery and vein are divided in the same manner used for distal pancreatectomy with splenectomy. Once the posterior dissection in the retroperitoneum progresses past the end of the pancreas, the splenic vessels are then divided again utilizing a stapling device. This allows the pancreatic specimen to be delivered. The spleen should be visually inspected for any evidence of segmental infarction or global perfusion abnormality. If the spleen is not viable, it should be removed at this point by dividing the short gastric vessels and mobilizing it from the retroperitoneum.

Pancreatic Cancer Resections

In the management of pancreatic adenocarcinoma, staging laparoscopy is generally accepted as a method to decrease operative morbidity rates for patients found to have laparoscopic evidence of unresectable disease.

Since there is no survival benefit to performing palliative resections for adenocarcinoma in the head of the pancreas, laparoscopy can save patients the morbidity of an open laparotomy that reveals an unresectable tumor. Laparoscopic resection of the head of the pancreas has been performed, but to date there is no information that this approach yields a decreased morbidity rate to the patients.[8] Operative times are excessively long and there is no apparent benefit of reduced length of hospital stay or complication rates. Additionally, the added cost of a lengthy laparoscopic operation cannot be justified without improvements in patient outcomes.

In our series of laparoscopic distal pancreatic resections, 3 patients with pancreatic adenocarcinoma have been identified. Two patients were suspected preoperatively to have pancreatic adenocarcinoma and 1 patient had a large cystic lesion. All lesions were in the tail of the pancreas. The 3 resections were performed utilizing a hand access port, since a large specimen was being removed. Our standard port positioning places a hand access port in the upper midline (see Figure 4b). This allows for retraction in a cephalad direction and generally keeps the hand out of the video field. In many cases the placement of the hand access port is delayed until dissection at the pancreatic neck is complete, because the intra-abdominal hand can diminish visualization. The mean surgical time for these 3 procedures was 278 ± 29 minutes. In-hospital stays in these 3 patients were 3, 4, and 11 days, respectively. One complication occurred in the patient with the 11-day hospital stay; bleeding from the staple line used to transect the pancreas occurred in the first patient and required re-exploration on the third postoperative day. After this complication occurred, all subsequent pancreatic transections were performed utilizing the TissueLink™ EndoSH with no further episodes of bleeding.

All 3 patients with adenocarcinoma of the pancreatic tail had node-positive disease. All retroperitoneal and pancreatic margins were free of tumor. The patient with the cystic lesion required an en bloc resection of the fundus of the stomach and left adrenal gland (Figure 5). To date, there have been no local recurrences in this anecdotal set of patients. One patient succumbed from liver metastases 176 days after distal pancreatectomy. Another patient was noted to have lung metastases on his first postoperative CT scan, which was done prior to consideration of adjuvant therapy. He remains alive with disease at 456 days. The third patient is alive without disease 296 days after operation. The 2 patients who had uncomplicated resections were back to normal functional status within 2 weeks of surgery.

Laparoscopic Palliation

For most patients with unresectable pancreatic malignancies, relief of biliary obstruction can be achieved with endoscopic manipulations. Rarely do patients with metastatic tumor require palliative operations.[2] For this group of patients, the majority who require surgical palliation are indicated for the management of gastric outlet obstruction. With malignant gastric outlet obstruction, the endoscopic management of biliary obstruction can be technically impossible. In these cases laparoscopic management of biliary and gastric outlet obstruction can be accomplished. This group of patients has a significantly short life span and any improvement in recovery time after a palliative surgical procedure should lead to significant improvement in quality of life.

Patients with malignant gastric outlet and biliary tract obstruction can be managed in different ways. Open biliary and gastric bypass can be performed. Significant wound-related complications and pneumonia occur frequently after open laparotomy in these debilitated patients. Laparoscopy offers the potential to reduce the incidence of both of these complications. Laparoscopic gastro-jejunostomy can be performed readily in experi-

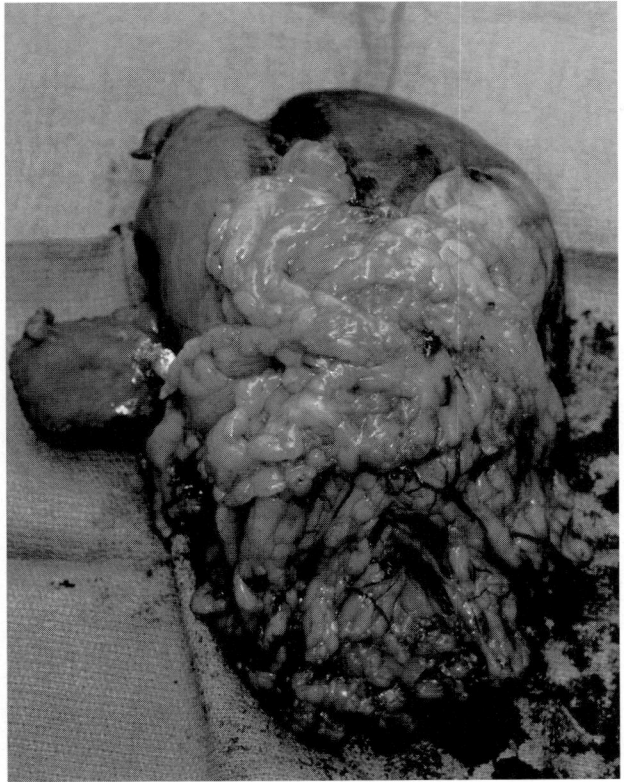

Figure 5 Resected distal pancreatic cancer en bloc with fundus of the stomach.

enced hands. Since these patients generally have a short life expectancy, biliary obstruction can be managed in selected patients with a laparoscopic cholecysto-jejunostomy. For those with extensive malignant disease involving regional lymph nodes or infiltrating directly into the porta hepatis with occlusion of the cystic duct, an open biliary bypass is probably warranted. When the cystic duct is absent because of a prior cholecystectomy, and when the dilated common bile duct can be identified, laparoscopic choledocho-jejunostomy can be performed, but requires significantly more laparoscopic skills.

Palliative laparoscopic bypass can be performed from the straight supine position, but a split-leg position offers more flexibility for the operating surgeon. There are a variety of trocar positions that can be used. In cases of isolated gastric outlet obstruction without the need for biliary bypass, a camera port can be placed at the umbilicus or the left paramedian position. A 12 mm working port is placed in the left subcostal position. This port positioning can be difficult as the obstructed, distended stomach extends lower in the abdomen. Port positions placed too high in the abdomen make the application of laparoscopic staplers used to perform the gastrojejunal anastomosis difficult. The anastamosis can be performed on the anterior or posterior wall of the stomach. The enterotomy produced by the linear stapler to create the gastrojejunal anastomosis can either be closed with sutures or with additional applications of the linear cutting stapler.

Care must be exercised in patients with widely disseminated carcinomatosis. In patients with carcinomatosis and ascites, prudent consideration should be given to attempting placement of an endoscopic duodenal stent for palliation, as the operative complication rate, even with a laparoscopic approach, is substantial.

After completion of the gastro-jejunostomy, a cholecysto-jejunostomy can be performed using the distal jejunal limb (Figure 6). This anastomosis can also be performed utilizing a linear cutting stapling device or can be hand sewn. If a cholecysto-jejunostomy cannot be performed, then laparoscopic choledocho-jejunostomy can be considered. This procedure requires meticulous port positioning to allow adequate angles to suture the anastamosis. This procedure should be reserved for surgeons with significant laparoscopic experience with intracorporeal suturing techniques.

In the immediate postoperative period, patients should continue nasogastric decompression. The minimally invasive approach does not diminish the delayed gastric emptying that many of these patients develop because of chronic gastric outlet obstruction. Hospital stay will depend on how quickly delayed gastric emptying resolves, thus allowing patients to resume oral alimentation.

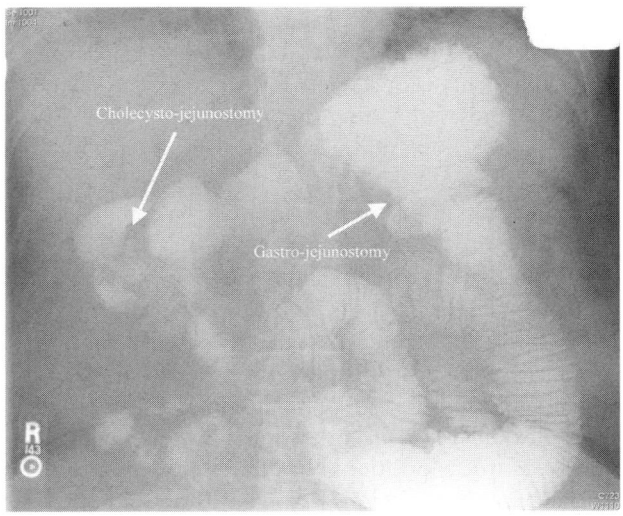

Figure 6 Upper gastrointestinal contrast radiographs after laparoscopic gastro-jejunostomy and cholecysto-jejunostomy.

Conclusions

Laparoscopy offers a new approach in the management of solid organ tumors. For select procedures in the hands of experienced surgeons, these procedures offer potential benefits to patients when considering short-term outcomes. There remains little long-term outcome information for these procedures, which continues to promote skepticism in the utility of laparoscopy in surgical oncology from the standpoint of a method for resection. It is unlikely that a randomized trial of open versus laparoscopic resection will be performed for hepatic and pancreatic tumors. In the absence of randomized trials, all patients undergoing this form of therapy should be followed long term for any evidence of suboptimal therapy. A consensus on specific outcomes measures should be agreed on, and those involved in performing these procedures should work together to standardize the surgical techniques.

References

1. Conlon KC. Value of laparoscopic staging for upper gastrointestinal malignancies. J Surg Oncol 1999;71:71–3.

2. Espat NJ, Brennan MF, Conlon KC. Patients with laparoscopically staged unresectable pancreatic adennocarcinoma do not require subsequent surgical biliary or gastric bypass. J Am Coll Surg 1999;188:649–55.

3. Raut CP, Izzo F, Marra P, et al. Significant long-term survival after radiofrequency ablation of unresectable hepatocellular carcinoma in patients with cirrhosis. Ann Surg Oncol 2005;12:616–28.

4. Learn PA, Bowers SP, Watkins KT. Initial experience with laparoscopic hepatic resection utilizing saline enhanced lectrocautery leads to significantly short hospital stays. J Gastrointest Surg 2006. [In press].

5. Cuschieri A, Jakimowicz JJ, van Spreeuwel J. Laparoscopic distal 70% pancreatectomy and splenectomy for chronic pancreatitis. Ann Surg 1996;223:280–5.

6. Assalia A, Gagner M. Laparoscopic pancreatic surgery for islet cell tumors of the pancreas. World J Surg 2004;28:1239–47.

7. Fernandez-Cruz L, Martinez I, Gilabert R, et al. Laparoscopic distal pancreatectomy combined with preservation of the spleen for cystic neoplasms of the pancreas. J Gastrointest Surg 2004;8:493–501.

8. Gagner M, Inabnet WB, Biertho L, Salky B. Laparoscopic pancreatectomy: a series of 22 patients. Ann Chir 2004;129:2–7.

9. Watkins KT. A novel approach to sealing the cut pancreatic duct during distal resection. J Gastrointest Surg 2003;7:314–5.

10. Learn PA, Bowers SP, Watkins KT. Elimination of pancreatic fistula in distal resection utilizing topical radiofrequency energy. [In preparation].

CHAPTER 17

SURGICAL TREATMENT OF GALLBLADDER CANCER

CHRISTINA BERTOCCHI, MD

MARK S. ROH, MD

Though relatively rare, gallbladder cancer is the fifth most common malignancy of the gastrointestinal tract and is the most common cancer of the biliary tree. In the United States, approximately 5,000 new cases are diagnosed each year, accounting for an incidence of 1 to 2 cases per 100,000. Gallbladder cancer occurs more commonly in later life, with most patients presenting in their seventh or eighth decade, and affects females 3 to 4 times more frequently than males. The incidence varies among ethnic groups, with Native and Hispanic Americans having a higher incidence when compared with the general population, and whites more frequently affected than blacks.[1,2]

The precise etiology of gallbladder cancer is not known; however, chronic irritation and inflammation of the gallbladder mucosa plays an important role. Patients at risk of developing the disease suffer from chronic cholecystitis or choleliathiasis. Approximately 1% of gallbladders resected for benign disease contain a focus of carcinoma, and over 75% of gallbladder carcinomas are associated with gallstones.[2]

The prognosis for gallbladder cancer remains poor. Historically, the 1-year survival rate is 14%, with median survival ranging from 3 to 8 months.[3–5] This dismal outcome is due to the slow and asymptomatic nature of this malignancy. Signs and symptoms specific for gallbladder cancer are absent in the early stages, and the diagnosis is frequently made as an incidental finding following cholecystectomy for benign disease. Symptoms occur with invasion of surrounding structures. Complete surgical resection at this point, if possible, is difficult and can be associated with significant morbidity and mortality rates.

Staging

Physicians caring for patients with gallbladder cancer must have a thorough understanding of the staging classification. This knowledge is necessary to offer a realistic and optimal treatment strategy. The current staging system is based on the depth of penetration and extent of metastatic spread (Table 1).

The classification of primary tumor (T) is determined by the depth of penetration into the gallbladder wall and invasion into adjacent organs. The majority of patients with in situ T1 and T2 tumors are staged on pathological examination following cholecystectomy for presumed benign disease. T2 tumors invade the perimuscular connective tissue, but cannot be optimally treated with a simple cholecystectomy. Patients with T3 and T4 tumors are usually symptomatic and are diagnosed preoperatively through radiologic testing. The hepatic surface of the gallbladder does not have a serosa, so cancer will spread through direct local invasion of the liver parenchyma (Couinaud segments IV and V). T3 and T4 tumors can extend beyond the gallbladder into adjacent organs (stomach, duodenum, pancreas, or colon) or portal vascular structures. Patients with T3 tumors are frequently amenable to an en bloc resection, but T4 tumors are considered unresectable owing to involvement of the portal vein and/or hepatic artery. The recent edition of the *AJCC Cancer Staging Handbook* differs from the previous staging system that defined T3 and T4 in terms of the depth of liver invasion. The current T3 designation includes tumors penetrating the serosa of the gallbladder; included in the category are tumors that invade any adjacent organ and not

Table 1 AJCC TNM Staging for Gallbladder Carcinoma

Primary Tumor (T)

TX	Primary tumor cannot be assessed
T0	No evidence of primary tumor
Tis	Carcinoma in situ
T1	Tumor invades lamina propria or muscle layer
T1a	Tumor invades lamina propria
T1b	Tumor invades muscle layer
T2	Tumor invades perimuscular connective tissue; no extension beyond serosa or into liver
T3	Tumor perforates serosa (visceral peritoneum) and/or directly invades the liver and/or other adjacent organ or structure, such as the stomach duodenum, colon, or pancreas, omentum, or extrahepatic bile ducts
T4	Tumor invades main portal vein or hepatic artery or invades two or more extrahepatic organs or structures

Regional Lymph Nodes (N)

NX	Regional lymph nodes cannot be assessed
N0	No regional lymph node metastasis
N1	Regional lymph node metastasis

Distant Metastasis (M)

MX	Presence of distant metastasis cannot be assessed
M0	No distant metastasis
M1	Distant metastasis

Stage Grouping

Stage 0	Tis	N0	M0
Stage IA	T1	N0	M0
Stage IB	T2	N0	M0
Stage IIA	T3	N0	M0
Stage IIB	T1	N1	M0
	T2	N1	M0
	T3	N1	M0
Stage III	T4	Any N	M0
Stage IV	Any T	Any N	M1

Reproduced with permission from Springer-Verlag, New York 2002

exclusively the liver. T4 tumors are those that involve multiple local organs or the structures of the porta hepatis.[6]

Gallbladder cancer spreads through predictable patterns based on the lymphatic drainage of the gallbladder. The first nodal basin includes the porta hepatis (cystic duct, common bile duct, hepatic artery, and portal vein). The second nodal area is the retroportal region, posterior pancreas, and to the celiac and superior mesenteric axis. The first and second nodal areas are classified as regional nodes and defined as N1. Lymphatic metastases to the aortocaval and peripancreatic nodes along the body and tail are classified as distant metastases (M1).[7,8]

Distant metastases involve hematogenous spread to distant locations in the liver, lung, bone, and brain.[1,9] Peritoneal seeding is considered distant disease and occurs when a tumor perforates the gallbladder. Perforation occurs with progressive tumor growth or iatrogenic spillage during laparoscopic cholecystectomy.

Gallbladder cancer is classified into 4 stages. In most cases, patients with stage I and II are eligible for curative resections. Stage I is divided into tumors that require a simple cholecystectomy (stage IA), and stage IB tumors, which require a more extensive surgical procedure (hepatic resection and portal lymphadenectomy). Stage II is subdivided into T3 tumors not associated with nodal disease (IIA) and all T classifications with lymph node metastases (IIB). Stages III and IV tumors are unresectable and differ only in whether distant metastatic disease is present at diagnosis.

Diagnostic Evaluation

Ultrasonography is usually the first imaging modality used to assess gallbladder disease with a 70 to 90% sensitivity rate for cancer.[1,10] However, this sensitivity applies for more advanced carcinomas. The ability of ultrasound to diagnose early carcinomas involving only the mucosa or muscular layers is limited. Common findings to raise suspicion of a malignant process include discontinuity of gallbladder mucosa, wall thickening, or calcification. Submucosal echolucency, a fixed mass within the gallbladder or protruding into the lumen from the gallbladder wall, especially if greater than 1cm, loss of the interface between the gallbladder wall and liver, and a heterogeneous mass replacing part of the gallbladder or infiltrating into liver parenchyma, are clear signs of a likely malignant process.[1,10] With addition of Doppler imaging, delineation of biliary, vascular, and nodal involvement can be achieved for clinical staging purposes in advanced cancers.[11]

Computed tomography (CT) can be useful in the diagnosis and preoperative assessment of patients with gallbladder cancer. Although not as sensitive as ultrasonography at identifying T1 lesions, helical CT has been shown to be accurate in defining T stage for more advanced lesions, with a common finding of a polypoid mass filling the gallbladder lumen.[12] The correlation between findings on preoperative helical CT scanning and final pathology demonstrates a high sensitivity and specificity for T2, T3, and T4 lesions. Sensitivity for T1 lesions is limited because of poor differentiation of the mucosal and muscular layers of the gallbladder.[13] CT is not reliable in identifying early lymphatic metastases. Only 38% of pathologically positive nodes are correctly identified on preoperative CT scan, with the lowest sensitivity being for cystic duct and aortocaval nodes. In more advanced disease, certain features on CT are more accurate in predicting nodal metastases. Common findings include anteroposterior lymph node dimensions of 1 cm or greater, and heterogeneous or ring-like contrast enhancement of the affected lymph nodes.[14] Helical CT can define the extent of hepatic disease and, using dual-phase helical modes, can delineate biliary and vascular involvement at the hilar level that could preclude resection.[15]

Magnetic resonance imaging (MRI) is valuable in the preoperative evaluation of gallbladder cancer. As compared with CT, it is more accurate in defining the depth of direct liver invasion and the presence of biliary dilatation, and is more sensitive in identifying peritoneal and omental disease.[16,17] MR cholangiography (MRCP) can assess the extent of tumor within the bile duct and the accuracy is comparable with endoscopic retrograde cholangiopancreatography. MRCP is noninvasive and provides the opportunity to review isolated segments of the bile duct in greater detail. Contrast-enhanced dual-phase MR angiography (MRA) is more accurate in identifying hepatic vascular invasion and the relationship to an extraluminal tumor mass than conventional angiography.[18] The combined use of MRI, MRCP, and MRA provides a noninvasive and accurate method for staging and the preoperative determination of respectability.[18]

The role of positron emission tomography (PET) in the evaluation of gallbladder cancer is not yet defined. Since most patients with gallbladder cancer are diagnosed on pathological review of a presumably benign cholecystectomy specimen, a PET scan is not routinely obtained preoperatively. In addition, accurate interpretation of a positive study in the presence of active inflammation and postoperative changes at the operative site is difficult.[9]

Treatment

EARLY-STAGE CARCINOMA (T1)

Early-stage carcinomas are frequently found during pathological examination of gallbladders resected for presumed benign disease. For T1a tumors, without invasion beyond the lamina propria or muscular layer, a simple cholecystectomy is adequate therapy as long as margins are free of cancer. Five-year survival rates for T1a tumors ranges from 85 to 100%, with an extremely low incidence of metastases.[19] Patients with T1b tumors, which involve the muscular layer, can be adequately treated with a cholecystectomy and do not require an extensive resection. No survival benefit is derived for radical resection for T1b tumors as these patients rarely have lymph node metastases and the 10-year survival rate is 87%.[19] Patients with T1 tumors found on postoperative review of cholecystectomy specimen do not require additional therapy. However, if carcinoma is suspected intraoperatively, the cystic and common bile duct lymph nodes should be biopsied. The presence of nodal metastases for a T1 tumor changes the stage from IA to IIB and the patient will require a more extensive resection for cure.[19]

Although the majority of tumors originate in the fundus and the body of the gallbladder, the cystic duct may be involved with cancer.[20] If the cystic duct margin is positive for carcinoma, a common bile duct resection with a biliary-enteric anastamosis is necessary. Ideally, this diagnosis would be made on frozen analysis at the time of cholecystectomy. Therefore, a positive cystic duct margin would be the only time that a T1 or stage IA tumor would warrant reoperation for a curative resection.

INTERMEDIATE-STAGE DISEASE (T2)

Patients with T2 disease have invasion into the perimuscular connective tissue of the gallbladder without extension into the liver. Since the incidence of metastases in gallbladder carcinoma is directly correlated with depth of tumor invasion, an extensive resection is warranted for T2 disease.[21,22] Curative surgical treatment for T2 tumors should include hepatic resection of the gallbladder fossa,

Couinaud segments IVB and V, and lymph node dissection of cholecystic, pericholedochal, porta hepatis, and posterior-superior pancreatic-duodenal nodes.[23] Occasionally, a bile duct resection may be necessary for a tumor-free margin lymphadenectomy.[11] Performing an extensive procedure in the early postoperative period has mortality, morbidity, and long-term survival rates that are equivalent to patients undergoing a curative resection as the first procedure.[22]

LATE-STAGE DISEASE (T3/T4)

In patients with T3 and T4 tumors, the tumor penetrates the serosa with invasion into the organs adjacent to the gallbladder. A direct correlation exists between tumor stages and the incidence of lymphatic and distant metastases. Up to 79% of T3 tumors that appear to be resectable on preoperative evaluation studies will be unresectable at laparotomy because of the finding of diffuse intra-abdominal metastases.[22] The only chance for cure requires an en bloc resection of the gallbladder and the involved organs with a tumor-free margin. Growth into the liver requires resection of the liver, segments IVB and V, and possibly an extended hepatectomy. Involvement of the right hepatic artery or right portal vein mandates an extended right hepatectomy for a curative resection. Tumors that involve the main portal vein or hepatic artery are unresectable.

Patients with lymph node metastases in hilar regions and regional nodal basins may achieve an improved survival rate with a regional lymphadenectomy. Resection of all regional lymph nodes can produce a 5-year survival rate of 45 to 60% and usually requires a common bile duct resection for a curative resection.[25,26] Lymph node metastases beyond this region are considered distant metastases and incurable. Pancreaticoduodenectomy with regional lymphadenectomy, including the aortocaval and peripancreatic nodes, can be curative in highly selected patients.[27,28]

LAPAROSCOPIC CHOLECYSTECTOMY

With the advent of laparoscopic cholecystectomy as a routine procedure for benign gallbladder disease, iatrogenic tumor dissemination is possible during the surgery. Multiple mechanisms exist for tumor spread during laparoscopic cholecystectomy. Surgical manipulation of the gallbladder and perforation of the gallbladder with spillage of bile can disseminate cancer cells. In addition, port sites are at risk of seeding by instruments that are contaminated by tumor cells. Aerosolization of tumor cells by pneumoperitoneum can cause diffuse peritoneal metastases. In patients who experienced a gallbladder perforation during the laparoscopic cholecystectomy, 43% developed a port site recurrence.[24]

All laparoscopic procedures should be converted to open cholecystectomy if cancer is suspected on direct visualization of the gallbladder. However, as diagnosis at such early stages is rarely possible, precautions should be taken to minimize bile spillage in all patients undergoing a laparoscopic cholecystectomy. If a specimen is positive for carcinoma and staged as a T1 tumor, no further treatment is necessary. Patients with T2 or higher require an extensive resection with excision of the port sites from the original laparoscopic procedure. In the unusual occasion when a gallbladder cancer is diagnosed on preoperative evaluation, a laparotomy is necessary.[29–31]

RADIATION THERAPY AND CHEMOTHERAPY

The only chance for cure or long-term survival in gallbladder cancer is complete surgical resection. Radiation therapy and systemic chemotherapy have been used in an attempt to decrease recurrence or to treat unresectable disease. Intraoperative radiotherapy can accurately target select areas and improve survival in patients with microscopic and gross residual disease.[32]

The benefit of radiotherapy is limited since gallbladder cancer is more likely to recur at distant sites rather than locally.[33] Despite a curative resection with tumor-free margins, up to 66% of patients will develop recurrent disease. Only 15% of the recurrences are local and 85% occur at distant sites with or without concomitant regional disease.[33] The value of adjuvant radiotherapy remains to be defined.

Systemic chemotherapy may provide benefit in select patients. A phase III trial evaluated the impact of adjuvant systemic mitomycin C and 5-fluorouracil, without radiotherapy, following primary resection of stage II-IV gallbladder cancer. The chemotherapy significantly improved overall 5-year (26% vs 14%) and disease-free (20% vs 12%) survival rates when compared with patients who did not receive adjuvant therapy. However, the improved survival was limited only to patients who had undergone noncurative resections.[34]

Numerous small studies have reported potential benefits of chemotherapy and external beam radiation in resected patients as means of controlling local and distant disease and recurrence. Unfortunately, most of these are retrospective reviews using historical controls, and it is difficult to detect a genuine benefit in long-term survival. Nevertheless, with the safety of external beam radiation and intraoperative radiation therapy having been shown, consideration should be given to the use of combined modality treatment.[35–37] Despite the difficulty

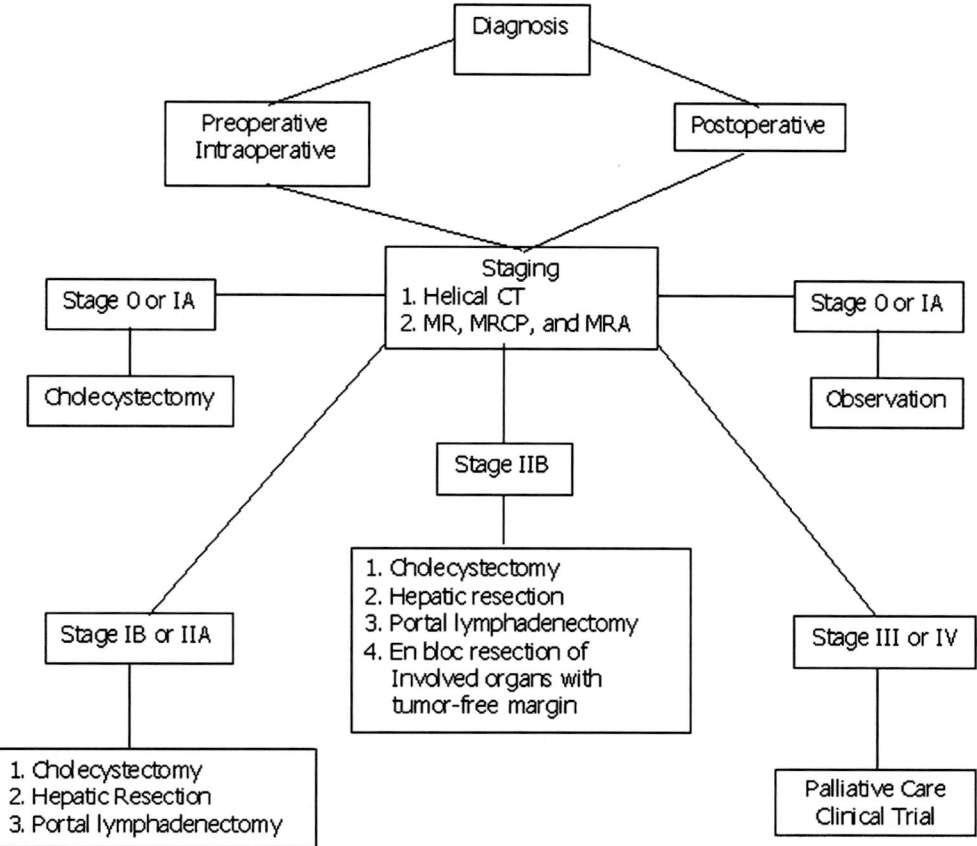

Figure 1 Treatment Algorithm for Gallbladder Cancer.

imposed by the rarity of this disease, prospective controlled studies are required to provide definitive guidance in treatment regimens.

Conclusion

In conclusion, gallbladder cancer, though rare, remains an aggressive disease with a dismal prognosis. A clear understanding of its pattern of spread supports the need for adequate surgical resection to allow the best chance for a cure. A treatment algorithm is presented in Figure 1.

References

1. Rajagopalan V, Daines WP, Grossbard ML, Kozuch P. Gallbladder and biliary tract carcinoma: a comprehensive update, Part 1. Oncology 2004;18:889–96.

2. Ahmad SA, Abdalla EK, Spitz FR, et al. Hepatobiliary cancers. In: Feig BW, Berger DH, Fuhrman GM, editors. The M. D. Anderson surgical oncology handbook. 3rd ed. Philadelphia: Lippincott Williams and Wilkins; 2003. p. 266–302.

3. Cubertafond P, Gainant A, Cucchiaro G. Surgical treatment of 724 carcinomas of the gallbladder: results of the French Surgical Association Survey. Ann Surg 1994;219: 275–80.

4. Piehler JM, Crichlow RW. Primary carcinoma of the gallbladder. Surg Gynecol Obstet 1978;147:929–42.

5. Cubertafond P, Mathonnet M, Gainant A, Launois B. Radical surgery for gallbladder cancer. Results of the French Surgical Association Survey. Hepatogastroenterology 1999;46:1567–71.

6. American Joint Committee on Cancer. AJCC cancer staging handbook. 6th ed. New York: Springer-Verlag; 2002.

7. Lin HT, Liu GJ, Wu D, Lou JY. Metastasis of primary gallbladder carcinoma in lymph node and liver. World J Gastroenterol 2005;11:748–51.

8. Shirai Y, Yoshida K, Tsukada K, et al. Identification of the regional lymphatic system of the gallbladder by vital staining. Br J Surg 1992;79:659–62.

9. Anderson CD, Rice MH, Pinson CW, et al. Fluorodeoxyglucose PET imaging in the evaluation of gallbladder carcinoma and cholangiocarcinoma. J Gastrointest Surg 2004;8:90–7.

10. Wibbenmeyer LA, Sharafuddin MJ, Wolverson MK, et al. Sonographic diagnosis of unsuspected gallbladder cancer: imaging findings in comparison with benign gallbladder conditions. AJR Am J Roentgenol 1995;165:1169–74.

11. Fong Y, Malhotra S. Gallbladder cancer: recent advances and current guidelines for surgical therapy. Adv Surg 2001;35:1–20.

12. Kumar A, Aggarwal S. Carcinoma of the gallbladder: CT findings in 50 cases. Abdom Imaging 1994;19:304–8.

13. Yoshimitsu K, Honda H, Shinozaki K, et al. Helical CT of the local spread of carcinoma of the gallbladder: evaluation according to the TNM system in patients who underwent surgical resection. Am J Radiol 2002;179:423–8.

14. Ohtani T, Shirai Y, Tsukada K, et al. Carcinoma of the gallbladder: CT evaluation of lymphatic spread. Radiology 1993;189:875–80.

15. Kumaran V, Gulati MS, Paul SB, et al. The role of dual-phase helical CT in assessing respectability of carcinoma of the gallbladder. Eur Radiol 2002;12:1993–9.

16. Schwartz LH, Black J, Fong Y, et al. Gallbladder carcinoma: findings at MR imaging with MR cholangiopancreatography. J Comput Assist Tomogr 2002;26:405–10.

17. Tseng JW, Wan YL, Jung CF, et al. Diagnosis and staging of gallbladder carcinoma: evaluation with dynamic MR imaging. Clin Imaging 2002;26:177–82.

18. Kim JG, Kim TK, Wun HW, et al. Preoperative evaluation of gallbladder carcinoma: efficacy of combined use of MR imaging, MR cholangiography, and contrast-enhanced dual-phase three dimensional MR angiography. J Magn Reson Imaging 2002;16:676–84.

19. Wakai T, Shirai Y, Yokoyama N, et al. Early gallbladder carcinoma does not warrant radical resection. Br J Surg 2001;88:675–8.

20. Albores-Saavedra J, Henson DE. Tumors of the gallbladder and extrahepatic bile ducts. In: Anonymous atlas of tumor Pathology. 2nd Series. Bethesda: Armed Forces Institute of Pathology; 1986.

21. Nevin JE, Moran TJ, Kay S, King R. Carcinoma of the gallbladder: staging, treatment and prognosis. Cancer 1976;37:141–8.

22. Fong Y, Jarnagin WR, Blumgart LH. Gallbladder cancer: comparison of patients presenting initially for definitive operation with those presenting after prior noncurative intervention. Ann Surg 2000;232:557–69.

23. Donohue JH, Nagorney DM, Grant CS, et al. Carcinoma of the gallbladder: does radical resection improve outcome? Arch Surg 1990;125:237–41.

24. Wakai T, Shirai Y, Hatakeyama K. Radical second resection provides survival benefit for patients with T2 gallbladder carcinoma first discovered after laparoscopic cholecystectomy. World J Surg 2002;26:867–71.

25. Shirai Y, Yoshida K, Tsukada K, et al. Radical surgery for gallbladder carcinoma. Ann Surg 1992;216:565–8.

26. Onoyama H, Yamamoto M, Tseng A, et al. Extended cholecystectomy for carcinoma of the gallbladder. World J Surg 1995;19:758–63.

27. Sasaki R, Takahashi M, Funato O, et al. Hepatopancreatoduodenectomy with wide lymph node dissection for locally advanced carcinoma of the gallbladder—long-term results. Hepatogastroenterology 2002;49:912–5.

28. Todokori T, Kawamoto T, Takahashi H, et al. Treatment of gallbladder cancer by radical resection. Br J Surg 1999;86:622–7.

29. Fong Y, Heffernana N, Blumgart LH. Gallbladder carcinoma discovered during laparoscopic cholecystectomy: aggressive reresection is beneficial. Cancer 1998;83:423–7.

30. Antonakis P, Alexakis N, Mylonaki D, et al. Incidental finding of gallbladder carcinoma detected during or after laparoscopic cholecystectomy. Eur J Surg Oncol 2003;29:358–60.

31. Shirai Y, Ohtani T, Hatakeyama K. Laparoscopic cholecystectomy may disseminate gallbladder carcinoma. Hepatogastroenterology 1998;45:81–2.

32. Todoroki T, Iwasaki Y, Orii K, et al. Resection combined with intraoperative radiation therapy for stage IV (TNM) gallbladder carcinoma. World J Surg 1991;15:357–66.

33. Jarnagin WR, Ruo L, Little SA, et al. Patterns of initial disease recurrence after resection of gallbladder carcinoma and hilar cholangiocarcinoma: implications for adjuvant therapeutic strategies. Cancer 2003;98:1689–700.

34. Takada T, Amano H, Yasuda H, et al. Is postoperative adjuvant chemotherapy useful for gallbladder carcinoma? Cancer 2002;95:1685–95.

35. Daines WP, Rajagopalan V, Grossbard ML, Kozuch P. Gallbladder and biliary tract carcinoma: a comprehensive update, part 2. Oncology 2004;18:1049–68.

36. Sasson AR, Hoffman JP, Ross E, et al. Trimodality therapy for advanced gallbladder cancer. Am Surg 2001;67:277–84.

37. Kresl JJ, Schild SE, Henning GT, et al. Adjuvant external beam radiation therapy with concurrent chemotherapy in the management of gallbladder carcinoma. Int J Radiat Oncol Biol Phys 2002;50:167–75.

CHAPTER 18

SURGICAL TREATMENT OF CHOLANGIOCARCINOMA

JOHN T. MULLEN, MD

DARIA ZORZI, MD

JEAN-NICOLAS VAUTHEY, MD

Introduction

Cholangiocarcinomas are malignant neoplasms arising from the epithelium of the intrahepatic or extrahepatic bile ducts. Cholangiocarcinoma is a relatively rare malignancy, with an incidence of only 3,000 cases each year in the United States, although the worldwide incidence of this disease is steadily increasing.[1] Cholangiocarcinomas can arise at any site along the intrahepatic or extrahepatic biliary tree; a review by Nakeeb and colleagues[2] demonstrated that two-thirds of these tumors are perihilar, 27% are in the distal bile duct, and only 6% are intrahepatic.

Cholangiocarcinomas typically present during the fifth and sixth decades of life, although those patients with risk factors such as primary sclerosing cholangitis, hepatolithiasis, liver flukes, and choledochal cysts can develop this malignancy as much as 2 decades earlier. The clinical presentation of a patient with cholangiocarcinoma is nonspecific and depends on the location of the lesion. More than 90% of patients with hilar cholangiocarcinoma present with jaundice, but weight loss, pain, and anorexia are common symptoms as well.[1] Cholangiocarcinomas that arise in the peripheral bile ducts within the liver parenchyma typically reach a large size before they become clinically evident. These patients often present with upper abdominal and back pain associated with hepatomegaly, and in advanced cases patients present with jaundice and ascites. Elevations in the serum tumor markers carcinoembryonic antigen (CEA) and carbohydrate antigen (CA) 19-9 are common, occurring in 40 to 60% and in nearly 80% of patients with cholangiocarcinoma, respectively. However, these markers have been shown to have a sensitivity of only 70% and a specificity of approximately 80% for the diagnosis of cholangiocarcinoma.[3]

Surgical Treatment of Intrahepatic Cholangiocarcinoma

The majority of patients with intrahepatic cholangiocarcinoma (IHCC) present with advanced disease, with evidence of regional lymph node, pulmonary, and/or bone metastases. In addition, patients who present with jaundice are rarely candidates for an attempt at curative resection, given the high likelihood of hepatic artery and/or portal vein invasion, bilobar liver involvement, and regional lymph node and distant metastases. Only 30 to 40% of patients with IHCC will present without evidence of jaundice or metastatic disease, and may thus be candidates for curative hepatic resection.[4] An aggressive intraoperative approach to achieve a margin-negative (R0) resection, including an extended hepatectomy with or without bile duct and major vascular resections, is warranted, as these patients have a median survival of 46 months compared with 5 months for patients who undergo an R1 resection.[5] The poor outcome after R1 resection in conjunction with the high morbidity rate of an extensive surgical procedure does not justify palliative resections. Although lymph node involvement is common in IHCC, performing an extended lymphadenectomy at the time of hepatic resection has not been shown to improve survival.[6] The 5-year overall survival rates for patients who undergo a margin-negative hepatic resection range from 13 to 44%.[7-9] Poor prognostic factors

157

include large primary tumor size (> 5 cm diameter), as this factor is frequently associated with lymphatic and vascular invasion, the presence of satellite tumor nodules, vascular invasion, regional lymph node metastases, and a positive resection margin.[8–10] After curative resection of IHCC, recurrence is common,[10] with the most frequent sites including the liver, regional nodes, peritoneum, lung, and bone.

Orthotopic liver transplantation for IHCC has resulted in rather disappointing outcomes. Post-transplant recurrence is nearly universal and long-term survivors rare. Some studies have reported a median survival of only 5 months for patients who underwent transplantation compared with 13 to 17 months for those who underwent resection of IHCC.[7,11] However, in the highly selected group of patients in whom the major predictors of poor outcome are excluded, including positive margins, multiple tumors, and lymph node metastases, the 5-year survival rate is greater than 60% after liver transplantation.[12] Likewise, prolonged disease-free survival after orthotopic liver transplantation in combination with preoperative chemoradiation has been reported by investigators at the Mayo Clinic.[13] At this time, however, liver resection is the treatment of choice for IHCC, and liver transplantation for IHCC should be performed only in the context of a clinical trial.

Surgical Treatment of Hilar Cholangiocarcinoma

Cholangiocarcinomas arising at the confluence of the left and right hepatic ducts are commonly referred to as Klatskin's tumors. However, the initial report describing three patients with hilar cholangiocarcinomas was actually made by Altemeier in 1957.[14] Early reports of resection of hilar cholangiocarcinoma consisted primarily of isolated bile duct resections.[15,16] However, advances in liver surgery over the past several decades have enabled a more aggressive approach to this disease, including extended hepatic and bile duct resection in order to obtain negative margins and improved outcomes.

Resection with negative margins (R0 resection) is the only potentially curative treatment for hilar cholangiocarcinoma. In contrast to most gastrointestinal cancers, in which clear margins are common, hilar cholangiocarcinomas develop in a confined space between the portal vein, hepatic artery, liver, and pancreas, allowing for only limited surgical clearance margins.[17] Despite recent advances in the surgical treatment of this disease to increase the percentage of patients who are candidates for R0 resection, including the addition of extended hepatic and portal vein resections, nearly two-thirds of patients who are referred to major hepatobiliary centers

are deemed unresectable.[18] These patients rarely survive more than 6 months, and palliative, nonsurgical options should be entertained, as surgical resection of hilar cholangiocarcinoma is associated with significant morbidity. Accordingly, proper patient selection for surgery is paramount and should include a thoughtful, detailed preoperative evaluation.

CRITERIA OF UNRESECTABILITY AND THE ROLE FOR STAGING LAPAROSCOPY

In order to determine resectability, the preoperative evaluation must provide information regarding the following: (1) the anatomic extent of bile duct involvement; (2) the radial extent of tumor spread (i.e., involvement of the vasculature and the extent of hepatic lobar hypertrophy/atrophy); and (3) the presence or absence of metastatic disease. This information is best attained by (1) cholangiography, which can be invasive (percutaneous or endoscopic), or noninvasive (magnetic resonance cholangiopancreatography [MRCP]); and (2) multiphasic intravenous contrast-enhanced helical computed tomography (CT) with thin cuts (1.5–3 mm) in an oblique coronal plane. This CT scan is also used to obtain a three-dimensional volumetric reconstruction of the future liver remnant to assess the need for preoperative portal vein embolization (PVE).

Standard criteria of unresectability include the following:[19]

- Bilateral intrahepatic bile duct spread to secondary or segmental biliary radicles
- Bilobar involvement of hepatic arterial and/or portal venous branches
- Encasement or occlusion of the main portal vein proximal to its bifurcation
- Unilateral segmental duct extension with contralateral vascular involvement
- Lobar atrophy with contralateral segmental duct extension or vascular involvement
- Lymph node metastases outside the hepatoduodenal ligament (N2 lymph nodes)
- Distant metastases

High quality cross-sectional imaging studies are increasingly capable of detecting metastatic disease. However, staging laparoscopy remains a powerful tool to identify those patients with occult unresectable or metastatic disease for a variety of hepatobiliary malignancies, including hilar cholangiocarcinoma.[20,21] Laparoscopy with laparoscopic ultrasound is quite accurate for identifying peritoneal disease and noncontiguous hepatic metastases, but less accurate for identifying vascular invasion and lymph node metastases.[21]

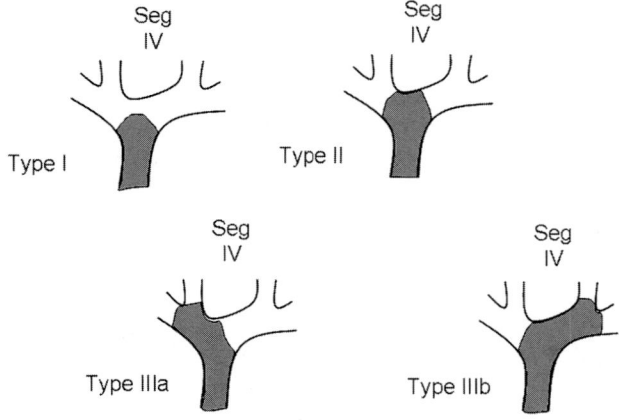

Figure 1 Bismuth-Corlette classification of potentially resectable (excludes type IV) hilar cholangiocarcinoma.

Overall, staging laparoscopy spares approximately 20% of patients with hilar cholangiocarcinoma the morbidity of an unnecessary laparotomy, and so should be considered routine in the preoperative staging evaluation of these patients.[20,21]

CLASSIFICATION OF HILAR CHOLANGIOCARCINOMA AND THE EXTENT OF RESECTION

In most cases, the resection strategy is determined by the location and the longitudinal extent of the tumor within the biliary tree, as defined by the Bismuth-Corlette classification[22] (Figure 1). Local or hilar resections of the extrahepatic biliary tract represent the least extensive resection, and in our opinion should largely be abandoned except perhaps in the rare case of an isolated mid-bile duct cholangiocarcinoma. Although no prospective randomized trials comparing common bile duct versus combined liver and common bile duct resection for hilar cholangiocarcinoma have been conducted, several large retrospective studies have demonstrated improved R0 resection rates and survival outcomes with combined resections.[23–25] In addition, perioperative

morbidity and mortality rates after major hepatectomy have declined over the past several years with refinements in surgical technique and an increased awareness of the importance of remnant liver function.[26–29] The extent of resection, perioperative mortality, and survival data from several recent series of patients who underwent resection of hilar cholangiocarcinoma are presented in Table 1.

A thorough knowledge of hepatic ductal anatomy and its variants is essential in planning the surgical resection. The right hepatic duct is inconstant and short ($<$ 1 cm). In contrast, the left hepatic duct is present in 97% of patients and is longer (1–5 cm).[30] In order to achieve a negative margin for a type I, II, or IIIa tumor, we recommend an extended right hepatectomy with partial or complete resection of segment IV (Figure 2). The relatively long, extrahepatic course of the left hepatic duct permits a longer proximal bile duct margin, and thus offers a better chance for long-term survival. Indeed, previous investigators have shown that a surgical margin of greater than 5 mm confers a significant survival benefit compared with a narrow margin of less than 5 mm.[28,31] In contrast, for a type IIIb hilar cholangiocarcinoma, we recommend a left hepatectomy with resection of segment IV (see Figure 2).

PREVENTION OF POSTOPERATIVE LIVER FAILURE: THE ROLE FOR PREOPERATIVE BILIARY DRAINAGE AND PORTAL VEIN EMBOLIZATION

A significant concern regarding major hepatic resection for hilar cholangiocarcinoma is the potential for postoperative hepatic insufficiency, reported in up to 32% of patients after combined resections.[32] Liver resection in the setting of biliary obstruction with or without cholangitis is associated with an increased risk of postoperative complications.[33] Preoperative biliary drainage of the *remnant* liver can lead to an improvement in hepatic function and resolution of cholangitis, and thereby reduce the risk of postoperative hepatic insufficiency.[26,28,34] Although preoperative biliary stent place-

Table 1 Results of Resection for Hilar Cholangiocarcinoma

Author	Year	Patients Resected (N)	Hepatic Resection (%)	Operative Mortality (%)	5-year Survival after R0 Resection (%)
Launois[55]	1999	40	62	12	NA
Kosuge[24]	1999	65	88	9	52
Miyazaki[56]	1999	93	86	10	38
Neuhaus[43]	1999	95	84	6	37
Nimura[26]	2000	142	90	6	26
Jarnagin[18]	2001	80	78	10	30
Seyama[28]	2003	67	87	0	46
Hemming[57]	2005	53	98	9	45

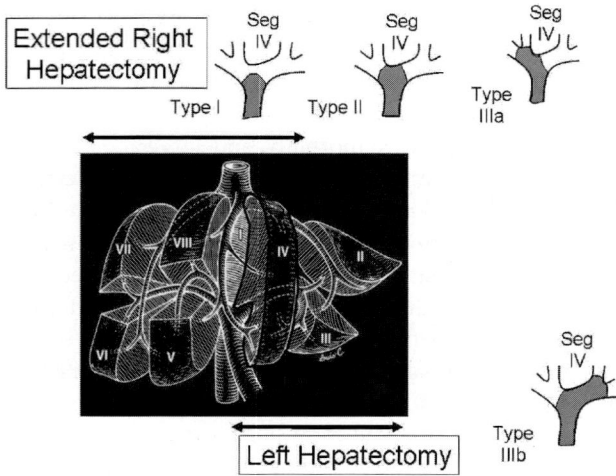

Figure 2 Extent of hepatic resection for types I to IIIb hilar cholangiocarcinoma.

ment may increase the incidence of wound infections,[35] most authors now recommend the placement of biliary drains in patients with a bilirubin level greater than 3 mg/dL or with dilated bile ducts in the future remnant liver.[23,28,36] Ideally, patients with hilar cholangiocarcinoma should be referred to a center specializing in the management of this disease such that preoperative lobar or sectoral biliary drainage can be appropriately directed in anticipation of resection.

Although survival following resection of more than 80% of the hepatic parenchyma is possible, such extensive resections are associated with an increased risk of complications.[37,38] The importance of the concept of lobar atrophy and subsequent contralateral lobar hypertrophy in patients with hilar cholangiocarcinoma became apparent as patients who had lobar hypertrophy induced by contralateral portal vein involvement by tumor were less likely to die in the postoperative period. This finding emphasizes the importance of sufficient remnant liver function after extended hepatectomy. Thus, in patients in whom an extensive liver resection is planned such that the anticipated future liver remnant volume is less than 20% of the total estimated liver volume, we recommend preoperative portal vein embolization (PVE). Though preoperative PVE has not been compared with resection alone in a prospective, randomized trial, there are significant data supporting the safety and efficacy of this technique.[27,29,39,40] In a recent series of 58 patients undergoing major hepatectomy for hilar cholangiocarcinoma, Seyama and colleagues[28] performed preoperative PVE in all patients ($n = 31$) undergoing resection of $> 50\%$ of initial liver volume and reported a 0% operative mortality and no cases of postoperative liver failure.

CAUDATE LOBE RESECTION

Resection of the caudate lobe (segment I) at the time of hepatic resection for hilar cholangiocarcinoma remains somewhat controversial. Proponents argue that pathologic specimens demonstrate direct tumor invasion into the parenchyma or bile ducts of the caudate lobe in a significant percentage of patients. Indeed, the bile duct draining the caudate lobe joins within 1 cm of the confluence of the main left and right hepatic ducts in the vast majority of patients, and the caudate lobe is a frequent site of recurrence within the liver after resection.[23,41] Proponents also argue that improved margins can be achieved with the addition of minimal morbidity with routine caudate lobe resection. Others suggest that the caudate lobe should be removed selectively based on tumor location and extent.

Resection of the caudate lobe requires a thorough understanding of its anatomy and its relationship to the hepatic vasculature and ductal system (Figure 3). The caudate lobe is divided into three subsegments. To the right of the inferior vena cava (IVC) and portal structures is situated the caudate process, and to the left of these structures and visible beneath the lesser omentum is situated Spiegel's lobe, or the papillary process of the caudate lobe. The paracaval portion of the caudate lobe is situated between these two processes and drapes the IVC.[42] We recommend resection of the caudate process and the paracaval subsegment with all hepatic resections for hilar cholangiocarcinoma because of their proximity to the hepatic duct confluence. Moreover, we recommend resection of Spiegel's lobe (papillary process) in addition to the caudate process and paracaval caudate at the time of left hepatectomy for Bismuth-Corlette type IIIb tumors.

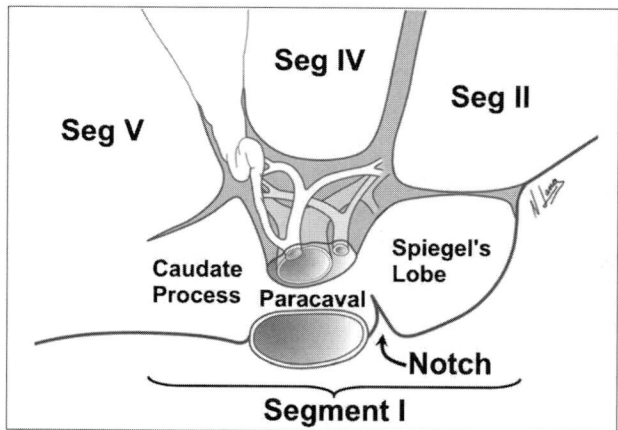

Figure 3 Anatomy of the caudate lobe (segment I). Reproduced with permission from Abdalla EK et al.[42]

PORTAL VEIN RESECTION

Invasion of the portal vein by tumor has long been deemed a contraindication to surgical resection in patients with hilar cholangiocarcinoma. In the past, portal vein resection and reconstruction was performed only in those cases in which gross invasion was noted at the time of resection or on preoperative imaging studies.[23] More recently, portal vein resection has been proposed as part of a "no-touch" technique in the resection of hilar cholangiocarcinoma.[43] In this study, portal vein resection was performed in both left ($n = 6$) and right ($n = 17$) hepatectomies, but histologically confirmed tumor infiltration was identified in only 22% of the specimens, including only 12% of the right-sided hepatectomies. In a multivariate analysis of patient survival after R0 resection, portal vein resection was identified as the only significant factor; however, this was evident only when deaths within 60 days of operation were excluded. The overall postoperative mortality rate after portal vein resection was 17% compared with less than 6% for all other patients who did not undergo portal vein resection.[43] Considering the lack of portal vein infiltration in the majority of specimens and the mortality associated with this procedure, routine portal vein resection as part of a "no-touch" technique cannot be recommended. However, in cases of "macroscopic" portal vein invasion by tumor, in which the portal vein is discovered to be adherent to the tumor during the dissection of the hepatoduodenal ligament, portal vein resection should be performed. Ebata and colleagues[44] have shown in their audit of 52 consecutive cases of portal vein resection for hilar cholangiocarcinoma that macroscopic (not microscopic) portal vein involvement is a significant predictor of survival, and that long-term survival can be achieved with combined hepatic and portal vein resection in some patients with advanced hilar cholangiocarcinomas who were previously deemed inoperable.

LYMPH NODE METASTASIS

Nodal status is an important predictor of survival after resection of hilar cholangiocarcinoma.[24,45] The incidence of nodal involvement in resected specimens has been reported to range from 25% to more than 50%,[2,46,47] and a range of 5-year survival rates from 0%[46,48] to more than 30%[24] have been reported for patients with regional lymph node metastasis. It is not clear whether an extended lymph node dissection, including the para-aortic lymph nodes, provides a survival benefit. Kitagawa and colleagues[49] audited 110 patients who underwent regional and para-aortic lymph node dissections at the time of surgical resection of hilar cholangiocarcinoma.

This study is interesting in that it details the pattern of lymph node spread from the pericholedochal nodes (43% with metastatic disease), to the periportal nodes (31%), to the common hepatic artery nodes (27%), to the posterior pancreaticoduodenal nodes (14.5%), and lastly to the para-aortic lymph nodes (17%). However, in this series, among 110 patients who underwent extended lymphadenectomies, including 58 patients with positive lymph nodes, only 5 patients survived for more than 5 years. Likewise, several other authors have shown that 0 to 5% of patients with positive lymph nodes will survive 5 years, including no patient with para-aortic node metastases.[2,24,43,50,51] These data suggest that lymph node dissection may add valuable staging and prognostic information, but that any survival benefit as a result of the dissection itself is minimal at best. Accordingly, routine lymphadenectomy beyond the hepatoduodenal ligament cannot be recommended.

ADJUVANT THERAPY

Given that hilar cholangiocarcinomas are rare tumors, no large-scale randomized trials have evaluated the role of adjuvant chemotherapy and/or radiotherapy following curative resection. Thus, there is no conclusive evidence that adjuvant treatment improves survival compared with surgical treatment alone. Nonetheless, 68% of patients with hilar cholangiocarcinoma develop recurrent disease at a median of 24 months, and the first site of recurrence is locoregional in nearly 60% of patients.[52] Therefore, in an effort to reduce locoregional recurrence rates and to improve survival after resection, we commonly administer postoperative radiation therapy in combination with radiosensitizing chemotherapy, particularly to those patients with positive resection margins (R1 resections). Pitt and colleagues[53] reported that postoperative radiation therapy did not improve survival, yet most of the patients in this series underwent palliative or R2 resections. Todoroki and colleagues[51] demonstrated that adjuvant radiotherapy for patients with stage IV hilar cholangiocarcinoma who underwent R1 resections significantly prolonged survival compared with resection alone. We have reported our experience at The University of Texas M. D. Anderson Cancer Center with the use of preoperative (neoadjuvant) chemoradiation therapy in patients with cholangiocarcinoma, initiated in an effort to increase the resectability rate as well as the rate of R0 resections.[54] Nine patients (5 with hilar and 4 with distal common bile duct cholangiocarcinomas) were treated with 5-FU-based chemoradiation, and all 9 patients had a margin-negative resection and 3 of the patients had a pathologic complete response.

Summary

The surgical treatment of hilar cholangiocarcinoma demands a detailed and thoughtful preoperative evaluation and operative strategy in order to maximize the opportunity for long-term survival while minimizing the perioperative risk. The majority of patients with hilar cholangiocarcinoma are deemed unresectable at the time of diagnosis, and staging laparoscopy can identify another 20% of patients thought to be resectable on the basis of preoperative imaging studies. The single most important prognostic factor for long-term survival in patients with hilar cholangiocarcinoma is the ability to achieve a margin-negative (R0) resection. A formal hepatic resection in addition to resection of the common bile duct and hepatoduodenal lymph nodes is recommended for all hilar cholangiocarcinomas. Given that extended hepatectomies are frequently required to achieve an R0 resection, preoperative biliary drainage and portal vein embolization should be considered to improve liver remnant function and to minimize the incidence of postoperative hepatic insufficiency and death. Routine resection of at least portions of the caudate lobe is recommended, whereas routine portal vein resection as part of a "no-touch" technique cannot be recommended. Extended lymphadenectomy to include lymph nodes outside the hepatoduodenal ligament does not confer a survival advantage and should not be performed routinely.

References

1. Olnes MJ, Erlich R. A review and update on cholangiocarcinoma. Oncology 2004;66:167–79.

2. Nakeeb A, Pitt HA, Sohn TA, et al. Cholangiocarcinoma. A spectrum of intrahepatic, perihilar, and distal tumors. Ann Surg 1996;224:463–75.

3. Qin XL, Wang ZR, Shi JS, et al. Utility of serum CA19-9 in diagnosis of cholangiocarcinoma: in comparison with CEA. World J Gastroenterol 2004;10:427–32.

4. Roayaie S, Guarrera JV, Ye MQ, et al. Aggressive surgical treatment of intrahepatic cholangiocarcinoma: predictors of outcomes. J Am Coll Surg 1998;187:365–72.

5. Lang H, Sotiropoulos GC, Fruhauf NR, et al. Extended hepatectomy for intrahepatic cholangiocellular carcinoma (ICC): when is it worthwhile? Single center experience with 27 resections in 50 patients over a 5-year period. Ann Surg 2005;241:134–43.

6. Shimada M, Yamashita Y, Aishima S, et al. Value of lymph node dissection during resection of intrahepatic cholangiocarcinoma. Br J Surg 2001;88:1463–6.

7. Weimann A, Varnholt H, Schlitt HJ, et al. Retrospective analysis of prognostic factors after liver resection and transplantation for cholangiocellular carcinoma. Br J Surg 2000;87:1182–7.

8. Uenishi T, Hirohashi K, Kubo S, et al. Clinicopathological factors predicting outcome after resection of mass-forming intrahepatic cholangiocarcinoma. Br J Surg 2001;88:969–74.

9. Hanazaki K, Kajikawa S, Shimozawa N, et al. Prognostic factors of intrahepatic cholangiocarcinoma after hepatic resection: univariate and multivariate analysis. Hepatogastroenterology 2002;49:311–6.

10. Weber SM, Jarnagin WR, Klimstra D, et al. Intrahepatic cholangiocarcinoma: resectability, recurrence pattern, and outcomes. J Am Coll Surg 2001;193:384–91.

11. Pichlmayr R, Lamesch P, Weimann A, et al. Surgical treatment of cholangiocellular carcinoma. World J Surg 1995;19:83–8.

12. Casavilla FA, Marsh JW, Iwatsuki S, et al. Hepatic resection and transplantation for peripheral cholangiocarcinoma. J Am Coll Surg 1997;185:429–36.

13. De Vreede I, Steers JL, Burch PA, et al. Prolonged disease-free survival after orthotopic liver transplantation plus adjuvant chemoirradiation for cholangiocarcinoma. Liver Transpl 2000;6:309–16.

14. Altemeier WA, Gall EA, Zinninger MM, Hoxworth PI. Sclerosing carcinoma of the major intrahepatic bile ducts. AMA Arch Surg 1957;75:450–61.

15. Launois B, Campion JP, Brissot P, Gosselin M. Carcinoma of the hepatic hilus. Surgical management and the case for resection. Ann Surg 1979;190:151–7.

16. Tompkins RK, Thomas D, Wile A, Longmire WP Jr. Prognostic factors in bile duct carcinoma: analysis of 96 cases. Ann Surg 1981;194:447–57.

17. Nagorney DM, Donohue JH, Farnell MB, et al. Outcomes after curative resections of cholangiocarcinoma. Arch Surg 1993;128:871–9.

18. Jarnagin WR, Fong Y, DeMatteo RP, et al. Staging, resectability, and outcome in 225 patients with hilar cholangiocarcinoma. Ann Surg 2001;234:507–19.

19. Vauthey JN, Blumgart LH. Recent advances in the management of cholangiocarcinomas. Semin Liver Dis 1994;14:109–14.

20. Weber SM, DeMatteo RP, Fong Y, et al. Staging laparoscopy in patients with extrahepatic biliary carcinoma. Analysis of 100 patients. Ann Surg 2002;235:392–9.

21. D'Angelica M, Fong Y, Weber S, et al. The role of staging laparoscopy in hepatobiliary malignancy: prospective analysis of 401 cases. Ann Surg Oncol 2003;10:183–9.

22. Bismuth H, Corlette MB. Intrahepatic cholangioenteric anastomosis in carcinoma of the hilus of the liver. Surg Gynecol Obstet 1975;140:170–8.

23. Nimura Y, Hayakawa N, Kamiya J, et al. Hepatic segmentectomy with caudate lobe resection for bile duct carcinoma of the hepatic hilus. World J Surg 1990;14:535–44.

24. Kosuge T, Yamamoto J, Shimada K, et al. Improved surgical results for hilar cholangiocarcinoma with procedures including major hepatic resection. Ann Surg 1999;230:663–71.

25. Lee SG, Lee YJ, Park KM, et al. One hundred and eleven liver resections for hilar bile duct cancer. J Hepatobiliary Pancreat Surg 2000;7:135–41.

26. Nimura Y, Kamiya J, Kondo S, et al. Aggressive preoperative management and extended surgery for hilar cholangiocarcinoma: Nagoya experience. J Hepatobiliary Pancreat Surg 2000;7:155–62.

27. Abdalla EK, Barnett CC, Doherty D, et al. Extended hepatectomy in patients with hepatobiliary malignancies with and without preoperative portal vein embolization. Arch Surg 2002;137:675–80.

28. Seyama Y, Kubota K, Sano K, et al. Long-term outcome of extended hemihepatectomy for hilar bile duct cancer with no mortality and high survival rate. Ann Surg 2003;238:73–83.

29. Vauthey JN, Pawlik TM, Abdalla EK, et al. Is extended hepatectomy for hepatobiliary malignancy justified? Ann Surg 2004;239:722–32.

30. Couinaud C. Le foie. Etudes anatomiques et chirurgicales. Paris: Masson, 1957, 469–79.

31. Sakamoto E, Nimura Y, Hayakawa N, et al. The pattern of infiltration at the proximal border of hilar bile duct carcinoma: a histologic analysis of 62 resected cases. Ann Surg 1998;227:405–11.

32. Nagino M, Ando M, Kamiya J, et al. Liver regeneration after major hepatectomy for biliary cancer. Br J Surg 2001;88:1084–91.

33. Cherqui D, Benoist S, Malassagne B, et al. Major liver resection for carcinoma in jaundiced patients without preoperative biliary drainage. Arch Surg 2000;135:302–8.

34. Kawasaki S, Imamura H, Kobayashi A, et al. Results of surgical resection for patients with hilar bile duct cancer: application of extended hepatectomy after biliary drainage and hemihepatic portal vein embolization. Ann Surg 2003;238:84–92.

35. Hochwald SN, Burke EC, Jarnigan WR, et al. Association of preoperative biliary stenting with increased postoperative infectious complications in proximal cholangiocarcinoma. Arch Surg 1999;134:261–6.

36. Makuuchi M, Thai BL, Takayasu K, et al. Preoperative portal embolization to increase safety of major hepatect-omy for hilar bile duct carcinoma: a preliminary report. Surgery 1990;107:521–7.

37. Abdalla EK, Hicks ME, Vauthey JN. Portal vein embolization: rationale, technique and future prospects. Br J Surg 2001;88:165–75.

38. Shoup M, Gonen M, D'Angelica M, et al. Volumetric analysis predicts hepatic dysfunction in patients undergoing major liver resection. J Gastrointest Surg 2003;7:325–30.

39. Nagino M, Nimura Y, Kamiya J, et al. Right or left trisegment portal vein embolization before hepatic trisegmentectomy for hilar bile duct carcinoma. Surgery 1995;117:677–81.

40. Nagino M, Kamiya J, Kanai M, et al. Right trisegment portal vein embolization for biliary tract carcinoma: technique and clinical utility. Surgery 2000;127:155–60.

41. Baer HU, Stain SC, Dennison AR, et al. Improvements in survival by aggressive resections of hilar cholangiocarcinoma. Ann Surg 1993;217:20–7.

42. Abdalla EK, Vauthey JN, Couinaud C. The caudate lobe of the liver: implications of embryology and anatomy for surgery. Surg Oncol Clin N Am 2002;11:835–48.

43. Neuhaus P, Jonas S, Bechstein WO, et al. Extended resections for hilar cholangiocarcinoma. Ann Surg 1999;230:808–19.

44. Ebata T, Nagino M, Kamiya J, et al. Hepatectomy with portal vein resection for hilar cholangiocarcinoma: audit of 52 consecutive cases. Ann Surg 2003;238:720–7.

45. Klempnauer J, Riddre GJ, von Wasielewski R, et al. Resectional surgery of hilar cholangiocarcinoma: a multivariate analysis of prognostic factors. J Clin Oncol 1997;15:947–54.

46. Iwatsuki S, Todo S, Marsh JW, et al. Treatment of hilar cholangiocarcinoma (Klatskin tumors) with hepatic resection or transplantation. J Am Coll Surg 1998;187:358–64.

47. Ogura Y, Mizumoto R, Tabada M, et al. Surgical treatment of carcinoma of the hepatic duct confluence: analysis of 55 resected carcinomas. World J Surg 1993;17:85–93.

48. Ogura Y, Kawarada Y. Surgical strategies for carcinoma of the hepatic duct confluence. Br J Surg 1998;85:20–4.

49. Kitagawa Y, Nagino M, Kamiya J, et al. Lymph node metastasis from hilar cholangiocarcinoma: audit of 110 patients who underwent regional and paraaortic node dissection. Ann Surg 2001;233:385–92.

50. Iwasaki M, Takada Y, Hayashi M, et al. Noninvasive evaluation of graft steatosis in living donor liver transplantation. Transplantation 2004;78:1501–5.

51. Todoroki T, Kawamoto T, Koike N, et al. Radical resection of hilar bile duct carcinoma and predictors of survival. Br J Surg 2000;87:306–13.

52. Jarnagin WR, Ruo L, Little SA, et al. Patterns of initial disease recurrence after resection of gallbladder carcinoma and hilar cholangiocarcinoma: implications for adjuvant therapeutic strategies. Cancer 2003;98:1689–700.

53. Pitt HA, Nakeeb A, Abrams RA, et al. Perihilar cholangio-carcinoma. Postoperative radiotherapy does not improve survival. Ann Surg 1995;221:788–98.

54. McMasters KM, Tuttle TM, Leach SD, et al. Neoadjuvant chemoradiation for extrahepatic cholangiocarcinoma. Am J Surg 1997;174:605–9.

55. Launois B, Terblanche J, Lakehal M, et al. Proximal bile duct cancer: high resectability rate and 5-year survival. Ann Surg 1999;230:266–75.

56. Miyazaki M, Ito H, Nakagawa K, et al. Parenchyma-preserving hepatectomy in the surgical treatment of hilar cholangiocarcinoma. J Am Coll Surg 1999;189:575–83.

57. Hemming AW, Reed AI, Fujita S, et al. Surgical management of hilar cholangiocarcinoma. Ann Surg 2005;241:693–702.

CHAPTER 19

SURGICAL TREATMENT OF PANCREATIC ADENOCARCINOMA

KEITH D. AMOS, MD

DEBRA L. KENNAMER, MD

CHUSILP CHARNSANGAVEJ, MD

HUAMIN WANG, MD, PhD

DOUGLAS B. EVANS, MD

Introduction

Pancreatic cancer is the fourth leading cause of cancer-related death for both men and women (following lung, colorectal, and breast cancer), being responsible for 6% of all cancer-related deaths.[1] An estimated 33,730 people were diagnosed with pancreatic cancer in the United States in 2006.[1] Exocrine pancreatic cancer is characterized by early vascular dissemination and spread to regional lymph nodes. Subclinical liver or lung metastases are present in most patients at the time of diagnosis, even when findings from imaging studies suggest localized disease. Survival duration depends on the extent of disease and the patient's performance status at diagnosis. The extent of disease is best categorized as resectable (stage I or II), locally advanced (stage III), or metastatic (stage IV). The TNM (tumor-nodes-metastasis) staging system has been modified in the last edition of the *AJCC Cancer Staging Manual* to allow staging to be determined by CT images and to reflect the emphasis on stage-specific treatment planning.[2] Patients who undergo surgical resection for localized adenocarcinoma of the pancreatic head without metastasis have a long-term survival rate of approximately 20% and a median survival of 18 to 24 months.[3,4] It is common for disease to recur following pancreaticoduodenectomy. The most common sites of recurrence include the liver and lung (distant recurrence), the peritoneal cavity (regional recurrence), and the pancreatic tumor bed (local recurrence). In patients who undergo an incomplete surgical resection or surgery without adjuvant therapy, local recurrence may occur in up to 50% of patients. When multimodality therapy is combined with good technical surgery and appropriate patient selection for operation, local-regional tumor control is improved and distant disease in the liver (and less commonly in lung and bone) becomes the dominant form of tumor recurrence.[3]

Approximately 50% of patients with pancreatic cancer have jaundice at diagnosis as the result of extrahepatic biliary obstruction. Tumors arising in the ampulla of Vater or within the intrapancreatic portion of the common bile duct cause biliary obstruction early in the disease course and, therefore, may be associated with a better prognosis. Small tumors of the pancreatic head strategically located near the intrapancreatic portion of the bile duct also may obstruct the bile duct and cause the patient to seek medical attention while the tumor is still localized and potentially resectable. In contrast, adenocarcinomas arising in the pancreas that do not obstruct the intrapancreatic portion of the bile duct are often not diagnosed until they are locally advanced or metastatic. If jaundice is not present, patient complaints are often nonspecific and include pain, fatigue, weight loss, hyperglycemia, and pancreatic exocrine insufficiency. The pain typical of locally advanced pancreatic cancer is a dull, fairly constant pain localized to the middle and upper back owing to tumor invasion of the celiac and mesenteric plexus. Pancreatic exocrine insufficiency, when present, is due to obstruction of the pancreatic duct and commonly results in malabsorption, steatorrhea, and mild changes in stool frequency. Fatigue, weight loss, and anorexia are common even in the absence of mechanical gastric outlet obstruction or steatorrhea.

In this chapter, we will review our current approach to the diagnosis and surgical treatment of patients with localized pancreatic cancer. Our diagnostic algorithm emphasizes the use of computed tomography (CT) and the rapidly evolving technique of endoscopic ultrasound (EUS). Good surgical outcomes require proper patient selection, detailed surgical technique, and attention to all aspects of patient care, especially anesthetic management. We will not comment on the expanding field of adjuvant and neoadjuvant therapy, and refer the reader to recent reviews by our group.[4,5]

Epidemiology

The risk of pancreatic cancer is low in the first 3 to 4 decades of life, but increases sharply after age 50 years. Only 10% of patients develop pancreatic cancer below age 50.[6] Although pancreatic cancer is uncommon in patients under 40 years of age, apparently, sporadic adenocarcinoma of pancreatic origin does occur in patients younger than 30 years. In the past, pancreatic cancer was more common in men than women, but now the incidence is about the same for both sexes in the United States, probably as a result of the increased use of tobacco by women.[1]

Pancreatic cancer incidence and mortality statistics are similar throughout the world. Incidence rates are highest in industrialized societies and western countries. In Europe, rates are highest in the Nordic countries.[6] In the United States, rates are particularly high in native Hawaiians, African Americans, and Korean Americans, with the highest rates in blacks. The fact that the rates in African Americans are considerably higher than in native Africans suggests an environmental influence. The reasons for the slight regional and ethnic differences in the incidence of pancreatic cancer are unknown, but this may be due to changes in tobacco use in certain groups and regions. Unfortunately, these broad epidemiologic categories do little to identify specific individuals at high risk of pancreatic cancer.

Diagnostic Evaluation

Biliary obstruction is usually evaluated with abdominal ultrasonography to confirm the mechanical nature of the obstruction and to determine whether the site of obstruction is the intrahepatic or extrahepatic portion of the biliary tree. Obstruction of the intrapancreatic portion of the bile duct is then evaluated with a combination of CT, EUS, and endoscopic retrograde cholangiopancreatography (ERCP). High-quality CT can identify most pancreatic tumors and accurately define the relationship of the tumor to the celiac axis and superior mesenteric vessels.[7] The development of multislice or multidetector CT (MDCT) allows imaging of the entire pancreas during the bolus phase of contrast enhancement. In addition, scan data can be processed to display images in three-dimensional and multiplanar formats. This allows accurate pretreatment staging using objective (and reproducible) radiologic criteria. The CT findings defining a potentially resectable pancreatic cancer (American Joint Committee on Cancer [AJCC] stages I or II) are (1) the absence of extrapancreatic disease, (2) a patent superior mesenteric-portal vein (SMPV) confluence (assuming it is technically possible to resect isolated involvement of the superior mesenteric vein [SMV] or SMPV confluence), and (3) no direct tumor extension to the celiac axis or superior mesenteric artery (SMA). A patient is deemed to have locally advanced, unresectable disease (AJCC stage III) when CT images demonstrate tumor extension to the SMA or celiac axis or occlusion of the SMPV confluence. Limited arterial abutment (often referred to as borderline or marginally resectable) may be amenable to a multimodality treatment approach to include eventual surgery.[8] In general, tumor extension to the celiac axis, common hepatic artery, or SMA should be considered a contraindication to immediate surgery. The accuracy of CT in predicting unresectability is well established; it is not necessary to perform a laparotomy to assess local tumor resectability when arterial involvement is clearly present.

If a low-density mass is not seen on CT scan, a patient with suspected pancreatic cancer should undergo upper endoscopy and EUS. Endoscopic evaluation may discover an ampullary tumor or related pathology, and EUS may define a mass in the pancreas or distal bile duct not seen on CT. When possible, upper endoscopy, EUS, and ERCP should always be performed after CT, because if endoscopy (ERCP or EUS-guided biopsy)-induced pancreatitis occurs, it may interfere with accurate assessment of the extent of disease. At the time of ERCP, a malignant obstruction can often be accurately differentiated from choledocholithiasis and the long, smooth, tapering bile duct stricture seen in chronic pancreatitis. We routinely place endoscopic stents to prevent cholangitis in patients with extrahepatic biliary obstruction who undergo diagnostic ERCP. We also place endoscopic stents in patients with elevated bilirubin levels in whom surgery is expected to be delayed, including those who are enrolled in preoperative chemoradiation therapy protocols.[9]

EUS-guided fine-needle aspiration (FNA) is currently the procedure of choice for obtaining a cytologic diagnosis of a malignancy in patients with nonmetastatic pancreatic tumors.[10] Confirmation of malignancy is required in all patients with locally advanced disease prior to treatment with systemic therapy or external beam radiation therapy (EBRT) and is being done more commonly in patients with localized, potentially resectable disease because of the growing popularity of neoadjuvant therapy. When FNA material is examined by an experienced cytopathologist, false-positive results should not occur; however, false-negative results may occur, especially when small tumors are involved. Therefore, negative results from EUS-guided FNA should not be considered definite proof that a malignancy does not exist. Importantly, as discussed above, high-quality CT imaging should be performed before an FNA (or an ERCP) is attempted because of the risk of the biopsy inducing pancreatitis, which would distort the pancreatic anatomy. Further, FNA biopsy should, in general, be performed only if a mass is identified; a blind biopsy of the pancreas is rarely considered.

At present, laparoscopy is rarely performed as a separate staging procedure under general anesthesia in patients with presumed resectable pancreatic cancer. However, most surgeons do routinely perform laparoscopy at the same anesthesia induction as a planned laparotomy when considering major pancreatic resection for presumed localized, resectable pancreatic cancer. Laparoscopy can be performed fairly quickly and may prevent the occasional patient from undergoing a nontherapeutic laparotomy. Importantly, the rapidly expanding body of literature on laparoscopic staging has drawn attention to the need to avoid nontherapeutic laparotomy. A fortunate consequence of the recent emphasis on minimally invasive surgery is the realization by clinicians that it is no longer acceptable to perform a major laparotomy in patients with presumed pancreatic cancer just to "explore" the possibility of resection. There is now general consensus that resectability be assessed prior to laparotomy.

Anesthetic Management for Pancreaticoduodenectomy

All patients receive epidural analgesia combined with a general anesthetic unless an epidural catheter is contraindicated. A mid to low thoracic epidural catheter is placed prior to induction of general anesthesia. The patient is then anesthetized and intubated, and continuous arterial and central venous pressure monitoring catheters are placed. The central venous line is used for both monitoring and venous access. Patients also receive at least one large bore peripheral intravenous catheter. The epidural catheter is activated with a local anesthetic (20 mL of 0.125% bupivacaine) prior to the surgical incision. This is followed by a continuous infusion of local anesthetic (0.075% bupivacaine) at a rate of 10 mL/ hour for the remainder of the case. General anesthesia is maintained with an inhalational agent (usually isoflurane or desflurane), in combination with an opiate infusion (sufentanil), and muscle relaxant titrated to provide adequate surgical relaxation. Forced warm air is used to maintain the patient's body temperature at 37°C. The patient's volume status is closely monitored and replacement consists of a mixture of plasmalyte, 5% albumin, and blood if necessary. Urine output of 1 to 2 mL/kg/hour is acceptable. It has been observed that some patients have a remarkable diuresis during this surgical procedure, which is not related to glucosuria or any identifiable hormone abnormality. Unless the patient has a severe pre-existing cardiopulmonary comorbidity, the patient is extubated at the end of the operation and remains in a monitored bed overnight prior to transfer to the surgical ward. Patient-controlled epidural analgesia (PCEA) is maintained with a mixture of low concentration local anesthetic (bupivacaine or ropivacaine) and opiate (fentanyl or hydromorphone). PCEA is maintained for 3 to 5 days postoperatively. Epidural local anesthetics produce neuraxial blockade of the afferent and efferent signals, resulting in inhibition or blunting of the endocrine responses to surgery. This results in lower plasma concentrations of cortisol, glucagon, and catecholamines.[11]

Patient satisfaction scores have been shown to be higher in patients receiving PCEA compared with patient-controlled analgesia (PCA).[12] Patients receiving PCEA following major abdominal surgery have demonstrated improved pain relief at rest and after coughing, with a lower incidence of side effects. In addition, PCEA is associated with shorter times to extubation, improved pulmonary function with a decreased incidence of respiratory failure and more rapid return of bowel activity.[12–14] Combined epidural and general anesthesia followed by postoperative PCEA has been shown to significantly increase wound tissue oxygenation when compared with general anesthesia and intravenous PCA.[15] This may be due to the intrinsic vasodilatory properties of the local anesthetics as well as the decreased physiologic stress response to surgery associated with epidural anesthesia. Tissue oxygen tension is an important determinant of wound healing because the bactericidal ability of neutrophils is directly related to the tissue oxygen tension.[16] It is difficult to define the relative contributions of postoperative pain and the surgical procedure in general to the immunosuppression associated with the perioperative period. It is clear that the nervous and immune systems influence each other.[17] Patients receiving a mixture of opiates and local anesthetics via PCEA exhibited reduced suppression of lymphocyte proliferation as well as an attenuated proinflammatory cytokine response.[17] Such data suggest a physiologic and clinical benefit to PCEA beyond that of just improved pain control.

Pancreaticoduodenectomy

Pancreaticoduodenectomy involves removal of the pancreatic head, duodenum, gallbladder, and bile duct with or without removal of the gastric antrum. It represents the standard surgical procedure for neoplasms of the pancreatic head and periampullary region. Our recommended technique for pancreaticoduodenectomy utilizes a midline, or occasionally, a bilateral subcostal incision. The abdomen is carefully explored to exclude extrapancreatic metastatic disease. The liver and peritoneal surfaces are examined as we would not proceed with tumor resection in the presence of biopsy-proven liver or peritoneal metastases. The issue of lymph node biopsy for frozen-section analysis remains controversial. Lymph node metastasis is a negative prognostic factor predictive of decreased survival duration. However, the majority (60–90%) of resected specimens contain microscopic metastases in regional lymph nodes.[18] In a good-risk patient with localized, resectable pancreatic cancer, we do not (at this time) view lymph node metastases as an absolute contraindication to pancreaticoduodenectomy when performed as part of a multimodality approach to pancreatic cancer. Therefore, in general, we do not perform random lymph node sampling for frozen-section analysis at the time of pancreaticoduodenectomy. However, each case should be considered individually. For example, in a high-risk patient (owing to medical comorbidities or oncologic concerns) with suspicious adenopathy, a positive regional lymph node may be viewed as a contraindication to proceeding with pancreaticoduodenectomy.

The surgical resection can be divided into 6 defined steps that may facilitate the organization of such a complex operation and minimize operative time.

The purpose of step 1 is to enter the lesser sac, mobilize the hepatic flexure of the colon and separate the colon (and its mesentery) from the duodenum and pancreatic head, and isolate the infrapancreatic SMV. Anatomic and technical considerations important to remember include the following:

1. The middle colic vein may enter directly into the anterior surface of the infrapancreatic SMV or arise as a common trunk with the gastroepiploic vein (gastrocolic trunk). If the middle colic vein and gastroepiploic vein share a common trunk, the common trunk is divided; otherwise, the gastroepiploic vein is left intact and divided later in the operation following pancreatic transection.

2. When necessary, the middle colic vein is divided proximal to its junction with the SMV. Division of the middle colic vein allows greater exposure of the infrapancreatic SMV and prevents iatrogenic traction injury to the SMV during dissection of the middle colic vein-SMV junction.

3. Occasionally, when there is extensive inflammatory change or scarring at the root of mesentery, we may not identify the SMV early in the operation. In such a case, the SMV will be exposed during step 6 when the pancreas is divided in a caudal direction from the level of the portal vein. This can be a dangerous maneuver because of the lack of vascular control; however, it is a valuable technique for the experienced surgeon who deals with more complicated pancreatic resections, often in the reoperative setting.

The purpose of step 2 is to perform a Kocher maneuver. This dissection is begun at the transverse portion (third portion) of the duodenum by identifying the inferior vena cava. All fibrofatty and lymphatic tissue medial to the right ureter and anterior to the inferior vena cava is elevated, along with the pancreatic head and duodenum. The Kocher maneuver is continued to the left lateral edge of the aorta, with care to identify the left renal vein. Anatomic and technical considerations important to remember include the following:

1. The right gonadal vein is usually preserved and serves as a good landmark to help prevent inadvertent injury to the ureter, which is usually lateral and slightly posterior to the gonadal vein.

2. Incision of the leaf of peritoneum that is posterior to the mesenteric vessels is often performed at this time and is necessary prior to performing the SMA dissection. Otherwise, the SMA can be tethered to the retroperitoneum, making the SMA dissection more difficult.

The purpose of step 3 is to complete the portal dissection by first exposing the common hepatic artery (CHA) proximal and distal to the right gastric artery and the gastroduodenal artery (GDA). The CHA is exposed by removing the large lymph node that lies directly anterior to this vessel. The right gastric artery, and then the GDA, are ligated and divided. Division of the GDA allows mobilization of the hepatic (common-proper) artery off the underlying PV, which can be found within the triangle formed by the CHA, GDA, and superior border of the pancreas. Cholecystectomy is then performed and the common hepatic duct is transected at its junction with the cystic duct. Anatomic and technical considerations important to remember include the following:

1. If tumor extension to within a few millimeters of the GDA is present, one should obtain proximal and distal control of the hepatic artery and divide the GDA flush at its origin. Dissection of the hepatic artery should be performed with gentle, sharp dissection, especially in patients who have received prior external beam radiation therapy, and in those with extensive scar formation from prior surgery. Intimal dissection of the hepatic artery can result from overly aggressive blunt dissection and inadequate vascular control of the proximal and distal hepatic artery.
2. The PV should always be exposed prior to dividing the common hepatic duct.
3. Review of the preoperative CT scan and careful palpation of the porta hepatis prior to division of the bile duct should alert one to the possibility of anomalous hepatic arterial circulation. A replaced or accessory right hepatic artery arising from the proximal SMA may course posterolateral to the PV.
4. When possible, we place a gentle vascular-type bulldog clamp on the transected bile duct to prevent bile spillage until the time of bile duct reconstruction.

The purpose of step 4 is to divide the stomach or duodenum. Anatomic and technical considerations important to remember include the following:

1. Pylorus preservation should not be performed in patients with bulky pancreatic head tumors, duodenal tumors involving the first or second portions of the duodenum, or lesions associated with grossly positive pyloric or peripyloric lymph nodes.
2. When opening the lesser omentum, be aware that an accessory left hepatic artery may be present arising from the left gastric artery.

The purpose of step 5 is to divide the mesentery of the proximal jejunum and the distal duodenum. The loose attachments of the ligament of Treitz are taken down with care to avoid injury to the inferior mesenteric vein (IMV). We prefer to tie the mesenteric side (staying side) of the proximal jejunum and duodenum and use the harmonic scalpel on the serosal (bowel) side.

The purpose of step 6 is to divide the pancreas and separate the specimen from the superior mesenteric-portal vein (SMPV) confluence and the SMA. Proper mobilization of the SMV involves identification of the jejunal branch of the SMV (referred to by some as the first jejunal branch); this branch originates from the right posterolateral aspect of the SMV (at the level of the uncinate process), travels posterior to the SMA, and enters the medial (proximal) aspect of the jejunal mesentery. Very rarely, the jejunal branch may course anterior to the SMA. The jejunal branch usually gives off one or two venous tributaries to the uncinate process; these tributaries should be divided. Medial retraction of the SMPV confluence allows one to expose the SMA. The specimen is then separated from the right lateral wall of the SMA, which is dissected to its origin at the aorta (Figure 1). Anatomic and technical considerations important to remember include the following:

1. Complete removal of the uncinate process from the SMV is required for full mobilization of the SMPV confluence and subsequent identification of the SMA. Failure to fully mobilize the SMPV confluence risks injury to the SMA and usually results in a positive margin of resection owing to incomplete removal of the uncinate process and the mesenteric soft tissue adjacent to the SMA.
2. Exposure of the SMA is necessary for direct ligation of the inferior pancreaticoduodenal arteries (usually two of them). Mass ligation of this vessel (or vessels) with mesenteric soft tissue is the major cause of postoperative retroperitoneal hemorrhage, as this vessel retracts from its poorly placed tie or ligature.
3. Injury to the distal SMV at the level of the jejunal branch (usually a tangential laceration as it courses posterior to the SMA) is hard to control and probably represents the most frequent cause of iatrogenic SMA injury, as one attempts to suture a venous injury prior to full exposure of the SMA.
4. The perineural and mesenteric tissue along the proximal SMA represents the SMA margin. A grossly positive SMA margin should not occur if high-quality preoperative imaging is performed. A microscopically positive margin will occur in 10 to 20% of cases; margin positivity can result from tumor spread along perineural sheaths and does not always result from direct extension of the primary tumor.

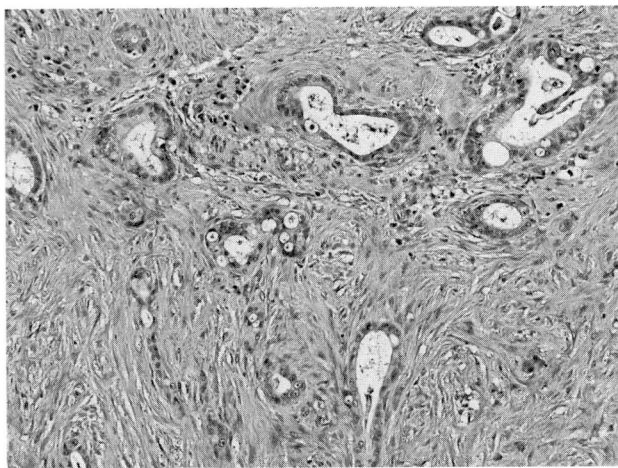

Figure 1 Illustration of the final step in resection of the pancreaticoduodenectomy specimen. Medial retraction of the superior mesenteric-portal vein confluence facilitates dissection of the soft tissues adjacent to the lateral wall of the proximal superior mesenteric artery (SMA); this site represents the SMA or retroperitoneal margin. The inferior pancreaticoduodenal artery (or arteries) is identified at its origin from the SMA—ligated and divided. SMV, superior mesenteric vein.

Pathology

GROSS EXAMINATION AND MARGIN ANALYSIS

Frozen-section evaluation of the pancreaticoduodenectomy specimen includes analysis of the pancreatic and common hepatic duct transection margins. Positive resection margins on the hepatic or pancreatic duct should be resected to a negative margin if possible. Complete permanent-section analysis of the pancreaticoduodenectomy specimen (Figure 2) requires that it be oriented for the pathologist to enable accurate assessment of the SMA margin (also termed retroperitoneal, mesenteric, or uncinate margin) of excision and other standard pathologic variables. Because we remove all tissue to the right of the SMA, further resection at the SMA/retroperitoneal margin is not possible. However, this margin must be identified and inked with the pathologist, it cannot be assessed retrospectively. All pancreatic resections should be classified according to residual disease status (termed "R" factor): R0, no gross or microscopic residual disease; R1, microscopic residual disease (microscopically positive surgical margins with no gross residual disease); and R2, grossly evident residual disease. The pathologist cannot usually differentiate an R1 (microscopically positive) from an R2 (grossly positive) SMA/retroperitoneal margin in the absence of information regarding the retroperitoneal

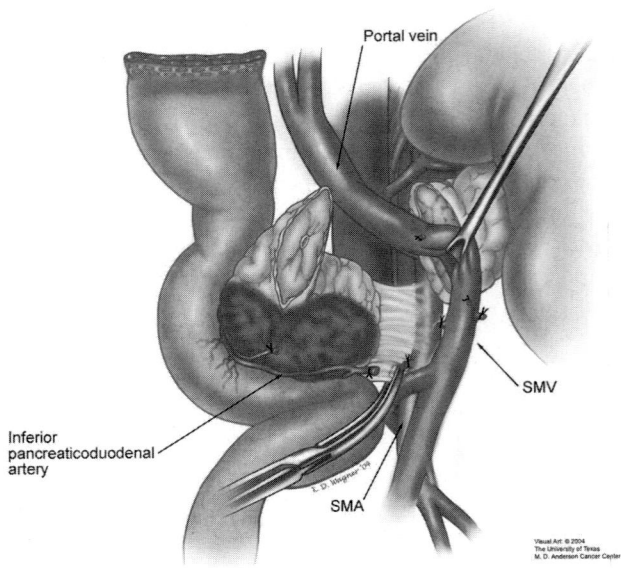

Figure 2 Illustration of a pancreaticoduodenectomy specimen. The superior mesenteric artery (SMA) margin (also termed retroperitoneal, mesenteric, or uncinate margin) is the perineural and soft tissue adjacent to the superior mesenteric artery and should be inked for evaluation of margin status. Complete permanent-section analysis of the pancreaticoduodenectomy specimen requires that the specimen be oriented to enable the pathologist to accurately assess the SMA margin to determine the adequacy of resection (R status).

dissection, which should be included in the operative dictation. The R designation should always be listed in the dictated operative report (we do not sign-off on the operative note until the pathology report is available for review, and we therefore know the status of the SMA margin). For example, if the surgeon states that gross tumor was encountered when completing the retroperitoneal dissection, a positive histologic margin should result in the R2 designation in the operative report and the medical record. If the surgeon states (in the operative report) that there was no gross evidence of tumor extension to the SMA margin, then a positive histologic margin should result in the R1 designation in the operative report and the medical record. The difficulty in differentiating R1 from R2 resections has significant implications for the conduct of clinical trials examining the potential advantage of nonsurgical therapies, especially in patients with borderline resectable tumors.

HISTOLOGIC EXAMINATION

The normal architecture of the pancreas is typical of the architecture of a secretory gland, and consists mainly of 3 epithelial components: the acini, the ducts, and the islets of Langerhans. The acinar cells account for approximately 85% of the cell number and volume of the gland,

and the endocrine component (islet cells) makes up only 1 to 2% of the volume of adult pancreas.[19] The rest of the pancreas is composed of pancreatic ducts lined by single-layered, cuboidal ductal cells and a sparse interlacing network of blood vessels, lymphatics, nerves, and connective tissue.

Infiltrating ductal adenocarcinoma is the most common histologic type of pancreatic cancers. Grossly, ductal adenocarcinomas form firm, poorly defined masses with yellow to white cut surfaces, which obliterate the lobular architecture of the normal pancreas. Necrosis or hemorrhage is uncommon. Adenocarcinomas in the pancreatic head typically involve the intrapancreatic portion of common bile duct and/or pancreatic duct and lead to stenosis or obstruction of these ducts. Microscopically, well-differentiated ductal adenocarcinomas are characterized by well-formed large- or medium-sized glands, often with a haphazard growth pattern. The glands are lined by cuboidal or columnar epithelial cells with basally located nuclei. Cytologic atypia and nuclear pleomorphism are often minimal. Distinguishing well-differentiated duct adenocarcinoma from benign reactive glands can be extremely difficult. Close attention must be given to growth pattern and location of the glands and the cytologic details (nuclear pleomorphism within individual glands). Findings of vascular invasion, perineural invasion, or glands next to muscular arteries without intervening pancreatic parenchyma are diagnostic for carcinoma. Other helpful features in establishing the diagnosis of an adenocarcinoma include incomplete glandular formation, intraluminal necrotic debris, and loss of DPC4 expression, which is detected in about half of pancreatic ductal adenocarcinomas, but not in reactive benign ductal epithelium. Compared with well-differentiated ductal adenocarcinomas, incomplete glandular formation, greater variation in nuclear size, chromatin pattern and prominence of nucleoli, and mitosis are more commonly seen in moderately differentiated ductal carcinomas. The neoplastic glands vary in size and shape with abundant desmoplastic stroma (Figure 3). Poorly differentiated ductal carcinomas are composed of poorly formed glands, individual infiltrating tumor cells in desmoplastic stroma, and solid nests and sheets of tumor cells. The neoplastic cells often show marked pleomorphism, brisk mitotic activities with little or no mucin production. According to World Health Organization Classification of tumors of the digestive system (WHO 2000), variants of pancreatic ductal adenocarcinoma include adenosquamous carcinoma, mucinous noncystic carcinoma, signet-ring cell carcinoma and undifferentiated (anaplastic) carcinoma, and undifferentiated carcinoma with osteoclast-like giant cells.

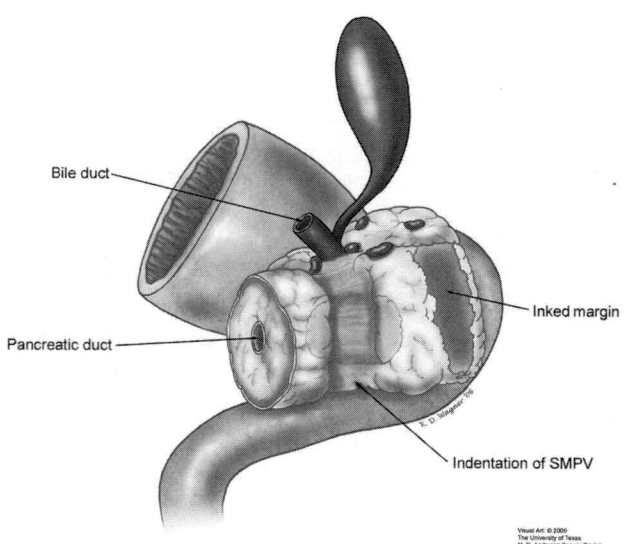

Figure 3 Histologic section of a moderately-differentiated adenocarcinoma of the pancreas. The infiltrating tumoral glands vary in size and shape within desmoplastic stroma (H & E stain, original magnification 100×).

The infiltration of perineural spaces is commonly seen in pancreatic adenocarcinoma. This is an important consideration because the superior mesenteric artery (SMA) is surrounded by a neural plexus that provides visceral innervation to the small intestine. This neural plexus extends proximally to the celiac ganglion (see Case Study 3 below), which surrounds the aorta at and above the level of the celiac artery. Infiltration of this mesenteric neural plexus is characteristic of pancreatic adenocarcinoma once it involves the SMA. For this reason, extended pancreatic resection that requires arterial resection typically fails to achieve a negative margin and has not been demonstrated to improve survival duration.[20]

Careful and complete histologic examination and detailed pathology reports on pancreatoduodenectomy specimens are not only critical for accurate tumor staging, but also facilitate prospective clinical studies. The pathology template currently used in all pathology reports at our institution appears in Table 1. Such templates are necessary to allow accurate transfer of pathologic data to prospective databases.

Pancreatic, Biliary, and Gastrointestinal Reconstruction

Reconstruction after pancreaticoduodenectomy proceeds first with the pancreatic anastomosis. The goal in performing the pancreatic anastomosis is to create a secure anastomosis that minimizes the risk of an

Table 1 Pathology Template Used at The University of Texas M. D. Anderson Cancer Center for Reporting of Pancreaticoduodenectomy Specimens

SYNOPTIC REPORT:

Specimen: Pancreaticoduodenectomy
Tumor Diagnosis: Histologic type of the tumor
Degree of Differentiation: well/moderate/poor
The tumor size (diameter in cm):
Extrapancreatic extension: present/absent
Lymphovascular invasion: present/absent
Perineural invasion: present/absent
Retroperitoneal (SMA) margin status: positive/negative (if negative, the distance to inked margin in mm)
Bile duct margin status: positive/negative
Pancreatic transection margin status: positive/negative
Proximal stomach or duodenum margin status: positive/negative
Distal duodenum or jejunum margin status: positive/negative
Regional Lymph Nodes:
    Total number positive:
    Total number examined:
Name of the vessel removed: presence or absence of vessel invasion and vascular resection margin status (if performed).
Degree of treatment effect (if patient received preoperative therapy): reported as a percentage of viable tumor cells, classified as < 10%, 10–50%, 50–90%, > 90%[21]
Final pTNM Staging (AJCC 6th edition):
    ypT: T1/T2/T3
    ypN: N0/N1
    ypMX: Distant metastasis cannot be assessed

anastomotic leak. The pancreatic remnant is mobilized from the retroperitoneum and splenic vein for a distance of 2 to 3 cm. The transected jejunum is brought through a generous incision in the transverse mesocolon to the left of the middle colic vessels. We prefer to bring the jejunum retrocolic rather than retroperitoneal (posterior to the mesenteric vessels in the bed of the resected duodenum). A two-layer, end-to-side, duct-to-mucosa panceaticojejunostomy is performed using 4-0 or 5-0 monofilament suture. If the pancreatic duct is not dilated, a Silastic stent (Dow Corning, Midland, MI) is used. Anatomic and technical considerations important to remember include the following:

1. Injury to the proximal splenic artery can occur when mobilizing the pancreatic remnant if one does not appreciate the location of this vessel.
2. Failure to adequately mobilize the pancreatic remnant results in poor suture placement at the pancreaticojejunal anastomosis.
3. When the pancreatic parenchyma is soft, we often use pledgets for the anterior row of sutures to prevent them from causing a tear in the pancreatic tissue.

When the pancreatic duct is not dilated and/or the pancreatic substance is soft (not fibrotic), one can perform a two-layer anastomosis that invaginates the cut end of the pancreas into the jejunum. However, we rarely use this technique because even a nondilated pancreatic duct can often be anastomosed using the duct-to-mucosa technique.

A single-layer biliary anastomosis is performed using interrupted 4-0 absorbable monofilament sutures. It is important to align the jejunum with the bile duct to avoid tension on the pancreatic and biliary anastomoses. A stent is rarely used in the construction of the hepaticojejunostomy.

An antecolic, end-to-side gastrojejunostomy is constructed in two layers. Starting from the greater curvature, 6 to 8 cm of the gastric staple line is removed. The distance between the biliary and gastric anastomoses should be at least 50 cm, thereby allowing the jejunum to assume its antecolic position (for the gastrojejunostomy) without tension, and also preventing bile reflux cholangitis. We prefer an antecolic gastrojejunostomy to prevent possible outlet obstruction caused by the colonic mesentery. A 10 French feeding jejunostomy tube may be placed distal to the gastrojejunostomy. We rarely utilize a gastrostomy tube for postoperative gastric decompression.

Prior to abdominal closure, the abdomen is carefully irrigated in all four quadrants. In patients with a previous indwelling endobiliary stent or a previous biliary bypass (contaminated bile), we often place one drain in the right upper quandrant; we no longer place a drain near the pancreatic anastomosis. The use of drains remains an active area of controversy in the field of pancreatic surgery, and many surgeons still drain the pancreaticojejunostomy. Importantly, we place the mobilized falciform ligament (carefully preserved when the abdomen was opened) between the hepatic artery, at the level of the GDA stump, and the afferent jejunal limb to cover the GDA stump. This is one technique used to prevent pseudoaneurysm formation at the site of the GDA stump in the event of a pancreatic anastomotic leak and resulting abscess formation.

Case Studies

CASE 1. IMPORTANCE OF ACCURATE ASSESSMENT OF THE SMA MARGIN

A 47-year-old man underwent pancreaticoduodenectomy for what returned as moderately differentiated adenocarcinoma of the pancreas. The patient was then referred to our institution for consideration of protocol-based postoperative adjuvant therapy. Review of the histopathology confirmed pancreatic adenocarcinoma. The original pathology report stated that the pancreatic transection margin was felt to be positive for invasive adenocarcinoma; there was no mention of the status of the SMA or retroperitoneal margin of resection. One of 10 lymph nodes examined contained metastatic adenocarcinoma. The patient recovered uneventfully from surgery and, prior to being considered for protocol-based therapy, underwent restaging evaluation. CT scan performed at our institution to assess protocol eligibility (Figures 4A and B) demonstrated retained tumor adjacent to the origin of the superior mesenteric artery and remaining in the root of mesentery encasing the more distal SMA. This patient was therefore not eligible for protocol-based postoperative adjuvant therapy.

This case illustrates a number of factors that should be considered in the design of adjuvant therapy trials, including (1) central review of preoperative CT images to assess the extent of local tumor and to provide an objective way of staging patients prior to surgery; (2) a standardized system for pathologic assessment of the pancreaticoduodenectomy specimen, which is critically important. In the case of this patient, no mention was made of the status of the SMA or retroperitoneal margin. While the pancreatic transection margin was positive, there clearly was gross tumor left behind at the level of the proximal superior mesenteric artery as seen in Figures 4A and B; and (3) surgeons performing pancreaticoduodenectomy need to provide an accurate description of the completeness of resection performed at the time of pancreaticoduodenectomy. In this patient's operative note, there was no mention of the adequacy of tumor resection, especially at the level of the SMA. The pathologist cannot differentiate a grossly complete·from a grossly incomplete resection. This information must be contained in the operative note. This surgeon's operative dictation should not have been finalized until the pathology report was available to provide the histologic status of the resection margins. The R2 designation

should have been clearly visible in the operative report and the medical record—easily retrievable by all physicians and data managers.

CASE 2. THE IMPORTANCE OF ACCURATE ASSESSMENT OF THE PRETREATMENT CT SCAN: LYMPH NODE METASTASES

A 66-year-old woman was referred to The University of Texas M. D. Anderson Cancer Center after developing obstructive jaundice following a laparoscopic cholecystectomy performed for right upper quadrant discomfort, dyspepsia, and a general feeling of anorexia. While the cholecystectomy was performed without complication, a few weeks later the patient developed obvious signs and symptoms of biliary obstruction with scleral icterus, pruritis, and visible jaundice. CT imaging demonstrated a mass in the head of the pancreas and endobiliary decompression was performed with placement of a polyethylene stent. She was then referred to our institution for further management and underwent repeat CT imaging that demonstrated an obvious mass in the pancreatic head and metastatic adenopathy at the root of mesentery (Figures 5A and B). She received a program of systemic therapy followed by chemoradiation. While the lymph nodes responded radiographically (images not shown), she unfortunately developed distant tumor progression in the form of liver metastases. This case demonstrates that occasionally patients with adenocarcinoma of pancreatic origin may have metastatic-appearing adenopathy that is visible on CT imaging. In general, this is an uncommon finding, but one that should be looked for when evaluating pretreatment

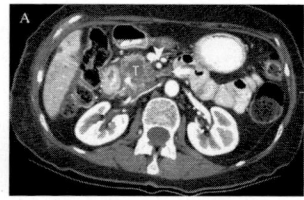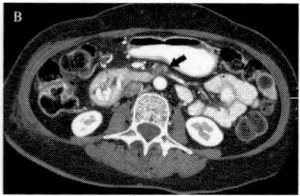

Figure 5 *A,* Computed tomography axial image demonstrating a low-density tumor (T) in the pancreatic head that is separated from the superior mesenteric artery (SMA, arrowhead) and the superior mesenteric vein (just anterior and to the right of the SMA) by a normal tissue plane. However, there is a metastatic-appearing lymph node (white arrow) anterior to the aorta and posterior and slightly to the left of the SMA. This metastatic-appearing node could easily be left behind if this patient were to undergo up-front surgery and the surgeon were unaware of the location of this metastatic lymph node. *B,* Computed tomography axial image of the same patient demonstrating an additional metastatic lymph node (black arrow) anterior to the aorta at the level transverse portion of the duodenum lying just posterior to a branch of the superior mesenteric artery.

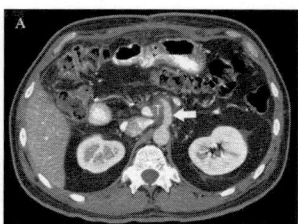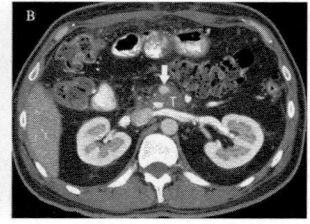

Figure 4 *A,* Computed tomography axial image demonstrating residual low-density tumor (T) at the level of the superior mesenteric artery origin (arrow). The superior mesenteric vein can be seen to the right side of the residual tumor and just anterior to the inferior vena cava.
B, Computed tomography axial image demonstrating persistent tumor (T) encasing the proximal superior mesenteric artery (arrow). The jejunal branch of the superior mesenteric vein can be seen encased with tumor lying directly anterior to the left renal vein coursing anterior to the aorta.

imaging studies. Typically, lymph node metastases from pancreatic adenocarcinoma are small and only appreciated by the pathologist. To what degree metastatic lymph nodes posterior and to the left of the superior mesenteric artery may contribute to local recurrence is not known. A standard pancreaticoduodenectomy removes all soft tissue and perineural tissue to the right of the SMA. This usually results in removal of some of the mesentery posterior to the SMA, but the extent of mesenteric resection at that level is usually somewhat variable. Most surgeons are hesitant to skeletonize the entire superior mesenteric artery because of the concern for denervation of the small bowel, resulting in hyperperistalsis and nutritional depletion. Therefore, the standard SMA dissection involves removal of perineural and soft tissue on the right 180° of the circumference of the vessel, while attempting to preserve the autonomic nerve along the left side of the SMA. This case illustrates that patients may occasionally have metastatic adenopathy that can be appreciated on CT imaging. Equally important is the practice of palpating the left supraclavicular fossa when examining all patients with upper abdominal malignancies to detect metastatic adenopathy by palpation. Occasionally, patients with what appears to be localized pancreatic adenocarcinoma will have a metastatic Virchow's node in the left supraclavicular fossa; such patients have metastatic disease not amenable to surgical resection.

CASE 3. THE IMPORTANCE OF ACCURATE ASSESSMENT OF THE PRETREATMENT CT SCAN: PERINEURAL INFILTRATION

A 59-year-old man was noted to have a slight elevation of liver function tests thought to be secondary to the use of cholesterol-lowering medication. This, however, was further evaluated with transabdominal ultrasound, which demonstrated slight intra- and extrahepatic biliary ductal dilatation. He therefore underwent CT imaging followed by ERCP, which suggested a malignant obstruction of the intrapancreatic portion of the bile duct. There was no visible mass seen on CT images. Because of the absence of an obvious mass in the pancreas and the concern for a malignant biliary stricture, he was referred to our institution for further evaluation. On repeat CT imaging, there was again no visible mass in the pancreatic head. However, there was subtle low-density change adjacent to the right lateral border of the celiac axis (Figure 6A) and similar low density change adjacent to the right lateral border of the proximal SMA (Figure 6B). Endoscopic ultrasound failed to demonstrate an obvious pancreatic mass. The patient was therefore brought to the operating room and underwent pancreaticoduodenect-

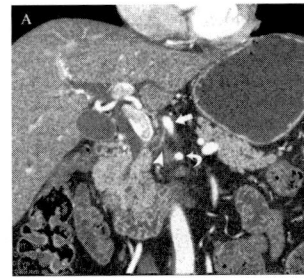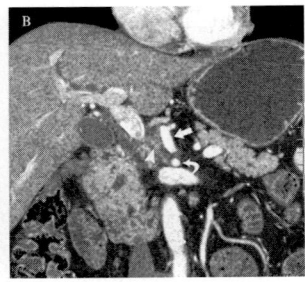

Figure 6 *A,* Computed tomography coronal image, reconstructed from axial image data, demonstrating a stricture of the common bile duct with tumor infiltrate (arrowhead) medial to the head of the pancreas along the right side of the superior mesenteric artery (curved arrow) and the celiac axis (arrow).
B, Computed tomography coronal image at the level posterior to image 6A demonstrating tumor infiltrate (arrowhead) on the right side of the celiac axis (arrow). Note the superior mesenteric artery (curved arrow) above the horizontal segment of the left renal vein.

omy. At the time of surgery, there was firm infiltration of the right celiac ganglion. This was completely excised with the pancreatic head and associated tissues. However, final pathology demonstrated diffuse infiltration of the celiac ganglion with adenocarcinoma (Figure 7). The exact focus of the primary tumor within the pancreatic head could not be identified grossly as an obvious tumor mass. There was microscopic infiltration of the pancreatic head extending into the autonomic plexus and diffusely involving the celiac ganglion; this extensive perineural invasion from ductal adenocarcinoma of the pancreatic head without a visible primary tumor mass either on CT or on gross inspection of the surgical specimen. This case emphasizes the predisposition for ductal pancreatic adenocarcinoma to spread along perineural sheaths to the origins of the SMA and celiac

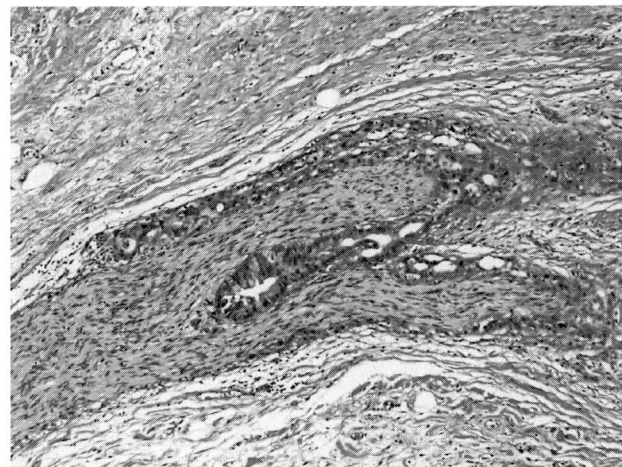

Figure 7 Perineural infiltration in a moderately differentiated pancreatic ductal adenocarcinoma (H & E stain, original magnification 100×).

axis and, therefore, the importance of accurate preoperative imaging and careful intraoperative attention to the SMA dissection.

CASE 4. THE IMPORTANCE OF ACCURATE ASSESSMENT OF THE PRETREATMENT CT SCAN: ARTERIAL ANATOMY

A 57-year-old woman developed painless jaundice and underwent operation for a presumed pancreatic head cancer. At the time of surgery, it was the opinion of the operating surgeon that her tumor was unresectable owing to involvement of the common hepatic artery. He performed a biliary and gastric bypass and the patient then received systemic chemotherapy. Following 4 months of systemic chemotherapy, there was no evidence of disease progression, and, therefore, her treatment was consolidated with chemoradiation. She was then referred to our institution for consideration of reoperation. CT images demonstrated encasement of the left hepatic artery arising from the celiac axis. However, there was a replaced right hepatic artery arising from the SMA (Figure 8). Successful pancreaticoduodenectomy was performed with ligation of the common hepatic artery at its origin from the celiac axis without reconstruction of this vessel owing to the large dominant replaced right hepatic artery arising from the SMA. Histologic assessment of the resected tumor demonstrated that approximately 50% of the primary tumor appeared nonviable. Margins of resection were negative (R0 resection) as were all 25 regional lymph nodes.

CASE 5. THE EMERGING ROLE FOR MULTIMODALITY THERAPY

A 63-year-old woman initially developed steatorrhea and underwent gastrointestinal evaluation. When this returned negative, her very perceptive family physician recognized the possible association of steatorrhea with pancreatic duct obstruction and pursued further imaging evaluations. CT scans suggested a mass in the pancreatic head that was thought to be unresectable owing to involvement of the SMV. She was referred to our institution where EUS-guided fine-needle aspiration biopsy confirmed the cytologic diagnosis of adenocarcinoma. Repeat CT scan demonstrated segmental occlusion of the SMV (Figures 9A and B). Segmental occlusion of the SMV with an adequate vein above and below the region of occlusion (so that resection remains a possibility) is one criteria used to define a borderline resectable pancreatic cancer. This woman received systemic chemotherapy for 4 months; there was no evidence of disease progression and treatment was then consolidated with chemoradiation. Restaging evaluation

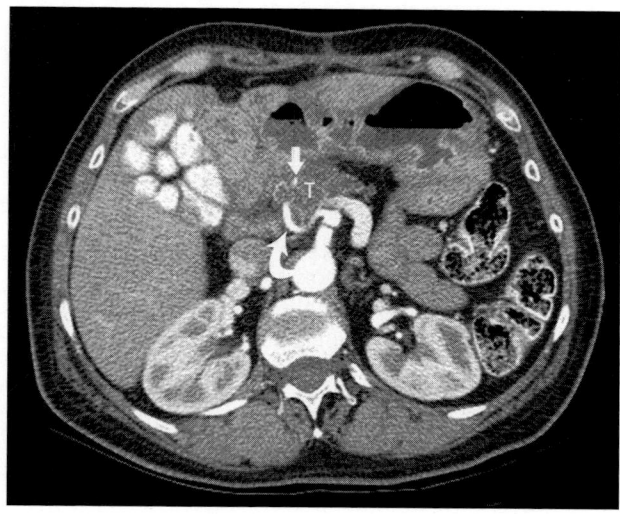

Figure 8 Computed tomography axial image demonstrating a low-density tumor (T) in the pancreatic head encasing the gastroduodenal artery (arrow), arising from the left hepatic artery. The large replaced right hepatic artery (curved arrow) arising from the superior mesenteric artery can be seen coursing posterior to the tumor. The splenic vein can be seen just anterior and to the left of the superior mesenteric artery. This patient also required venous resection and reconstruction.

after chemoradiation and approximately 5 months following initial diagnosis demonstrated marked improvement in the caliber of the SMV and a reduction

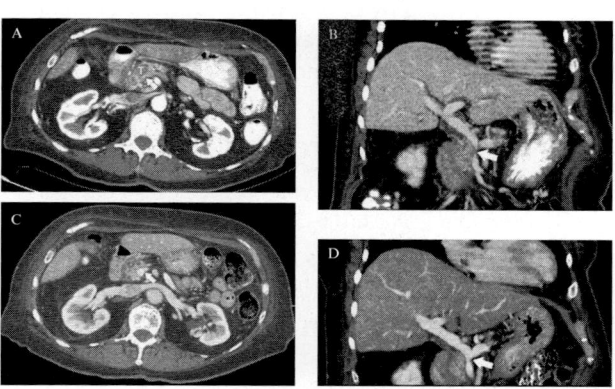

Figure 9 *A,* Computed tomography axial image demonstrating a low-density tumor (T) in the pancreatic head with perhaps a thin, poorly opacified rim of contrast material in the expected region of the superior mesenteric vein (arrow). The superior mesenteric artery directly adjacent and to the left of the arrow is not involved by the tumor. *B,* Computed tomography coronal image demonstrating short segmental occlusion of the superior mesenteric vein (arrow), prior to initial therapy.
C, Computed tomography axial image following all treatment demonstrating marked tumor reduction resulting in reconstitution of the superior mesenteric vein (arrow).
D, Computed tomography coronal image following all treatment demonstrating reconstitution of the superior mesenteric vein (arrow).

in overall tumor size (Figures 9C and D). This degree of response at the site of the primary tumor is uncommon, but now being seen more frequently with the advent of more effective systemic therapies and more sophisticated radiation therapy treatment planning. This patient underwent successful pancreaticoduodenectomy with segmental resection of the SMPV confluence. Venous reconstruction was with a primary end-to-end anastomosis. Final pathology demonstrated extensive treatment effect with less than 50% viable tumor, negative margins, and negative regional lymph nodes (0 of 21).

Summary

Detailed preoperative assessment of resectability and precise attention to surgical technique will maximize the benefit that can be achieved from surgery. At present, the best option for physicians to improve the care of patients with pancreatic cancer is to accurately stage the extent of disease and apply stage-specific therapies that are protocol-based whenever possible. Future progress in the treatment of pancreatic cancer will involve techniques for early diagnosis, to allow more patients to undergo potentially curative surgery, and the development of more effective systemic therapies, which may be combined with surgery and radiation therapy. The advent of targeted therapies that are based on an improved understanding of the molecular basis for pancreatic cancer growth and development will enhance the therapeutic options available to patients with localized and metastatic pancreatic cancer.

References

1. Jemal A, Siegel R, Ward E, et al. Cancer statistics, 2006. CA Cancer J Clin 2006;56:106–30.

2. American Joint Committee on Cancer. Exocrine pancreas. In: Greene FL, Page DL, Fleming ID, et al, editors. AJCC cancer staging manual. 6th ed. New York: Springer; 2002. p. 157–64.

3. Wolff RA, Abbruzzese JL, Evans DB, et al. Neoplasms of the exocrine pancreas. In: Kufe DW, Pollock RE, Weichelbaum RR, et al, editors. Holland-Frei cancer medicine. 7th ed. Ontario: B.C. Decker; 2006. p. 1331–58.

4. Pisters PWT, Wolff RA, Crane CH, Evans DB. Combined-modality treatment for operable pancreatic adenocarcinoma. Oncology 2005;19:393–404.

5. Raut CP, Evans DB, Crane CH, et al. Neoadjuvant therapy for resectable pancreatic cancer. Surg Oncol Clin N Am 2004;4:639–61.

6. Lowenfels AB, Maisonneuve P. Epidemiology and risk factors for pancreatic cancer. Best Pract Res Clin Gastroenterol 2006;20:197–209.

7. Tamm E, Charnsangavej C. Pancreatic cancer: current concepts in imaging for diagnosis and staging. Cancer J 2001;7:298–311.

8. Varadhachary GR, Tamm EP, Crane C, et al. Borderline resectable pancreatic cancer. Curr Treat Options Gastroenterol 2005;8:377–84.

9. Mullen JT, Lee JH, Gomez HF, et al. Pancreaticoduodenectomy after placement of endobiliary metal stents. J Gastrointest Surg 2005;9:1094–105.

10. Raut CP, Grau AM, Staerkel GA, et al. Diagnostic accuracy of endoscopic ultrasound-guided fine-needle aspiration in patients with presumed pancreatic cancer. J Gastrointest Surg 2003;7:118–28.

11. Kehlet H. Modification of responses to surgery by neural blockade. In: Cousins MJ, Bridenbaugh PO, editors. Neural blockade I clinical anesthesia and management of pain. Philadelphia: Lippincott-Raven; 1988. p. 129–75.

12. Mann C, Pouzeratte Y, Boccara G, et al. Comparison of intravenous or epidural patient-controlled analgesia in the elderly after major abdominal surgery. Anesthesiology 2000;92:433–41.

13. Norris EJ, Beattie C, Perler BA, et al. Double-masked randomized trial comparing alternate combinations of intraoperative anesthesia and postoperative analgesia in abdominal aortic surgery. Anesthesiology 2001;95:1054–67.

14. Rigg J, Jamrozik K, Myles P, et al. Epidural anaesthesia and analgesia and outcome of major surgery: a randomized trial. Lancet 2002;359:1276–82.

15. Buggy D, Doherty W, Hart E, Pallett E. Postoperative wound oxygen tension with epidural or intravenous analgesia. Anesthesiology 2002;97:952–8.

16. Allen D, Maguire J, Mahdavian M, et al. Wound hypoxia and acidosis limit limit neutrophil bacterial killing mechanisms. Arch Surg 1997;132:991–6.

17. Beilin B, Shavit Y, Trabekin E, et al. The effects of postoperative pain management on immune response to surgery. Anesth Analg 2003;97:822–7.

18. Pawlik TM, Abdalla EK, Barnett CC, et al. Feasability of a randomized trial of extended lymphadenectomy for pancreatic cancer. Arch Surg 2005;140:584–9.

19. Cubilla AL, Fitzgerald PJ. Tumors of the exocrine pancreas. Washington DC: Armed Forces Institute of Pathology; 1984. p. 118–28.

20. Yen TWF, Abdalla EK, Pisters PWT, Evans DB. Pancreaticoduodenectomy. In: VonHoff DD, Evans DB, Hruban RH, editors. Pancreatic cancer. Sudbury, MA: Jones and Bartlett; 2005. p. 265–85.

21. Evans DB, Rich TA, Byrd DR, et al. Preoperative chemoradiation and pancreaticoduodenectomy for adenocarcinoma of the pancreas. Arch Surg 1992;127:1335–9.

CHAPTER 20

PALLIATIVE MANAGEMENT OF LOCALLY ADVANCED PANCREATIC CANCER

ANDREAS KARACHRISTOS, MD, PhD

ALEXANDER A. PARIKH, MD

Introduction

It is estimated that 32,800 new cases of pancreatic cancer will be diagnosed in 2005 in the United States. During the same year, there will be approximately 31,800 deaths from pancreatic cancer, making it the fourth most common cause of cancer death. Despite advances in understanding the pathogenesis of pancreatic cancer, as well as improved diagnostic and therapeutic modalities, pancreatic cancer is curable in only a minority of cases. Approximately 80 to 85% of patients are unresectable at presentation and, therefore, providing adequate palliation of tumor-related symptoms is of critical importance. The primary issues that face clinicians include palliation of pain and management of obstructive jaundice and gastric outlet obstruction.

Management of Pain

Since the vast majority of pancreatic cancer patients will succumb to their disease, adequate and sustained pain relief is of paramount importance. In recently diagnosed pancreatic cancer patients, pain is present in up to 70%,[1] and nearly 30% complain of severe or moderate pain, a figure that increases with the stage of their disease. Ultimately, more than 80% of patients with pancreatic cancer will experience significant pain at some point during the course of the disease that will directly impair their functional ability and compromise their quality of life.[2]

In addition to the obvious emotional and physical burden, pain has been adversely related to prognosis and outcome. In a prospective, randomized study of patients with unresectable pancreatic cancer, comparing intraoperative chemical splachnicectomy with alcohol versus placebo, patients with significant preoperative pain who had splachnicectomy had markedly improved survival.[4] However, a recent randomized prospective trial of percutaneous neurolytic celiac plexus block (NCPB) did not demonstrate a significant difference in survival, although the intervention did improve pain scores.[5] Nevertheless, improved functional ability and mood provided by pain relief may lead to modification of psychosocial behavior, and thus, patients may become more active, adhere to palliative therapy, and have better nutritional status, which potentially affects survival.

Multiple treatment modalities are currently available for relieving pain in patients with unresectable pancreatic cancer and include local and systemic approaches. Oral analgesics, ranging from nonsteroidals to oral or transdermal opioids are the mainstay of therapy. Unfortunately, many patients develop tolerance to narcotic therapy and increasing doses are associated with significant side effects, including constipation, cognitive impairment, and dependence. Simultaneous treatment with local or regional approaches, including celiac plexus blocks, has therefore been proposed and, in general, has been very successful. Another advantage of the early use of these of interventional procedures is that regional anatomy often becomes distorted by tumor invasion of the celiac plexus in later stages. Neurolysis of the celiac plexus has been extensively studied, and several procedures, intraoperative, percutaneous or endoscopic, attempting to disrupt the transmission of pain by interfering with the sympathetic fibers, have been described. However, randomized trials are rare.

A randomized study from Johns Hopkins of 139 patients showed that intraoperative injection of 50% alcohol along both sides of the aorta at the level of the celiac axis provided significant pain relief with no increased incidence in mortality or morbidity rates.[4] Even in patients without preoperative pain, alcohol injection significantly reduced postoperative pain scores and delayed the onset of pain. The effect of the alcohol seemed to diminish after 6 months, and both groups eventually required additional therapy, although the interval was significantly longer in the alcohol injection group.

Percutaneous neurolytic celiac plexus block (NCPB), initially described in 1914, has been used widely for pain control in pancreatic cancer. Under radiologic guidance, or more recently with endoscopic ultrasound (EUS) guidance, a needle is inserted into each side of the anterolateral aspect of the superior portion of the first lumbar vertebrae and a local anesthetic agent and alcohol is infused. The technique has been reported to provide satisfactory short-term pain relief in approximately 87% of patients with pancreatic cancer, and pain control is maintained until death in 60 to 75% of patients.[6] Unfortunately, pain symptoms increase progressively after 4 to 5 weeks, and the percentage of pain-free patients decreases significantly with time.[7] The procedure is safe, and the most common adverse effects are transient and include procedure-related local pain, diarrhea, and hypotension. No mortality related to NCPB has been reported, and severe morbidity such as lower extremity weakness, pneumothorax, hematuria, and pleuritic pain is rare. A large randomized study compared the efficacy of NCPB with placebo in 100 patients with pancreatic cancer followed for at least 1 year or until death.[5] Both treatment groups received optimal systemic analgesic therapy according to a specific analgesic ladder. Although baseline pain decreased in both groups, moderate or severe pain was significantly less (14% vs 40%) in the NCPB group within 6 weeks of the procedure. About 20% of the placebo group required "rescue" NCPB. NCPB had no effect on opioid consumption, quality of life, or length of survival over the group with placebo and systemic analgesic therapy alone, however. The beneficial effect of NCPB decreased gradually with time.

Thoracoscopic sympathetic splanchnicectomy is another technique to abolish the afferent sympathetic signals from the pancreas. This technique disrupts the afferent sympathetic nerves within the thorax. The technique was initially described via a thoracotomy, but is now more commonly performed via video-assisted thoracoscopy (VATS).[8] The procedure can be performed unilaterally or bilaterally and involves transection of the greater and lesser splachnic nerves, lateral to the azygous vein on the right side and lateral of the descending aorta as it leaves the thorax at the left side. In a study of 23 patients with pancreatic cancer, bilateral thoracoscopic splanchnicectomy decreased pain scores by 50%, and more than half of the patients were palliated with nonopioid analgesics for a mean of 4 months.[8] Although there was no mortality, 9% of patients required thoracotomy because of bleeding.

Finally, palliative treatment with systemic chemoradiation may also provide significant pain relief in some patients. Concurrent chemoradiation with gemcitabine has been reported to control pain in up to 39% of patients with locally advanced pancreatic cancer.[9] In addition, hypofractionated, short-term irradiation may have significant analgesic effects in up to 75% of patients.[10]

In summary, pain control in patients with unresectable pancreatic cancer is a challenging problem. In patients who are discovered to be unresectable at the time of operation, chemical splanchnicectomy with alcohol is safe and provides adequate pain control, particularly in the short term. In patients who are known to be unresectable preoperatively, percutaneous or EUS-guided neurolytic celiac plexus block (NCPB) is a viable option if traditional opioid and nonopioid analgesics are ineffective. For those who have failed NCPB or those with suspicion that the celiac plexus is involved by tumor, thoracoscopic splanchnicectomy might be a valuable alternative. In general, a multifaceted approach to pain management will likely be the most successful strategy for these unfortunate patients.

Management of Obstructive Jaundice

Since the majority of pancreatic adenocarcinomas arise in the head and uncinate process, obstructive jaundice is a common problem. Biliary obstruction results in a variety of problems that not only impair quality of life, but also can lead to serious morbidities and even mortality. These sequelae include pruritus, liver dysfunction, coagulopathy, malnutrition, renal failure, and biliary sepsis.

Biliary decompression can be accomplished by several methods including percutaneous drainage, operative biliary diversion, or insertion of an endoprosthesis (stent) placed percutaneously or via endoscopy. Percutaneous or T-tube decompression is helpful in the acute setting of cholangitis or as a temporizing measure, but is seldom used for definitive therapy secondary to the significant associated electrolyte abnormalities and malnutrition. Surgical bypass of the obstructed biliary tree is often performed when a periampullary cancer is found to be unresectable intraoperatively. Since being introduced in 1979, endobiliary stents placed via endoscopy or percutaneously have been evaluated extensively. This approach is currently the most common form of biliary decompression in inoperable patients or in patients who are candidates for neoadjuvant therapy.

OPERATIVE BILIARY DECOMPRESSION

Several techniques of biliary bypass have been used to relieve jaundice: These include cholecystojejunostomy (CJ), hepaticojejunostomy or choledochojejunostomy (HJ), cholecystoduodenostomy (CD), hepaticoduodenostomy (HD), and cholecystogastrostomy (CG). Techniques incorporating the stomach are no longer recommended because of high incidence of bile gastritis. Procedures using the duodenum should also be avoided because of high postoperative morbidity and increased frequency of persistent or recurrent jaundice.[1]

The choice between utilizing the gallbladder (CJ) or bile duct (HJ) has been evaluated in several studies (Table 1). Proponents of CJ state that the procedure is technically easier, faster, associated with less blood loss, and results in adequate palliation. Advocates of HJ believe that this method is associated with better long-term results and acceptable morbidity in experienced hands. In a small, retrospective study of 36 patients with biliary obstruction owing to pancreatic cancer, mortality was actually higher in the CJ group as compared with the HJ group, although morbidity rates were similar. Successful short- and long-term palliation was also achieved more often in the HJ group (93% and 83%) than in the CJ group (50% and 50%).[11] In contrast, Singh and colleagues in a retrospective study found no difference in the palliative ability of these two procedures, but CJ was associated with significantly less morbidity and mortality, and thus

cholecystojejunostomy was their procedure of choice. These authors emphasize that cystic duct patency should be confirmed by inspection and/or operative cholangiogram.[1] Similarly, in a collective review by Sarr and Cameron of more than 1,600 patients with unresectable pancreatic cancer, there were no significant differences in mortality or morbidity between the two procedures, although they noticed a small difference in favor of HJ in the incidence of recurrent jaundice.[12] A more recent retrospective study of 1,919 patients who underwent operative biliary bypass found that patients who initially had a cholecystojejunostomy were 4.4 times more likely to have additional biliary surgery and 2.9 times more likely to have any subsequent biliary intervention than patients who initially underwent choledocho- or hepaticojejunostomy.[13] Finally, a small prospective randomized study from 1988 compared the two methods in 31 patients with malignant and benign biliary obstruction and found that those who had CJ had significantly reduced operative time and intraoperative blood loss, but increased mortality, morbidity, and inferior relief of biliary obstruction.[14]

Most failures after biliary bypass are thought to be caused by progression of disease with subsequent invasion of the anastomosis by the tumor. Consequently, the proximity of the tumor to the cystic duct is critical if one is considering cholecystojejunostomy. If the tumor is within 1 cm of the hepatocystic junction, the chances of recurrent jaundice after a cholecystojejunostomy are high and would not be recommended. Using these criteria, a retrospective study of 218 patients with locally advanced periampullary tumors found that only 21% of patients would be candidates for a cholecystojejunostomy. This study not only revealed the importance of accurate evaluation of the patency and location of the hepatocystic junction prior of using the gallbladder as bypass conduit, but also suggests that CJ would be a reasonable approach in only a fraction of patients with obstructive jaundice from pancreatic cancer. In our opinion, HJ is the preferred

Table 1 Comparison between Cholecystojejunostomy (CJ) and Choledochojejunostomy (HS)

Authors	Sarfeh[14] 1988†		Rosemurgy[11] 1989		Singh[1] 1990		Urbach[13] 2003	
Procedures	CJ	HJ	CJ	HJ	CJ	HJ	CJ	HJ
Patients	15	16	22	15	74	60	945	974
Morbidity (%)	53.3	18.75*	59.1	53.3	27*	38.3	–	–
Mortality (%)	13.3	0*	22.7	6.7	5.4*	11.7	14.1	9.7
Palliation (%)	53.3	87.5*	50	93.3	74.32	76.6	–	–
Hospital stay (d)	19	14	–	–	–	–	15.6	15.7
Survival (m)	4.9	6.6	–	–	–	–	4.4	6.3
Additional biliary intervention (%)	–	–	–	–	–	–	26*	13.3
Operative time (h)	2.6*	3.7	–	–	–	–	–	–

*$p < 0.05$; †prospective randomized study.

approach for operative biliary bypass if technically feasible, and CJ is reserved for patients with higher operative risk or for those with lower expected survival times and with tumors located away from the hepatocystic junction.

Surgical bypass using the common bile duct and jejunum can be accomplished by constructing a Roux-en-Y limb or a loop choledocho- or hepaticojejunostomy. Utilization of a Roux-en-Y limb has traditionally been preferred as it prevents reflux of intestinal contents into the biliary tree, thus reducing the risk cholangitis. Disadvantages of this method include the additional anastomosis, longer operative time, and the inability to allow secondary endoscopic access to the anastomosis if needed. The last problem can be overcome with construction of a "siphon" Roux by bringing the end of the Roux limb to the abdominal wall, thus making it accessible to percutaneous intervention. In contrast, a loop hepaticojejunostomy is technically easier to construct, provides easier endoscopic access, and in the small minority of patients who may eventually become candidates for resection, a pancreaticoduodenectomy is easier to perform. In the retrospective study by Sarr and Cameron discussed earlier, similar outcomes were noted with either technique.[12] We believe that both techniques can result in adequate palliation, and the decision should be individualized according the anatomy and taking into account the possibility of future surgical explorations.

In summary, operative palliative biliary and duodenal bypass can be accomplished with acceptable perioperative mortality (2–3.1%) and morbidity (22–27%)[17] and may actually provide a small survival benefit in select patients versus exploration alone.[12] Although nonoperative decompression has become very common, for patients found to be unresectable at exploration, operative biliary bypass should be considered.

NONOPERATIVE DECOMPRESSION

Nonoperative decompression of obstructive jaundice includes percutaneous drainage and/or placement of an indwelling biliary stent (percutaneously or endoscopically). A prospective, randomized study in patients with biliary obstruction owing to malignancy revealed that endoscopic placement via an endoscopic retrograde cholangiopancreatography (ERCP) procedure has a significantly higher success rate (81%) for relieving the obstruction than the percutaneous method (61%).[18] Furthermore, the early complication rate was significantly lower in the endoscopic group (19% vs 67%), as was the 30-day mortality rate (15% vs 33%). The higher morbidity and mortality rates were secondary to a higher incidence of biliary leak, bleeding, and abscess formation after percutaneous drain placement. In general, we recommend ERCP-placed biliary stents whenever possible and reserve percutaneous-placed stents only when the endoscopic route fails or is not possible.

Two types of stents are available: Plastic (polyethylene) and metal stents. Plastic stents have a fixed diameter, and therefore a larger endoscope is needed to introduce an adequate size stent (10 or 12 French [F]). The metal stents are self-expandable, flexible, and usually expand from an outer diameter of 9F to 30F. In general plastic stents cost less and are easier to remove but occlude faster, have higher incidence of cholangitis, migrate more often, and result in overall longer hospital stay after ERCP. In contrast, metallic stents stay open longer but are expensive, become shorter after deployment, and are permanent. There is also some evidence, however, that metallic stents might offer a survival benefit in patients with locally advanced pancreatic carcinoma by decreasing the septic complications and need for subsequent interventions.[19] Whereas the most common cause of occlusion of plastic stents is an accumulation of debris, metallic stents are more commonly occluded secondary to tumor ingrowth through the stent. Polyethylene-covered metallic stents might overcome that problem; however, an increased risk of acute cholecystitis and pancreatitis have been reported owing to cystic or pancreatic duct obstruction when using covered metal stents.

A prospective, randomized trial by Davids and colleagues compared metal and plastic stents in patients with malignant biliary obstruction.[20] The initial relief of obstruction was equally successful in both groups, but the median patency of the metallic stent was significantly prolonged (273 vs 126 days). Stent occlusion occurred in 33% of patients with metallic stents after a median follow-up of 273 days compared with 54% of the plastic stent group after a median follow-up of only 126 days. After re-intervention, none of the metallic stents occluded, whereas 48% of the plastic stents occluded a second time. The median survival was comparable in both groups.

Two other prospective, randomized trials[21,22] confirmed that metallic stents have longer patency rates, require less diagnostic or therapeutic interventions, and decrease the need for hospitalization. The major disadvantage of these stents is the increased cost. Patients with unresectable pancreatic cancer typically have median survival times of 4 to 12 months, which varies widely according to the presence of metastatic disease, the response to therapy, and the overall performance status of the patient. Metallic stents, despite their increased initial cost, become cost-effective by decreasing repeated interventions and readmissions. In one prospective trial, it was noted that plastic stents were preferable in patients with hepatic metastases because of a significantly shorter patient survival time. In patients without hepatic metastases, however, initial placement of a metallic stent resulted in lower overall cost.[22] In another study that analyzed the cost of different treatment strategies, plastic stents were shown to be preferable as the initial treatment for patients expected to survive less than 4 months.[23]

OPERATIVE VERSUS NONOPERATIVE PALLIATION.

Four prospective, randomized trials comparing placement of an endoprosthesis versus operative biliary bypass in patients with a distal malignant biliary obstruction are listed in Table 2. All of these trials compared the use of plastic stents, however, rather than expandable metal stents.

The largest of these trials randomized a total of 201 patients to either decompression by an endoscopic stent or operative bypass.[24] A plastic (Teflon) 10F endoprosthesis was used in the stent group and the bypass technique selected was hepatoduodenostomy (HD), hepaticojejunostomy (HJ), or cholecystojejunostomy (CJ). The surgical group had significantly more procedure-related morbidity and mortality as well as length of stay; however, there was no difference in 30-day mortality rates. The preferred operative biliary bypass technique used in this study was HD, which has been found to significantly increase the incidence of perioperative complications.[1] The initial therapeutic outcome was equally successful in both groups; however, recurrent jaundice and cholangitis occurred significantly more frequently in the stent group (34% vs 2%) and the median stent patency was 4.5 months. A smaller study by Andersen and colleagues randomized 50 patients and found that both techniques provide adequate initial

palliation.[25] The incidence of cholangitis was not significantly different in either group. The stent that was most commonly used in this study was 7F, which has generally been accepted to have increased the risk of obstruction compared with the larger 10F. In addition, the operative bypass most commonly used was cholecystojejunostomy rather than hepaticojejunostomy. A small study by Shepherd and colleagues also showed that both techniques were equally effective in relieving jaundice.[26] Although the endoscopic group had significantly more episodes of recurrent jaundice, the overall hospital stay was shorter. Mortality and morbidity rates were not statistically different in either group. Finally, Bornman and colleagues reported adequate palliation and comparable morbidity and mortality rates with transhepatic stent placement or surgical decompression.[27]

The main limitation of all of these randomized studies is the use of plastic stents, which are known to have lower patency rates than expandable metallic stents, as discussed previously.[21,22] There is only one randomized study comparing metallic stents with surgical decompression; this study allocated 13 patients with unresectable pancreatic cancer to laparoscopic surgical palliation (HJ and gastrojejunostomy) and 14 patients to endoscopic palliation with an expandable metallic stent.[28] There was no procedure-related mortality in either group and the morbidity rate was 7% for the laparoscopy group and 8% for the endoscopic group. The endoscopic group had a shorter initial hospital stay (3 days vs 12 days) but the readmission rate and the complication rate during follow-up were comparable. Taking into consideration that the number of patients in both groups was small, surgical palliation did not seem to offer any benefit over current endoscopic palliation techniques, although there was a marginally improved survival rate for patients undergoing surgical bypass.

Table 2 Prospective, Randomized Trials Comparing Biliary Stents versus Operative Decompression

Author	Bornman[27] 1986		Shepherd[26] 1988		Andersen[25] 1989		Smith[24] 1994	
Procedure	Surgery	Percutaneous	Surgery	Endoscopy	Surgery	Endoscopy	Surgery	Endoscopy
Patients	25	25	25	23	25	25	101	100
Decompression (%)	76	84	92	82	96	84	91.1	92
Mortality (%)	20	8	20	9	0	0	14	3*
Morbidity (%)	32	28	14	7	20	36	29	11*
Median Stay (d)	35	27	13	8*	27	26	26	20*
Recurrent jaundice / cholangitis (%)	16	38	0	30	16	28	2*	34
Duodenal Obstruction (%)	0	14.3	4	9	0	0	7(1)	17
Survival (weeks)	15	19	17.8	21	14	12	26	21

(1) Gastrojejunostomy was done in 45/101 patients

*$p < 0.05$.

In light of very little prospective data comparing metal stents with operative bypass, selection of technique should be individualized. The advantages of endoscopically placed stents is the obvious less invasive nature of the procedure and associated lower morbidity rates and shorter length of hospital stay. The median duration of patency of metal stents is approximately 8.3 months, and the incidence of occlusion is about 40% in 1 year. The advantages of operative bypass include less need for subsequent interventions as well as the ability to bypass both the obstructed bile duct and duodenum (as discussed in the next section). In our opinion, patients with metastatic pancreatic cancer or poor performance status generally have median survival times of less than 6 months and should be treated with an endoscopic placement of an endoprosthesis, either plastic or metal. In patients with locally advanced, unresectable tumors without clinically evident distant metastases, median survival is approximately 11 months. In these patients, an expandable coated or uncoated metallic stent should be the initial treatment of choice, particularly if adverse prognostic factors are present, such as poor performance status, high serum tumor markers, and enlarged, likely metastatic regional lymph nodes. In younger patients with good performance status, or in whom expandable metallic stents fail, operative decompression should be considered. Patients who are noted to be unresectable during exploratory laparotomy should also be considered for operative bypass if the volume of disease is minimal, their expected survival is reasonable, and particularly if established gastric outlet obstruction is also present.

LAPAROSCOPIC DECOMPRESSION

Within the last 20 years laparoscopy has been extensively utilized in the staging of pancreatic cancer. Many centers use laparoscopy in patients with potentially resectable and even locally advanced pancreatic cancer to identify those with occult metastatic disease (thus avoiding laparotomy) or to guide treatment plans. Advances in technology and increased experience in laparoscopy have expanded its role in the palliation and resection of pancreatic tumors. Patients with obstructive jaundice who are found unresectable during diagnostic laparoscopy may also be candidates for laparoscopic palliative

biliary decompression, thereby obviating the need for laparotomy or endoscopy.

Recently, several studies utilizing minimally invasive techniques for the palliation of jaundice have been reported (Table 3). Rhodes and colleagues reported on a series of 16 patients with unresectable pancreatic cancer, including 11 patients with biliary obstruction. Successful laparoscopic cholecystojejunostomy (CJ) was performed in 10 patients (1 patient underwent open bypass), and 3 of them also had laparoscopic gastrojejunostomy performed. Mean operative time was 75 minutes and mean hospital stay was 4 days.[30] There was no mortality and the morbidity rate was 13.3%. None of the patients needed any further intervention during their remaining lifespan. In this study, the operative time, morbidity rate, and hospital stay compares favorably with reported outcomes in open surgery. In another study by Kuriansky and colleagues, laparoscopic CJ and retrocolic gastro-jejunostomy was performed in 12 patients with unresectable pancreatic cancer. None of these patients had to be converted to open laparotomy. There was 1 death—a patient with cirrhosis developed postoperative bleeding at the CJ site and subsequently died on postoperative day 2. The overall morbidity rate was 30%. All patients eventually succumbed to their disease, but without evidence of recurrent jaundice.[31] Rothlin and colleagues compared 14 patients who underwent laparoscopic palliative procedures with 14 patients who had open palliation. Four of the 14 in the laparoscopy group underwent diagnostic laparoscopy and stenting (via ERCP), 7 underwent gastrojejunostomy only, and 3 underwent a double bypass using a hepaticojejunostomy (HJ).[32] Compared with conventional open surgical palliation, laparoscopic palliation resulted in shorter operative time (129 min vs 175 min), less mortality (0 vs 28.5%), less morbidity (7% vs 42.9%), and a shorter hospital stay (9.4 vs 21.1 days). No follow-up information was provided. Although these results suggest superiority of laparoscopic palliation over conventional surgical palliation, it should be noted that only 3 patients underwent HJ in the laparoscopic group, and the mortality and morbidity rates reported in the open group is higher than in most recent reports.

Most surgeons performing laparoscopic decompression for malignant obstructive jaundice use the gall-

Table 3 Results of Laparoscopic Biliary Palliation in Patients with Unresectable Pancreatic Cancer

Author	Patients	Biliary bypass	Gastric bypass	Operative time (min)	Conversion to open	Mortality rate (%)	Morbidity rate (%)	Hospital stay (d)	Recurrence of jaundice
Rhodes[30] 1995	16	10/11	8	75	1	0	13.3	4	0
Rothlin[32] 1999	14	3	10	129	–	0	7	9.4	–
Kuriansky[31] 2000	12	12	12	89	0	0.8	30	6.4	0

bladder as a conduit, as this approach is technically easier than laparoscopic hepaticojejunostomy. As discussed earlier, however, HJ usually provides a better chance of long-term operative biliary decompression than CJ. Although the advocates of laparoscopic CJ emphasize the importance of examining the confluence of cystic and hepatic ducts with intraoperative cholangiogram, few patients with distal common hepatic duct obstruction owing to pancreatic cancer are suitable for CJ.[15] The evaluation of a laparoscopic approach should ideally be compared with the optimal open technique, which we, as others, believe is hepaticojejunostomy.[33] Furthermore, the applicability of minimally invasive decompression should also be compared against endoscopic stenting, since these methods also provide adequate palliation without the need for laparotomy or laparoscopy.

Moreover, there is evidence that patients with pancreatic cancer who are deemed unresectable by diagnostic laparoscopy may not even need any further operative palliation. In a systematic follow-up of 155 patients who were laparoscopically staged and found to have unresectable pancreatic adenocarcinoma (65% involving the head), only 2% of those ever required surgery for biliary or gastric outlet obstruction (4% of those with tumors of the head of the pancreas).[34] This study suggests that the majority of patients with advanced disease identified by laparoscopy can be adequately managed by nonoperative means, although data regarding the complications of these nonsurgical means are not provided. It is evident that laparoscopic palliative procedures should be tested in prospective, randomized trials with nonoperative methods of palliation, including quality of life parameters, before laparoscopic palliative bypass procedures can be generally recommended.

Management of Gastric Outlet Obstruction

Although approximately 30% of patients with pancreatic cancer present with nausea and vomiting, less than 5% of pancreatic cancers present with duodenal obstruction.[12] Functional duodenal dysmotility probably accounts for a significant portion of these symptoms, and these patients are best managed by promotility agents such as erythromycin and metoclopramide. Other patients, particularly those with tumors of the uncinate process, have a higher risk of mechanical obstruction, particularly at the third and fourth portions of the duodenum. Tumors arising from the head of the gland, however, tend to invade the second portion of the duodenum and are less likely to cause duodenal obstruction.

Patients with radiographic or endoscopic evidence of gastric outlet obstruction (GOO) should have some form of decompression. Those found to be unresectable at exploration, but with gastric outlet obstruction and without diffuse systemic metastases should have a palliative gastrojejunostomy (GJ). A retrocolic isoperistaltic gastrojejunostomy, either stapled or hand-sewn at the most dependent portion of the stomach is usually the preferred method. We do not routinely perform vagotomy because of the risk of delayed gastric emptying. In addition, these patients typically have a short median survival time. The main questions that merit discussion are (1) is there a role for prophylactic gastrojejunostomy in patients with unresectable pancreatic cancer? and (2) how should a patient with GOO and unresectable pancreatic cancer as detected by preoperative radiographic imaging be treated?

The first question applies only to patients without evidence of GOO who were found to be unresectable on exploratory laparotomy. A clinical review by Sarr and Cameron analyzing data from 8,000 patients suggested that the incidence of subsequent duodenal obstruction requiring GJ after initial laparotomy ranges from 2 to 50%, and in their own series of 1,800 patients, it was 13%. Additionally, 10 to 20% of patients died with symptoms of duodenal obstruction that may have been prevented if GJ, when patients became symptomatic, had been performed at the initial exploration. Furthermore, the mortality of *subsequent* GJ was between 14% and 40%, whereas the addition of GJ to the initial operation did not add significant morbidity or mortality.[12] Similarly, Singh and colleagues found no difference in mortality between a double bypass (GJ and biliary bypass) versus biliary bypass alone (8.6% vs 6.3%), although the morbidity rate associated with the GJ was approximately 20%.[1] One-quarter of patients who underwent biliary bypass alone required a GJ during the course of their disease, and an additional 20% had significant vomiting at the terminal stages of their disease. The authors concluded that a GJ probably should be performed in all cases of pancreatic cancer coming to laparotomy if estimated duration of patient survival is beyond a few weeks. In contrast, Egrari and O'Connell reviewed 50 patients with unresectable pancreatic adenocarcinoma who underwent biliary bypass without GJ and found that only 8% of patients developed GOO. Furthermore, the mean time that GOO developed after the initial operation was 15.75 months, with only 1 patient developing obstruction within 10 months. The mean survival of all patients in the study was 13 months, and therefore the authors concluded that the vast majority of patients will succumb to their disease before GOO occurs.[35] Additionally, none of the patients who subsequently required GJ died during the perioperative period and actually had a surprisingly long mean survival of 16.5 months after the second operation performed to create a GJ.

Two prospective randomized trials have been published addressing the role of prophylactic GJ in patients with unresectable periampullary cancer discovered during the initial operation (Table 4). Lillemoe and colleagues identified 87 patients with periampullary tumors found to be unresectable at laparotomy, but without any evidence of GOO. These patients were randomized to have prophylactic gastrojejunostomy or no gastrojejunostomy. The morbidity, mortality, and mean hospital stay were similar in both groups. The rate of delayed gastric emptying between the two groups was also similarly low. Nineteen percent of patients without prophylactic GJ developed GOO, requiring therapeutic intervention, whereas none of the patients who had prophylactic GJ developed GOO. None of the patients who required delayed GJ died in the hospital, but 1 died within 30 days of the operation (12.5%).[36] Another multicenter prospective study randomized patients to biliary or double bypass and led to similar results. Morbidity, mortality, length of hospital stay, and survival was similar in both groups. Forty-one percent of patients who did not have GJ eventually developed GOO, versus 5% for the double bypass group. The quality of life scores were similar in both groups, however.[37] Both studies strongly suggest that double bypass is preferable to biliary bypass alone in patients with unresectable pancreatic cancer undergoing exploratory laparotomy.

More recently, laparoscopic gastrojejunostomy has showed some promising results in small studies.

Laparoscopic GJ can be performed safely in either an antecolic or retrocolic fashion.[31,32] Median time to postoperative oral intake is 3 to 4 days, and median postoperative length of stay about 7 to 9 days.[31] Postoperative delayed gastric emptying appears to be less frequent than with the open method, and obstruction of the gastrojejunostomy appears rare.[32]

A variety of expanding metallic endoprostheses have also been used for palliation of GOO. These devices were used initially in patients with malignant GOO who were poor surgical candidates, but during the last several years they have been used increasingly for primary palliation. A review by Mauro and colleagues reported that expandable metallic stents relieved the obstructive symptoms and allowed rapid recovery to oral intake in 89% of patients with inoperable GOO, mostly owing to malignancy. In those who failed, approximately half also had distal small bowel obstructions that were difficult to diagnose, since the GOO precluded evaluation of the small bowel. Tumor ingrowth through the stent leading to reobstruction occurred in 15% of patients, and an additional 3% experienced stent migration.[38] Others have reported that approximately 25% of patients develop clinical symptoms related to recurrent GOO, and most are successfully managed by reendoscopy, although in some of these patients advanced or metastatic disease precluded further attempts. Retrospective comparisons of endoscopic and surgical palliation in patients with malignant GOO have also revealed that the hospital stay and costs are significantly less for endoscopic palliation. Recently, Mittal and colleagues retrospectively evaluated patients with malignant GOO who underwent palliation by endoscopic, laparoscopic, or open means.[39] Endoscopic therapy resulted in a significantly shorter time to resumption of an oral diet, a shorter length of hospital stay, and fewer complications compared with laparoscopic or open palliation. In order to overcome the problems of tumor ingrowth within the stent or stent migration, a novel dual expandable nitinol stent has been recently used with promising results. Another problem that may be encountered in patients with advanced pancreatic cancer is difficulty in providing biliary drainage after placement of a duodenal stent. Although rarely necessary, this can usually be managed by percutaneous biliary drainage.

In general, we perform a prophylactic gastrojejunostomy in selected patients with pancreatic cancer found to be unresectable at exploratory laparotomy. Patients with evidence of a tumor near the third or fourth portion of the duodenum or those with symptoms of imminent gastric outlet obstruction undergo prophylactic gastrojejunostomy. In those patients in whom GOO eventually develops, endoscopic stenting or surgical bypass (laparo-

Table 4 Prospective Randomized Studies Addressing Prophylactic Gastrojejunostomy

Authors	Lillemoe[36] 1999		Van Heek[37] 2003	
Procedure	With GJ	Without GJ	With GJ	Without GJ
Patients	44	43	36	29
Mortality (%)	0	0	3	0
Morbidity (%)	32	33	11	9
Delayed gastric emptying (%)	2	2	17	3
Operative time (min)	254	209*		
Hospital stay (d)	8.5	8.0	11	9
Survival (m)	8.3	8.3	7.2	8.4
GOO (%)	0*	19	5.5*	41.4
30-day mortality after late GJ (%)	—	12.5		
Survival after late GJ (m)	—	5.1		
Interval between procedures (m)	—	5.1		3.5

GOO = gastric outlet obstruction.

scopic or open) will result in significant palliation, and the choice usually depends on expertise of clinicians in the institution. Patients presenting with malignant GOO secondary to advanced pancreatic cancer usually have a short survival duration, and endoscopic palliation should be attempted if possible. If adequate palliation is not achieved, laparoscopic or open bypass should be considered.

Palliative Pancreatoduodenectomy

While the mortality rate of pancreatoduodenectomy during the 1970s was in the range of 17%, this number was reduced to less than 10% in the 1980s and now ranges between 0 and 5% at specialized centers. Similarly, the morbidity after pancreatic resection has also decreased significantly. These improved results have led to examining the role of pancreatoduodenectomy as palliative therapy for patients with locally advanced pancreatic cancer. To date, there are no prospective randomized studies evaluating pancreatic resection for palliation. The results for palliative pancreatoduodenectomy, therefore, comes from those patients found unresectable intraoperatively secondary to macroscopically unresectable disease after pancreatic resection, or postoperatively after the pathology report describes positive microscopic margins. In both circumstances, resection was planned with curative intent.

A report by Reinders and colleagues retrospectively compared outcomes between patients found with positive margins after pancreaticoduodenectomy with patients who underwent surgical bypass for unresectable pancreatic cancer. Patient characteristics and tumor diameter were matched for both groups. In-hospital mortality and perioperative morbidity rates were similar in both groups, although the only death occurred in the resection group. Postoperative hospital stay was significantly longer for the group that underwent resection (25 vs 18 days). The 2-year survival rate of the resection group was 24%, whereas, in contrast, the rate was only 2% for the bypass group.[40] Similarly, another study by Lillemoe and colleagues addressing the same issue found that perioperative mortality rate (1.6%), morbidity rate, and the number of readmissions were similar in both groups. Postoperative length of stay was shorter for the bypass group. Median survival of the resected group was significantly longer (12 months) versus the bypass group (9 months). Patients who received chemoradiation after pancreatoduodenectomy had significantly longer survival versus resected patients who did not receive postoperative therapy and those undergoing bypass who received postoperative therapy.[41]

Several studies have established that patients with negative margins after pancreatoduodenectomy have significantly improved survival compared with those with positive margins.[42] Survival of those in the latter group mimic the survival duration of patients with locally advanced, unresectable disease. Since both of these studies are retrospective, the survival advantage of pancreatoduodenectomy over bypass may be attributed to patient selection. Patients who underwent resection may have had less tumor burden, since they underwent resection with curative intent. Details of the tumor, including size and lymph node status, were also not compared. Although patients who had chemoradiation after resection had the longest survival in the study by Lillemoe, there is no evidence in the literature to support the idea that reducing the tumor burden affects response to chemoradiation in locally advanced pancreatic cancer. With no definitive randomized data available, a planned palliative pancreaticoduodenectomy for patients with locally advanced disease cannot be recommended.

Conclusions

The majority of patients who present with pancreatic cancer are unresectable, and therefore, improving the quality of life of these patients is of paramount importance. Considering the short median survival time of these patients, this becomes even more crucial. For those with locally advanced disease, there are several options that currently exist. For the control of pain, the use of opioids and other analgesics as well as celiac blocks and splanchnicectomy are viable options and should be individualized. The management of obstructive jaundice is also challenging and therapy should also be individualized. For patients found to be locally advanced at exploration, operative biliary bypass should certainly be considered. For patients deemed to be unresectable prior to exploration, however, endoscopically placed metallic stents are usually a better option. For patients who present with gastric outlet obstruction, endoscopic placement of an expandable metallic stent can be considered depending on local expertise. If this fails, laparoscopic or open gastrojejunostomy should be offered. Routine prophylactic gastrojejunostomy should be reserved for those select patients with evidence of imminent obstruction or those at high risk of subsequent obstruction. Finally, although the results after pancreaticoduodenectomy for resectable patients continue to improve, there is no evidence that palliative pancreaticoduodenectomy affords better palliation than less aggressive techniques and cannot be recommended. Certainly, additional well-designed prospective randomized trials are needed to answer many of these questions.

References

1. Singh SM, Longmire WP Jr, Reber HA. Surgical palliation for pancreatic cancer. The UCLA experience. Ann Surg 1990;212:132–9.

2. Ihse I. Pancreatic pain. Br J Surg 1990;77:121–2.

3. Kelsen DP, Portenoy R, Thaler H, et al. Pain as a predictor of outcome in patients with operable pancreatic carcinoma. Surgery 1997;122:53–9.

4. Lillemoe KD, Cameron JL, Kaufman HS, et al. Chemical splanchnicectomy in patients with unresectable pancreatic cancer. A prospective randomized trial. Ann Surg 1993;217:447–55.

5. Wong GY, Schroeder DR, Carns PE, et al. Effect of neurolytic celiac plexus block on pain relief, quality of life, and survival in patients with unresectable pancreatic cancer: a randomized controlled trial. JAMA 2004;291:1092–9.

6. Eisenberg E, Carr DB, Chalmers TC. Neurolytic celiac plexus block for treatment of cancer pain: a meta-analysis. Anesth Analg 1995;80:290–5.

7. Polati E, Finco G, Gottin L, et al. Prospective randomized double-blind trial of neurolytic coeliac plexus block in patients with pancreatic cancer. Br J Surg 1998;85:199–201.

8. Ihse I, Zoucas E, Gyllstedt E, et al. Bilateral thoracoscopic splanchnicectomy: effects on pancreatic pain and function. Ann Surg 1999;230:785–90.

9. Li CP, Chao Y, Chi KH, et al. Concurrent chemoradiotherapy treatment of locally advanced pancreatic cancer: gemcitabine versus 5-fluorouracil, a randomized controlled study. Int J Radiat Oncol Biol Phys 2003;57:98–104.

10. Morganti AG, Trodella L, Valentini V, et al. Pain relief with short-term irradiation in locally advanced carcinoma of the pancreas. J Palliat Care 2003;19:258–62.

11. Rosemurgy AS, Burnett CM, Wasselle JA. A comparison of choledochoenteric bypass and cholecystoenteric bypass in patients with biliary obstruction due to pancreatic cancer. Am Surg 1989;55:55–60.

12. Sarr MG, Cameron JL. Surgical management of unresectable carcinoma of the pancreas. Surgery 1982;91:123–33.

13. Urbach DR, Bell CM, Swanstrom LL, Hansen PD. Cohort study of surgical bypass to the gallbladder or bile duct for the palliation of jaundice due to pancreatic cancer. Ann Surg 2003;237:86–93.

14. Sarfeh IJ, Rypins EB, Jakowatz JG, Juler GL. A prospective, randomized clinical investigation of cholecystoenterostomy and choledochoenterostomy. Am J Surg 1988;155:411–4.

15. Tarnasky PR, England RE, Lail LM, et al. Cystic duct patency in malignant obstructive jaundice. An ERCP-based study relevant to the role of laparoscopic cholecystojejunostomy. Ann Surg 1995;221:265–71.

16. Moraca RJ, Lee FT, Ryan JA Jr, Traverso LW. Long-term biliary function after reconstruction of major bile duct injuries with hepaticoduodenostomy or hepaticojejunostomy. Arch Surg 2002;137:889–93.

17. van Wagensveld BA, Coene PP, van Gulik TM, et al. Outcome of palliative biliary and gastric bypass surgery for pancreatic head carcinoma in 126 patients. Br J Surg 1997;84:1402–6.

18. Speer AG, Cotton PB, Russell RC, et al. Randomised trial of endoscopic versus percutaneous stent insertion in malignant obstructive jaundice. Lancet 1987;2:57–62.

19. Hammarstrom LE. Endobiliary stents for palliation in patients with malignant obstructive jaundice. J Clin Gastroenterol 2005;39:413–21.

20. Davids PH, Groen AK, Rauws EA, et al. Randomised trial of self-expanding metal stents versus polyethylene stents for distal malignant biliary obstruction. Lancet 1992;340:1488–92.

21. Prat F, Chapat O, Ducot B, et al. A randomized trial of endoscopic drainage methods for inoperable malignant strictures of the common bile duct. Gastrointest Endosc 1998;47:1–7.

22. Kaassis M, Boyer J, Dumas R, et al. Plastic or metal stents for malignant stricture of the common bile duct? Results of a randomized prospective study. Gastrointest Endosc 2003;57:178–82.

23. Yeoh KG, Zimmerman MJ, Cunningham JT, Cotton PB. Comparative costs of metal versus plastic biliary stent strategies for malignant obstructive jaundice by decision analysis. Gastrointest Endosc 1999;49:466–71.

24. Smith AC, Dowsett JF, Russell RC, et al. Randomised trial of endoscopic stenting versus surgical bypass in malignant low bile duct obstruction. Lancet 1994;344:1655–60.

25. Andersen JR, Sorensen SM, Kruse A, et al. Randomised trial of endoscopic endoprosthesis versus operative bypass in malignant obstructive jaundice. Gut 1989;30:1132–5.

26. Shepherd HA, Royle G, Ross AP, et al. Endoscopic biliary endoprosthesis in the palliation of malignant obstruction of the distal common bile duct: a randomized trial. Br J Surg 1988;75:1166–8.

27. Bornman PC, Harries-Jones EP, Tobias R, et al. Prospective controlled trial of transhepatic biliary endoprosthesis versus bypass surgery for incurable carcinoma of head of pancreas. Lancet 1986;1:69–71.

28. Nieveen van Dijkum EJ, Romijn MG, Terwee CB, et al. Laparoscopic staging and subsequent palliation in patients with peripancreatic carcinoma. Ann Surg 2003;237:66–73.

29. Taylor MC, McLeod RS, Langer B. Biliary stenting versus bypass surgery for the palliation of malignant distal bile duct obstruction: a meta-analysis. Liver Transpl 2000;6:302–8.

30. Rhodes M, Nathanson L, Fielding G. Laparoscopic biliary and gastric bypass: a useful adjunct in the treatment of carcinoma of the pancreas. Gut 1995;36:778–80.

31. Kuriansky J, Saenz A, Astudillo E, et al. Simultaneous laparoscopic biliary and retrocolic gastric bypass in patients with unresectable carcinoma of the pancreas. Surg Endosc 2000;14:179–81.

32. Rothlin MA, Schob O, Weber M. Laparoscopic gastro- and hepaticojejunostomy for palliation of pancreatic cancer: a case controlled study. Surg Endosc 1999;13:1065–9.

33. Date RS, Siriwardena AK. Laparoscopic biliary bypass and current management algorithms for the palliation of malignant obstructive jaundice. Ann Surg Oncol 2004;11: 815–7.

34. Espat NJ, Brennan MF, Conlon KC. Patients with laparoscopically staged unresectable pancreatic adenocarcinoma do not require subsequent surgical biliary or gastric bypass. J Am Coll Surg 1999;188:649–55.

35. Egrari S, O'Connell TX. Role of prophylactic gastroenterostomy for unresectable pancreatic carcinoma. Am Surg 1995;61:862–4.

36. Lillemoe KD, Cameron JL, Hardacre JM, et al. Is prophylactic gastrojejunostomy indicated for unresectable periampullary cancer? A prospective randomized trial. Ann Surg 1999;230:322–8.

37. Van Heek NT, De Castro SM, van Eijck CH, et al. The need for a prophylactic gastrojejunostomy for unresectable periampullary cancer: a prospective randomized multi-center trial with special focus on assessment of quality of life. Ann Surg 2003;238:894–902.

38. Mauro MA, Koehler RE, Baron TH. Advances in gastro-intestinal intervention: the treatment of gastroduodenal and colorectal obstructions with metallic stents. Radiology 2000;215:659–69.

39. Mittal A, Windsor J, Woodfield J, et al. Matched study of three methods for palliation of malignant pyloroduodenal obstruction. Br J Surg 2004;91:205–9.

40. Reinders ME, Allema JH, van Gulik TM, et al. Outcome of microscopically nonradical, subtotal pancreaticoduode-nectomy (Whipple's resection) for treatment of pancreatic head tumors. World J Surg 1995;19:410–4.

41. Lillemoe KD, Cameron JL, Yeo CJ, et al. Pancreaticoduodenectomy. Does it have a role in the palliation of pancreatic cancer? Ann Surg 1996;223:718–25.

42. Neoptolemos JP, Stocken DD, Dunn JA, et al. European Study Group for Pancreatic Cancer. Influence of resection margins on survival for patients with pancreatic cancer treated by adjuvant chemoradiation and/or chemotherapy in the ESPAC-1 randomized controlled trial. Ann Surg 2001;234:758–68.

CHAPTER 21

ISLET CELL TUMORS OF THE PANCREAS

WILLIAM E. FISHER, MD

DAVID H. BERGER, MD

Introduction

Pancreatic endocrine tumors occur with an incidence of only 5 cases per million annually, but oncologists in busy urban referral centers will occasionally encounter patients with one of these interesting and heterogeneous group of tumors.[1] Pancreatic endocrine tumors have a variety of clinical presentations related to excess hormone release. These tumors can also vary in their prognosis and treatment. Pancreatic endocrine tumors include insulinomas, gastrinomas, vasoactive intestinal peptide (VIPomas), glucagonomas, somatostatinomas, adrenocorticotropic hormone-secreting tumors (ACTHomas), growth hormone releasing factor-secreting tumors (GRFomas), and nonfunctioning pancreatic endocrine tumors.

Pancreatic endocrine tumors resemble carcinoid tumors in producing products characteristic of neuroendocrine differentiation such as neuron specific enolase, chromogranins, and synaptophysin. In fact, plasma chromogranin A is elevated in 60 to 100% of both functional and nonfunctional pancreatic endocrine tumors, and serum levels are useful in individual patients to assess tumor progression, relapse, and relative tumor burden. Most pancreatic endocrine tumors express somatostatin receptors and can be localized with somatostatin receptor scintigraphy, (octreoscan). There is no absolute agreement on the best name for this group of neoplastic endocrine tumors, and although referred to as "islet cell tumors," it is unproven if they actually originate from pancreatic islets. Pancreatic endocrine tumor is also a misnomer because some of these tumors (ie, gastrinomas, VIPomas, somatostatinomas) can arise outside the pancreas. In all of these tumors, treatment is directed not only against the tumor, but also the hormone-excess state. This chapter summarizes recent advances made in the diagnosis, localization, and treatment of islet cell, or pancreatic endocrine, tumors.

Insulinoma

Approximately 75% of all pancreatic endocrine neoplasms are insulinomas.[2,3] Therefore, the most common presentation of a pancreatic endocrine neoplasms is a clinical syndrome known as Whipple's triad. About 60% of the patients are women who present with symptomatic fasting hypoglycemia, a documented serum glucose level less than 50 mg/dL, and relief of symptoms with the administration of glucose. Patients often present with a profound syncopal episode and admit to similar less severe episodes in the recent past. They may also complain of other neuroglycopenic symptoms such as headache, visual disturbances, dizziness, lightheadedness, confusion, and weakness. The catecholamine response to hypoglycemia causes diaphoresis, tremulousness, palpitations, irritability, and hunger. Insulinoma patients typically develop hypoglycemic symptoms during fasting or exercise; these symptoms resolve or improve after carbohydrate ingestion. Obesity frequently is present because of habitual overeating as an adaptation to recurrent hypoglycemic symptoms. Family members may report that the patient has undergone a personality change. Since the patients present with syncopal episodes, it is not uncommon for cases of insulinoma to be mistaken for a primary neurologic disease or epilepsy. Routine laboratory work will uncover a low blood sugar, the cause of all of these symptoms. The diagnosis is clinched with a monitored fast in which blood is sampled every 4 to 6 hours for glucose and insulin levels until the patient becomes symptomatic. The plasma glucose level during symptomatic hypoglycemia is usually less than 45 mg/dL and the insulin level is greater then 5 U/mL. Elevated C-peptide levels ($>$ 1.7 ng/mL) rule out the unusual case of surreptitious administration of insulin or oral hypoglycemic agents, because excess endogenous insulin production leads to excess C-peptide.

Once the diagnosis is secured, hypoglycemia is managed medically during the preoperative phase by frequent meals combined with diazoxide to suppress insulin release. An oral diazoxide dosage of 100 to 150 mg every 8 hours maintains euglycemia in approximately 60% of patients. Refractory patients may require admission and continuous intravenous infusion of 10% glucose solution.

Unlike most other islet cell tumors of the pancreas, most sporadic insulinomas can be resected for cure once localized. Insulinomas are usually localized with computed tomography (CT) or magnetic resonance imagery (MRI) scans and endoscopic ultrasound (EUS). The sensitivity of CT and MRI scanning for localizing insulinomas is only about 50% because it is difficult to detect lesions less than 1 cm in diameter. Technical advances in EUS have led to preoperative identification of about 90 to 94% of insulinomas. Visceral angiography with injection of calcium and hepatic venous sampling may rarely be required to localize the insulinoma to a region of the pancreas when the above modalities fail. Injection of calcium solution results in an increased tumor blush angiographically and a 2-fold rise in serum insulin levels. A positive result with injection of the gastroduodenal or superior mesenteric arteries indicates the tumor is in the head or neck of the pancreas, whereas response to injection of the splenic artery indicates the tumor is in the tail of the pancreas. In contrast to most other islet cell tumors, insulinomas contain somatostatin receptors in only 60% of cases. Thus, the sensitivity of the octreotide scan is relatively limited in insulinomas and is used only when routine tests fail to localize the tumor. In a clear-cut clinical case of insulinoma, in which the tumor cannot be localized after all of the above techniques have been exhausted, surgical exploration is warranted because the experienced surgeon, especially with the use of intraoperative ultrasound, can localize the tumor in 90 to 95% of cases.

Insulinomas are evenly distributed throughout the pancreas with a third of the tumors occurring in the head, a third in the body, and a third in the tail. Unlike most endocrine pancreatic tumors, the majority (90%) of insulinomas are benign, whereas only 10% are malignant. Approximately 80% of insulinomas occur singly, with a mean tumor size of 1 to 3 cm. They are typically cured by simple surgical enucleation, which is possible in half the cases (Figure 1). However, tumors located close to the main pancreatic duct and large ($>$ 2 cm) tumors may require a distal pancreatectomy or pancreaticoduodenectomy.[4–6] This is also the approach to tumors that are localized only to a region of the pancreas and cannot be visualized pre- or intraoperatively. Intraoperative ultrasound is useful to determine the tumor's proximity to the main pancreatic duct or distal common bile duct and to guide intraoperative decision making. It is also useful to exclude multiple tumors, particularly in cases of multiple endocrine neoplasia (MEN) syndrome. Although most insulinomas are benign, any enlarged regional lymph nodes should be removed and hepatic metastases, if found, are excised by wedge or formal hepatic resection if feasible. In general, debulking of large unresectable insulinomas involving the pancreas, lymph nodes, or liver is indicated to attenuate hypoglycemia. Since these tumors are usually benign and solitary, enucleation of isolated solitary insulinomas and distal pancreatectomy for insulinoma has been performed in some centers using a minimally invasive technique. Ninety percent of insulinomas are sporadic and 10 percent are associated with the MEN-1 syndrome. Insulinomas associated with the MEN-1 syndrome are more likely to be multifocal and have a higher rate of recurrence.

The results of chemotherapy for widely metastatic insulinoma have been disappointing. Streptozotocin alone or in combination with 5-fluorouracil (5-FU) and/or doxorubicin are typically used. About half the patients obtain an objective response, but this response is generally of short duration. Other agents such as chlorozotocin and alpha-interferon have recently been tried. Octreotide may stabilize tumor growth in the short

Insulinoma enucleated from pancreatic neck

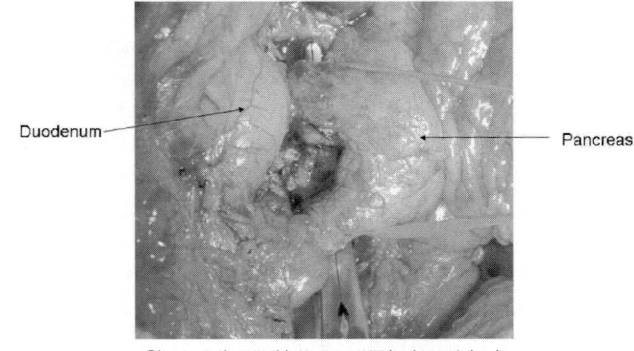

Clamp and vessel loop are anterior to portal vein

Figure 1 Site in the neck of pancreas where an insulinoma has been enucleated.

term for some patients in which the tumors can be localized with octreoscan, indicating that the tumor cells express specific somatostatin receptors. Chemoembolization is a viable option to address liver metastases and may present a superior approach to debulking surgery in some patients. Radiofrequency ablation is another modality that is currently being evaluated for hepatic metastases.

Gastrinoma

Approximately 20% of all endocrine pancreatic neoplasms are gastrin-producing tumors. Zollinger-Ellison syndrome (ZES) is caused by gastrinomas—endocrine tumors that secrete gastrin, leading to acid hypersecretion and peptic ulceration. Patients with ZES can present with abdominal pain, peptic ulcer disease, and severe esophagitis. However, in the era of a reliable radioimmunoassay for gastrin to assist with diagnosis, and effective antacid therapy, the presentation can be less dramatic. Although most of the ulcers are solitary, multiple ulcers in atypical locations that fail to respond to antacids should raise suspicion for ZES and prompt a work-up. However, many patients in the era of improved antacids have presented with ulcers in typical locations. Twenty percent of patients with gastrinoma have diarrhea at the time of diagnosis caused by acid hypersecretion.

The diagnosis of ZES is made by measuring the serum gastrin level. It is important that patients stop taking proton pump inhibitors for this test. In most patients with gastrinomas, the serum gastrin level is greater than 1,000 pg/mL (normal < 100 pg/mL). Gastrin levels can be elevated in conditions other than ZES. Common causes of hypergastrinemia include pernicious anemia, treatment with proton pump inhibitors, renal failure, G-cell hyperplasia, atrophic gastritis, retained or excluded antrum, and gastric outlet obstruction. In equivocal cases, when the gastrin level is not markedly elevated, or when other causes of hypergastrinemia are suspected, a secretin stimulation test is helpful. Acid suppression does not have to be stopped for this test. Secretin injection (2 U/kg) causes a paradoxic rise in the plasma gastrin level of 200 pg/mL or greater above the basal level in patients with gastrinomas. Operation for intractable peptic ulcer disease is now uncommon after aggressive antacid therapy, eradication of *Helicobacter pylori* infection, and elimination of ingestion of all nonsteroidal anti-inflammatory drugs. Therefore, a serum gastrin level and secretin stimulation test should be performed to rule out gastrinoma before considering an operation for intractable peptic ulcer disease.

Once the diagnosis of gastrinoma is made, patients are placed on proton pump inhibitors, which provide complete symptomatic relief in 80%. The next step is to localize the tumor, which will be found in Passaro's triangle in 70 to 90% of affected individuals. This area is defined by a triangle with points located at the junction of the cystic duct and common bile duct, the second and third portion of the duodenum, and the neck and body of the pancreas. As many as two-thirds of gastrinomas are found outside the pancreas, usually in the duodenum. Since gastrinomas can be found outside the pancreas, whole body imaging is required. The test of choice is somatostatin receptor (octreotide) scintigraphy in combination with CT (Figure 2). Most gastrinomas are about 1 to 2 cm in diameter. The octreotide scan (octreoscan) is more sensitive than CT, locating about 85% of gastrinomas and detecting tumors smaller than 1 cm. With the octreoscan, the need for tedious and technically demanding selective angiography and measurement of gastrin gradients has declined. EUS is another new modality that assists in the preoperative localization of gastrinomas. It is particularly helpful in localizing tumors in the pancreatic head or duodenal wall where gastrinomas are often less than 1 cm in diameter. A combination of octreoscan and EUS localizes more than 90% of gastrinomas.

It is important to rule out MEN-1 syndrome by checking serum calcium levels prior to surgery. These

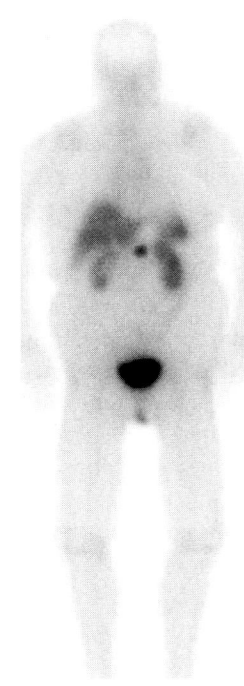

Figure 2 Octreoscan demonstrating gastrinoma in the pancreatic body.

patients have multiple pancreatic and duodenal tumors that are small, often microscopic, and an attempt at resection of the gastrinomas in these patients rarely results in normalization of serum gastrin concentrations or a prolongation of survival. Most of these patients are treated medically unless a tumor is readily identified on preoperative imaging studies. Fortunately, only one-fourth of gastrinomas occur in association with the MEN-1 syndrome. In patients with MEN-1 syndrome, the parathyroid hyperplasia and its associated hypercalcemia exacerbate hypergastrinemia and gastric acid hypersecretion. The preferred approach to control hypercalcemia is total parathyroidectomy and implantation of parathyroid tissue in the forearm. Aggressive surgical treatment aimed at complete resection of the gastrinoma is justified in patients with sporadic gastrinomas.

The appropriate goal of surgical therapy for gastrinoma is control of the hormonal syndrome and prevention or treatment of malignant disease by complete tumor excision. Routine intraoperative localization techniques include the use of ultrasound, transduodenal illumination, and routine duodenotomy, which result in localization of the tumor in 90% of patients (Figures 3 and 4). Overall, approximately 60% of gastrinomas are malignant, but the biologic behavior of tumors metastatic only to lymph nodes is distinctly indolent, with infrequent progression to liver metastases on long-term follow-up. In contrast, gastrinomas metastatic to the liver behave in a much more aggressive manner and inevitably result in patient fatality. Patients

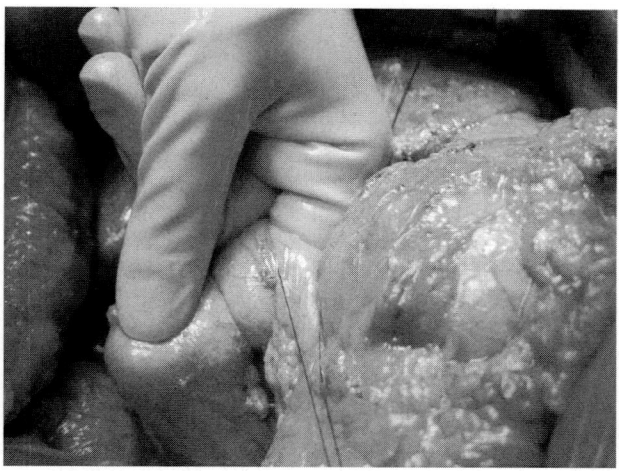

Figure 4 A duodenotomy is performed to facilitate thorough palpation of the duodenum to localize a gastrinoma located in the duodenum wall.

who meet criteria for operability should undergo exploration for possible removal of the primary tumor. An aggressive approach is warranted in the absence of unresectable metastatic disease, those with MEN-1 syndrome without preoperative localization of any tumor, and in patients who are medically fit for surgery.

Most gastrinomas within the pancreas are amenable to enucleation but large invasive tumors require distal pancreatectomy or pancreaticoduodenectomy.[4–6] The first step in surgery for gastrinoma is a systematic general abdominal exploration using intraoperative ultrasound. A generous Kocher maneuver is performed so that the entire head of the pancreas is palpable. The lesser sac is entered and the retroperitoneum along the inferior border of the pancreas is incised. It is sometimes helpful to mobilize the spleen so that the body and tail of the pancreas can be lifted anteriorly and palpated. Proper exposure should allow full bimanual palpation and visual inspection of both the anterior and posterior pancreatic surfaces. The duodenal wall is also carefully examined and intraoperative ultrasound is utilized to examine the duodenum, pancreas, and liver. If the tumor is still not localized, intraoperative esophagogastroduodenoscopy is performed. If the tumor is still not localized, a duodenotomy is made in the second portion of the duodenum or through the pylorus and first portion of the duodenum. The index finger is placed in the duodenal lumen with the thumb on the serosal surface as the duodenal wall is palpated. Approximately 70% of duodenal gastrinomas are found in the first portion of the duodenum and the frequency decreases as one

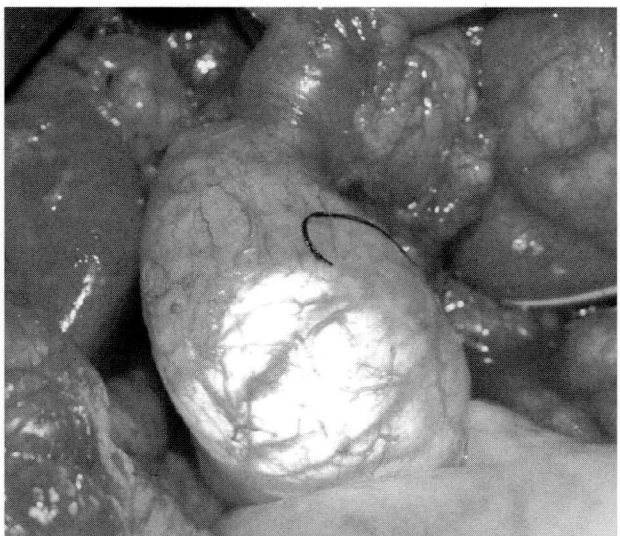

Figure 3 Intraoperative transillumination of the duodenum.

proceeds distally. Although the tumors are submucosal, an elliptical full-thickness excision of the duodenal wall is performed if a duodenal gastrinoma is found. In all cases, the lymph nodes in Passaro's triangle are excised and sent for pathologic analysis. If the gastrinoma is found in the pancreas, and does not involve the main pancreatic duct, it is enucleated. For gastrinomas that involve the main pancreatic duct or distal common bile duct, a pancreaticoduodenectomy is performed for tumors in the pancreatic head or uncinate process, and a distal pancreatectomy is performed for tumors located in the body or tail of the gland. Large or multiple duodenal tumors also require pancreaticoduodenectomy. Some surgeons perform a highly selective vagotomy if unresectable disease is identified or if the gastrinoma cannot be localized. This may reduce the requirement for expensive proton pump inhibitors. In cases where hepatic metastases are identified, resection is justified only if the primary gastrinoma is controlled and the metastases can be safely and completely removed. Debulking or incomplete removal of multiple hepatic metastases is not generally helpful.

The application of new modalities such as radiofrequency ablation (RFA) seems reasonable, but data to support this approach are limited. Postoperatively, patients are followed with fasting serum gastrin levels, secretin stimulation tests, octreoscans, and CT scans. In patients found to have inoperable disease, chemotherapy with streptozotocin, doxorubicin, and 5-FU is used. Results are similar to those in patients with inoperable insulinoma. Only 40% of patients have a partial response, but there are no complete responses and minimal impact on long-term survival. Other approaches such as somatostatin analogs, interferon, and chemoembolization also have been used in metastatic gastrinoma with some palliative success.

Unfortunately, a long-term biochemical cure is achieved in only about one-third of the patients operated on for ZES, despite apparent complete surgical resection and initial biochemical cure. Despite the lack of success, long-term survival rates are good, even in patients with liver metastases. The 15-year survival rate for patients without liver metastases is about 80%, whereas the 5-year survival rate for patients with liver metastases is 20 to 50%. Pancreatic tumors are usually larger than tumors arising in the duodenum and more often have lymph node metastases. In gastrinomas, liver metastases decrease survival rates, but lymph node metastases do not. The best results are seen after complete excision of small sporadic tumors originating in the duodenum. Large tumors associated with liver metastases or with disease spread located outside of Passaro's triangle have the worst prognosis.

The remaining 10% of pancreatic endocrine neoplasms are quite rare and are malignant in about 90% of the cases. The diagnosis is made in most cases by recognition of the typical clinical syndrome and confirmation by measuring the relevant excess hormone in the serum. The same localization procedures apply, but frequently the tumors are found to be advanced and unresectable. They often metastasize to the lymph nodes and the liver.

VIPoma

In 1958, Verner and Morrison first described the syndrome associated with a pancreatic neoplasm secreting vasoactive intestinal polypeptide (VIP). The classic clinical syndrome associated with this pancreatic endocrine neoplasm consists of severe intermittent watery diarrhea leading to dehydration, and weakness from fluid and electrolyte losses. Large amounts of potassium are lost in the stool. The VIPoma syndrome is also called the WDHA syndrome because of the presence of watery diarrhea, hypokalemia, and achlorhydria. The massive (5 L/day) and episodic nature of the diarrhea associated with the appropriate electrolyte abnormalities should raise suspicion of the diagnosis. Serum VIP levels must be measured on multiple occasions because the excess secretion of VIP is episodic and single measurements might be normal and misleading. Fasting plasma VIP levels greater than 300 pg/mL are diagnostic in the setting of secretory diarrhea. A CT scan localizes most VIPomas, although as with all islet cell tumors, EUS is the most sensitive imaging method. Electrolyte and fluid balance is sometimes difficult to correct preoperatively and must be pursued aggressively. Somatostatin analogs are helpful in controlling the diarrhea and allowing replacement. VIPomas are more commonly located in the distal pancreas and most have metastasized outside the pancreas at the time of diagnosis. Palliative debulking operations can sometimes improve symptoms for a period of time, particularly when combined with somatostatin analogs. Hepatic artery embolization has also been reported as a potentially beneficial palliative treatment to reduce symptoms in patients with hepatic metastases.

Glucagonoma

Diabetes in association with a recent onset of dermatitis should raise the suspicion of a glucagonoma. The diabetes usually is mild. The classic necrolytic migratory erythema associated with glucagonoma manifests as cyclic migrations of lesions with spreading margins and healing centers, typically on the lower abdomen, perineum, perioral area, and feet. The diagnosis is confirmed by measuring serum glucagon levels, which are usually over 500 pg/mL (normal < 100 pg/mL). Glucagon is a catabolic hormone and most patients present with malnutrition. The rash associated with glucagonoma is thought to be caused by low circulating levels of amino acids. Preoperative treatment usually includes control of the diabetes, parenteral nutrition, and octreotide. Octreotide usually improves the rash, reduces weight loss, and decreases diarrhea and abdominal cramping, but does not improve the diabetes. Like VIPomas, glucagonomas are more often in the body and tail of the pancreas and tend to be large tumors with metastases easily detected by CT. The average size is about 6 cm and 70% have metastatic disease at the time of diagnosis. Again, debulking operations are recommended in good operative candidates to relieve symptoms, and complete resection results in rapid resolution of the syndrome. Although most tumors are incurable, the average survival is 5 years.

Somatostatinoma

Because somatostatin inhibits pancreatic and biliary secretions, patients with a somatostatinoma present with gallstones owing to bile stasis, diabetes owing to inhibition of insulin secretion, and steatorrhea owing to inhibition of pancreatic exocrine secretion and bile secretion. Most somatostatinomas originate in the proximal pancreas or the pancreatoduodenal groove, with the ampulla and periampullary area as the most common site (60%). The most common presentations are abdominal pain (25%), jaundice (25%), and cholelithiasis (19%). This rare type of pancreatic endocrine tumor is diagnosed by confirming elevated serum somatostatin levels, which are usually above 10 ng/mL. Most tumors are large and metastases are typically present. Although most reported cases of somatostatinoma involve metastatic disease, an attempt at complete excision of the tumor (pancreaticoduodenectomy that includes cholecystectomy) is warranted in fit patients.

Nonfunctioning islet cell tumors

Most pancreatic endocrine neoplasms do secrete one or more hormones and are associated with characteristic clinical syndromes. After insulinoma, however, the most common islet cell tumor is the "nonfunctioning" islet cell neoplasm. Because it is clinically silent until its size and location produce symptoms, it is usually malignant when first diagnosed. Some presumably nonfunctional pancreatic endocrine neoplasms stain positive for pancreatic polypeptide (PP), and elevated PP levels are

therefore a marker for the lesion. Since clinical manifestations are absent, the tumors are usually large and metastatic at the time of diagnosis, unless they are detected serendipitously on CT scan or sonogram. Nonfunctioning islet cell tumors are also seen in association with other multiple neoplasia syndromes, such von Hippel-Lindau syndrome. The tumors grow slowly and 5-year survival is common as opposed to pancreatic exocrine tumors where 5-year survival is extraordinarily rare.

Rare Islet Cell Tumors

Rarely, carcinoid tumors are localized to the pancreas, but these account for < 1% of all carcinoids. Most are large and malignant. These tumors secrete serotonin, histamines, and prostaglandins, which result in characteristic diarrhea and facial flushing, the so-called carcinoid syndrome. Pancreatic endocrine tumors secreting growth hormone-releasing factor (GRF) or adrenocorticotropic hormone (ACTH) have also been reported. Pancreatic ACTHomas account for 4 to 16% of all cases of ectopic Cushing's syndrome. These tumors can be associated with gastrinomas and the MEN-1 syndrome.

Conclusion

Although relatively rare, pancreatic endocrine tumors are encountered on occasion in oncologic practice, and a knowledge of the various clinical syndromes and some index of suspicion allows for diagnosis of these interesting lesions. Serum radioimmunoassay of the appropriate peptide confirms the diagnosis in most cases. Immediate medical therapy is provided and localization is pursued usually with abdominal CT and EUS. An aggressive approach is undertaken in most patients fit for major surgery who are not found to have advanced metastatic disease (or MEN-1 without a definable tumor). Insulinomas and gastrinomas can be treated with enucleaion or local resection, but the other islet cell tumors are usually large, malignant, and require a radical resection. Unlike other pancreatic cancers, palliative debulking and resection of liver metastases is often indicated to control the hormonal syndromes. The standard chemotherapy agents used are streptozotocin and 5-FU, but they are not particularly effective. Chemoembolization can be useful as a palliative technique to control hepatic metastases. Patients with tumors that are localized with octreoscan, or demonstrate somatostatin receptors on immunohistochemical stains may benefit from octreotide to control symptoms and perhaps even slow tumor growth, but this is controversial.

References

1. Brentjens R, Saltz L. Islet cell tumors of the pancreas: the medical oncologist's perspective. Surg Clin North Am 2001; 81:527–42.

2. Arnold R, Kloppel G, Rothmund M, et al, editors. Endocrine tumors of the pancreas. Berlin: Karger; 1994.

3. Von Hoff DD, Evans DB, Hruban RH, editors. Pancreatic cancer. Boston: Jones & Bartlett: 2005.

4. Udelsman R, Yeo CJ, Hruban RH, et al. Pancreaticoduodenectomy for selected pancreatic endocrine tumors. Surg Gynecol Obstet 1993;177:269–78.

5. Townsend CM Jr, Thompson JC. Surgical management of tumors that produce gastrointestinal hormones. Annu Rev Med 1985;36:111–24.

6. Assalia A, Gagner M. Laparoscopic pancreatic surgery for islet cell tumors of the pancreas. World J Surg 2004;28:1239–47.

CHAPTER 22

SURGICAL MANAGEMENT OF CYSTIC NEOPLASMS OF THE PANCREAS

WADDAH B. AL-REFAIE, MD

JEFFREY E. LEE, MD

Introduction

Surgeons are increasingly called upon to evaluate patients with cystic lesions of the pancreas. In particular, the widespread availability and application of high-quality cross-sectional imaging studies have resulted in the identification of many more cystic pancreatic neoplasms incidentally in patients undergoing abdominal imaging for reasons unrelated to their pancreatic tumor process.[1] Appropriate evaluation and surgical treatment of patients with cystic lesions of the pancreas take into account the typical clinical and radiographic presentations of the inflammatory and neoplastic processes that give rise to such lesions, the natural histories of the various pancreatic cystic neoplasms, and the indications and limitations of available preoperative diagnostic tests, including computed tomography (CT) imaging as well as upper endoscopy with endoscopic ultrasound (EUS) and cyst aspiration. Surgeons operating on patients with cystic pancreatic neoplasms should have technical experience with the various surgical options for pancreatic resection, and be familiar with the details of postoperative care and follow-up evaluation for these patients.

Cystic Pancreatic Tumors

As a group, cystic tumors are the third most common group of pancreatic neoplasms, following ductal adenocarcinomas of the pancreas and pancreatic neuroendocrine tumors (PNET). The most common cystic pancreatic tumors and their associated radiographic appearances, cyst fluid biochemical and cytologic findings, and clinical implications are summarized in Table 1.

PSEUDOCYSTS

Pseudocysts are non-neoplastic, inflammatory fluid-filled lesions of the pancreas occurring in the setting of acute or chronic pancreatitis. Patients usually, but not always, have a history of clinical pancreatitis (abdominal pain, vomiting, elevated serum amylase and lipase levels) and clinical or radiographic factors suggesting an underlying etiology (gallstones, alcohol abuse, trauma, family history, hypertriglyceridemia). Abdominal imaging of the pancreas may show evidence for acute (edema, peripancreatic fluid or phlegmon) or chronic (calcifications, alternating strictures and dilation of the pancreatic duct) pancreatitis. Radiographically, pancreatic pseudocysts are usually solitary and unilocular. Communication of the pseudocyst with the pancreatic duct can sometimes be identified on abdominal imaging, by EUS, or by endoscopic retrograde cholangiopancreatography (ERCP). An occasional patient may present with a solitary pancreatic pseudocyst without a history suggestive of pancreatitis (Figure 1). Internal drainage (preferably endoscopic) or surgical resection are appropriate in patients with chronic, symptomatic pseudocysts that do not respond to conservative management. Surgical resection is preferred when the diagnostic evaluation is indeterminate (as in the patient illustrated in Figure 1). On the other hand, observation of the patient with a pancreatic pseudocyst is appropriate when the clinical presentation and the radiographic features establish the

Table 1 Cystic Ttumors of the Pancreas

Diagnosis	CT Appearance	Cyst Fluid	Cytology	Clinical Implications
Pseudocyst	Unilocular cyst	Amylase high (> 5000 IU/L), CEA low (< 192 ng/mL)	Inflammatory cells and debris	Benign
Serous cystadenoma	Small, multilocular cysts; occasionally macrocystic	Amylase and CEA low	Benign epithelial cells	Almost always benign
Lymphoepithelial cyst	Single unilocular cyst	No data (likely amylase and CEA low)	Benign squamous epithelial cells	Benign
Solid pseudopapillary tumor	Large, unilocular cyst with associated enhancing mass	No data	Monomorphic cells and debris	Indolent but potentially malignant
Mucinous cystic neoplasm	Unilocular	Amylase variable, CEA high, thick mucin	Benign, dysplastic, or malignant	Potentially malignant
IPMN-associated	Unilocular or multiple, associated with pancreatic duct ectasia	Amylase variable, CEA high, thick mucin		Potentially malignant
Ductal adenocarcinoma-associated	Unilocular, associated hypodense mass	Amylase low, CEA high	Malignant	Malignant
Acinar cell adenocarcinoma-associated	Unilocular, associated hypodense mass	No data (likely amylase low, CEA high)	Malignant	Malignant
Neuroendocrine tumor-associated	Unilocular, associated enhancing mass	Amylase variable, CEA low	Neuroendocrine cells	Potentially malignant

CEA = carcinoembryonic antigen; IPMN = intraductal papillary mucinous neoplasm.

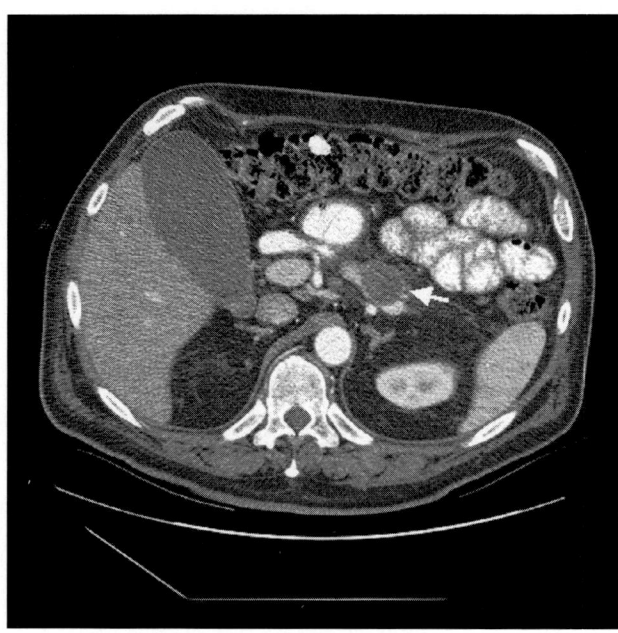

Figure 1 Computed tomography (CT) image of a patient with an incidentally identified pancreatic pseudocyst (arrow). The patient had no history of pancreatitis, cholecystitis, or heavy alcohol use. The radiographic findings are nonspecific; the radiographic differential diagnosis includes pseudocyst as well as mucinous cystic neoplasm. Endoscopic ultrasound-guided cyst fluid analysis revealed scant mucin and epithelial cells; fluid analysis for amylase and carcinoembryonic antigen (CEA) was not performed. Distal pancreatectomy and splenectomy revealed a pancreatic pseudocyst.

diagnosis, and the lesion is either acute or is relatively small and symptoms are resolving, mild, or absent.

SEROUS CYSTADENOMAS

Serous cystadenomas are more commonly identified in the head of the pancreas, and are most common in patients of advanced age. Serous cystadenomas are usually identified incidentally or in patients with vague abdominal complaints; it is relatively uncommon for patients to present with weight loss or obstructive jaundice.[2] On CT, these neoplasms appear as well-circumscribed lesions, usually composed of multiple small cysts (*microcystic serous cystadenoma*, Figure 2); a macrosystic variety occurs occasionally. A central calcification with radiating septa giving a "sunburst" appearance is seen in 10 to 20% of patients. EUS can also effectively delineate these features. Cyst fluid analysis characteristically reveals both low amylase and low carcinoembryonic antigen (CEA) values.[3–6] However, the small size of the individual cysts and the multiple septations present can limit the volume of cyst fluid obtained, and therefore limit one's ability to perform accurate biochemical analysis. Serous cystic tumors are almost uniformly benign; rare serous cyst adenocarcinomas have been reported.[7–10] Pancreatectomy is suggested when the diagnosis is uncertain or when patients are symptomatic. Size has been suggested as a predictor of tumor growth, and therefore may be considered in the selection of relatively young but otherwise asymptomatic

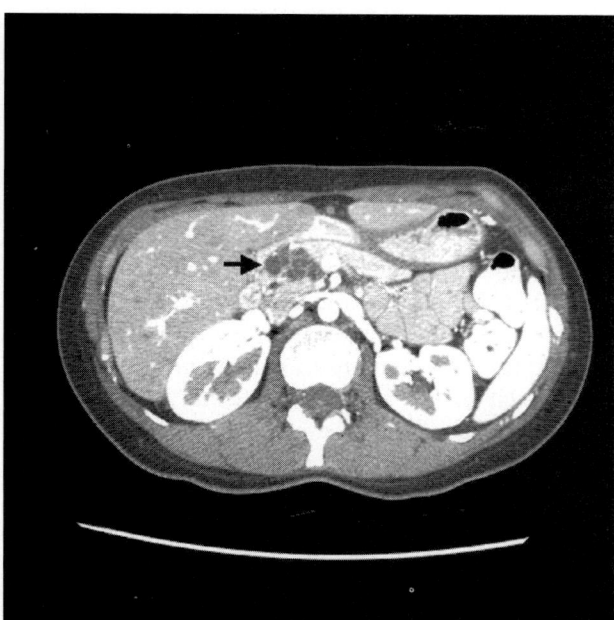

Figure 2 CT image of a patient with a microcystic serous cystadenoma. A multiloculated cystic lesion is demonstrated in the head of the pancreas (arrow). The radiographic differential diagnosis includes microcystic serous cystadenoma, mucinous cystic neoplasm, and intraductal papillary mucinous neoplasm. Endoscopic ultrasound-guided cyst fluid analysis revealed scant mucin and ductal epithelial cells; fluid analysis for amylase and CEA was not performed. Pylorus-preserving pancreatectomy revealed a microcystic serous cystadenoma.

patients for resection over observation. Patients with a tumor size larger than 4 cm appear to be more likely to be symptomatic and to display a more rapid growth rate compared with patients with tumors less than 4 cm.[11] Relatively small, asymptomatic and radiographically typical serous cystadenomas may safely be observed.

LYMPHEPITHELIAL CYSTS

Lymphepithelial cysts of the pancreas are rare lesions that may be identified incidentally or in patients presenting with abdominal pain.[12,13] Radiographic features classically demonstrate a unilocular cystic mass that extends beyond the surface of the pancreas. Lymphoepithelial cysts are benign lesions composed of squamous epithelium surrounded by lymphoid tissue. Conservative excision, sparing pancreatic parenchyma, may be considered when the diagnosis is suggested by the clinical, radiographic, and intraoperative findings.[13]

SOLID PSEUDOPAPILLARY TUMORS

Solid pseudopapillary tumors are predominantly identified in young women who present with abdominal pain. These tumors are characteristically large, well demar-

cated, hypervascular, and composed of both solid and macrocystic components containing degenerated tumor and blood. These are indolent tumors that carry a low potential for malignancy. Occasional patients present with established metastatic disease, usually involving the liver. Even in patients with metastatic spread, long-term survival has been reported.[14,15] Resection is recommended for localized solid pseudopapillary tumors, and may also be indicated in selected patients when limited metastatic disease is present.

MUCINOUS CYSTIC NEOPLASMS (MCNS)

MCNs are usually found in the body or tail of the pancreas; the peak incidence occurs in patients in their early 50s. More than 50% of patients present with vague abdominal pain. A history of pancreatitis has been reported in up to 20% of patients. MCNs are the most common cystic neoplasms of the pancreas; histologically, these lesions may be benign (Figure 3), preinvasive but malignant, or invasive (Figure 4).[16,17] This variability in histology highlights the difficulty in excluding the presence of malignancy preoperatively in patients with such tumors. Radiographically, these tumors appear as a

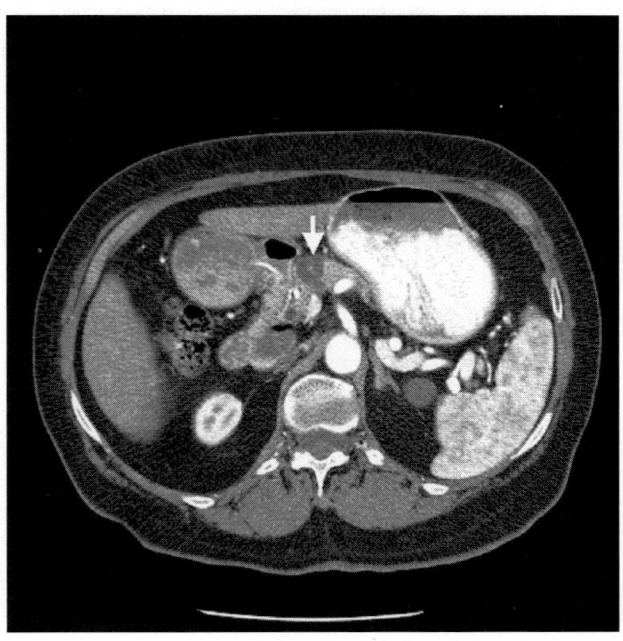

Figure 3 CT Image of a patient with a mucinous cystic neoplasm. There is a complex cystic structure involving the neck of the pancreas; the image is consistent with, but not diagnostic of, a mucinous cystic neoplasm (arrow). Endoscopic ultrasound-guided biopsy revealed gross mucin, cytology revealed a few atypical cells, and fluid analysis revealed a CEA of 430.7 ng/mL; cyst fluid analysis for amylase was not performed. Pylorus-preserving pancreatectomy revealed a mucinous cystic lesion with low-grade dysplasia.

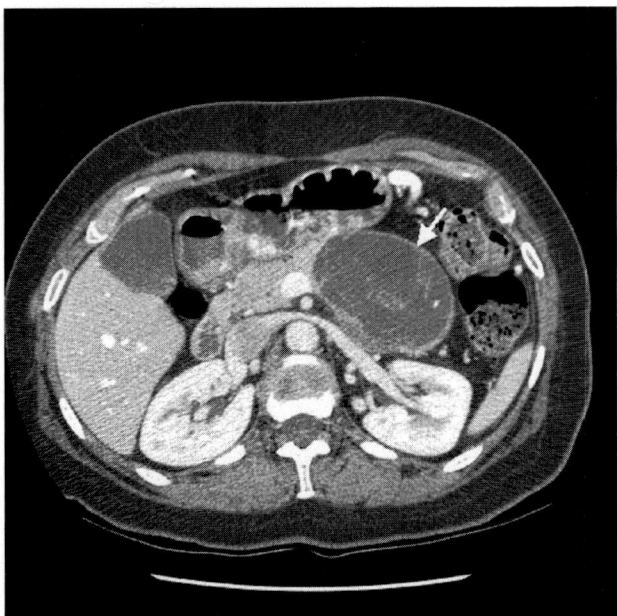

Figure 4 CT image of a patient with a mucinous cystadenocarcinoma. This image demonstrates a complex macrocystic mass containing septations and foci of calcifications (arrow). The tumor process has resulted in thrombosis of the splenic vein. The radiographic picture is consistent with a mucincous cystadenocarcinoma. Endoscopic ultrasound-guided biopsy revealed mucin and glandular epithelium consistent with a mucinous cystic neoplasm without evidence for carcinoma. Cyst fluid analysis revealed an amylase of less than 26 IU/L; cyst fluid analysis for CEA was not performed. Distal pancreatectomy and splenectomy revealed an invasive, poorly differentiated mucinous cystadenocarcinoma arising in a mucinous cystic neoplasm with associated low- and high-grade dysplasia.

solitary unilocular or multilocular cysts; loculations are characteristically larger and fewer in number than those seen in patients with serous tumors. A rim of calcification may be present around the MCN and suggests malignancy. Cyst fluid analysis typically reveals a high CEA and a low amylase level. The presence of an ovarian-type stroma and the absence of cyst communication with the pancreatic duct distinguish these tumors from intraductal papillary mucinous neoplasms (IPMN).[18,19] All MCNs are considered potentially malignant tumors, and therefore pancreatic resection is the standard treatment. Observation rather than resection is reasonable in selected patients with advanced age or severe medical comorbidities, especially when the suspected or confirmed MCN is asymptomatic, small (< 2 cm), and lacks a solid component or rim calcification, suggesting it is a noninvasive tumor. Patients with resected, invasive MCNs may exhibit a more favorable prognosis when

compared with patients with pancreatic ductal adeno-carcinoma.[20]

INTRADUCTAL PAPILLARY MUCINOUS NEOPLASMS (IPMNS)

IPMNs have also been identified as mucin-secreting carcinomas, villous adenomas of the Wirsung's duct, diffuse intraductal papillary adenocarcinomas, intraductal cystadenomas, and mucinous duct ectasia. IPMNs demonstrate a wide spectrum of epithelial changes, ranging from adenoma to carcinoma in situ to invasive adenocarcinoma.[21–27] Patients with IPMN typically present in their sixth to seventh decade of life; patients with malignant IPMNs are on average 6 years older than patients with adenomas or borderline lesions.[28,29] Approximately 50% of patients with IPMN present with abdominal pain; acute pancreatitis has been reported in up to 20%. A sizeable fraction of patients with IPMN are asymptomatic. Characteristic radiographic features of IPMN include a dilated pancreatic duct with associated macroscopic cysts of varying sizes (Figure 5). The multiplicity of cysts, cyst communication with the pancreatic duct, and the associated dilatation of the pancreatic duct can distinguish IPMN from MCN. EUS, ERCP, and magnetic resonance cholangiopancreatography (MRCP) are often helpful in the evaluation of patients with suspected IPMN; these studies help identify mural nodules and assist in pretreatment differentiation of main duct from branch-duct IPMN (which may have a less aggressive clinical behavior).[30,31] At the time of ERCP, the finding of thick, viscid mucin oozing from a patulous Vater's ampulla is characteristic of IPMN. Results of cyst fluid analysis are similar to those seen in MCNs. Pancreatectomy is generally recommended for patients with main-duct IPMN or large (> 3 cm) or symptomatic branch-duct IPMN. A recent consensus conference has recommended observation for patients with asymptomatic, small (< 3 cm) branch-duct IPMN without associated nodularity.[32] Surveillance rather than immediate resection in such patients is reasonable, as the risk of malignancy appears to be low, and most patients are elderly; the time required to develop invasive malignancy is often longer than the patient's life expectancy.[31] We favor partial over total pancreatectomy when anatomically feasible. We discuss the management of the pancreatic margin with the IPMN patient preoperatively and advise them that approximately 15% of patients require total pancreatectomy to achieve a negative parenchymal resection margin. We assess the surgical margin in patients with IPMN intraoperatively with frozen section; additional margins are obtained if carcinomas in situ or invasive cancer is identified at the

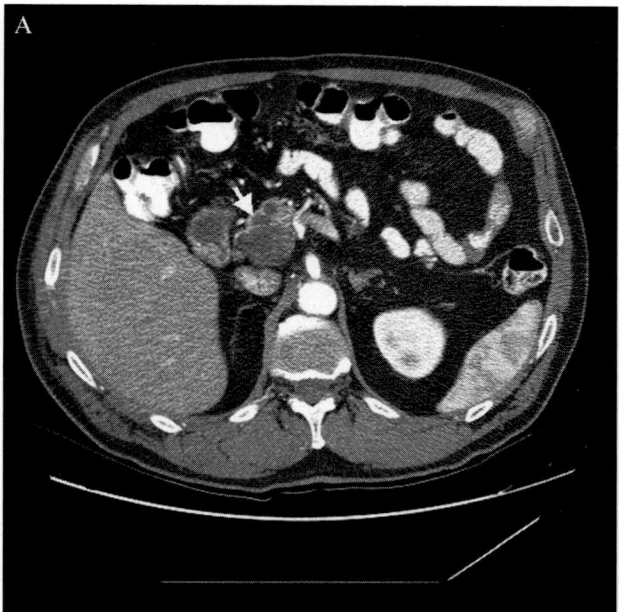
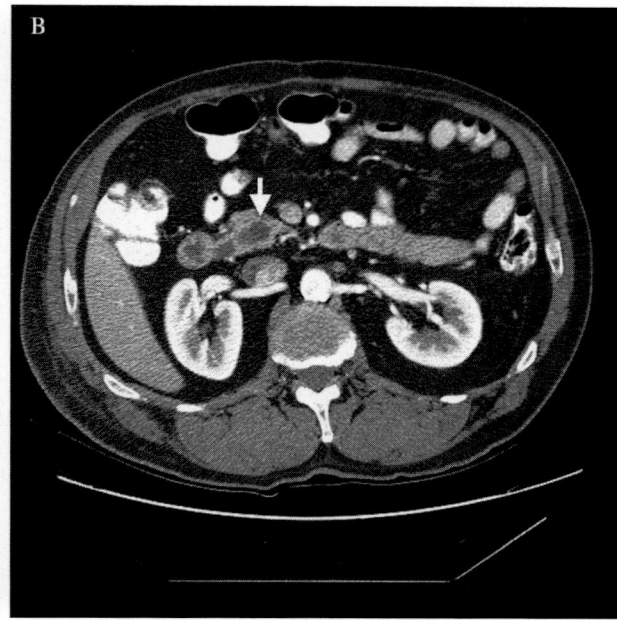

Figure 5 CT images of a patient with an intraductal papillary mucinous neoplasm (IPMN). *A*, cystic component (arrow); *B*, duct ectasia component (arrow). The appearance of the CT images is characteristic, but not diagnostic, of main-duct IPMN. Endoscopic ultrasound-guided cytology revealed a mucinous neoplasm; fluid analysis for amylase and CEA was not performed. Pancreatectomy revealed a noninvasive IPMN.

margin. Survival of patients with resected, invasive IPMN is generally better than for patients with ductal adenocarcinoma of the pancreas, at least when regional lymph nodes are uninvolved.[28,29,33]

CYSTIC DUCTAL ADENOCARCINOMAS

Cystic ductal adenocarcinomas are uncommon variants of ductal adenocarcinoma of the pancreas. Presentation, evaluation, staging, treatment, and prognosis are the same as for the more common type of pancreatic adenocarcinoma, except that the cystic component of the tumor may make the cystic variant easier to confuse clinically and radiographically with a pancreatic pseudocyst, especially if the solid component of the tumor is not evident on cross-sectional imaging (Figure 6). Treatment includes surgical resection in the absence of distant metastatic disease for patients without major vascular involvement. As for patients with solid ductal adenocarcinoma, we consider patients with cystic ductal adenocarcinoma candidates for segmental venous resection and reconstruction when vascular involvement is limited to the superior mesenteric vein-portal vein confluence (see Figure 6).[34]

ACINAR CELL CYSTADENOCARCINOMAS

Acinar cell cystadenocarcinomas are uncommon variants of acinar cell adenocarcinoma of the pancreas. Patients with acinar cell adenocarcinomas occasionally present

with subcutaneous fat necrosis related to an elevated serum lipase level; the serum alpha-fetoprotein level may also be elevated.[35] The prognosis of patients with this type of pancreatic adenocarcinoma appears to be slightly better than that of patients with the more common ductal adenocarcinoma of the pancreas.[35,36] Treatment is identical to solid acinar cell adenocarcinoma, and includes surgical resection when technically possible in patients without metastatic disease.

CYSTIC NEUROENDOCRINE TUMORS

Cystic neuroendocrine tumors are an uncommon variant of pancreatic neuroendocrine tumors (PNET). Patients may present with signs and symptoms related to a mass lesion (eg, jaundice), hormone overproduction (eg, insulin), or the tumors may be discovered incidentally (nonfunctioning tumors).[37–41] Aside from the cystic component, the radiographic features can resemble those of other neuroendocrine tumors, with contrast enhancement and calcifications (Figure 7). Cyst fluid analysis demonstrates a low CEA, variable amylase, and nonviscous fluid. Hormone markers in the cyst fluid may be elevated (eg, insulin). Cytology demonstrates neuroendocrine epithelial cells; chromogranin and synaptophysin staining can help distinguish these cells histologically. These tumors are considered malignant or potentially malignant. Prognosis for patients with pancreatic neuroendocrine carcinoma is better than for similar-stage

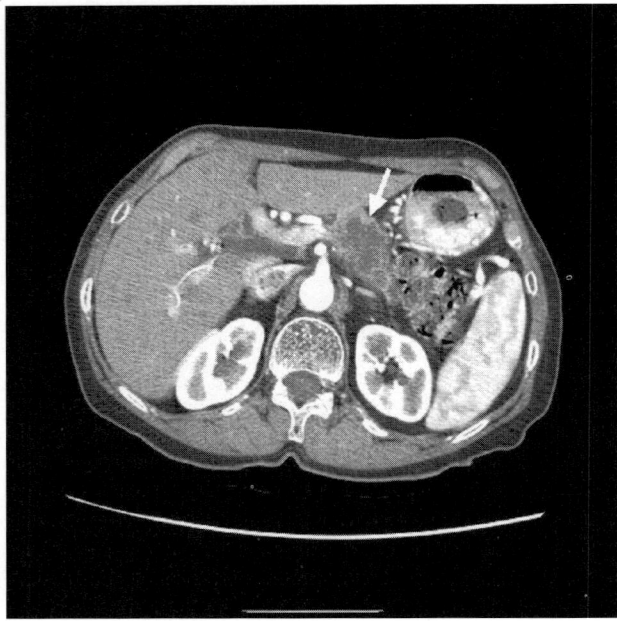

Figure 6 CT image of a patient with ductal adenocarcinoma of the pancreas with associated cystic degeneration. The image demonstrates a hypodense mass in the body of the pancreas with associated cystic change (arrow). The pancreatic tail is atrophied. The tumor abuts the superior mesenteric vein-portal vein confluence (SMV-PV). The differential diagnosis based on these images includes mucinous cystic neoplasm and pancreatic adenocarcinoma with cystic degeneration. No preoperative biopsy was performed. Resection of the tumor was performed via distal subtotal pancreatectomy and splenectomy. Segmental resection and reconstruction of the SMV-PV via direct anastamosis was required because of direct tumor invasion of this structure. Final pathology revealed an infiltrating moderately to poorly differentiated ductal adenocarcinoma of the pancreas.

patients with ductal adenocarcinoma of the pancreas.[42] Resection is recommended for patients with localized tumors that do not involve major vascular structures. Resection is generally not recommended for patients with established distant metastatic disease, but may be considered in highly selected patients with low-volume distant disease when combined resection of the primary and the metastasis can be performed, or when the patient has symptoms related to their primary tumor (hormone production, bleeding, or obstruction).

Patient Evaluation

A thorough history and physical examination are performed in all patients, with special attention to risk factors of pancreatitis (alcohol abuse, cholelithiasis, family history, dyslipidemia) or a pancreatic tumor process (smoking, obesity, family history suggesting multiple endocrine neoplasia). Bloodwork should include evaluation for amylase, lipase, CEA, and carbohydrate antigen (CA) 19-9. In selected patients with clinical or radiographic features suggesting PNET, preoperative hormone evaluation should include measurement of serum pancreatic neuroendocrine markers (pancreatic polypeptide, chromogranin, insulin, gastrin, glucagon, somatostatin, vasoactive intestinal peptide, neurotensin). Because these tumors frequently occur in patients of relatively advanced age, attention to comorbidity is essential, and frequently guides the surgeon in deciding the extent of evaluation indicated, the decision for operation versus observation, and the follow-up interval.

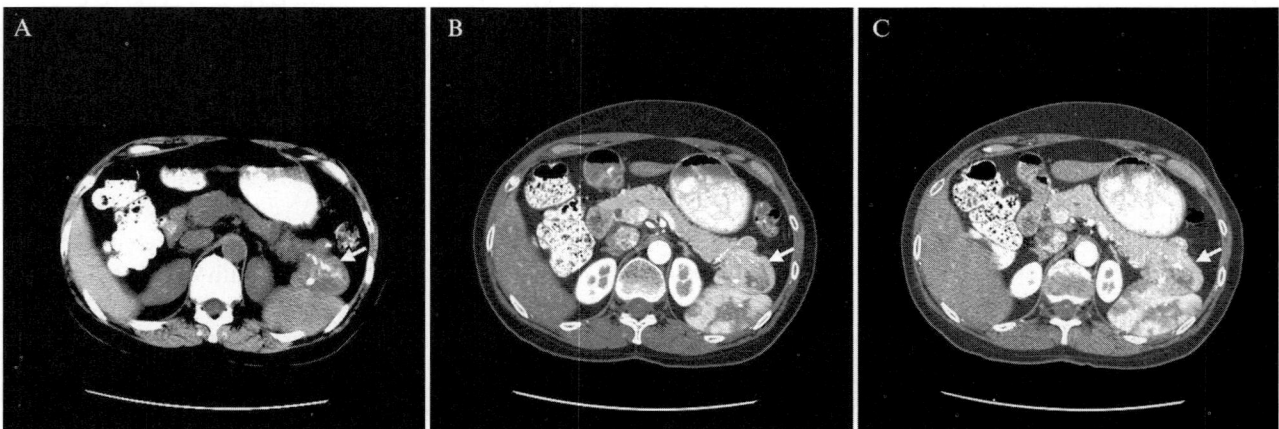

Figure 7 CT images of a patient with a nonfunctioning pancreatic neuroendocrine tumor with cystic degeneration. *A*, precontrast; *B*, arterial phase; *C*, venous phase. These images demonstrate a heterogenous, partially cystic mass in the tail of the pancreas that contains calcifications and enhances with intravenous contrast (arrows). These findings are consistent with pancreatic neuroendocrine tumor. Distal pancreatectomy with splenectomy confirmed this diagnosis.

Imaging

Preoperative evaluation in all patients includes high-quality CT of the abdomen. The development of multislice or multidetector CT allows imaging of the entire pancreas during peak contrast enhancement. In addition, scan data can be processed to display images in three-dimensional and multiplanar formats. Helical CT performed with contrast enhancement and a thin-section technique can accurately assess details of the cystic structure of the tumor, identify solid components of the tumor, reveal communication of the cyst with the pancreatic duct, accurately assess resectability, and screen for the presence of intra-abdominal metastatic disease. Magnetic resonance imaging (MRI) and MRCP can be helpful in selected patients with IPMN in delineating the anatomy of the cystic tumor within the pancreas, as described above.

Role of Upper Endoscopy with Ultrasound and Cyst Aspiration

EUS with or without cyst aspiration is a useful diagnostic tool in patients with cystic tumors of the pancreas, and is complementary to CT imaging. EUS can identify details of cyst structure, cyst communication with the pancreatic duct, the presence of associated pancreatic parenchymal changes (solid tumor component, pancreatitis), the extent of the process within the pancreas, the relationship of the primary tumor to critical vascular structures, and the presence of regional lymphadenopathy.[43] EUS-guided cyst aspiration for biochemical analysis and cytology is used selectively. It can be helpful in situations in which the clinical and radiographic picture is atypical, and when findings suggesting a benign process (pseudocyst, serous tumor) would result in a decision for observation rather than surgical resection. Cyst aspiration is not necessary if the biopsy results will not influence the resulting treatment plan. The results of cyst aspiration must be interpreted with caution; whereas the finding of abundant mucin on cyst aspiration has been considered diagnostic for a mucinous neoplasm, scant mucin suggests contamination carried into the EUS aspiration biopsy specimen from the wall of the gastrointestinal tract.[44] In addition, cyst fluid biochemical analysis can sometimes be misleading. A recent cooperative study found cyst fluid CEA (with a cutoff of 192 ng/mL) to be the best single tumor marker distinguishing mucinous from nonmucinous cystic pancreatic lesions.[6] When possible, upper endoscopy, EUS, and cyst aspiration should always be performed after CT, because if EUS-guided biopsy-induced pancreatitis occurs, it may interfere with accurate assessment of the tumor process and extent of disease.

Extent of Preoperative Evaluation and Patient Selection for Surgery

When a diagnosis is confirmed preoperatively by a combination of the clinical presentation, the radiographic features, and the results of EUS with cyst aspiration (if performed), the decision for surgical resection versus observation in an individual patient can be based on the considerations outlined above for the individual tumor types. However, results of evaluation in many patients are indeterminate. Furthermore, surgeons evaluating patients with cystic processes in the pancreas may elect not to perform cyst aspiration if the results are likely to be unreliable or unlikely to influence treatment recommendations. For example, cyst aspiration may be unreliable for very small cysts (1 cm or less), and a small cyst (even a small MCN) is unlikely to represent a malignant process if there is not an associated solid component. Additionally, it is reasonable to adopt a policy of observation rather than surgery for patients of advanced age or significant comorbidity and cysts without features suggestive of malignancy that are identified incidentally. Finally, surgery can be recommended to relatively young healthy patients without cyst aspiration when the clinical features demand treatment for symptoms, or the radiographic picture is characteristic (large serous cyst, MCN, cystic neuroendocrine tumor) (see Figure 7).

Operative Technique

A segmental pancreatic resection of the head, body, or tail of the pancreas represents the most appropriate strategy for most patients chosen for surgical treatment and is favored over enucleation for almost all tumors.[2] Pancreaticoduodenectomy (Whipple) is the appropriate resection strategy for most patients with cystic tumors involving the head and uncinate process of the pancreas. We currently perform a pylorus-preserving procedure in most patients when technically possible.[45] Pylorus preservation is not performed for bulky tumors of the pancreatic head, or if there are associated grossly positive pyloric or peripyloric lymph nodes; these situations are uncommon in patients with cystic tumors. Preservation of the antropyloric pump mechanism may result in improved long-term upper gastrointestinal tract function with enhanced weight gain and fewer nutritional sequelae. These long-term advantages come at the expense of an increased incidence of early postoperative delayed gastric emptying.[46] Surgeons performing a pylorus-preserving procedure must be careful to preserve sufficient blood supply to the proximal duodenum as well as vagal innervation to the antrum and pylorus;

caution must be exercised during the portal dissection to avoid unnecessary injury to the Latarjet's nerve. This is essential to minimize postoperative gastroparesis.

When dealing with cystic tumors involving the pancreatic neck, surgeons should be mindful that preservation of islet cell function in patients with benign or low-grade tumors is particularly important in younger individuals who have a relatively long life expectancy. When a tumor arises in the pancreatic neck or proximal body of the pancreas, a subtotal distal pancreatectomy may leave only a small portion of pancreatic head and uncinate process; the patient may not have adequate islet cell mass for normal glucose metabolism, and therefore may require insulin injections. Therefore, in patients with cystic tumors of the pancreatic neck with relatively favorable histology (eg, neuroendocrine tumor, serous cystic neoplasm, MCN), segmental resection of the pancreatic neck with preservation of the splenic artery and vein (when possible) is preferred to ensure adequate islet cell reserve.[47,48] Reconstruction requires Roux-en-Y pancreaticojejunostomy to the remaining segment of distal pancreas.

Distal pancreatectomy can often be performed with splenic preservation in patients with relatively small, histologically favorable cystic tumors. Following distal pancreatic resection, it is important that the transected pancreatic duct be identified and suture ligated to minimize the risk of postoperative pancreatic leak.[49] Spleen-preserving distal pancreatectomy for cystic neoplasms has been reported, and represents an alternative surgical approach for highly selected patients.[50]

Postoperative Management and Complications

As with all complex surgery, a good outcome after pancreatectomy for cystic neoplasms of the pancreas depends in part on meticulous postoperative care. We no longer routinely place intra-abdominal drains, feeding tubes, or gastrostomy tubes in patients at the time of pancreatectomy. Postoperative fevers occurring after postoperative days 3 to 4 in patients who have undergone pancreatectomy demand careful evaluation. Potential sources of fever include those common to all major abdominal surgery (pneumonia, deep venous thrombosis, central line sepsis, urinary tract infection, and wound infection); patients who undergo pancreatic resection are also at risk of the development of intra-abdominal abscess as a result of leakage from the pancreatic anastomosis (pancreaticoduodenectomy, central pancreatectomy) or pancreatic stump closure (central or distal pancreatectomy). Intra-abdominal sepsis in a postoperative pancreatectomy patient is considered to be due to a pancreatic leak until proven otherwise. The study of choice for evaluation of presumed intra-abdominal sepsis following pancreatectomy is CT of the abdomen and pelvis with oral and intavenous administration of contrast material. Patients found to have a localized fluid collection in the region of pancreatic resection should be considered for CT-guided aspiration and drainage.

Adjuvant Therapy and Follow-Up Evaluation

For patients who undergo surgical resection of cystic pancreatic tumors, postoperative restaging and follow-up evaluation is based on the histopathologic findings. Patients with resected cystic pancreatic carcinoma (mucinous cystadenocarcinoma, ductal adenocarcinoma, acinar cell adenocarcinoma, or neuroendocrine carcinoma) should undergo regular clinical and radiographic reevaluation and follow-up similar to that recommended to patients with the solid varieties of these cancers.[51] Although there is no single standard adjuvant therapy yet available for patients with any type of pancreatic cancer, patients with cystic adenocarcinoma in particular are eligible for consideration for protocol-based and off-protocol systemic adjuvant therapy.[52] Off-protocol recommendations for adjuvant local-regional radiation therapy in such patients must be individualized. Patients with resected benign cystic pancreatic tumors do not need follow-up restaging CT imaging, except in the case of patients with IPMN; even in the setting of an uninvolved pancreatic transaction margin and a radiographically normal residual pancreas, patients with resected IPMN are at life-long risk for the development of additional lesions within the remaining pancreas.[22,25,28,53] Interval annual CT imaging is therefore indicated.

For patients selected for observation rather than surgical resection, interval reimaging is indicated. Although appropriate repeat imaging intervals for a patient with an indeterminate lesion, a small MCN, or side-branch IPMN have not been established, it is reasonable to repeat an initial imaging study in such a patient in 6 months, and then perform annual reimaging. Because the growth rate of serous cystadenomas is low (median 6 mm per year), follow-up imaging in such patients can be limited to every 1 to 2 years.[11]

Summary and Conclusions

Patients with cystic tumors of the pancreas present unique diagnostic and treatment challenges. Optimal evaluation of patients with these tumors integrates information from the patient's clinical presentation with results of an individualized diagnostic strategy that includes high-quality abdominal imaging in all patients. Surgical resection is indicated for patients with documented or suspected localized malignant and premalignant cystic tumors. Total pancreatectomy is avoided when possible. In contrast, patients with benign, asymptomatic lesions are candidates for observation without immediate resection, and selected patients with indeterminate lesions may also be observed.

References

1. Fernandez-del Castillo C, Targarona J, Thayer SP, et al. Incidental pancreatic cysts: clinicopathologic characteristics and comparison with symptomatic patients. Arch Surg 2003;138:427–4.

2. Pyke CM, van Heerden JA, Colby TV, et al. The spectrum of serous cystadenoma of the pancreas. Clinical, pathologic, and surgical aspects. Ann Surg 1992;215:132–9.

3. Lewandrowski KB, Southern JF, Pins MR, et al. Cyst fluid analysis in the differential diagnosis of pancreatic cysts. A comparison of pseudocysts, serous cystadenomas, mucinous cystic neoplasms, and mucinous cystadenocarcinoma. Ann Surg 1993;217:41–7.

4. Hammel P, Levy P, Voitot H, et al. Preoperative cyst fluid analysis is useful for the differential diagnosis of cystic lesions of the pancreas. Gastroenterology 1995;108:1230–5.

5. Pinto MM, Meriano FV. Diagnosis of cystic pancreatic lesions by cytologic examination and carcinoembryonic antigen and amylase assays of cyst contents. Acta Cytol 1991;35:456–63.

6. Brugge WR, Lewandrowski K, Lee-Lewandrowski E, et al. Diagnosis of pancreatic cystic neoplasms: a report of the cooperative pancreatic cyst study. Gastroenterology 2004;126:1330–6.

7. Yoshimi N, Sugie S, Tanaka T, et al. A rare case of serous cystadenocarcinoma of the pancreas. Cancer 1992;69:2449–53.

8. Bassi C, Salvia R, Molinari E, et al. Management of 100 consecutive cases of pancreatic serous cystadenoma: wait for symptoms and see at imaging or vice versa? World J Surg 2003;27:319–23.

9. Matsumoto T, Hirano S, Yada K, et al. Malignant serous cystic neoplasm of the pancreas: report of a case and review of the literature. J Clin Gastroenterol 2005;39:253–6.

10. Strobel O, Z'Graggen K, Schmitz-Winnenthal FH, et al. Risk of malignancy in serous cystic neoplasms of the pancreas. Digestion 2003;68:24–33.

11. Tseng JF, Warshaw AL, Sahani DV, et al. Serous cystadenoma of the pancreas: tumor growth rates and recommendations for treatment. Ann Surg 2005;242:413–21.

12. Adsay NV, Hasteh F, Cheng JD, et al. Lymphoepithelial cysts of the pancreas: a report of 12 cases and a review of the literature. Mod Pathol 2002;15:492–501.

13. Truong LD, Stewart MG, Hao H, et al. A comprehensive characterization of lymphoepithelial cyst associated with the pancreas. Am J Surg 1995;170:27–32.

14. Papavramidis T, Papavramidis S. Solid pseudopapillary tumors of the pancreas: review of 718 patients reported in English literature. J Am Coll Surg 2005;200:965–72.

15. Klimstra DS, Wenig BM, Heffess CS. Solid-pseudopapillary tumor of the pancreas: a typically cystic carcinoma of low malignant potential. Semin Diagn Pathol 2000;17:66–80.

16. Compagno J, Oertel JE. Microcystic adenomas of the pancreas (glycogen-rich cystadenomas): a clinicopathologic study of 34 cases. Am J Clin Pathol 1978;69:289–98.

17. Sarr MG, Carpenter HA, Prabhakar LP, et al. Clinical and pathologic correlation of 84 mucinous cystic neoplasms of the pancreas: can one reliably differentiate benign from malignant (or premalignant) neoplasms? Ann Surg 2000;231:205–12.

18. Thompson LD, Becker RC, Przygodzki RM, et al. Mucinous cystic neoplasm (mucinous cystadenocarcinoma of low-grade malignant potential) of the pancreas: a clinicopathologic study of 130 cases. Am J Surg Pathol 1999;23:1–16.

19. Zamboni G, Scarpa A, Bogina G, et al. Mucinous cystic tumors of the pancreas: clinicopathological features, prognosis, and relationship to other mucinous cystic tumors. Am J Surg Pathol 1999;23:410–22.

20. Wilentz RE, Albores-Saavedra J, Zahurak M, et al. Pathologic examination accurately predicts prognosis in mucinous cystic neoplasms of the pancreas. Am J Surg Pathol 1999;23:1320–7.

21. Sohn TA, Yeo CJ, Cameron JL, et al. Intraductal papillary mucinous neoplasms of the pancreas: an increasingly recognized clinicopathologic entity. Ann Surg 2001;234:313–22.

22. Falconi M, Salvia R, Bassi C, et al. Clinicopathological features and treatment of intraductal papillary mucinous tumour of the pancreas. Br J Surg 2001;88:376–81.

23. Jang JY, Kim SW, Ahn YJ, et al. Multicenter analysis of clinicopathologic features of intraductal papillary mucinous tumor of the pancreas: is it possible to predict the malignancy before surgery? Ann Surg Oncol 2005;12:124–32.

24. Rivera JA, Fernandez-del Castillo C, Pins M, et al. Pancreatic mucinous ductal ectasia and intraductal papillary neoplasms. A single malignant clinicopathologic entity. Ann Surg 1997;225:637–46.

25. Shimamura H, Furukawa T, Kodama T, et al. Mucin-producing tumor of the pancreas—surgical treatment. J Hepatobiliary Pancreat Surg 1997;4:168–72.

26. D'Angelica M, Brennan MF, Suriawinata AA, et al. Intraductal papillary mucinous neoplasms of the pancreas: an analysis of clinicopathologic features and outcome. Ann Surg 2004;239:400–8.

27. Wada K, Kozarek RA, Traverso WL. Outcomes following resection of invasive and noninvasive intraductal papillary mucinous neoplasms of the pancreas. Am J Surg 2005;189:632–7.

28. Sohn TA, Yeo CJ, Cameron JL, et al. Intraductal papillary mucinous neoplasms of the pancreas: an updated experience. Ann Surg 2004;239:788–99.

29. Salvia R, Fernandez-del Castillo C, Bassi C, et al. Main-duct intraductal papillary mucinous neoplasms of the pancreas: clinical predictors of malignancy and long-term survival following resection. Ann Surg 2004;239:678–87.

30. Tanaka M, Kobayashi K, Mizumoto K, et al. Clinical aspects of intraductal papillary mucinous neoplasm of the pancreas. J Gastroenterol 2005;40:669–75.

31. Terris B, Ponsot P, Paye F, et al. Intraductal papillary mucinous tumors of the pancreas confined to secondary ducts show less aggressive pathologic features as compared with those involving the main pancreatic duct. Am J Surg Pathol 2000;24:1372–7.

32. Tanaka M, Chari S, Adsay V, et al. International consensus guidelines for management of intraductal papillary mucinous neoplasms and mucinous cystic neoplasms of the pancreas. Pancreatology 2005;6:17–32.

33. Maire F, Hammel P, Terris B, et al. Prognosis of malignant intraductal papillary mucinous tumours of the pancreas after surgical resection. Comparison with pancreatic ductal adenocarcinoma. Gut 2002;51:717–22.

34. Tseng JF, Raut CP, Lee JE, et al. Pancreaticoduodenectomy with vascular resection: margin status and survival duration. J Gastrointest Surg 2004;8:935–50.

35. Klimstra DS, Heffess CS, Oertel JE, et al. Acinar cell carcinoma of the pancreas. A clinicopathologic study of 28 cases. Am J Surg Pathol 1992;16:815–37.

36. Holen KD, Klimstra DS, Hummer A, et al. Clinical characteristics and outcomes from an institutional series of acinar cell carcinoma of the pancreas and related tumors. J Clin Oncol 2002;20:4673–8.

37. Schwartz RW, Munfakh NA, Zweng TN, et al. Nonfunctioning cystic neuroendocrine neoplasms of the pancreas. Surgery 1994;115:645–9.

38. Weissmann D, Lewandrowski K, Godine J, et al. Pancreatic cystic islet-cell tumors. Clinical and pathologic features in two cases with cyst fluid analysis. Int J Pancreatol 1994;15:75–9.

39. Ahrendt SA, Komorowski RA, Demeure MJ, et al. Cystic pancreatic neuroendocrine tumors: is preoperative diagnosis possible? J Gastrointest Surg 2002;6:66–74.

40. Thompson NW, Eckhauser FE, Vinik AI, et al. Cystic neuroendocrine neoplasms of the pancreas and liver. Ann Surg 1984;199:158–64.

41. Iacono C, Serio G, Fugazzola C, et al. Cystic islet cell tumors of the pancreas. A clinico-pathological report of two nonfunctioning cases and review of the literature. Int J Pancreatol 1992;11:199–208.

42. Solorzano CC, Lee JE, Pisters PW, et al. Nonfunctioning islet cell carcinoma of the pancreas: survival results in a contemporary series of 163 patients. Surgery 2001;130:1078–85.

43. Cellier C, Cuillerier E, Palazzo L, et al. Intraductal papillary and mucinous tumors of the pancreas: accuracy of preoperative computed tomography, endoscopic retrograde pancreatography and endoscopic ultrasonography, and long-term outcome in a large surgical series. Gastrointest Endosc 1998;47:42–9.

44. Stelow EB, Bardales RH, Stanley MW. Pitfalls in endoscopic ultrasound-guided fine-needle aspiration and how to avoid them. Adv Anat Pathol 2005;12:62–73.

45. Traverso LW, Longmire WP Jr. Preservation of the pylorus in pancreaticoduodenectomy a follow-up evaluation. Ann Surg 1980;192:306–10.

46. Lin PW, Lin YJ. Prospective randomized comparison between pylorus-preserving and standard pancreaticoduodenectomy. Br J Surg 1999;86:603–7.

47. Warshaw AL, Rattner DW, Fernandez-del Castillo C, et al. Middle segment pancreatectomy: a novel technique for conserving pancreatic tissue. Arch Surg 1998;133:327–31.

48. Efron DT, Lillemoe KD, Cameron JL, et al. Central pancreatectomy with pancreaticogastrostomy for benign pancreatic pathology. J Gastrointest Surg 2004;8:532–8.

49. Bilimoria MM, Cormier JN, Mun Y, et al. Pancreatic leak after left pancreatectomy is reduced following main pancreatic duct ligation. Br J Surg 2003;90:190–6.

50. Fernandez-Cruz L, Martinez I, Gilabert R, et al. Laparoscopic distal pancreatectomy combined with preservation of the spleen for cystic neoplasms of the pancreas. J Gastrointest Surg 2004;8:493–501.

51. Tamm EP, Silverman PM, Charnsangavej C, et al. Diagnosis, staging, and surveillance of pancreatic cancer. AJR Am J Roentgenol 2003;180:1311–23.

52. Pisters PW, Wolff RA, Crane CH, et al. Combined-modality treatment for operable pancreatic adenocarcinoma. Oncology (Williston Park) 2005;19:393–404, 409–10, 412–6.

53. Chari ST, Yadav D, Smyrk TC, et al. Study of recurrence after surgical resection of intraductal papillary mucinous neoplasm of the pancreas. Gastroenterology 2002;123:1500–7.

CHAPTER 23

CHEMORADIATION FOR LOCALIZED PANCREATIC CANCER

CHRISTOPHER H. CRANE, MD

MARC E. DELCLOS, MD

Introduction

Pancreatic cancers (adenocarcinomas) are typically resistant to the effects of chemotherapy and radiotherapy. The median survival is usually less than 1 year from the time of diagnosis owing to high rates of local and distant progression. Most patients who present with pancreatic cancer have some combination of host-related factors, such as advanced age, poor performance status, and medical comorbidities; and tumor-related factors, such as anorexia or exocrine insufficiency, which make them relatively poor candidates for aggressive therapy. The challenge for clinicians who care for these patients is to use therapies that address the pattern of disease recurrence without causing a significant negative impact on quality of life. Although significant limitations remain, the use of novel chemotherapeutic agents and targeted molecular therapies that selectively enhance the effects of radiotherapy and chemotherapy seem to be the most promising avenue of clinical research in this disease. Fortunately, investigators have placed more emphasis on pancreatic cancer in recent years than in the past, and clinical trials of novel treatments are ongoing. It is hoped that these efforts will lead to gradual improvements in outcome for patients with pancreatic cancer. In this chapter, the principles surrounding the dose and technique of radiotherapy for pancreatic cancer will be discussed for both locally advanced and resectable disease.

Diagnosis, Staging, and Initial Management of Pancreatic Adenocarcinoma

The issues surrounding diagnosis, staging, and initial management of pancreatic cancer are addressed elsewhere in this book, and so are only summarized here. The initial goals in the evaluation and treatment of symptomatic patients are to determine resectability, establish a histologic diagnosis, and reestablish biliary tract outflow. Pancreatic cancer is diagnosed, clinically evaluated, and managed differently from center to center in the United States, and the definition of resectability after clinical evaluation varies from surgeon to surgeon.

The various diagnostic approaches include preoperative imaging; laparoscopy, or laparotomy; and attempted resection. Abdominal computed tomography (CT) is the most common diagnostic imaging technique used to determine the stage of suspected pancreatic malignancies. In many centers, endoscopic ultrasonographically guided fine-needle biopsy of the pancreas is the procedure of choice for the diagnosis of pancreatic malignancies. Biliary outflow can be reestablished with the endoscopic placement of an endobiliary stent in most patients.

Determining resectability is the most important aspect of clinical staging. Changes in the most recent American Joint Committee on Cancer staging system for exocrine pancreatic cancer reflect a clinical definition of resectability based on CT assessment. The T-stage designation classifies T1 through T3 tumors as potentially resectable and T4 tumors as locally advanced (unresectable). Tumors with any involvement of the superior mesenteric artery (SMA) or celiac artery are classified as T4; however, tumors that involve the superior mesenteric, splenic, or portal veins are classified as T3, since these veins can be resected and reconstructed provided that they are patent.[1] Therefore, three criteria are necessary for resectability: (1) localized disease only, (2) lack of involvement of the celiac axis or superior mesenteric artery, and (3) patency of the superior mesenteric/portal venous confluence.

Chemoradiation as a Component of Multidisciplinary Management

Chemoradiation appears to improve median survival duration modestly in both resectable and locally advanced disease. However, the impact of surgical resection, adjuvant locoregional therapy, and definitive nonsurgical local therapy is limited by the competing high risk of the development of distant metastatic disease in pancreatic cancer patients. Chemoradiation is an important component of therapy for locally advanced disease, but even if chemoradiation were as effective as surgery for resectable disease, the development of distant metastatic disease would still undermine its impact on survival. In fact, studies that have attempted to increase the radiotherapeutic dose through novel means have improved local tumor control, but have not made a significant impact on overall patient survival.[2,3] Therefore, the rationale for radiotherapy dose intensification studies is less appealing than the investigation of strategies that include standard doses of radiotherapy with novel radiosensitizers that also address systemic disease spread. However, the importance of local disease control from chemoradiation in both resectable and locally advanced disease will be considerably greater if systemic therapies improve substantially, because reliable control of local disease would then become a greater component of the overall problem.

Normal Tissue Constraints of Radiation Dose

ACUTE EFFECTS OF RADIOTHERAPY

The acute effects of radiotherapy to the upper abdomen are most commonly caused by depletion of the rapidly dividing cells that make up the mucosal lining of the stomach or gastric remnant (in surgically treated patients). The common clinical manifestations of acute mucosal radiation injury in the upper abdomen are nausea, vomiting, anorexia, and, in severe cases, upper abdominal pain. Significant toxicity commonly results in dehydration and anorexia, which compounds the nutritional deficiency that patients with pancreatic cancer typically face. Severe acute radiation mucosal toxicity can lead to ulceration of the stomach or duodenum. Known as a consequential reaction, this type of radiation injury usually occurs within a few months of therapy. Nausea can also result from hepatic irradiation, but the volume of irradiated liver is rarely significant when appropriate treatment volumes are planned. Antiemetics can be used as needed initially, but if persistent nausea is observed, they should be used prophylactically. The use of proton pump inhibitors or H-2 blockers during radiotherapy may reduce the risk of significant mucosal injury. Diarrhea seldom results from pancreatic radiotherapy because typically only a relatively small volume of ileum and jejunum is within the radiation field. When diarrhea does occur, pancreatic exocrine insufficiency resulting from pancreatic duct obstruction is usually the cause.

LATE EFFECTS OF RADIOTHERAPY

The late effects of radiotherapy are permanent effects on tissues that limit the dose of radiation that can be given safely. The dose-limiting organs surrounding the pancreas include the stomach, duodenum, small bowel, kidneys, spinal cord, and liver. Each of these organs has known manifestations related to late radiation injury. The dose of radiotherapy that can be safely given to pancreatic tumors is limited by the proximity of the pancreas to the stomach and duodenum. The dose of conventional external beam radiotherapy that can be used safely in the upper abdomen is generally limited by the gastric and duodenal mucosa's tolerance to late radiation injury. This dose has been clinically established in patients receiving radiotherapy alone or in combination with 5-fluorouracil (5-FU). Given at 2 Gy per fraction, 50 Gy is well tolerated, even with large volumes of irradiated mucosa. However, doses between 55 Gy and 60 Gy appear to cause chronic radiation injury if large volumes of the gastric and duodenal mucosa are treated. It is unlikely that doses higher than 60 Gy will be routinely delivered in pancreatic cancer patients because of the proximity of pancreatic head lesions to the duodenum and pancreatic body and tail lesions to the stomach. The most common late radiation injury is ulceration of the mucosal surface, and in rare instances, perforation. Usually these complications can be managed medically unless perforation occurs.

With commonly used radiation techniques, the dose of radiation to the spinal cord, kidneys, and liver can easily be kept low enough to avoid late radiation injury. Even if an entire kidney is treated beyond the known tolerance (higher than 26 Gy), overall kidney function is not affected in clinically relevant ways. [4] Clinically relevant kidney function compromise rarely develops as long as at least one kidney is spared from the radiation field.

Radiation-induced liver disease, often referred to as radiation hepatitis, is characterized by the development of anicteric ascites approximately 2 weeks to 4 months after hepatic irradiation.[5] The whole liver has been treated safely with doses of up to 20 Gy in patients with pancreatic cancer,[6] but whole-liver doses more than 35 Gy have resulted in a significant risk of radiation-induced liver disease.[7] The risk can be predicted based on radiation dose and volume considerations.[8,9] It is now clear that only limited volumes of hepatic tissue can tolerate high doses of irradiation.[10]

Adjuvant Chemoradiation in Potentially Resectable Disease

Chemoradiation is used to reduce the probability of local tumor recurrence in patients who undergo potentially curative resection of pancreatic cancer. Based on limited data,[11,12] chemoradiation is the standard adjuvant treatment in patients with resected pancreatic cancer in the United States. Neoadjuvant chemoradiation has also been investigated, because this approach has theoretical biological advantages over postoperative chemoradiation, allows all patients access to multimodality therapy, and provides an opportunity for identifying patients with rapidly progressive metastatic disease so that they may be spared nontherapeutic surgery.[13]

Postoperative Adjuvant Chemoradiation

The current standard of care for resected pancreatic cancer patients is in part based on a single randomized trial of postoperative adjuvant chemoradiation verses surgical resection alone conducted by the Gastrointestinal Tumor Study Group. Forty-three patients who had successfully recovered from pancreaticoduodenectomy were entered in the study over 8 years. In the combined modality arm, radiotherapy was delivered to the primary disease site and regional lymphatics in a split course of 40 Gy over 6 weeks with concurrent 5-fluorouracil (500 mg/m^2/day intravenous bolus on days 1 to 3 each 2-week radiotherapy course).

Weekly maintenance 5-fluorouracil was then given for 2 years or until disease recurrence. The survival results in the combined modality arm were statistically superior to the results in the observation arm (43% versus 18% at 2 years, and 14% versus 5% at 5 years, $p < 0.05$).[14] An additional 30 patients were subsequently registered to the experimental treatment with a duplication of the results.[12] Similar findings were reported by the European Organization for the Research and Treatment of Cancer.[15] Between 1987 and 1995, 218 patients who had undergone pancreaticoduodenectomy for adenocarcinoma of the pancreas or periampullary region were randomized to receive either chemoradiation (40 Gy in a split course along with 5-fluorouracil given as a continuous infusion at a dosage of 25 mg/kg/day during radiotherapy) or no further treatment. The median overall survival duration was 24.5 months for the group who received adjuvant therapy and 19 months for the group who received surgery alone ($p = 0.2$). The median disease-free survival duration was 17.1 months for patients with pancreatic cancer who received adjuvant therapy and 12.6 months for those who received surgery alone ($p = 0.099$). Twenty percent of 104 evaluable patients assigned to receive chemoradiation did not receive the intended therapy because of patient refusal, medical comorbidities, or rapid tumor progression. The low level of compliance and inadequate statistical power could explain the lack of a clear benefit. Both of these studies incorporated a suboptimal chemotherapy dose and schedule as well as an inadequate radiotherapy dose, equipment (supervoltage), and schedule (split course).

The current standard postoperative chemoradiation regimen for pancreatic cancer in the United States is radiotherapy (50.4 Gy in 28 fractions) delivered to the operative bed and regional lymphatics with concurrent protracted venous infusion 5-fluorouracil. There is typically a field reduction after 45 Gy in 25 fractions. The tumor bed, including the retroperitoneal margin, is then typically treated for an additional 5.4 Gy in 3 fractions. A multi-institutional assessment of treatment efficacy using modern doses, schedules, equipment, and techniques will be available when the results of the Radiation Therapy Oncology Group (RTOG)-led Gastrointestinal Intergroup Protocol 97-04 are reported. In that study, 538 patients, after undergoing pancreaticoduodenectomy, were randomized to receive either gemcitabine or protracted venous infusion 5-fluorouracil (250 mg/m^2/day) before and after concurrent chemoradiation (50.4 Gy with protracted venous infusional 5-fluorouracil at 250 mg/m^2/day). The chemoradiation component of the trial was not a randomized variable, but since locoregional control is one of the end points that will be evaluated, an assessment of the adequacy of current locoregional treatment will be possible.

The results of the European Study Group of Pancreatic Cancer (ESPAC-1) study raise questions about the benefit of radiotherapy in resected pancreatic cancer patients.[16,17] An analysis of all patients treated showed no benefit from postoperative chemoradiation, but showed a survival benefit from adjuvant 5-fluorouracil and leucovorin chemotherapy without radiotherapy. However, interpreting the data from this study is problematic because of the lack of quality control, the use of off-study therapies in addition to the randomized therapy, and the use of an outdated chemoradiation dose and schedule. The recent update of this trial provided some new information regarding a possible explanation for the lack of a benefit. Sixty-two percent of patients had local recurrence (35% were isolated) as a component of the first site of failure.[17] This can be compared with less than a 10% local recurrence rate among patients resected at The University of Texas M. D. Anderson Cancer Center.[18] The results were not detailed by treatment arm, but this high degree of local disease recurrence/persistence raises concerns about oncologically inadequate surgical resections. Since there was no effort to stratify patients by surgeon or by center, there may have been an imbalance in the number of incompletely resected (R2), incurable tumors in the chemoradiation arm. Although this study contains the largest number of resected pancreatic cancer patients randomized to treatment with and without chemoradiation, the limitations described above have prevented it from changing standard practice in the United States, and chemoradiation had been included in the major adjuvant trials (Table 1).

Neoadjuvant Chemoradiation

Neoadjuvant chemoradiation has been used as a strategy to improve tumor control rates in patients who have resectable disease at the time of clinical evaluation. The rationale for the use of neoadjuvant therapy, as opposed to postoperative adjuvant therapy, has been discussed in detail elsewhere by investigators from M. D. Anderson.[13] The initial preoperative regimen evaluated at our institution was 50.4 Gy over 5.5 weeks (standard fractionation) with concurrent protracted venous infusional 5-fluorouracil. In addition, intraoperative radiotherapy was used in selected cases. However, because of the significant acute toxicity seen,[19] the higher radiation dose was abandoned in favor of a short course of "rapid fractionation" radiotherapy (30 Gy in 10 fractions over 2 weeks), with a supplemental 10 Gy dose of intraoperative

Table 1 Ongoing and completed adjuvant trials in the United States

Study	Design	Arms
GI Intergroup	Randomized phase II (Adjuvant/Postop)	Gem + C-225
		Cape + XRT (50.4 Gy / 5.5 weeks)
		Gem + C-225
		Gem + Bev
		Cape + XRT (50.4 Gy/5.5 weeks)
		Gem + Bev
ACOSOG Z05031	Phase II	XRT (50.4 Gy/5.5 weeks) + PVI 5-FU + IFN + CDDP weekly

ACOSOG = American College of Surgical Oncologists; Bev = bevacizumab; Cape = capecitabine; CDDP = cisplatin; C-225 = cetuximab; 5-FU = 5-fluorouracil; Gem = gemcitabine; GI = gastrointestinal; IFN = interferon alpha; OS = overall survival; PVI = protracted venous infusion; XRT = radiotherapy.

radiotherapy delivered at the time of surgical resection. The effective dose delivered to the tumor bed with the latter approach is comparable with that delivered with the former approach, based on linear quadratic modeling.[20] Initially, protracted venous infusional 5-fluorouracil, subsequently paclitaxel,[21] and most recently, gemcitabine,[22] have been investigated in consecutive phase II studies of neoadjuvant chemoradiation. Further details of this neoadjuvant approach are discussed elsewhere in this book.

Current Clinical Trials in the Adjuvant Treatment of Pancreatic Cancer (see Table 1)

The successful completion of the (RTOG)-led Gastrointestinal Intergroup Protocol 97-04 has generated momentum for future trials in resectable pancreatic cancer. The proposed replacement study by the GI intergroup is evaluating the role of the addition of cetuximab or bevacizumab to gemcitabine given before and after chemoradiation in patients with resected pancreatic cancer. Capecitabine (oral prodrug of 5-FU) will be given concurrently with radiation. The American College of Surgeons Oncology Group (ACOSOG) Z05031 trial is a single-arm phase II study evaluating postoperative radiotherapy, infusional 5-FU, interferon alpha, and cisplatin given concurrently in the postoperative setting. This trial is based on very promising data from a single institution. Patients with resected pancreatic cancer that were treated with this regimen had a 5-year survival rate of 55%.[23]

Radiotherapy Technique and Dose

POSTOPERATIVE RADIOTHERAPY

The standard dose of radiotherapy in the postoperative setting is typically 50.4 Gy in 28 fractions. Field reductions are often made after 45 Gy. A 4-field technique using anterior, posterior, and opposed lateral fields allows critical tissues such as the liver, kidneys, stomach, spinal cord, and small bowel to be spared. Fields are weighted so that the dose contribution from the lateral fields is restricted to 20 Gy. This prevents the liver and kidney tissue in the lateral fields that are not also in the anterior and posterior fields from being treated beyond the known tolerance.

At the time of radiotherapy simulation, the patient is positioned supine with a treatment device that stabilizes the arms overhead. Barium is given at the time of simulation. After simulation films are taken, the preoperative tumor volume, duodenum, and kidneys are drawn on all films based on the preoperative images. CT-based treatment planning with dose-volume histograms is helpful to verify the dose to the target and to limit the dose to critical structures.

For lesions located in the pancreatic head, the anterior and posterior fields typically cover the T11-L3 vertebral bodies. The celiac axis should be covered with a 2 cm margin superiorly. Inferiorly, the goal is to cover the tumor and duodenal bed with a 2 cm margin. The left border is located 2 cm to the left of the vertebral body edge, as long as there is adequate coverage of the preoperative tumor volume. The preoperative tumor volume and preoperative location of the duodenum defines the right field border and the anterior extent of the lateral fields as well. The porta hepatis should be identified on the CT scans and included in all fields. This usually means that the upper right border of the anterior and posterior fields is located 4 to 5 cm to the right of the vertebral body edge and the anterior aspect of the lateral field is 5 to 6 cm from the anterior vertebral body edge. Blocking is placed over the inferior pole of the right kidney in the anterior and posterior fields, bisecting the vertebral bodies in the lateral fields. Corner blocks are typically placed in the anterior aspect of the lateral fields as well. Care should be taken not to block the preoperative tumor volume or porta hepatis.

For lesions of the pancreatic body and tail, similar fields are used, except that the splenic hilum is covered, and the porta hepatis and duodenal bed are not covered. The right field border is typically located 2 cm from the right vertebral body edge. Similar fields are recommended for patients with an intact pancreas if the goal is neoadjuvant therapy with planned or likely surgical resection.

Radiotherapy Technique for Patients with Locally Advanced Disease

Since patients with locally advanced tumors probably do not benefit from regional nodal irradiation, radiotherapy fields should be confined to the gross tumor alone. This strategy reduces the gastrointestinal toxicity of chemoradiation. It is important, therefore, to identify the pancreatic tumor correctly. On contrast-enhanced CT scans, pancreatic tumors are typically hypodense compared with the surrounding pancreatic parenchyma. When there is doubt about the location of the primary tumor, the CT images should be reviewed with a diagnostic radiologist. Administration of an oral contrast agent at the time of simulation illuminates the duodenal "C-loop." Endobiliary biliary stents can also be visualized, which facilitates identifying the common bile duct.

The pancreas and duodenum move a median of 1 cm with respiratory excursion.[24] If the gross tumor alone is to be treated, respiratory motion must be either controlled or accounted for in radiation treatment planning. The most common way that this is accomplished is by simply adding an additional margin in the cranial and caudal directions to the planned radiation fields. However, since axial tumor motion is negligible, an additional margin for motion in the axial directions is not necessary. Radiation treatment that is gated to the respiratory cycle (respiratory gating)[25,26] is a necessary component of radiation dose escalation studies that seek to deliver > 60 Gy to the primary tumor while sparing the duodenum. Thus, radiation fields designed to spare the duodenum that are tightly confined to the primary tumor without correction for organ motion could lead to underdosing the tumor target, or "marginal miss." A 4-field technique is recommended with equally weighted anterior, posterior, and opposed lateral fields. A 2 cm block margin is used in the radial directions, and a 3 cm margin is used in the cranial and caudal directions (Figure 1).

The median survival in patients with locally advanced pancreatic cancer treated with concurrent protracted venous infusional 5-fluorouracil and radiotherapy to a dosage of 30 Gy in 10 fractions over 2 weeks is similar to that achieved with a dosage of 50.4 Gy in 28 fractions over 5.5 weeks with the same chemotherapy.[27] Although 50.4 Gy is a more commonly prescribed dose, it probably does not significantly improve outcome and has a slightly higher risk of acute toxicity. However, patients with minimal arterial abutment ("marginally

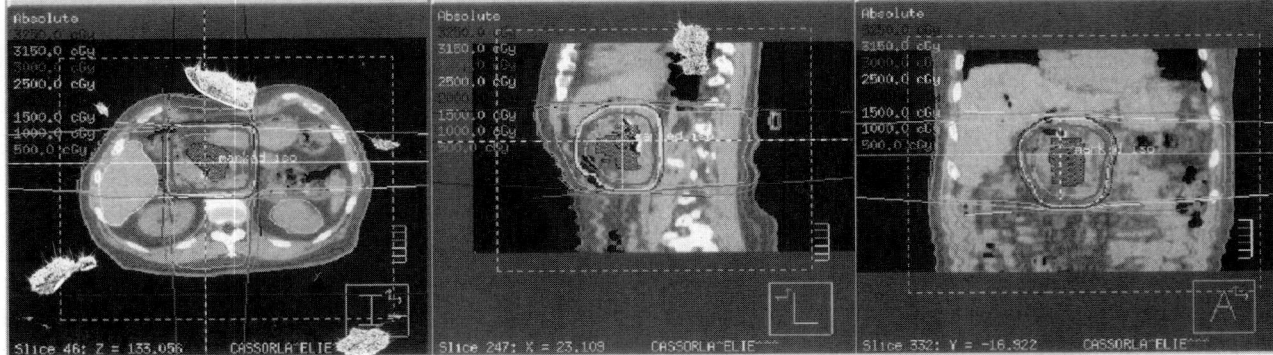

Figure 1 Computed tomography planning images in a patient with a locally advanced pancreatic adenocarcinoma. The radiation isodose lines to the tumor and surrounding tissues are displayed in these multiplanar treatment planning images.

resectable" patients) should be treated with 50.4 Gy to maximize the possibility of surgical resection. Prospective studies that evaluate novel radiosensitizers should administer 50.4 Gy to maximize the opportunity for radiosensitization.

Principles of Chemoradiation in Locally Advanced Disease

Although it has significant limitations, chemoradiation for locally advanced disease is considered a standard treatment. 5-fluorouracil-based chemoradiation has led to an improvement in median survival as compared with either chemotherapy or radiotherapy alone[28] in randomized trials. Since the median survival in patients with locally advanced disease is generally less than 1 year and the benefit of treatment is limited, therapy should be planned to minimize negative impact on quality of life. Severe toxicity can usually be avoided, regardless of the radiosensitizing chemotherapy that is used if the radiation fields are confined to the gross primary tumor and clinically enlarged lymph nodes. Treating uninvolved regional lymph nodes with larger radiation fields is not likely to improve outcome, but may increase the risk of gastrointestinal toxicity.

All patients with locally advanced pancreatic cancer should be considered for protocol-based therapy. If they refuse or are ineligible, they are probably best served by a treatment strategy that takes advantage of the best available therapies. Patients should receive a well-tolerated chemoradiation regimen, either preceded or followed by systemic gemcitabine-based chemotherapy. A strategy that starts with 2 to 4 months of gemcitabine-based systemic therapy, followed by consolidation with chemoradiation, probably takes advantage of the best available established therapies for this disease.

Gemcitabine-Based Chemoradiation

The introduction of gemcitabine was a modest step forward in the treatment of pancreatic cancer. It prolongs median survival and leads to clinical benefit in patients with advanced disease.[29] The recognition of its radiosensitizing properties[30] stimulated the clinical investigation of concurrent gemcitabine and radiotherapy in patients with locally advanced pancreatic cancer. Initially, many different approaches were used to combine gemcitabine with radiotherapy in pancreatic cancer.[31] In a novel study, investigators at the University of Michigan combined full-dose gemcitabine with limited field radiotherapy. They reported acceptable toxicity,[32] but other studies have reported more significant toxicity with this approach. Unfortunately, concurrent gemcitabine as compared with 5-fluorouracil has generally not led to dramatic improvement in median survival.[33] What has become clear from studies of gemcitabine combined with radiotherapy is that the extent of mucosal irradiation correlates with gastrointestinal toxicity.[34] For this reason, radiation fields for all patients with locally advanced disease who are treated with concurrent gemcitabine should be confined to the gross tumor and any enlarged lymph nodes, sparing as much mucosa as possible.

In addition to the single institutional studies, 3 multi-institution studies have evaluated concurrent gemcitabine and radiotherapy in locally advanced pancreatic cancer. Of these, the only published randomized trial compared gemcitabine with an unconventional regimen of biweekly intravenous bolus of 5-fluorouracil, each given concurrently with radiotherapy to patients with locally advanced pancreatic cancer.[35] The results demonstrate that the toxicity was unacceptably high in both groups. Among all patients, a median of 25% of the patients' time alive was spent in the hospital, and only 75% of patients were able to complete the 50.4 Gy planned radiotherapy dose. Protracted venous infusional 5-fluorouracil[33] or capecitabine[36] probably would have been much better tolerated by the control group and would likely have emphasized the significant toxicity of the gemcitabine arm. In addition, the median survival difference (14.5 months versus 6.7 months, $p = 0.027$) that was reported has to be interpreted with caution because of the poor results in the control group. Similarly, a phase II study conducted in locally advanced pancreatic cancer patients by the Cancer and Leukemia Group B (CALGB) evaluated gemcitabine given at 40 mg/m^2 twice weekly. In that study, there were 35% and 50% grade 3 or 4 gastrointestinal and hematologic toxicities, respectively, and the median survival was only 8.5 months.[37] Not surprisingly, the Cancer and Leukemia Group B has abandoned this approach in locally advanced pancreatic cancer. Both of these studies used expanded regional nodal radiation fields that likely contributed to the significant gastrointestinal toxicity. In contrast, the approach that was developed at the University of Michigan delivers the manufacturer's recommended dose of gemcitabine (1 gm/m^2) and a slightly lower radiotherapy dose (36 Gy in 15 fractions over 3 weeks) with conformal radiation fields encompassing the gross tumor volume alone. At that institution, the irradiation of a smaller volume of normal tissue was reported to be well tolerated.[32] Investigators have since embarked on a multi-institution phase II study evaluating the same regimen. Preliminary results indicate that approximately 25% of patients experience grade 3 or 4 gastrointestinal toxicity (McGinn, Oral Presentation, European Cancer Conference, 2003).

Several points about gemcitabine-based chemoradiation are worth emphasizing. All chemoradiation regimens that have been studied in patients with locally advanced disease, including regimens that contain gemcitabine, have significant efficacy limitations. Similar to its value as a systemic agent,[29] gemcitabine is probably only modestly better than 5-fluorouracil when used with radiotherapy,[33,35] but it is not tolerated as well. The gastrointestinal toxicity reported in the 3 multi-institution studies using gemcitabine calls into question whether the combination of gemcitabine and radiotherapy will be tolerated well enough for future studies that try to build on these experiences. Finally, compared with radiotherapy fields that target the gross tumor only,[32] elective regional nodal irradiation results in increased gastrointestinal toxicity.[31] Since currently available chemoradiation regimens cannot control the primary tumor, it is unlikely that irradiation of microscopic regional nodal metastases contributes anything positive to the outcome of patients with locally advanced pancreatic cancer, regardless of the concurrent

chemotherapeutic agent that is used. Certainly, if gemcitabine is used in combination with the irradiation of esophageal, gastric, or duodenal mucosa, the volume of mucosa being treated should be minimized or there will be a significant risk of severe acute toxicity.

Capecitabine-Based Chemoradiation

Protracted venous infusional 5-fluorouracil (225–300 mg/m^2/day) is well tolerated with radiotherapy. Acute gastrointestinal toxicity that results in hospitalization or a prolonged need for intravenous rehydration occurs in less that 10% of patients.[33] Capecitabine is an oral fluoropyrimidine prodrug that is converted to 5-FU more efficiently in tumors than in normal tissue because of the presence of increased thymidine phosphorylase activity in tumor cells.[38] Single-agent capecitabine has an increased response rate, equivalent progression-free and overall survival, and a more favorable toxicity profile than bolus 5-fluorouracil and leucovorin in metastatic colorectal cancer.[39] It also has a clinical benefit response similar to gemcitabine in patients with locally advanced or metastatic pancreatic cancer.[40] Furthermore, since capecitabine is administered orally, patients are not at risk of deep venous thrombosis and infections that occur with indwelloing central venous lines. Additionally, the dose-limiting toxicity of capecitabine is hand-and-foot syndrome, which can serve as a signal to reduce the dose before gastrointestinal or hematologic toxicity occurs. At doses that are known to be systemically active, capecitabine is extremely well tolerated with radiotherapy. In a phase I study conducted in rectal cancer patients, there were no grade 3 hematologic or gastrointestinal toxicities.[36] In contrast to gemcitabine with radiotherapy, the favorable acute toxicity profile of capecitabine and radiotherapy makes it an attractive platform upon which to build.

Future studies will combine molecular targeted therapies with capecitabine-based chemoradiation. For example, a recently completed phase I study at M. D. Anderson evaluated capecitabine, bevacizumab (a monoclonal antibody against vascular endothelial growth factor), and radiotherapy in locally advanced pancreatic cancer. The gastrointestinal toxicity was minimal, with only 2 of 47 (4%) requiring hospitalization for grade 3 gastrointestinal toxicity and no hospitalizations for hematologic toxicity.[41] There have been 6 of 12 patients with a partial response to therapy at the 5 mg/kg bevacizumab dose level. This study is the basis of RTOG PA 04-11, a phase II study evaluating concurrent capecitabine, radiotherapy, and bevacizumab followed by gemcitabine in combination with bevacizumab (Table 2). Based on the responses, the 5mg/kg dose level of

Table 2 Recent trials in locally advanced disease

Study	Eligiblity	Design	Arms
ECOG 1200	SMA or Celiac arterial involvement without encasement	Randomized Phase II	Gem/Cisplatin/5-FU, followed by 5-FU/XRT 50.4 Gy/5.5 weeks (Patients considered for surgical resection) Gem weekly $\times$ 5 + XRT 50.4 Gy/5.5 weeks (Patients considered for surgical resection)
ECOG/RTOG 4201	Unresectable based on SMA or celiac arterial encasement or SMV or portal vein occlusion	Randomized Phase III	Gem Days 1, 8, 21 (repeat monthly, max 7 cycles) XRT 50.4 Gy/5.5 weeks + Gem followed by Gem 1gm/m^2 weekly $\times$ 3 (max 5 cycles)
RTOG PA 0411	Unresectable by institutional criteria	Phase II	XRT 50.4 Gy/5.5 weeks + Cape + Bev followed by Gem Days 1, 8, 21 + Bev D1, 14 (repeat monthly until progression)

Bev = Bevacizumab; BID = twice daily; Cape = capecitabine; ECOG = Eastern Cooperative Oncology Group; 5-FU = fluorouracil; Gem = gemcitabine; Gy = Gray; kg = kilogram; mg/m^2 = milligrams per meter squared; RTOG = Radiation Therapy Oncology Group; SMA = superior mesenteric artery; SMV= superior mesenteric vein.

bevacizumab was selected. Capecitabine will be administered at 825 mg/m^2 orally twice daily on days of radiation. The incorporation of targeted molecular therapy with well-tolerated chemoradiation is a promising avenue of future investigation in pancreatic cancer.

Important Considerations Regarding "Downstaging"

The term "downstaging" in pancreatic cancer is used to describe the conversion of an unresectable tumor to resectable using cytotoxic therapy. However, the interpretation of whether true downstaging actually occurs is limited by inconsistent and subjective definitions of resectability and by inadequate preoperative radiographic assessments of resectability. Probably the most variable factor in determining respectability, and thus interpreting whether downstaging has occurred, is the description of arterial involvement by the tumor. Although most surgeons would agree that tumor encasement of either the celiac artery or the superior mesenteric artery constitutes unresectable disease, opinions vary with regard to more limited arterial involvement. It is probably in this group of patients that, theoretically, active cytotoxic therapy could lead to downstaging. At M. D. Anderson, patients having locally advanced tumors who have undergone margin-negative resections have typically had tumors with very limited arterial involvement (< one-third the circumference and < 1 cm along the length of the artery) that have responded to chemoradiation.[34] These patients are sometimes referred to as "marginally resectable" patients.

Another factor that affects the determination of resectability and the determination of whether downstaging has occurred is the evaluation and extent of tumor involvement of venous structures (superior

mesenteric/portal venous confluence). Tumor extension to a venous structure without occlusion is not an absolute contraindication to resection. Involved veins can be resected successfully and reconstructed at the time of pancreaticoduodenectomy, and in fact, the long-term outcome of these patients is not compromised by vein involvement.[42] However, many surgeons would consider this type of tumor extension, seen either intraoperatively or on preoperative imaging, as evidence of unresectability. Thus, the attribution of increased resectability to chemoradiation in some studies could be simply the result of a difference in surgical opinion and practice. The existence of broad definitions of locally advanced pancreatic cancer can give the impression that downstaging occurs more commonly than it actually does.

Another variable that frequently affects the interpretation of whether downstaging has occurred is the lack of reproducible imaging before and after chemoradiation. Imaging that is not designed to address vascular involvement may not provide sufficient resolution for making an assessment. Thus, CT scans of the same patient at different times may result in different interpretations, with or without any therapy being administered.

Strictly defined, true downstaging must include an objective definition of resectability as well as reproducible imaging before and after chemoradiation. Although many studies have reported that downstaging occurred, very few fulfilled these criteria of objectivity and reproducibility. Nonetheless, reports of downstaging after 5-fluorouracil-based chemoradiation are uncommon. Review of the available literature suggests that only a small percentage (8–16%) of clinically unresectable patients treated with 5-fluorouracil-based chemoradiation have eventually undergone margin-negative resection.[43]

The use of novel, more active regimens is anticipated in the future. To document the occurrence of downstaging more accurately, all studies evaluating novel chemoradiation regimens should adhere to a strict CT-based definition of locally advanced pancreatic cancer that includes arterial involvement (ie, a low-density tumor inseparable from the superior mesenteric artery or celiac axis on contrast-enhanced CT) or occlusion of the superior mesenteric/portal venous confluence.

Current Radiotherapy-Based Clinical Trials in Locally Advanced Pancreatic Cancer

The importance of enrolling pancreatic cancer patients in clinical trials cannot be overstated. Table 2 outlines the features of selected ongoing clinical trials that are evaluating radiation-based therapies in locally advanced pancreatic cancer. The Eastern Cooperative Oncology Group (ECOG) is currently conducting a randomized phase II trial (ECOG 1200) evaluating pancreaticoduodenectomy after 1 of 2 novel chemoradiation regimens in patients with locally advanced pancreatic cancer (see Table 2). Eligible patients must have involvement but not encasement of the SMA or celiac axis. This trial was designed to evaluate the value of surgical resection in patients who have direct tumor extension involving the artery. Hopefully, this study will generate prospective data regarding the possibility of downstaging patients and the value of resection in patients with locally advanced disease. Two other trials are worth mentioning. ECOG/RTOG 4201 is a phase III trial evaluating the benefit of adding radiotherapy to gemcitabine. Eligible patients must either have SMA or celiac arterial encasement or occlusion of superior mesenteric or portal veins. Finally, RTOG PA 0411 is a single-arm phase II study evaluating the role of adding bevacizumab to a cytotoxic backbone of concurrent capecitabine and radiation, followed by gemcitabine until progression.

Conclusion

Improving the treatment outcomes in patients with pancreatic cancer is a challenge. Whenever possible, patients should be enrolled in investigational studies that evaluate novel therapies. Outside of a clinical trial, postoperative chemoradiation is the current standard adjuvant treatment following pancreaticoduodenectomy. The results of RTOG 97-04 will provide information about the use of gemcitabine in the adjuvant setting compared with 5-fluorouracil, and will also provide multi-institution-based data regarding the outcomes and patterns of failure with modern radiotherapy doses and techniques. For locally advanced disease, patients probably benefit from using gemcitabine-based chemotherapy as well as chemoradiation. A strategy that starts with gemcitabine-based systemic therapy for 2 to 4 months, followed by chemoradiation takes advantage of the best available established therapies. Radiation dose-intensification studies are probably of minimal value until distant disease is better controlled. The incorporation of targeted molecular therapy with well-tolerated chemoradiation regimens is a promising approach that addresses the limitations of conventional therapy without introducing unacceptable toxicity, and radiation-based clinical trials are underway that include targeted agents. Fortunately, investigators have placed more emphasis on pancreatic cancer in recent years than in the past, and many more clinical trials evaluating novel treatments are available to patients. As clinicians caring for pancreatic cancer patients, it our responsibility to enroll patients in these studies.

References

1. AJCC. Exocrine pancreas. In Greene F, Page D, Irvin D, et al, editors. AJCC cancer staging manual. 6th ed. New York: Springer; 2002. p. 157–64.

2. Garton GR, Gunderson LL, Nagorney DM, et al. High-dose preoperative external beam and intraoperative irradiation for locally advanced pancreatic cancer. Int J Radiat Oncol Biol Phys 1993;27:1153–7.

3. Mohiuddin M, Rosato F, Barbot D, et al. Long-term results of combined modality treatment with I-125 implantation for carcinoma of the pancreas. Int J Radiat Oncol Biol Phys 1992;23:305–11.

4. Willett CG, Tepper JE, Orlow EL, Shipley WU. Renal complications secondary to radiation treatment of upper abdominal malignancies. Int J Radiat Oncol Biol Phys 1986;12:1601–4.

5. Lawrence TS, Robertson JM, Anscher MS, et al. Hepatic toxicity resulting from cancer treatment. Int J Radiat Oncol Biol Phys 1995;31:1237–48.

6. Komaki R, Wilson JF, Cox JD, Kline RW. Carcinoma of the pancreas: results of irradiation for unresectable lesions. Int J Radiat Oncol Biol Phys 1980;6:209–12.

7. Ingold J, Reed G, Kaplan H, Bagshaw M. Radiation hepatitis. Am J Roentgenol 1965;93:200–8.

8. Lawrence TS, Ten Haken RK, Kessler ML, et al. The use of 3-D dose volume analysis to predict radiation hepatitis. Int J Radiat Oncol Biol Phys 1992;23:781–8.

9. McGinn CJ, Ten Haken RK, Ensminger WD, et al. Treatment of intrahepatic cancers with radiation doses

based on a normal tissue complication probability model. J Clin Oncol 1998;16:2246–52.

10. Dawson LA, McGinn CJ, Normolle D, et al. Escalated focal liver radiation and concurrent hepatic artery fluorodeoxyuridine for unresectable intrahepatic malignancies. J Clin Oncol 2000;18:2210–8.

11. Yeo CJ, Abrams RA, Grochow LB, et al. Pancreaticoduodenectomy for pancreatic pancreatic adenocarcinoma: postoperative adjuvant chemoradiation improves survival. A prospective, single-institution experience. Ann Surg 1997;225:621–36.

12. Anonymous. Further evidence of effective adjuvant combined radiation and chemotherapy following curative resection of pancreatic cancer. Gastrointestinal Tumor Study Group. Cancer 1987;59:2006–10.

13. Wayne JD, Abdalla EK, Wolff RA, et al. Localized adenocarcinoma of the pancreas: the rationale for preoperative chemoradiation. Oncologist 2002;7:34–45.

14. Kalser MH, Ellenberg SS. Pancreatic cancer. Adjuvant combined radiation and chemotherapy following curative resection [published erratum appears in Arch Surg 1986;121:1045]. Arch Surg 1985;120:899–903.

15. Klinkenbijl JH, Jeekel J, Sahmoud T, et al. Adjuvant radiotherapy and 5-fluorouracil after curative resection of cancer of the pancreas and periampullary region: phase III trial of the EORTC gastrointestinal tract cancer cooperative group. Ann Surg 1999;230:776–84.

16. Neoptolemos JP, Dunn JA, Stocken DD, et al. Adjuvant chemoradiotherapy and chemotherapy in resectable pancreatic cancer: a randomised controlled trial. Lancet 2001; 358:1576–85.

17. Neoptolemos JP, Stocken DD, Friess H, et al. A randomized trial of chemoradiotherapy and chemotherapy after resection of pancreatic cancer. N Engl J Med 2004;350: 1200–10.

18. Breslin TM, Hess KR, Harbison DB, et al. Neoadjuvant chemoradiotherapy for adenocarcinoma of the pancreas: treatment variables and survival duration. Ann Surg Oncol 2001;8:123–32.

19. Evans DB, Rich TA, Byrd DR, et al. Preoperative chemoradiation and pancreaticoduodenectomy for adenocarcinoma of the pancreas. Arch Surg 1992;127:1335–9.

20. Rich TA, Janjan NA, Abbruzzese JL, Evans DB. Preoperative and postoperative chemoradiation strategies in patients treated with pancreaticoduodenectomy for adenocarcinoma of the pancreas [Comment]. J Clin Oncol 1997;15:3292–3.

21. Pisters P, Wolff R, Janjan N, et al. Preoperative paclitaxel and concurrent rapid-fractionation radiation for resectable pancreatic adenocarcinoma: toxicities, histologic response rates, and event-free outcome. J Clin Oncol 2002;20:2537–44.

22. Wolff RA, Evans DB, Gravel DM, et al. Phase I trial of gemcitabine combined with radiation for the treatment of locally advanced pancreatic adenocarcinoma. Clin Cancer Res 2001;7:2246–53.

23. Picozzi VJ, Kozarek RA, Traverso LW. Interferon-based adjuvant chemoradiation therapy after pancreaticoduodenectomy for pancreatic adenocarcinoma. Am J Surg 2003; 185:476–80.

24. Bussels B, Goethals L, Feron M, et al. Respiration-induced movement of the upper abdominal organs: a pitfall for the three-dimensional conformal radiation treatment of pancreatic cancer. Radiother Oncol 2003;68:69–74.

25. Ramsey CR, Scaperoth D, Arwood D, Oliver AL. Clinical efficacy of respiratory gated conformal radiation therapy. Med Dosim 1999;24:115–9.

26. Balter JM, Lam KL, McGinn CJ, et al. Improvement of CT-based treatment-planning models of abdominal targets using static exhale imaging. Int J Radiat Oncol Biol Phys 1998;41:939–43.

27. Wong AA, Delclos ME, Wolff RA, et al. Radiation dose considerations in the palliative treatment of locally advanced adenocarcinoma of the pancreas. Am J Clin Oncol 2005;28:227–33.

28. Anonymous. Treatment of locally unresectable carcinoma of the pancreas: comparison of combined-modality therapy (chemotherapy plus radiotherapy) to chemotherapy alone. Gastrointestinal Tumor Study Group. J Natl Cancer Inst 1988;80:751–5.

29. Burris HA III, Moore MJ, Andersen J, et al. Improvements in survival and clinical benefit with gemcitabine as first-line therapy for patients with advanced pancreas cancer: a randomized trial [see comments]. J Clin Oncol 1997;15: 2403–13.

30. Mason KA, Milas L, Hunter NR, et al. Maximizing therapeutic gain with gemcitabine and franctionated radiation. Int J Radiat Oncol Biol Phys 1999;44:1125–35.

31. Crane CH, Wolff RA, Abbruzzese JL, et al. Combining gemcitabine with radiation in pancreatic cancer: understanding important variables influencing the therapeutic index. Semin Oncol 2001;28:25–33.

32. McGinn CJ, Zalupski MM, Shureiqi I, et al. Phase I trial of radiation dose escalation with concurrent weekly full-dose gemcitabine in patients with advanced pancreatic cancer. J Clin Oncol 2001;19:4202–8.

33. Crane CH, Abbruzzese JL, Evans DB, et al. Is the therapeutic index better with gemcitabine-based chemoradiation than with 5-fluorouracil-based chemoradiation in locally advanced pancreatic cancer? Int J Radiat Oncol Biol Phys 2002;52:1293–302.

34. Crane C, Janjan N, Evans D, et al. Concurrent gemcitabine and rapid-fraction radiotherapy for unresectable pancreatic cancer: toxicity, local control and survival. Int J Pancreatol 2001;29:59–68.

35. Li CP, Chao Y, Chi KH, et al. Concurrent chemoradiotherapy treatment of locally advanced pancreatic

cancer: gemcitabine versus 5-fluorouracil, a randomized controlled study. Int J Radiat Oncol Biol Phys 2003;57:98–104.

36. Dunst J, Reese T, Sutter T, et al. Phase I trial evaluating the concurrent combination of radiotherapy and capecitabine in rectal cancer. J Clin Oncol 2002;20:3983–91.

37. Blackstock A, Tempero M, Niedwiecki D, et al. Cancer and Leukemia Group B (CALGB) 89805: phase II chemoradiation trial using gemcitabine in patients with localoregional adenocarcinoma of the pancreas [abstract 49]. Int J Radiat Oncol Biol Phys 2001;51:31.

38. Schuller J, Cassidy J, Dumont E, et al. Preferential activation of capecitabine in tumor following oral administration to colorectal cancer patients. Cancer Chemother Pharmacol 2000;45:291–7.

39. Hoff PM, Ansari R, Batist G, et al. Comparison of oral capecitabine versus intravenous fluorouracil plus leucov-orin as first-line treatment in 605 patients with metastatic colorectal cancer: results of a randomized phase III study. J Clin Oncol 2001;19:2282–92.

40. Cartwright TH, Cohn A, Varkey JA, et al. Phase II study of oral capecitabine in patients with advanced or metastatic pancreatic cancer. J Clin Oncol 2002;20:160–4.

41. Crane C, Ellis L, O'Reilly M, et al. RhuMab VEGF (Bevacizumab) with concurrent radiotherapy and capecitabine in locally advanced pancreatic cancer: an active, well tolerated regimen. Int J Radiat Oncol Biol Phys 2004;60 Suppl 1:S149.

42. Tseng JF, Raut CP, Lee JE, et al. Pancreaticoduodenectomy with vascular resection: margin status and survival duration. J Gastrointest Surg 2004;8:935–50.

43. Crane C, Evans D, Wolff R, et al. The pancreas. In: Cox J, Kian K, Ang K, editors. Radiation oncology: rationale, technique, results. 8th ed. St. Louis, MO: Mosby; 2003. p. 465–80.

CHAPTER 24

SPLENECTOMY FOR HEMATOLOGIC MALIGNANCY

MATTHEW H. G. KATZ, MD

BARRY W. FEIG, MD

MICHAEL BOUVET, MD

The value of splenectomy in the treatment of patients with many benign hematologic disorders, such as idiopathic thrombocytopenia purpura (ITP) and hereditary spherocytosis, is well established. In contrast, the indications for splenectomy in the setting of hematologic malignancy are both controversial and evolving.[1] Although splenectomy for treatment of hairy cell leukemia and the diagnosis of Hodgkin's disease has become less common, its role in other malignancies, including the chronic myeloid disorders and chronic lymphocytic leukemia, has expanded. In these disorders, splenectomy may be employed to relieve bulk symptoms of massive splenomegaly, to reverse cytopenias owing to hypersplenism and marrow failure, to decrease the incidence of constitutional symptoms, and to allow more aggressive dosing of myelosuppressive therapy. In some cases, the procedure may also prolong survival.

Given that patients with hematologic malignancy may be compromised by both their underlying disease and associated treatment, the use of splenectomy in these patients must be balanced against a risk of morbidity and mortality that is somewhat higher than when the procedure is performed for other routine indications (Table 1).[2] Special considerations, such as massive splenomegaly and profound thrombocytopenia, must be addressed as they may influence operative strategy and the overall therapeutic course. Nonetheless, a progressive experience with both the open and, now, laparoscopic approaches to splenectomy has led to a reduction in its associated morbidity, allowing it to be effectively performed as part of a palliative and, occasionally, curative strategy in many patients with hematologic malignancy.

The Leukemias

THE CHRONIC MYELOID DISORDERS

Chronic myelogenous leukemia (CML), myeloid metaplasia, essential thrombocythemia, and polycythemia vera, each of which is characterized by a clonal neoplastic proliferation of multipotent myeloid stem cells, together comprise a group of related chronic myeloid disorders.[3] The members of this group share several pathophysiological and clinical similarities, including a propensity for myelofibrosis and splenomegaly. In some cases, conversion between these disorders may occur. Despite their apparent relatedness, however, each disease is associated

Table 1 Indications for Splenectomy

Trauma
Iatrogenic Injury
Hematologic Disorders
  Idiopathic Thrombocytopenic Purpura (ITP)
  Hereditary Spherocytosis
  Autoimmune Hemolytic Anemia
  Sickle Cell Disease
  Thalassemia Major
Hematologic Malignancies
  Chronic Myeloid Disorders
  Chronic Lymphocytic Leukemia
  Hairy Cell Leukemia
  Non-Hodgkin's Lymphoma
  Hodgkin's Disease
Primary Splenic Tumors
Splenic Abscess/Cysts
Sinistral Portal Hypertension
Felty's Syndrome
Gaucher's Disease

with a unique clinical course and requires a distinct treatment strategy in which the role and efficacy of splenectomy varies.

Chronic Myelogenous Leukemia (CML)

CML is a malignant clonal hematopoetic disorder identified by the Philadelphia (Ph) chromosome, which is characterized by a translocation of genetic material leading to fusion of the *BCR* gene on chromosome 22 to the *ABL1* gene on chromosome 9. The gene product that results from this translocation, the BCR-ABL fusion protein, is a constituitively active tyrosine kinase that functions as an oncogene and results in leukemogenesis. The Philadelphia chromosome is detectable in up to 95% of patients with this disease, and may be used clinically as a marker to assess therapeutic progress.[4]

Most patients with CML are diagnosed in an indolent chronic phase, which lasts an average of 4 to 6 years. In this phase of the disease, approximately 50% of patients are asymptomatic, although nonspecific constitutional symptoms such as fatigue, weight loss, and night sweats are also common. Splenomegaly is present in up to 75% of patients and may lead to associated complaints of abdominal pain or early satiety. The peripheral white blood cell (WBC) count is typically greater than 50 $\times$ 10^9/L, with anemia, basophilia, and eosinophilia common findings.

The chronic phase of this disease is generally well controlled with systemic medical therapy. Nonetheless, patients with CML typically progress to an accelerated phase, characterized by an increase in both clinical symptoms and the number of circulating blast cells, in which the disease may become difficult to control despite more aggressive therapy. Progressive splenic enlargement may lead to massive splenomegaly and hypersplenism; painful splenic infarcts may occur, and complications of thrombocytopenia and anemia may necessitate frequent transfusions of blood products. A blastic phase leading to death within 3 to 6 months typically follows, although it may begin abruptly after the chronic phase in up to 50% of patients.

Standard treatment for CML patients in the chronic phase is medical, with imatinib now forming the cornerstone of treatment. Interferon-alpha, cytotoxic agents, and stem cell transplant may also be employed in selected patients. The role of splenectomy in CML has historically been controversial. Although early reports seemed to suggest that early splenectomy could positively affect survival, no relationship between splenectomy and overall survival could be demonstrated in a prospective, randomized, multicenter trial in which CML patients received either standard chemotherapy or chemotherapy followed immediately by splenectomy.[5] Moreover, patients in this trial who received early splenectomy were found to have a small but significantly increased risk of thromboembolic complications associated with thrombocytosis.

In contrast, the use of stem cell transplant in selected patients clearly does confer a survival advantage to selected patients with chronic-phase CML, and in some, may well be curative. Early stem cell transplants were performed only after splenectomy or splenic irradiation, the goal being eradication of residual disease prior to transplantation. These procedures directed at the spleen have since been shown to be ineffective.[6,7]

While splenectomy does not appear to have a role in the treatment of patients in the chronic phase, selected patients in the accelerated or blastic phases of disease may benefit from the procedure. Advances in both surgical technique and postoperative care now allow splenectomy to be performed with acceptable morbidity and mortality in this population in whom massive splenomegaly and profound thrombocytopenia have, in the past, prohibited its use. In this setting, the operation may be used effectively in a palliative role to ameliorate mechanical symptoms of splenomegaly or to reduce blood product transfusions and bleeding episodes in patients with severe anemia or thrombocytopenia.[8] Even in severely thrombocytopenic patients, the procedure produces a significant and durable restoration of normal platelet levels in the majority of patients by the seventh postoperative day.[9] Unfortunately, these benefits do not appear to translate into a survival advantage.

In summary, the role of splenectomy in patients with CML appears to be palliative, with relief of symptoms of organomegaly and hypersplenism in patients with advanced disease being the major indications for surgical intervention.

Myelofibrosis with Myeloid Metaplasia (MMM)

This chronic myeloproliferative disorder is characterized by progressive fibroblast proliferation and marrow fibrosis secondary to stimulation by a clonal proliferation of neoplastic megakaryocytes or monocytes. Ineffective hematopoiesis in the fibrotic marrow, combined with extramedullary hematopoesis in the spleen and liver, typically leads to massive splenomegaly and hepatomegaly with resulting pancytopenia, abdominal pain, early satiety, portal hypertension, and severe constitutional symptoms.[10] MMM is the least common of the myeloproliferative disorders and has a median age of diagnosis of 60 years. In contrast to CML, no biologic or genetic marker has been found that is specific for MMM, and therefore, its diagnosis rests on characteristic findings on the peripheral blood smear and bone marrow biopsy. The prognosis of patients with this disease is generally poor—survival of approximately 3 to 5 years is typical before the disease progresses into an acute leukemic phase.

While autologous stem cell transplantation offers patients with MMM their only hope for cure, most patients are not eligible for transplantation because of their advanced age and comorbid medical conditions. Therefore, treatment of this disease is focused primarily on palliation of the symptoms associated with organomegaly and cytopenia.[11] Steroids, androgens, and erythropoietin are used in an attempt to reduce the number of blood product transfusions prescribed for anemia, whereas cytotoxic agents such as hydroxyurea may be used treat splenomegaly.

Although it has been employed sporadically for almost a century, splenectomy has only recently become a well-accepted procedure in the treatment of patients with MMM. Early series described extraordinarily high rates of postoperative morbidity and mortality attributed in large part to the premorbid condition of these patients. No beneficial effect on survival was demonstrated with its use, but splenectomy was shown to have a favorable effect on symptoms related to organomegaly.

Further experience with splenectomy in these patients has led to a reduction in the mortality rate associated with its use to 10% or less. Therefore, the procedure is now recognized as a reasonable palliative option. Its greatest success is achieved in this patient population when used to relieve mechanical symptoms of splenomegaly or severe constitutional symptoms.[12] The procedure may therefore play an important role in improving the quality of life of these chronically ill patients. Additional indications for its use include transfusion-dependent anemia and symptomatic portal hypertension, in which clinical benefit can be expected in a smaller, yet significant, number of patients. Splenectomy may also be used prior to stem cell transplantation; early reports suggest that it may hasten engraftment in this capacity. It is important to note that the procedure appears to have little efficacy in improving transfusion-dependent thrombocytopenia.

Despite a decrease in mortality rates, splenectomy still carries a rate of perioperative morbidity rate from 35 to 75%, with early complications including bleeding, infection, and thrombosis. As an alternative to splenectomy, external beam radiation therapy has been shown to be clinically effective in relieving the mechanical symptoms of splenomegaly, but its effect is not as durable as that of splenectomy, and it is associated with its own set of complications.[13]

In addition to its immediate risks, several important long-term complications of splenectomy must be considered.[14] Progressive postoperative hepatomegaly owing to extramedullary hematopoiesis may occur, occasionally resulting in hepatic dysfunction. Postsplenectomy thrombocytosis may also occur, requiring platelet pheresis or further therapy to avoid thrombotic complications. Finally, splenectomy may be associated with an increased risk of leukemic transformation, although a cause and effect relationship between the two has not been established conclusively.

In summary, splenectomy is a valuable palliative option in for patients with MMM. Although the mortality rate associated with this procedure has declined in recent years, it still carries a high morbidity rate in this patient population, and therefore should be performed only after a thorough analysis of the risks and benefits associated with its use.

Essential Thrombocythemia and Polycythemia Vera

Both polycythemia vera (PV) and essential thrombocythemia (ET) are rare, chronic myeloid disorders with trilineage myeloid involvement. In PV, proliferation of erythroid elements is predominant; an absolute increase in red cell mass is the most obvious laboratory finding, but leukocytosis and thrombocytosis are also typical. In contrast, isolated thrombocytosis is the hallmark of ET. Patients with both diseases are prone to both thrombotic and hemorrhagic complications. In time, both diseases may transition to an advanced phase clinically similar to MMM, in which splenomegaly is a common feature; a smaller number of patients transition to an acute leukemic phase similar to acute myelogenous leukemia (AML). Treatment of patients with PV is primarily medical, and includes phlebotomy and cytotoxic agents. Many with ET can be managed expectantly, but cytoreductive agents can be offered to high-risk patients. Splenectomy plays little role in the treatment of either disorder, although it has been used in isolated cases to palliate symptoms associated with massive splenomegaly or to treat thrombosis of the portal system.

CHRONIC LYMPHOCYTIC LEUKEMIA (CLL)

Accounting for almost one-quarter of all leukemias, CLL is the most common leukemia of adults in the western hemisphere. More than 95% of patients have a B-cell phenotype, in which a progressive accumulation of morphologically mature yet functionally incompetent B-lymphocytes occurs. The diagnosis of CLL is suggested in patients with $> 5 \times 10^9$/L lymphocytes in the circulation and at least 30% lymphocytes in the bone marrow. The disorder is one of the elderly, and is more common in men.

Patients with CLL are often asymptomatic, although constitutional symptoms such as fevers, night sweats, fatigue, and unexplained weight loss are described. Lymphadenopathy is the most common physical finding. Splenomegaly is not as prevalent as in the chronic myeloid disorders, but may be identified in up to 40% of patients. A diagnostic work-up is often initiated only after an incidental laboratory finding of leukocytosis. Laboratory tests may also reveal anemia and/or thrombocytopenia, especially in patients with advanced disease. Cytopenias may arise secondary to bone marrow failure, an autoimmune phenomenon, hypersplenism, or the effects of therapy.

Prognosis of patients with CLL is assessed using a modified clinical staging system devised by Rai.[15] In the original Rai system, patients with lymphocytosis as their only manifestation of disease are defined as stage 0. Stage I includes the presence of lymphadenopathy, stage II includes organomegaly, stage III includes anemia, and stage IV includes thrombocytopenia. In a simplified modification, stage 0 disease is classified as low risk; stages I and II are combined into an intermediate-risk category, and stages III and IV are labeled high risk. Stage is correlated with prognosis; low-risk patients have a median survival over 12 years, but the median survival of high-risk patients is under 2 years.

Low-risk, asymptomatic patients may be managed expectantly. Therapy should be initiated in higher-risk patients to treat severe constitutional symptoms, mechanical effects of splenomegaly, or complications of cytopenia such as episodic infection or bleeding. First-line therapy for patients with high-risk CLL consists of fludarabine, but patients must be observed for signs of myelosupression and immunosuppression, which may be severe. Other cytoreductive therapies may be used in select groups of patients.

The role of splenectomy in patients with CLL is incompletely defined. Certainly, splenectomy is useful to relieve mechanical symptoms of organomegaly, but a significant hematologic response in patients with high-risk disease can also be achieved with this procedure. Several reports demonstrate a significant and durable effect of splenectomy on cytopenias in these patients. An excellent hematologic response to splenectomy can be expected in those with isolated anemia or thrombocytopenia, but patients with both appear to have a poorer response, suggesting that an adequate hematopoetic reserve is required to support recovery after the procedure.[16] Reversal of cytopenia may lead to a reduction in transfusion requirements in those patients requiring them, and may also allow the administration of increased doses of myelosuppressive chemotherapy.

While the effect of splenectomy on patient survival has been controversial historically, recent evidence suggests that the survival of two groups of patients may be significantly enhanced by splenectomy over conventional therapy: those with anemia (hemoglobin $\leq$ 10g/dL) or with profound thrombocytopenia (platelets $\leq$ 50 $\times$ 10^9/L). With regard to CLL, therefore, the use of splenectomy is most relevant to those patients with high-risk disease.

HAIRY CELL LEUKEMIA (HCL)

HCL is a chronic B-cell lymphoproliferative disorder named for the characteristic irregularly shaped cells that are found in the peripheral blood and bone marrow of affected patients. The disease is uncommon, representing only 2 to 5% of leukemias, and is primarily one of older males. Splenomegaly is the clinical hallmark of disease, with up to 90% of patients having splenic enlargement, often massive, owing to infiltration of the organ with neoplastic cells. Bone marrow infiltration is also common, but lymphadenopathy is conspicuously absent. Hepatomegaly is found in approximately 20% of patients. Pancytopenia is seen in approximately 50% and is secondary to both hypersplenism and marrow infiltration, but most patients present with suppression of at least one cell line. Although many patients are asymptomatic, symptoms related to splenomegaly or complications of cytopenia such as infection or hemorrhage may be noted and necessitate treatment.

Until recently, splenectomy was the cornerstone of management in patients with HCL.[17] The procedure is highly effective at relieving mechanical symptoms associated with splenomegaly. Moreover, partial to complete cytologic response and improvement in cytopenia is seen in up to 80% of patients after splenectomy, and several studies suggest a survival advantage may result. Despite these benefits, however, therapeutic advances have limited the use of splenectomy. Interferon-alpha is associated with a cytologic response rate in up to 90% of patients and has been shown to be a more effective first-line treatment for patients with HCL than splenectomy. Unfortunately, complete remissions are rare and early relapse is common after the drug is discontinued. In contrast, administration of the purine analogs pentostatin or cladribine results in a complete and durable response in 80 to 90% of patients. These drugs now represent first-line treatment for patients with HCL. Splenectomy may still be considered in rare cases, such as in cases of splenic rupture, as a diagnostic modality in difficult cases, or to relieve refractory symptoms of splenomegaly.

The Lymphomas

NON-HODGKIN'S LYMPHOMA

Non-Hodgkin's lymphoma (NHL) refers to a group of related disorders that includes all lymphoid malignancies except Hodgkin's disease. The disease is relatively common, ranking fifth among adult cancers in the United States. In this country, approximately 90% are of B-cell origin. While several classification systems have been used and appear in the literature, the World Health Organization (WHO) classification is currently the most widely used. This system differentiates between the numerous subtypes of NHL on the basis of the cell of origin, cell morphology, and immunophenotype.

Many patients with indolent disease are asymptomatic, but in advanced disease constitutional symptoms ("B symptoms") predominate. Symptoms may also result from extranodal deposits of disease, such as abdominal pain or bowel obstruction owing to involvement of the gastrointestinal system. In the majority of patients, lymphadenopathy is the major presenting feature. Painless lymphadenopathy in the cervical, supraclavicular, axillary, and inguinal regions is found in the majority of patients, and should be sought in all patients suspected of having the disease. In contrast to Hodgkin's disease, progressive lymph node involvement is characteristically disorderly and extranodal disease is common. Splenomegaly, identified in 35 to 80% of patients, may result in hypersplenism, and isolated splenic disease may rarely occur.

Hemogram findings may be nonspecific or may show cytopenia; other laboratory studies are typically nonspecific. The diagnosis is secured by surgical excision of an involved node or malignant focus. Subsequent imaging studies and bone marrow biopsy may then be used to stage the disease. Staging laparotomy plays no role in patients with NHL.

Cytotoxic agents are currently the treatment of choice for most patients with NHL. Radiation therapy may be employed in selected patients. Asymptomatic patients with early disease may often be managed expectantly. The role of splenectomy in these patients is not well defined, and, for the majority of patients, splenectomy is not required. Splenectomy may be used effectively in patients with splenomegaly and hypersplenism as a palliative therapy to correct cytopenias temporarily, thereby reducing the risk of hemorrhagic or infectious complications.[18] The procedure may also be required, though rarely, to assist in diagnosis in the absence of peripheral lymphadenopathy. Finally, splenectomy is often successful in relieving the bulk symptoms of massive splenomegaly that may be experienced by patients with advanced disease.[19] The benefits achieved from this therapy must be balanced against moderate morbidity (20–37%) and mortality (< 5%) rates.

HODGKIN'S DISEASE

Hodgkin's Disease (HD) is an uncommon disorder, primarily of younger patients, characterized by the presence of pathognomonic, neoplastic Reed-Sternberg cells in the lymphatic tissues. Most patients with the disease present with painless enlargement of the cervical, axillary, or mediastinal lymph nodes. Extranodal spread of disease is characteristically orderly, and may be found in the bone marrow, lungs, liver, and bones. Approximately one-quarter of patients complain of significant B symptoms, including weight loss, persistent fever, and lethargy, which are often associated with advanced disease.

Overall prognosis is related to disease stage, and has been steadily improving over the past few decades. Stage by the Ann Arbor system depends on the number of involved lymphatic regions, location of disease either above or below the diaphragm, and the presence or absence of extranodal disease. The presence of B symptoms also has staging and prognostic value. In past years, stage was most reliably assessed surgically using staging laparotomy. This procedure involves thorough exploration and biopsy of all intra-abdominal nodal groups and the liver, with splenectomy. Bone marrow biopsy is performed simultaneously. The procedure is rarely performed today, because reliable clinical staging data can be acquired less invasively using diagnostic imaging techniques and laboratory studies. The decline in the number of splenectomies performed as part of staging laparotomy for Hodgkin's disease over the past decades accounts in large part for a reduction in the number of splenectomies performed annually in general.[1]

Treatment with brief multiagent chemotherapy followed by external beam irradiation has been shown to be a highly effective curative treatment for patients with limited-stage disease. Aggressive systemic chemotherapy is the treatment of choice for most patients with advanced-stage disease. Stem cell transplant may be employed in some patients with recurrent or refractory disease. Therapeutic splenectomy does not play a role in treatment.

Technical Points of Open Splenectomy

In all of the hematologic malignancies, open splenectomy becomes a particularly demanding procedure technically. Much of the difficulty associated with the operation is related to the massive splenomegaly often seen in such patients (Figure 1); in fact, splenic size has been shown to be the single most important factor predicting the

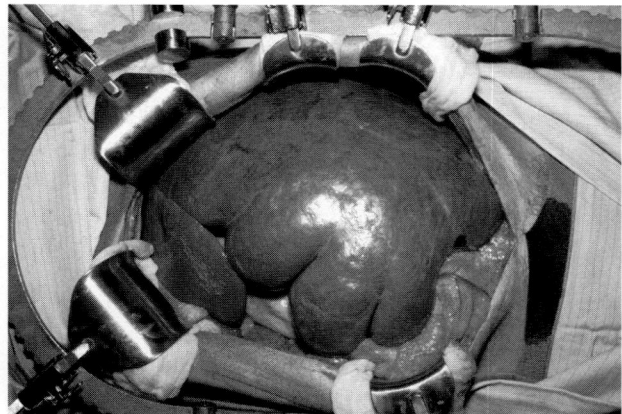

Figure 1 Open splenectomy performed for bulk symptoms secondary to massive splenomegaly.

likelihood of postoperative complications.[2] Other confounding variables include qualitative or quantitative platelet dysfunction, which may predispose to intraoperative or postoperative hemorrhage. An experienced surgical team is mandatory.

The procedure begins with a midline incision, which both provides excellent exposure and avoids dividing the rectus abdominus muscles, thereby decreasing the risk of abdominal wall hemorrhage.[20,21] A thorough exploration and identification of any accessory splenic tissue follows. The splenic artery should be ligated early in the procedure, and is approached through the lesser omental sac. Once this has been performed, shrinkage of the spleen from autotransfusion through the splenic vein typically occurs, allowing easier mobilization of the enlarged organ. Platelet transfusion may be performed at this point without risk of splenic platelet sequestration. The spleen can then be divided from its retroperitoneal and intraperitoneal attachments. It is passed off the table after ligation and division of the splenic and short gastric vessels at the hilum. Drainage of the splenic bed is reserved for cases of suspected injury to the pancreatic tail. Preoperative vaccination against postsplenectomy infection, including S. Pneumoniae (streptococcus), *Haemophilus Influenzae*, and N. Meningitidis (nisseria), is recommended.

Laparoscopic Splenectomy

Laparoscopic splenectomy has quickly evolved into the treatment of choice for patients with benign hematologic disease, in which the characteristically normal-sized spleen lends itself well to this approach. In contrast, the massive splenomegaly often seen in association with hematologic malignancy has slowed its adoption in this group of patients. Nonetheless, accumulating evidence demonstrates that laparoscopic splenectomy for hematologic malignancy is not only technically feasible, but is also a highly effective therapeutic approach in select cases.

The theoretical advantages of laparoscopic compared with open splenectomy in general include less postoperative pain, a shorter length of hospital stay, and faster recovery. This appears to be true in patients with hematologic malignancy as well. Conversion rates as high as 40% from the laparoscopic to open approach are common, however, and laparoscopic splenectomy is typically associated with a longer operative time and greater operative blood loss then open splenectomy. Nonetheless, this does not translate into an increase in intraoperative transfusion rates nor an increase in procedure-related morbidity or mortality rates compared with the open approach.[22] Splenic weight certainly has an impact on outcomes, with massive splenomegaly increasing intraoperative blood loss, length of stay, and rates of conversion. A hand-assisted laparoscopic technique, with advantages over open splenectomy similar to those of the laparoscopic procedure, may be useful in cases of massive splenomegaly.[23]

Technical points regarding the procedure for laparoscopic splenectomy in these patients include the following: An open Hasson approach is used for placement of the first trocar in the infraumbilical position, and a 5-trocar set-up is employed. When the laparoscopic hand-assist device is used, it is placed in the upper midline position through an incision approximately 7.5 cm in length. After port placement, the stomach is retracted downward and to the right. The gastrocolic ligament is sharply divided after coagulation of its vessels. The peritoneum is then opened to the level of the lienorenal ligament. The splenic artery is identified in its course along the superior border of the pancreas. The artery is then ligated with a suture or vascular clip to provide shrinkage of the spleen, as described previously with open splenectomy. After the vessels to the lower pole of the spleen are individually ligated, the lateral retroperitoneal splenic attachments are divided, and the tail of the pancreas is carefully dissected free from the hilum of the spleen. Use of the harmonic scalpel facilitates division of the short gastric vessels (Figure 2). The splenic artery and vein are identified at the splenic hilum and divided with an endoscopic linear vascular stapling device (Figure 3). Finally, the spleen is placed into a large laparoscopic bag that is partially exteriorized through an enlarged port site or through the hand-assist device incision.

Conclusion

In summary, open or laparoscopic splenectomy plays an important diagnostic and therapeutic role in several

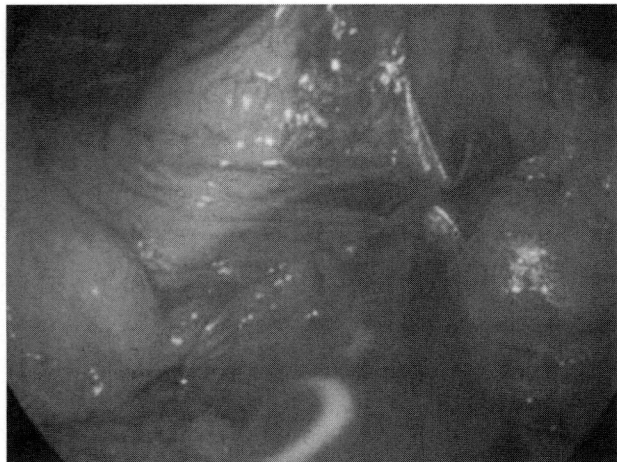

Figure 2 Division of the short gastric vessels using the harmonic scalpel in laparoscopic splenectomy.

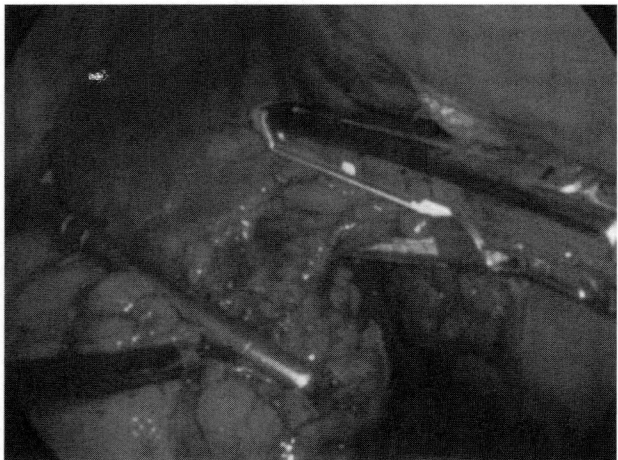

Figure 3 An endovascular linear cutting stapler facilitates ligation and division of the splenic vessels at the hilum.

hematologic malignancies. Although the mortality rate associated with splenectomy in this setting has fallen over the past several decades, it is still associated with a significant rate of morbidity. When performed by a skilled and experienced surgical team, however, the procedures may be effective in improving the quality, and occasionally the quantity, of life of patients with these hematologic diseases.

References

1. Wilhelm MC, Jones RE, McGehee R, et al. Splenectomy in hematologic disorders. The ever-changing indications. Ann Surg 1988;207:581–9.

2. Horowitz J, Smith JL, Weber TK, et al. Postoperative complications after splenectomy for hematologic malignancies. Ann Surg 1996;223:290–6.

3. Dameshek W. Some speculations on the myeloproliferative syndromes. Blood 1951;6:372–5.

4. Sawyers CL. Chronic myeloid leukemia. N Engl J Med 1999;340:1330–40.

5. Results of a prospective randomized trial of early splenectomy in chronic myeloid leukemia. The Italian Cooperative Study Group on Chronic Myeloid Leukemia. Cancer 1984;54:333–8.

6. Gratwohl A, Goldman J, Gluckman E, Zwaan F. Effect of splenectomy before bone-marrow transplantation on survival in chronic granulocytic leukaemia. Lancet 1985;2:1290–1.

7. Kalhs P, Schwarzinger I, Anderson G, et al. A retrospective analysis of the long-term effect of splenectomy on late infections, graft-versus-host disease, relapse, and survival after allogeneic marrow transplantation for chronic myelogenous leukemia. Blood 1995;86:2028–32.

8. Bouvet M, Babiera GV, Termuhlen PM, et al. Splenectomy in the accelerated or blastic phase of chronic myelogenous leukemia: a single-institution, 25-year experience. Surgery 1997;122:20–5.

9. Berman RS, Feig BW, Hunt KK, et al. Platelet kinetics and decreased transfusion requirements after splenectomy for hematologic malignancy. Ann Surg 2004;240:852–7.

10. Tefferi A. Myelofibrosis with myeloid metaplasia. N Engl J Med 2000;342:1255–65.

11. Tefferi A. Treatment approaches in myelofibrosis with myeloid metaplasia: the old and the new. Semin Hematol 2003;40(1 Suppl 1):18–21.

12. Tefferi A, Mesa RA, Nagorney DM, et al. Splenectomy in myelofibrosis with myeloid metaplasia: a single-institution experience with 223 patients. Blood 2000;95:2226–33.

13. Elliott MA, Tefferi A. Splenic irradiation in myelofibrosis with myeloid metaplasia: a review. Blood Rev 1999;13:163–70.

14. Barosi G, Ambrosetti A, Buratti A, et al. Splenectomy for patients with myelofibrosis with myeloid metaplasia: pretreatment variables and outcome prediction. Leukemia 1993;7:200–6.

15. Rai KR, Sawitsky A, et al. Clinical staging of chronic lymphocytic leukemia. Blood 1975;46:219–34.

16. Cusack JC Jr, Seymour JF, Lerner S, et al. Role of splenectomy in chronic lymphocytic leukemia. J Am Coll Surg 1997;185:237–43.

17. Zakarija A, Peterson LC, Tallman MS. Splenectomy and treatments of historical interest. Best Pract Res Clin Haematol 2003;16:57–68.

18. Lehne G, Hannisdal E, Langholm R, Nome O. A 10-year experience with splenectomy in patients with malignant

non-Hodgkin's lymphoma at the Norwegian Radium Hospital. Cancer 1994;74:933–9.

19. Xiros N, Economopoulos T, Christodoulidis C, et al. Splenectomy in patients with malignant non-Hodgkin's lymphoma. Eur J Haematol 2000;64:145–50.

20. Pollock RE, Hohn DC. Splenectomy. In: Roh MS, Ames FC, editors. Advanced oncologic surgery. London: Mosby; 1994.

21. Danforth DN Jr, Fraker DL. Splenectomy for the massively enlarged spleen. Am Surg 1991;57:108–13.

22. Berman RS, Yahanda AM, Mansfield PF, et al. Laparoscopic splenectomy in patients with hematologic malignancies. Am J Surg 1999;178:530–6.

23. Knauer EM, Ailawadi G, Yahanda A, et al. 101 laparoscopic splenectomies for the treatment of benign and malignant hematologic disorders. Am J Surg 2003;186:500–4.

CHAPTER 25

SMALL BOWEL ADENOCARCINOMA DISTAL TO THE LIGAMENT OF TREITZ

COURTNEY L. SCAIFE, MD

Background

Beyond the Ligament of Treitz, the small bowel is divided into the jejunum and ileum, without distinct anatomic landmarks to delineate the transition from jejunum to ileum. Generally, the proximal third of the small bowel is considered the jejunum, whereas the distal two-thirds comprise the ileum. It is rare for a primary neoplasm to develop in this segment of the midgut; the *2005 Cancer Facts and Figures* estimated approximately 5,500 new cancers of the small bowel in 2005, with an estimated 1,000 cancer-related deaths.[1] Of these tumors of the small bowel, only 40% are adenocarcinomas.[2]

The histology of the small bowel consists of a 4-layered hollow organ made of an external serosa, muscularis propria, submucosa, and internal mucosa. The blood supply to the jejunum and ileum arises from the superior mesenteric artery, which arborizes into extensive branches within the small bowel mesentery. The lymphatic drainage of the small bowel follows the arterial vasculature in an extensive arcade, which coalesces into a main lymphatic trunk leading to the cisterna chyli along the abdominal aorta. The jejunum and ileum function to absorb the majority of ingested fluids, electrolytes, carbohydrates, proteins, fats, minerals, vitamins, and bile salts. Vitamin B12 is absorbed selectively in the terminal ileum by the cobalamin-intrinsic factor brush-border receptors.

Epidemiology

Neoplasms of the small bowel are rare, despite the fact that the small bowel constitutes over 60% of the intestinal tract.[3] Ninety percent of small bowel neoplasms are benign lesions, the majority of which are leiomyomas (41%).[4] Malignant lesions of the small bowel include adenocarcinomas, sarcomas, neuroendocrine tumors, lymphomas, and metastatic lesions. The dominant malignant lesion of the small bowel is an adenocarcinoma, which accounts for 37 to 40% of small intestinal malignancies.[5,6]

Risk factors of developing small intestinal adenocarcinoma are not well defined. Several implicated factors include smoking, alcohol consumption, and low-fiber, low-antioxidant dietary intake.[7] Comorbid medical conditions that may have an associated increased risk of small intestinal adenocarcinoma include Crohn's disease, familial adenomatous polyposis, celiac sprue, cystic fibrosis, and chronic peptic ulcer disease.[7,8] Additionally, an analysis of several international cancer registries implies that a history of a previous intestinal, uterine, ovarian, prostate, or renal carcinoma increases the risk of developing a primary small bowel carcinoma.[6] The reasons for the low incidence of carcinoma of the midgut are not well understood, but are felt to be related to a short transit time of potentially carcinogenic lumen contents, low bacterial flora load, an alkaline environment, and a low rate of activated precarcinogenic enzymes.[7]

Presentation

Adenocarinomas of the small bowel most commonly present with patients complaining of vague abdominal pain syndromes.[9,10] Other presenting symptoms include nausea and vomiting, weight loss, gastrointestinal bleeding, obstruction, and fatigue caused by anemia.[9–11] The majority of patients are men in most series (52–67%).[10–12] The mean age at presentation is 52 to 65 years of age, ranging from 4 to 85 years of age.[10–12] Eighty to 85% of patients are white.[11,12] The mean time from onset of symptoms to diagnosis is approximately 4 months (range < 1 month to 1.2 years).[10]

Diagnosis

Diagnosis of neoplasms of the small bowel remains challenging, as direct visual endoscopic access to the midgut lumen is limited. The most common physical exam abnormality in patients with a neoplasm of the small bowel is a palpable abdominal mass, followed by abdominal distention and tenderness on examination.[10] Physical examination established a diagnosis in only 4% of patients in 1 series.[11] Surgical exploration, including laparotomy and laparoscopy, was diagnostic in 26% of cases after 1988, in The University of Texas M. D. Anderson Cancer Center series.[11] The majority of lesions are diagnosed by radiographic imaging. Diagnostic radiographic studies include enteroclysis, ultrasound, computed tomography (CT), and capsule endoscopy. In the M. D. Anderson case series, an upper intestinal barium study was the most frequent radiographic diagnostic modality to demonstrate a probable neoplasm (diagnostic in 22% of cases), but this series predates the use of capsule endoscopy and modern helical-CT imaging.[11] CT enteroclysis utilizes spiral and multi-detector row CT technology with a volume challenge of 2 liters of enteral contrast agent administrated through a nasojejunal catheter (Figure 1). This technique has become the radiographic diagnostic tool of choice for suspected small bowel neoplasms, with a sensitivity and specificity rate of 100% and 95%, respectively.[13,14]

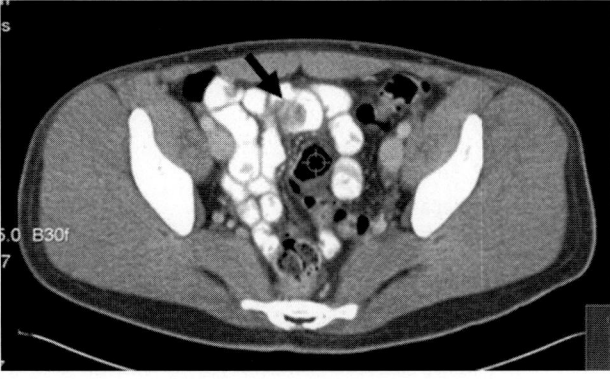

Figure 1 Computed tomography (CT) enteroclysis of small bowel adenocarcinoma. Arrow indicates the intraluminal neoplasm.

Recent advances in endoscopic techniques have improved the diagnostic yield for the evaluation of midgut neoplasms. Double-balloon endoscopy is the most recent endoscopy technique that allows direct visualization of the midgut from a transanal and transoral approach.[15] More recent experience with capsule endoscopy has shown this technique to have a higher diagnostic yield than push enteroscopy.[16,17] Other series have shown improved diagnostic rates for capsule endoscopy compared with radiographic contrast studies, as well.[18,19]

Rarely, a diagnostic biopsy is considered or necessary for the evaluation of a small intestinal tumor. Only in the unique scenario of a suspected small bowel lymphoma would one consider a pretreatment biopsy (see Chapter 27, "Lymphoma of the Small Bowel"). The primary resection of a suspicious lesion remains the diagnostic and treatment approach of choice.

Staging

The American Joint Committee on Cancer (AJCC) distant staging of small intestinal tumors is based on the tumor-nodes-distant metastases (TNM) classification, summarized in Table 1. Metastatic disease from a small bowel adenocarcinoma is found most commonly in the regional lymph nodes and the liver. The most common site for recurrent disease following curative resection of the primary tumor is in the peritoneal cavity, the liver, and the lungs.[11,20]

Treatment

Few series have been published on the experience with the treatment and outcomes of patients with small bowel adenocarcinoma. The largest series include Bauer and colleagues, 38 patients from Roswell Park Cancer Center; DiSario and colleagues, 80 patients from the Utah Cancer Registry; Veyrieres and colleagues, 100 patients from the French Associations for Surgical Research; Cunningham and colleagues, 29 patients from Mount Sinai Medical Center; Howe and colleagues, 4,995 cases from the National Cancer Data Base; and finally, Dabaja and colleagues, 217 patients from M. D. Anderson.[9,11,12,20–22]

The primary treatment for adenocarcinoma of the small bowel remains wide surgical resection. Table 1 summarizes the survival outcomes published in these series. The mean overall survival is 13 months, with a 30% 5-year survival rate. Factors that reduce long-term survival probability include metastases at diagnosis, unresectability, positive regional lymph nodes, and poorly differentiated tumors.[9,11,20] Cunningham and colleagues reported a 23-month median survival in

Table 1 TNM Staging System for Small Intestine Cancer[26]

Staging		0	1	2	3	4	X
Primary Tumor (T)	Tis — carcinoma in situ	No tumor	Invades lamina propria	Invades muscularis propria	Invades into subserosa, mesentery, or retroperitoneum; extension $\leq$ 2cm	Perforates visceral peritoneum or invades surrounding structure	Tumor cannot be assessed
Lymph nodes (N)		Negative regional nodes	Nodal metastases				
Distant metastases (M)		None	Metastatic disease				
STAGE		Tis, N0, M0	T1, N0, M0 T2, N0, M0	T3, N0, M0 T4, N0, M0	Any T, N1, M0	Any T, Any N, M1	

patients who underwent complete resection of a small bowel adenocarcinoma compared with only a 7-month median survival in patients undergoing incomplete or palliative resection.[9] Howe and colleagues found a 2.19-fold increased risk of cancer-related death in patients who did not undergo a curative surgical resection.[12] Dabaja and colleagues documented a 78-month versus a 22-month survival advantage for node-negative compared with node-positive disease, respectively.[11]

The role of chemotherapy for small intestine adenocarcinoma is poorly defined. There are no well-established treatment regimens for small bowel adenocarcinoma, and most commonly, colorectal cancer regimens are applied. Two series evaluated the benefit of adjuvant therapy following surgical resection. Howe and colleagues found that patients who underwent a potentially curative operation without adjuvant chemotherapy had a 47.8-month mean survival compared with a mean of 23.6 months for patients who received chemotherapy following surgical resection.[12] The M. D. Anderson series also found that chemotherapy did not improve survival following surgical resection. This series, however, did show a survival advantage for chemotherapy in patients who did not undergo curative surgery, with chemotherapy-treated patients having a mean survival of 12 months versus a mean of 2 months for those patients who received no treatment. The selection

biases for the treatment modality in these retrospective reviews must be considered, though, when interpreting these results (Table 2).

There are no current trials for primary chemotherapy or adjuvant therapy following surgical resection of a small bowel primary adenocarcinoma, whereas several phase I and II trials are currently open for the treatment of advanced, metastatic, or refractory intestinal adenocarcinomas. The results of these large multidisease trials will remain difficult to interpret for the treatment of small bowel adenocarcinomas.

There is no evidence demonstrating a benefit for radiation therapy for small bowel adenocarcinomas. The use of radiation therapy should be considered for palliative control of locally advanced or metastatic disease only.

Surgical resection of hepatic metastases of gastrointestinal primary neoplasms has become more aggressive and common in the past 10 years. Evidence of improved patient survival following resection of colorectal hepatic metastases is encouraging. Unfortunately, there is no evidence that this approach translates to the treatment of small bowel primary adenocarcinomas. In reviews of noncolorectal, non-neuroendocrine hepatic metastatectomies several institutions show no benefit of resection of noncolorectal gastrointestinal adenocarcinoma metastases.[23–25]

Table 2 Summary of Reported Patient Survival Rates with Small Intestinal Adenocarcinoma

Study	Number of patients	Mean overall 5-year survival	Mean survival
Bauer et al 1994[20]	38	23%	3.6–9 months
DiSario et al 1994[22]	80	25%	N/A
Veyrieres et al 1997[21]	100	38%	N/A
Cunnignham et al 1997[9]	29	30%	13 months
Howe et al 1999[12]	4,995	30%	19.7 months
Dabaja et al 2004[11]	217	26%	20 months

Technical Aspects of Resection

Surgery remains the primary treatment for small bowel adenocarcinomas, with a curative resection of locally contained disease significantly improving overall survival.[11,12] Although many primary neoplasms of the small bowel are diagnosed at the time of resection, the surgeon should consider intraoperative analysis by the pathologist to determine a benign versus a malignant neoplasm. At the time of primary resection, the confirmation of an adenocarcinoma of the small bowel should change the operative approach to include a wide regional nodal resection in the form of resection of the associated small bowel mesentery. A laparoscopic approach for adenocarcinoma of the small bowel has not been studied in a prospective manner, but if adequate oncologic principles are applied, including a wide resection margin and adequate lymph node resection, a laparoscopic approach may be considered. The advantage of a laparoscopic approach lies in the fact that 90% of small bowel neoplasms are benign and are nicely amenable to a minimally invasive surgical approach.[4] If an aggressive resection of the terminal ileum is necessary, postsurgery replacement of vitamin B should be considered.

The surgical treatment of metastatic disease requires case-by-case review. The poor prognostic outcome with advanced small bowel adenocarcinoma indicates that aggressive resection of locally advanced or metastatic disease may not change a patient's quality of life and overall survival. Palliative surgical interventions for obstructive, bleeding, or painful lesions should be considered individually.

References

1. Jemal A, Murray T, Ward E, et al. American Cancer Society. Cancer statistics 2005.

2. Serour F, Dona G, Birkenfeld S, et al. Primary neoplasms of the small bowel. J Surg Oncol 1992;49:29–34.

3. Ahrens EH Jr, Blankenhorn DH, Hirsch J. Measurement of the human intestinal length in vivo and some causes of variation. Gastroenterology 1956;31:274–84.

4. Ciresi DL, Scholten DJ. The continuing clinical dilemma of primary tumors of the small intestine. Am Surg 1995;61:698–703.

5. Martin RG. Malignant tumors of the small intestine. Surg Clin North Am 1986;66:779–85.

6. Scelo G, Boffetta P, Hemminki K, et al. Associations between small intestine cancer and other primary cancers: an international population-based study. Int J Cancer 2006;118:189–96.

7. Neugut AI, Jacobson JS, Suh S, et al. The epidemiology of cancer of the small bowel. Cancer Epidemiol Biomarkers Prev 1998;7:243–51.

8. Persson PG, Bernell O, Leijonmarck CE, et al. Crohn's disease and cancer: a population-based cohort study. Gastroenterology 1994;107:1675–9.

9. Cunningham JD, Aleali R, Aleali M, et al. Malignant small bowel neoplasms: histopathologic determinants of recurrence and survival. Ann Surg 1997;225:300–6.

10. Garcia Marcilla JA, Sanchez Bueno F, Aguilar J, et al. Primary small bowel malignant tumors. Eur J Surg Oncol 1994;20:630–4.

11. Dabaja BS, Suki D, Pro B, et al. Adenocarcinoma of the small bowel: presentation, prognostic factors, and outcome of 217 patients. Cancer 2004;101:518–26.

12. Howe JR, Karnell LH, Menck HR, Scott-Conner C. The American College of Surgeons Commission on Cancer and the American Cancer Society. Adenocarcinoma of the small bowel: review of the National Cancer Data Base, 1985–1995. Cancer 1999;86:2693–706.

13. Schmidt S, Felley C, Meuwly JY, et al. CT enteroclysis: technique and clinical applications. Eur Radiol 2006;16:648–60.

14. Boudiaf M, Jaff A, Soyer P, et al. Small-bowel diseases: prospective evaluation of multi-detector row helical CT enteroclysis in 107 consecutive patients. Radiology 2004;233:338–44.

15. May A, Nachbar L, Ell C. Double-balloon enteroscopy (push-and-pull enteroscopy) of the small bowel: feasibility and diagnostic and therapeutic yield in patients with suspected small bowel disease. Gastrointest Endosc 2005;62:62–70.

16. Chong AK, Taylor A, Miller A, et al. Capsule endoscopy vs. push enteroscopy and enteroclysis in suspected small-bowel Crohn's disease. Gastrointest Endosc 2005;61:255–61.

17. Mylonaki M, Fritscher-Ravens A, Swain P. Wireless capsule endoscopy: a comparison with push enteroscopy in patients with gastroscopy and colonoscopy negative gastrointestinal bleeding. Gut 2003;52:1122–6.

18. Eliakim R, Fischer D, Suissa A, et al. Wireless capsule video endoscopy is a superior diagnostic tool in comparison to barium follow-through and computerized tomography in patients with suspected Crohn's disease. Eur J Gastroenterol Hepatol 2003;15:363–7.

19. Voderholzer WA, Ortner M, Rogalla P, et al. Diagnostic yield of wireless capsule enteroscopy in comparison with computed tomography enteroclysis. Endoscopy 2003;35:1009–14.

20. Bauer RL, Palmer ML, Bauer AM, et al. Adenocarcinoma of the small intestine: 21-year review of diagnosis, treatment, and prognosis. Ann Surg Oncol 1994;1:183–8.

21. Veyrieres M, Baillet P, Hay JM, et al. Factors influencing long-term survival in 100 cases of small intestine primary adenocarcinoma. Am J Surg 1997;173:237–9.

22. DiSario JA, Burt RW, Vargas H, McWhorter WP. Small bowel cancer: epidemiological and clinical characteristics from a population-based registry. Am J Gastroenterol 1994; 89:699–701.

23. Laurent C, Rullier E, Feyler A, et al. Resection of noncolorectal and nonneuroendocrine liver metastases: late metastases are the only chance of cure. World J Surg 2001;25:1532–6.

24. Yedibela S, Gohl J, Graz V, et al. Changes in indication and results after resection of hepatic metastases from non-colorectal primary tumors: a single-institutional review. Ann Surg Oncol 2005;12:778–85.

25. Weitz J, Blumgart LH, Fong Y, et al. Partial hepatectomy for metastases from noncolorectal, nonneuroendocrine carcinoma. Ann Surg 2005;241: 269–76.

26. AJCC. Small intestine. In: American Joint Committee on Cancer: AJCC Cancer staging manual. 6th ed. New York: Springer; 2002. p. 107–12.

CHAPTER 26

DUODENAL ADENOCARCINOMA

CHARLES R. SCOGGINS, MD

ROBERT C.G. MARTIN, MD

KELLY M. MCMASTERS, MD, PhD

Primary duodenal adenocarcinoma is an uncommon disease; it represents less than 0.05% of all malignancies[1] and less than 0.5% of gastrointestinal (GI) malignancies, yet accounts for the majority (45%) of small bowel adenocarcinomas.[2–4] Despite the fact that duodenal carcinoma is usually diagnosed in an advanced stage, long-term survival is possible. Diagnostic imaging and endoscopy remain the optimal methods for preoperative diagnosis, and extirpative surgery is the treatment of choice. Patients treated with palliative surgery (GI and/or biliary bypass) have a very short median survival, usually 7 to 9 months,[5,6] compared to 5-year survival rates of over 40% for resected patients.[5] The preferred surgical approach is dictated by tumor location, with most duodenal carcinomas being treated with pancreaticoduodenectomy. Selected distal duodenal lesions may be adequately treated with segmental duodenectomy and lymphadenectomy.

Presentation and Diagnosis

Duodenal cancer typically presents in an advanced stage, and nodal metastases are common upon diagnosis. These tumors do not produce symptoms for extended periods of time, only causing obstruction of the duodenal lumen when they have achieved a substantial size. When the tumor is located at the ampulla of Vater, obstructive jaundice may be present and, in fact, may lead to earlier detection. Preoperative assessment of these tumors should include triple-phase computed tomography (CT) (Figure 1) of the abdomen and pelvis as well as chest radiography to allow for accurate staging. (Table 1) Serum tumor markers (including carcinoembryonic antigen, carbohydrate antigen (CA)19-9 and CA-125 should be assessed because levels may be elevated in these patients. CT not only offers reliable data regarding

staging, but also allows for preoperative determination of resectability. (Table 2) A thorough search for distant metastases should be performed, as well as determination of any neighboring viscera that may be involved by tumor. Important tumor-vessel relationships that should be evaluated include assessment of venous (vena cava and superior mesenteric-portal venous [SMPV] confluence, including patency of the vein) and arterial (hepatic and superior mesenteric artery [SMA]) involvement. CT is extremely accurate in predicting the need for venous resection.[7] As with pancreatic cancer, arterial involvement represents unresectable disease; once the 2 to 4 mm thick neural plexus that ensheathes the mesenteric arteries becomes infiltrated with tumor cells, there is little chance of a margin-negative (R0) resection.[8–10] Isolated venous involvement by itself does not preclude resection, and data from the pancreatic cancer literature

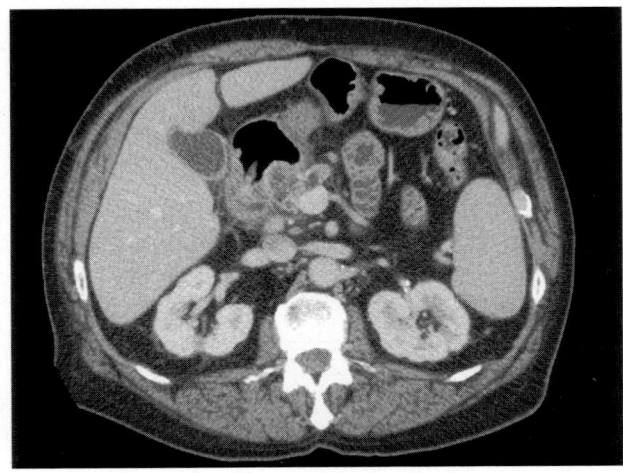

Figure 1 Staging computed tomography demonstrating thickening of the proximal duodenum. Endoscopic biopsy demonstrated duodenal adenocarcinoma.

Table 1 Staging System for Small Intestine Adenocarcinoma, Including Duodenum

Primary Tumor	
TX	Primary tumor cannot be assessed
T0	No evidence of primary tumor
Tis	Carcinoma in situ
T1	Tumor invades lamina propria or submucosa
T2	Tumor invades muscularis propria
T3	Tumor invades through muscularis propria into the subserosa or into the nonperitonealized perimuscular tissue (mesentery of retroperitoneum) with extension 2 cm or less
T4	Tumor perforates visceral peritoneum or directly invades other organs or structures

Regional Lymph Nodes	
NX	Regional lymph nodes cannot be assessed
N0	No regional lymph node metastasis
N1	Regional lymph node metastasis

Distant Metastasis	
MX	Distant metastasis cannot be assessed
M0	No distant metastasis
M1	Distant metastasis

Stage Grouping			
Stage 0	Tis	N0	M0
Stage I	T1-2	N0	M0
Stage II	T3-4	N0	M0
Stage III	Any T	N1	M0
Stage IV	Any T	Any N	M1

Reprinted with permission from Greene FL, et al.[45]

demonstrate the oncologic rationale and potential survival benefit of en bloc resection of involved venous structures, providing it allows for negative margins.[11,12] When the SMPV confluence is involved by tumor, venous thrombosis represents advanced disease and a remote chance for a margin-negative resection.[13] Thrombosis rarely occurs with less than 50% of the venous circumference involved by tumor; when the vein is encased with tumor, and thrombosis has occurred, the SMA margin is also likely involved, thus precluding an R0 resection.

Endoscopic evaluation usually includes esophagogastroduodenoscopy (EGD) with biopsy, and possibly endoscopic ultrasound. EGD is less reliable with distal (third or fourth portion of the duodenum [D3 or D4]) lesions. Endoscopic ultrasound (EUS) is extremely accurate in predicting the depth of tumor penetration; however, it is less than 70% accurate in determining the status of regional nodes.[14] EUS may aid in determining resectability, as vascular invasion may be determined;[15] however, these data should be correlated with CT and may not provide additional information. Presently, we do not routinely obtain EUS as part of the staging evaluation in patients with duodenal cancer. Fluorodeoxyglucose-positron emission tomography (PET) accurately detects both the primary and metastatic lesions in upper GI malignancies, including duodenal adenocarcinoma.[16] The role of PET in duodenal cancer is not fully defined, and most patients do not require a PET scan preoperatively. PET may be most useful in situations where preoperative imaging suggests metastatic disease, and the additional information provided by PET may obviate a nontherapeutic laparotomy.

Table 2 Criteria for Resectability of Duodenal Adenocarcinomas Determined on Preoperative Computed Tomography

Resectable	Unresectable
No evidence of distant metastasis*	Distant metastasis
Lack of arterial involvement†	Arterial involvement
Patent SMPV confluence	Thrombosed SMPV confluence

*Enlarged lymph nodes seen on preoperative imaging that may be included within the lymphadenectomy should not be considered a contraindication for resection. †Arterial involvement, direct tumor extension to or around the superior mesenteric artery or common hepatic artery. SMPV= superior mesenteric-portal vein.

Surgical Treatment of Duodenal Adenocarcinoma

Surgery offers the only chance at long-term survival for patients with duodenal cancer. General oncologic surgical principles that should be followed include meticulous hemostasis and complete margin-negative tumor extirpation. The peritoneal cavity may be entered either via a bilateral subcostal or midline incision, although the midline incision provides excellent exposure and ease of closure. A thorough exploration should be performed, with careful assessment of the peritoneal surfaces and the liver. With modern thin-section CT, there should be a low rate of nontherapeutic laparotomy. In cases where the staging CT suggests metastatic disease or peritoneal carcinomatosis but is nondiagnostic, a laparoscopic exploration is extremely useful because it adds minimal time to the operation should there be no distant disease, and it may avoid a laparotomy in an incurable patient. Resection of the tumor should proceed in an orderly fashion, and utilizing careful operative technique will minimize blood loss. For carcinomas arising in the proximal duodenum, pancreaticoduodenectomy (PD) is the procedure of choice. The operative technique for PD is detailed in Chapter 19. When the tumor is remote from the SMA, and there is little concern for the status of the perimesenteric (retroperitoneal) margin along the medial border of the SMA, a vascular stapler may be used to take this tissue, providing special care is taken to avoid bowing the artery into the stapler while retracting the specimen laterally. This maneuver allows for rapid dissection of the retroperitoneum while providing excellent hemostasis. When the tumor is close to the artery, or when the SMPV confluence requires resection, meticulous dissection of the medial SMA border should be performed. Because the pancreatic duct is usually not obstructed in cases of duodenal cancer, the pancreatic parenchyma is usually soft. This places the patient at significant risk for postoperative pancreatic leak, thus mandating extreme care when performing the pancreaticojejunostomy. Although there is no consensus on the routine use of somatostatin postoperatively, it may be helpful in cases when the pancreas is soft.

Special mention is made of carcinomas arising in the distal duodenum (distal D3 or D4). Among duodenal cancers, tumors of the distal duodenum are uncommon, comprising about 20% of duodenal carcinomas.[17] When the tumor is distal to the ampulla and there is no evidence of pancreatic involvement, segmental duodenectomy and lymphadenectomy may be the optimal treatment. (Figure 2) Segmental resection offers excellent survival results[18–20] and avoids the risks of pancreatic and biliary fistula. A retropancreatic and proximal mesenteric (along the inferior border of the pancreas at the root of the mesentery) lymphadenectomy should be performed. Any enlarged nodes seen on preoperative imaging should also be dissected and removed. A primary duodenojeju-

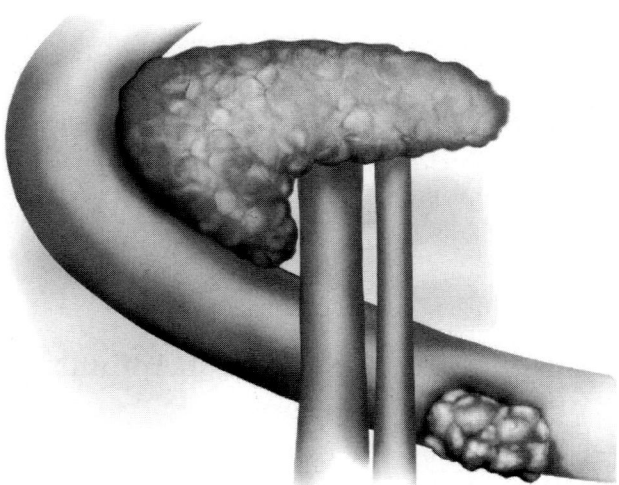

Figure 2 Duodenal carcinomas distal to the uncinate process, especially those to the left of the mesenteric vessels, may be resected with segmental duodenectomy and regional lymphadenectomy.

nostomy may then be performed, either side-to-side or end-to-end in a single layer with absorbable sutures.

Primary tumor location within the duodenum does not appear to influence outcome.[21] Because of the duodenum's anatomical relationships with the pancreas and bile duct, tumor location may, however, influence the surgical plan. For patients with proximal duodenal cancers (D1, D2, and possibly large, more proximal D3 lesions), the operation of choice is PD. Pancreaticoduodenectomy provides properly selected patients with negative margins (67 to 73% of patients),[17,21] and permits an adequate regional lymphadenectomy.

There are several clinicopathological factors that have been shown to impact survival in patients resected for duodenal cancer (Table 3). Completeness of resection is critically important. In fact, this is the single most important surgeon-controlled factor. The margin status influences survival,[21–25] and a margin-negative (R0) resection should be the goal of surgery. There is no role for debulking in duodenal carcinoma, and patients who undergo noncurative surgery probably derive minimal benefit as compared to patients in whom negative margins are achieved. For this reason, every effort should

Table 3 Factors Shown to Influence Outcome Following Surgery for Duodenal Carcinoma

Impact on Outcome	No Impact on Outcome
Node metastases	Tumor size (in cm)
Tumor stage	Location within the duodenum
Resection margin	
Tumor grade	

be made preoperatively to stage the disease accurately and determine resectability. Additionally, lymph node status has been shown to affect survival.[21,25,26] There are patients with this disease that enjoy long-term survival despite nodal metastasis, and the 5-year survival rate for node-positive patients is 17 to 44%,[26,27] far better than that of node-positive pancreas cancer patients. For resected patients without nodal involvement, the 5-year survival rate is 35 to 76%.[6,21,26–28]

Transduodenal Resection of Ampullary Tumors

First described by Halstead in 1899, transduodenal resection of ampullary tumors has received much attention. Many small, benign ampullary adenomas may be resected endoscopically; however, some adenomas will be too large for this approach. Ampullary tumors have a high incidence of malignancy, with invasive carcinoma found in approximately 35 to 60%.[29–31] Following transduodenal resection of an ampullary adenoma, especially in the presence of dysplasia, close endoscopic surveillance is mandatory, as there is a low but real chance of developing an invasive recurrence.[32,33] Additionally, patients with villous tumors of the duodenum and ampulla that have anemia, jaundice, and weight loss have a higher incidence of invasive carcinoma,[32] and thus should be considered for more radical surgery.

Careful patient selection may permit successful transduodenal resection of ampullary adenomas. For benign adenomas, including those with low-grade dysplasia, transduodenal resection of the ampulla of Vater is curative.[34] However, the presence of high-grade dysplasia or carcinoma within an ampullary adenoma places the patient at a very high risk for recurrence following local resection.[34] Therefore, intraoperative pathological analysis is mandatory with conversion to PD should these high-risk histologies be identified. The technique of transduodenal resection of ampullary adenomas is detailed in Figure 3. Following complete exploration, a wide Kocher maneuver permits a lateral duodenotomy. Submucosal injection of saline aids the dissection, which is done with electrocautery for hemostasis. A narrow margin is taken around the adenoma, and with gentle retraction, the distal bile duct and pancreatic duct can be identified and divided. A probe or Fogarty catheter placed into the bile duct via the cystic duct stump may guide identification. Closure of the mucosal defect is performed with interrupted 4-0 absorbable monofilament sutures between the duodenal mucosa and the ductal mucosa. Spatulating a small bile or pancreatic duct by opening it longitudinally for 2 to 3

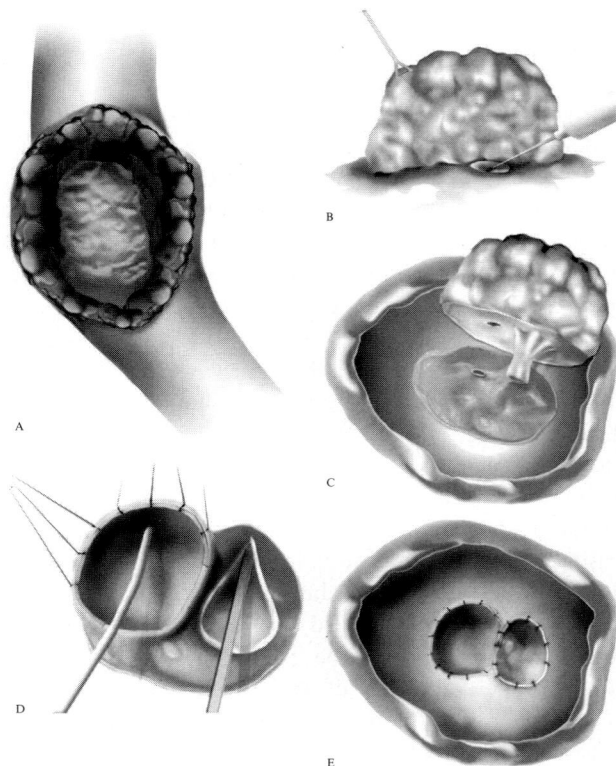

Figure 3 *A,* Lateral duodenotomy demonstrating a papillary tumor. *B,* Submucosal injection of epinephrine solution may facilitate resection of the ampullary tumor. *C,* Submucosal resection of the tumor with division of the biliary and pancreatic ducts. *D,* 4-0 monofilament sutures are used to reapproximate the duodenal mucosa to the ductal mucosa. *E,* Completed resection with widely patent biliary and pancreatic ducts.

mm aids in this step. Once completed, the duodenotomy is carefully closed and a closed suction drain is placed near the duodenotomy.

Neoadjuvant Chemotherapy and Radiation

Preoperative chemotherapy and radiotherapy are attractive theoretically for several reasons. First, many patients experience recurrences and ultimately succumb to their disease despite "curative" surgery.[35] Additionally, there is a substantial population of patients who undergo surgery and due to various reasons (eg, postoperative complications) will not be able to receive a full course of adjuvant therapy. Data from other tumor types have shown that neoadjuvant chemotherapy can result in significant tumor downsizing, thus permitting less aggressive surgery; this has been suggested in duodenal cancer but not proven.[36] Lastly, neoadjuvant therapy provides the clinician with an in-situ gauge of response to treatment.

Currently, the role for neoadjuvant chemotherapy and radiation therapy for patients with duodenal carcinoma is not defined. This approach has been demonstrated to be safe,[36] and needs further study. At this time, there is no proven role for preoperative therapy in duodenal cancer.

Adjuvant Therapy for Duodenal Carcinoma

There are no randomized trials of adjuvant therapy for patients with duodenal cancer, and firm conclusions cannot be drawn at this time. Most reports of adjuvant therapy include a heterogeneous patient population with periampullary cancer (including duodenal, ampullary, pancreatic and distal biliary cancers) with small numbers of patients. Data from these studies have shown mixed results, with most authors suggesting improved local control and possibly increased survival rates with adjuvant therapy, especially in those patients with adverse pathological factors.[35,37–39] Without firm data to state otherwise, it is reasonable to recommend adjuvant chemotherapy, and possible radiation therapy, to a resected patient with adverse pathological features, such as involved lymph nodes and neurovascular invasion.

Duodenal Tumors and Polyposis Syndromes

Patients with genetic disorders that result in GI polyps (Familial adenomatous polyposis (FAP), Gardner's syndrome, and Peutz-Jegher's syndrome) are commonly affected with duodenal tumors. Similar to the situation in the colon, the entire duodenal mucosa may be at risk for malignant transformation. In fact, since the wide-spread adoption of prophylactic colectomy for FAP patients, duodenal carcinoma is now the leading cause of cancer-related death in FAP patients.[40,41] These patients may have multiple villous tumors scattered within the duodenum, but there seems to be a predominance of ampullary villous adenomas. Aggressive regimens of endoscopic surveillance in patients with these syndromes, especially FAP, will allow for early detection of duodenal adenomas while it is still possible to perform successful endoscopic therapy. Certainly, villous tumors with histologic evidence of malignancy should be treated with PD, even when the tumor arises distal to the ampulla. Since the entire mucosa is at risk in these patients, standard PD should be performed because recurrent cancer in the duodenal remnant has been reported

following pylorus-preserving PD performed for FAP-related carcinoma of the ampulla.[42]

Palliation for Unresectable Duodenal Carcinoma

Many patients with duodenal cancer will not be resectable at the time of diagnosis. Accurate staging CT should detect distant (non-nodal) metastases, and thus avoid a nontherapeutic operation. Once distant metastases develop from duodenal cancer, the median survival is dismal and is generally less than 12 months. Additionally, patients deemed unresectable due to locally advanced tumors invading the mesenteric arteries have a universally poor prognosis. Efforts to palliate symptoms and improve quality of life should take precedence because cure is not possible in these situations. Palliative procedures that effectively improve symptoms with minimal morbidity are ideal. For patients with malignant duodenal obstruction, endoscopic duodenal stenting with expandable metallic stents can restore the luminal passage. Biliary stenting is also very effective in relieving obstructive jaundice, and the long-term patency rates for metallic biliary stents is excellent.[43,44] Palliative surgical bypass should be reserved for stenting failures and kept as simple as possible. There is no role for palliative PD in patients with stage IV disease.

References

1. Sarma DP, Weilbaecher TG. Adenocarcinoma of the duodenum. J Surg Oncol 1987;34:262–3.

2. Moss WM, McCart PM, Juler G, Miller DR. Primary adenocarcinoma of the duodenum. Arch Surg 1974;108:805–7.

3. Spira IA, Ghazi A, Wolff WI. Primary adenocarcinoma of the duodenum. Cancer 1977;39:1721–6.

4. van Ooijen B, Kalsbeek HL. Carcinoma of the duodenum. Surg Gynecol Obstet 1988;166:343–7.

5. Scott-Coombes DM, Williamson RC. Surgical treatment of primary duodenal carcinoma: a personal series. Br J Surg 1994;81:1472–4.

6. Memon MA, Shiwani MH, Anwer S. Carcinoma of the ampulla of Vater: results of surgical treatment of a single center. Hepatogastroenterology 2004;51:1275–7.

7. Bold RJ, Charnsangavej C, Cleary KR, et al. Major vascular resection as part of pancreaticoduodenectomy for cancer: Radiologic, intraoperative, and pathologic analysis. J Gastrointest Surg 1999;3:233–43.

8. Scoggins CR, Meszoely IM, Leach SD, Pearson AS. Vascular resection and reconstruction for localized pancreatic

cancer. In: Evans DB PPAJ, editor. Pancreatic cancer. New York: Springer-Verlag; 2002. p. 161–9.

9. Nagakawa T, Konishi I, Ueno K, et al. The results and problems of extensive radical surgery for carcinoma of the head of the pancreas. Jpn J Surg 1991;21:262–7.

10. Takahashi S, Ogata Y, Tsuzuki T. Combined resection of the pancreas and portal vein for pancreatic cancer. Br J Surg 1994;81:1190–3.

11. Leach SD, Lee JE, Charnsangavej C, et al. Survival following pancreaticoduodenectomy with resection of the superior mesenteric-portal vein confluence for adenocarcinoma of the pancreatic head. Br J Surg 1998;85:611–7.

12. Tseng JF, Raut CP, Lee JE, et al. Pancreaticoduodenectomy with vascular resection: margin status and survival duration. J Gastrointest Surg 2004;8:935–49.

13. Fuhrman GM, Charnsangavej C, Abbruzzese JL, et al. Thin-section contrast-enhanced computed tomography accurately predicts the resectability of malignant pancreatic neoplasms. Am J Surg 1994;167:104–11.

14. Rosch T, Lorenz R, Zenker K, et al. Local staging and assessment of resectability in carcinoma of the esophagus, stomach, and duodenum by endoscopic ultrasonography. Gastrointest Endosc 1992;38:460–7.

15. Ishida H, Konno K, Sato M, et al. Duodenal carcinoma: sonographic findings. Abdom Imaging 2001;26:469–73.

16. Watanabe N, Hayashi S, Kato H, et al. FDG-PET imaging in duodenal cancer. Ann Nucl Med 2004;18:351–3.

17. Santoro E, Sacchi M, Scutari F, et al. Primary adenocarcinoma of the duodenum: treatment and survival in 89 patients. Hepatogastroenterology 1997;44:1157–63.

18. Lowell JA, Rossi RL, Munson JL, Braasch JW. Primary adenocarcinoma of third and fourth portions of duodenum. Favorable prognosis after resection. Arch Surg 1992;127:557–60.

19. Barnes G Jr, Romero L, Hess KR, Curley SA. Primary adenocarcinoma of the duodenum: management and survival in 67 patients. Ann Surg Oncol 1994;1:73–8.

20. Kaklamanos IG, Bathe OF, Franceschi D, et al. Extent of resection in the management of duodenal adenocarcinoma. Am J Surg 2000;179:37–41.

21. Bakaeen FG, Murr MM, Sarr MG, et al. What prognostic factors are important in duodenal adenocarcinoma? Arch Surg 2000;135:635–41.

22. Allema JH, Reinders ME, van Gulik TM, et al. Results of pancreaticoduodenectomy for ampullary carcinoma and analysis of prognostic factors for survival. Surgery 1995;117:247–53.

23. Sohn TA, Lillemoe KD, Cameron JL, et al. Adenocarcinoma of the duodenum: factors influencing long-term survival. J Gastrointest Surg 1998;2:79–87.

24. Schutz G, Aleksic M, Ulrich B. Surgical treatment of non-ampullary duodenal cancer: good long term survival after radical tumour resection including lymphadenectomy. Int J Surg Investig 2000;1:525–9.

25. Howe JR, Klimstra DS, Moccia RD, et al. Factors predictive of survival in ampullary carcinoma. Ann Surg 1998;228:87–94.

26. Bauer RL, Palmer ML, Bauer AM, et al. Adenocarcinoma of the small intestine: 21-year review of diagnosis, treatment, and prognosis. Ann Surg Oncol 1994;1:183–8.

27. Ohigashi H, Ishikawa O, Tamura S, et al. Pancreatic invasion as the prognostic indicator of duodenal adenocarcinoma treated by pancreatoduodenectomy plus extended lymphadenectomy. Surgery 1998;124:510–5.

28. Ryder NM, Ko CY, Hines OJ, et al. Primary duodenal adenocarcinoma: a 40-year experience. Arch Surg 2000;135:1070–4.

29. Galandiuk S, Hermann RE, Jagelman DG, et al. Villous tumors of the duodenum. Ann Surg 1988;207:234–9.

30. Farouk M, Niotis M, Branum GD, et al. Indications for and the technique of local resection of tumors of the papilla of Vater. Arch Surg 1991;126:650–2.

31. Rattner DW, Fernandez-del Castillo C, Brugge WR, Warshaw AL. Defining the criteria for local resection of ampullary neoplasms. Arch Surg 1996;131:366–71.

32. Farnell MB, Sakorafas GH, Sarr MG, et al. Villous tumors of the duodenum: reappraisal of local vs. extended resection. J Gastrointest Surg 2000;4:13–21.

33. Posner S, Colletti L, Knol J, et al. Safety and long-term efficacy of transduodenal excision for tumors of the ampulla of Vater. Surgery 2000;128:694–701.

34. Branum GD, Pappas TN, Meyers WC. The management of tumors of the ampulla of Vater by local resection. Ann Surg 1996;224:621–7.

35. Willett CG, Warshaw AL, Convery K, Compton CC. Patterns of failure after pancreaticoduodenectomy for ampullary carcinoma. Surg Gynecol Obstet 1993;176:33–8.

36. Coia L, Hoffman J, Scher R, et al. Preoperative chemoradiation for adenocarcinoma of the pancreas and duodenum. Int J Radiat Oncol Biol Phys 1994;30:161–7.

37. Lee JH, Whittington R, Williams NN, Berry MF, et al. Outcome of pancreaticoduodenectomy and impact of adjuvant therapy for ampullary carcinomas. Int J Radiat Oncol Biol Phys 2000;47:945–53.

38. Mehta VK, Fisher GA, Ford JM, et al. Adjuvant chemoradiotherapy for "unfavorable" carcinoma of the ampulla of Vater: preliminary report. Arch Surg 2001;136:65–9.

39. Sikora SS, Balachandran P, Dimri K, et al. Adjuvant chemo-radiotherapy in ampullary cancers. Eur J Surg Oncol 2005;31:158–63.

40. Offerhaus GJ, Giardiello FM, Krush AJ, et al. The risk of upper gastrointestinal cancer in familial adenomatous polyposis. Gastroenterology 1992;102:1980–2.

41. Belchetz LA, Berk T, Bapat BV, et al. Changing causes of mortality in patients with familial adenomatous polyposis. Dis Colon Rectum 1996;39:384–7.

42. Murakami Y, Uemura K, Sasaki M, et al. Duodenal cancer arising from the remaining duodenum after pylorus-preserving pancreatoduodenectomy for ampullary cancer in familial adenomatous polyposis. J Gastrointest Surg 2005;9:389–92.

43. Taylor MC, McLeod RS, Langer B. Biliary stenting versus bypass surgery for the palliation of malignant distal bile duct obstruction: a meta-analysis. Liver Transpl 2000;6: 302–8.

44. Dormann A, Meisner S, Verin N, Wenk LA. Self-expanding metal stents for gastroduodenal malignancies: systematic review of their clinical effectiveness. Endoscopy 2004;36: 543–50.

45. Greene FL, Page DL, Fleming ID, et al, editors. In: AJCC Cancer Staging Manual. 6th ed. 2002. New York: Springer Verlag; 2002;11:119–26.

CHAPTER 27

LYMPHOMA OF THE SMALL BOWEL

CHANDRAJIT P. RAUT, MD, MSC

ANN S. LA CASCE, MD

In 1832, Thomas Hodgkin, a pathologist at Guy's Hospital in London, first described the disease now called lymphoma.[1] In 1871, Billroth reported the first case of non-Hodgkin's lymphoma localized to the gastrointestinal (GI) tract.[2] Lymphoma is generally managed by medical oncologists. Traditionally, surgeons performed staging laparotomies or laparoscopies, but now do so less frequently. More commonly, surgeons provide support with lymph node biopsies.[3] However, one exception is primary small bowel lymphoma, which frequently requires surgical management.

Definition

Dawson and colleagues[4] originally defined primary GI lymphoma by several criteria eliminate, which must be met at presentation:

1. demonstration at surgery that the disease is predominantly a bowel lesion, with or without regional nodal involvement;
2. absence of palpable lymphadenopathy on physical exam;
3. absence of mediastinal lymphadenopathy on chest radiography; and
4. normal white blood cell count and differential peripheral blood smear.

This precludes involvement of the liver and spleen except via direct extension from a primary bowel lesion. Bone marrow biopsy should also be normal.[5] The definition was subsequently modified by others to encompass a broader range of presentations.[6,7] In particular, Lewin and colleagues[7] proposed that the term "primary GI lymphoma" should refer to a predominantly GI lesion or to symptoms attributable to the GI tract.

Epidemiology and Demographics

EPIDEMIOLOGY AND DISTRIBUTION OF GASTROINTESTINAL LYMPHOMA

Primary GI lymphoma accounts for 4 to 20% of all lymphomas and 30 to 40% of all primary extranodal lymphomas, making the GI tract the most common site for extranodal lymphoma.[8] The incidence of primary intestinal lymphoma in the US has nearly doubled between 1985 and 1990.[3] Contributing factors include the increase in number of immunocompromised individuals from both acquired immunodeficiency syndrome (AIDS) and organ transplantation, and the rise in immigration from developing nations.

Primary adult GI lymphoma is found most frequently in the stomach (50 to 75%), followed by small bowel (20 to 30%) and colon (10%).[9,10] Unlike adult GI lymphomas, 67% of pediatric GI lymphomas involve the small intestine.[11] In a contemporary, comprehensive, multi-institution review of 371 adult patients with primary GI lymphoma treated in Germany, Koch and colleagues[12,13] identified the stomach as the site of origin in 74.7% of cases. Small bowel sites included jejunum/ileum in 8.6% of patients, the ileocecal region in 7.0%, and duodenum in less than 1%. Multiple GI sites were seen in 6.5% of cases.

Primary small intestine lymphoma represents 1 to 4% of all GI malignancies and 15 to 20% of all malignant small bowel neoplasms. Lymphoma is the third most common small bowel malignancy after adenocarcinoma and carcinoid.[5,14] In patients under the age of 10 years, lymphoma is the most common malignant lesion of the small intestine.[15] Small bowel lymphomas present as either primary neoplasms without systemic nodal disease or as secondary tumors as part of disseminated disease.[8] The incidence of lymphoma increases along the course of the small intestine distally.[14] The ileum, where bowel wall lymphoid tissue predominates, is the most common small bowel site.

GEOGRAPHIC VARIATION

The term "primary small bowel lymphoma" encompasses several distinct entities, including adult lymphoma in Western developed countries, pediatric lymphoma, immunoproliferative small intestinal disease (IPSID, formerly Mediterranean lymphoma), and enteropathy-associated T-cell lymphoma (EATL). The majority of adult lymphomas in Western countries are B-cell, non-Hodgkin's type.[16] Primary small bowel Hodgkin's lymphoma is exceedingly rare.

Lymphoma is a more common malignancy of the small bowel in developing countries than adenocarcinoma, which predominates in industrialized nations.[17] In most industrialized countries, small bowel lymphomas predominantly arise in the ileum.[4,18] They usually present in the fifth and sixth decades of life, have a slight male predominance, and are multifocal in 15% of patients.[19–21] Such lymphomas are associated with a relatively longer survival than adenocarcinoma.[4,18] In developing countries, lymphoma is distributed more evenly across the small bowel, affects young adults, and has a relatively poor prognosis.[22–24] IPSID is the small bowel lymphoma variant more common in under-developed countries and in the Mediterranean region.[22,25,26] EATL is most often seen in the Middle East.[27] Each of the clinically distinct variants is discussed in more detail below.

RISK FACTORS

There is a greater predominance of small bowel lymphoma in patients with malabsorptive or inflammatory conditions or with immunosuppression. Malabsorptive and inflammatory conditions identified as risk factors include regional enteritis and Crohn's disease. EATL arises in patients with celiac sprue, which is typically longstanding but may be diagnosed concomitantly. Immunosuppression may arise congenitally (agammaglobulinemia, ataxia-telangiectasia, Wiskott-Aldrich syndrome, Sjogren's syndrome), through pharmacological induction (after organ or bone marrow transplantation), or through immunologic dysfunction (rheumatoid arthritis, systemic lupus erythematosus, Wegener's granulomatosis, AIDS).

Clinical Features

PRESENTATION

In studies by Koch and colleagues,[12,13] the most common presenting symptom for small bowel lymphoma was abdominal pain (75%), followed by loss of appetite (41%), weight loss (34%), vomiting (31%), and constipation (25%). Pain may be related to partial small bowel obstruction and patients may present with a palpable abdominal mass.[19–21] Other typical symptoms include general fatigue and weight loss.[8] Diffuse lymphadenopathy is generally absent.[8] The other "B" symptoms, fever and night sweats, characteristically seen with nodal lymphoma, are uncommon unless the intestinal lymphoma is secondary to a disseminated process.[13] Malabsorption is usually indicative of lymphoma associated with celiac disease.[27] Complications requiring surgery, such as hemorrhage, perforation, or obstruction/intussusception, are identified in 25% of patients.[8] Small bowel perforation is more common with lymphoma than with adenocarcinoma.[3]

Physical examination findings include a palpable abdominal mass in 40 to 60% of patients, particularly in pediatric patients.[3,28] Peripheral lymphadenopathy and hepatosplenomegaly occur in up to 25% of cases.[3,20]

Histologic Classification and Staging

HISTOLOGIC CLASSIFICATION

The first morphological classification for lymphoma was proposed by Gall and Mallory in 1942.[29] The first classification of non-Hodgkin's lymphoma (NHL) based on cellular morphology was proposed by Rappaport and colleagues in 1956.[30] The classification of lymphoma was further refined by identifying the morphology of the follicle center as either of B-cell or T-cell origin.[31] The subsequent Kiel classification incorporated both morphology and cell surface markers, which correlated best with prognosis.[32]

Based on the fact that the clinical course of primary intestinal lymphoma differs from primary nodal lymphomas, Isaacson and colleagues[33] proposed a new histologic classification that introduced the concept of mucosa-associated lymphatic tissue (MALT). Investigators at a Workshop convened during the 5th International Conference on Malignant Lymphoma (Lugano, June 6 to 9, 1993) agreed that the unique histology of GI lymphoma necessitated a new classification system and recommended adopting the Isaacson histological classification.[33,34] The currently accepted World Health Organization (WHO) histologic classification system was introduced in 1999 and is based on clinicopathologic, cytogenetic, and immunophenotypic characteristics (Table 1).[35]

The most common histology of primary GI lymphoma is diffuse large B-cell, followed by MALT lymphoma, Burkitt's/atypical Burkitt's lymphoma, mantle cell lymphoma, and less commonly, IPSID (which is now considered a subtype of MALT lymphoma) and follicular lymphoma. Apart from EATL, T-cell lymphomas are rare.[36]

Koch and colleagues[12] reported that over 70% of primary small bowel lymphomas were high-grade B-cell lymphomas while 25% were T-cell lymphomas. Shia and colleagues[37] reported that follicular lymphoma generally accounted for 1% to 3% of lymphomas arising from the

Table 1 WHO Classification of Non-Hodgkin's Lymphoma

Precursor B-cell neoplasm
Precursor B-lymphoblastic leukemia/lymphoma (precursor B-cell acute lymphoblastic leukemia)

Mature (peripheral) B-cell neoplasms

B-cell chronic lymphocytic leukemia/small lymphocytic lymphoma
B-cell prolymphocytic lymphoma
Lymphoplasmacytic lymphoma
Splenic marginal zone B-cell lymphoma (+/- villous lymphocytes)
Hairy cell leukemia
Extranodal marginal zone B-cell lymphoma of MALT type
Nodal marginal zone B-cell lymphoma (+/- monocytoid B cells)
Follicular lymphoma
Mantle cell lymphoma
Diffuse large B-cell lymphoma
  Mediastinal large B-cell lymphoma
  Primary effusion lymphomas
Burkitt's lymphoma/Burkitt cell leukemia

T-cell and NK-cell neoplasms

Precursor T-cell neoplasm
Precursor T-lymphoblastic leukemia/lymphoma (precursor T-cell acute lymphoblastic leukemia)

Mature (peripheral) T cell neoplasms
T-cell prolymphocytic leukemia T-cell granular lymphocytic leukemia Aggressive NK-cell leukemia Adult T-cell leukemia/lymphoma (HTLV1+) Extranodal NK/T-cell lymphoma, nasal type Enteropathy-type T-cell lymphoma Hepatosplenic gamma-delta T-cell lymphoma Mycosis fungoides/Sezary syndrome Anaplastic large-cell lymphoma, T/null cell, primary cutaneous type Peripheral T-cell lymphoma, not otherwise specified Angioimmunoblastic T-cell lymphoma Anaplastic large-cell lymphoma, T/null cell, primary systemic type

HTLV = human T-cell leukemia virus; MALT = mucosa-associated lymphoid tissue; NK = natural killer; WHO = World Health Organization.

GI tract. Amongst cases of primary follicular lymphoma of the GI tract, the small bowel was the primary site in 80% of cases.[37]

Burkitt's lymphoma not associated with human immunodeficiency virus (HIV) is a highly aggressive lymphoma.[38] It may be either sporadic or endemic (Africa). The sporadic form accounts for most childhood GI lymphomas and usually presents in the distal ileum, cecum, and mesentery.[39] It is rapidly fatal without treatment, but is responsive and potentially curable with aggressive chemotherapy.

STAGING

Several staging classification systems used for GI lymphomas are shown in Table 2. Traditionally, primary GI lymphoma was staged according to Musshoff's modification of the Ann Arbor staging system for Hodgkin's lymphoma, usually by designating extranodal lymphoma with the subscript "E." [5,40] The Ann Arbor system was replaced by one proposed by Blackledge and colleagues[41] and validated by Rao and colleagues[42] Other histologic classification systems that have been used for GI NHL include the Working Formulation and the Kiel classification.[43] Rohatiner and colleagues,[34] on behalf of investigators at the Workshop convened during the 5th International Conference on Malignant Lymphoma, recommended adopting a staging classification specific for extranodal lymphomas based on the framework of the Ann Arbor classification.

DIAGNOSTIC STUDIES

Complete staging requires physical examination and a variety of serum laboratory studies, including complete blood count with differential, lactate dehydrogenase level, and serum renal and liver function tests. Bone marrow aspirate, protein electrophoresis, and measurement of serum β2-microglobulin are necessary. Lumbar puncture should be performed in patients with Burkitt's lymphoma. Steps in the evaluation used at our institution are listed in Table 3.

The most common radiographic finding is a thickened segment of distal small bowel (on small bowel contrast study or computed tomography [CT]), though this may be confused with other segmental diseases of the distal small bowel, such as Crohn's disease.[44] On small bowel contrast radiographs, the morphologic changes of small bowel lymphoma may be variably described as polypoid or infiltrating, with thickened mucosa, ulcerations, aneurysmal dilatation, thickening of the valvulae conniventes, and/or submucosal nodular filling defects.[8,45] While 90% of patients with small bowel lymphoma may have an abnormal small bowel follow-

Table 2 Staging Systems for GI Lymphoma

Stage	Description
Ann Arbor Staging System	
I	Involvement of 1 nodal group
I$_E$	Involvement of 1 extranodal site
II	Involvement of > 1 nodal group on the same side of the diaphragm
II$_E$	Involvement of 1 extranodal site and ≥ 1 nodal group(s) on the same side of the diaphragm
III	Involvement of nodes on both sides of the diaphragm
III$_E$	Involvement of extranodal sites
III$_S$	Involvement of spleen
III$_{ES}$	Involvement of extranodal sites and spleen
IV	Diffuse involvement of viscera or bone marrow
Blackledge Staging System	
I	Tumor confined to GI tract
II	Tumor with local mesenteric nodal involvement
III	Tumor with perforation
IV	Tumor with distant (para-aortic and beyond) nodal involvement
V	Tumor with visceral or bone marrow involvement
International Workshop Staging of GI-NHL	
I	Tumor confined to GI tract
	Single primary site or multiple, noncontiguous lesions
II	Tumor extending into abdomen from primary GI site (nodal involvement)
II$_1$	Local nodes (paragastric for gastric lymphoma; paraintestinal for intestinal lymphoma)
II$_2$	Distant nodes (mesenteric for intestinal primary; otherwise para-aortic, paracaval, pelvic, inguinal)
IIE	Penetration of serosa to involve adjacent organs or tissues
	Enumeration of actual site of involvement:
	IIE$_{pancreas}$, IIE$_{large intestine}$, IIE$_{postabdominal wall}$
	If both nodal involvement and penetration to involve adjacent organs is present, stage may be denoted using both subscript ($_1$ or $_2$) and E
IV	Disseminated extranodal involvement or a GI tract lesion with supradiaphragmatic nodal involvement

GI = gastrointestinal; NHL = non-Hodgkin's lymphoma.
Ann Arbor Staging System[100,101]
Blackledge Staging System[41]
International Workshop Staging of Gastrointestinal Non-Hodgkin's Lymphoma[34]

through series, such a study is rarely diagnostic.[46] On CT, findings may include a discrete mass, diffuse bowel wall thickening, or mesenteric adenopathy.[8] There may be extraluminal tracking of contrast into a necrotic tumor mass.[3] The morphologic appearance is unrelated to the specific histology.[45] In general, all of these radiographic findings are nonspecific and insufficient to make the diagnosis.

PET (positron emission tomography) using [F-18] fluorodeoxyglucose (FDG), identifies areas of disease with high sensitivity, particularly in aggressive and highly aggressive lymphomas, such as diffuse large B-cell lymphoma and Burkitt's lymphoma. Recent studies have shown that the resolution of FDG-avid disease on restaging studies during and following the completion of chemotherapy is predictive of a favorable outcome.[47]

For lesions in the duodenum or terminal ileum, endoscopy may yield diagnostic tissue.[8] Disease involving other areas of the small bowel may necessitate laparotomy or laparoscopy to establish a diagnosis. The emerging technology of capsule endoscopy may have a role in this disease, particularly in identifying the extent of disease, but no studies to date have described its utility.

Treatment

The optimal management of the distinct variants of lymphoma involving the small bowel has not been evaluated by randomized, controlled trials. Suggested therapy, based on mostly retrospective case series, is discussed below. Proposed treatment regimens for each variant are summarized in Table 4. The applicability of the different treatment modalities to specific lymphoma histologies is listed in Table 5.

Table 3 Pretreatment Evaluation of Patients with Small Bowel Lymphoma

History, physical examination	Performance status
	B symptoms (presence or absence)
	Complete physical exam
Laboratory studies	Complete blood count with differential
	Liver function tests
	Renal function tests (BUN, creatinine)
	Protein electrophoresis (under certain circumstances)
	Immunoelectrophoresis
	Electrolytes, uric acid
	Lactate dehydrogenase
	β2-microglobulin
Radiographic studies	CT scan—chest, abdomen, pelvis
	Contrast radiographs—upper GI series, small bowel follow-through, barium enema as needed
	PET scan—aggressive lymphomas
Tissue diagnosis	Endoscopy
	Image guided
	Laparoscopy/laparotomy
Staging studies	Bone marrow biopsy
	Lumbar puncture (Burkitt's lymphoma)

BUN = blood urea nitrogen; B symptoms = fever, weight loss, night sweats; CT = computed tomography; GI = gastrointestinal; PET = positron emission tomography.

EXTRANODAL MARGINAL ZONE B-CELL LYMPHOMA

MALT lymphoma is an indolent lymphoma classified as a subtype of marginal zone lymphoma in the WHO classification. Gastric MALT lymphomas are often associated with *Helicobacter pylori* (*H. pylori*) infection. The majority of patients will respond to antibiotic therapy to eradicate *H. pylori*. For patients who fail antibiotic therapy or are negative for *H. pylori*, long-term local control may be achieved with involved-field radiation therapy, typically with doses of approximately 30 Gy.

MALT lymphoma involving the small bowel is managed in an analogous manner with antibiotic therapy for *H. pylori*-positive cases. Radiation therapy for chemotherapy-resistant or *H. pylori*-negative cases may be administered depending on the location and extent of disease. For instance, for patients with localized duodenal involvement, radiation is often feasible since the position of the duodenum is relatively fixed in the retroperitoneum. On the other hand, for more distal disease, where the radiation field may be too large and the target lesion in the bowel is mobile within the peritoneal cavity, treatment options include chemotherapy directed at indolent lymphoma, such as alkylating agent-based therapy including CVP (cyclophosphamide, vincristine, prednisone) or nucleoside analog-based therapy with or without rituximab, an antibody directed at CD20 on the surface of B-cells. Response rates for rituximab as a single agent are high, but the reported duration of response has been variable.[48,49]

IPSID

IPSID is the variant more common in underdeveloped countries in the Middle East, Africa, and the Mediterranean.[22,25,26] In the WHO classification, IPSID is considered a variant of marginal zone B-cell lymphoma. Recent evidence has linked IPSID with *Campylobacter jejuni* infection.[50,51]

IPSID frequently affects younger adults (median age, 30 years) and has a slight male predominance. The triad of presenting symptoms are colicky abdominal pain, malabsorption (diarrhea, steatorrhea, weight loss), and clubbing of the nails.[22] Approximately 50% of affected patients have a palpable abdominal mass.[14]

IPSID diffusely involves the entire small bowel.[8] The diagnosis is often made by peroral jejunal biopsy, with surgery reserved for cases in which the diagnosis is unclear or when there are complications (obstruction or perforation). Macroscopically, the bowel appears thickened, with some nodularity. Lymph node metastases are present in 85% of cases. Approximately 30% have free alpha heavy-chain protein in serum and jejunal fluid; this is neither specific nor diagnostic. Microscopically, the small bowel shows evidence of villous atrophy and an intense lymphoplasmacytoid infiltrate in the lamina propria.[14]

Patients with early-stage disease often respond to antibiotic therapy (usually tetracycline-based).[52,53] Patients with advanced stage disease may respond to anthracycline-based combination therapy such as CHOP (cyclophosphamide, adriamycin, vincristine, prednisone). Prognosis is typically poor, although one study reported a 5-year survival rate of 70% with combination chemotherapy plus antibiotics for the control of diarrhea.[22,54] Surgery is typically reserved for complications such as obstruction. Responses to whole abdominal radiation have also been reported.[55]

DIFFUSE LARGE B-CELL LYMPHOMA

Diffuse large B-cell lymphoma (DLBCL) is the most common lymphoma affecting adults and may present primarily in the small bowel. Patients with indolent forms of lymphoma, such as MALT or follicular lymphoma, can transform into DLBCL. DLBCL involving the small bowel is managed with anthracycline-based combination chemotherapy, such as CHOP-rituximab, similar to large cell lymphoma arising in other nodal or extranodal sites.[56] Approximately half of

Table 4 Suggested Treatment Regimens for Patients with Small Bowel Lymphoma on Histology

Lymphoma Histology	Therapeutic Options
MALT lymphoma	
H. pylori-positive	Antibiotic therapy
H. pylori-negative or antibiotic resistant	Localized radiation therapy
	Chemotherapy (CVP, fludarabine-based regimen +/- rituximab)
IPSID	Antibiotic therapy
	Aggressive combination therapy (eg, CHOP, if unresponsive to antibiotics)
DLBCL	Chemotherapy (R-CHOP)
Mantle cell lymphoma	Chemotherapy (R-CHOP, R-HyperCVAD)
	Consider upfront stem cell transplant
Burkitt's lymphoma	Chemotherapy (Magrath regimen, HyperCVAD)
Follicular lymphoma	Chemotherapy (CVP, fludarabine-based regimen +/- rituximab)
EATL	Chemotherapy (anthracycline-containing combination chemotherapy, eg, CHOP)
Hodgkin's lymphoma	Chemotherapy (ABVD, Stanford V)
	Occasionally radiation therapy in addition to chemotherapy

ABVD = doxorubicin, bleomycin, vinblastine, dacarbazine; CHOP = cyclophosphamide, doxorubicin, vincristine, prednisone; CVP = cyclophosphamide, vincristine, prednisone; DLBCL = diffuse large B-cell lymphoma; EATL = enteropathy-associated T-cell lymphoma; *H. pylori* = *Helicobacter pylori*; HyperCVAD = cyclophosphamide, vincristine, doxorubicin, dexamethasone, methotrexate, cytarabine; IPSID = immunoproliferative small intestine disease; Magrath regimen = cyclophosphamide, doxorubicin, vincristine, methotrexate, ifosfamide, etoposide, cytarabine; MALT = mucosa-associated lymphoid tissue; R = rituximab; Stanford V = doxorubicin, vinblastine, mechlorethamine, etoposide, vincristine, bleomycin, prednisone.

Table 5 Indications for Different Treatment Modalities in Patients with Small Bowel Lymphoma

Therapeutic Modality	Situation
Antibiotic therapy	MALT lymphoma (*H. pylori*-positive)
	IPSID
Chemotherapy	MALT lymphoma (*H. pylori*-negative or antibiotic resistant)
	IPSID (unresponsive to antibiotics)
	DLBCL
	Mantle cell lymphoma
	Burkitt's lymphoma
	EATL
	Hodgkin's lymphoma
	Localized indolent disease not amenable to or unresponsive to radiation therapy
Stem cell transplant	Mantle cell lymphoma
Radiotherapy	Localized indolent lymphoma (follicular, MALT-*H. pylori*-negative)
	Aggressive disease unresponsive to combination chemotherapy
	Hodgkin's lymphoma (in combination with chemotherapy)
Surgery	Diagnostic evaluation
	Palliation for disease unresponsive to other modalities
	Perforation
	Obstruction

DLBCL = diffuse large B-cell lymphoma; EATL = enteropathy-associated T-cell lymphoma; *H. pylori* = *Helicobacter pylori*; IPSID = immunoproliferative small intestine disease; MALT = mucosa-associated lymphoid tissue.

patients with DLBCL will be cured of their disease with initial chemotherapy. The additional benefit of radiation therapy for localized disease, which responds completely to chemotherapy, is unclear. Surgical resection is typically reserved for obstruction or for cases refractory to other therapy.

MANTLE CELL LYMPHOMA

Mantle cell lymphoma (MCL) is an uncommon type of B-cell lymphoma, typically affecting older males. MCL has a median survival of 3 to 5 years and is incurable with combination chemotherapy. Patients typically present with advanced stage disease and the GI tract is frequently involved, often with numerous small polyps, termed "lymphomatous polyposis." Multiple sites within the small bowel may be involved. The optimal management of mantle cell lymphoma is controversial but typically consists of aggressive combination chemotherapy, such as CHOP with rituximab or R-HyperCVAD (rituximab with hyperfractionated cyclophosphamide, vincristine, doxorubicin, and dexamethasone alternating with high dose methotrexate and cytarabine), often followed by

stem cell transplantation for suitable patients.[57–63] Surgery may be of benefit in managing complications such as bleeding or perforation.

BURKITT'S/ATYPICAL BURKITT'S LYMPHOMA

Burkitt's and Burkitt's-like lymphomas represent less than 5% of all NHL in adults in the US. In children, however, these tumors comprise approximately half of all cases.[64,65] Three subtypes of Burkitt's lymphoma are recognized: (1) endemic, (2) sporadic, and (3) immunodeficiency-associated.[66] Endemic Burkitt's lymphoma is found in specific geographic areas in Africa and is highly associated with Epstein-Barr virus (EBV) infection. Sporadic Burkitt's lymphoma occurs in other geographic locations and is less frequently linked with EBV. Immunodeficiency-associated Burkitt's lymphoma is seen primarily in association with HIV infection; only a subset of these tumors is EBV-positive. Sporadic Burkitt's lymphoma commonly presents in children and young adults with involvement of the GI tract and extranodal disease sites. In contrast, Burkitt's-like lymphomas are rare under the age of 18 and typically involve nodal areas with or without extranodal disease sites.

Initial treatment regimens for Burkitt's and Burkitt's-type lymphomas were developed in Africa and were based on intravenous high-dose, single-agent cyclophosphamide. Intrathecal therapy was added later to address the observed high rates of central nervous system (CNS) relapse.[67] Based on the success of combination chemotherapy in other lymphoid malignancies, vincristine and methotrexate were subsequently added to Burkitt's lymphoma regimens. Such combination chemotherapy resulted in improved response rates and overall survival (OS) rates. Later studies demonstrated the superiority of shorter duration, lymphoma-type regimens that included other active agents such as etoposide and cytarabine.[68,69] In children with Burkitt's/Burkitt's-type lymphomas, such short duration, high-intensity regimens have resulted in long-term survival rates of over 80%. In adults, similar regimens have resulted in complete response rates of 70 to 80% and progression-free survival (PFS) rates of 60% to 70%.[70–73]

FOLLICULAR LYMPHOMA

Follicular lymphoma is the second most common form of NHL in Western countries. Primary involvement of the GI tract is extremely uncommon.[36,74] Patients typically present with abdominal pain and obstruction. Though few reports of management have been published, management is similar to that used in patients presenting with nodal disease. Asymptomatic patients may be observed carefully off therapy. Localized disease may be amenable to involved-field radiation therapy. Chemotherapy is used in disseminated disease. Regimens are similar to those used in *H. pylori*-negative MALT lymphoma with CVP or nucleoside analog (such as fludarabine)-based therapy with or without rituximab.

EATL

EATL is an uncommon form of aggressive T-cell NHL most often seen in the Middle East and associated with an antecedent history of malabsorption or celiac disease.[27] This type of lymphoma arises from the unrestricted proliferation of T-cell clones from the reactive T-cell population in the enteropathic bowel.[75] The peak incidence is in the sixth decade of life. In contrast, no cases were identified in a series of celiac disease-associated malignancies in children. EATL usually develops 5 to 10 years after the diagnosis of celiac disease, though intervals of up to 60 years have been reported.[76] Disease is usually disseminated in the bowel at presentation, often with significant malnutrition. In fact, lymphoma may account for 10 to 20% of deaths in patients with known celiac disease.[77–79] Approximately 50% of patients with EATL require

laparotomy for hemorrhage, perforation, or obstruction.[80] Patients are typically managed with anthracycline-containing chemotherapy regimens, such as CHOP. Prognosis is poor despite multi-agent chemotherapy with 5-year OS rates of less than 20%.[81,82]

PEDIATRIC LYMPHOMA

Pediatric GI lymphoma is clinically distinct from adult GI lymphoma. Usually identified in children under the age of 15, pediatric GI lymphomas often present with right lower quadrant pain and a palpable mass. Half of the cases resemble Burkitt's-type lymphoma.[83] Unlike adult GI lymphomas, 67% of pediatric GI lymphomas involve the small intestine (usually ileum) while only 2.5% involve the stomach.[11] Pediatric lymphomas require resection before systemic therapy because perforation while on therapy is not uncommon. The 5-year OS rate is approximately 76%, with most deaths occurring within 10 months of diagnosis.[83] Outcome depends on stage at presentation and resectability.[22,26,46]

HODGKIN'S LYMPHOMA

Primary Hodgkin's lymphoma of the small bowel is extremely unusual, accounting for 3% of all small bowel lymphomas.[46,84] Symptoms in many cases may represent impingement of mesenteric lymphadenopathy on the bowel rather than primary visceral involvement.[85] Diagnostic and/or palliative surgery is followed by systemic chemotherapy, such as ABVD (doxorubicin, bleomycin, vinblastine, dacarbazine) or Stanford V (doxorubicin, vinblastine, mechlorethamine, etoposide, vincristine, bleomycin, prednisone) with or without radiotherapy.[86,87]

AIDS-RELATED LYMPHOMA

The AIDS-related lymphoma variant was not defined until 1985.[3] These tumors commonly arise in the rectum and present with bleeding, pain on defecation, and mucous rectal discharge. Affected AIDS patients may also have "B" symptoms (fever, weight loss, night sweats). These tumors are usually Burkitt's lymphoma or diffuse large B-cell lymphoma. In older studies, prognosis was generally no worse than for similarly advanced AIDS without lymphoma; due to the concomitant immunocompromised state, median survival was under one year.[3] With the advent of highly active antiretroviral therapy, however, some patients may be effectively treated with standard dose combination anthracycline-based chemotherapy used in immunocompetent patients (as above) with CNS prophylaxis, given the propensity for early dissemination.[88]

ROLE FOR SURGERY

Traditionally, lymphoma of the small bowel was managed primarily with surgical resection with or without postoperative radiation therapy, but the rate of distant involvement was high.[3] Several series reported that 50 to 80% of patients are amenable to surgical resection.[19,20,89,90] Others reported that only 30% could be resected with curative intent.[91] As a result, chemotherapy with or without radiation therapy is the currently favored initial treatment approach.

The role of primary surgical therapy in patients with localized lymphoma (stages I and II) still remains controversial.[92] Most of the information on the efficacy of surgery in early GI lymphoma is based on limited, retrospective reviews that do not specifically compare primary surgical therapy with primary nonsurgical management (chemotherapy, radiation therapy, or both).[93] Localized disease is often managed with surgical excision, usually requiring bowel resection with wide resection of the adjacent mesentery. Pancreaticoduodenectomy may be necessary for proximal duodenal lesions. Unlike other oncologic operations, microscopically negative surgical margins are less critical because prognosis is independent on completeness of resection when adjuvant therapy is used.[94]

In patients with advanced lymphoma not amenable to complete surgical resection, the role of surgery is limited to diagnosis and palliation.[92]

RECURRENCE AND SURVIVAL RATES

The published studies of GI lymphoma use different clinical and histologic classification systems, making comparison difficult.[3] Furthermore, because few studies have distinguished cases of primary small bowel lymphoma in sufficient volume from other GI lymphoma or secondary small bowel lymphoma, identifying consistent prognostic factors is difficult. Several factors are listed in Table 6.

Table 6 Negative Prognostic Factors Identified in Small Bowel Lymphomas

Stage greater than IIE$_2$
Involvement of para-aortic lymph nodes
Tumor size > 10 cm
Serosal involvement
Adjacent organ involvement
Immunoblastic histology
Aneuploidy
T-cell origin
Presentation with acute abdomen

Data adapted from Gill SS, et al[5] and Rohatiner A, et al.[34]

Contreary and colleagues[20] reported a recurrence rate of 25% for small bowel lymphoma. Specific histology is prognostically significant. Follicular lymphomas have a better prognosis.[3] B-cell lymphomas have better median survival than T-cell lymphomas. Domizio and colleagues[81] reported a 5-year OS rate of 75% for patients with B-cell intestinal lymphoma and only 25% for those with T-cell lymphoma.

The distinction between stages II$_{E1}$ and II$_{E2}$ on the modified Ann Arbor staging system is prognostically significant. The 5-year OS rate is 50% in patients with disease involving local, contiguous lymph nodes (II$_{E1}$) and 0% in those with disease involving noncontiguous lymph nodes (II$_{E2}$).[91,93,95] Using this same classification system, Weingrad and colleagues[95] reported no survivors at 1 year with stage III or IV disease.

Two studies of primary small bowel lymphoma cases reported the results of multivariate analyses performed to identify prognostic factors for survival. Domizio and colleagues[81] from St. Bartholomew's Hospital (UK) reviewed a series of 119 cases of primary small bowel lymphoma presenting over four decades. Approximately 66% were a B-cell phenotype and 34% were T-cell lymphomas. The former were generally annular or polypoid masses in the distal and terminal ileum, whereas the latter were ulcerated plaques or strictures in the proximal small bowel. Low-grade B-cell lymphomas had better survival than T-cell lymphomas. On multivariate analysis, perforation, location in the terminal ileum, histologic grade, and clinical stage were independent prognostic factors.

Nakamura and colleagues[96] from Kyushu University reported a retrospective analysis of 80 cases of primary small bowel lymphoma classified using the schema proposed by Isaacson and colleagues.[33] This study specifically addressed the clinicopathologic significance of MALT-derived lymphoma. Patients were treated with antibiotics, chemotherapy, surgery, or radiation therapy alone or in combination or with no specific therapy. Univariate analysis identified a significantly higher probability of survival for patients with B-cell lymphomas (as compared to T-cell lymphomas), early stage disease (I$_E$/II$_{E1}$), resectable disease, and benign lymphoid follicular hyperplasia. Survival rates were worse with stomach or colon involvement, macroscopic diffuse-infiltrating type, perforation, or fever. Among those with a B-cell phenotype, low histologic grade, marginal zone tumors, and MALT features were favorable prognostic factors. Age, gender, tumor number and size, depth of invasion, and adjuvant chemotherapy or radiation therapy did not affect survival. On multivariate analysis, MALT-derived tumors ($p = .0257$) and early stage disease (p = .0009) were the only independent predictors of improved survival.

Prognosis for pediatric small bowel lymphoma is better than for adult small bowel lymphoma. Cure rates of 90 to 95% have been reported after resection plus aggressive adjuvant therapy for stage I and II disease.[97] Tumor burden at the time of diagnosis is the strongest predictor of survival.[98]

Koch and colleagues[13] reported that patients with small bowel lymphoma had an event-free survival (EFS) rate of 52% and OS rate of 56%, significantly worse than for gastric (EFS 77%, OS 83%) and ileocecal (EFS 78%, OS 76%) lymphomas.

Ha and colleagues[99] reported a retrospective analysis of 61 patients from the M. D. Anderson Cancer Center. Complete resection of small bowel disease was achieved in 75% of patients; another 15% underwent partial resection of their disease. Intermediate- or high-grade lymphoma accounted for 72% of all cases, with 10-year relapse-free survival (RFS) and OS rates of 53% and 47%, respectively. For patients with low-grade lymphoma, RFS and OS rates were 62% and 81%, respectively. Recurrence rates within the abdomen and pelvis were 11% after radiation therapy with or without chemotherapy versus 25% after chemotherapy alone (p = .21). In contrast, recurrence rates outside of the abdomen and pelvis were 33% after radiation therapy alone versus 3% after chemotherapy alone or combined modality therapy (p = .003). The authors concluded that chemotherapy reduced the incidence of recurrence outside of the abdomen and pelvis.

In another retrospective study, Talamonti and colleagues[92] identified small bowel lymphoma in 19% of the 129 patients with small bowel tumors treated surgically. The 5-year OS rate among the lymphoma patients was only 29%, compared to 37% for those with adenocarcinoma, 64% for those with carcinoid tumors, and 22% for those with sarcoma. Using the Ann Arbor classification, stage-specific median OS was 65 months for stages I and II, 43 months for stage III, and 18 months for stage IV. 5-year OS rates were 42% (stage I and II), 28% (stage III), and 0% (stage IV).

In a recent retrospective study from France, Lee and colleagues[73] reviewed 25 cases of primary follicular lymphoma of the GI tract. Follicular lymphoma and mantle cell lymphoma of the GI tract had a similar endoscopic and clinical presentation but unique immunohistochemical and molecular profiles. While the former had a more indolent course similar to nodal follicular lymphoma, the latter had a worse prognosis. In this study, median time to progression was similar for patients with follicular lymphoma treated with surgery with or without adjuvant therapy and those managed expectantly.[73] Based

on these data, follicular lymphoma of the GI tract may not necessitate treatment in the absence of clinical symptoms or disease progression. On the other had, mantle cell lymphoma requires aggressive therapy.

Conclusion

Nonoperative therapy (chemotherapy or, in selected cases, antibiotics) has replaced surgery as the primary course of treatment for small bowel lymphoma. Treatment regimens are based on specific tumor histology. Radiation is reserved for localized lymphoma or lymphoma unresponsive to chemotherapy. Patients rarely require therapeutic surgery as first-line therapy. Surgery is still required is some cases for diagnosis and may need to be performed emergently for perforation or obstruction. In patients with untreatable disease, surgery may be needed for palliation.

References

1. Hodgkin T. On some morbid appearances of the absorbent glands and spleen. Med Chir Trans 1832;17:68–114.

2. Bilroth T. Multiple lymphoma. Erfolgreiche behandlung mit aresnik. Wien Med Wochenschr 1871;21:1066.

3. Turowski GA, Basson MD. Primary malignant lymphoma of the intestine. Am J Surg 1995;169:433–41.

4. Dawson IM, Cornes JS, Morson BC. Primary malignant lymphoid tumours of the intestinal tract. Report of 37 cases with a study of factors influencing prognosis. Br J Surg 1961;49:80–9.

5. Gill SS, Heuman DM, Mihas AA. Small intestinal neoplasms. J Clin Gastroenterol 2001;33:267–82.

6. Herrmann R, Panahon AM, Barcos MP, et al. Gastrointestinal involvement in non-Hodgkin's lymphoma. Cancer 1980;46:215–22.

7. Lewin KJ, Ranchod M, Dorfman RF. Lymphomas of the gastrointestinal tract: a study of 117 cases presenting with gastrointestinal disease. Cancer 1978;42:693–707.

8. Campbell KA. Small bowel tumors. In: Cameron JL, editors. Current surgical therapy. 7th ed. St. Louis: Mosby; 2001. p. 139–44.

9. Rosenfelt F, Rosenberg SA. Diffuse histiocytic lymphoma presenting with gastrointestinal tract lesions. The Stanford experience. Cancer 1980;45:2188–93.

10. Zucca E, Roggero E, Bertoni F, et al. Primary extranodal non-Hodgkin's lymphomas. Part 1: Gastrointestinal, cutaneous and genitourinary lymphomas. Ann Oncol 1997;8:727–37.

11. Malpas JS. Lymphomas in children. Semin Hematol 1982;19:301–14.

12. Koch P, del Valle F, Berdel WE, et al. Primary gastrointestinal non-Hodgkin's lymphoma: II. Combined surgical and conservative or conservative management only in localized gastric lymphoma--results of the prospective German Multicenter Study GIT NHL 01/92. J Clin Oncol 2001;19:3874–83.

13. Koch P, del Valle F, Berdel WE, et al. Primary gastrointestinal non-Hodgkin's lymphoma: I. Anatomic and histologic distribution, clinical features, and survival data of 371 patients registered in the German Multicenter Study GIT NHL 01/92. J Clin Oncol 2001;19:3861–73.

14. Coit DG. Cancer of the small intestine. In: DeVita VTJ, Hellman S, Rosenberg SA, editors. Cancer: principles and practice of oncology. 6th ed. Philadelphia: Lippincott Williams & Wilkins; 2001. p. 1204–16.

15. Mestel AL. Lymphosarcoma of the small intestine in infancy and childhood. Ann Surg 1959;149:87–94.

16. Chan JK. Gastrointestinal lymphomas: an overview with emphasis on new findings and diagnostic problems. Semin Diagn Pathol 1996;13:260–96.

17. Neugut AI, Jacobson JS, Suh S, et al. The epidemiology of cancer of the small bowel. Cancer Epidemiol Biomarkers Prev 1998;7:243–51.

18. Sweetenham JW, Mead GM, Wright DH, et al. Involvement of the ileocaecal region by non-Hodgkin's lymphoma in adults: clinical features and results of treatment. Br J Cancer 1989;60:366–9.

19. Auger MJ, Allan NC. Primary ileocecal lymphoma. A study of 22 patients. Cancer 1990;65:358–61.

20. Contreary K, Nance FC, Becker WF. Primary lymphoma of the gastrointestinal tract. Ann Surg 1980;191:593–8.

21. Gray GM, Rosenberg SA, Cooper AD, et al. Lymphomas involving the gastrointestinal tract. Gastroenterology 1982;82:143–52.

22. Al-Bahrani ZR, Al-Mondhiry H, Bakir F, et al. Clinical and pathologic subtypes of primary intestinal lymphoma. Experience with 132 patients over a 14-year period. Cancer 1983;52:1666–72.

23. Azar HA. Cancer in Lebanon and the Near East. Cancer 1962;15:66–78.

24. Khojasteh A, Haghighi P. Immunoproliferative small intestinal disease: portrait of a potentially preventable cancer from the Third World. Am J Med 1990;89:483–90.

25. Chandran RR, Raj EH, Chaturvedi HK. Primary gastrointestinal lymphoma: 30-year experience at the Cancer Institute, Madras, India. J Surg Oncol 1995;60:41–9.

26. Haghighi P, Nasr K. Primary upper small intestinal lymphoma (so-called Mediterranean lymphoma). Pathol Annu 1973;8:231–55.

27. Catassi C, Bearzi I, Holmes GK. Association of celiac disease and intestinal lymphomas and other cancers. Gastroenterology 2005;128:S79–86.

28. Al-Mondhiry H. Primary lymphomas of the small intestine: east-west contrast. Am J Hematol 1986;22:89–105.

29. Gall EA, Mallory TB. Malignant lymphoma: a clinico-pathologic survey of 618 cases. Am J Pathol 1942;18:381–329.

30. Rappaport H, Winter WJ, Hicks E. Follicular lymphoma: a reevaluation of its position in the scheme of malignant lymphoma based on the survey of 253 cases. Cancer 1956;9:792–821.

31. Lukes RJ, Collins RD. Immunologic characterization of human malignant lymphomas. Cancer 1974;34:suppl:1488–503.

32. van Krieken JH, Otter R, Hermans J, et al. Malignant lymphoma of the gastrointestinal tract and mesentery. A clinico-pathologic study of the significance of histologic classification. NHL Study Group of the Comprehensive Cancer Center West. Am J Pathol 1989;135:281–9.

33. Isaacson PG, Spencer J, Wright DH. Classifying primary gut lymphomas. Lancet 1988;2:1148–9.

34. Rohatiner A, d'Amore F, Coiffier B, et al. Report on a workshop convened to discuss the pathological and staging classifications of gastrointestinal tract lymphoma. Ann Oncol 1994;5:397–400.

35. Harris NL, Jaffe ES, Diebold J, et al. World Health Organization classification of neoplastic diseases of the hematopoietic and lymphoid tissues: report of the Clinical Advisory Committee meeting-Airlie House, Virginia, November 1997. J Clin Oncol 1999;17:3835–49.

36. Chim CS, Loong F, Leung AY, et al. Primary follicular lymphoma of the small intestine. Leuk Lymphoma 2004;45:1463–6.

37. Shia J, Teruya-Feldstein J, Pan D, et al. Primary follicular lymphoma of the gastrointestinal tract: a clinical and pathologic study of 26 cases. Am J Surg Pathol 2002;26:216–24.

38. Parente F, Anderloni A, Greco S, et al. Ileocecal Burkitt's lymphoma. Gastroenterology 2004;127:8368.

39. Takahashi H, Hinuma Y. Nature of antigens of cultured Burkitt lymphoma cells, as revealed by membrane immunofluorescence. Gann 1970;61:337–46.

40. Musshoff K. [Clinical staging classification of non-Hodgkin's lymphomas (author's transl)]. Strahlentherapie 1977;153:218–21.

41. Blackledge G, Bush H, Dodge OG, et al. A study of gastrointestinal lymphoma. Clin Oncol 1979;5:209–19.

42. Rao AR, Kagan AR, Potyk D, et al. Management of gastrointestinal lymphoma. Am J Clin Oncol 1984;7:213–9.

43. Stansfeld AG, Diebold J, Noel H, et al. Updated Kiel classification for lymphomas. Lancet 1988;1:292–3.

44. Sartoris DJ, Harell GS, Anderson MF, et al. Small-bowel lymphoma and regional enteritis: radiographic similarities. Radiology 1984;152:291–6.

45. Nagi B, Verma V, Vaiphei K, et al. Primary small bowel tumors: a radiologic-pathologic correlation. Abdom Imaging 2001;26:474–80.

46. Cooper BT, Read AE. Small intestinal lymphoma. World J Surg 1985;9:930–7.

47. Kostakoglu L, Leonard JP, Coleman M, et al. The Role of FDG-PET imaging in the management of lymphoma. Clin Adv Hematol Oncol 2004;2:115–21.

48. Conconi A, Martinelli G, Thieblemont C, et al. Clinical activity of rituximab in extranodal marginal zone B-cell lymphoma of MALT type. Blood 2003;102:2741–5.

49. Martinelli G, Laszlo D, Ferreri AJ, et al. Clinical activity of rituximab in gastric marginal zone non-Hodgkin's lymphoma resistant to or not eligible for anti-Helicobacter pylori therapy. J Clin Oncol 2005;23:1979–83.

50. Al-Saleem T, Al-Mondhiry H. Immunoproliferative small intestinal disease (IPSID): a model for mature B-cell neoplasms. Blood 2005;105:2274–80.

51. Peterson MC. Immunoproliferative small intestinal disease associated with Campylobacter jejuni. N Engl J Med 2004;350:1685–6; author reply 1685–6.

52. el Saghir NS. Combination chemotherapy with tetracycline and aggressive supportive care for immunoproliferative small-intestinal disease lymphoma. J Clin Oncol 1995;13:794–5.

53. el Saghir NS, Jessen K, Mass RE, et al. Combination chemotherapy for primary small intestinal lymphoma in the Middle East. Eur J Cancer Clin Oncol 1989;25:851–6.

54. Akbulut H, Soykan I, Yakaryilmaz F, et al. Five-year results of the treatment of 23 patients with immunoproliferative small intestinal disease: a Turkish experience. Cancer 1997;80:8–14.

55. Shepherd FA, Evans WK, Kutas G, et al. Chemotherapy following surgery for stages IE and IIE non-Hodgkin's lymphoma of the gastrointestinal tract. J Clin Oncol 1988; 6:253–60.

56. Coiffier B, Lepage E, Briere J, et al. CHOP chemotherapy plus rituximab compared with CHOP alone in elderly patients with diffuse large-B-cell lymphoma. N Engl J Med 2002;346:235–42.

57. Howard OM, Gribben JG, Neuberg DS, et al. Rituximab and CHOP induction therapy for newly diagnosed mantle-cell lymphoma: molecular complete responses are not predictive of progression-free survival. J Clin Oncol 2002;20:1288–94.

58. Hiddemann W, Dreyling M, Unterhalt M. Rituximab plus chemotherapy in follicular and mantle cell lymphomas. Semin Oncol 2003;30:16–20.

59. Jacobsen E, Freedman A. An update on the role of high-dose therapy with autologous or allogeneic stem cell transplantation in mantle cell lymphoma. Curr Opin Oncol 2004;16:106–13.

60. Vigouroux S, Gaillard F, Moreau P, et al. High-dose therapy with autologous stem cell transplantation in first response in mantle cell lymphoma. Haematologica 2005; 90:1580–2.

61. Lenz G, Dreyling M, Hoster E, et al. Immunochemotherapy with rituximab and cyclophosphamide, doxorubicin, vincristine, and prednisone significantly improves response and time to treatment failure, but not long-term outcome in patients with previously untreated mantle cell lymphoma: results of a prospective randomized trial of the German Low Grade Lymphoma Study Group (GLSG). J Clin Oncol 2005;23: 1984–92.

62. Dreyling M, Lenz G, Hoster E, et al. Early consolidation by myeloablative radiochemotherapy followed by autologous stem cell transplantation in first remission significantly prolongs progression-free survival in mantle-cell lymphoma: results of a prospective randomized trial of the European MCL Network. Blood 2005;105: 2677–84.

63. Romaguera JE, Fayad L, Rodriguez MA, et al. High rate of durable remissions after treatment of newly diagnosed aggressive mantle-cell lymphoma with rituximab plus hyper-CVAD alternating with rituximab plus high-dose methotrexate and cytarabine. J Clin Oncol 2005;23:7013–23.

64. Magrath IT, Haddy TB, Adde MA. Treatment of patients with high grade non-Hodgkin's lymphomas and central nervous system involvement: is radiation an essential component of therapy? Leuk Lymphoma 1996;21:99–105.

65. Soussain C, Patte C, Ostronoff M, et al. Small noncleaved cell lymphoma and leukemia in adults. A retrospective study of 65 adults treated with the LMB pediatric protocols. Blood 1995;85:664–74.

66. Hecht JL, Aster JC. Molecular biology of Burkitt's lymphoma. J Clin Oncol 2000;18:3707–21.

67. Burkitt D. Long-term remissions following one and two-dose chemotherapy for African lymphoma. Cancer 1967; 20:756–9.

68. Anderson JR, Jenkin RD, Wilson JF, et al. Long-term follow-up of patients treated with COMP or LSA2L2 therapy for childhood non-Hodgkin's lymphoma: a report of CCG-551 from the Childrens' Cancer Group. J Clin Oncol 1993;11:1024–32.

69. Patte C, Philip T, Rodary C, et al. High survival rate in advanced-stage B-cell lymphomas and leukemias without CNS involvement with a short intensive polychemotherapy: results from the French Pediatric Oncology Society of a randomized trial of 216 children. J Clin Oncol 1991;9: 123–32.

70. Magrath I, Adde M, Shad A, et al. Adults and children with small non-cleaved-cell lymphoma have a similar excellent outcome when treated with the same chemotherapy regimen. J Clin Oncol 1996;14:925–34.

71. Mead GM, Sydes MR, Walewski J, et al. An international evaluation of CODOX-M and CODOX-M alternating with IVAC in adult Burkitt's lymphoma: results of United Kingdom Lymphoma Group LY06 study. Ann Oncol 2002;13:1264–74.

72. Thomas DA, Cortes J, O'Brien S, et al. Hyper-CVAD program in Burkitt's-type adult acute lymphoblastic leukemia. J Clin Oncol 1999;17:2461–70.

73. Lee EJ, Petroni GR, Schiffer CA, et al. Brief-duration high-intensity chemotherapy for patients with small non-cleaved-cell lymphoma or FAB L3 acute lymphocytic leukemia: results of cancer and leukemia group B study 9251. J Clin Oncol 2001;19:4014–22.

74. Damaj G, Verkarre V, Delmer A, et al. Primary follicular lymphoma of the gastrointestinal tract: a study of 25 cases and a literature review. Ann Oncol 2003;14:623–9.

75. Murray A, Cuevas EC, Jones DB, et al. Study of the immunohistochemistry and T cell clonality of enteropathy-associated T cell lymphoma. Am J Pathol 1995;146:509–19.

76. Howdle PD, Jalal PK, Holmes GK, et al. Primary small-bowel malignancy in the UK and its association with coeliac disease. Qjm 2003;96:345–53.

77. Holmes GK, Stokes PL, Sorahan TM, et al. Coeliac disease, gluten-free diet, and malignancy. Gut 1976;17:612–9.

78. Logan RF, Rifkind EA, Turner ID, et al. Mortality in celiac disease. Gastroenterology 1989;97:265–71.

79. Swinson CM, Slavin G, Coles EC, et al. Coeliac disease and malignancy. Lancet 1983;1:111–5.

80. Egan LJ, Walsh SV, Stevens FM, et al. Celiac-associated lymphoma. A single institution experience of 30 cases in the combination chemotherapy era. J Clin Gastroenterol 1995;21:123–9.

81. Domizio P, Owen RA, Shepherd NA, et al. Primary lymphoma of the small intestine. A clinicopathological study of 119 cases. Am J Surg Pathol 1993;17:429–42.

82. Gale J, Simmonds PD, Mead GM, et al. Enteropathy-type intestinal T-cell lymphoma: clinical features and treatment of 31 patients in a single center. J Clin Oncol 2000;18:795–803.

83. Fleming ID, Turk PS, Murphy SB, et al. Surgical implications of primary gastrointestinal lymphoma of childhood. Arch Surg 1990;125:252–6.

84. Morgan DR, Holgate CS, Dixon MF, et al. Primary small intestinal lymphoma: a study of 39 cases. J Pathol 1985;147:211–21.

85. Monco A, Sartori C. Hodgkin's primary lymphoma of the small intestine. Haematologica 1984;69:568–71.

86. Bonadonna G, Zucali R, Monfardini S, et al. Combination chemotherapy of Hodgkin's disease with adriamycin, bleomycin, vinblastine, and imidazole carboxamide versus MOPP. Cancer 1975;36:252–9.

87. Horning SJ, Hoppe RT, Breslin S, et al. Stanford V and radiotherapy for locally extensive and advanced Hodgkin's disease: mature results of a prospective clinical trial. J Clin Oncol 2002;20:630–7.

88. Levine AM. Acquired immunodeficiency syndrome-related lymphoma. Blood 1992;80:8–20.

89. O'Rourke MG, Lancashire RP, Vattoune JR. Lymphoma of the small intestine. Aust N Z J Surg 1986;56:351–5.

90. Williamson RC, Welch CE, Malt RA. Adenocarcinoma and lymphoma of the small intestine. Distribution and etiologic associations. Ann Surg 1983;197:172–8.

91. Dragosics B, Bauer P, Radaszkiewicz T. Primary gastrointestinal non-Hodgkins lymphomas: a retrospective clinicopathological study of 150 cases. Cancer 1985;55:1060–73.

92. Talamonti MS, Goetz LH, Rao S, et al. Primary cancers of the small bowel: analysis of prognostic factors and results of surgical management. Arch Surg 2002;137:564–70; discussion 570–1.

93. Talamonti MS, Dawes LG, Joehl RJ, et al. Gastrointestinal lymphoma. A case for primary surgical resection. Arch Surg 1990;125:972–6; discussion 976–7.

94. Rackner VL, Thirlby RC, Ryan JA Jr. Role of surgery in multimodality therapy for gastrointestinal lymphoma. Am J Surg 1991;161:570–5.

95. Weingrad DN, DeCosse JJ, Sherlock P, et al. Primary gastrointestinal lymphoma: a 30 year review. Cancer 1982;49:1258–63.

96. Nakamura S, Matsumoto T, Takeshita M, et al. A clinicopathologic study of primary small intestine lymphoma: prognostic significance of mucosa-associated lymphoid tissue-derived lymphoma. Cancer 2000;88:286–94.

97. Murphy SB, Hustu HO. A randomized trial of combined modality therapy of childhood non-Hodgkin's lymphoma. Cancer 1980;45:630–7.

98. Magrath IT, Lee YJ, Anderson T, et al. Prognostic factors in Burkitt's lymphoma: importance of tumor burden. Cancer 1980;45:1507–15.

99. Ha CS, Cho MJ, Allen PK, et al. Primary non-Hodgkin lymphoma of the small bowel. Radiology 1999;211:183–7.

100. Carbone PP, Kaplan HS, Musshoff K, et al. Report of the Committee on Hodgkin's Disease Staging Classification. Cancer Res 1971;31:1860–1.

101. Rosenberg SA, Boiron M, DeVita VT Jr, et al. Report of the Committee on Hodgkin's Disease Staging Procedures. Cancer Res 1971;31:1862–3.

CHAPTER 28

SURGICAL TREATMENT OF CARCINOID TUMORS OF THE GASTROINTESTINAL TRACT

MARK ONAITIS, MD

DOUGLAS TYLER, MD

Carcinoid tumors are neoplasms arising from the amine precursor uptake and decarboxylation (APUD) cells of the gastrointestinal (GI) tract and bronchial tree. Oberdorfer first used the term karzinoid (carcinoid) in 1907 to describe atypical pathologic characteristics of a tumor that was thought to be a primary carcinoma of the ileum.[1] Masson found that carcinoids arise from enterochromaffin cells and described their uptake and reduction of silver.[2] Lembech and Page described the serotonin production of carcinoid cells[3] and resulting presence of the serotonin metabolite 5-hydroxyindoleacetic acid (5-HIAA) in the urine of these patients.[4]

In addition to serotonin and its metabolites, carcinoid cells secrete many other peptides. The presence of neuron-specific enolase, chromogranin, and synaptophysin has been identified in carcinoid cells, and these have become indispensible to the pathologist diagnostically.[5-7] Other products of carcinoids cells include growth hormone, growth hormone releasing hormone, gastrin, calcitonin, substance P, insulin, and neurotensin.[6-9]

Differences in patterns of production of these peptides as well as in clinical behavior have led most to adopt the classification system first put forth by Williams and Sandler in 1963.[10] This system breaks down carcinoids by region of origin: foregut, midgut, and hindgut. Foregut carcinoids arise from stomach, pancreas, duodenum, and the respiratory tract; secrete low levels of serotonin and serotonin precursors; and may metastasize to bone. Midgut carcinoids arise from the jejunum, ileum, cecum, and right colon; secrete larger amounts of serotonin and serotonin precursors; and rarely metastasize to bone.

They most often produce the classical carcinoid syndrome when metastatic. Hindgut carcinoids arise from the left colon and rectum, rarely secrete serotonin and serotonin precursors, and rarely metastasize to bone. Foregut and hindgut carcinoids tend to produce non-serotonergic hormones such as substance P, kallikrein, tumor necrosis factor-alpha, and histamine. Carcinoids are far more likely to originate in the midgut region than in the foregut or hindgut regions. Within the midgut region, the frequency of carcinoids varies directly with distance from the ligament of Treitz.

Incidence

The incidence of carcinoid tumors is difficult to discern. Series in the US and Europe have estimated the incidence to be between 1 and 2 per 100,000 population.[11-13] However, subclinical disease may cause these estimates to be low. Data from both surgical specimens and autopsy studies from the Mayo clinic and from Sweden reveal much higher subclinical incidences.[14,15] More recently, a large population-based study of 11,427 carcinoid patients from the Surveillance, Epidemiology, and End Results (SEER) national cancer registry demonstrated an overall incidence of carcinoids of 38.4 cases per one million individuals in the year 1997. This figure dwarfs the 8.5 cases per million incidence from the same database in 1973. Thus, the incidence of carcinoid has increased 6.3% per year over this period. This increase has been primarily noted in rectal, gastric, and small intestinal carcinoids. The causes for the increased incidence are unclear.[16]

Considering site of origin, one large study demonstrated that the appendix is the most common site, followed by the rectum, ileum, lungs and bronchi, and stomach.[12] This too has recently been called into question. The recent SEER database review found the predominant site to be the small intestine (44.7%) followed by the rectum (19.6%), appendix (16.7%), colon (10.6%), and the stomach (7.2%).[16] In our series from Duke University, which excludes appendiceal and bronchial carcinoids, ileal carcinoids were by far the most common, followed by those originating in the rectum, pancreas, stomach, other areas of the small bowel, and cecum (Figure 1).[17]

Presentation

Carcinoid tumors are relatively indolent in growth, local invasion, and metastasis. In fact, up to one-fifth of carcinoid tumors may be discovered only at autopsy.[18] Possibly because of this indolence, many studies have revealed 40 to 60% of carcinoids to be asymptomatic.[18,19] This is especially true of appendiceal carcinoids, which, as a rule, are found incidentally. However, symptoms are more common at other sites. Small bowel carcinoids tend to produce the nonspecific symptoms of intestinal obstruction, vague abdominal pain, or diarrhea. Because of this, small bowel carcinoids are a challenge to diagnose/localize before operative exploration.[18, 20, 21] Rectal carcinoids, because they most often are located between 4 and 13 centimeters from the dentate line[22, 23], are discovered incidentally by digital or proctoscopic

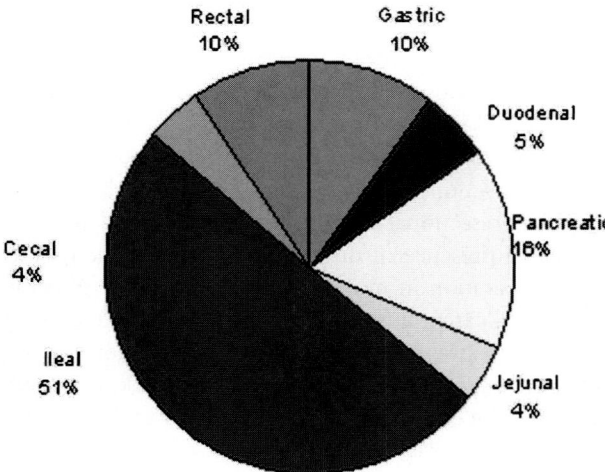

Figure 1 Frequency of carcinoid tumors arising in different locations in a series of 336 patients treated at the Duke University Medical Center.

examination. Other symptoms of rectal carcinoids include bleeding, pain, and pruritis ani. Gastric carcinoids most often present with abdominal pain.

Perhaps the most famous set of presenting symptoms is that of the carcinoid syndrome, which occurs most often with disseminated (metastatic) midgut carcinoid tumors. The classical symptoms include diarrhea, flushing, bronchoconstriction/wheeze, and right-sided heart disease.[18,19,24] The cause of these symptoms has been thought to be related to persistent excess serotonin release. Evidence for this comes from studies of patients with carcinoid syndrome in which 18 to 84% had elevated serum serotonin levels.[24,25] and 88% had elevated urinary 5-HIAA levels.[26] Others have noted increased serotonin levels in the platelets of these patients.[27] Studies of foregut carcinoids reveal an atypical carcinoid syndrome of flushing, headache, edema, bronchoconstriction, and lacrimation.[25,28] These symptoms may be histamine-related.

Diagnosis/Localization

Carcinoid tumors are rarely suspected at the time of initial symptoms in the large majority of patients. They are most often either an incidental finding or picked up as part of a larger work-up for either GI bleeding or abdominal pain. Gastric and rectal carcinoids should be included among the differential diagnoses for upper and lower GI bleeds, respectively. Small gastric, duodenal, and rectal carcinoids can be suspected based upon appearance of a small nodular lesion detected during endoscopy. These lesions are frequently biopsied for diagnosis, and if the pathology demonstrates a neuroendocrine tumor, then an evaluation for additional sites of disease is undertaken. In some patients with chronic abdominal complaints who have vague abdominal pain or obstructive symptoms in the absence of prior operations or hernias, the diagnosis of carcinoid tumor should be entertained. Because they are inexpensive, serum or urinary biochemical tests can be useful in suggesting a diagnosis. However, most physicians will usually order an abdominal computed tomography (CT) scan as the initial diagnostic test in an attempt to assess other causes included in the differential diagnosis. Urinary 5-HIAA is about 70% sensitive and 80 to 100% specific in the diagnosis of midgut carcinoid.[25,29] However, false-positive test results may be obtained when foods with high serotonin content are eaten.[30] Because of this, many also advocate measurement of serum, urine, and platelet serotonin levels.[31,32] Others have studied the serum markers neurotensin, substance P, and the chromogranins,[8,31] but these have limited accuracy and are not performed in all hospitals.

Once a carcinoid tumor has been diagnosed bio-chemically or by a tissue biopsy, the next step is defining the extent of the tumor locally and whether there is any regional or distant metastatic disease. Gastric and hindgut carcinoids usually have caused symptoms necessitating upper or lower endoscopy. Upper and lower GI contrast studies are generally poor at visualizing these lesions.[21,33,34] Endoscopic ultrasound is a useful tool in determining the local extent of these lesions and deciding if they are amenable to local or endoscopic resection. Midgut carcinoids are difficult to localize, which explains the finding that 40% of carcinoid tumors may not be visualized radiologically.[35] As with carcinoids arising in other locations, contrast studies are disap-pointing.[36] The localization rate of CT scanning for the primary tumor is about 50%,[37] but is more useful in defining nodal disease, liver metastases, and response to therapy.[38,39] Angiography has also been used in order to visualize mesenteric vessels and to map blood supply to the bowel or liver, particularly to assess for characteristic neovascularity, or "tumor blush," indicating the location of a lesion.[40,41] Abdominal ultrasound appears to be most beneficial for diagnosing liver metastases and for biopsy of liver masses.[42,43] Scintigraphic techniques can be complementary to CT scans and are useful in defining the extent of disease. Iodine-131 metaiodobenzylguani-dine (MIBG) is concentrated in carcinoids and localizes 68% of midgut carcinoids. However, it is better at diagnosing metastases than in localizing the primary tumor.[44] Finally, taking advantage of the fact that the majority of carcinoid tumors possess the somtatostatin receptor, octreotide scanning has become a popular imaging tool. One study has shown a 75% sensitivity, 100% specificity, and 100% positive predictive value for indium-labeled octreotide scanning.[45] Other groups have also had success with this method.[46,47] Because of the success with this technique, many consider it the test of choice for over MIBG scanning for localization and staging of carcinoid tumors.[37]

Treatment

SURGICAL MANAGEMENT

As with most solid tumors, surgical excision is the only curative treatment for carcinoid tumors.[20,48–50] Because tumors arising in different locations behave somewhat differently and may have differing extents of disease at presentation (Figure 2), we will discuss each site of origin in turn. Appendiceal carcinoids have been well-studied. Size of the primary tumor is the main issue in decisions regarding extent of excision for appendiceal carcinoids. Moertel's work revealed that these tumors have low

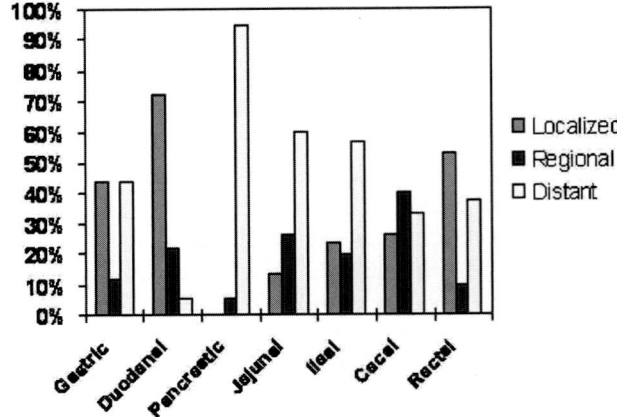

Figure 2 Extent of disease at the time of diagnosis of carcinoid tumors arising at different locations.

metastatic potential when they are small (< 1 cm).[51] Of 103 patients with appendiceal carcinoids this small, none had either regional or distant metastasis at 5 years. However, close follow-up is indicated because others have noted metastasis with small appendiceal carcinoid tumors.[52] For tumors greater than 2 centimeters, most agree that formal right hemicolectomy with regional lymphadenectomy is indicated.[20,48] Controversy arises over appropriate treatment for size-intermediate carci-noids (between 1 and 2 cm). Many advocate appendect-omy with close follow-up in this group.[15,48] However, others point to factors that necessitate right hemicolect-omy: location at the base of the appendix/invasion of the mesoappendix,[21] mucinous histology,[53] or cellular pleo-morphism/high mitotic rate.[54] However, the lack of prospective data precludes definitive recommendations on this issue.

Size has also been demonstrated to be important in hindgut carcinoids. Most advocate local or endoscopic resection of those tumors less than 1 centimeter in diameter.[55,56] For tumors greater than 2 cm in diameter, most perform either abdominoperineal resection or low anterior resection. However, retrospective studies reveal that larger resectional approaches do not extend survival due to the presence of distant metastatic disease by the time of operation in most of these patients.[57,58] As with appendiceal carcinoids, controversy exists over treatment of intermediate size hindgut carcinoid tumors. Most authors treat these patients with full-thickness local excision with definitive excision for invasion of the muscularis propria, symptomatic disease, or ulcera-tion.[23,48,56,59,60] As with rectal adenocarcinoma in this area, the patient's age and coexisting medical conditions should be taken into account when planning surgical procedures for carcinoids in this area.[61]

For foregut carcinoids, much depends upon the setting of the tumor. In up to 75% of gastric carcinoids, chronic atrophic gastritis type A is present.[23,62,63] The hypergastrinemia associated with this disorder is thought to cause hyperplasia of the enterocromaffin-like cells, which may then develop into carcinoids. Most of these tumors are small and can be treated with endoscopic resection.[28,64] Others have also described antrectomy in this situation in order to attenuate the hypergastrinemia.[65,66] No long-term studies on this strategy have been performed. Another subset of gastric carcinoids (5 to 10%) is associated with Zollinger-Ellison syndrome/ multiple endocrine neoplasia type I and is also thought to arise from gastrin-induced enterocromaffin-like cell hyperplasia. Because of this, treatment also involves local resection with gastrin control. Finally, 15 to 25% of gastric carcinoids are sporadic. Unlike the other subsets, these tumors are aggressive and usually metastatic at the time of diagnosis.[63] Radical resection is attempted for early-stage tumors of this type. Treatment of duodenal carcinoids is similar to that of this last group. Pancreatic carcinoids are rare and are almost always metastatic at the time of presentation.[17,67] For this reason, most are managed palliatively.

Midgut carcinoid tumors, as stated above, often present late due to nonspecific symptoms and difficulty in localization, and they are more often than not metastatic at the time of diagnosis. However, because the desmoplastic reaction that often involves the mesentery may lead to mesenteric ischemia[18,69] (because they often lead to small bowel obstruction), and because they have relatively indolent courses,[17] small bowel resection with the associated mesentery is the accepted treatment whether metastatic disease is present or not.[21,50,69] Two important facts to be remembered about midgut carcinoids is their association with colon cancer and their propensity to be multifocal. As such, all patients with midgut carcinoids should undergo a colonoscopy preoperatively and be placed on a colon surveillance program. In addition, at the time of surgery, the entire small bowel should be examined to determine if multiple lesions are present that should be removed.

Metastatic disease may also be treated surgically. In patients with regional lymph node metastases, resection may offer a chance for a cure.[20,49] Symptomatic improvement may be achieved with resection of liver metastases.[48,70–72] One large study suggests that if 90% of the cumulative tumor mass in the liver can be resected, marked alleviation of symptoms results.[73] However, other groups' experiences suggest that only 5% of these patients have liver lesions amenable to surgery.[11,21] A recent retrospective study of 60 patients with metastatic neuroendocrine tumors (including carcinoids) revealed symptom, and thus quality of life, improvement and survival advantage for aggressive treatment (either liver resection or liver resection and chemoembolization) when compared with medical management.[74] However, the medically managed group had greater disease burden. Finally, some groups have performed orthotopic liver transplantation in these patients.[75–77] This is highly controversial and should be undertaken only as part of an experimental protocol.

MEDICAL MANAGEMENT

Medical management of carcinoid tumors involves palliative treatment of metastatic disease as well as symptomatic treatment of the carcinoid syndrome. For treatment of the latter, octreotide has been shown successful. Octreotide is specific for the type 2 serotonin receptor and leads to reduction in peripheral serotonin levels.[78] When administered subcutaneously either twice or three times a day, one study revealed that 50% of patients had improvement in diarrhea and 82% had improvement in flushing.[79] Long-acting forms of octreotide given monthly by intramuscular injection are similarly effective. Other agents that have been administered to patients with carcinoid syndrome include antidiarrheals, bronchodilators, and diuretics, all with modest success. More recently, the serotonin receptor antagonists ketanserin, methylsergide, cyproheptadine, ondansetron, and tropisetron have been used with variable degrees of success.[80–82]

Interferon-α has been used to treat both symptoms of the carcinoid syndrome as well as metastatic disease. One study revealed transient improvements in 39% of patients as measured by 5-HIAA secretion, in 33% with reduced diarrhea, and in 65% with decreased flushing.[83] Antitumor responses may also occur with interferon, but this is controversial. One study found prolonged survival in patients treated with interferon when compared to another group treated with streptozotocin and 5-fluorouracil (5-FU).[84] Partly because of this, interferon was given in combination with streptozotocin/doxorubicin and with 5-fluorouracil, but no added effect was seen with addition of the interferon.[85,86] Regardless of tumor effect, the use of interferon is limited by its adverse side effects, which include fatigue, nausea, myalgias, pruritis, depression, and hair loss.

Other cytotoxic conventional chemotherapeutic agents have also been used to treat metastatic carcinoid without a great deal of success. Single-agent regimens include doxorubicin, cyclophosphamide, streptozotocin, dacarbazine, and 5-FU, with the latter three of these giving the best response rates (but none greater than 40%).[87] Combinations of these agents, most commonly streptozotocin/5-FU, streptozotocin/cyclophosphamide, or streptozotocin/dozorubicin, have met with similar low success rates.[88,89]

Additional nonoperative options have become more popular in recent years. Hepatic artery embolization of liver metastases is now performed in a large number of centers. This technique is attractive due to the fact that metastatic liver tumors receive almost all of their blood supply via the hepatic arteries.[90,91] Studies have used oil emulsion and gelfoam to occlude the hepatic arteries supplying carcinoid liver metastases with subsequent improvement in symptoms and reductions in urinary 5-HIAA levels.[92–96] Building on this experience, chemoembolization using gelfoam in combination with chemotherapeutic agents has been studied. These studies revealed impressive response rates of 35 to 100%[73,97,98] One study compared embolization with chemoembolization and found similar rates of response, but significantly increased duration of response in the chemoembolization group.[72] Another nonoperative approach to patients with metastatic disease that have failed optimal medical management is I^{131} MIBG. In a recent study, patients received a median dose of approximately 400 millicuries I^{131} MIBG. Many patients in this study had an improvement in symptoms and prolonged survival, but predicting who would benefit proved difficult; toxicity included pancytopenia, thrombocytopenia, nausea, and emesis.[99] Finally, radiofrequency ablation of liver metastasis may be another invasive option to destroy smaller carcinoid liver lesions to help decrease symptoms associated with excess hormonal production.

Prognosis

Prognosis of patients presenting with carcinoid disease varies according to several factors. Size of the primary tumor is an important predictor of metastasis and survival. Many studies have shown that carcinoid tumors greater than 2 centimeters in diameter portend a worse prognosis than those less than 2 centimeters.[100] However, this is probably related to propensity to metastasize and not to any increased biologic aggressiveness of these larger tumors. In our series, we found a direct correlation between size of the primary tumor and extent of disease at presentation.[17] (Figure 3). This correlation was mirrored by the recent large SEER database review.[16] This study also found gender and race to be important in survival: males had a hazard ratio for death of 1.30 when compared to women, and black patients had a hazard ratio of 1.53 when compared to white patients.

The presence of metastatic tumor, either locally or in distant locations, has been shown to be an independent predictor of survival in these patients.[101] However, after controlling for stage of disease, region of origin of the

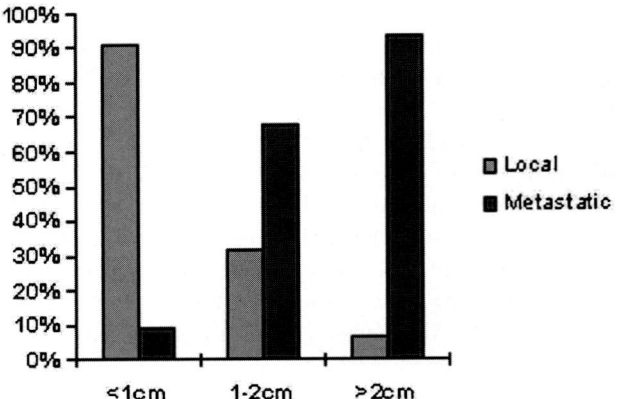

Figure 3 Extent of disease at diagnosis as a function of size of the primary carcinoid tumor.

primary tumor predicted prognosis in our series of patients. In those with distant metastases at presentation, those with midgut tumors had markedly better prognoses than those with foregut or hindgut tumors (Figure 4). The reasons for the relative indolence of metastatic midgut carcinoid tumors are unclear.

Summary

Carcinoid tumors remain challenging for the surgeon in terms of early diagnosis and appropriate treatment of both the primary tumor and metastatic disease. Despite these challenges, the prognosis of these patients is often good and aggressive therapy should be considered. Further study of these tumors is necessary to define therapeutic strategies to afford these patients optimal outcomes.

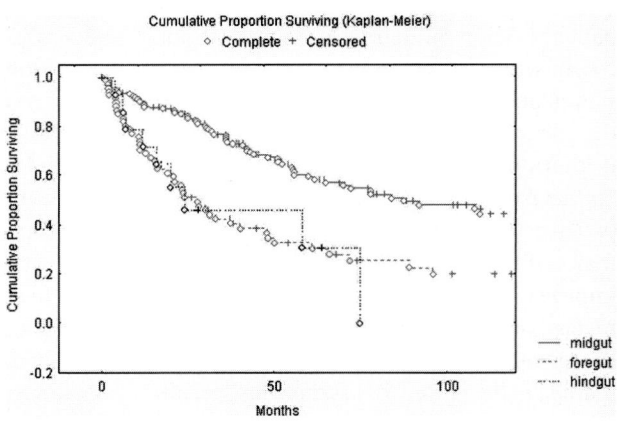

Figure 4 Patients with metastatic midgut carcinoid tumors have a significantly better prognosis than those with foregut or hindgut tumors ($p < .01$).

References

1. Obendorfer S. Karzinoide tumoren des Dunndarms. Frankfurt Zeitschr Pathol 1907;1:426–32.

2. Masson P. Cacinoids (argentaffin-cell tumors) and nerve hyperplasia of appendicular mucosa. Am J Pathol 1928;4:181–212.

3. Lembech F. 5-hydroxytryptamine in carcinoid tumor. Nature 1953;172:910–1.

4. Page IH, Corcoran AC, Vollenfrend S, et al. Argentaffinoma as an endocrine tumor. Lancet 1955;1:198–9.

5. Creutzfeld W. Carcinoid tumors: development of our knowledge. World J Surg 1996;20:126–31.

6. Kloppel G, Heitz PU. Classification of normal and neoplastic neuroendocrine cells. Ann NY A Sci 1994;733:18–24.

7. Wilander E, Sceibenpflug L, Ericksson B, et al. Diagnostic criteria of classical carcinoids. Acta Oncol 1991;30:469–76.

8. Eriksson B, Oberg K. Peptide hormones as tumor markers in neuroendocrine gastrointestinal tumors. Acta Oncol 1991;30:477–85.

9. Wilander E. Diagnostic pathology of gastrointestinal and pancreatic neuroendocrine tumors. Acta Oncol 1989;28:363.

10. Williams E, Sandler M. The classification of carcinoid tumors. Lancet 1963;1:238–9.

11. Buchanan KD, Johnston CF, O'Hare MM, et al. Neuroendocrine tumors. A European view. Am J Surg 1986;81(6B):14–22.

12. Godwin J. Carcinoid tumors: an analysis of 2837 cases. Cancer 1975;36:560–9.

13. Modlin I, Sandor A. An analysis of 8305 cases of carcinoid tumors. Cancer 1997;79:813–29.

14. Berge T, Linell F. Carcinoid tumors. Frequency in a defined population during a 12 year period. Acta Pathol Microbiol Scand 1976;84:322–30.

15. Moertel C. An odyssey in the land of small tumors. J Clin Oncol 1987;5:1503–22.

16. Maggard MA, O'Connell JB, Ko CY. Updated population-based review of carcinoid tumors. Ann Surg 2004;240:117–22.

17. Onaitis MW, Kirshbom PM, Hayward TZ, et al. Gastrointestinal carcinoids: a characterization by site of origin and hormone production. Ann Surg 2000;232:542–56.

18. Moertel C, Sauer WG, Dockerty MB, Baggenstoss AH. Life history of the carcinoid tumor of the small intestine. Cancer 1961;14:901–12.

19. Eller R, Frazee R, Roberts J. Gastrointestinal carcinoid tumors. Am Surg 1991;57:434–7.

20. Rothmund M, Kisker O. Surgical treatment of carcinoid tumors of the small bowel, appendix, colon, and rectum. Digestion 1994;55(Suppl 3):86–91.

21. Thompson G, van Heerden J, Martin JJ, et al. Carcinoid tumors of the gastrointestinal tract: presentation, management, and prognosis. Surgery 1985;98:1054–63.

22. Caldarola VT, Jackman RJ, Dockerty MB, et al. Carcinoid tumors of the rectum. Am J Surg 1964;107:844–9.

23. Jetmore AB, Ray JE, Gathright JB, et al. Rectal carcinoids: the most frequent carcinoid tumor. Dis Colon Rectum 1992;35:717–25.

24. Davis Z, Moertel CG, McIlrath DC. The malignant carcinoid syndrome. Surg Gynecol Obstet 1973;137:637–42.

25. Feldman JM. Carcinoid tumors and the carcinoid syndrome. Curr Probl Surg 1989;26:835–85.

26. Norheim I, Oberg K, Theodorsson-Norheim E, et al. Malignant carcinoid tumors. Ann Surg 1987;206:373–8.

27. Kema I, Vries E, Schellings A, et al. Improved diagnosis of carcinoid tumors by measurement of platelet serotonin. Clin Chem 1992;38:534–40.

28. Rindi G, Luinetti O, Cornaggia M, et al. Three subtypes of gastric argyrophil carcinoid and the gastric neuroendocrine carcinoma: a clinicopathologic study. Gastroenterology 1993;104:994–1006.

29. Tormey WP, Fitzgerald RJ. The clinical and laboratory correlates of an increased urinary 5-hydroxyindoleacetic acid. Postgrad Med 1995;71:542–5.

30. Feldman JM, Lee EM. Serotonin content of foods: effect on urinary excretion of 5–hydroxyindoleacetic acid. Am J Clin Nutr 1985;42:639–43.

31. Feldman JM, O'Dorisio TM. The role of neuropeptides and serotonin in the dignosis of carcinoid tumors. Am J Med 1986;81:41.

32. Kema IP, de Vries GE, Sloof MJH, et al. Serotonin, catecholamines, histamine, and their metabolites in urine, platelets, and tumor tissue of patients with carcinoid tumors. Clin Chem 1994;40:86–91.

33. Davies MG, O'Dowd GO, MoEutee GP, et al. Primary gastric carcinoid tumors: a view on management. Br J Surg 1990;77:1013.

34. Gough DB, Thompson GB, Crotty TB, et al. Diverse clinical and pathologic features of gastric carcinoid and the relevance of hypergastrinemia. World J Surg 1994;18:473–8.

35. Kisker O, Weinel RJ, Geks J, et al. Value of somatostatin receptor scintigraphy for preoperative localization of carcinoids. World J Surg 1996;20:162–7.

36. Sugimoto E, Lorelius LE, Ericksson B, et al. Midgut carcinoid tumors. Acta Radiol 1995;36:367–74.

37. Dolan JP, Norton JA. Neuroendocrine tumors of the pancreas and gastrointestinal tract and carcinoid disease. In Surgery: Basic Science and Clinical Evidence, Norton JA, Bollinger RR, Chang AE, et al, editors. Springer, New York; 2000. p. 919–52.

38. Cockey BM, Fishman EK, Jones B, et al. Computed tomography of abdominal carcinoid tumor. J Comput Assist Tomogr 1985;9:38–42.

39. Makridis C, Oberg K, Juhlin C, et al. Surgical treatment of midgut carcinoid tumors. World J Surg 1990;14:377–83.

40. Andersson T, Ericksson B, Hemmingson A, et al. Angiography, computed tomography, magnetic resonance imaging, and ultrasonography in detection of liver metastases from endocrine gastrointestinal tumors. Acta Radiol 1987;28:535–9.

41. Collatz-Christianson S, Stage JG, Henrikson FW. Angiography in the diagnosis of carcinoid syndrome. Scand J Gastroenterol 1979;(1 Suppl 53):11–14.

42. Andersson T, Ericksson B, Lindgren PG, et al. Percutaneous ultrasonography-guided cuttin biopsy from liver metastases of endocrine gastrointestinal tumors. Ann Surg 1987;206:728–32.

43. Rioux M, Langis P, Naud F. Sonographic appearance of small bowel carcinoid tumor. Abdom Imaging 1995;20: 37–43.

44. Hanson MW, Feldman JM, Blinder RH, et al. Carcinoid tumors: iodine 131 MIBG scintigraphy. Radiology 1989; 172:699.

45. Modlin M, Cornelius E, Lawton GP. Use of an isotopic somatostatin probe to image gut endocrine tumors. Arch Surg 1995;130:367–73.

46. Ahlman H, Wangberg B, Tisell LE, et al. Clinical efficacy of octreotide scintigraphy in patients with midgut carcinoid tumors and evaluation of intraoperative scintillation detection. Br J Surg 1994;81:1144–9.

47. Meunier B, Le Cloirec J, Dazord L, et al. Perioperative localization of a carcinoid tumor of the breast using indium-111 pentreotide and a nuclear surgical probe. Eur J Nucl Med 1995;22:281–3.

48. Loftus JP, van Heerden JA. Surgical management of gastrointestinal carcinoid tumors. Adv Surg 1995;28:317–36.

49. Norton J. Surgical management of carcinoid tumors: role of debulking and surgery for patients with advanced disease. Digestion 1994;(55 suppl 3):98–103.

50. Stinner B, Kisker O, Zielke A, et al. Surgical management of carcinoid tumor of small bowel, appendix, colon, and rectum. World J Surg 1996;20:183–8.

51. Moertel CG, Docherty MB, Judd ES. Carcinoid tumors of the vermiform appendix. Cancer 1968;21:270.

52. MacGillivray DC, Heaton RB, Rushin JM, et al. Distant metastases from a carcinoid tumor of the appendix less than one centimeter in size. Surgery 1992;111:466–71.

53. Gouzi JL, Laigneau P, Delalande JP, et al. Indication for right hemicolectomy in carcinoid tumor of the appendix: the French Association for Surgical Research. Surg Gynecol Obstet 1993;176:543–7.

54. Deans GT, Spence RA. Neoplastic lesions of the appendix. Br J Surg 1995;82:299–306.

55. Federspiel BH, Burke AP, Sokin LH, et al. Rectal and colonic carcinoids. Cancer 1990;65:135–9.

56. Sauven P, Ridge J, Quan S, et al. Anorectal carcinoid tumors: is aggressive surgery warranted? Ann Surg 1990; 211:67–71.

57. Burke M, Shepherd N, Mann CV. Carcinoid tumours of the rectum and anus. Br J Surg 1987;74:358–61.

58. Koura AN, Giacco GG, Curley SA, et al. Carcinoid tumors of the rectum: effect of size, histopathology, and surgical treatment on metastasis-free survival. Cancer 1997;79: 294–8.

59. Naunheim KS, Zeitels J, Kaplan EL, et al. Rectal carcinoid tumors—treatment and prognosis. Surgery 1983;94:670–6.

60. Soga J. Carcinoids of the rectum. Acta Med Biol 1982;29: 157–201.

61. Kulke MH, Mayer RJ. Carcinoid tumors. N Eng J Med 1999;340:858–68.

62. Modlin I, Gilligan CJ, Lawton GP, et al. Gastric carcinoids: the Yale experience. Arch Surg 1995;130:255–6.

63. Rindi G, Bordi C, Rappel S, et al. Gastric carcinoids and neuroendocrine carcinomas: pathogenesis, pathology, and behavior. World J Surg 1996;20:168–72.

64. Borch K, Renvall H, Kullman E, et al. Gastric carcinoid associated with the syndrome of hypergastrinemic atrophic gastritis. Am J Surg 1987;11:435–44.

65. Eckhauser FE, Lloyd RV, Thompson NW, et al. Antrectomy for multicentric, argyrophil gastric carcinoids: a preliminary report. Surgery 1988;104:1046–53.

66. Hirschowitz BI, Griffith J, Pellegrin D, et al. Rapid regression of enterocromaffinlike cell gastric carcinoids in pernicious anemia after antrectomy. Gastroenterology 1992;102:1409–18.

67. Kirshbom P, Kherani AR, Onaitis MW, et al. Foregut carcinoids: a clinical and biochemical analysis. Surgery 1999;126:1105–10.

68. Eckhauser FE, Argenta LC, Strodel WE, et al. Mesenteric angiopathy, intestinal gangrene, and midgut carcinoids. Surgery 1981;90:720–8.

69. Akerstrom G, Makridis C, Johansson H. Abdominal surgery in patients with midgut carcinoid tumors. Acta Oncol 1991;30:547–53.

70. Dousset B, Saint-Marc O, Pitre J. Metastatic neuroendocrine tumors: medical treatment, surgical resection, or liver transplantation. World J Surg 1996;20:908–15.

71. McEntee GP, Nagorney DM, Kvols LK, et al. Cytoreductive hepatic surgery for neuroendocrine tumors. Surgery 1990;108:1091–6.

72. Moertel CG, Johnson CM, McKusick MA, et al. The management of patients with advanced carcinoid tumors and islet cell carcinomas. Ann Intern Med 1994;120:302.

73. Foster JH, Berman MM. Solid liver tumors. Major Probl Surg 1977;22:1–342.

74. Touzios JG, Kiely JM, Pitt SC, et al. Neuroendocrine hepatic metastases: does aggressive management improve survival? Ann Surg 2005;241:776–85.

75. Bechstein WO, Neuhaus P. Liver transplantation for hepatic metastases of neuroendocrine tumors. Ann NY A Sci 1994;733:507–14.

76. Lang H, Oldhafer KJ, Weimann A, et al. Liver transplantation for metastatic neuroendocrine tumors. Ann Surg 1997;225:347–54.

77. LeTreut YP, Delpero JR, Dousset B, et al. Results of liver transplantation in the treatment of metastatic neuroendocrine tumors: a 31-case French multicentric report. Ann Surg 1997;225:355–64.

78. Reichlin S. Somatostatin. N Eng J Med 1983;309:1495–501.

79. Arnold R, Frank M, Kajdan U. Management of gastroenteropancreatic endocrine tumors: the place of somatostatin analogues. Digestion 1994;55:107.

80. Gregor M. Therapeutic principles in the management of metastasizing carcinoid tumors: drugs for symptomatic treatment. Digestion 1994;55:60.

81. Robertson JIS. Carcinoid syndrome and serotonin: therapeutic effect of ketanserin. Cardiovasc Drugs Therapy 1990;4:53–6.

82. Schworer H, Munke H, Stockmann F, et al. Treatment of diarrhea in carcinoid syndrome with ondansetron, tropisetron, and clonidine. Am J Gastroenterol 1995;90:645–8.

83. Ramage JK, Catnach SM, Williams R. Overview: the management of metastatic carcinoid tumors. Liver Transplant Surg 1995;1:107.

84. Oberg K, Ericksson B. The role of interferons in the management of carcinoid tumors. Acta Oncol 1991;30:519.

85. Janson ET, Ronnblom L, Ahlstrom H, et al. Treatment with alpha interferon versus alpha interferon in combination with streptozocin and doxorubicin in patients with malignant carcinoid syndrome. Ann Oncol 1992;3:635–8.

86. Saltz L, Kemeny N, Schwartz G, et al. A phase-II trial of alpha-interferon and 5-fluorouracil in patients with advanced carcinoid and islet cell tumors. Cancer 1994;74:958–61.

87. Maton PN, Hodgson HJF. Carcinoid tumors and the carcinoid syndrome. In: Bouchier IAD, editors. Textbook of gastroenterology. London: Balliere-Tindall; 1984. p. 620.

88. Kelsen DG, Cheng E, Kemeny N, et al. Streptozotocin and adriamycin in the treatment of APUD tumors (carcinoid, islet cell, and medullary thyroid). Proc Am Assoc Cancer Res 1982;23:433.

89. Moertel CG, Hanley JA. Combination chemotherapy trials in metastatic carcinoid and malignant carcinoid syndrome. Cancer Clin Trials 1979;2:327–30.

90. Ahlman H, Westherg G, Wangberg B, et al. Treatment of liver metastases of carcinoid tumors. World J Surg 1996;20:196–202.

91. Idema AA, Tjiong HS, Oldhoff J. Improvements of hepatic dearterialisation: a case report. J Surg Onc 1980;13:197–205.

92. Marlink RG, Lakich JJ, Robins JR, et al. Hepatic arterial embolization for metastatic hormone secreting tumors. Cancer 1991;65:2227–31.

93. Maton PN, Camillieri M, Griffin G, et al. Role of hepatic artery embolization in the carcinoid syndrome. Br J Med 1983;287:932–5.

94. Mitty HA, Warner RR, Newman LH, et al. Control of carcinoid syndrome with hepatic artery embolization. Radiology 1985;155:623–6.

95. Norbin A, Mansson B, Lunderquist A. Evaluation of temporary liver dearterialisation and embolization in patients with metastatic carcinoid tumors. Acta Oncol 1989;28:419.

96. Winklebauer FW, Niederle B, Pietschmann F, et al. Hepatic artery embolization of hepatic metastases from carcinoid tumors: value of using a cranacrylate and ethodized oil. Am J Roentgenol 1995;165:323–7.

97. Stokes KR, Stuart K, Clouse ME. Hepatic artery chmeoembolization for metastatic endocrine tumors. J Vasc Interventional Radiol 1993;4:341.

98. Therasse E, Breittmayer F, Roche A, et al. Transcatheter chemoembolization of progressive carcinoid liver metastasis. Radiology 1993;189:541.

99. Safford SD, Coleman RE, Gockerman JP, et al. Iodine-131 metaiodobenzylguanidine treatment for metastatic carcinoid. Results in 98 patients. Cancer 2004;101:1987.

100. Zeitels J, Naunheim K, Kaplan E, et al. Carcinoid tumors: a 37 year experience. Archives of Surgery 1982;117:732–7.

101. McDermott E, Guduric B, Brennan M. Prognostic variables in patients with gastrointestinal carcinoid tumors. British J Surg 1994;81:1007–9.

CHAPTER 29

SURGICAL MANAGEMENT OF NONCARCINOID EPITHELIAL NEOPLASMS OF THE APPENDIX AND THE PSEUDOMYXOMA PERITONEI SYNDROME

LAURA A. LAMBERT, MD

PAUL F. MANSFIELD, MD

Epithelial neoplasms of the appendix constitute a rare group of tumors that account for less than 1% of all gastrointestinal epithelial tumors.[1,2] Within this group, carcinoid tumors are the most frequent (85%), and the remaining 15% is divided among adenocarcinomas (12%), adenocarcinoids (2%), and others (1%). Like epithelial neoplasms of the colon, these lesions follow an adenoma-to-carcinoma progression, and their natural history is highly dependent on histology. A unique combination of anatomy and physiology within the vermiform appendix, however, predisposes these patients to a characteristically prolonged, morbid clinical course of peritoneal carcinomatosis with or without the pseudomyxoma peritonei syndrome of mucinous ascites.

Surgery is the current mainstay of treatment for appendiceal neoplasms. Because of the indolent nature of this disease process and its extremely low rate of metastases outside the peritoneal cavity, there is no standard role for systemic chemotherapy. Unfortunately, once peritoneal spread has occurred, the incidence of disease recurrence is high when surgery is the only treatment. Recent efforts to decrease the rate of tumor recurrence and prolong survival have focused on intraperitoneal administration of chemotherapy in addition to complete surgical extirpation.

This chapter reviews the clinical features of neoplastic processes of the appendix and discusses the current understanding of the pathology of this disease process. Our approach to the surgical treatment of patients with appendiceal neoplasms is detailed and common management issues are described.

Clinical and Pathological Characteristics

Because of the rarity of primary appendiceal neoplasms and the protean clinical symptoms, most cases are diagnosed at the time of laparotomy. A series of 410 patients described by Esquivel and Sugarbaker indicates that the most common presenting clinical signs or symptoms of appendiceal tumors are right lower quadrant abdominal pain (27%), abdominal distention (23%), or a new hernia (14%).[3] The most common age at presentation is the late forties to early fifties, although the range is from the early twenties to the late eighties. While some earlier reports suggested a female predominance, most recent and larger studies show a near equal incidence by sex, likely owing to improvements in pathologic differentiation of appendiceal neoplasms from ovarian cancer.

Up to 50% of newly diagnosed appendiceal neoplasms are accompanied by mucinous ascites, a condition commonly referred to as "pseudomyxoma peritonei" (PMP). PMP was first reported in 1884 by Werth, who described the pathological findings in a patient with a ruptured ovarian cystadenoma and copious gelatinous intraperitoneal ascites.[4] This term has subsequently been applied to any process (benign or malignant) of any etiology (small or large bowel, peritoneum, stomach, etc.) that results in the intraperitoneal accumulation of mucin. Unfortunately, the indiscriminant use of this term has generated considerable confusion among clinicians and patients regarding the natural history, clinical significance, and management of this condition.

Although indolent in nature and rarely metastasizing outside the peritoneal cavity, the natural history of mucinous appendiceal tumors is not benign. Long-term survival is poor; 5- and 10-year survival rates of 50% and 10 to 30%, respectively, have been reported.[5] Patients with the PMP syndrome can experience relentless reaccumulation of the mucin or mucinous ascites, which is associated with an insidious fibrotic process. These patients typically undergo multiple exploratory laparotomies and frequent debulking procedures, resulting in further adhesion formation and eventual entrapment of segments of intestine within recurrent fibrosing tumor and mucin. Over time, repeated surgeries become less effective and increasingly risky. Ultimately, the patient dies of the increasing burden of the mucinous ascites and malnutrition, often following a prolonged period of intravenous hyperalimentation.

Multiple recent studies by independent investigators have determined that the histopathology of the primary appendiceal tumor (low-grade mucinous neoplasm, mucinous adenocarcinoma, or nonmucinous adenocarcinoma) is a significant prognostic factor. In 1995, Carr and colleagues analyzed the correlation of clinicopathologic factors with prognosis in 184 patients with noncarcinoid appendiceal neoplasms–the first report encompassing more than a score of patients.[6] Retrospective follow-up data were obtained on 82 patients whose tumor was either of low histologic grade (n = 18) or carcinoma (n = 64). The 5-year overall survival (OS) rate for all 82 patients was 65%; the carcinoma group had a significantly higher mortality rate than the low-grade histology group ($p \leq .01$). Further multivariate analysis revealed that the presence of epithelial cells outside the appendix and the presence of mucin outside the right lower quadrant were independent and interchangeable prognostic variables (relative risk of shortened survival = 3.3).

In 2001, results of a long-term follow-up study by Ronnett and colleagues confirmed the utility of a

pathologic classification system based on primary tumor pathology in patients with appendiceal neoplasms.[7] In this series, 109 patients with an appendiceal neoplasm and multifocal peritoneal involvement were classified into three groups on the basis of the pathologic features of their peritoneal lesions: disseminated peritoneal adenomucinosis (DPAM) (scant, histologically bland to low-grade adenomatous, mucinous epithelium within abundant extracellular mucin associated with fibrosis); peritoneal mucinous carcinomatosis (PMCA) (mucinous epithelium forming glands and/or signet ring cells with sufficient cytologic atypia and architectural complexity warranting a diagnosis of mucinous carcinoma) and peritoneal mucinous carcinomatosis with intermediate or discordant features (PMCA-I/D) (peritoneal lesions with predominant features of DPAM but also with focal areas of well-differentiated mucinous carcinoma). Unlike most available studies evaluating prognosis within this patient population, all 109 patients were treated surgically by one surgeon. Five- and 10-year survival rates for patients with DPAM (n = 65) were 75% and 68%, respectively, which were significantly higher than the 5- and 10-year survival rates for patients with PCMA (14% and 3%, respectively; (n = 30; $p < .001$). The PCMA-I/D group had intermediate 5- and 10-year survival rates of 50% and 21%, respectively, which were also significantly lower than those of the DPAM group (n = 14; $p < .001$). Mean survival duration for the DPAM group was 112 months, and the median survival had not been reached despite mean and median follow-up intervals of 96 and 104 months, respectively. The mean and median survival times were 27 and 16 months, respectively, for PMCA and 46 and 21 months, respectively, for PMCA-I/D. The authors concluded that there is an inherent biologic difference between DPAM and PMCA and that the biological behavior of PMCA-I/D is more closely related to that of PMCA than that of DPAM. They also argued that the histopathology of either the primary tumor or the peritoneal lesions provided a better prognostic indicator than the presence or absence of epithelial cells within the mucinous ascites. These findings also raise the potential for planning more patient-specific therapeutic approaches.

A review of 107 patients with appendiceal mucinous neoplasms by Misdraj and colleagues confirmed the prognostic utility of a system of classification by histopathologic features.[8] In this series, patients were classified into three groups based upon architectural and cytological features of the primary tumor or peritoneal lesions: low-grade appendiceal mucinous neoplasms (LAMN), mucinous adenocarcinomas (MACA), or discordant type. The LAMN patients were further divided according to the presence or absence of extra-appendiceal spread. No recurrences were seen in patients with LAMN confined to the appendix at a median follow-up interval of 6 years. Three-, 5-, and 10-year survival rates in patients with LAMN with extra-appendiceal spread were 100%, 86%, and 45%, respectively. Similar to the findings in the study by Ronnett and colleagues,[7] these rates were significantly higher than those for patients with MACA (3- and 5-year survival rates 90% and 44%, respectively; $p = .04$). Furthermore, the clinical course in patients with a primary LAMN but high-grade peritoneal lesions (discordant) more closely resembled that of the patients with MACA. On the basis of these studies, use of the term PMP as a pathologic diagnosis suggesting stage IV adenocarcinoma has been discouraged, and it has been suggested that the term be restricted to use as a clinical description only.

Occurring less frequently, nonmucinous or colonic-type adenocarcinomas of the appendix feature a significantly different natural history. These tumors often are less differentiated and more aggressive than the mucinous variety (contrary to what is seen in the colon). In a study comparing the clinicopathological features of 30 mucinous and nonmucinous appendiceal adenocarcinomas, Kabbani and colleagues found that 86% of the patients with nonmucinous adenocarcinoma presented with appendicitis while 70% of the patients with mucinous adenocarcinoma presented with PMP syndrome.[9] Omental metastases were identified in 62% of the patients with mucinous adenocarcinomas and in 0% of those with nonmucinous disease; 43% of the patients with nonmucinous disease had evidence of systemic metastases (liver or lung). Patients with mucinous carcinoma had significantly better OS and disease-free survival (DSF) rates than those with nonmucinous tumors. Unlike patients with mucinous appendiceal neoplasms, patients with the colonic-type appendiceal carcinoma either die of metastatic disease or, in the setting of peritoneal spread, experience a course more characteristic of carcinomatosis from other colorectal sources.

Management

The primary treatment of appendiceal cancer with peritoneal spread is surgery; optimal therapy is considered to be complete tumor extirpation leaving no residual tumor deposits greater than 2.0 mm in diameter. Because of the frequently extensive peritoneal spread, the operation required to achieve this goal can be long and challenging for both the surgeon and the patient. Maximal cytoreductive procedures often involve removal of the appendix and/or right colon, general intraperitoneal tumor debulking, resection of multiple abdom-

inal and pelvic organs afflicted with peritoneal tumor studding, and stripping of involved parietal peritoneum. Despite such a comprehensive surgical approach, disease recurrence is common. Evidence is currently amassing that administration of perioperative intraperitoneal heated chemotherapy (IPHC) may provide a survival advantage in patients with peritoneal involvement by appendiceal neoplasms.[10–12] Successful management of these neoplasms, in which a patient undergoes a major abdominal operation combined with concurrent chemotherapy and the physiologic sequelae of intraperitoneal hyperthermic perfusion, demands both surgeon and institutional experience and careful patient selection.

PREOPERATIVE EVALUATION

Once the diagnosis is established, a thorough evaluation must be performed to determine the extent of the tumor, tumor resectability, the presence of primary colonic tumors, and the appropriateness and fitness of the patient for aggressive definitive treatment. It has been our experience that treatment of most patients older than 70 years must be approached with caution because the risks of cytoreduction and IPHC may be greater than the potential benefits. Similarly, because of the relative sensitivity of the liver to hyperthermia, patients with evidence of cirrhosis are not offered IPHC at our institution.

To determine the extent of the tumor and potential for complete cytoreduction, computed tomography (CT) scans of the chest, abdomen, and pelvis are the most reliable and widely used preoperative evaluative techniques. In a retrospective review of preoperative CT scans of 45 patients with mucinous peritoneal carcinomatosis who underwent cytoreduction and intraperitoneal chemotherapy, Jacquet and colleagues identified specific CT findings that help predict which patients are likely to achieve complete cytoreduction.[13] In comparing patients who had complete cytoreduction (n = 25) with those who had incomplete cytoreduction (n = 20), findings that were significantly different included volume of tumor in the small bowel mesentery, volume of tumor on the small bowel excluding the distal ileum, gathering together of the small bowel mesentery ("cauliflowering"), and obstructed segments of bowel. Patients with both obstruction of bowel segments by tumor and tumor diameter greater than 5 mm on small bowel surfaces (excluding the distal ileum) had an 88% probability of incomplete resection, while patients without these two findings had a 92% probability of complete resection. Although magnetic resonance imaging (MRI) can show the morphological features seen by CT scan, and T2-weighted images may differentiate between mucinous and fluid ascites, there are no significant data supporting the routine use of MRI for preoperative assessment of resectability in this patient population. One exception, however, may be patients with significant pelvic disease—MRI may help to better delineate the anatomic relationships in this region. Finally, given the relatively slow-growing nature and extremely low rate of distant metastases of appendiceal neoplasms, there is no known role for positron emission tomography.

Preoperative laboratory studies that should be checked in all patients being considered for cytoreduction and IPHC include a complete blood count, electrolytes, blood urea nitrogen, creatinine, prothrombin time, partial thromboplastin time, liver function tests, and prealbumin. All abnormal test results must be addressed prior to surgery. In addition, given the incidence of synchronous colonic primary tumors (up to 15%), preoperative colonoscopy is essential for all appendiceal cancer patients prior to definitive surgery.[14]

Tumor markers, including carbohydrate antigen 19.9 (CA19.9), carcinoembryonic antigen (CEA), and carbohydrate antigen 125 (CA 125) are frequently tested and may be monitored in patients with appendiceal neoplasms. The prognostic values of baseline and serial CA19.9 and CEA in 63 patients with PMP of appendiceal origin who underwent cytoreduction and IPHC were assessed by van Ruth and colleagues[15] In this study, preoperative CEA and CA19.9 levels were increased in 75% and 58% of patients, respectively. Within 3 months of cytoreduction and IPHC, CEA and CA19.9 normalized in 73% and 57% of patients, respectively. No relationship between preoperative CEA and extent of tumor or OS or DFS rate was identified. With respect to predicting disease recurrence, a weak correlation between the pattern of CEA change and tumor recurrence was found. Because of the short follow-up period in this study, changes in serial tumor marker levels were not correlated with OS.

The absolute CA19.9 level at baseline appeared to be attributable to the volume of disease and, like baseline CEA, was not prognostic with respect to OS or DFS interval. The pattern of postoperative CA19.9 change was, however, significantly different in patients who experienced tumor recurrence and in those who did not. Increasing CA19.9 levels on three successive occasions predicted imminent clinical or radiographic recurrence (based on CT scan or histology) with a median lead time of 9 months. Earlier elevation of CA19.9 correlated with a higher risk of recurrence. Furthermore, patients who never attained a normal postoperative CA19.9 level had higher recurrence rates than those who did, while patients who maintained a normal postoperative CA19.9 level rarely experienced disease recurrence. Tumor recurrence in patients with a normal preoperative

CA19.9 was not associated with increased CA19.9 tumor marker levels when recurrent disease was diagnosed.

SURGERY

In our practice, patients are routinely admitted to the hospital 1 day prior to surgery to receive aggressive intravenous hydration while undergoing a supervised mechanical bowel preparation and to review the surgical plan. Informed consent is obtained following a discussion of the potential resection of all involved and potentially involved organs (most commonly the right colon, other segments of bowel, greater and lesser omenta, gallbladder, spleen, and involved peritoneum, as well as the uterus and ovaries in women), review of the rationale for the heated chemotherapy perfusion, description of its common side effects, and discussion of the placement of a gastrostomy tube and feeding jejeunostomy tube. If splenectomy is considered a reasonable possibility, the patient typically receives vaccines against Haemophilus influenzae, Meningococcus, and Pneumococcus infections at least 2 weeks prior to operation.

Scheduled surgical time is usually at least 8 hours (range of operations in our experience is 6 to 17 hours). At the time of surgery, appropriate preoperative antibiotics are given in the operating room within 1 hour of making the initial incision. Placement of an epidural catheter is encouraged to assist with postoperative pain management. Once general anesthesia is established, a central venous catheter, arterial line, Foley catheter with a temperature probe, esophageal temperature probe, and nasogastric tube are placed in addition to adequate peripheral venous access catheters. The patient is positioned supine on a cooling blanket on the operating table with the arms extended at right angles to the torso.

Because success in terms of survival benefit depends upon the completeness of cytoreduction,[12,16] the primary objective of the procedure is to resect and debride all visible tumor, minimizing any residual implants to less than 2.0 mm thickness. Achievement of this level of cytoreduction is important to optimize drug penetration into residual tumor deposits (approximately 5 mm for mitomycin-C [MMC], one of the most commonly used intraperitoneal chemotherapeutic agents) and adequately treat any residual disease. This degree of cytoreduction can often require both resection of encased organs and debridement of isolated tumor implants or plaques. The organs most frequently resected include the greater and lesser omenta, the right colon, gallbladder, spleen, sigmoid colon, and uterus with salpinx and ovaries. Less frequently, the pancreatic tail, stomach, segments of small bowel, or the total abdominal colon are also removed.

Resection of the right hemicolon is often advocated, not only to remove encasing disease, but also to effect a dissection of the appendiceal nodal basin, which has been suggested to prolong median survival.[14] A recent review by Gonzalez-Moreno and Sugarbaker of 501 patients with peritoneal seeding from epithelial malignancy of the appendix did not find a significant survival advantage for right hemicolectomy over appendectomy in the setting of IPHC.[17] The authors suggest that appendectomy alone, although controversial, may be adequate treatment for some patients provided that the appendix can be removed with clear margins and there is little to no risk of lymph node involvement. Settings in which it would be necessary to perform a right hemicolectomy include inability to clear the primary tumor or to achieve complete cytoreduction by appendectomy alone, known lymph node involvement, and a primary tumor of nonmucinous or signet ring cell histology.

Parietal peritoneal implants can either be removed from the peritoneum or be treated by stripping the peritoneum covering the posterior surface of the rectus sheaths in continuity with the peritoneum covering each hemidiaphragm–areas that are frequently involved with plaques of tumor. Involvement of the surface of the liver can be managed with a combination of partial stripping of Glisson's capsule if necessary (although efforts are made to avoid this owing to resultant blood loss) and cautery ablation of discontinuous tumor deposits. Argon beam coagulation is helpful in maintaining hemostasis. The colon must be mobilized bilaterally and the peritoneum stripped at the lateral gutters when involved with tumor. The pelvic parietal peritoneum can be stripped anteriorly off the inferior portion of the rectus sheath and bladder and laterally off the iliac vessels and ureters to the level of the vagina in women and the seminal vesicles in men when tumor deposits are present. Visceral peritoneal involvement of the uterus or rectosigmoid can be managed by en-bloc resection with the involved peritoneum if necessary. Some have argued against extensive peritoneal stripping in combination with IPHC, noting that exposure of subperitoneal tissue may increase not only the absorption of perfusate and systemic toxic effects from the chemotherapy but also the surgical morbidity.[16] Alternatively, it has been argued that extensive peritoneal stripping without IPHC may contribute to tumor implantation in exposed tissue.[18] We typically use peritonectomy when necessary to remove visible disease, particularly from the diaphragm, in combination with IPHC. Lysis of all adhesions is performed during the procedure to allow maximal exposure of the peritoneal surfaces to the perfusate.

Bowel anastomoses are generally performed after the hyperthermic perfusion is completed in order to minimize sequestration of tumor deposits in the suture line, thus limiting their exposure to the perfusate.

INTRAPERITONEAL HYPERTHERMIC PERFUSION

Several perfusion methods have been described; these can generally be classified as open or closed techniques. The open, or "Coliseum," technique involves suturing a silastic sheet over a self-retaining retractor and to the patient's skin over the abdominal incision, effectively lifting the abdominal wall and creating a "coliseum" of the abdominal wall to serve as a reservoir for the perfusate. An incision is made in the middle of the sheet to allow manual manipulation of the intra-abdominal contents. Proponents of the open technique argue that the principal benefit is the assurance that the heated chemotherapy is distributed adequately throughout the abdominal cavity. Disadvantages of this technique include heat dissipation, making it difficult to obtain the desired degree of hyperthermia, and the theoretical risk of increased exposure of the operating room personnel to chemotherapy, though this has not been reported.

The alternate approach is the closed technique, which is used as frequently as the open technique. The main advantage of this approach is the ability to achieve and maintain hyperthermia rapidly; the principal disadvantage is the lack of assurance of uniform distribution of the heated chemotherapy. We use the closed technique with continuous intra-abdominal thermal monitoring in multiple sites to ensure uniform intraperitoneal heating and, by extrapolation, perfusate distribution. This is performed by placing eight thermistor probes in different regions throughout the abdominal cavity. Four wire probes are inserted under the peritoneum (or directly into the muscle if the peritoneum has been removed) of the bilateral upper and lower quadrants of the abdominal wall and temporarily secured with chromic suture. Another two probes are positioned under the peritoneum at the bases of the small bowel and sigmoid colon mesenteries. Finally, two needle probes are placed into the substance of each half of the liver. The probes are labeled and connected to a computer for monitoring during the procedure.

Next, efferent and afferent cannulae are placed within the peritoneal cavity. Starting inferiorly, the first few centimeters of the abdominal wall incision are closed at the level of the skin using a heavy nylon suture in a running fashion. A custom-made collector is then placed in the pelvis with an outflow channel exiting through the lower portion of the midline wound. The skin is closed tightly around the collector to prevent leakage of perfusate. The wires connected to the temperature probes are brought through the incision as the running suture is continued superiorly. A few centimeters below the superior end of the incision, a catheter with a Y-shaped connector is placed into the abdominal cavity to establish inflow into each subdiaphragmatic space. Again the skin is closed tightly around the catheter with the nylon suture, and the remainder of the incision is closed. Additional purse-string or single sutures may be required to prevent perfusate leakage around the inflow catheter and outflow collector (Figure 1).

Circulation and heating of the chemotherapy is established with a circuit composed of a reservoir, roller pump, heat exchanger, and the inflow and outflow cannulae. Prior to starting the perfusion, the patient's temperature is cooled to 34° to 36° Celsius. The heated chemotherapy solution is circulated for 90 minutes as two assistants manually agitate (shake) the abdomen for the duration of the perfusion. The temperatures within the various regions of the abdomen are typically maintained above 40° Celsius. The patient's core temperature is carefully monitored and maintained below 39.5 ° Celsius through the use of the cooling blanket, nonheated intravenous fluids and inspired gases, low ambient temperature, a circulating air cooling blanket, and, if necessary, packing the patient in ice.

MMC and cisplatin are the most commonly used intraperitoneal chemotherapeutic agents because of their synergistic cell kill effect when combined with hyperther-

mia.[19] The synergism between hyperthermia and MMC has been found to be effective against tumors with low growth rates and high chemotherapy resistance, such as appendiceal cancer. This factor, in addition to its pharmacokinetic profile and relatively low systemic absorption, has made MMC our chemotherapy agent of choice. Chemotherapy dosing, degree of hyperthermia, flow rates, volumes of perfusate, and duration of perfusion vary from center to center. We base these parameters upon the patient's weight and previous chemotherapy exposure. For single-agent MMC, we administer a total dose between 37.5 and 65 mg in a volume of 5.0 to 6.5 liters of electrolyte solution at a flow rate of 3.0 to 3.5 L/minute.

Intraoperative hemodynamic and thermal monitoring and management are essential in the care and outcome of the perfusion patient. Profound insensible and third-space fluid losses are anticipated because of the combined effects of a lengthy duration operation, a large abdominal wound, extensive tumor debulking and visceral resections, drainage of ascites, and hyperthermic exposure. Furthermore, during the course of the actual perfusion, a reduction in systemic vascular resistance due to warming, with compensatory tachycardia and increased cardiac output, is characteristic. Early hydration helps minimize these effects, and maintenance of urine output should be used as a guide for optimal hydration. During the perfusion, an intravenous fluid rate of 1,500 cc/hour may sometimes be necessary to keep the urine output greater than 100 cc/hour. When the closed technique is used, extensive motion artifact may interrupt electrocardiographic monitoring, making a reliable arterial waveform essential for monitoring blood pressure and cardiac rhythm.

Hyperthermia in the treatment field has been implicated in causing a "scald injury" to the peritoneal surface, resulting in increased microvascular permeability, peritoneal edema, increased third-space losses, and hypoalbuminemia. Preclinical animal studies suggest that the H2 blocker cimetidine may inhibit ultrastructural changes in the microvasculature associated with cutaneous scald injuries and decrease the amount of fluid resuscitation required.[20,21] In a clinical study of pre-perfusion intravenous cimetidine in gastric cancer patients, Fujimoto and colleagues found protein losses to be lower in patients receiving cimetidine.[22] Further studies also showed lower levels of catecholamines thought to be secondary to elevated levels of histamine.[23] We routinely administer a large dose of cimetidine (40 mg/kg up to a total dose of 3.2 grams), given as a slow intravenous infusion prior to beginning the perfusion. We have sometimes noted hypotension, likely due to the increased histamine, at the initiation of the infusion; this

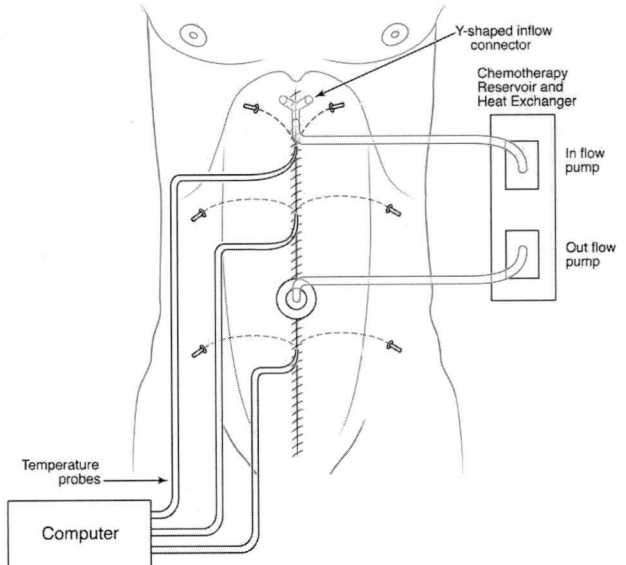

Figure 1 Intraoperative set-up of intraperitoneal hyperthermic perfusion.

can be controlled by administration of intravenous fluids and adjusting the flow rate of the cimetidine.

All patients undergoing IPHC experience modest loss of perfusate or absorption of drug. In our experience, following a 90-minute perfusion, approximately 75% of the perfusate volume is recovered. A dramatic loss of perfusate from the circuit in patients who have had peritoneal stripping of the diaphragm may, however, indicate injury to the diaphragm with loss of perfusate into the pleural space. Maintaining a slight positive end-expiratory pressure (10 to 15 mmHg) during the perfusion can help minimize any leakage. If an intrathoracic loss of perfusate is suspected, a chest radiograph should be obtained immediately. In the event that a pleural effusion is found, there are two management options. First, the perfusion can be halted, the patient placed in reverse Trendelenburg position, the pleural space evacuated, and the diaphragm repaired prior to resuming the perfusion. Alternatively, a chest tube can be placed with connective tubing to return the perfusate to the circuit. Repairing the diaphragm may be preferable if the leak is observed early in the perfusion and the rate of loss of the perfusate is high.

If perfusate is not being lost into the thoracic cavity, poor return of the perfusate to the reservoir may be due to loss of perfusate at the level of the skin, inadequate intra-abdominal circulation, or excessive absorption through raw surfaces, though this is not common. Significant perfusate leakage at the level of the skin can be addressed with additional sutures. Adequate agitation of the abdomen is essential to ensure proper circulation of the perfusate throughout the abdomen and through the outflow collector.

At the conclusion of the perfusion, the perfusate is drained back to the reservoir and the catheters and temperature probes are removed. Bowel anastomoses are then performed and a gastrotomy tube and feeding jejunostomy tube are placed. Average estimated blood loss ranges from 500 to 1000 cc, but they can be greater if extensive disease is present.

POSTOPERATIVE MANAGEMENT

Because of the length and magnitude of the surgery, most patients are admitted intubated and sedated to the surgical intensive care unit for immediate postoperative care. While time to extubation depends on individual patient characteristics and operative issues, most are extubated within the first 24 hours. In the initial postoperative period, patients who receive intraperitoneal MMC often develop a spontaneous and inappropriate diuresis, which requires careful monitoring and fluid replacement to avoid significant dehydration. For the first 24 hours, fluid resuscitation should be targeted to

maintain a central venous pressure of 6 to 12 mmHg. Because nephrotoxicity can occur following treatment with MMC (though this has not been reported after IPHC), aggressive hydration (establishing central venous pressure greater than 12 mmHg) prior to and during the perfusion, as well as forced diuresis if necessary to maintain urine output greater than 100 cc/hour, may help minimize this toxic effect. Cisplatin has a greater nephrotoxicity and may require maintenance of urine output at 200 cc/hour. Similar hydration should be continued during the initial postoperative period, with maintenance of the urine output at 200 cc/hour for 12 hours, then 100 cc/hour for the next 12 hours. Intravenous sodium thiosulfate should be administered prior to cisplatin IPHC to help minimize renal injury. Early postoperative intravenous fenoldopam may be considered.

Other routine initial postoperative orders include the administration of perioperative antibiotics for 24 hours. Prophylaxis against deep venous thrombosis is administered in the form of compression stockings and sequential compression devices. Low-molecular-weight heparin is administered in the absence of any bleeding concerns, but given the magnitude of the surgery and the large raw surface areas, this is not typically started before surgery and may be delayed for several days after surgery. Early patient ambulation is strongly encouraged.

Postoperative nutrition is one of the most important and challenging aspects of clinical care following IPHC because gastric and/or small bowel ileus is frequent. Variations in the literature regarding the frequency and duration of ileus may be related to differences in chemotherapy regimens, degree of hyperthermia, and duration of treatment. Patients receiving MMC have been shown to have the highest incidence of ileus, and approximately 50% of our patients experience a protracted gastric ileus—some for as long as 6 weeks. For this reason, we routinely place a gastrostomy tube at the end of the procedure. Prolonged gastric drainage and multiple clamping trials may be necessary before oral nutrition is tolerated. Nearly all patients are discharged with the gastric tube in place, even with little drainage. Placement of a gastrostomy tube offers an additional benefit. Because the stomach is permanently fixed to the anterior abdominal wall, easy placement of a subsequent palliative gastrostomy tube is facilitated in the event of disease recurrence and intestinal obstruction.

Intestinal ileus tends to be less severe, and low-rate elemental tube feedings can be attempted as early as postoperative day 2. Some patients require total parenteral nutrition prior to tolerating complete enteral nutritional support. With this approach, most patients are discharged receiving full nutritional and hydration support through the jejunostomy tube, supplemented by a small amount of oral intake (median hospitalization: 17 days). A gradual transition to full oral nutrition and hydration is often made on an outpatient basis. Early and regular involvement of a registered dietician is invaluable.

Complications

Performing cytoreduction and IPHC incurs significant risks, of which both the operating surgeon and patient need to be cognizant. The literature reviewing the morbidity and mortality of this procedure clearly demonstrates a technical learning curve, with morbidity rates of over 50% and mortality rates greater than 10% reported in early experience series. A number of centers have gained more experience, and these rates have decreased significantly in those high-total-volume institutions. Since 1993, five centers have published eight series of over 100 patients undergoing IPHC. The mortality rates in these series range from 1 to 8%, while the surgical morbidity rates range from 16 to 35%.[24,25] The most common complications reported include enteric fistula, anastomotic leak, bowel perforation, abscess, and pancreatitis (Table 1).[12,24–28] The most common risk factors for increased morbidity include extent of disease, duration of the surgery, and extent of resection and peritonectomy procedures. Although it is difficult to separate the effects of hyperthermia and chemotherapy in these procedures, we believe that hyperthermic perfusion doubles the risk of leak from a bowel anastomosis to about 5%.

Another potentially life-threatening morbidity associated with MMC IPHC is bone marrow suppression. Rates of neutropenia and thrombocytopenia as high as 50% have been reported, including some neutropenia-related deaths.[16,29] In our experience, the thrombocytopenia associated with MMC-based IPHC is infrequent and characteristically self-limiting. On the other hand, approximately 30 to 50% of patients develop some degree of neutropenia. This usually begins around postoperative day 7 to 10. Granulocyte-macrophage colony-stimulating factor (GM-CSF) is administered and neutropenic precautions are instituted in those patients who develop an absolute neutrophil count (ANC) less than 1,000, or those who exhibit a precipitous rate of decline of the ANC (approximately 20 to 30%). Neutropenic fevers are not uncommon during this period.

Postperfusion pulmonary complications, although common, are rarely severe or life threatening. The most frequent pulmonary complication following the closed technique is pleural effusion (incidence close to 100%), of which only a minority require intervention. If recovery-limiting dyspnea develops, a single therapeutic thoracentesis is often sufficient treatment. Because of the high incidence of this complication, however, some advocate routine placement of chest tubes if the diaphragm is stripped at the time of surgery. The second most common pulmonary complication is atelectasis (incidence greater than 75%), which is usually self-limiting and, with adequate pain control, resolves with routine postoperative pulmonary toilet. Other less commonly reported complications include pneumothorax, adult respiratory distress

Table 1 Most Frequent Complications of Intraperitoneal Hyperthermic Perfusion and Associated Risk Factors

Source	Patients	Primary Site(s)	Chemotherapy Agent	Mortality/Morbidity (%)	Most Frequent Complication (%)	Complication Associated Risk Factors
Sugarbaker[24]	181	Colon, appendix	MMC, 5-FU	1.5/17	Fistula (12)	Bowel obstruction; h/o radiation; h/o intraperitoneal chemotherapy
Stephens[28]	200	Multiple GI	MMC	1.5/27	Pancreatitis (6) Marrow suppression (4)	Duration of surgery; Number of peritonectomies; Number of suture lines
Sugarbaker[12]	385	Appendix	MMC, 5-FU	2.5/27	Pancreatitis (7.1) Fistula (4.7) Anastomotic leak (2.4)	Not assessed
Glehen[26]	216	Multiple GI and non-GI	MMC and/or cisplatin	3.2/24.5	Fistula (6.5) Marrow suppression (4.6)	Extent of disease; Duration of surgery; Extent of resection and peritonectomy
Verwaal[25]	102	Colorectal	MMC	8/35	Fistula (18)	>6 liter blood loss; >3 anastomoses
Schmidt[27]	67	Multiple GI and non-GI	MMC or cisplatin or mitoxantrone	4.5/34	Fistula (13) Abscess (7) Postoperative bleeding (7)	Extent of resection

5-FU = 5-fluorouracil; GI = gastrointestinal; h/o = ; MMC = mitomycin-C.

syndrome, and pulmonary embolus. MMC can cause pulmonary toxic effects, though this is unusual (we have only recently seen our first case). Finally, patients need to be aware of the possibility of temporary alopecia, renal failure, and hemolytic-uremic syndrome associated with MMC IPHC.

Outcomes

The IPHC technique has been applied to patients with a variety of tumor histologies who develop a pattern of peritoneal spread including malignancies of the stomach, colon, small bowel, and appendix, as well as sarcomatosis and peritoneal mesothelioma. While there are few randomized trials, some retrospective and prospective studies suggest a significant survival advantage after cytoreduction and IPHC in both gastric[30,31] and colon cancer.[32] IPHC has also been shown to be very effective in the management of malignant ascites; over 80% of patients experience relief.

Although there are no randomized trials of IPHC in patients with appendiceal neoplasms, Sugarbaker and Chang have reported on 385 appendiceal cancer patients treated with IPHC.[12] These investigators found that patients who underwent complete tumor resection for DPAM histology achieved a 5-year survival rate of 86%, as compared with 50% for patients with higher grade tumors and 20% for patients who did not have complete cytoreduction. Similarly, Loggie and colleagues, in a phase II study, demonstrated a 52% 3-year survival rate in patients treated for appendiceal cancer, which was also related to the completeness of cytoreduction.[16] Two additional studies of IPHC for appendiceal neoplasm have yielded 3-year survival rates of greater than 75%.[11,29] Although these series lack control study cohorts and are not directly comparable owing to differences in surgical and perfusion techniques and chemotherapy regimens, the results are comparable to our experience of a 5-year actuarial survival rate of 75% following IPHC for DPAM and PMCA evaluated together.

Summary

Although not considered aggressive in terms of distant metastatic potential, appendiceal neoplasms with peritoneal spread do not exhibit a benign natural history. Maximal cytoreduction accompanied by IPHC has been suggested to prolong the survival of patients suffering from this disease process. Unfortunately, this course of treatment is not without significant morbidity and mortality risks. Minimizing these risks requires careful patient selection and significant surgeon and institutional experience. Studies are currently underway to assess more completely the true benefit of this approach to peritoneal carcinomatosis as well as to identify more effective and less toxic chemotherapeutic agents for intraperitoneal administration.

References

1. Hesketh KT. The management of primary adenocarcinoma of the vermiform appendix. Gut 1963;4:158–68.

2. Connor SJ, Hanna GB, Frizelle FA. Appendiceal tumors: retrospective clinicopathologic analysis of appendiceal tumors from 7,970 appendectomies. Dis Colon Rectum 1998;41:75–80.

3. Esquivel J, Sugarbaker PH. Clinical presentation of the Pseudomyxoma peritonei syndrome. Br J Surg 2000;87:1414–8.

4. Werth R. Klinische and anatomische Unteruschungen Zur Lehre Von den Bauchgeschwilsten und der Laparotomie. Arch Gynecol Obstet 1884;42:100–18.

5. Hinson FL, Ambrose NS. Pseudomyxoma peritonei. Br J Surg 1998;85:1332–9.

6. Carr NJ, McCarthy WF, Sobin LH. Epithelial noncarcinoid tumors and tumor-like lesions of the appendix. A clinicopathologic study of 184 patients with a multivariate analysis of prognostic factors. Cancer 1995;75:757–68.

7. Ronnett BM, Zahn CM, Kurman RJ, et al. Disseminated peritoneal adenomucinosis and peritoneal mucinous carcinomatosis. A clinicopathologic analysis of 109 cases with emphasis on distinguishing pathologic features, site of origin, prognosis, and relationship to "pseudomyxoma peritonei." Am J Surg Pathol 1995;19:1390–408.

8. Misdraji J, Yantiss RK, Graeme-Cook FM, et al. Appendiceal mucinous neoplasms: a clinicopathologic analysis of 107 cases. Am J Surg Pathol Aug 2003;27:1089–103.

9. Kabbani W, Houlihan PS, Luthra R, et al. Mucinous and nonmucinous appendiceal adenocarcinomas: different clinicopathological features but similar genetic alterations. Mod Pathol 2002;15:599–605.

10. Mansfield PF. Appendiceal malignancy: where do we stand? Ann Surg Oncol 1999;6:715–6.

11. Piso P, Bektas H, Werner U, et al. Improved prognosis following peritonectomy procedures and hyperthermic intraperitoneal chemotherapy for peritoneal carcinomatosis from appendiceal carcinoma. Eur J Surg Oncol 2001;27:286–90.

12. Sugarbaker PH, Chang D. Results of treatment of 385 patients with peritoneal surface spread of appendiceal malignancy. Ann Surg Oncol 1999;6:727–31.

13. Jacquet P, Jelinek JS, Chang D, et al. Abdominal computed tomographic scan in the selection of patients with mucinous peritoneal carcinomatosis for cytoreductive surgery. J Am Coll Surg 1995;181:530–8.

14. Nitecki SS, Wolff BG, Schlinkert R, Sarr MG. The natural history of surgically treated primary adenocarcinoma of the appendix. Ann Surg 1994;219:51–7.

15. van Ruth S, Hart AA, Bonfrer JM, et al. Prognostic value of baseline and serial carcinoembryonic antigen and carbohydrate antigen 19.9 measurements in patients with pseudomyxoma peritonei treated with cytoreduction and hyperthermic intraperitoneal chemotherapy. Ann Surg Oncol 2002;9:961–7.

16. Loggie BW, Fleming RA, McQuellon RP, et al. Cytoreductive surgery with intraperitoneal hyperthermic chemotherapy for disseminated peritoneal cancer of gastrointestinal origin. Am Surg 2000;66:561–8.

17. Gonzalez-Moreno S, Sugarbaker PH. Right hemicolectomy does not confer a survival advantage in patients with mucinous carcinoma of the appendix and peritoneal seeding. Br J Surg 2004;91:304–11.

18. Sugarbaker PH. Peritonectomy procedures. Cancer Treat Res 1996;82:235–53.

19. Barlogie B, Corry PM, Drewinko B. In vitro thermo-chemotherapy of human colon cancer cells with cis-dichlorodiammineplatinum(II) and mitomycin C. Cancer Res 1980;40:1165–8.

20. Boykin JV Jr, Eriksson E, Sholley MM, Pittman RN. Histamine-mediated delayed permeability response after scald burn inhibited by cimetidine or cold-water treatment. Science 1980;209:815–7.

21. Boykin JV Jr, Crute SL, Haynes BW Jr. Cimetidine therapy for burn shock: a quantitative assessment. J Trauma 1985; 25:864–70.

22. Fujimoto S, Kokubun M, Shrestha RD, et al. Prevention of scald injury on the peritoneo-serosal surface in advanced gastric cancer patients treated with intraperitoneal hyperthermic perfusion. Int J Hyperthermia 1991;7:543–50.

23. Fujimoto S, Takahashi M, Kobayashi K, et al. Metabolic changes in cimetidine treatment for scald injury on the peritoneo-serosal surface in far-advanced gastric cancer patients treated by intraperitoneal hyperthermic perfusion. Surg Today 1993;23:396–401.

24. Sugarbaker PH, Jablonski KA. Prognostic features of 51 colorectal and 130 appendiceal cancer patients with peritoneal carcinomatosis treated by cytoreductive surgery and intraperitoneal chemotherapy. Ann Surg 1995;221: 124–32.

25. Verwaal VJ, van Tinteren H, Ruth SV, Zoetmulder FA. Toxicity of cytoreductive surgery and hyperthermic intraperitoneal chemotherapy. J Surg Oncol 2004;85:61–7.

26. Glehen O, Osinsky D, Cotte E, et al. Intraperitoneal chemohyperthermia using a closed abdominal procedure and cytoreductive surgery for the treatment of peritoneal carcinomatosis: morbidity and mortality analysis of 216 consecutive procedures. Ann Surg Oncol 2003;10:863–9.

27. Schmidt U, Dahlke MH, Klempnauer J, et al. Perioperative morbidity and quality of life in long-term survivors following cytoreductive surgery and hyperthermic intraperitoneal chemotherapy. Eur J Surg Oncol 2005;31:53–8.

28. Stephens AD, Alderman R, Chang D, et al. Morbidity and mortality analysis of 200 treatments with cytoreductive surgery and hyperthermic intraoperative intraperitoneal chemotherapy using the coliseum technique. Ann Surg Oncol 1999;6:790–6.

29. Witkamp AJ, de Bree E, Kaag MM, et al. Extensive surgical cytoreduction and intraoperative hyperthermic intraperitoneal chemotherapy in patients with pseudomyxoma peritonei. Br J Surg 2001;88:458–63.

30. Fujimoto S, Takahashi M, Mutou T, et al. Successful intraperitoneal hyperthermic chemoperfusion for the prevention of postoperative peritoneal recurrence in patients with advanced gastric carcinoma. Cancer 1999; 85:529–34.

31. Yonemura Y, de Aretxabala X, Fujimura T, et al. Intraoperative chemohyperthermic peritoneal perfusion as an adjuvant to gastric cancer: final results of a randomized controlled study. Hepatogastroenterology 2001;48:1776–82.

32. Verwaal VJ, van Ruth S, Witkamp A, et al. Long-term survival of peritoneal carcinomatosis of colorectal origin. Ann Surg Oncol 2005;12:65–71.

CHAPTER 30

OPEN AND LAPAROSCOPIC SURGERY FOR COLON CANCER

GEORGE J. CHANG, MD

Background

Colorectal cancer (CRC) is the fourth most common cancer and the second-leading cause of cancer deaths overall in men and women in the US. The past decade has been witness to improvements in the understanding, diagnosis, and treatment of CRC. These have included advances in our knowledge of the molecular pathways of carcinogenesis and the genetic alterations in inheritable CRC syndromes, the establishment of screening guidelines, and the rapid evolution of cytotoxic and biologic agents for chemotherapy. Advances have also been achieved in surgical therapy with the evolution of surgical standards for both sporadic and familial colon cancer, postoperative management protocols, and the development and validation of laparoscopic approaches to colectomy for cancer.

EPIDEMIOLOGY

It has been estimated that in 2005, 145,000 new cases of CRC will be diagnosed and 104,950 of these will be colon cancer. CRC incidence and mortality rates have continued to decline since 1985; however, CRC still accounts for 10% of cancer deaths in the US. Estimates for the year 2005 indicate that, combined, 54,290 people will die from colon and rectal cancer.[1]

The cumulative lifetime risk of developing CRC is about 6%, with a mean age at onset of 65 years, and this risk increases with age. Except in the setting of hereditary forms of CRC, this disease is rare before age 40. After age 50 there is a rapid increase in the rate of its occurrence, and 90% of the cases of sporadic CRC occur in patients older than 50. During the past several decades there has been a shift from left-sided cancers to more right-sided tumors.

When diagnosed, approximately 77% of patients have localized or regional disease and 23% have distant metastasis. The overall survival (OS) rates for local, regional, and distant disease at 5 years are 90%, 66%, and 9.0%, respectively. Approximately 75% of CRC cases are sporadic, with the remainder of cases occurring in patients considered to be at increased risk. The patients at increased risk include those with inflammatory bowel disease, familial adenomatous polyposis (FAP), hereditary nonpolyposis colorectal cancer (HNPCC), and the mutY homolog (MYH)-associated polyposis, and those with a strong family history of CRC. Men are at slightly increased risk when compared to women, with age-adjusted incidence rates of 58.5 per 100,000 and 44.2 per 100,000, respectively.

RISK FACTORS

Geographic and ethnic variations exist in the incidence of CRC, with the highest rates found in the more industrialized countries. In the US, African Americans have the highest incidence and mortality rates; in fact the incidence of CRC among African Americans has not changed since 1985, while it has declined 2.9% per year in white men and 1.7% per year in white women.

A number of observational studies have demonstrated that the increased intake of fats and red meat along with the decreased intake of fruits and vegetables in the Western diet are associated with an increased risk for CRC. Furthermore, rather than the total fat intake, saturated animal fat appears to be a stronger risk factor, and polyunsaturated fats and fish oils may be protective. Dietary fiber has a beneficial effect on CRC risk, although the mechanism for this association remains elusive. Although far from definitive, calcium, vitamin D, and folate intake have been variably associated with reduced CRC risk.

Both decreased physical activity and obesity have been related to an increased risk for CRC in both men and women, and a body mass index > 30 kg/m^2 in premenopausal women has been associated with a hazard ratio of 1.88 (95% confidence interval 1.24 to 2.86) for the risk of CRC.[2]

GENETIC PATHWAYS

The majority of CRCs develop through an orderly progression from normal mucosa to adenomas to carcinomas, the polyp-cancer sequence. In 1990, Fearon and Vogelstein described a model for CRC and provided a framework to elucidate the mutations in the genetic regulatory elements that lead to uncontrolled cell growth.[3] Further studies have elaborated this multistep pathway, commonly referred as loss of heterozygosity (LOH), which can be observed in inherited and sporadic CRC. Three major categories of genes have been implicated in the development of CRC, namely oncogenes such as K-*ras;* tumor suppressor genes such as *adenomatous polyposis coli (APC), deleted in colorectal cancer (DCC), p53, mutated in colon cancer (MCC);* and the *mismatch repair (MMR)* genes *hMSH2, hMLH1, hPMS,* and *hPMS2.*

Microsatellite instability (MSI) is another pathway of cancer development that consists of insertions or deletions of simple repeated sequences causing defects within the mismatch repair genes. In such cases replication errors increase, leading to MSI and gene malfunction. These tumors are biologically different from those acquired through LOH. MSI, also called replication error (RER), is found in the majority of HNPCC tumors and in approximately 10 to 20% of sporadic cancers.

INFLAMMATORY BOWEL DISEASE

Patients with chronic ulcerative colitis (CUC) have a 30-fold greater risk for CRC than the general population. The risk for cancer in this patient group is approximately 2% after 10 years, with active disease and increases 0.5 to 1% per year thereafter. In contrast to sporadic CRCs, CUC-related cancers are more often multiple, broadly infiltrating, poorly differentiated tumors that are often difficult to distinguish endoscopically from the chronic inflammatory changes. Therefore, random surveillance biopsies should be routinely performed in patients with CUC, and prophylactic colectomy or proctocolectomy should be recommended in cases of high-grade dysplasia and considered in cases of low-grade dysplasia. Crohn's disease is also associated with an increased risk for CRC, and the risk is related to the duration and severity of the Crohn's disease. The risk for CRC in patients with Crohn's disease is similar to that in patients with CUC. The risk associated with inflammatory bowel disease

underscores the importance of surveillance in this patient population.

INHERITABLE CRC SYNDROMES

Three hereditary CRC syndromes have been characterized and are discussed here: FAP, MYH-associated polyposis, and HNPCC.

Familial Adenomatous Polyposis

FAP is the best characterized of the inheritable CRC syndromes; 1 to 2% of patients diagnosed with colon carcinoma will have FAP. Germline mutations in the *APC* gene on chromosome 5q leading to truncation are characteristic of FAP. The pattern of inheritance is autosomal dominant with 90% penetrance, but approximately 25% of all cases of FAP are the result of a de novo mutation. Patients with FAP have thousands of polyps throughout the colon and the gastrointestinal tract. Without prophylactic colectomy, CRC will develop in virtually all affected individuals by the end of the third decade of life. A milder phenotype, known as attenuated FAP, is associated with fewer polyps and the typical age at onset for CRC is the early fifties. Patients with FAP may also have extracolonic manifestations, including gastric polyps, duodenal adenomas and carcinomas, desmoid tumors, thyroid carcinoma, mandibular osteomas, congenital hypertrophy of the retinal pigmented epithelium (CHRPE), sebaceous and epidermoid cysts and fibromas in Gardner's syndrome, or central nervous system tumors in Turcot's syndrome. Genetic testing and counseling should be offered to all patients in whom FAP is suspected.

The primary treatment for FAP is prophylactic colectomy. Surgical options include abdominal colectomy with ileorectal anastamosis (IRA) for those with low rectal polyp burdens, restorative proctocolectomy with ileal-pouch anal anastomosis (IPAA), and less commonly, proctocolectomy with end ileostomy. After prophylactic colectomy or proctocolectomy, patients must continue life-long surveillance because they are still at risk for cancer in the remaining rectum after IRA or at the anastomosis or within the ileal pouch after IPAA.

MYH-Associated Polyposis Syndrome

MYH-associated polyposis syndrome has recently been identified in subgroups of patients in FAP registries who have tested negative for *APC* gene mutations. The pattern or inheritance is autosomal recessive, and the phenotype demonstrates multiple colorectal polyps (> 10) but typically fewer than in individuals with classic FAP. The age at onset of CRC in patients with biallelic MYH mutations has been reported to be less than 50 years. CRCs in MYH polyposis syndrome are associated with G:C to T:A transversions resulting from defects in base excision repair. This CRC-associated polyposis syndrome continues to be defined.

HNPCC Syndrome

HNPCC, also classically known as the Lynch I and II syndromes, is a nonpolyposis autosomal dominant disease that occurs five times more frequently than FAP. HNPCC accounts for 5 to 7% of colon cancers. It is associated with early-onset CRC as well as tumors of the endometrium, ovary, stomach, small bowel, hepatobiliary tract, pancreas, ureter, and renal pelvis. Penetrance is between 30 and 70%. Patients with HNPCC have an estimated 85% lifetime risk to develop colon cancer. Compared with sporadic colon cancer, HNPCC cancers are more often right-sided (60 to 70% are proximal to the splenic flexure), occur at an earlier age (about 45 years), are lower stage tumors, portend a better survival, and are associated with a high rate of metachronous and synchronous tumors (20%).

The genetic mutations causing HNPCC are in *MMR* genes (*hMSH2*, *hMLH1*, *hMSH6*, *hPMS1*, and *hPMS2*). Mutations in tumor suppressor genes such as p53, *DCC*, and *APC* can be associated with HNPCC because replication errors are produced in them. Patients with HNPCC are at a high risk for synchronous and metachronous tumors, and prophylactic colectomy may be offered in selected cases.

Other Hereditary CRC-Associated Syndromes

Less commonly occurring hereditary CRC-associated syndromes include hamartomatous polyposis such as Peutz Jeghers Syndrome (PJS), Juvenile Polyposis Syndrome (JPS), Cowden syndrome, and Bannanyan-Ruvalcaba-Riley syndrome. Germline mutations in STK11/LKB1 are associated with PJS, mutations in *SMAD4* and *BMPR1-A* are associated with JPS, and *PTEN* mutations are associated with Cowden syndrome and Bannanyan-Ruvalcaba-Riley syndrome. Hamartomatous polyposis syndromes are associated with a significantly high risk for CRC and occur in less than 1% of CRC in cases in North America.

People with a first-degree relative with CRC have a 1.8- to 8-fold higher risk for CRC than the general population. The risk increases if there is more than one affected relative, and is further increased if cancer developed in that relative at a young age (< 45 years). The role of inheritable genetic defects in predisposition to CRC in such people is not well understood.

ANATOMY

The colon extends from the end of the ileum to the rectum. The ascending colon and descending colon are fixed in the retroperitoneal space, and the transverse colon and sigmoid colon are suspended in the peritoneal cavity by the mesocolon. The junction end of the sigmoid colon is defined by the spreading fibers of the taeniae coli on the rectum.

The arterial supply and the venous drainage to each segment of the colon generally run together within the mesocolon along with the associated lymphatic drainage. In addition, the existence of a collateral circulation principally through the highly variable marginal artery of Drummond permits preservation of the blood supply to the cut ends of the bowel during oncologic resection. There are two watershed regions that include Griffith's point at the splenic flexure and Sudeck's point at the junction between the sigmoid colon and rectum.

The arterial supply to the ascending and transverse colon come from the superior mesenteric artery (SMA) through its ileocolic, right colic, and middle colic branches. The right colic anatomy is highly variable. It may be absent or arise directly from the SMA in approximately 10% of individuals. The descending and sigmoid colon and the upper rectum obtain their blood supply through the inferior mesenteric artery (IMA). The IMA gives rise to the arc of Riolan, the left colic, and the superior rectal arteries. The superior rectal artery gives rise to several sigmoidal branches before supplying the rectum. The venous drainage parallels the arterial supply but drains principally into the portal venous system through the superior and inferior mesenteric veins, providing a direct route for hematogenous metastasis to the liver.

The sympathetic nerves originating at T10–12 travel to the preaortic and superior mesenteric plexuses, from which postganglionic fibers are distributed along the SMA and its branches to the right colon. The left colon is supplied by sympathetic fibers that arise in L1–3, synapse in the paravertebral ganglia, and accompany the inferior mesenteric artery to the colon. The parasympathetic nerves to the right colon come from the right vagus and travel with the sympathetic nerves. The parasympathetic supply to the left colon comes from S2–4. These fibers emerge from the spinal cord as the nervi erigentes, which form the pelvic plexus and send branches to the transverse, descending, and pelvic portions of the large bowel.

The curative resection and staging of colon cancer includes resection of the lymphatic drainage basin of the primary tumor site. Thus, the extent of bowel resection is determined by the relationship between the blood supply to the affected bowel and the associated draining lymphatics. The epicolic lymph nodes run between the intestinal wall and the vascular arcades and drain into the paracolic nodes, which follow the routes of the marginal arteries. The epicolic and paracolic nodes represent the majority of the colonic lymph nodes and are the most likely sites of regional metastatic disease. The drainage then follows the main colic vessels to para-aortic chain.

STAGING

In 1932, Dukes proposed a classification system for CRC that was based upon the extent of direct tumor extension into the bowel wall along with the presence or absence of regional lymphatic metastases. Dukes' A lesions are tumors in which the depth of penetration is confined to the bowel wall. Dukes' B tumors penetrate the full thickness of the bowel to include serosa or pericolic fat. Dukes' C lesions have local (C_1) or regional (C_2) nodal involvement. However, the American Joint Committee on Cancer and International Union Against Cancer (AJCC/UICC) tumor-node-metastasis (TNM) system is presently the internationally preferred standard method of staging colon cancer and has largely replaced the traditional Dukes system and the Astler-Coller modification (Table 1). The AJCC/UICC TNM system provides

prognostic information based on depth of bowel-wall penetration, extent of lymph node involvement, and presence of distant metastases. It currently requires that at least 12 lymph nodes be evaluated in the surgical specimen for adequate nodal staging. Furthermore, it provides additional histopathologic information such as tumor grade (G0-4) and lymphatic or vascular invasion designated by the letters L and V.

CLINICAL PRESENTATION

Colon cancer is most commonly identified during screening in asymptomatic individuals or during the work-up for hematochezia or anemia. Less commonly, presenting symptoms include abdominal pain, alteration in bowel habits, weight loss, anorexia, nausea, and indications of obstruction or perforation. Patients with pulmonary metastases may present with a solitary lung nodule or hemoptysis. Bacteremia with Streptococcus bovis is uncommon but has an important association with colorectal malignancy.

PREOPERATIVE EVALUATION

Preoperative evaluation of the patient with CRC begins with a detailed family history and a thorough physical

Table 1 AJCC/TNM Staging System, 6th edition, Comparison to Dukes and Modified Aster-Coller (MAC) Classification

TX	Primary tumor cannot be assessed
T0	No evidence of primary tumor
Tis	Carcinoma in situ; intraepithelial or invasion of lamina propria with no extension through the muscularis mucosae into the submucosa
T1	Tumor invades submucosa
T2	Tumor invades muscularis propria
T3	Tumor invades through the muscularis propria into the subserosa, or into nonperitonealized pericolic or perirectal tissues
T4	Tumor directly invades other organs or structures and/or perforates visceral peritoneum
NX	Regional lymph nodes cannot be assessed
N0	No regional lymph node metastasis
N1	Metastasis in 1–3 regional lymph nodes
N2	Metastasis in 4 or more regional lymph nodes
MX	Distant metastasis cannot be assessed
M0	No distant metastasis
M1	Distant metastasis

Stage	Depth	Nodal Status	Distant Metastasis	Dukes	MAC
0	Tis	N0	M0		
I	T1	N0	M0	A	A
	T2				B1
IIA	T3	N0	M0	B	B2
IIB	T4				B3
IIIA	T1-2	N1	M0	C	C1
IIIB	T3-4	N1			C2/C3
IIIC	Any T	N2			C1/C2/C3
IV	Any T	Any N	M1		D

Note: **V** and **L** substaging are used to denote the presence or absence of vascular or lymphatic invasion but do not impact the overall stage. The prefix **p** denotes pathologic evaluation (For example: if the involved segment of bowel is macroscopically adherent to adjacent organs, the classification is T4 but if no tumor is microscopically present within the adhesion, the classification is pT3.)
AJCC/TMN = American Joint Committee on Cancer and International Union Against Cancer/ tumor-node-metastasis.

examination. Laboratory investigations include complete blood count, chemistry panel, liver function tests, carcinoembryonic antigen, albumin, urinalysis, and coagulation profile. Essential diagnostic examinations include a complete colonoscopy if obstruction does not exist, chest radiograph, and computed tomography (CT) scan. Magnetic resonance imaging may be helpful in circumstances when intravenous contrast-enhanced CT scanning is contraindicated. Positron emission tomography (PET), and now PET-CT, has emerged as a potentially important imaging modality for patients with CRC. The technique utilizes the glucose analog fluorodeoxyglucose, which accumulates in metabolically active tissues. The standardized uptake value can provide a semiquantitative determination to help discriminate benign disease from malignant disease. Although potentially useful in recurrent cancer, it has not been helpful in the primary evaluation of patients with colon cancer because of false positives and high costs, and its routine use for screening should be discouraged.

A complete evaluation is essential to identify comorbidities and suitability for surgery, risk for inheritable cancer syndromes, synchronous colon lesions, involvement of adjacent organs, and presence of metastatic disease. Approximately 20% of patients will have synchronous liver metastasis at the time of initial diagnosis. Preoperative identification of liver metastasis is necessary when planning combined resections of the primary tumor and liver metastasis or for the treatment of tumors involving contiguous organs. Even in cases of advanced metastatic colon cancer, surgical resection of the primary lesion may be indicated for palliation.

Treatment

The surgical principles for the curative resection of colon cancer are the same for both conventional open surgery and laparoscopic surgery. These principles are discussed in this section.

General considerations for patients with malignancy include the increased risk for deep venous thrombosis, and prophylaxis should include the use of pneumatic compression devices for the legs and subcutaneous heparin at the induction of anesthesia unless otherwise contraindicated. Preoperative parenteral antibiotic prophylaxis should be given to reduce the incidence of infectious complications as with all open-bowel surgeries. Although the utility of the mechanical bowel preparation has recently been called into question, it is likely to remain standard practice until prospective randomized data are available.

ABDOMINAL EXPLORATION

A thorough exploration of the abdomen should include inspection and palpation, when possible, of the liver, peritoneal surface, omentum, retroperitoneum, and ovaries, if present. The primary tumor should be evaluated for local adherence. If suspicious lesions are identified within the liver, intraoperative ultrasound has been shown to be the most accurate method of evaluating the liver and can be performed with either open or laparoscopic approaches. The small bowel and the remaining colon should be examined for the presence of synchronous lesions.

EXTENT OF BOWEL RESECTION

The extent of bowel resection should include the primary tumor along with the adjacent bowel supplied by the primary feeding arterial vessel. When the primary tumor is between two feeding vessels, both vessels should be excised at their origin. This includes proximal ligation of the ileocolic artery at the duodenum, the middle colic artery at its origin from the SMA, the left colic artery at its origin from the IMA, and the superior rectal artery (IMA) just distal to the origin of the left colic artery. At least 5 to 10 cm of normal bowel on either side of the primary lesion appears to be adequate to prevent anastomotic recurrences.[4]

EXTENT OF LYMPHADENECTOMY

Lymph node resection in CRC has both therapeutic and prognostic implications. A subset of patients with lymph node-positive disease can be cured by surgery alone; therefore, the importance of an adequate lymphadenectomy cannot be overemphasized. An appropriate radical lymph node resection extends to the level of the origin of the primary feeding vessel and is removed en bloc. Suspicious lymph nodes outside the field of resection should also be sampled. Adequate lymphadenectomy has previously been defined as the evaluation of a minimum of 12 lymph nodes.[5] However, more recent evidence from the randomized trials of adjuvant chemotherapy for stages II and III colon cancer demonstrate improved overall, cause-specific, and disease-free survival rates with an increase in the number of lymph nodes evaluated. In the Intergroup 0089 trial of adjuvant 5-fluorouracil and leucovorin, after controlling for the number of nodes involved, survival increased as more nodes were evaluated ($p = .0001$ for all three end points). Even when no nodes were involved, the overall and cause-specific survival rates improved as more lymph nodes were evaluated ($p = .0005$ and $p = .007$, respectively)[6] (Table 2). Clearly, improved survival is associated with improved lymph node evaluation and adequate lymph

Table 2 Overall, Cause-Specific, and DFS Rates at 5 and 10 Years After Curative Resection for Colon Cancer: Summary of Data from INT 0089

Stage	Number LN	5-year			10-year		
		OS	CSS	DFS	OS	CSS	DFS
N0	1-10	73%	80%	72%	59%	74%	70%
	11-20	80%	85%	79%	73%	81%	77%
	>20	87%	92%	83%	79%	97%	77%
N1	1-10	67%	74%	65%	56%	67%	62%
	11-40	74%	78%	70%	64%	72%	67%
	>40	90%	93%	93%	90%	93%	93%
N2	1-35	51%	55%	48%	43%	49%	45%
	>35	71%	71%	69%	71%	71%	67%

Adapted from Le Voyer, et al.[6]
CSS = cause-specific survival; DFS =disease-free survival; LN = lymph nodes; OS = overall survival.

node evaluation may require at least 14 to 20 lymph nodes in the resected specimen.[6–8]

CONTIGUOUS ORGAN INVOLVEMENT

The preoperative evaluation, including history, physical examination, and CT scan, can help to identify contiguous organ involvement for surgical planning. When tumors are identified to be adherent to adjacent organs, the adhesions should not be taken down. Rather, all or at least the affected part of the adjacent organ should be resected en bloc because the adhesions will contain carcinoma in $\geq$ 40% of cases.[9] Furthermore, after resection of locally advanced CRC, the 5-year survival rate has been reported to be 61% with a local recurrence rate of 36% with en bloc resection compared with 5-year survival rate of 23% with a local recurrence rate of 77% for those who did not undergo en bloc resection.[10] If the tumor is transected at the site of local adherence, the resection is not complete. If the abdominal wall is involved, it should be resected en bloc as well.

OOPHORECTOMY

Because ovarian metastases subsequently develop in 1 to 8% of women who undergo potentially curative resections, prophylactic oophorectomy at the time of colectomy has been considered. However, prophylactic oophorectomy has not been shown to improve survival and data does not support this approach. The preliminary results of a prospective randomized trial of 155 patients treated at the Mayo Clinic showed an initial trend towards improved survival with prophylactic oophorectomy; however, this difference did not persist at 5 years and the trial results have not since been updated.[11] When isolated metastatic disease to one ovary is identified, a bilateral oophorectomy should be performed because of the high risk for bilateral involvement.

SPECIAL MANAGEMENT PROBLEMS

Obstruction

Obstructing CRCs are usually treated with a two-stage approach initially, with resection and Hartmann's procedure followed by subsequent colostomy takedown and anastomosis. An alternative treatment is a one-stage procedure with either subtotal colectomy and primary ileorectostomy or, for carefully selected patients, a segmental resection and intraoperative colonic lavage. These two treatment strategies were compared in a prospective randomized trial conducted by the Subtotal Colectomy versus On-table Irrigation and Anastomosis (SCOTIA) study group. Ninety-one patients with malignant left-sided colonic obstruction were randomized and the morbidity and mortality rates were similar.[12] Laser fulguration and endoscopic stenting of obstructive lesions can be used for palliation to allow for bowel preparation and subsequent single-step resection. Obstructing right-sided cancers can be effectively treated with resection and anastomosis in one stage. Regardless of the treatment approach, data from the National Surgical Adjuvant Breast and Bowel Project (NSABP) shows this group to have an increased risk for treatment failure.[13]

Perforation

Colon perforation caused by carcinoma can occur either at the site of the primary tumor or in the colon proximal to the tumor. Many of these patients have locally advanced disease at the time of presentation. They may also present with peritonitis and may require emergency treatment. If the perforation is contained, an en bloc resection of the abscess cavity and any involved organs should be performed when possible. In some instances it may be safer to perform percutaneous drainage and await resolution of the inflammation rather than to embark on an unsafe operation. If this approach is required, it is important to resect all affected tissues, including the drainage tract, at the time of definitive resection to prevent local tumor recurrence. Patients with perforation may benefit from adjuvant radiation; therefore, the metal clips should be placed at the time of resection in the areas at risk.[14]

Synchronous Tumors

A complete preoperative colonoscopic examination is essential for identification and evaluation of synchronous neoplasms including polyps within the colon. At presentation in patients with colon cancer, synchronous carcinoma occurs in 3 to 5% and synchronous polyps occur in 30 to 40%. Treatment should be tailored to the patient; partial colectomies will require surveillance for metachronous but a subtotal colectomy will have the functional consequences of an ileorectostomy and still leave the rectum at risk. The prognosis of the patient with synchronous colon malignancies will be similar to that for the more advanced stage lesion alone. Finally, patients with synchronous malignancies should be evaluated for the presence of HNPCC syndrome.

Open Colectomy

The anatomic extent of the typical colon resections based on tumor location are shown in Figure 1. The technical principles are similar regardless of the segment of bowel removed.

RIGHT HEMICOLECTOMY

Right hemicolectomy is indicated for cecal, ascending colonic, and proximal hepatic flexure lesions. The approach is through a midline incision with the patient in supine position. Although a right transverse incision has been described for right colectomy, a midline incision allows more flexibility and improved exposure should a more extensive operation be required (such as with unsuspected abdominal wall or adjacent organ involvement or metastatic disease to the liver or ovaries). After the placement of a self-retaining Bookwalter or similar retractor, the abdomen is explored. The colon and its mesentery are mobilized beginning with sharp electrocautery dissection of the cecum away from the retroperitoneal plane. It is important to identify this avascular plane in order to avoid injury to the underlying retroperitoneal structures, including the gonadal vessels, ureter, and duodenum. In most cases the ureter can be

seen through a thin veil of connective tissue. Direct visualization of the ureter indicates that the plane of dissection is too deep and should be avoided. The terminal ileal mesentery must also be mobilized to permit identification for proximal ligation of the ileocolic vessels at the level of the duodenum. The hepatic flexure is also mobilized with a combination of electrocautery and ligatures because there may be small vessels running within the hepatocolic attachments. T4 tumors can involve the abdominal wall, small bowel, or retroperitoneal structures, including the duodenum or kidney, which should be resected en bloc with the colon.

Once the bowel has been mobilized, the vessels are identified by incising the medial aspect of the peritoneum at the base of the mesentery. There may be significant variation in the ileocolic vascular anatomy, so this region should be carefully examined prior to ligation at the base of the mesentery. The right colic artery may arise directly from the SMA or be absent. It should be noted that there is generally a vascular clear space in the mesentery between the ileocolic artery and the right branch of the middle colic artery. Proximal ligation of the ileocolic trunk will include the right colic arterial pedicle in most cases. This can be done between clamps and ties or with a vascular stapler. The venous anatomy may, however, run separately and should be ligated separately. The ileocolic trunk is divided between clamps and ties. The right branch of the middle colic artery is then divided just distal to its bifurcation.

The author's preference is to construct the anastomosis between the ileum and the proximal transverse colon with two fires of the 100 mm intestinal stapler with the specimen in continuity with the remaining bowel. The first application creates the anastomosis along the antimesenteric aspect of the two limbs of bowel, and the second application is placed across both the ileum and the colon at the point of transection. Thus, the anastomosis is completed and the specimen is delivered. The apex of the stapled anastomosis is reinforced with a seromuscular suture. The corners of the staple line are inverted, as is the intersection of the two staple lines. An alternative approach is a two-layered end-to-end hand-sewn anastomosis, which is easily performed by either transecting the ileum at an angle or creating a Cheatle slit to minimize the size mismatch. The inner layer of mucosa and submucosa is approximated with a simple running 3-0 monofilament absorbable suture that is locked at the corners. The outer seromuscular layer is performed to invert the anastomosis with 3-0 absorbable braided suture such as vicryl. A very large mesenteric defect will now remain and does not need to be closed.

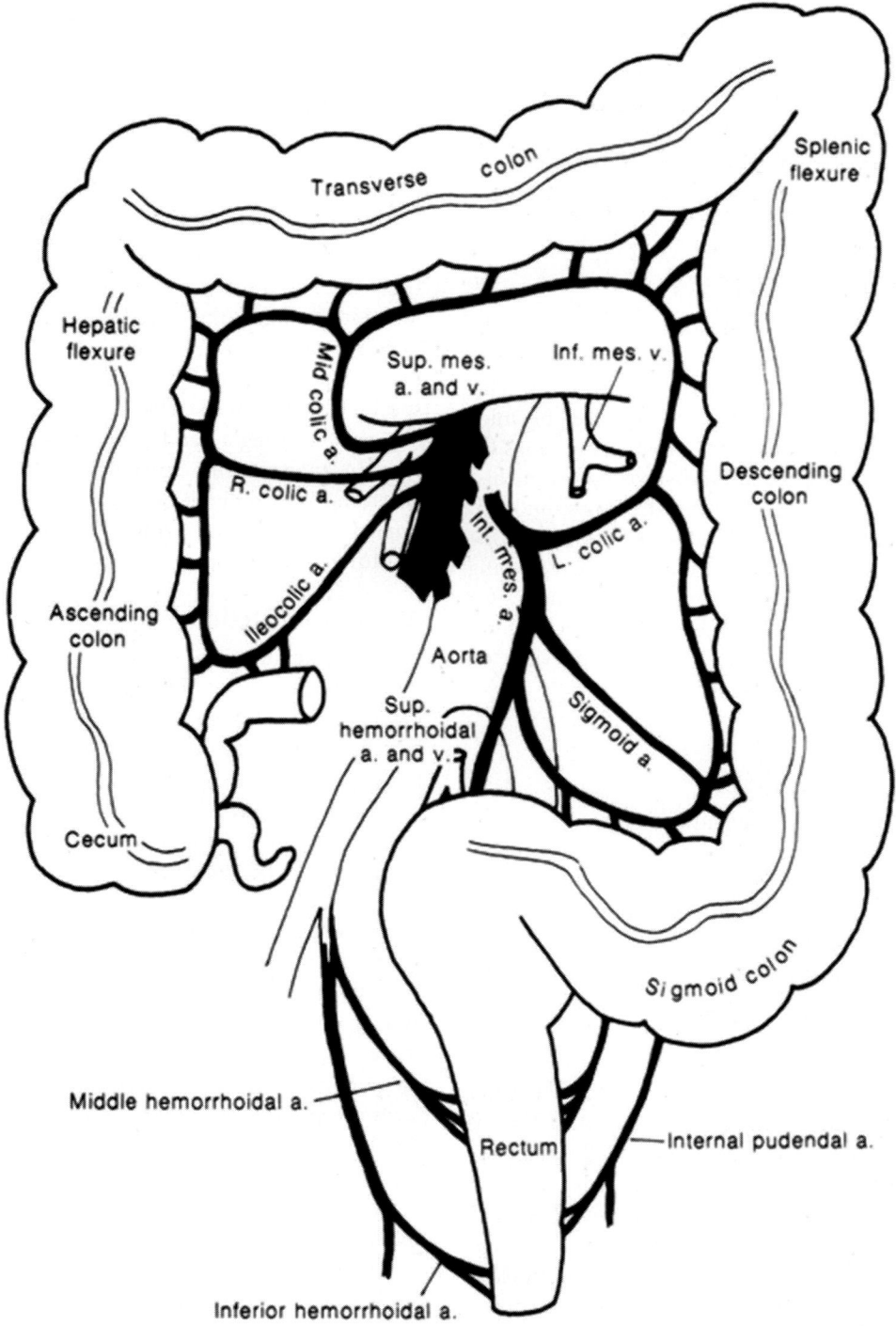

Figure 1 Vascular anatomy of the colon.

EXTENDED RIGHT HEMICOLECTOMY

The extended right hemicolectomy is an extension of the right colectomy to include resection of the transverse colon (including proximal ligation of the middle colic artery at its origin) in addition to the structures removed in the right hemicolectomy. Indications for the procedure are hepatic flexure or select transverse colon lesions. Mobilization of the splenic flexure is generally required to allow a tension free anastomosis. For lesions in the transverse colon, the omentum should be resected en bloc with the colon, noting the location of the gastroepiploic vessels. Care should be taken during the dissection of the transverse mesocolon because the lesser sac is not well developed in some patients. The middle colic vein is taken at the border of the pancreas, taking care to avoid injury to the collaterals from the pancreaticoduodenal vein. The ileocolic anastomosis is constructed as has been described for right colectomy.

TRANSVERSE COLECTOMY

A transverse colectomy is indicated for select middle transverse colon lesions. It removes the transverse colon with proximal ligation of the middle colic vessels. This operation is infrequently performed because the mid-transverse colon is one of the least common locations for primary colon cancers. To prevent anastomotic dehiscence, a well-vascularized and tension-free anastomosis is mandated. This requires mobilization of both the right and left colon along with both flexures, and an ascending to descending colon anastomosis. Various techniques for the anastomosis exist, but the author's preference is for a hand-sewn end-to-end anastomosis, which provides an anatomic and tension-free reconstruction.

LEFT HEMICOLECTOMY

Tumors of the splenic flexure and descending colon are resected by a left colectomy that includes transection of the transverse colon distal to the right branch of the middle colic and proximal sigmoid colon. With the patient in the modified low lithotomy position, the left side of the colon and the transverse colon are completely mobilized in order to achieve a tension-free anastomosis between the transverse colon and sigmoid colon. This is best achieved by initiating mobilization along the sigmoid colon and mesentery, beginning with an incision in the left peritoneal reflection along the white line of Toldt. The avascular plane posterior to the sigmoid mesentery is carefully developed using sharp electrocautery dissection. The ureter and gonadal vessels should be visible but undissected and covered by the loose areolar tissue of the retroperitoneum. By taking this approach along the retroperitoneum, the correct plane of dissection is identified and maintained. A laterally based approach increases the risk for developing the wrong plane that typically is too deep. The mobilization is then carried up along the descending colon. For tumors within the descending colon, entry into the lesser sac by elevating the omentum away from the transverse colon can facilitate splenic flexure mobilization. For lesions involving the distal transverse colon or the splenic flexure, the omentum should be resected en bloc and

the lesser sac should be entered through the omentum above the colon. The splenic flexure mobilization should be performed under careful direct vision to avoid an inadvertent injury to the spleen.

Once the bowel has been mobilized, the vessels are isolated by taking advantage of the avascular windows within the mesentery. The left colic artery should be ligated at its origin from the IMA. The left branch of the middle colic should be divided at its origin for distal transverse colon lesions. For tumors located in the junction between the descending and sigmoid colon, division of the IMA trunk simplifies the vascular dissection. The bowel is divided and the surgical specimen is removed. The resultant colo-colostomy is best created using a hand-sewn end-to-end technique to provide an anatomic, tension-free anastomosis. If the anastomosis is to the distal sigmoid or rectum, a double-stapled anastomosis using the circular end-to-end anastomosis (EEA) stapler is preferred.

Anterior Resection

Resection of tumors of the sigmoid colon and proximal rectum is performed using the approach as previously described for left colectomy. The sigmoid colon should be removed with the affected rectum and reconstruction performed between the descending colon and the rectum. Complete mobilization of the splenic flexure is essential to provide a tension-free anastomosis if an adequate resection has been performed. The mesenteric dissection is performed as described above such that the origin of the IMA and its bifurcation to the left colic artery and the superior rectal artery are clearly visualized. Distally, the upper rectum should be sharply mobilized away from the sacrum in the avascular plane between the fascia propria of the mesorectum and the presacral fascia. The sympathetic nerve trunks run in the retroperitoneum deep to the superior rectal vascular pedicles and should be protected. Lesions in the proximal sigmoid colon should be treated as previously described for lesions at the junction of the descending and sigmoid colons. Lesions in the mid-sigmoid to proximal rectum should be treated with a proximal ligation of the superior rectal artery at its origin from the IMA. The distal point of resection should be on the proximal rectum and incorporate at least 5 cm of uninvolved bowel and mesorectum. This can be done using a linear stapling device 45 to 60 mm in length. The temptation to "cone-down" during the mesorectal transection resulting in an inadequate mesorectal excision should be avoided. If necessary, mobilization of the rectum along the mesorectal planes releases the rectum to reach higher in the pelvis to facilitate the bowel anastomosis.

The anastomosis is most easily performed using the circular EEA stapler. The anvil is secured to the proximal bowel with a purse-string suture. Excessive devascularization of the bowel in preparation for the anastomosis should be avoided because it will increase the risk for stricture or dehiscence. After serially dilating the anus using the EEA sizers, the shaft of the stapler is inserted through the rectum. The spike is deployed just distal to the rectal staple line and the anvil engaged and the stapler is then closed and fired. The tissue "donuts" are checked for completeness. A completion proctoscopy with air insufflation is performed with the pelvis filled with saline irrigation to identify anastomotic incompetence. A small leak, demonstrated by air bubbles arising from the anastomosis, may be easily repaired by over-sewing the anastomosis with inverting Lembert sutures of 3-0 vicryl. An alternative approach is a two-layered hand-sewn anastomosis.

SUBTOTAL COLECTOMY

Subtotal colectomy involves the removal of the entire colon to the rectum with IRA. This procedure is indicated in cases of multiple synchronous colonic tumors that are not confined to a single anatomic distribution; obstructing left-sided tumors; and in select patients with HNPCC, colon cancer, and FAP with minimal rectal involvement. The operation is performed with the patient in a modified lithotomy position and through a midline incision. Proximal vascular ligation of the principal vessels simplifies the resection and is essential for tumors. The anastomosis is performed in an end-to-end fashion using the circular EEA stapler. The ileal mesentery should be carefully oriented to avoid inadvertent twisting. The author avoids the alternative approach of performing a side-to-end circular EEA stapled anastomosis, which may result in dysfunction and stasis due to dilation of the blind limb. Finally, every surgeon should be prepared to perform a hand-sewn anastomosis in the event a stapled anastomosis is not appropriate. Although an excellent quality of life can be achieved after IRA, frequent loose bowel movements are the norm and occasional incontinence may occur in 5 to 20% of patients. Patients should be counseled preoperatively regarding bowel regimens and about perianal care. In a study by the Cleveland Clinic, the risk of cancer in the retained rectum after IRA for FAP was 12.9% at a median follow-up of 212 months. By selecting only those patients with low rectal polyp burdens for IRA, no patient has developed rectal cancer in the remaining rectum at a median follow-up of 60 months.[15] Restorative proctocolectomy with ileal J-pouch anal anastomosis has the advantage of removing all or nearly all of the large intestine mucosa at risk for cancer while preserving some transanal defecation sensation and function. It is the preferred approach in patients with FAP and more than 20 to 30 rectal polyps. Complication and pouch failure rates are low when this procedure is done in experienced centers.[16]

Laparoscopic Colectomy

The appeal of laparoscopic colon surgery is simple: minimally invasive techniques result in faster recovery and may therefore result in improved quality of life and lower health care costs when compared to open laparotomy. These benefits have been dramatically realized with surgery at other sites, such as for benign gallbladder disease. When considering colectomy, reduction in postoperative pain and narcotic use, faster resolution of ileus, and shorter duration of hospitalization are unifying features of the laparoscopic approach. Added benefits may include the potential for reduced short- and long-term complication rates as well as costs. However, owing to the relative complexity of laparoscopic colectomy and the ongoing evolution of the techniques, the magnitude of these benefits is still being determined. Furthermore, the importance of these effects may, in part, depend on the underlying diagnosis.

Most patients with colon cancer are candidates for laparoscopic-assisted techniques. Transverse colon tumors require extensive bilateral colonic mobilization and are technically more difficult to treat laparoscopically. Factors associated with an increased need for conversion include tumor-related factors such as proximal left-sided lesions, large bulky tumors, as well as patient obesity, adhesions, and the presence of an associated abscess. Cancers with perforation, obstruction, or invasion of the retroperitoneum or abdominal wall are not approached laparoscopically.

Recent studies have confirmed that laparoscopy for colorectal carcinoma resection is technically feasible and safe and that the number of resected lymph nodes and length of resected bowel are equivalent to that of open colectomy. Despite early reports of port-site recurrence rates of up to 21%, no series has reported a rate greater than 1.4% since 1996.

Concerns regarding oncologic adequacy have been addressed by two major single-institution trials and four major multi-institution randomized control trials that compared laparoscopic-assisted resection to open colon resection in patients with colon cancer. Only one of the multinational trials has reported final results; the others are still underway.

The Barcelona study was the first adequately powered randomized trial of laparoscopic colectomy for colon cancer.[17] In this trial, 219 patients were randomized to laparoscopic versus open colectomy for cancer, and oncologic equivalency was demonstrated. Only 1 patient in the laparoscopy group and no patients in the open group developed a surgical wound recurrence. Considerable discussion was sparked by this trial because an unexpected oncologic benefit with improvement in cancer-related survival when compared to open colectomy was observed for a small subset of patients with stage III disease[17]. An additional single-institution trial from Hong Kong demonstrated oncologic equivalency with laparoscopy in 403 patients with sigmoid and rectosigmoid tumors randomized to open or laparoscopic approaches with intracorporeal vascular ligation and anastomosis.[18]

The National Cancer Institute sponsored multicentered Clinical Outcomes of Surgical Therapy (COST) trial opened in 1994 and randomized 872 patients to open or laparoscopic colectomy for colon cancer. Laparoscopic-assisted colectomy for cancer was associated with equivalent recurrence-free and OS rates when compared to open surgery, with no increase in wound recurrences; 0.5% in the laparoscopy group and 0.2% in the open group ($p = .50$)[17,19]. Patient-related benefits of the laparoscopic approach included reduced length of hospital stay, decreased pain, faster resolution of ileus, improved cosmesis, and an improvement in short-term quality of life.[19]

The Medical Research Council-sponsored Conventional versus Laparoscopic-Assisted Surgery In patients with CRC (CLASICC) multicenter trial, which was conducted in the UK, randomized 794 patients to open or laparoscopic surgery for CRC. Short-term oncologic results were equivalent for laparoscopic versus open colectomy. Similar patient-related benefits favoring laparoscopy, as were observed in the COST trial, were reported.[20]

The European multicenter Colon carcinoma Laparoscopic or Open Resection (COLOR) trial began enrollment from 27 European centers in 1997[21]. An additional Australasian multi-institution trial began accrual in 1998. The long-term oncologic results of the randomized trials are summarized in Table 3.

Laparoscopic colectomy for CRC is one of the best examples of the use of a rigorous approach in the evaluation of the safety and efficacy of a new technique in the surgical literature. With data from the reported randomized trials and the anticipated reports from additional large trials, laparoscopic colectomy for CRC has been validated and established as an important treatment modality for colorectal malignancies. It should be noted, however, that the results shown in these trials were obtained by experienced surgeons who have demonstrated proficiency in performing laparoscopic colectomy for cancer. To achieve these results, laparoscopic approaches to colon cancer must adhere to the same oncologic principles that guide open surgery, as were outlined above.

PREOPERATIVE CONSIDERATIONS

The preoperative evaluation of the patient for laparoscopic surgery is the same as that performed for conventional surgery. Because tactile identification of the lesion is typically limited, emphasis is placed on the preoperative localization of lesions utilizing anatomic landmarks or India ink tattoo at the time of colonoscopy. Identifying patients who are good candidates for the laparoscopic approach depends in part on the expertise of the surgeon. The surgeon should have a thorough knowledge of and experience in performing open colectomy for malignant disease and demonstrable advanced laparoscopic experience. The American Society of Colon and Rectal Surgeons has issued a position statement establishing that a surgeon must have performed at least 20 laparoscopic resections for benign or metastatic disease before performing a laparoscopic resection for a primary malignancy with curative intent.

The laparoscopic approach is contraindicated in patients with tumor infiltration into adjacent structures; a large phlegmon mass; acute complications, such as obstruction or perforation; or an underlying bleeding

Table 3 Long-Term Oncologic Results of the Randomized Trials of Laparoscopic versus Conventional Open Surgery for Colon Cancer

STUDY	N	Median Follow-up (mos)	Recurrence LAP	OPEN	p	Survival LAP	OPEN	p
Barcelona 2002[17]	219	43	17%	28%	.07 5-year actuarial	82% / 91%	74% / 79%	.14 5-year actuarial / .03 cancer specific
Hong-Kong[18]	403	52.7 lap / 49.2 open	25%	22%	.37 5-year actuarial	76% / 75%	73% / 78%	.61 5-year actuarial / .45 cancer specific
COST[19]	872	48	18%	20%	.32 3-year actual	86%	85%	.51 3-year actual

LAP = laparoscopic.

disorder. Relative contraindications include morbid obesity and multiple prior abdominal surgeries. Patients with cardiac or pulmonary disease should be carefully monitored intraoperatively due to the requirements for positional changes, as well as the potential for carbon dioxide (CO_2) absorption and for hemodynamic effects of the pneumoperitoneum. However such patients stand to benefit most from the improved recovery time after a minimally invasive approach.

TECHNICAL CONSIDERATIONS

Laparoscopic colectomy is performed utilizing standard laparoscopic video equipment and instruments after a pneumoperitoneum has been established to 12 to 14 mm Hg with CO_2. Gastric decompression with a nasogastric tube is requisite. Laparoscopic colectomy for cancer is a technically demanding procedure. Some of the difficulty comes from the need to operate in multiple quadrants of the abdomen and the mobility of the colon. This requires not only the skill of the operating surgeon, but of the camera operator as well. Most laparoscopic colectomy procedures are performed in the following general steps: 1) port placement and establishment of the working space, 2) vascular division, 3) colon mobilization, 4) specimen retrieval, and 5) intestinal reconstruction. However, these steps are performed in a variety of different ways with respect to the method and location of port placement, the sequence and the approach to the dissection, and the method of reconstruction. The operating surgeon must have the facility with multiple approaches in order to tailor the operation to individual patient differences. Thus the terminology "laparoscopic colectomy" may refer to totally laparoscopic approaches, laparoscopic-assisted approaches with extracorporeal anastomosis, and hand-assisted laparoscopic surgery (HALS). This variability of techniques is due in part to the necessity for specimen removal as well as the mobile nature of the colon in contrast to other fixed intra-abdominal organs such as the gallbladder or kidneys. Specimen retrieval is usually performed through a 4 to 8 cm incision; however, the location of this incision can vary.

The hand-assist devices have led to an increased appeal of the laparoscopic technique to a broader audience of surgeons adequately trained to perform HALS. The patient-related benefits of HALS appear to be similar to those achieved with standard laparoscopic colectomy.[22] Moreover, in the appropriate setting, HALS may have the advantage of decreased operative times and lower conversion rates compared to standard laparoscopic colectomy. The site used for bowel exteriorization determines where the hand-assist port is placed. For lesions on the left side or those requiring total colectomy, the suprapubic site is the ideal location to place the hand-assist port. This site can be moved cephalad to accommodate splenic flexure and descending colon lesions that require an anastomosis involving the transverse colon. For lesions proximal to the splenic flexure, the incision should be periumbilical; however, in that location the hand-assist port will be located centrally within the operative field.

Conversion from laparoscopic to conventional surgery can be an important factor in determining outcomes after laparoscopy. Most large series report conversion rates ranging from 5 to 25% with a trend towards improvement with experience.[23–25] In the COST trial, a conversion rate of 21% was reported and is comparable to rates observed in other trials for cancer.[19] Risk factors for conversion include obesity; tumor factors, such as advanced lesions or location on the left colon or splenic flexure; and surgeon and operating team experience. The need to convert to an open procedure should not be considered failure. Rather, it is determined by sound judgment, but every effort should be made to make that determination as early as possible during the procedure.

Right Colectomy

The patient is placed in the supine position with the left arm tucked. Chest and Trendelenburg ankle straps are used after appropriate padding to secure the patient. The monitors are placed on the patient's right side and the surgeon and assistant stand on the patient's left side. Although multiple approaches to port placement have been described, the author prefers a simplified approach using 3 or 4 ports that can be used regardless of the operation being performed (Figure 2).

Once the ports have been placed, a thorough exploration is performed as with open surgery. The presence of excessive adhesions, altered anatomy, or adverse tumor characteristics should prompt conversion to the open approach. The next step is the identification and division of the ileocolic pedicle. This is done most easily prior to colonic mobilization because the normal attachments of the colon facilitate exposure. With the table tilted to the left and in slight Trendelenburg to allow the small bowel to fall away, the cecal mesentery is gently grasped and retracted away from the duodenum, which will cause the ileocolic vessels to tent-up the mesentery. Dissection is then sharply performed on the proximal vessel, which is divided. After further dissection distally along the ileocolic mesentery, the patient is repositioned into steep Trendelenburg position with the left side down. The small bowel is moved out of the pelvis to expose the base of the cecum and terminal ileal mesentery. The avascular retroperitoneal plane behind the colon and ileal mesentery is sharply developed until

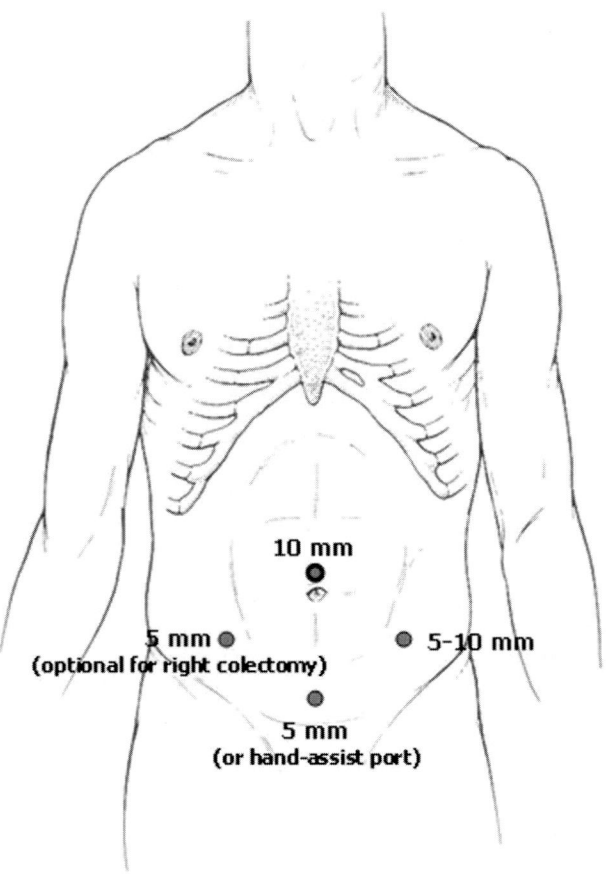

Figure 2 Port site placement for laparoscopic colectomy.

the plane of previous dissection on the ileocolic pedicle is encountered. The patient is then repositioned to steep reverse Trendelenburg position. The omentum overlying the proximal transverse colon is grasped, and the hepatocolic ligament is divided with electrocautery. Small vessels may run through this tissue but can easily be controlled with electrocautery. The plane of dissection along the posterior aspect of the colon mesentery is easily encountered if the posterior dissection along the colon mesentery has been performed appropriately.

Once mobilization has been completed, the pneumoperitoneum should be released through the ports to minimize the risk for port-site recurrences. The umbilical port is removed and the incision is extended to 4 to 6 cm to exteriorize the bowel. The mesenteric division is completed as needed, and the anastomosis is constructed as for open surgery.

Left-Sided Resection

With the patient in the modified lithotomy position with the right arm tucked at the side, complete mobilization of the left side of the colon and the splenic flexure is

performed as for open surgery. It is important that the legs are positioned low enough to permit a full range of motion of the instruments through lateral ports. This operation can be performed with complete laparoscopic mobilization or with the use of a hand-assist port placed in the suprapubic position. The hand-assist port is particularly useful in obese patients in whom exposure and visualization is made difficult by the thick mesentery. The vascular dissection is best performed from the right side of the patient first, allowing the natural attachments of the bowel to facilitate retraction. This is best accomplished by placing a trochar through the hand-assist port. The patient is placed in Trendelenburg with the right side down, and the superior rectal vessel is identified at the sacral promontory. The vascular dissection is continued proximally until the IMA and the left colic artery are identified. The appropriate vessels are then divided, and the posterior dissection of the colon mesentery is initiated from the medial aspect. In this position, exposure is also good for performing the proximal rectal dissection.

The surgeon then moves between the legs to complete mobilization of the sigmoid colon and its mesentery along the avascular plane as described for open surgery. It is important to avoid the temptation to move on to the next step in the procedure or to take down the lateral attachments prior to completing the retroperitoneal dissection on the colon mesentery. Such maneuvers are commonly performed by inexperienced surgeons and inevitably result in more difficulty in completing the subsequent steps and may lead to the operation being converted to an open procedure. Once the splenic flexure is approached from this aspect, the patient is repositioned in reverse Trendelenburg and the lesser sac is entered by detaching the omentum from the distal transverse colon. For splenic flexure lesions, the gastrocolic omentum should be divided to enter the lesser sac. If the posterior dissection has been performed adequately, coming around the lienocolic ligament in this fashion should cause the splenic flexure to fall completely down into the lower aspect of the abdomen. The dissection is carefully completed with additional transverse colic mesenteric mobilization as needed, taking care to avoid inadvertent injury to the middle colic vessels or the IMV.

The pneumoperitoneum is released through the ports and the bowel is exteriorized, either through the hand-assist port site or a small incision (4 to 8 cm) that is made in the suprapubic location for distal lesions, or by extending the supraumbilical port site for splenic flexure lesions. The suprapubic position (either as a Pfannenstiel or midline incision) has the advantage of allowing exposure of the rectum for dissection in treating lesions located in the distal sigmoid or proximal rectum. The remaining mesenteric attachments of the proximal bowel are ligated and the proximal bowel is divided. This is easily performed through the small incision if adequate mobilization has been performed. The distal dissection, including mesorectal transection, is then completed. The author prefers this approach over performing the mesorectal transection intracorporeally because it is simpler and faster and can be performed with a less experienced assistant. The anastomosis can then be performed using standard techniques under direct vision.

Transverse Colectomy

The transverse colectomy is the most difficult colon resection to perform laparoscopically because it requires complete mobilization of the intra-abdominal colon, using the techniques described above, so that a tension-free anastomosis can be constructed. The vessels are exposed and divided just prior to exteriorization of the bowel and completion of the distal peripheral mesenteric division and bowel transection with anastomosis. In thin patients, the entire colon, once mobilized, can be exteriorized through a small periumbilical incision. Proximal vascular ligation can also be performed through this small incision because it directly overlies the origin of the middle colic vessels.

POSTOPERATIVE CARE

Patients are encouraged to ambulate on the evening of surgery and multiple times daily throughout the remainder of their hospitalization. A clear liquid oral diet may be initiated on the first postoperative day for most patients. If liquids are well tolerated and the patient does not develop distension, a soft diet can be initiated and parenteral narcotics can be discontinued on the second postoperative day. Most patients will pass flatus on the second to third day and may be discharged on the third or fourth postoperative day.

Based on the lessons learned from patients after laparoscopic surgery, a fast-track program of post-operative rehabilitation has been increasingly used for patients who undergo open colectomy. The data are mixed, and although one blinded randomized trial demonstrated no difference in the duration of hospitalization between laparoscopic colectomy and fast-track open colectomy, nearly twice as many patients in the fast-track arm and their family members expressed that they felt that the hospital stay was too short (30% and 41% fast track versus 17% and 21% laparoscopic, respectively, $p < .05$). Furthermore, the nursing staff correctly identified those patients who had undergone laparoscopic surgery in 79% of cases and open surgery in 68% ($p < .05$), indicating significant differences in

patient recovery despite the fast-track protocol achieving a similar length of stay.[26] Supporting this observation, others have shown a significant decrease in the duration of hospitalization with laparoscopic colectomy when compared to fast-track open colectomy.[27]

COMPLICATIONS

Anastomotic dehiscence remains a major complication of colorectal surgery; however, most authors report clinically evident anastomotic leak rates of approximately 3% or less after colectomy. This is true for both open and laparoscopic approaches and is independent of the anastomotic technique employed. The European Laparoscopic Colorectal Surgery Study Group (LCSSG) recently reported the results of a multi-institution review of complications in 4,834 consecutive cases of laparoscopic colorectal surgery. Approximately 35% of the cases were for cancer. Intraoperative complications occurred in 5.4% of patients and included bleeding and inadvertent bowel injuries as the leading complications occurring in 1.7% and 1.3% of cases, respectively.[28]

Conclusions

The development and validation of the laparoscopic approach to colon cancer is a significant recent advance and addition to the surgeon's armamentarium. Early fears of port-site metastases and poor oncologic outcome have been put to rest. However, good outcomes depend on the surgeon's adherence to the principles of cancer surgery of the colon as well as skill and experience in performing advanced laparoscopic surgery. Regardless of the approach to colon cancer, either open or laparoscopic, the standards for surgical resection—thorough exploration, adequate bowel resection, proximal vascular ligation with lymphadenectomy, and en bloc resection—should be strictly applied.

References

1. Jemal A, Murray T, Ward E, et al. Cancer statistics, 2005. CA Cancer J Clin 2005;55:10–30.

2. Terry PD, Miller AB, Rohan TE. Obesity and colorectal cancer risk in women. Gut 2002;51:191–4.

3. Fearon ER, Vogelstein B. A genetic model for colorectal tumorigenesis. Cell 1990;61:759–67.

4. Nelson H, Petrelli N, Carlin A, et al. Guidelines 2000 for colon and rectal cancer surgery. J Natl Cancer Inst 2001;93: 583–96.

5. Fielding LP, Arsenault PA, Chapuis PH, et al. Clinicopathological staging for colorectal cancer: an International Documentation System (IDS) and an

International Comprehensive Anatomical Terminology (ICAT). J Gastroenterol Hepatol 1991;6:325–44.

6. Le Voyer TE, Sigurdson ER, Hanlon AL, et al. Colon cancer survival is associated with increasing number of lymph nodes analyzed: a secondary survey of intergroup trial INT-0089. J Clin Oncol 2003;21:2912–9.

7. Goldstein NS, Sanford W, Coffey M, Layfield LJ. Lymph node recovery from colorectal resection specimens removed for adenocarcinoma. Trends over time and a recommendation for a minimum number of lymph nodes to be recovered. Am J Clin Pathol 1996;06:209–16.

8. Wong JH, Severino R, Honnebier MB, et al. Number of nodes examined and staging accuracy in colorectal carcinoma. J Clin Oncol 1999;17:2896–900.

9. Lopez MJ, Monafo WW. Role of extended resection in the initial treatment of locally advanced colorectal carcinoma. Surgery 1993;113:365–72.

10. Hunter JA, Ryan JA Jr, Schultz P. En bloc resection of colon cancer adherent to other organs. Am J Surg 1987;154:67–71.

11. Young-Fadok TM, Wolff BG, Nivatvongs S, et al. Prophylactic oophorectomy in colorectal carcinoma: preliminary results of a randomized, prospective trial. Dis Colon Rectum 1998;41:277–83; discussion 283–5.

12. Single-stage treatment for malignant left-sided colonic obstruction: a prospective randomized clinical trial comparing subtotal colectomy with segmental resection following intraoperative irrigation. The SCOTIA Study Group. Subtotal Colectomy versus On-table Irrigation and Anastomosis. Br J Surg 1995;82:1622–7.

13. Wolmark N, Wieand HS, Rockette HE, et al. The prognostic significance of tumor location and bowel obstruction in Dukes B and C colorectal cancer. Findings from the NSABP clinical trials. Ann Surg 1983;198:743–52.

14. Willett CG, Goldberg S, Shellito PC, et al. Does postoperative irradiation play a role in the adjuvant therapy of stage T4 colon cancer? Cancer J Sci Am 1999;5:242–7.

15. Church J, Burke C, McGannon E, et al. Risk of rectal cancer in patients after colectomy and ileorectal anastomosis for familial adenomatous polyposis: a function of available surgical options. Dis Colon Rectum 2003;46:1175–81.

16. Chapman JR, Larson DW, Wolff BG, et al. Ileal pouch-anal anastomosis: does age at the time of surgery affect outcome? Arch Surg 2005;140:534–9; discussion 539–40.

17. Lacy AM, Garcia-Valdecasas JC, Delgado S, et al. Laparoscopy-assisted colectomy versus open colectomy for treatment of non-metastatic colon cancer: a randomised trial. Lancet 2002;359:2224–9.

18. Leung KA, Kwok SP, Lam SCW, et al. Laparoscopic resection of rectosigmoid carcinoma: prospective randomized trial. Lancet 2004;363:1187–92.

19. A comparison of laparoscopically assisted and open colectomy for colon cancer N Engl J Med 2004;350:2050–9.

20. Guillou PJ, Quirke P, Thorpe H, et al. Short-term endpoints of conventional versus laparoscopic-assisted surgery in patients with colorectal cancer (MRC CLASICC trial): multicentre, randomized controlled trial. Lancet 2005;365:1718–26.

21. Group CS. COLOR: a randomized clinical trial comparing laparoscopic and open resection for colon cancer. Dig Surg 2000;17:617–22.

22. Chang YJ, Marcello PW, Rusin LC, et al. Hand-assisted laparoscopic sigmoid colectomy: helping hand or hindrance? Surg Endosc 2005;19:656–61.

23. Marusch F, Gastinger I, Schneider C, et al. Importance of conversion for results obtained with laparoscopic colorectal surgery. Dis Colon Rectum 2001;44:207–14; discussion 214–6.

24. Scheidbach H, Schneider C, Rose J, et al. Laparoscopic approach to treatment of sigmoid diverticulitis: changes in the spectrum of indications and results of a prospective, multicenter study on 1,545 patients. Dis Colon Rectum 2004;47:1883–8.

25. Tekkis PP, Senagore AJ, Delaney CP. Conversion rates in laparoscopic colorectal surgery: a predictive model with 1,253 patients. Surg Endosc 2005;19:47–54.

26. Basse L, Jakobsen DH, Bardram L, et al. Functional recovery after open versus laparoscopic colonic resection: a randomized, blinded study. Ann Surg 2005;241:416–23.

27. Zutshi M, Delaney CP, Senagore AJ, Fazio VW. Shorter hospital stay associated with fastrack postoperative care pathways and laparoscopic intestinal resection are not associated with increased physical activity. Colorectal Dis 2004;6:477–80.

28. Rose J, Schneider C, Yildirim C, et al. Complications in laparoscopic colorectal surgery: results of a multicentre trial. Tech Coloproctol 2004;8Suppl 1:s25–8.

Chapter 31

Management Issues in Patients Presenting with Stage IV Colorectal Cancers

Scott Kopetz, MD

Paulo M. Hoff, MD

The increased use of colorectal screening has improved the survival for patients diagnosed with early colorectal cancer (CRC), but half of these patients eventually develop distant metastases. Outcomes for those patients have not improved greatly; however, recent advances in therapies for metastatic CRC, including new cytotoxic agents and molecular-targeted therapies, aim to improve this situation. Regional therapies, such as surgery, offer additional means of managing metastatic disease and the opportunity for curing it in a small subset of patients.

Although CRC can metastasize to almost any location in the body, the most common places are the liver, lung, and peritoneum. Less common are the brain, bone, and the thyroid. Routine staging of CRC is usually directed to the most common sites. Staging includes abdominal and pelvic imaging, usually by computed tomography (CT). Practice guidelines state that chest radiography is sufficient for evaluation of the lungs.[1] However, because resection of single lung metastasis has recently been associated with a higher chance for cure than once thought, in our practice at The University of Texas M. D. Anderson Cancer Center, we also routinely obtain a CT scan of the chest at baseline. Bone scans and brain images are obtained only if symptoms dictate. The level of the nonspecific tumor marker carcinoembryonic antigen (CEA) is measured before the start of therapy in order to follow the cancer's response to therapy. Staging should be completed as close to the initiation of therapy as possible.

The optimal timing of surgery and chemotherapy for patients with high-volume metastatic disease is still under debate. Patients who present with a perforation, significant bleeding, or impending obstruction should undergo hemicolectomy. Asymptomatic patients, however, can either be referred for surgery on the primary tumor first or undergo chemotherapy before surgery. The latter approach is usually favored in our group. There are pros and cons for each approach, and the decision should be individualized.

During systemic treatment, we usually repeat disease staging every 8 to 12 weeks with appropriate imaging and laboratory studies. Carcinoembryonic antigen levels are commonly monitored but should not be the deciding factor in treatment changes because transiently increased levels may occur after initiation of therapy.

Systemic Treatment Strategies

The median survival for patients treated with the best available supportive care from the time of diagnosis of metastatic disease from CRC is only around 6 months, but the most recently introduced chemotherapeutic regimens have increased overall survival (OS) to a median of more than 20 months. The systemic treatments currently used for CRC are usually well tolerated and rarely lead to a significant decline in functional status. In fact, the longer survival times achieved with these therapies is usually associated with very good quality of life. The major chemotherapeutic agents used in stage IV CRC are 5-fluorouracil (5-FU), capecitabine, irinotecan, and oxaliplatin; details of the particular regimens using these agents are given in Table 1. The role of the two monoclonal antibodies bevacizumab and cetuximab in the management of metastatic CRC will be discussed.

CHEMOTHERAPEUTIC AGENTS

5-FU

5-FU is the most commonly used chemotherapeutic agent for CRC. It was developed almost 50 years ago and, until the 1990s, was the standard of care as a single agent

with or without modulating agents. 5-FU has two different mechanisms of action. One is the binding of thymidylate synthetase by its active metabolite, 5-dUMP, which depletes the pool of uracil available for deoxyribonucleic acid (DNA) duplication. The second mechanism incorporates 5-FU metabolites into ribonucleic acid, resulting in disrupted protein synthesis.

The most successful modulator used with 5-FU is leucovorin (also called folinic acid), which increases the availability of reduced folate within cancer cells. Reduced folate is a cofactor necessary for 5-dUMP to inhibit thymidylate synthetase. In a meta-analysis that compared 5-FU to 5-FU and leucovorin, the addition of leucovorin to 5-FU resulted in a response rate of 21%, whereas 5-FU alone resulted in a rate of 11%. The combination also resulted in a slight improvement in OS.[2]

Table 1 Commonly Used Chemotherapeutic Agents and Regimens for the Treatment of Patients with Stage IV Colorectal Cancers

Regimen Name	Leucovorin	Bolus 5-FU	Infusion 5-FU	Repeated
Mayo	LV 20 mg/m^2, days 1–5	5-FU 425 mg/m^2, days 1–5		Every 4–5 weeks
Roswell-Park	LV infusion 500 mg/m^2 over 2 hours	5-FU IV bolus 600 mg/m^2 weekly		Weekly × 6, with 2 weeks rest
DeGramont or LV5FU2	LV 200 mg/m^2 over 2 hours	5-FU bolus 400 mg/m^2, days 1 and 2	5-FU 600 mg/m^2 over 22 hours, days 1 and 2	Days 1 and 2, every 2 weeks
AIO	LV 500 mg/m^2 over 2 hours, day 1		5-FU 2600 mg/m^2 over 24 hours	Weekly × 6, with 2 weeks rest

Regimen Name	Leucovorin	5-FU	Irinotecan	Repeat
IFL	LV 20 mg/m^2 over 2 hours, day 1	5-FU 425-500 mg/m^2 bolus, day 1	Irinotecan 100–125 mg/m^2, day 1	Every 4 weeks, with 2 weeks rest
FOLFIRI	LV 200 mg over 2 hours, days 1 and 2	5-FU 400 mg/m^2 bolus, days 1 and 2; 600 mg infusion over 22 hours, days 1 and 2	Irinotecan 180 mg/m^2, day 1	Every 2 weeks
XELIRI (CapIri) [caps as ir Figure 3?]		Capecitabine 1000 mg/m^2/day orally, twice a day, days 1–14	Irinotecan 200–250 mg IV, day 1, or 80 mg IV, days 1 and 8	Every 3 weeks

Regimen Name	Leucovorin	5-FU	Oxaliplatin	Repeat
FOLFOX 4	LV 200 mg IV over 2 hours, days 1 and 2	5-FU 400 mg/m^2 IV bolus, days 1 and 2; 600 mg/m^2 infusion over 22 hours, days 1 and 2	Oxaliplatin 85 mg/m^2, day 1	Every 2 weeks
FOLFOX 6	LV 400 mg IV over 2 hours, day 1	5-FU 400 mg/m^2 IV bolus, day 1; 2,400–3,000 mg/m^2 infusion over 46 hours	Oxaliplatin 100 mg/m^2, day 1	Every 2 weeks
Modified FOLFOX 6	LV 400 mg IV over 2 hours, day 1	5-FU 400 mg/m^2 IV bolus, day 1; 2,400–3,000 mg/m^2 infusion over 46 hours	Oxaliplatin 85 mg/m^2, day 1	Every 2 weeks
FOLFOX 7 (OPTIMOX)	LV 400 mg IV over 2 hours, day 1	5-FU 400 mg/m^2 IV bolus, day 1; 2,400 mg/m^2 infusion over 46 hours	Oxaliplatin 130 mg/m^2, day 1	Every 2 weeks
XELOX (CAPOX)		Capecitabine 1,000 mg/m^2/day orally, twice a day, days 1–14	Oxaliplatin 130 mg/m^2 IV, day 1	Every 3 weeks

5-FU = 5-fluorouracil; IV = intravenous; LV = Leucovorin.

5-FU can be delivered as an intravenous bolus or continuous intravenous infusion. The dosage and rate of its administration correlate with both clinical response and toxic effects. Bolus regimens, such as the Mayo and Roswell Park regimens, attempt to maximize the total dose of 5-FU given (see Table 1). These regimens are, however, considered difficult for patients to tolerate because they result in a 30 to 40% occurrence of grade 3/4 toxicities.

The use of different continuous 5-FU infusion regimens can achieve protracted inhibition of thymidylate synthase. High doses can also be administered via infusion, and the bone marrow suppression, mucositis, and diarrhea associated with bolus administration occur less commonly with these regimens. A meta-analysis that compared intravenous bolus and infusion regimens showed that patients who received the prolonged infusion programs had a better response rate (22% versus 14%) and a small but significant prolongation of survival.[3] Because of their greater response rates and better toxicity profiles, prolonged infusion regimens are progressively replacing bolus regimens in clinical practice.

The adverse effect profile of 5-FU depends on the dose and administration schedule. Bolus regimens are associated with higher rates of mucositis and neutropenia than are prolonged infusion regimens. A large meta-analysis confirmed this clinical observation; whereas 31% of the patients given a 5-FU bolus experienced grade 3 or 4 hematologic toxicities, only 4% of those who received prolonged infusion regimens experienced grade 3 or 4 hematologic toxicities.[4] In contrast, hand-foot syndrome, or palmar-plantar erythrodysesthesia, which is characterized by erythematous, painful swelling of the palms and soles (Figure 1), was seen more frequently with continuous infusion than with bolus administration

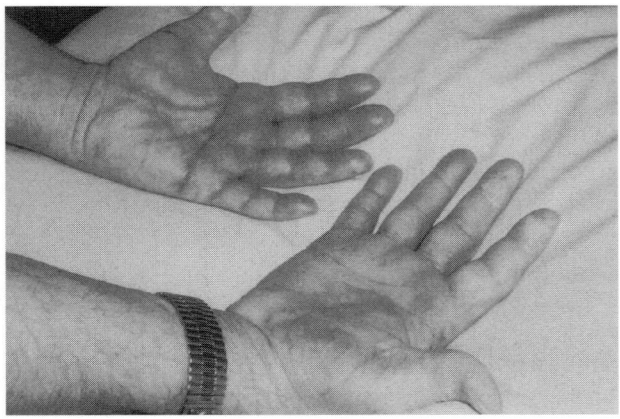

Figure 1 Severe hand-foot syndrome in a patient treated with capecitabine.

(34% versus 13%).[4] This syndrome can occur within days of initiation of 5-FU but usually resolves within a week after discontinuation of therapy. Management of hand-foot syndrome focuses on the use of emollients and appropriate 5-FU dosage reductions.

Ischemic chest pain due to coronary vasoconstriction can occur after infusion of 5-FU in patients with or without a history of cardiac problems. Symptoms usually occur within hours of the infusion, typically after the second or third dose. The presence of angina should trigger a full cardiac evaluation to rule out coronary artery disease. If the angina is due to vasoconstriction alone, the use of nitrates has been shown to control the problem successfully in most patients.

Severe myelosuppression, gastrointestinal toxicity, mucositis, diarrhea, alopecia, and/or neurotoxicity can result from a low level of dihydropyrimidine dehydrogenase, the main catabolic enzyme in the 5-FU catabolism pathway. Unfortunately, although this enzyme's activity is low in 3 to 5% of the population, screening is not performed routinely because of technical difficulties associated with enzyme activity assays.

5-FU as a single agent to treat metastatic CRC increases OS and improves patients' quality of life. Although 5-FU remains the backbone of most first-line regimens for the treatment of metastatic CRC, major advances have resulted from its combination with newer classes of chemotherapeutic and molecular-targeted agents. The next few sections review these chemotherapeutic agents.

Capecitabine

Capecitabine is an oral prodrug of 5-FU that is active against metastatic CRC. It is administered twice a day for an approved total daily dose of 2500 mg/m^2.

In a study comparing the capecitabine regimen with the Mayo bolus 5-FU regimen, capecitabine yielded a better response rate (22% versus 13%) and a similar OS time.[5] In phase II trials, capecitabine plus oxaliplatin or irinotecan produced results similar to those of 5-FU and leucovorin plus oxaliplatin or irinotecan.[6] The toxicity profile of capecitabine is similar to that of continuously infused 5-FU except that hand-foot syndrome occurs more commonly with capecitabine. Capecitabine is commonly offered as a therapeutic option for patients who wish to avoid intravenous chemotherapy.

Irinotecan

Irinotecan, a topoisomerase I inhibitor, was approved in 1997 on the basis of single-agent response rates of 26% in untreated CRC patients and 13% in patients who experienced disease progression after treatment with 5-

FU.[7] The clinical benefit of irinotecan is most apparent when it is combined with 5-FU. Two such combination regimens are in clinical use. The IFL regimen, which combines bolus 5-FU and leucovorin with irinotecan, has resulted in a better survival rate than that achieved with combined 5-FU and leucovorin. However, this regimen has high reported toxicity rates, with 54% grade 3 or 4 neutropenia and a 60-day mortality rate of up to 4.8% due to sepsis and profound diarrhea.[8] A second regimen, called FOLFIRI, was developed in Europe and is based on a prolonged intravenous infusion 5-FU regimen. It is apparently more effective and better tolerated than the IFL regimen.[9] As a result, the FOLFIRI regimen has become a common front-line treatment and has largely replaced IFL, even in the US.

Irinotecan's most significant adverse effect is diarrhea. Early-onset diarrhea occurs within 24 hours of the infusion and is manifest with a cholinergic syndrome of flushing, abdominal cramping, miosis, diaphoresis, and excessive salivation. This is attributed to irinotecan's incidental inhibition of cholinesterase. Anticholinergic drugs such as atropine can be effective in palliating these symptoms.

Late-onset diarrhea is ubiquitous after treatment with irinotecan, with grade 3 or 4 toxicity in more than 30% of patients on the IFL regimen. This type of diarrhea is attributed to the bowel's exposure to SN-38, the active metabolite of irinotecan. An inactive metabolite, SN-38G is excreted via the biliary system; enzymes present in the intestines then re-form the active drug SN-38, which damages the mucosal lining and induces diarrhea. Early treatment with high-dose loperamide is effective in reducing the severity of diarrhea and preventing complications. At the University of Texas M. D. Anderson Cancer Center, we initiate therapy with an initial dose of two 2 mg tablets of loperamide, followed by one tablet every 2 hours until the patient is free from diarrhea for at least 12 hours. Patients are encouraged to wake themselves up every 4 hours during the night to take two tablets. They are also instructed to drink 2 to 3 liters of fluids daily to avoid dehydration. A dosage reduction of irinotecan is warranted for grade 3 or 4 diarrhea (more than six stools a day). Interestingly, the incidence of diarrhea is considerably lower with the FOLFIRI regimen than with single-agent irinotecan or the IFL regimen.

Oxaliplatin

Oxaliplatin is a platinum-containing agent that has yielded only modest response rates as a single agent. However, when given in combination with 5-FU, it has considerable synergistic activity and results in very high response rates. Oxaliplatin acts by forming DNA cross-links that inhibit DNA replication and transcription. Several pivotal comparative trials have shown the clinical superiority of oxaliplatin regimens over single-agent 5-FU regimens or IFL. One trial evaluated use of the FOLFOX4 regimen intravenous bolus 5-FU and leucovorin followed by prolonged infusion 5-FU with or without oxaliplatin in 420 patients. FOLFOX4 resulted in an impressive 50% response rate and prolonged the time to progression; unfortunately, it failed to produce a statistically significant improvement in OS.[10]

A larger trial of 795 patients compared front-line use of FOLFOX4, IFL, and a combination of irinotecan and oxaliplatin (IROX).[11] The final analysis revealed a better OS with FOLFOX4 than with IFL or IROX. The median survival time of patients treated with FOLFOX4 was 19.5 months, and the response rate was 45%, whereas the IFL and IROX regimens produced response rates of 31% and 35% and median survival times of 15.0 months and 17.4 months, respectively. FOLFOX4 was the best tolerated of the three regimens, with roughly half the incidence of severe nausea and vomiting, diarrhea, and febrile neutropenia than noted for the other regimens. However, 20% of the patients receiving FOLFOX4 developed grade 3 neuropathy, which was usually reversible but typically limited further oxaliplatin therapy.[11]

A similar regimen, known as FOLFOX6, uses a smaller bolus dose of 5-FU and a slightly larger dose of oxaliplatin. FOLFOX6 improves the convenience compared to FOLFOX4 by replacing the second-day bolus of 5-FU with a longer infusion of 5-FU. The efficacy of this regimen was similar to that of FOLFOX4, but patients experienced considerable neurotoxicity. To reduce the incidence of peripheral neuropathy, the dose of oxaliplatin was decreased. This modified FOLFOX6 regimen is now the most commonly used FOLFOX regimen among American cooperative groups and academic institutions.

In one study, a combination regimen of capecitabine and oxaliplatin, XELOX, produced results similar to those of FOLFOX, with a response rate of 55% and a 19.5-month median OS time.[12] Although these results need to be evaluated in additional trials, this regimen provides an additional option for patients with metastatic CRC.

Neuropathies seen with oxaliplatin include cold-induced pharyngolaryngeal dysesthesia and cumulative sensory neuropathies. Pharyngolaryngeal dysesthesia is a rare reaction in which patients have difficulty breathing after drinking cold liquids but show no evidence of desaturation or actual laryngospasm. The condition resolves rapidly but can be distressing if patients are not forewarned about its possible occurrence. The cumulative sensory neuropathy is commonly described as a painful numbness and tingling in the extremities that is exacerbated by cold temperatures. This adverse effect is most profound shortly after each treatment cycle. The symptoms, which last longer after each dose of oxaliplatin, may eventually lead to discontinuation of oxaliplatin.

Classically, patients begin to experience dose-limiting neuropathies after the cumulative oxaliplatin dose reaches 700 to 800 mg/m^2, although the interpatient variability is considerable. At M. D. Anderson, we commonly stop administering oxaliplatin after patients report experiencing neuropathic pain that does not resolve between cycles or that interferes considerably with their activities of daily living. These neuropathies are usually reversible in 4 to 6 months. In one small retrospective study, an infusion of calcium gluconate and magnesium sulfate (1 g each) administered over 30 minutes before and after oxaliplatin infusion reduced the incidence of these neuropathies and shortened the time to pain resolution.[13]

MONOCLONAL ANTIBODIES

Bevacizumab

Bevacizumab is a humanized monoclonal antibody directed against circulating vascular endothelial growth factor (VEGF), a potent angiogenic signaling molecule. It interrupts the angiogenesis signaling pathway and prevents endothelial cell proliferation and migration. The reduction in neovascularization that results is thought to deprive a tumor of the nutrition and oxygen necessary for its continued growth. However, bevacizumab's mechanism of action may be more complicated when it is used in combination regimens and may involve improvements in intratumoral chemotherapy delivery.

VEGF is overexpressed in 70 to 80% of CRCs, providing a scientific rational for using bevacizumab for these tumors. However, because bevacizumab has resulted in similar clinical benefit for patients whose tumors express normal levels of VEGF, the level of expression of VEGF cannot be used to determine whether the treatment is given.

In a small, phase II randomized trial, patients given a combination of bevacizumab at 5 mg/m^2, bolus 5-FU, and leucovorin every 2 weeks showed a nonsignificant trend toward improved median survival time compared with patients given bolus 5-FU and leucovorin (21.5 months versus 13.8 months). The group given bevacizumab experienced thrombosis and hypertension more often than the group given 5-FU and leucovorin.[14]

A larger, phase III randomized trial evaluated the addition of bevacizumab to the IFL combination regimen as a first-line treatment for patients with metastatic CRC.[15] The patients given bevacizumab plus IFL had a higher response rate than the patients given the IFL regimen alone (45% versus 35%), a slower time to tumor progression (10.4 months versus 7.1 months), and a longer median OS (20.3 months versus 15.6 months), results that led to the FDA's approval of the drug as a first-line regimen for CRC.[15]

Bevacizumab combined with FOLFOX has also been investigated as a second-line treatment for patients whose disease progresses after treatment with IFL. Like the IFL-bevacizumab combination, the FOLFOX-bevacizumab combination improved survival time (12.5 months versus 10.7 months) without significant additional toxicity.[16] Interestingly, the bevacizumab-only treatment was considered inferior to both FOLFOX and FOLFOX plus bevacizumab and was discontinued at the first interim analysis. Although bevacizumab was effective in a combination regimen as a second-line treatment, whether it would be effective for patients previously exposed to bevacizumab as part of their first-line regimen is not known.

Bevacizumab is generally well tolerated. Hypertension is a common adverse effect: 60 to 70% of patients develop some degree of elevated blood pressure, and around 15% develop grade 3 hypertension. Although common, the hypertension usually responds well to antihypertensive agents. Proteinuria is sometimes seen, although it only rarely (< 0.5%) progresses to nephrotic syndrome. Patients should be screened with a urinalysis, and if proteinuria is found, with a 24-hour urine test. If more than 2 g of protein is seen in the 24-hour urine, treatment should be held until the proteinuria decreases to less than 2 g per 24 hours.

In phase IV studies, patients treated with bevacizumab have experienced a twofold increase in serious arterial thromboembolic events, mainly cerebrovascular or cardiovascular events, increasing the overall risk of such events in bevacizumab-treated patients to 5%. Older age and previous arterial thromboembolic events are risk factors for this adverse effect. Colonic perforations have also occurred at a reported rate of up to 2%, and patients given bevacizumab should be carefully monitored for this problem.

Because of a possible association between bevacizumab and impaired wound healing, therapy with bevacizumab should not begin until at least 28 days after major surgery. At M. D. Anderson, we provide a 6- to 8-week window between bevacizumab therapy and elective surgery because of the long half-life of this antibody.

Cetuximab

Cetuximab is a chimeric monoclonal antibody targeted to the epidermal growth factor receptor (EGFR), which is expressed in most CRCs. The EGFR signaling pathway has been implicated in cell growth, invasion, metastasis, and survival in vitro.

Cetuximab is given at an initial intravenous loading dose of 400 mg/m^2, followed by 250 mg/m^2 weekly.[17] In a study of patients with metastatic CRC that was refractory to irinotecan, single-agent cetuximab resulted in a response rate of 9%, with a 6-month median OS.[18] Greater benefit, however, was seen when cetuximab combined with irinotecan was given to patients whose disease had progressed after treatment with irinotecan alone. In approximately half of the patients with previously refractory disease, the cancer was controlled, with a response rate that was higher than that in the patients given cetuximab as a single agent (23% versus 11%, respectively).[18]

One reported adverse effect of cetuximab therapy is an acneiform rash, seen in about 80% of treated patients, usually during the first 3 weeks of therapy. This rash can usually be controlled with topical antibiotics. It tends to improve with continued treatment, but it occasionally becomes more severe and requires discontinuation of treatment (Figure 2).The rash's severity appears to be associated with the overall response rate of cetuximab: in one large study of patients heavily pretreated with cetuximab, those who did not develop the rash did not respond to treatment. This subgroup survived a median of only 1.7 months, compared with 11.5 months for patients who developed a grade 3 rash.[19]

Early studies of cetuximab were conducted only in patients whose tumors were immunohistochemically positive for EGFR; however, because evidence now suggests that EGFR-negative tumors also respond to cetuximab,[20] it appears that EGFR expression status does not correlate with clinical response. A similar lack of correlation between expression level and clinical response to therapy has been seen with the use of EGFR tyrosine kinase inhibitors in lung cancer.

The exact role of cetuximab in patients with stage IV CRC is still being investigated, but currently it is recommended for use in combination with irinotecan as a second- or third-line treatment in patients whose disease has progressed after the use of any other irinotecan-containing regimen. Preclinical data suggest that combined inhibition of VEGF and EGFR signaling is synergistic. This finding has prompted further studies on regimens containing bevacizumab and cetuximab combined with standard first-line cytotoxic drug regimens.

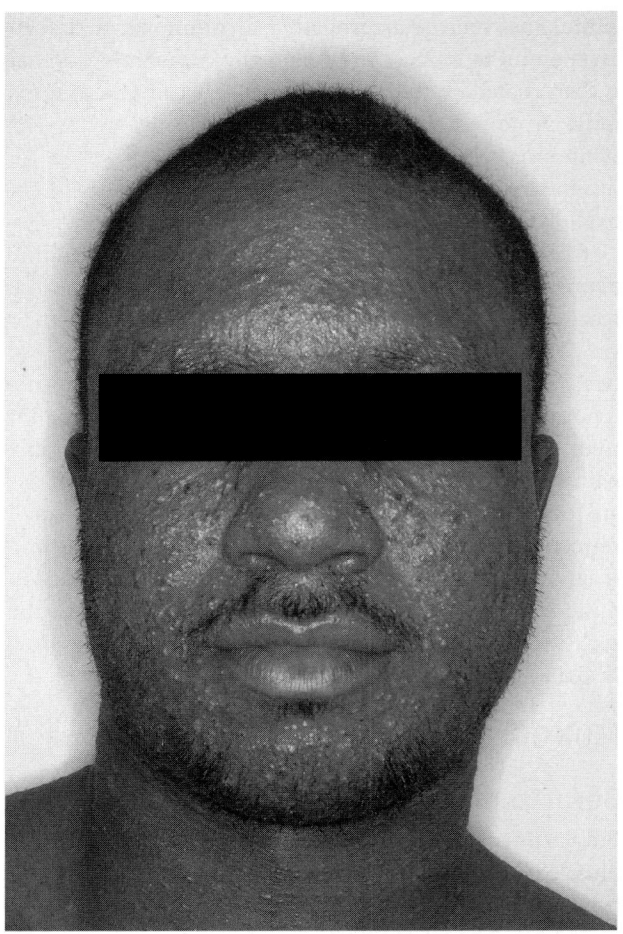

Figure 2 Severe acneiform rash in a patient treated with cetuximab.

OUR RECOMMENDATIONS FOR SYSTEMIC TREATMENTS

At the M. D. Anderson Cancer Center, we recommend that patients with stage IV CRC be treated with FOLFOX or FOLFIRI because these two regimens have produced similar clinical benefits as first-line therapies for metastatic CRC in at least two clinical trials. In the Tournigand trial, patients were randomly assigned to one of the two regimens.[21] If their disease progressed after the first regimen, they were crossed over to the second regimen as the second-line therapy, eliminating the possible impact of exposure to different active agents. The response rates were similar for the two regimens, with a median OS time of approximately 21 months.[21]

Whichever regimen is chosen, the initial treatment program should be individualized and based on the expected toxicity profile and the patient's preference. For example, oxaliplatin-containing regimens should be avoided as first-line treatment for patients who have long-standing diabetes and neuropathy at baseline and for patients whose professions require fine motor skills. Similarly, irinotecan-containing regimens should be avoided as long as possible for patients who have Gilbert syndrome or significant diarrhea at baseline.

We also strongly recommend that bevacizumab be considered as a first-line therapy unless a patient has a contraindication to it. A subgroup analysis of patients treated with bevacizumab plus IFL followed by a second-line oxaliplatin-containing regimen revealed a remarkable 25-month median OS time.[22] In addition, a review of reports of several large trials found that the median OS is directly related to the number of active agents that a patient receives[23] (Figure 3).

For patients intolerant of intensive regimens, either capecitabine plus bevacizumab or infusional 5-FU/leucovorin plus bevacizumab is a possible therapeutic option. The exact sequence of administration is less critical than exposure to all the agents that are active against CRC. Our recommended approach to therapy with FOLFOX or FOLFIRI is outlined in Figure 3.

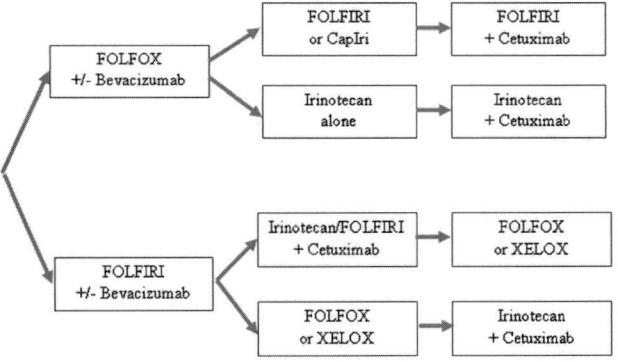

Figure 3 Diagram of recommended chemotherapy approach for patients with metastatic colorectal cancer.

Localized Treatment Strategies

METASTASECTOMY

The latest advances in chemotherapy and the introduction of monoclonal antibodies for treating stage IV CRC have produced improvements in disease control. A result of this, aggressive localized treatment strategies, such as metastasectomy, are more frequently considered. Because the majority of isolated metastases are to the liver and lung, most of the research has focused on these areas. Whether these principles can be extended to other sites of metastases is not known.

Some 10 to 20% of patients who initially present with stage IV CRC have isolated metastatic lesions in the liver, and are thus candidates for surgical resection with curative intent. In two large retrospective studies, long-term 10-year survival rates for patients who underwent resection of liver metastases ranged from 22 to 32%.[24,25] In carefully selected patients, the perioperative mortality rates associated with metastasectomy have been minimal.

One large retrospective study included 1,001 consecutive patients seen from 1985 to 1998 who had undergone at least a lobectomy with curative intent to treat CRC liver metastases.[24] Five preoperative factors were found to predict a poor long-term outcome after metastasectomy in this large study: a disease-free interval of less than 12 months between the diagnosis of the primary disease and that of metastases, a carcinoembryonic antigen level of greater than 200 ng/mL, the presence of a node-positive primary tumor, more than one hepatic metastatic lesion, or a hepatic metastatic tumor larger than 5 cm in diameter. The length of survival was based on the number of preoperative factors present (Table 2).[24]

A second large retrospective study reviewed the records of more than 1,500 patients seen in French hospitals before 1990.[26] Most of these patients had low-volume disease and had not received adjuvant therapy. In this study, six preoperative factors were found to be

Table 2 Preoperative Factors that Predict Disease Recurrence after Resection of Liver Metastases of Colorectal Cancers

Score	Survival (%)					
	1-yr	2-yr	3-yr	4-yr	5-yr	Median (mo)
0	93	79	72	60	60	74
1	91	76	66	54	44	51
2	89	73	60	51	40	47
3	86	67	42	25	20	33
4	70	45	38	29	25	20
5	71	45	27	14	14	22

Each risk factor is one point: node-positive primary, disease-free interval < 12 months, > 1 tumor, size > 5 cm, carcinoembryonic antigen > 200 ng/mL.
Reprinted with permission from *Annals of Surgery*, 1999;230:309-318.

predictive of disease relapse: age greater than 60 years, a disease-free interval of more than 24 months, the presence of a metastatic tumor larger than 5 cm in diameter, lymphatic spread, extension of the primary tumor into the serosa, or the presence of more than three metastatic nodules in the liver. Patients were categorized into three risk groups on the basis of how many risk factors they had: 0 to 2, 3 to 4, or 5 to 6. The 2-year survival rates for the respective groups were 78%, 59%, and 35%. Neither the number of lobes involved nor the volume of liver resected was a prognostic factor.[26]

The results of another large-scale study involving a population-based tumor registry of 2,280 CRC patients in Sweden suggested that many opportunities for tumor resection are missed in clinical practice.[27] Liver metastases had been present in 537 patients in that population, yet only 21 (4%) of them had undergone resection with curative intent. Retrospective analysis of the clinical history and imaging studies of this subpopulation showed that one-third of the patients did not undergo imaging studies that could have helped determine the resectability of the metastatic lesions. On the basis of the imaging studies that were obtained, twice as many patients could have undergone metastasectomy, even after excluding patients with poor performance status and comorbidities. The authors concluded that even using conservative criteria for resectability, physicians missed many opportunities for surgery with curative intent.[27] No clear consensus guidelines exist for identifying which hepatic colorectal metastases are resectable. However, some absolute contraindications to resection do exist: the presence of an unresectable extrahepatic tumor or metastases at the liver hilum, involvement of more than 70% of the liver, and involvement of more than six hepatic segments. One international consensus panel recently developed a computerized decision model that analyzes individual cases on the basis of expert opinion and suggests whether resection is advisable (this free resource can be found at http://www.kgu.de/alm/oncosurge/).[28]

Pulmonary metastases from CRC may also be resected in carefully selected patients. A study of the International Registry of Lung Metastases identified 4,572 patients with lung metastases from any primary cancer.[29] These patients had OS rates after metastasectomy of 36% at 5 years and 26% at 10 years. The subset of patients with pulmonary metastases from primary CRCs had similar survival rates after metastasectomy.[29] In a smaller series of 159 CRC patients who had undergone pulmonary metastasectomy, the reported survival rate was similar— 41% at 5 years.[30]

Pulmonary metastases of CRCs can occur synchronously with hepatic metastases. In that case, the presence of pulmonary metastases is not necessarily a contraindication for performing a hepatic metastasectomy. In one report of 58 patients who had undergone surgical resection of both hepatic and pulmonary metastases, 55% were disease free 5 years later.[31]

HEPATIC ARTERY INFUSION

A localized means of administering chemotherapeutic agents, hepatic artery infusion (HAI), has been evaluated as both neoadjuvant and adjuvant treatment in an attempt to improve outcome and expand the pool of patients suitable for undergoing curative resection. HAI delivers the chemotherapeutic agents continuously from a reservoir and requires surgical placement of a pump and selective cannulization of the hepatic artery. Theoretically, HAI is more beneficial than systemic therapy for hepatic metastases because those metastases are selectively perfused by the hepatic artery, whereas the normal liver is perfused predominantly by the portal vein. HAI thus allows more targeted delivery to the metastases and administration of a higher concentration of chemotherapeutic agents with a more acceptable level of hepatic toxicity than can be accomplished with systemic chemotherapy. Lesions that are initially believed to be unresectable rarely become operable after treatment with neoadjuvant HAI. In a retrospective review conducted at M. D. Anderson, only 22 of 383 patients with initially unresectable hepatic metastases of CRC were able to undergo resection or ablation of their metastatic lesions after they were given HAI therapy.[32] In addition, the relapse rate was high, with only one patient disease free 1 year later. Moreover, half the patients subsequently developed extrahepatic metastases.[32] Because of this poor response, we do not routinely advocate the use of neoadjuvant HAI for unresectable liver metastases.

Various agents have been investigated for administration by HAI, including 5-FU, floxuridine (FUDR), carmustine (BCNU), cisplatin, doxorubicin, and newer agents such as irinotecan.

The use of FUDR for HAI after curative resection of hepatic lesions has been evaluated in several studies, with mixed results. In one single-institution study of adjuvant systemic 5-FU with or without HAI of FUDR after liver resection, the length of progression-free survival of the patients who were also treated with FUDR by HAI was much longer than that for those who were not (31.3 months versus 17.2 months, $p = .02$).[33] Despite this difference, however, the OS did not change. This discrepancy may have been due to the difference in the longer total treatment length in patients randomized to the HAI arm.

A recent meta-analysis that included six other studies of adjuvant 5-FU and FUDR administered by HAI found no survival benefit at 1 or 2 years.[34] The studies analyzed, however, did not compare the use of the newer systemic combination therapies with HAI. A small phase II study of 28 patients with inoperable liver metastases evaluated oxaliplatin by HAI plus systemic 5-FU. This study demonstrated a remarkable 27-month median progression-free survival.[35] A separate phase I/II study of patients win inoperable liver metastases noted a 90% response rate to FUDR by HAI with concurrent systemic treatment with modern combinations of oxaliplatin, irinotecan, and 5-FU.

NEOADJUVANT CHEMOTHERAPY

The fact that only a small subset of patients can benefit from resection of metastatic lesions provides the rationale for using neoadjuvant chemotherapy to reduce the tumor burden first. With a smaller tumor burden, more liver tissue can be spared—a factor that has been inversely correlated with postoperative morbidity. Neoadjuvant chemotherapy is also useful because micrometastatic disease can theoretically be controlled early in the natural history of the disease. This approach allows time to identify patients with aggressive tumors who would not benefit from surgery. Neoadjuvant chemotherapy may allow subsequent metastasectomy to be performed in 15 to 35% of patients whose liver metastases were initially unresectable.

No results from randomized trials have been reported, but in one large retrospective series of patients with liver metastases only, 14% of the patients given infusional 5-FU, leucovorin, and oxaliplatin as therapy for initially unresectable liver metastases were able to undergo subsequent resections, and their median survival time was 4 years after the resection.[36] Although the definitions of unresectable lesions used in this study are debatable, the concept of performing curative resections after neoadjuvant systemic chemotherapy has been accepted. In a separate analysis of the patients who underwent treatment in the trial of IFL, FOLFOX4, and IROX,[11] the investigators found that a curative resection had been attempted in only 3% of the patients. These resections had mostly been partial hepatectomies, but some also involved radiofrequency ablation and lung resection.[37] The inclusion of all patients who had undergone first-line therapy for metastatic disease in the analysis might more closely reflect the true percentage of patients whose metastases could be converted from unresectable to resectable.

Even in patients whose tumors are initially resectable, the response to neoadjuvant chemotherapy can predict long-term outcomes. For example, in one retrospective analysis, the response to neoadjuvant chemotherapy was evaluated in 131 patients who subsequently underwent resection.[38] The 5-year survival rates after resection were 37% for patients whose tumors had responded, 30% for those whose tumors had remained stable, and only 8% for those whose tumors had progressed.[38] These results suggest that the response to neoadjuvant therapy can help physicians differentiate which patients would and would not benefit from surgery (Figure 4).

OUR RECOMMENDATIONS FOR LOCAL THERAPY

At the University of Texas M. D. Anderson, our clinical practice is to consider patients as candidates for metastasectomy if resection is technically feasible and they are responding well to neoadjuvant chemotherapy. Patients with both hepatic and pulmonary metastatic lesions are considered for staged resections if they meet the same criteria of surgical feasibility and chemotherapy-sensitive disease. Whether the primary tumor or the metastases are resected first depends on numerous factors, including symptoms of bleeding or obstruction by the primary tumor, volume of metastatic disease, location of metastatic tumors near key intrahepatic structures where disease progression could render a lesion unresectable, and the overall health of the patient. Occasional patients may undergo resection of the primary and metastatic disease during a single operation. In most, these procedures are staged and performed anywhere from 6 weeks to 6 months apart. If there is excellent downsizing and no symptoms related to the

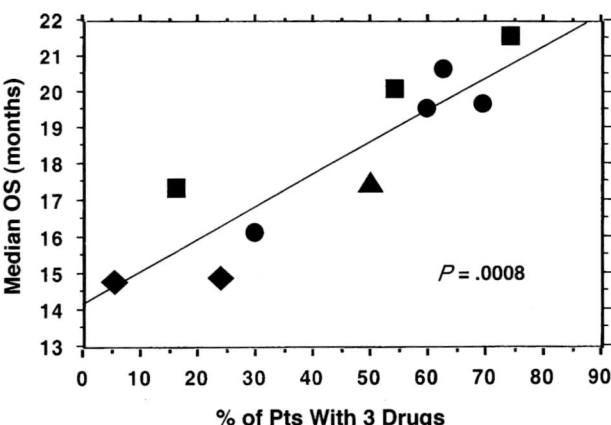

Figure 4 Summary of 14 studies that correlate the percentage of patients receiving modern combination chemotherapy and the reported median overall survival Modern combination therapies were defined as 5-FU/LV plus oxaliplatin or irinotecan for first line, or a second-line regimen including oxaliplatin or irinotecan. (Grothey, *J Clin Oncol*, 2004;22:1209-1214. Copyright 2004, Grothey, *Journal of Clinical Oncology.*)

primary CRC, liver or lung metastases may be resected first. Importantly, some patients with advanced disease at multiple sites who will succumb to their metastatic disease may never require an operation for their primary tumor if it remains asymptomatic. In our experience with current regimens, 13% percent of patients with metastatic disease undergo a resection with curative intent (unpublished data). This percentage is expected to rise as chemotherapy regimens improve. Additional systemic chemotherapy is commonly given after metastasectomy. Because of the high extrahepatic relapse rate with HAI of FUDR, we limit the use of HAI to a select group of refractory patients.

Conclusion

Despite important advances in chemotherapy, metastasectomy remains the only curative therapy for stage IV CRC and should always be considered when resection is technically possible. Multimodality management of metastatic CRC necessitates an understanding of medical and surgical treatment approaches. Identifying the opportunities for metastasectomy and the means of prolonging survival when surgery is not possible requires close coordination within the oncology team.

References

1. Group, NCCW, Colon Cancer, Vol 4. In NCCN Clinical Practice Guidelines in Oncology. 2005.

2. Thirion P, et al. Modulation of fluorouracil by leucovorin in patients with advanced colorectal cancer: an updated meta-analysis. [erratum appears in J Clin Oncol 2005;20; 23:1337–8]. J Clin Oncol 2004;22:3766–75.

3. Cancer M.-A.G.i. Efficacy of intravenous continuous infusion of fluorouracil compared with bolus administration in advanced colorectal cancer. Meta-analysis Group In Cancer. J Clin Oncol 1998;16(1):301–8.

4. Cancer M.-A.G.i. Toxicity of fluorouracil in patients with advanced colorectal cancer: effect of administration schedule and prognostic factors. Meta-Analysis Group In Cancer. J Clin Oncol 1998;16(11):3537–41.

5. Seitz JF. 5-fluorouracil/leucovorin versus capecitabine in patients with stage III colon cancer. Semin Oncol 2001;28(1 Suppl 1):41–4.

6. Walko CM, Lindley C. Capecitabine: a review. Clin Ther 2005;27:23–44.

7. Pitot HC, et al. Phase II trial of irinotecan in patients with metastatic colorectal carcinoma. J Clin Oncol 1997;15: 2910–9.

8. Saltz LB, et al. Irinotecan plus fluorouracil and leucovorin for metastatic colorectal cancer. Irinotecan Study Group. N Engl J Med 2000;343:905–14.

9. Douillard JY, et al. Irinotecan combined with fluorouracil compared with fluorouracil alone as first-line treatment for metastatic colorectal cancer: a multicentre randomised trial. [erratum appears in Lancet 2000;15;355: 1372] Lancet 2000;355:1041–7.

10. de Gramont A, et al. Leucovorin and fluorouracil with or without oxaliplatin as first-line treatment in advanced colorectal cancer. J Clin Oncol 2000;18:2938–47.

11. Goldberg RM, et al. A randomized controlled trial of fluorouracil plus leucovorin, irinotecan, and oxaliplatin combinations in patients with previously untreated metastatic colorectal cancer. J Clin Oncol 200422, 23–30.

12. Cassidy J, et al. XELOX (capecitabine plus oxaliplatin): active first-line therapy for patients with metastatic colorectal cancer. J Clin Oncol 2004;22:2084–91.

13. Gamelin L, et al. Prevention of oxaliplatin-related neurotoxicity by calcium and magnesium infusions: a retrospective study of 161 patients receiving oxaliplatin combined with 5-Fluorouracil and leucovorin for advanced colorectal cancer. Clin Cancer Res 2004;10(12 Pt 1):4055–61.

14. Kabbinavar F, et al. Phase II, randomized trial comparing bevacizumab plus fluorouracil (FU)/leucovorin (LV) with FU/LV alone in patients with metastatic colorectal cancer. J Clin Oncol 2003;21:60–5.

15. Hurwitz H, Fehrenbacher L, Novotny W, et al. Bevacizumab plus irinotecan, fluorouracil, and leucovorin for metastatic colorectal cancer. N Engl J Med 2004;350: 2335–42.

16. Giantonio B, et al. High-dose bevacizumab improves survival when combined with FOLFOX4 in previously treated advanced colorectal cancer: Results from the Eastern Cooperative Oncology Group (ECOG) study E3200. In 2005 ASCO Annual Meeting. 2005. Orlando, FL.

17. Saltz LB, et al. Phase II trial of cetuximab in patients with refractory colorectal cancer that expresses the epidermal growth factor receptor. J Clin Oncol 2004;22:1201–8.

18. Cunningham D, et al. Cetuximab monotherapy and cetuximab plus irinotecan in irinotecan-refractory metastatic colorectal cancer. N Engl J Med 2004;351:337–45.

19. Lenz HM, RJ, Gold P, Van Cutsem E. Activity of erbitux (cetuximab) in patients with colorectal cancer refractory to a fluoropyrimidine, irinotecan, and oxaliplatin. In ASCO 2005 Gastrointestinal Cancers Symposium. 2005. Ft. Lauderdale, FL.

20. Chung KY, et al. Cetuximab shows activity in colorectal cancer patients with tumors that do not express the epidermal growth factor receptor by immunohistochemistry. J Clin Oncol 2005;23:1803–10.

21. Tournigand C, et al. FOLFIRI followed by FOLFOX6 or the reverse sequence in advanced colorectal cancer: a randomized GERCOR study. J Clin Oncol 2004;22:229–37.

22. Hendrick E, et al. Post-progression therapy (PPT) effect on survival in AVF2107, a phase III trial of bevacizumab in first-line treatment of metastatic colorectal cancer (mCRC). In 2004 ASCO Annual Meeting. 2004. New Orleans, LA.

23. Grothey A, et al. Survival of patients with advanced colorectal cancer improves with the availability of fluor-ouracil-leucovorin, irinotecan, and oxaliplatin in the course of treatment. J Clin Oncol 2004;22:1209–14.

24. Fong Y, et al. Clinical score for predicting recurrence after hepatic resection for metastatic colorectal cancer: analysis of 1001 consecutive cases. Ann Surg 1999;230:309–18; discussion 318–21.

25. Scheele J, et al. Resection of colorectal liver metastases. World J Surg 1995;19:59–71.

26. Nordlinger B, et al. Surgical resection of colorectal carcinoma metastases to the liver. A prognostic scoring system to improve case selection, based on 1568 patients. Association Francaise de Chirurgie. Cancer 1996;77:1254–62.

27. Sjovall A, et al. The potential for improved outcome in patients with hepatic metastases from colon cancer: a population-based study. Eur J Surg Oncol 2004;30:834–41.

28. Haller DA, S, Adam R, Poston G. ONCOSURGE: a therapeutic decision model to optimize the management of colorectal liver metastases. In ASCO 2005 Gastrointestinal Cancers Symposium. 2004. Ft. Lauderdale, FL.

29. Group I.R.o.L.M.W. Long-term results of lung metasta-sectomy: prognostic analyses based on 5206 cases. J Thorac Cardiovasc Surg 1997;113:37–49.

30. Okumura S, et al. Pulmonary resection for metastatic colorectal cancer: experiences with 159 patients. J Thorac Cardiovasc Surg 1996;112:867–74.

31. Headrick JM, DL, Nagorney DM. Surgical treatment of hepatic and pulmonary metastases from colon cancer. Ann Thorac Surg 2001;71:975–9.

32. Meric F, et al. Surgery after downstaging of unresectable hepatic tumors with intra-arterial chemotherapy. Ann Surg Oncol 2000;7:490–5.

33. Kemeny NE, Gonen M. Hepatic arterial infusion after liver resection. N Engl J Med 2005;352:734–5.

34. Clancy TE, et al. Hepatic arterial infusion after curative resection of colorectal cancer metastases: a meta-analysis of prospective clinical trials. J Gastrointest Surg 2005;9:198–206.

35. Ducreux M, et al. Hepatic arterial oxaliplatin infusion plus intravenous chemotherapy in colorectal cancer with inoperable hepatic metastases: a trial of the gastrointestinal group of the Federation nationale des centres de lutte contre le cancer. J Clin Oncol 2005;23:4881–7.

36. Adam R, et al. Five-year survival following hepatic resection after neoadjuvant therapy for nonresectable colorectal. Ann Surg Oncol 2001;8:347–53.

37. Delaunoit T, et al. Chemotherapy permits resection of metastatic colorectal cancer: experience from Intergroup N9741. Ann Oncol 2005;16:425–9.

38. Adam R, et al. Tumor progression while on chemotherapy: a contraindication to liver resection for multiple colorectal metastases? Ann Surg 2004;240:1052–61; discussion 1061–4.

CHAPTER 32

SURGICAL CONSIDERATIONS IN RECTAL ADENOCARCINOMA

JOHN M. SKIBBER, MD

Improving the outcomes of patients with resectable rectal cancer involves the optimization of disease management through (1) a detailed understanding of the pathology of rectal cancer and its relationship to surgical techniques; (2) multidisciplinary treatment; and (3) organ and function conservation. The goal of the treatment of rectal carcinoma is cure with maintenance of quality of life. The biology of the tumor is the most important factor in overall outcome. Adequate surgical removal of the tumor is the major treatment factor affecting local control and cure.[1] Appropriate adjuvant therapies can enhance local control, reduce systemic recurrence, and increase organ preservation rates.[2–4]

A major difference between colon cancer and rectal cancer outcomes is the difference in local recurrence.[5] Abdominoperineal resection (APR) has been used for the management of rectal cancer with excellent results. However, APR requires a permanent colostomy, which adversely affects patient quality of life.[6] Advances in rectal cancer management and surgical techniques have improved our ability to achieve oncologic control and optimal patient function without APR, even in patients with low rectal cancers.[7] Even in the absence of adjuvant therapy, 79 of 95 patients with T3 N0 rectal cancer who underwent sphincter-preserving procedures had a local recurrence rate of less than 10%.[8] This study, as well as others, demonstrates that there is no difference in local recurrence rates between appropriate sphincter-preserving surgery for rectal cancer and APR.[9]

Treatment of Local Disease

LOCAL EXCISION

Full-thickness local excision can be effective in the treatment of selected early low rectal cancers. Local excision can be curative in patients who have superficial tumors (Table 1). Transanal excision is the most common method of local excision. Factors such as tumor size and degree of circumferential involvement predict the success of transanal excision. Transanal endoscopic microsurgery also can be successfully performed with low complication rates.[10–12] Whichever method is selected, the full-thickness excision must have at least 1 cm margins of normal tissue surrounding the tumor; an inadequate margin is a predictor of failure.[13] Fragmentation of the tumor is associated with an increased incidence of local recurrence.[14] If the lesion cannot be adequately resected by local excision, a more standard surgical approach should be used. In cases where cure is possible, patients should be counseled to consider local excision as a form of definitive biopsy. Transmural penetration or adverse histologic characteristics can be found in the local excision specimen, and these findings should prompt a standard resection. In a retrospective review of 155 patients, 5-year disease-free survival (DFS) was 94.1% for patients undergoing immediate surgery for adverse findings after local excision, compared to 55% for the delayed salvage therapy group.[14]

Patient Selection

The criteria used to select patients for local excision are intended to make a negative-margin, full-thickness local

Table 1 Local Excision of Rectal Cancer without Adjuvant Radiotherapy

	N	Local Recurrence Rate
Mellgren, et al.[135]	108	28%
Balani, et al.[136]	20	0%
Garcia-Aguilar, et al.[137]	82	24%
Paty, et al.[138]	97	17%

Table 2 Indications for the Local Excision of Rectal Cancer

Tumor < 3 cm in greatest dimension
Invades only the submucosa or superficial muscularis
Favorable pathologic grade

Adapted from Nivatvongs S, et al.[139]

excision technically feasible and to ensure a low risk of lymph node metastasis (Table 2). Technical and biologic factors that can help identify patients who are at low risk for lymphatic metastasis include small tumors, absence of lymphatic and vascular invasion, well- or moderately differentiated tumor, and absence of clinical or radiologic evidence of enlarged lymph nodes. In patients where these factors are favorable, the risk of lymph node metastases in patients treated with local excision alone is considered low enough to be acceptable because such procedures do not involve resection of the mesorectal lymph nodes.

The major factor predicting patient survival and perirectal lymph node metastasis is the depth of penetration of the primary tumor. The most useful test for preoperatively demonstrating the depth of tumor penetration is endorectal ultrasonography.[15] In 1966, Morson reported that lymphatic metastasis occurred from 10% of tumors confined to the submucosa, 12% of tumors invading the muscularis propria, and 58% of tumors extending beyond the bowel wall.[16] In a study of tumors treated with radical resection, the incidence of lymphatic metastasis was 12% for T1 tumors and 22% for T2 tumors.[17]

The incidence of lymph node metastasis in patients with T1 tumors approximates the recurrence rate for T1 cancers treated by local excision alone. Studies describe a 3 to 10% rate of local recurrence after excision alone.[18] Survival rates in patients with T1 rectal carcinomas treated with local excision alone or with radical resection (APR) are 90 to 100%.[19] Local excision alone is a reasonable treatment for T1 carcinoma of the rectum if the tumor meets the previously stated selection criteria. A caveat is that blood vessel or lymphatic invasion detected on pathologic evaluation of the resected tumor is a significant predictor of lymph node involvement and poor survival. In such cases, standard surgical therapy, including total mesorectal excision should be performed. If the patient refuses or cannot tolerate standard surgical therapy, the use of adjuvant therapy after local excision should be considered. In patients with T2 rectal carcinomas, the risk of lymph node metastasis is 10 to 30%.[16,17] Recurrence rates after local excision range from 17 to 24% in patients with T2 tumors. Survival rates are 78 to 82% with excision alone in these patients.

Adjuvant Therapy

Many retrospective and single-institution studies have examined the results of local excision alone in the management of T1/T2 rectal cancer. Graham and colleagues found the local recurrence rate to be 5% (range = 0 to 12%) for T1 lesions and 18% (range = 8 to 27%) for T2 lesions.[18] These clinically significant rates of local recurrence, especially when compared with lower rates of local recurrence (0 to 10%) in historical series of similar patients treated with standard surgical approaches,[19–21] have led to multiple studies examining the use of postoperative radiotherapy and postoperative chemoradiation after local excision in selected patients.

In one of the first series with an sufficient follow-up, Bailey and colleagues reported their experience with local excision between 1978 and 1988.[22] Of the 65 patients studied, 34 (54%) received postoperative radiotherapy, and 2 of those (5.9%) had local recurrences. The crude 5-year survival rate in this series was 74.3%, and the 5-year disease-specific survival rate was 90.3%. This study provided some of the first indirect evidence of the long-term efficacy of adjuvant radiotherapy.

In a similar report from the Massachusetts General and Emory University hospitals, 52 patients were treated with local excision alone, while 47 patients were given postoperative adjuvant radiotherapy.[23] Although the patients chosen to receive postoperative radiotherapy were at higher risk of local failure because they had higher-stage lesions than the patients treated with local excision alone (70% T2 versus 15% T2, respectively), 5-year local recurrence-free survival (LRFS) and DFS rates were significantly better in the patients who received adjuvant therapy (LRFS 10% versus 28%; DFS 74% versus 66%). The authors concluded that adjuvant radiotherapy should be offered to all patients with T2 disease undergoing local excision as well as to all patients with T1 disease and high-risk histologic features (advanced grade or lymphatic or vascular invasion).

A prospective series from The University of Texas M. D. Anderson Cancer Center reported excellent local control rates for 46 patients treated with local excision and postoperative chemotherapy or radiotherapy.[24] In addition to T1 and T2 tumors, T3 tumors in patients who were medically compromised or refused standard therapy were also included in the study. All patients underwent negative-margin, full-thickness excisions. The overall survival (OS) rate at 3 years was 93%. Table 3 shows the pattern of treatment failure by the American Joint Committee on Cancer T stage. Local recurrence-free survival at 3 years was 90%. None of the patients with T1 tumors demonstrated treatment failure. An update of the M. D. Anderson Cancer Center experience

Table 3 Patterns of Failure by AJCC T Stage of Disease after Local Excision and Adjuvant Therapy for Rectal Cancer

	T1 (N=16)	T2 (N=15)	T3 (N=15)	Total (N=46)
Local recurrence only	0	0	2	2 (4%)
Distant recurrence only	0	0	4	4 (7%)
Combined recurrence	0	1	1	2 (4%)

AJCC = American Joint Committee on Cancer.
Adapted from Ota DM, et al.[24]

with local excision seems to support these findings, with 4-year LRFS rates of 90%, 80%, and 73% for T1, T2, and T3 tumors, respectively.[13]

The best data regarding a multidisciplinary approach to local excision for T1/T2 rectal cancer come from the initial results of a Cancer and Leukemia Group B (CALGB) prospective phase II trial.[25] This study enrolled patients who met the usual criteria for local excision of distal rectal cancer: mobile tumors confined to the rectal wall (T1/T2), less than 4 cm in size, less than 40% of the bowel wall circumference involved by tumor, and no evidence of lymph node involvement. Patients were registered after a negative-margin, full-thickness local excision. Patients with T1 tumors received no further treatment, while patients with T2 tumors received adjuvant chemoradiation. A total of 110 patients completed the study protocol (59 with T1 tumors and 51 with T2 tumors). The 6-year overall DFS rates were 85% and 78%, for patients with T1 and T2 tumors, respectively. Overall, 9 patients (2 with T1 tumors, 7 with T2 tumors) had local recurrence of disease, and 4 of them died of the disease.

Table 4 shows the timing of local recurrence in selected large series of patients who did or did not receive postoperative radiotherapy. As the data suggest, postoperative radiotherapy seems to result in a shift toward

Table 4 Timing of Local Recurrence Following Local Excision of Rectal Cancer with and without the Use of Postoperative Radiotherapy

Series	N	# LR	# LR > 2 years postop
Local Excision Alone			
Chakravarti et al.[23]	52	10	2 (20%)
Bailey et al.[22]	28	2	1 (50%)
Willett et al.[14]	40	6	1 (17%)
Biggers et al.[140]	141	36	4 (11%)
Local Excision + Postoperative Radiotherapy			
Chakravarti et al.[23]	47	8	6 (75%)
Bailey et al.[22]	34	2	1 (50%)
Willett et al.[14]	26	4	2 (50%)

LR = local recurrence.

later local failure when compared with local excision alone. In the combined experience of Massachusetts General and Emory University hospitals, the median time to local recurrence was 13.5 months for patients treated with local excision alone and 55 months for patients treated with postoperative radiotherapy.[23]

Salvage Surgery

Results of attempted surgical salvage in patients with local recurrence after local excision (with or without adjuvant therapy) are summarized in Table 5. In these combined series comprising 493 patients, 73 patients suffered local failure, alone or in combination with distant disease. In 44 (60%) of these patients, a potentially curative, margin-negative salvage procedure was performed, most often using APR. Of these 44 patients, 21 (48%) had no evidence of disease at last follow-up. Salvage surgery seems to be feasible in about half of patients with isolated local failure after local excision; however, more than 50% of those patients will eventually die of their recurrent disease. Therefore, it appears that the argument for a liberal approach to selecting patients for local excision on the basis of the likelihood of successful salvage therapy in patients with recurrent disease is not supported by the literature.

Baron and colleagues examined the issue of salvage surgery after local excision at Memorial Sloan-Kettering Cancer Center.[26] They compared the outcomes of 21 patients who had undergone local excision followed by immediate APR or low anterior resection (LAR) for tumors with adverse histologic features with the outcomes of 21 patients who underwent local excision followed by LAR or APR at the time of clinical local recurrence. The DFS rate was significantly higher in the patients undergoing immediate LAR or APR (94.1% versus 55.5%, $p < .05$), a finding that again emphasizes that salvage surgery after local excision does not seem to be an optimal strategy.

ALTERNATIVE LOCAL THERAPY

Alternative forms of local therapy for T1 and T2 rectal cancer include endocavitary irradiation, fulguration, cryosurgery, and Nd:YAG laser therapy.[27] Of these modalities, endocavitary irradiation has received the most attention. In Papillon's initial experience with this technique in 1972, the local recurrence rate was 7% and the 5-year OS rate was 72% among a selected low-risk group of patients.[28] The advantage of endocavitary irradiation over external-beam radiotherapy (EBRT) is its ability to deliver a higher dose of radiation in a more concentrated fashion to the tumor. Both Papillon and others have subsequently reported similar results, again

Table 5 Surgical Salvage of Locoregional Recurrence Following Local Excision of T1/T2 Rectal Carcinoma

Series	N	# LR *	# Salvaged †	Salvage Procedure	Outcome
Chakravarti et al.[23]	99	18	10 (56%)	9 − APR	5 − DOD
				1 - Exenteration	3 − DOC
					2 − NED
Wong et al.[97]	25	6	5 (83%)	4 −APR	3 − DOD
				1- Exenteration	2 − NED
Steele et al.[25]	59 (T1)	3	2 (67%)	All APR	1 - DOD
	51 (T2)	7	7 (100%)	All APR	1 − NED
					3 − DOD
					4 − NED
Bailey et al.[22]	53	4	3 (75%)	2 − APR	1 − DOD
				1 - LE	2 − NED
Bleday et al.‡[141]	48	4	3 (75%)	All APR	1 − DOD
					1 − AWD
					1 − NED
Valentini et al.[142]	21	3	2 (67%)	All APR	1 − DOD
					1 − NED
Taylor et al.[143]	47	17	7 (50%)	5 − APR	3 − DOD
				2 - LE	1 - AWD
					3 − NED
Bouvet et al.[13]	90	11	5 (45%)	All APR	5 - NED

*local recurrences alone and combined with distant recurrences.
†number of potentially curative (margin-negative) salvage procedures.
‡5 patients had T3 tumors.
APR = abdominoperineal resection; AWD = alive with disease; DOC = dead of other causes; DOD = dead of disease; LE = local excision; NED = no evidence of disease.

among carefully selected low-risk patients.[29–31] Birnbaum and colleagues identified characteristics of rectal lesions considered "ideal" for treatment with combination endocavitary and external-beam irradiation (Table 6).[32] Among 72 patients, they found that recurrence was significantly less likely in patients with "ideal" tumors than in those with "non-ideal" tumors (15% versus 48%, $p = .01$). These authors stressed the importance of careful clinical and endorectal ultrasonography (EUS) staging to identify patients ideally suited to this treatment approach.

Transanal endoscopic microsurgery (TEM), in which either submucosal excision (for adenomas) or full-thickness excision (for invasive carcinomas) is performed through an operating rectoscope, has recently emerged as an option for the local treatment of rectal cancer.[33,34] In a recent series, local recurrence occurred in 2 of 16 patients (12.5%) with T1 lesions undergoing TEM.[33]

Despretz and colleagues reported results in 25 patients with rectal cancer treated with preoperative EBRT (35 Gy) followed by local excision and brachytherapy.[35] Local recurrences developed in 5 of the 25 patients. Mohiuddin and colleagues reported results in 14 patients who underwent preoperative radiotherapy (45 Gy) followed by a full-thickness excision; local recurrences developed in 3 patients.[36] The preoperative use of chemotherapy and radiotherapy to downstage the disease and permit a more satisfactory local excision may be feasible.[37] In a series of 10 patients with T2/T3 primary tumors, such an approach demonstrated an absence of local recurrence and a 78% 2-year survival rate.[38]

Treatment of Locoregional Disease

PRETREATMENT LOCOREGIONAL STAGING

Pretreatment locoregional staging is important in the evaluation of patients with resectable rectal cancer. It can indicate which patients can be treated with surgical approaches alone, such as patients with tumors confined to the bowel wall. Second, and much more commonly, locoregional staging is used to select patients for

Table 6 Ideal Characteristics of Rectal Cancer Lesions for Combination Endocavitary and External Beam Radiation

Well or Moderately Differentiated
Mobile
Not ulcerated
< 3 cm in diameter
< 12 cm from the anal verge

Adapted from Birnbaum et al.[32]

preoperative chemoradiation, which is used in cases of high-risk transmural or node-positive rectal cancer. This pretreatment staging and preoperative chemoradiation approach has been favored in decision analysis.[39]

The modalities used for determining the depth of penetration of the primary tumor and enlargement of perirectal lymph nodes are computed tomography (CT), magnetic resonance imaging (MRI), and EUS. Digital rectal examination has been shown to be a poor selector of patients for preoperative treatment.[40] Table 7 shows the accuracy of EUS, MRI, and CT for the T and N classification of rectal cancer preoperatively. Overall, it appears that EUS is the most accurate way to determine the depth of penetration (T stage).

MRI has been shown to predict a positive circumferential margin after resection better than digital rectal examination or EUS.[40] In a treatment algorithm in which preoperative treatment was used for patients with deep mesorectal invasion or extension of the mesorectal fascia, MRI was the superior strategy over digital rectal examination or EUS in terms of cost effectiveness.[40] In another study of cost effectiveness, a strategy of CT and EUS was superior to CT- or MRI-only approaches in cases where the demonstration of transmural rectal cancer was the prompt for preoperative radiotherapy.[41]

In the staging of patients after neoadjuvant therapy, the dominant component of the lesion seen on EUS is fibrosis. Thus, the technique really determines the extent of fibrosis rather than that of the true residual tumor, which may be only microscopic.[42] The overall accuracy of pathologic T classification may drop to 48% in preoperatively treated patients who are restaged with EUS. From these data, it appears that EUS is unreliable for evaluating the degree of residual disease after neoadjuvant therapy.[43] CT and MRI have similar limitations in the restaging of irradiated rectal cancers.[44,45]

Positron emission tomography (PET) scanning has the potential to image clinically and radiologically inapparent foci of colorectal cancer. The presence of distant metastases can influence decisions about using specific treatment. In a preoperative study of primary rectal cancer staging where EUS or MRI/CT was also used, 78% of cases had no change in management due to PET results and an additional 4% of cases had changes in treatment independent of the PET results. The management changes appear to have been chiefly due to the detection or confirmation of metastatic disease.[46] After neoadjuvant chemoradiation, PET has been used to measure tumor response.[47] In a preoperative study of rectal cancer restaging using PET, macroscopic residual disease could not be distinguished from microscopic residual disease after chemoradiation.[48] A prospective study of PET restaging in 15 patients with resectable high-risk rectal cancer found that visual assessment of response on PET imaging correlated with pathologic response in 60% of cases.[49] PET appears to have limited usefulness for lymph node staging even prior to changes

Table 7 Accuracy of Locoregional Staging for Rectal Cancer

	DRE %	EUS %		MRI%		CT%	
		T	N	T	N	T	N
Harewood, et al.[15]		91	82			71	76
Brown, et al.[40]	40		48		88		
Panzironi, et al.[144]		100	72	92	76	75	88
Shami, et al.[145]		89	85			45	68
Mathur, et al.[146]				76		41	
Fuchsjager, et al.[147]		64	70	64	62		
Nesbakken, et al.[148]		74	65				
Marusch, et al.[149]		63					
Tobaruela, et al.[150]		72					
Gagliardi, et al.[151]				86	69		
Kim, et al.[152]		81	64				
Garcia-Aguilar, et al.[153]		69	64				
Gualdi, et al.[154]		77		84			
Beets-Tan, et al.[155]				83			
Hunerbein, et al.[156]		86	86				
Chiesura-Corona, et al.[157]						82	79
Civelli, et al.[158]						86	73
Akasu, et al.[159]		96	72				

CT = computed tomography; DRE = digital rectal examination; EUS = endoscopic ultrasonography; MRI = magnetic resonance imaging.

induced by chemoradiation, with a sensitivity of only 22 to 29%.[50,51]

LOCOREGIONAL RESECTION

Patients with stage II or III rectal cancer often have tumors that are large and biologically aggressive. Disease at this stage also carries a higher risk of local and systemic recurrence after surgical treatment. Therefore, strategies such as locoregional resection and multimodality therapy have been developed to address these issues.[52] However, adequate surgical resection and the proper choice of surgical technique are the most critical treatment factors determining patient outcome.[53,54]

The risk of spread to local lymph nodes and the risk of local recurrence increase as tumor penetration of the rectal wall increases. This has led to the development of operations such as APR that achieve tumor-free proximal and distal tissue margins and remove the upward pathways of lymphatic spread from rectal cancer.[55] The distal margin has been shown to be adequate when it is 2 cm from the edge of the tumor in unirradiated patients.[56,57]

The work of Quirke and colleagues has dramatically demonstrated the importance of lateral (radial) tumor spread in the local recurrence of resected rectal cancers.[58,59] Among patients with local recurrence, tumor involvement at the circumferential margin of resection has been found in 85% of cases.[58] Because of problems accessing the low pelvis and surrounding structures, circumferential margins around resected rectal cancers can be highly variable and minimal in many patients. In this regard, surgeon experience and surgical technique play key roles in the prevention of local recurrence.[60] Tumor extending to the circumferential resection margins can result from direct spread, mesenteric implants, vascular or lymphatic invasion, or cancer-bearing lymph nodes.[61] Primary tumor involvement of the circumferential margins of resection is frequently due to spread in the mesorectum distal to the tumor (Table 8).[59] The long-term outcome is poor in patients with a positive circumferential margin.[59] Total

mesorectal excision has been demonstrated to be effective in the surgical management of rectal cancer chiefly because it reduces the occurrence of positive circumferential margins.[62]

McAnena and colleagues described the long-term outcomes of 57 patients treated with total mesorectal excisions.[62] The mean follow-up was 4.8 years. Local recurrence was seen in only 3.5% of the patients, and the overall 5-year survival rate was 81%. It should also be noted that "serious" postoperative complications occurred in 17% of patients. Similar complication rates with total mesorectal excision have been confirmed by others.[63] In a subsequent larger review of their experience with total mesorectal excision for rectal cancer, MacFarlane and colleagues studied 135 patients with Dukes' B and C rectal cancers who were treated with surgery only, by one surgeon, over a 13-year period with a mean follow-up of 7.5 years.[64] None of the patients received adjuvant radiotherapy or chemotherapy, yet there was only a 5% local recurrence rate. Further long-term follow-up in a larger group of patients confirmed these findings by reporting a 10-year local recurrence rate of 4% and a 10-year DFS rate of 78%.[65] These results agree with the results from the North Central Cancer Treatment Group study that forms the basis for current recommendations for adjuvant rectal cancer therapy in the US.[66]

Similar results have been obtained, with high rates of LRFS, when a total mesorectal excision is done with meticulous sharp dissection along the pelvic sidewalls. Enker's report on this subject called for full rectal mobilization along anatomic planes to obtain a complete mesorectal excision.[67] In a series of 42 men who underwent sphincter-preserving surgery for low rectal cancer using this technique, only one had local recurrence (median follow-up, 20 months). Moreover, sexual function was preserved in 88% of the patients.

Wide pelvic lymphadenectomy has been proposed for the treatment of rectal cancer. Although there is little doubt that the presence of metastasis in pelvic lymph nodes is a highly significant negative prognostic factor,

Table 8 Efficacy of Bolus and Infusional Irinotecan/5-FU/LV in Advanced Colorectal Cancer

	N	RR	TTP	Median OS
Saltz, et al.[160]				
Bolus irinotecan/5-FU/LV (IFL), weekly x 4 of every 6 weeks	231	21%	4.3 M	12.6
Mayo Clinic 5-FU/LV	226	39%	7.0 M	14.8
Douillard, et al.[161]				
Infusional 5-FU/LV	187	22%	4.4 M	14.1 M
Irinotecan/infusional 5-FU/LV	198	41%	6.7 M	17.4 M

5-FU = 5-fluorouracil; LV = leucovorin; M = months; N = number of patients; OS = overall survival; RR = response rate; TTP = time to progression.

there is no evidence to support a therapeutic benefit of the routine addition of extensive lymphadenectomy to total mesorectal excision procedures.[68–70]

To address the effects of training and experience in rectal cancer surgery, a study conducted in a region of Sweden where all rectal cancer surgery has been performed in one colorectal treatment facility revealed that survival seems to have improved and local recurrence rates have dropped.[71] This appears to be due to a program for teaching total mesorectal excision. Several studies have suggested that the surgeon's experience is an important prognostic factor in rectal cancer. In a population-based study of 683 patients, Porter and colleagues found a significant local recurrence and survival advantage among the patients of surgeons with colorectal surgery fellowship training or a higher caseload.[72] In addition, a higher rate of sphincter preservation in low rectal cancer was also found to be associated with these experienced surgeon groups. Other studies suggest that hospital volume, hospital type (university versus community), and surgeon experience influence survival and recurrence outcomes.[73–75]

In general, three operative procedures, all of which conform to the principles of total mesorectal excision, can be performed for resectable rectal cancer: LAR, APR, and total proctectomy with coloanal anastomosis (CAA).[6,9,76]

LAR involves the resection of the tumor-bearing portion of the rectum and mesorectum with reconstruction to the remaining rectal stump. After complete mobilization of the rectum en bloc with the mesorectum, the rectum is divided at least 2 cm below the distal edge of the tumor. There is evidence that total mesorectal excision is not required for upper rectal cancers and that excision of the mesorectum 5 cm below the distal edge of the tumor is sufficient.[77] Reconstruction of the rectum is then carried out between the completely mobilized left colon and the remaining rectal stump. The double-staple technique has permitted an easier and lower anastomosis, with leak rates (clinical or radiographic) similar to or better than those obtained with hand-sewn techniques.[78–80] Five centimeters was previously thought to be the minimum acceptable distal margin, but acceptance of a 2-cm distal margin has allowed lower tumors to be resected by LAR.[4,57] APR involves a combined transabdominal and perineal approach to complete resection of the rectum, mesorectum, levator muscles, and anus with formation of a permanent colostomy. The rectum and mesorectum are mobilized via an abdominal approach. A perineal approach is used to widely resect the levator complex and anus along with an appropriate margin of perianal skin. A permanent end colostomy is then constructed. Because sphincter preservation has

increased, the overall proportion of rectal cancer patients undergoing APR has decreased.[71]

Proctectomy with CAA has emerged as a well-accepted surgical option in carefully selected patients. This approach can spare patients a permanent colostomy while still producing good functional and cancer-related outcomes. A review of 117 patients from the Mayo and Cleveland Clinics provides a perspective on the utility of proctectomy and CAA for patients with low rectal cancer.[81] The patients were treated over a 10-year period (1981 to 1991). The median distance of the tumor from the anal verge was 6 to 7 cm. The technique that was used required complete mobilization of the rectum to the levators, transanal transection of the rectum, complete mobilization of the left colon, and endoanal anastomosis. The authors recommended a diverting loop ileostomy for most patients. A local tumor recurrence rate of 7% was reported. Fecal continence was satisfactory in 78% of the cases. There were no surgery-related deaths. Early and late complications were related mainly to leaking of the anastomosis (10%) and healing with a stricture (21%).

Several groups have reported on patients who had a 6- to 10-cm colonic J pouch reservoir constructed with no additional risk or compromise of the anastomosis.[82] The formation of the colon pouch has been compared with CAA in randomized clinical trials.[83] Physiologic measures and short-term outcomes seem to be better with the pouch, although these findings are disputed by some,[84,85] and these differences in function may disappear with time.

Major long-term postoperative problems after CAA are related to rectal capacity and compliance, these are manifest as urgency and frequency of bowel movements. In a series from the Mayo Clinic described by Drake and colleagues, patients who had a CAA for malignancies had a stool frequency of 2.6 per 24 hours, and only 1 of 19 patients was incontinent.[86] Results from the Mayo and Cleveland Clinics study are similar to those of others describing proctectomy and CAA for rectal cancer.[87] In another study, even when combined with preoperative radiotherapy, coloanal anastomosis resulted in good to excellent bowel function in 77% of patients. The median number of bowel movements per day was 2 in the phase I/II trial.[88]

In a randomized clinical trial by the Gastrointestinal Tumor Study Group intended to examine the benefit of adjuvant therapy in rectal cancer, patients who underwent APR had a higher recurrence rate than did patients undergoing LAR ($p < .05$).[89] This result has also been seen in other studies[90]; however, it probably reflects the presence of larger, more advanced tumors in the patients undergoing APR. Several other studies involving large numbers of rectal cancer patients have shown no significant differences in local recurrence or survival rates between patients undergoing APR and those undergoing sphincter preservation.[91–94] In summary, there is no evidence that, in appropriately selected patients, sphincter-preserving locoregional procedures compromise oncologic outcome.

Postoperative Radiotherapy and Chemoradiation for Resectable Rectal Cancer

The first adjuvant treatment to be assessed for efficacy in patients with rectal cancer was postoperative radiotherapy. Both the Gastrointestinal Tumor Study Group and the National Adjuvant Breast and Bowel Project performed randomized clinical trials and found decreased local recurrence rates, but not improved survival, in patients with stage II and III rectal cancer receiving postoperative radiotherapy compared with patients undergoing surgery alone.[56,89]

The addition of chemotherapy to postoperative radiotherapy was an effort to prevent the development of systemic disease and increase the therapeutic effect of radiation. In 1991, Krook and colleagues reported a study conducted by the North Central Cancer Treatment Group.[66] This large, randomized trial for patients with high-risk (stage II and III) rectal cancer compared postoperative fluorouracil and radiotherapy with postoperative radiotherapy alone. Lower local and systemic recurrence rates and cancer-related death rates, as well as improved OS, were seen in patients randomly assigned to receive chemotherapy in addition to postoperative radiotherapy.

Another major step in adjuvant therapy for rectal cancer came from a report from an Intergroup trial testing the role of protracted or continuous intravenous infusion of 5-fluorouracil (5-FU) combined with radiotherapy as postoperative therapy. The rationale for this protocol was in vitro studies indicating that optimal cytotoxicity was obtained by continuous exposure of tumor cells to fluorouracil after irradiation.[95] A study by Rich and colleagues showed the regimen to be well tolerated during radiotherapy.[96] In another trial of 680 patients, significant reductions were seen in overall rates of tumor relapse and distant metastasis.[97] Also, survival was significantly increased in those who received the protracted infusion of 5-FU during radiotherapy. The National Institutes of Health Consensus Conference has recommended a standard approach for postoperative chemoradiation that is widely used in North America.[98]

Preoperative Radiotherapy and Chemoradiation

Although there have been many randomized clinical trials comparing preoperative radiotherapy with surgery alone, most did not use radiotherapy dosing strategies currently considered appropriate.[99–101] Local recurrence rates seemed to be reduced reproducibly, however, with preoperative radiotherapy compared to surgery alone.[102,103] More recently, the Swedish Rectal Cancer Study showed a significant improvement in local recurrence and survival rates with the use of a short course of radiotherapy followed by surgery versus surgery alone.[104] Notably, patients in this trial did not receive chemotherapy, and the delivery of radiotherapy (25 Gy, given over 5 days beginning 1 week preoperatively) differed substantially from the delivery strategy traditionally used in North America (45-50 Gy, given over 25 to 30 days ending 4 to 6 weeks preoperatively). A French study that examined the issue of the interval between completion of radiotherapy and surgery found that a longer interval was beneficial in terms of antitumor response and sphincter preservation.[105] The effect of short-course preoperative radiotherapy alone in an earlier randomized Swedish Rectal Cancer Trial was to reduce local recurrence rates from 27% with surgery alone to 12% in the group receiving surgery and radiotherapy.[106] In another study, short-course radiotherapy did not result in higher surgical morbidity rates.[107] The improvement in local recurrence rates with preoperative short-course radiotherapy is still seen when modern rectal cancer surgery techniques of total mesorectal excision and quality control of the circumferential margin are carried out.[108] The randomized Dutch trials indicate that radiotherapy is helpful when used with modern surgical techniques.[109,110]

In a meta-analysis by the Colorectal Cancer Collaborative Group, the results of 19 randomized trials of preoperative radiotherapy and nine trials of postoperative radiotherapy were considered. The absolute risks of any recurrence and local recurrence were reduced significantly by the use of radiotherapy, either preoperatively or postoperatively. Trials of preoperative radiotherapy appeared to have a greater effect on the reduction of local recurrence rates, at lower radiation doses, than did postoperative radiotherapy regimens. Early deaths from noncancer causes appeared to increase when radiotherapy was used.[111]

Minsky and colleagues reported on the efficacy and toxicity of preoperative radiotherapy with proctectomy and CAA for low rectal cancer in patients who otherwise would have required an APR.[87] Twenty-two patients with a diagnosis of invasive resectable T2 or T3 primary adenocarcinoma of the distal rectum (median distance from the anal verge, 4 cm) were treated. EBRT was given to a total dose of 50.4 Gy. Four to 5 weeks later, resection was performed in 21 of the 22 patients. Ten percent of patients had a complete response. Therapy was well tolerated, and the anastomotic leak rate was only 6%. Eighty-nine percent of patients had a good or excellent functional result. Local failure alone occurred in 5% of the patients. These data reveal acceptable local control, survival, and functional results in a small trial of selected patients treated with preoperative radiotherapy and proctectomy with CAA as an alternative to APR. Outstanding sphincter-preserving results in the treatment of low rectal cancers after preoperative radiotherapy have been described by Marks and colleagues at Thomas Jefferson University.[87] They demonstrated long-term adequate sphincter function in 91% of patients, with local recurrence rates of less than 13%. The addition of a preoperative endocavitary boost dose to low rectal cancers treated with EBRT improved sphincter preservation rates over those obtained with external-beam treatment alone.[112]

In another randomized trial, prolonging the interval between radiotherapy and surgery did not appear to affect the ability to perform sphincter preservation significantly, despite better tumor response rates with a longer interval between completion of radiation and performing surgery.[113] Similar results were seen when chemoradiation was used preoperatively.[114] Preoperative radiotherapy alone has produced complete pathologic response rates of 10 to 17%,[100,101,115] whereas preoperative chemoradiation has produced complete response rates of 20 to 30%.[116] Among patients who had tumors less than 7 cm from the anal verge and who underwent preoperative chemoradiation, Janjan and colleagues found a higher rate of sphincter preservation in patients who had a complete response compared with those who did not (53% versus 38%)[117]

The long-term significance of a pathologic complete response in a patient in long-term follow-up is unclear, although preliminary evidence suggests that it may be a prognostic factor for improved survival.[118] Moreover, the absence of mucosal tumor clearly does not ensure a complete response because residual tumor may be found within or beyond the rectal wall or within regional lymph nodes.[116,118] Among 41 patients with partial or complete primary tumor response to preoperative chemoradiation, 9 (16%) were found to have metastatic disease in mesorectal lymph nodes.[118] In a larger series of patients, similar results were seen despite an overall decrease in the number of patients with positive mesorectal nodes.[119] Obviously, shrinking the tumor preoperatively may allow for the achievement of acceptable negative margins and

may facilitate sphincter preservation. In a review of 94 patients treated with preoperative chemoradiation for low rectal cancers, distal margins of ≤ 1 cm did not compromise local control rates.[120] While overall these effects of preoperative chemoradiation tend to enable the performance of more sophisticated low rectal cancer operations that preserve sphincter function, they do not appear to support local excision, except in highly selected patients.[121,122]

Preoperative chemoradiation has been demonstrated to be less toxic than postoperative chemoradiation.[123] Minsky and colleagues[123] reported that when identical chemoradiation regimens were given preoperatively or postoperatively, significantly fewer patients experienced grade 3 or 4 toxic effects with preoperative therapy. In this study, 13% of patients treated preoperatively experienced gastrointestinal toxicity, whereas 48% of patients treated postoperatively had grade 3 to 5 gastrointestinal or genitourinary toxic treatment-related effects.

The addition of chemotherapy to preoperative radiotherapy for rectal cancer was studied across two different institutions. In a multivariate analysis of 403 patients, the use of concomitant 5-FU resulted in an increase in sphincter preservation rates for patients with tumors less than 6 cm from the anal verge.[124] Similar to the results of an endocavitary boost with radiotherapy alone, the combination of an external-beam boost dose to the tumor bed and 5-FU therapy increased sphincter preservation in patients with low rectal tumors.[125] Even among patients thought to require APR on initial assessment, up to 85% can be treated with sphincter-preserving surgery after such regimens.[126]

Rich and colleagues reported on the outcomes of 77 patients treated with preoperative chemoradiation who then underwent resection of low rectal T3 cancers staged by EUS.[127] The preoperative treatment was continuous intravenous infusion 5-FU (300 mg/m^2/day) given with daily radiotherapy (45 Gy in 25 fractions over 5 weeks). Sphincter preservation was accomplished in 67% of these patients, in whom the mean distance of the tumor from the anal verge was 5 cm. A complete pathologic response was found in 29% of patients, and only 4% had local recurrence detected during follow-up.

As previously mentioned, comparisons of preoperative and postoperative chemoradiation reveal that chemoradiation given preoperatively can result in high sphincter-preservation rates without compromising local recurrence rates. A preliminary report of the National Surgical Breast and Bowel Project Protocol R-03 randomized trial of 5-FU and leucovorin plus 50.4 Gy of radiotherapy given pre- or postoperatively indicated that sphincter preservation was increased from 33% to

50% in the group treated preoperatively.[128] Complications of surgery were similar in both groups. In a clinical trial of preoperative versus postoperative chemoradiation with continuous-infusion 5-FU and standardized surgery with total mesorectal excision, 628 patients with high-risk (T3/T4 or N+) cancer were randomized.[129] Postoperative complications were 12 to 13% in both arms, confirming that neoadjuvant therapy did not carry a higher risk of perioperative morbidity. In another report of this trial with a median follow-up of 43 months, pelvic and distant recurrence rates were lower in the preoperative treatment group, while OS rates were similar. Fewer patients were found to have anastomotic stenosis in the preoperative treatment group, while overall postoperative morbidity was equivalent between the two groups. In a randomized subgroup of patients with low-lying tumors, sphincter-preservation rates were significantly increased to 39% in the preoperatively treated group, compared with 19% in the other group. These results are a major step forward in confirming the value of preoperative conventional-dose chemoradiation in the management of high-risk rectal cancer.[130]

If function is poor after sphincter-preserving surgery, the patient's quality of life may be more impaired than with a permanent colostomy.[131] Kollmorgen and colleagues studied the long-term effects of postoperative chemoradiation on bowel function.[132] One hundred patients were studied after extensive exclusions were made to minimize the number of confounding variables that could affect outcomes. The group of patients that did not receive postoperative radiation treatment uniformly had fewer problems with bowel function. In contrast, clustering of bowel movements, stool frequency, and fecal soiling were all increased when the reconstructed rectum was postoperatively irradiated (Table 9). As is clear from this study, long-term detrimental effects on bowel function can result from postoperative chemoradiation. Further support for this conclusion can be drawn from the results of a study by Paty and colleagues on the outcomes of CAA treatment for rectal cancer.[133]

Sphincter preservation during multivisceral resections for locally advanced rectal cancer can be performed in patients who have involvement of adjacent pelvic organs. Selected patients may benefit from intraoperative radiotherapy or brachytherapy.[134]

References

1. Compton CC, Fielding LP, Burgart LJ, et al. Prognostic factors in colorectal cancer. College of American Pathologists Consensus Statement 1999. Arch Pathol Lab Med 2000;124:979–94.

2. Lipshultz SE, Colan SD, Gelber RD, et al. Late cardiac effects of doxorubicin therapy for acute lymphoblastic leukemia in childhood. N Engl J Med 1991;324:808–15.

3. Tveit KM, Guldvog I, Hagen S, et al. Randomized controlled trial of postoperative radiotherapy and short-term time-scheduled 5-fluorouracil against surgery alone in the treatment of Dukes B and C rectal cancer. Norwegian Adjuvant Rectal Cancer Project Group. Br J Surg 1997;84:1130–5.

4. Wolmark N, Wieand HS, Hyams DM, et al. Randomized trial of postoperative adjuvant chemotherapy with or without radiotherapy for carcinoma of the rectum: National Surgical Adjuvant Breast and Bowel Project Protocol R-02. J Natl Cancer Inst 2000;92:388–96.

5. Olson RM, Perencevich NP, Malcolm AW, et al. Patterns of recurrence following curative resection of adenocarcinoma of the colon and rectum. Cancer 1980;45:2969–74.

6. Dehni N, McFadden N, McNamara DA, et al. Oncologic results following abdominoperineal resection for adenocarcinoma of the low rectum. Dis Colon Rectum 2003;46:867–74; discussion 874.

7. Tocchi A, Mazzoni G, Lepre L, et al. Total mesorectal excision and low rectal anastomosis for the treatment of rectal cancer and prevention of pelvic recurrences. Arch Surg 2001;136:216–20.

8. Merchant NB, Guillem JG, Paty PB, et al. T3N0 rectal cancer: results following sharp mesorectal excision and no adjuvant therapy. J Gastrointest Surg 1999;3:642–7.

9. Nakagoe T, Ishikawa H, Sawai T, et al. Survival and recurrence after a sphincter-saving resection and abdominoperineal resection for adenocarcinoma of the rectum at or below the peritoneal reflection: a multivariate analysis. Surg Today 2004;34:32–9.

10. Nakagoe T, Sawai T, Tsuji T, et al. Local rectal tumor resection results: gasless, video-endoscopic transanal excision versus the conventional posterior approach. World J Surg 2003;27:197–202.

11. Neary P, Makin GB, White TJ, et al. Transanal endoscopic microsurgery: a viable operative alternative in selected patients with rectal lesions. Ann Surg Oncol 2003;10:1106–11.

Table 9 The Phase III MOSAIC Trial

	Infusional 5-FU/LV	FOLFOX4	Risk Reduction
Stage II (Dukes' B2)	83.9%	86.6%	18%
Stage III (Dukes' C)	65.5%	71.8%	24%
Overall 3-yr DFS	72.8%	77.9%	23% ($p < .01$)

5-FU = fluorouracil; DFS = disease-free survival; FOLFOX = fluorouracil, oxaliplatin, leucovorin; LV = leucovorin.
Adapted from Gramont et al.[162]

12. Sutton CD, Marshall LJ, White SA, et al. Ten-year experience of endoscopic transanal resection. Ann Surg 2002;235:355–62.

13. Bouvet M, Milas M, Giacco GG, et al. Predictors of recurrence after local excision and postoperative chemor-adiation therapy of adenocarcinoma of the rectum. Ann Surg Oncol 1999;6:26–32.

14. Willett CG, Tepper JE, Donnelly S, et al. Patterns of failure following local excision and local excision and post-operative radiation therapy for invasive rectal adenocarcinoma. J Clin Oncol 1989;7:1003–8.

15. Harewood GC, Wiersema MJ, Nelson H, et al. A prospective, blinded assessment of the impact of pre-operative staging on the management of rectal cancer. Gastroenterology 2002;123:24–32.

16. Morson BC. Factors influencing the prognosis of early cancer of the rectum. Proc R Soc Med 1966;59:607–8.

17. Minsky BD, Rich T, Recht A, et al. Selection criteria for local excision with or without adjuvant radiation therapy for rectal cancer. Cancer 1989;63:1421–9.

18. Graham RA, Garnsey L, Jessup JM. Local excision of rectal carcinoma. Am J Surg 1990;160:306–12.

19. McDermott FT, Hughes ES, Pihl E, et al. Local recurrence after potentially curative resection for rectal cancer in a series of 1008 patients. Br J Surg 1985;72:34–7.

20. Sticca RP, Rodriguez-Bigas M, Penetrante RB, Petrelli NJ. Curative resection for stage I rectal cancer: natural history, prognostic factors, and recurrence patterns. Cancer Invest 1996;14:491–7.

21. Wilson SM, Beahrs OH. The curative treatment of carcinoma of the sigmoid, rectosigmoid, and rectum. Ann Surg 1976;183:556–65.

22. Bailey HR, Huval WV, Max E, et al. Local excision of carcinoma of the rectum for cure. Surgery 1992;111:555–61.

23. Chakravarti A, Compton CC, Shellito PC, et al. Long-term follow-up of patients with rectal cancer managed by local excision with and without adjuvant irradiation. Ann Surg 1999;230:49–54.

24. Ota DM, Skibber J, Rich T. M. D. Anderson Cancer Center experience with local excision and multimodality therapy for rectal cancer. Surg Clin North Am 1992;1:147–52.

25. Steele GD Jr, Herndon JE, Bleday R, et al. Sphincter-sparing treatment for distal rectal adenocarcinoma. Ann Surg Oncol 1999;6:433–41.

26. Baron PL, Enker WE, Zakowski MF, Urmacher C. Immediate vs. salvage resection after local treatment for early rectal cancer. Dis Colon Rectum 1995;38:177–81.

27. Crile G Jr, Turnbull RB Jr. The role of electrocoagulation in the treatment of carcinoma of the rectum. Surg Gynecol Obstet 1972;135:391–6.

28. Papillon J. Endocavity irradiation of early rectal cancers for cure: a series of 123 cases. Proc R Soc Med 1973;66:1179–81.

29. Hull TL, Lavery IC, Saxton JP. Endocavitary irradiation. An option in select patients with rectal cancer. Dis Colon Rectum 1994;37:1266–70.

30. Myerson RJ, Ualz BJ, Kodner IJ, et al. Endocavitary radiation therapy for rectal cancer: results with and without external beam. Endocurie Hypertherm Oncol 1989;5:195–9.

31. Papillon J, Berard P. Endocavitary irradiation in the conservative treatment of adenocarcinoma of the low rectum. World J Surg 1992;16:451–7.

32. Birnbaum EH, Ogunbiyi OA, Gagliardi G, et al. Selection criteria for treatment of rectal cancer with combined external and endocavitary radiation. Dis Colon Rectum 1999;42:727–33; discussion 733–25.

33. Saclarides TJ. Transanal endoscopic microsurgery: a single surgeon's experience. Arch Surg 1998;133:595–8; discussion 598–9.

34. Buess G, Kipfmuller K, Hack D, et al. Technique of transanal endoscopic microsurgery. Surg Endosc 1988;2:71–5.

35. Despretz J, Otmezguine Y, Grimard L, et al. Conservative management of tumors of the rectum by radiotherapy and local excision. Dis Colon Rectum 1990;33:113–6.

36. Mohiuddin M, Marks G, Bannon J. High-dose preoperative radiation and full thickness local excision: a new option for selected T3 distal rectal cancers. Int J Radiat Oncol Biol Phys 1994;30:845–9.

37. Habr-Gama A, de Souza PM, Ribeiro U Jr, et al. Low rectal cancer: impact of radiation and chemotherapy on surgical treatment. Dis Colon Rectum 1998;41:1087–96.

38. Ruo L, Guillem JG, Minsky BD, et al. Preoperative radiation with or without chemotherapy and full-thickness transanal excision for selected T2 and T3 distal rectal cancers. Int J Colorectal Dis 2002;17:54–8.

39. Telford JJ, Saltzman JR, Kuntz KM, Syngal S. Impact of preoperative staging and chemoradiation versus post-operative chemoradiation on outcome in patients with rectal cancer: a decision analysis. J Natl Cancer Inst 2004;96:191–201.

40. Brown G, Davies S, Williams GT, et al. Effectiveness of preoperative staging in rectal cancer: digital rectal examination, endoluminal ultrasound or magnetic resonance imaging? Br J Cancer 2004;91:23–9.

41. Harewood GC, Wiersema MJ. Cost-effectiveness of endoscopic ultrasonography in the evaluation of proximal rectal cancer. Am J Gastroenterol 2002;97:874–82.

42. Gavioli M, Bagni A, Piccagli I, et al. Usefulness of endorectal ultrasound after preoperative radiotherapy in rectal cancer: comparison between sonographic and

histopathologic changes. Dis Colon Rectum 2000;43: 1075–83.

43. Vanagunas A, Lin DE, Stryker SJ. Accuracy of endoscopic ultrasound for restaging rectal cancer following neoadjuvant chemoradiation therapy. Am J Gastroenterol 2004; 99:109–12.

44. Watanabe M, Sugimura K, Kuroda S, et al. CT assessment of postirradiation changes in the rectum and perirectal region. Clin Imaging 1995;19:182–7.

45. Sugimura K, Carrington BM, Quivey JM, Hricak H. Postirradiation changes in the pelvis: assessment with MR imaging. Radiology 1990;175:805–13.

46. Heriot AG, Hicks RJ, Drummond EG, et al. Does positron emission tomography change management in primary rectal cancer? A prospective assessment. Dis Colon Rectum 2004;47:451–8.

47. Delrio P, Lastoria S, Avallone A, et al. Early evaluation using PET-FDG of the efficiency of neoadjuvant radiochemotherapy treatment in locally advanced neoplasia of the lower rectum. Tumori 2003;89(4 Suppl):50–3.

48. Calvo FA, Domper M, Matute R, et al. 18F-FDG positron emission tomography staging and restaging in rectal cancer treated with preoperative chemoradiation. Int J Radiat Oncol Biol Phys 2004;58:528–35.

49. Guillem JG, Puig-La Calle J Jr, Akhurst T, et al. Prospective assessment of primary rectal cancer response to preoperative radiation and chemotherapy using 18-fluorodeoxyglucose positron emission tomography. Dis Colon Rectum 2000;43:18–24.

50. Abdel-Nabi H, Doerr RJ, Lamonica DM, et al. Staging of primary colorectal carcinomas with fluorine-18 fluorodeoxyglucose whole-body PET: correlation with histopathologic and CT findings. Radiology 1998;206:755–60.

51. Mukai M, Sadahiro S, Yasuda S, et al. Preoperative evaluation by whole-body 18F-fluorodeoxyglucose positron emission tomography in patients with primary colorectal cancer. Oncol Rep 2000;7:85–7.

52. Gunderson LL, Sargent DJ, Tepper JE, et al. Impact of T and N stage and treatment on survival and relapse in adjuvant rectal cancer: a pooled analysis. J Clin Oncol 2004;22:1785–96.

53. Fernandez-Represa JA, Mayol JM, Garcia-Aguilar J. Total mesorectal excision for rectal cancer: the truth lies underneath. World J Surg 2004;28:113–6.

54. Martijn H, Voogd AC, van de Poll-Franse LV, et al. Improved survival of patients with rectal cancer since 1980: a population-based study. Eur J Cancer 2003;39: 2073–9.

55. Miles WE. A method of performing abdomino-perineal excision for carcinoma of the rectum and of the terminal portion of the pelvic colon (1908). CA Cancer J Clin 1971; 21:361–4.

56. Fisher B, Wolmark N, Rockette H, et al. Postoperative adjuvant chemotherapy or radiation therapy for rectal cancer: results from NSABP protocol R-01. J Natl Cancer Inst 1988;80:21–9.

57. Pollett WG, Nicholls RJ. The relationship between the extent of distal clearance and survival and local recurrence rates after curative anterior resection for carcinoma of the rectum. Ann Surg 1983;198:159–63.

58. Quirke P, Durdey P, Dixon MF, Williams NS. Local recurrence of rectal adenocarcinoma due to inadequate surgical resection. Histopathological study of lateral tumour spread and surgical excision. Lancet 1986;2:996–9.

59. Adam IJ, Mohamdee MO, Martin IG, et al. Role of circumferential margin involvement in the local recurrence of rectal cancer. Lancet 1994;344:707–11.

60. Stocchi L, Nelson H, Sargent DJ, et al. Impact of surgical and pathologic variables in rectal cancer: a United States community and cooperative group report. J Clin Oncol 2001;19:3895–902.

61. Quirke P, Scott N. The pathologist's role in the assessment of local recurrence in rectal carcinoma. Surg Oncol Clin N Am 1992;1:1–17.

62. McAnena OJ, Heald RJ, Lockhart-Mummery HE. Operative and functional results of total mesorectal excision with ultra-low anterior resection in the management of carcinoma of the lower one-third of the rectum. Surg Gynecol Obstet 1990;170:517–21.

63. Nesbakken A, Nygaard K, Westerheim O, et al. Audit of intraoperative and early postoperative complications after introduction of mesorectal excision for rectal cancer. Eur J Surg 2002;168:229–35.

64. MacFarlane JK, Ryall RD, Heald RJ. Mesorectal excision for rectal cancer. Lancet 1993;341:457–60.

65. Heald RJ, Moran BJ, Ryall RD, et al. Rectal cancer: the Basingstoke experience of total mesorectal excision, 1978–1997. Arch Surg 1998;133:894–9.

66. Krook JE, Moertel CG, Gunderson LL, et al. Effective surgical adjuvant therapy for high-risk rectal carcinoma. N Engl J Med 1991;324:709–15.

67. Enker WE. Potency, cure, and local control in the operative treatment of rectal cancer. Arch Surg 1992; 127:1396–401; discussion 1402.

68. Moreira LF, Hizuta A, Iwagaki H, et al. Lateral lymph node dissection for rectal carcinoma below the peritoneal reflection. Br J Surg 1994;81:293–6.

69. Hojo K, Koyama Y, Moriya Y. Lymphatic spread and its prognostic value in patients with rectal cancer. Am J Surg 1982;144:350–4.

70. Glass RE, Ritchie JK, Thompson HR, Mann CV. The results of surgical treatment of cancer of the rectum by radical resection and extended abdomino-iliac lymphadenectomy. Br J Surg 1985;72:599–601.

71. Dahlberg M, Glimelius B, Pahlman L. Changing strategy for rectal cancer is associated with improved outcome. Br J Surg 1999;86:379–84.

72. Porter GA, Soskolne CL, Yakimets WW, Newman SC. Surgeon-related factors and outcome in rectal cancer. Ann Surg 1998;227:157–67.

73. Holm T, Johansson H, Cedermark B, et al. Influence of hospital- and surgeon-related factors on outcome after treatment of rectal cancer with or without preoperative radiotherapy. Br J Surg 1997;84:657–63.

74. Hermanek P, Wiebelt H, Staimmer D, Riedl S. Prognostic factors of rectum carcinoma—experience of the German Multicentre Study SGCRC. German Study Group Colo-Rectal Carcinoma. Tumori 1995;81(3 Suppl):60–4.

75. Simons AJ, Ker R, Groshen S, et al. Variations in treatment of rectal cancer: the influence of hospital type and caseload. Dis Colon Rectum 1997;40:641–6.

76. Tiret E, Poupardin B, McNamara D, et al. Ultralow anterior resection with intersphincteric dissection—what is the limit of safe sphincter preservation? Colorectal Dis 2003;5:454–7.

77. Lopez-Kostner F, Lavery IC, Hool GR, et al. Total mesorectal excision is not necessary for cancers of the upper rectum. Surgery 1998;124:612–7; discussion 617–8.

78. Steichen FM, Ravitch MM. History of mechanical devices and instruments for suturing. Curr Probl Surg 1982;19:1–52.

79. Beart RW Jr, Kelly KA. Randomized prospective evaluation of the EEA stapler for colorectal anastomoses. Am J Surg 1981;141:143–7.

80. Docherty JG, McGregor JR, Akyol AM, et al. Comparison of manually constructed and stapled anastomoses in colorectal surgery. West of Scotland and Highland Anastomosis Study Group. Ann Surg 1995;221:176–84.

81. Cavaliere F, Pemberton JH, Cosimelli M, et al. Coloanal anastomosis for rectal cancer. Long-term results at the Mayo and Cleveland Clinics. Dis Colon Rectum 1995;38: 807–12.

82. Lazorthes F, Fages P, Chiotasso P, et al. Resection of the rectum with construction of a colonic reservoir and colo-anal anastomosis for carcinoma of the rectum. Br J Surg 1986;73:136–8.

83. Sailer M, Fuchs KH, Fein M, Thiede A. Randomized clinical trial comparing quality of life after straight and pouch coloanal reconstruction. Br J Surg 2002;89:1108–17.

84. Hallbook O, Pahlman L, Krog M, et al. Randomized comparison of straight and colonic J pouch anastomosis after low anterior resection. Ann Surg 1996;224:58–65.

85. Hida J, Yasutomi M, Maruyama T, et al. Indications for colonic J-pouch reconstruction after anterior resection for rectal cancer: determining the optimum level of anastomosis. Dis Colon Rectum 1998;41:558–63.

86. Drake DB, Pemberton JH, Beart RW Jr, et al. Coloanal anastomosis in the management of benign and malignant rectal disease. Ann Surg 1987;206:600–5.

87. Minsky BD, Cohen AM, Enker WE, Sigurdson E. Phase I/II trial of pre-operative radiation therapy and coloanal anastomosis in distal invasive resectable rectal cancer. Int J Radiat Oncol Biol Phys 1992;23:387–92.

88. Minsky BD, Cohen AM, Enker WE, Paty P. Sphincter preservation with preoperative radiation therapy and coloanal anastomosis. Int J Radiat Oncol Biol Phys 1995;31:553–9.

89. Prolongation of the disease-free interval in surgically treated rectal carcinoma. Gastrointestinal Tumor Study Group. N Engl J Med 1985;312:1465–72.

90. Law WL, Chu KW. Impact of total mesorectal excision on the results of surgery of distal rectal cancer. Br J Surg 2001;88:1607–12.

91. Nissan A, Guillem JG, Paty PB, et al. Abdominoperineal resection for rectal cancer at a specialty center. Dis Colon Rectum 2001;44:27–35; discussion 35–6.

92. Paty PB, Enker WE, Cohen AM, Lauwers GY. Treatment of rectal cancer by low anterior resection with coloanal anastomosis. Ann Surg 1994;219:365–73.

93. Zaheer S, Pemberton JH, Farouk R, et al. Surgical treatment of adenocarcinoma of the rectum. Ann Surg 1998;227:800–11.

94. Williams NS, Johnston D. Survival and recurrence after sphincter saving resection and abdominoperineal resection for carcinoma of the middle third of the rectum. Br J Surg 1984;71:278–82.

95. Byfield JE, Calabro-Jones P, Klisak I, Kulhanian F. Pharmacologic requirements for obtaining sensitization of human tumor cells in vitro to combined 5-Fluorouracil or ftorafur and X rays. Int J Radiat Oncol Biol Phys 1982; 8:1923–33.

96. Rich TA, Lokich JJ, Chaffey JT. A pilot study of protracted venous infusion of 5-fluorouracil and concomitant radiation therapy. J Clin Oncol 1985;3:402–6.

97. Wong CS, Stern H, Cummings BJ. Local excision and post-operative radiation therapy for rectal carcinoma. Int J Radiat Oncol Biol Phys 1993;25:669–75.

98. NIH consensus conference. Adjuvant therapy for patients with colon and rectal cancer. Jama 1990;264:1444–50.

99. Ghanem AN, Perry KC. Malignant lymphoma as a complication of ureterosigmoidostomy. Br J Surg 1985; 72:559–60.

100. Rider WD, Palmer JA, Mahoney LJ, Robertson CT. Preoperative irradiation in operable cancer of the rectum: report of the Toronto trial. Can J Surg 1977;20:335–8.

101. Roswit B, Higgins GA, Keehn RJ. Preoperative irradiation for carcinoma of the rectum and rectosigmoid colon: report of a National Veterans Administration randomized study. Cancer 1975;35:1597–602.

102. Gerard A, Buyse M, Nordlinger B, et al. Preoperative radiotherapy as adjuvant treatment in rectal cancer. Final results of a randomized study of the European Organization for Research and Treatment of Cancer (EORTC). Ann Surg 1988;208:606–14.

103. Martling A, Holm T, Johansson H, et al. The Stockholm II trial on preoperative radiotherapy in rectal carcinoma: long-term follow-up of a population-based study. Cancer 2001;92:896–902.

104. Improved survival with preoperative radiotherapy in resectable rectal cancer. Swedish Rectal Cancer Trial. N Engl J Med 1997;336:980–7.

105. Gerard JP. The use of radiotherapy for patients with low rectal cancer: an overview of the Lyon experience. Aust N Z J Surg 1994;64:457–63.

106. Initial report from a Swedish multicentre study examining the role of preoperative irradiation in the treatment of patients with resectable rectal carcinoma. Swedish Rectal Cancer Trial. Br J Surg 1993;80:1333–6.

107. Frykholm GJ, Glimelius B, Pahlman L. Preoperative or postoperative irradiation in adenocarcinoma of the rectum: final treatment results of a randomized trial and an evaluation of late secondary effects. Dis Colon Rectum 1993;36:564–72.

108. Kapiteijn E, Marijnen CA, Nagtegaal ID, et al. Preoperative radiotherapy combined with total mesorectal excision for resectable rectal cancer. N Engl J Med 2001; 345:638–46.

109. McCall JL, Cox MR, Wattchow DA. Analysis of local recurrence rates after surgery alone for rectal cancer. Int J Colorectal Dis 1995;10:126–32.

110. Hill GL, Rafique M. Extrafascial excision of the rectum for rectal cancer. Br J Surg 1998;85:809–12.

111. Adjuvant radiotherapy for rectal cancer: a systematic overview of 8,507 patients from 22 randomised trials. Lancet 2001;358:1291–304.

112. Gerard JP, Chapet O, Nemoz C, et al. Improved sphincter preservation in low rectal cancer with high-dose preoperative radiotherapy: the lyon R96-02 randomized trial. J Clin Oncol 2004;22:2404–9.

113. Francois Y, Nemoz CJ, Baulieux J, et al. Influence of the interval between preoperative radiation therapy and surgery on downstaging and on the rate of sphincter-sparing surgery for rectal cancer: the Lyon R90-01 randomized trial. J Clin Oncol 1999;17:2396.

114. Moore HG, Gittleman AE, Minsky BD, et al. Rate of pathologic complete response with increased interval between preoperative combined modality therapy and rectal cancer resection. Dis Colon Rectum 2004;47:279–86.

115. Cohen A, Minsky B, Schildky R. Cancer of the rectum. In: De Vita V, Hellman S, Rosenberg S, editors. Cancer: Principles and Practice of Oncology. 5th ed. Philadelphia: Lipincott Raven; 1997. p. 1197–234.

116. Meterissian S, Skibber J, Rich T, et al. Patterns of residual disease after preoperative chemoradiation in ultrasound T3 rectal carcinoma. Ann Surg Oncol 1994;1:111–6.

117. Janjan NA, Khoo VS, Abbruzzese J, et al. Tumor downstaging and sphincter preservation with preoperative chemoradiation in locally advanced rectal cancer: the M. D. Anderson Cancer Center experience. Int J Radiat Oncol Biol Phys 1999;44:1027–38.

118. Fleming J, Hunt K, Feig BW, et al. Primary tumor response to preoperative chemoradiation does not ensure the absence of regional lymph node metastases in patients with locally advanced rectal cancer. Paper presented at the 40th Meeting of the Society of Surgery of the Alimentary Tract; 1999 May 16–19; Orlando, FL.

119. Stipa F, Zernecke A, Moore HG, et al. Residual mesorectal lymph node involvement following neoadjuvant combined-modality therapy: rationale for radical resection? Ann Surg Oncol 2004;11:187–91.

120. Moore HG, Riedel E, Minsky BD, et al. Adequacy of 1-cm distal margin after restorative rectal cancer resection with sharp mesorectal excision and preoperative combined-modality therapy. Ann Surg Oncol 2003;10:80–5.

121. Pigot F, Dernaoui M, Castinel A, et al. Local excision with postoperative radiotherapy for T2 or T3 distal rectal cancer. Long-term results. Ann Chir 2001;126:639–43.

122. Kim CJ, Yeatman TJ, Coppola D, et al. Local excision of T2 and T3 rectal cancers after downstaging chemoradiation. Ann Surg 2001;234:352–8; discussion 358–9.

123. Minsky BD, Cohen AM, Kemeny N, et al. Combined modality therapy of rectal cancer: decreased acute toxicity with the preoperative approach. J Clin Oncol 1992;10: 1218–24.

124. Crane CH, Skibber JM, Birnbaum EH, et al. The addition of continuous infusion 5-FU to preoperative radiation therapy increases tumor response, leading to increased sphincter preservation in locally advanced rectal cancer. Int J Radiat Oncol Biol Phys 2003;57:84–9.

125. Janjan NA, Crane CN, Feig BW, et al. Prospective trial of preoperative concomitant boost radiotherapy with continuous infusion 5-fluorouracil for locally advanced rectal cancer. Int J Radiat Oncol Biol Phys 2000;47:713–8.

126. Grann A, Minsky BD, Cohen AM, et al. Preliminary results of preoperative 5-fluorouracil, low-dose leucovorin, and concurrent radiation therapy for clinically resectable T3 rectal cancer. Dis Colon Rectum 1997;40: 515–22.

127. Rich TA, Skibber JM, Ajani JA, et al. Preoperative infusional chemoradiation therapy for stage T3 rectal cancer. Int J Radiat Oncol Biol Phys 1995;32:1025–9.

128. Hyams DM, Mamounas EP, Petrelli N, et al. A clinical trial to evaluate the worth of preoperative multimodality therapy in patients with operable carcinoma of the rectum: a progress report of National Surgical Breast and Bowel Project Protocol R-03. Dis Colon Rectum 1997;40:131–9.

129. Sauer R, Fietkau R, Wittekind C, et al. Adjuvant versus neoadjuvant radiochemotherapy for locally advanced rectal cancer. A progress report of a phase-III randomized trial (protocol CAO/ARO/AIO-94). Strahlenther Onkol 2001;177:173–81.

130. Sauer R. Adjuvant versus neoadjuvant combined modality treatment for locally advanced rectal cancer: first results of the German rectal cancer study (CAO/ARO/AIO-94). Int J Radiat Oncol Biol Phys 2003;57(2 Suppl):S124–5.

131. Sprangers MA, Taal BG, Aaronson NK, te Velde A. Quality of life in colorectal cancer. Stoma vs. nonstoma patients. Dis Colon Rectum 1995;38:361–9.

132. Kollmorgen CF, Meagher AP, Wolff BG, et al. The long-term effect of adjuvant postoperative chemoradiotherapy for rectal carcinoma on bowel function. Ann Surg 1994; 220:676–82.

133. Paty PB, Enker WE, Cohen AM, et al. Long-term functional results of coloanal anastomosis for rectal cancer. Am J Surg 1994;167:90–4; discussion 94–5.

134. Weinstein GD, Rich TA, Shumate CR, et al. Preoperative infusional chemoradiation and surgery with or without an electron beam intraoperative boost for advanced primary rectal cancer. Int J Radiat Oncol Biol Phys 1995;32:197–204.

135. Mellgren A, Sirivongs P, Rothenberger DA, et al. Is local excision adequate therapy for early rectal cancer? Dis Colon Rectum 2000;43:1064–71; discussion 1071–64.

136. Balani A, Turoldo A, Braini A, et al. Local excision for rectal cancer. J Surg Oncol 2000;74:158–62.

137. Garcia-Aguilar J, Mellgren A, Sirivongs P, et al. Local excision of rectal cancer without adjuvant therapy: a word of caution. Ann Surg 2000;231:345–51.

138. Paty PB, Nash GM, Baron P, et al. Long-term results of local excision for rectal cancer. Ann Surg 2002;236:522–9; discussion 529–30.

139. Nivatvongs S, Wolff BG. Technique of per anal excision for carcinoma of the low rectum. World J Surg 1992;16: 447–50.

140. Biggers OR, Beart RW Jr, Ilstrup DM. Local excision of rectal cancer. Dis Colon Rectum 1986;29:374–7.

141. Bleday R, Breen E, Jessup JM, et al. Prospective evaluation of local excision for small rectal cancers. Dis Colon Rectum 1997;40:388–92.

142. Valentini V, Morganti AG, De Santis M, et al. Local excision and external beam radiotherapy in early rectal cancer. Int J Radiat Oncol Biol Phys 1996;35:759–64.

143. Taylor RH, Hay JH, Larsson SN. Transanal local excision of selected low rectal cancers. Am J Surg 1998;175:360–3.

144. Panzironi G, De Vargas Macciucca M, Manganaro L, et al. Preoperative locoregional staging of rectal carcinoma: comparison of MR, TRUS and Multislice CT. Personal experience. Radiol Med (Torino) 2004;107:344–55.

145. Shami VM, Parmar KS, Waxman I. Clinical impact of endoscopic ultrasound and endoscopic ultrasound-guided fine-needle aspiration in the management of rectal carcinoma. Dis Colon Rectum 2004;47:59–65.

146. Mathur P, Smith JJ, Ramsey C, et al. Comparison of CT and MRI in the pre-operative staging of rectal adenocarcinoma and prediction of circumferential resection margin involvement by MRI. Colorectal Dis 2003;5:396–401.

147. Fuchsjager MH, Maier AG, Schima W, et al. Comparison of transrectal sonography and double-contrast MR imaging when staging rectal cancer. AJR Am J Roentgenol 2003;181:421–7.

148. Nesbakken A, Lovig T, Lunde OC, Nygaard K. Staging of rectal carcinoma with transrectal ultrasonography. Scand J Surg 2003;92:125–9.

149. Marusch F, Koch A, Schmidt U, et al. Routine use of transrectal ultrasound in rectal carcinoma: results of a prospective multicenter study. Endoscopy 2002;34:385–90.

150. Tobaruela E, Arribas D, Mortensen N. Is endosonography useful to select patients for endoscopic treatment of rectal cancer? Rev Esp Enferm Dig 1999;91:614–21.

151. Gagliardi G, Bayar S, Smith R, Salem RR. Preoperative staging of rectal cancer using magnetic resonance imaging with external phase-arrayed coils. Arch Surg 2002;137: 447–51.

152. Kim NK, Kim MJ, Yun SH, et al. Comparative study of transrectal ultrasonography, pelvic computerized tomography, and magnetic resonance imaging in preoperative staging of rectal cancer. Dis Colon Rectum 1999;42:770–5.

153. Garcia-Aguilar J, Pollack J, Lee SH, et al. Accuracy of endorectal ultrasonography in preoperative staging of rectal tumors. Dis Colon Rectum 2002;45:10–5.

154. Gualdi GF, Casciani E, Guadalaxara A, et al. Local staging of rectal cancer with transrectal ultrasound and endorectal magnetic resonance imaging: comparison with histologic findings. Dis Colon Rectum 2000;43:338–45.

155. Beets-Tan RG, Beets GL, Vliegen RF, et al. Accuracy of magnetic resonance imaging in prediction of tumour-free resection margin in rectal cancer surgery. Lancet 2001;357: 497–504.

156. Hunerbein M, Totkas S, Ghadimi BM, Schlag PM. Preoperative evaluation of colorectal neoplasms by colonoscopic miniprobe ultrasonography. Ann Surg 2000;232:46–50.

157. Chiesura-Corona M, Muzzio PC, Giust G, et al. Rectal cancer: CT local staging with histopathologic correlation. Abdom Imaging 2001;26:134–8.

158. Civelli EM, Gallino G, Mariani L, et al. Double-contrast barium enema and computerised tomography in the preoperative evaluation of rectal carcinoma: are they still useful diagnostic procedures? Tumori 2000;86:389–92.

159. Akasu T, Kondo H, Moriya Y, et al. Endorectal ultrasonography and treatment of early stage rectal cancer. World J Surg 2000;24:1061–8.

160. Saltz LB, Cox JV, Blanke C, et al. Irinotecan plus fluorouracil and leucovorin for metastatic colorectal cancer. Irinotecan Study Group. N Engl J Med 2000;343:905–14.

161. Douillard JY, Cunningham D, Roth AD, et al. Irinotecan combined with fluorouracil compared with fluorouracil alone as first-line treatment for metastatic colorectal cancer: a multicentre randomised trial. Lancet 2000;355:1041–7.

162. Gramont Ad, Banzi M, Navarro M. Oxaliplatin/5-FU/LV in adjuvant colon cancer: results of the international randomized phase III "MOSAIC" trial. Proc Annu Meet Am Soc Clin Onc 2003;22:a1015.

CHAPTER 33

Neoadjuvant and Adjuvant Therapy for Rectal Adenocarcinoma

Prajnan Das, MD, MS, MPH

Miguel A. Rodriguez-Bigas, MD

Paulo M. Hoff, MD

Christopher H. Crane, MD

The Evidence for Adjuvant Chemoradiation

The role of adjuvant therapy in rectal cancer has been evaluated in a number of randomized clinical trials. The first such trial was conducted by the Gastrointestinal Tumor Study Group (GITSG). Patients with resected stage B2 or C (American Joint Committee on Cancer stage II and III) rectal cancer were randomized to one of four groups: no adjuvant therapy, adjuvant radiotherapy (40 to 48 Gy), adjuvant chemotherapy (bolus 5-fluorouracil [5-FU] and semustine), or concurrent radiotherapy and chemotherapy.[1] Patients treated with concurrent radiotherapy and chemotherapy had a higher rate of recurrence-free survival (RFS) than patients treated with surgery alone. Patients who received only radiotherapy had a lower rate of local failure, and those who received only chemotherapy had a lower rate of distant disease than those who received no adjuvant therapy. Subsequent analysis showed that adjuvant chemoradiation increased overall survival (OS). Patients treated with surgery alone had an OS rate of 45%, while those who received adjuvant chemoradiation had an OS rate of 58%.[2]

The Mayo/North Central Cancer Treatment Group (NCCTG) trial subsequently randomized a similar population of patients to receive postoperative radio-therapy (45 to 50.4 Gy in 25 to 28 fractions) alone or radiotherapy and concurrent bolus 5-FU, with a cycle of 5-FU and semustine before and after chemoradiation.[3] Adjuvant chemoradiation yielded significantly lower rates of both local recurrence and distant metastasis compared to radiation therapy alone. Moreover, adjuvant chemoradiation reduced the overall death rate by 29% compared to radiotherapy alone.

In the National Surgical Adjuvant Breast and Bowel Project (NSABP) R-01 trial, patients with resected Dukes B or C rectal cancer were randomized to one of three arms: no adjuvant therapy, postoperative radiotherapy (46 to 47 Gy in 26 to 27 fractions), or postoperative chemotherapy (semustine, vincristine, and 5-FU).[4] Chemotherapy yielded higher disease-free survival (DFS) and OS rates than no adjuvant therapy, but the effect was restricted to males. Radiotherapy decreased the locoregional recurrence rate from 25% to 16%, but did not improve DFS or OS compared to no adjuvant therapy. In the subsequent NSABP R-02 trial, patients were randomized to receive either postoperative chemotherapy alone or postoperative chemotherapy with radiation.[5] The addition of postoperative radiation to chemotherapy decreased the locoregional relapse rate from 13% to 8%, but did not increase DFS or OS.

In summary, these phase III studies showed that (1) adjuvant chemoradiation increases OS compared to no adjuvant treatment, (2) adjuvant chemoradiation improves OS compared to radiotherapy alone, and (3) adjuvant chemoradiation provides better locoregional control than chemotherapy alone. These randomized studies have clearly demonstrated the benefits of adjuvant chemoradiation in patients with resected stage T3/T4 and/or node-positive rectal cancer (Figure 1).

Chemotherapy Agents for Concurrent Chemoradiation

All of the initial trials evaluating concurrent chemoradiation used intravenous bolus 5-FU, with or without other drugs. The Gastrointestinal Intergroup trial compared protracted venous infusional 5-FU to bolus 5-FU in patients with resected stage II or III rectal cancer.[6] Patients were randomized to receive either bolus 5-FU (500 mg/m^2) for 3 consecutive days during weeks 1 and 5 of radiation therapy, or protracted venous infusional 5-FU (225 mg/m^2/day) 7 days every week during radiation therapy. In a 2 $\times$ 2 randomization design, patients were also randomized to receive either bolus 5-FU only or bolus 5-FU and semustine for two cycles before and after chemoradiation. The addition of semustine to bolus 5-FU did not produce any benefits. Protracted infusional 5-FU caused no significant change in local recurrence when compared to bolus 5-FU, but significantly increased the relapse-free survival rate, from 53% to 63%, and increased the OS rate, from 60% to 70%, compared to bolus 5-FU. On the basis of this trial, infusional 5-FU was accepted as the standard chemotherapy regimen for concurrent chemoradiation in patients with rectal cancer.

Subsequent trials have evaluated the biochemical modulation of 5-FU and the incorporation of infusional 5-FU before and after chemoradiation. The Intergroup 0114 trial investigated whether the effectiveness of combined postoperative radiation and bolus 5-FU could be enhanced by the addition of leucovorin and/or levamisole.[7,8] This trial showed that there was no statistically significant advantage for the addition of leucovorin or levamisole compared with bolus 5-FU alone.[7,8] The Intergroup 0144 trial compared three arms: bolus 5-FU before and after chemoradiation, protracted infusional 5-FU before and after chemoradiation, and 5-FU with leucovorin and levamisole before and after chemoradiation.[9] Preliminary results show no significant differences in RFS or OS between the three arms.[9]

Recent studies have evaluated capecitabine, an oral agent that pharmacologically mimics protracted venous infusional 5-FU. A phase III trial on adjuvant therapy for stage III colon cancer showed that capecitabine yielded at least equivalent DFS as bolus 5-FU/leucovorin, with

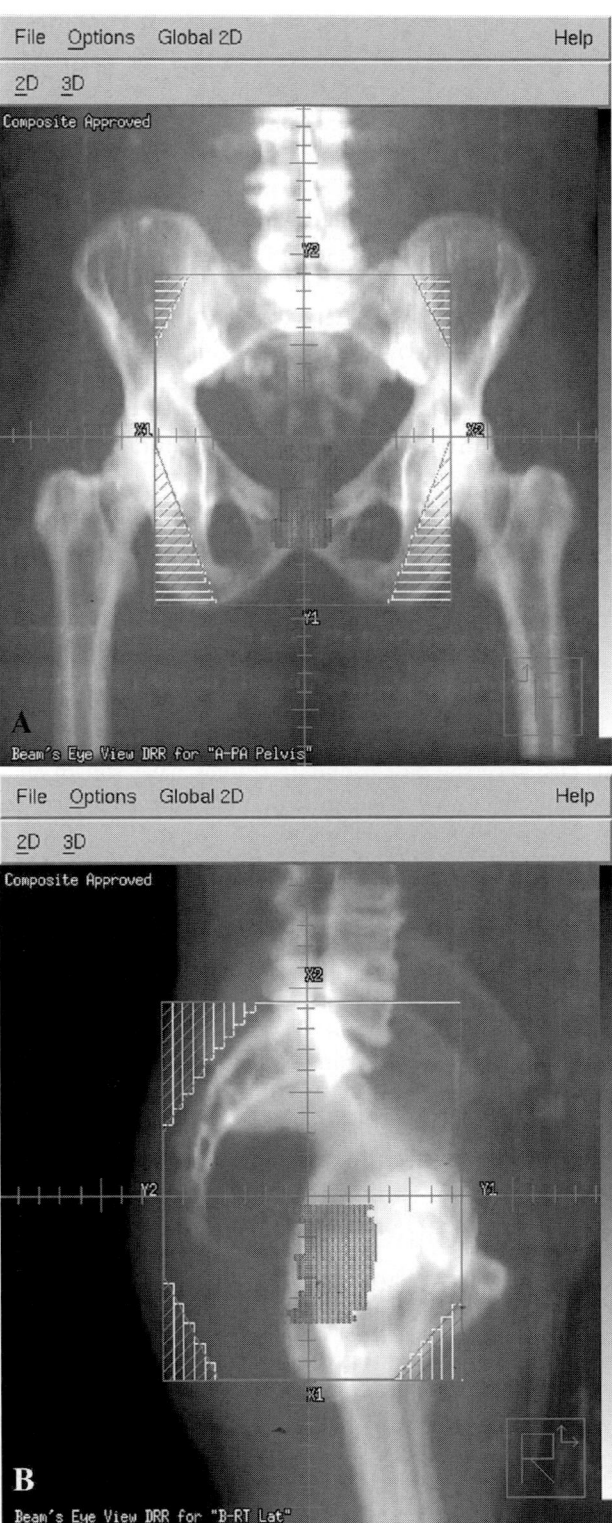

Figure 1 Digitally reconstructed radiographs showing typical posteroanterior (A) and lateral (B) radiotherapy fields for adjuvant radiotherapy for rectal carcinoma. These fields were used for preoperative chemoradiation in a male with T3N1 rectal cancer. The rectal tumor has been outlined and customized blocks drawn.

significantly longer relapse-free survival and fewer adverse events than intravenous 5-FU/leucovorin.[10] Phase I and phase II trials have shown that capecitabine is well tolerated with radiotherapy in rectal cancer patients and yields pathologic response rates comparable to those of 5-FU.[11,12] The dose-limiting toxicity of capecitabine is hand-foot syndrome, and this agent appears to cause less gastrointestinal and hematologic toxicity than intravenous bolus or infusional 5-FU. At the University of Texas M. D. Anderson Cancer Center, capecitabine is given concurrently with radiotherapy at a dose of 850-875 mg/m^2 by mouth twice daily, 5 days a week.

Oxaliplatin is a third-generation platinum analogue with radiosensitizing properties that has been approved by the US Food and Drug Administration for adjuvant treatment of colon cancers. In the randomized multi-institutional MOSAIC (Multicenter International Study of Oxaliplatin/FU-LV in the Adjuvant Treatment of Colon Cancer) trial, the addition of oxaliplatin to bolus 5-FU/leucovorin increased the DFS rate from 73% to 78% in patients with stage II or III colon cancer.[13] Oxaliplatin also may have a role in chemoradiation for rectal cancers. Phase I and II studies have shown that oxaliplatin is well tolerated in combination with radiation and either capecitabine or infusional 5-FU in rectal cancer patients.[14,15] Addition of oxaliplatin to the chemoradiation regimen could potentially benefit those at a high risk for relapse. The role of oxaliplatin needs to be further evaluated in randomized studies. Using a 2 × 2 factorial design, the NSABP plans to randomize patients in the R-04 trial to receive either oxaliplatin or no oxaliplatin and either infusional 5-FU or capecitabine concurrently with radiotherapy. This trial will help clarify the roles of capecitabine and oxaliplatin in chemoradiation for rectal cancer.

Neoadjuvant versus Adjuvant Chemoradiation

Neoadjuvant, or preoperative, chemoradiation has some potential advantages over adjuvant, or postoperative, chemoradiation. Neoadjuvant chemoradiation can downstage the tumor and lead to increased sphincter preservation. Neoadjuvant chemoradiation may sterilize the pelvis and decrease tumor seeding during surgery. Less small bowel is present in the radiation field, and small bowel can be mobilized more easily out of the field in patients treated preoperatively, thus reducing the risk of acute and chronic bowel toxicity from radiation. Tissue perfusion is uninterrupted in patients treated preoperatively, resulting in better drug perfusion and

better tissue oxygenation, which in turn enhances the effects of radiation.

The German Rectal Cancer Study Group conducted a phase III trial on patients with clinical stage T3 or T4 or node-positive disease, comparing preoperative and postoperative chemoradiation (50.4 Gy in 28 fractions with continuous infusional 5-FU, 1000 mg/m^2/day during weeks 1 and 5 of radiotherapy).[16] Patients received four cycles of bolus 5-FU, either after surgery in the preoperative group or after chemoradiation in the postoperative group. Patients in the postoperative group also received an additional radiotherapy boost of 540 cGy. The local recurrence rate was significantly lower in the preoperative group (6%) than in the postoperative group (13%). The rates of grade 3 or 4 acute and long-term toxicity were lower in the preoperative group than in the postoperative group. In particular, 12% of patients treated preoperatively and 18% of those treated postoperatively developed grade 3 or 4 diarrhea, while 4% of patients treated preoperatively and 12% of those treated postoperatively developed anastomotic strictures. Neoadjuvant chemoradiation also increased the rate of sphincter preservation. Prior to randomization, surgeons assessed the planned surgical procedure and determined that certain patients would require an abdominoperineal resection. Among these patients, 39% in the preoperative group and 19% in the postoperative group underwent sphincter-sparing surgery. Thus, this randomized trial demonstrated that preoperative chemoradiation yields higher rates of local control and sphincter preservation, and lower rates of acute and long-term toxicity, than postoperative chemoradiation.

A disadvantage of preoperative chemoradiation is that treatment is based on clinical and not pathologic staging. With postoperative chemoradiation, patients may be selected carefully for treatment based on their pathologic T and N stages and other predictive factors such as margin status and distance of tumor from the anal verge. Patients get selected for preoperative chemoradiation in the absence of such pathologic information, and some patients may be overtreated. Current preoperative staging procedures have led to improvements in patient selection for preoperative therapy. Endorectal ultrasound yields an accuracy rate of greater than 85% in identifying wall penetration (T stage) and greater than 70% in determining nodal involvement (N stage).[17] Magnetic resonance imaging with an endorectal coil produces an accuracy rate of greater than 80% in identifying either wall penetration or nodal involvement.[17] These imaging techniques can help minimize the number of patients being treated unnecessarily.

Preoperative hypofractionated radiotherapy may be an alternative to chemoradiation. The Swedish Rectal

Trial showed that a 1-week course of preoperative radiotherapy (25 Gy in 5 fractions) without chemotherapy increases local control and OS.[18] In some European countries, this short course of radiotherapy has been accepted as the standard regimen for neoadjuvant therapy for rectal cancer. Potential disadvantages of the short-course approach are that it leaves less time for tumor regression prior to surgery and may increase perioperative or late complications. In the United States, a longer course of radiation (45 to 54 Gy in 5 to 6 weeks) with concurrent fluoropyrimidine-based chemotherapy remains the standard for neoadjuvant treatment. A randomized trial in Poland is currently comparing these two approaches (Figure 2).

Neoadjuvant Therapy with Total Mesorectal Excision

Total mesorectal excision (TME) involves a sharp dissection of the plane between the endopelvic fascia and the mesorectum, with removal of the mesorectum with its intact fascia propria. Although TME produces a greater local control rate than conventional surgery, radiotherapy improves local control further in patients who undergo TME. In the Dutch Colorectal Cancer Group trial, patients were randomized to undergo preoperative radiotherapy (25 Gy in 5 fractions) and TME, or TME only.[19] Patients in the radiotherapy and TME arm had a local recurrence rate of 2.4%, while those in the TME only arm had a local recurrence rate of 8.2%. Radiotherapy therefore has a proven role in decreasing the rate of local failures, even in patients undergoing TME.

Patients at Low Risk for Local Recurrence

Patients who are at very low risk for recurrence may not need adjuvant radiotherapy. A pooled analysis from five randomized rectal cancer trials showed that the local relapse rate was 5% for stage T1-2N1 and 11% for stage T3N0 patients treated with surgery and chemotherapy, but no radiotherapy.[20] A retrospective study from Massachusetts General Hospital (MGH) found that the local control rate was 95% in patients with T3N0 tumors and favorable histologic features (well to moderately differentiated, < 2 mm invasion into perirectal fat, and no lymphovascular invasion) who underwent surgery without adjuvant chemotherapy or radiation.[21] Furthermore, the Dutch Colorectal trial showed that among patients undergoing surgery alone, those with high rectal tumors (> 10 cm from the anal verge) and

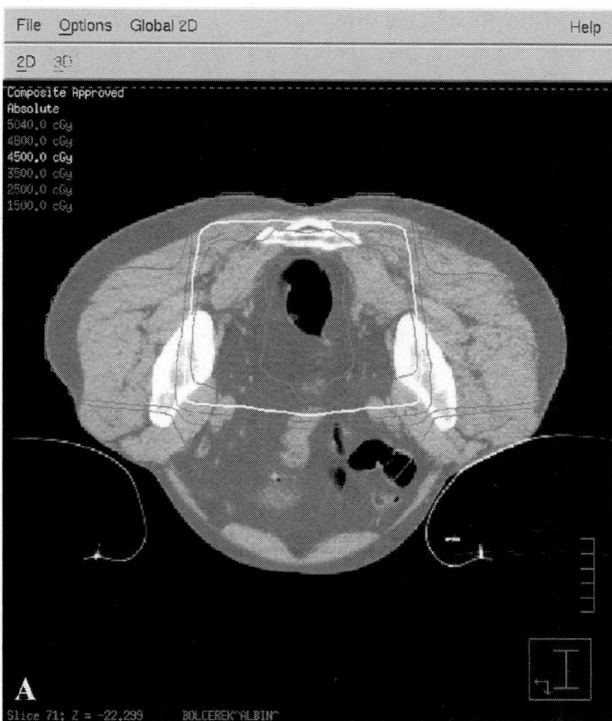

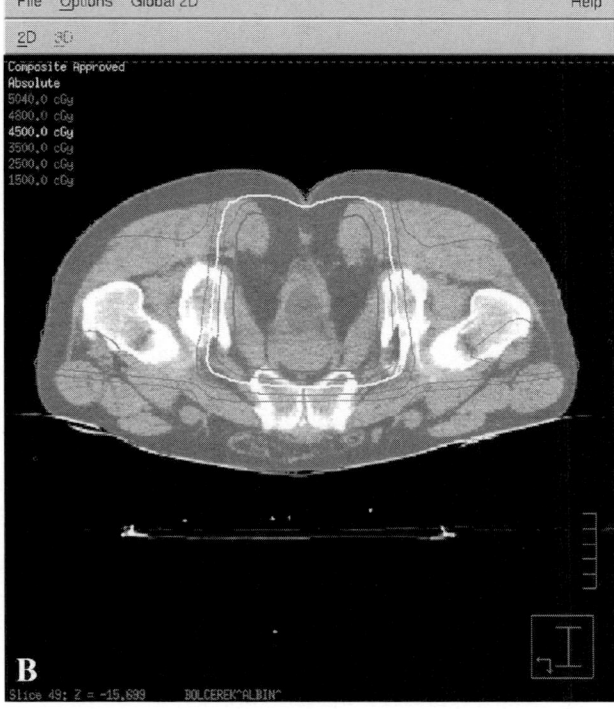

Figure 2 Representative axial CT sections of the mid (A) and low (B) pelvis showing dose distribution in a patient with T3N1 rectal cancer being treated with preoperative radiotherapy, using a three-field belly board technique. The small bowel appears displaced in A. The tumor has been outlined in B.

those with widely negative radial margins (> 2 mm) had a lower risk of locoregional recurrence.[19,22] The number of lymph nodes in the resected specimen has also been associated with the risk of relapse.[23] Thus, a selected subgroup of patients with T3N0 tumors with favorable pathologic features (well to moderate differentiation, minimal perirectal invasion, no lymphovascular invasion, > 10 cm from anal verge, widely negative radial margins, and adequate lymph node dissection) may have a low risk of local relapse with surgery and no radiotherapy. Prospective trials are needed to evaluate whether radiotherapy may be safely omitted for selected patients with T3N0 disease.

Adjuvant Chemotherapy after Surgery and Chemoradiation

The GITSG trial demonstrated that adjuvant chemotherapy reduces the rate of distant metastases, while the NSABP R-01 trial showed that adjuvant chemotherapy increases DFS and OS, at least in males.[1,4] Based on these trials, the current standard for postoperative treatment consists of 4 months of fluoropyrimidine-based chemotherapy in addition to pelvic chemoradiation. There is, however, no consensus regarding whether all rectal cancer patients require adjuvant chemotherapy following preoperative chemoradiation and surgery. In colon cancer, it appears that patients with node-positive disease and selected patients with node-negative disease benefit from adjuvant chemotherapy. On the basis of a meta-analysis, the American Society of Clinical Oncology (ASCO) recommended that only patients with high-risk stage II (node-negative) cancer be considered for adjuvant therapy, such as those with inadequately sampled nodes, T4 lesions, perforation at the primary tumor site, or poorly differentiated histology.[24] The ASCO recommendations did not address rectal cancers, and the selection of appropriate rectal cancer patients for adjuvant chemotherapy after treatment with preoperative chemoradiation has been controversial. This is partly due to the inherent inability of clinical staging to identify high-risk patients accurately in the same way that pathologic staging can. The pathologic T and N stages are frequently lowered ("down-staged") by preoperative chemoradiation, which complicates the decision about adjuvant chemotherapy. On the other hand, the degree of response to preoperative chemoradiation is prognostic. Patients treated at the M. D. Anderson Cancer Center who have had a complete response to chemoradiation have had excellent outcomes (5-year OS rate, 90%), and patients with pathologic T3/T4 disease or node-positive disease have had a poor prognosis (5-year OS rate, 60 to 70%, unpublished data).

Results from the European Organization for the Research and Treatment of Cancer (EORTC) 22921 trial were presented recently.[25] In this trial, patients were randomized to one of four arms: preoperative radiotherapy, preoperative chemoradiation (2 cycles of 5-FU and leucovorin), preoperative radiotherapy with adjuvant chemotherapy (4 cycles of 5-FU and leucovorin), and preoperative chemoradiation with adjuvant chemotherapy. Local control was significantly higher in the three chemotherapy-containing arms compared to the radiotherapy-alone arm. There were no significant differences in OS or progression-free survival (PFS) between the different arms, but there was a late divergence in the curves for OS and PFS in favor of adjuvant chemotherapy. Longer follow-up from this trial will be required to evaluate the effect of adjuvant chemotherapy on survival and PFS. Until that data are available, the use of adjuvant chemotherapy for rectal cancer can be supported on the basis of the GITSG and NSABP R-01 trials. Four cycles of either 5-FU-leucovorin or capecitabine could be used for otherwise healthy patients who have had a good response to chemoradiation (eg, microscopic residual disease or complete pathologic response). Conversely, the use of adjuvant FOLFOX (5-FU, leucovorin, and oxaliplatin) in patients who have had a poor response to chemoradiation (eg, gross residual or node-positive disease) is justifiable on the basis of their higher risk of recurrence.

Management of the Primary Tumor in Patients with Metastatic Disease

Patients with colorectal cancers and liver metastases can be treated aggressively with hepatic resection, radiofrequency ablation, and hepatic arterial infusion or systemic chemotherapy. The 5-year OS rate following resection of colorectal liver metastases has been found to be as high as 58%.[26] In patients with surgically curable metastatic disease, the primary rectal cancer should be treated definitively with resection and neoadjuvant or adjuvant chemoradiation, similar to the treatment recommended for those with nonmetastatic disease. The timing of liver resection and resection of the primary tumor must be individualized, but resection of the primary tumor should, in general, follow chemoradiation by no more than 5 to 10 weeks. For patients with surgically incurable metastases, chemotherapy is the mainstay of treatment. Radiotherapy can play a role in palliative care for these patients. A study on patients with metastatic rectal cancer treated at the M. D. Anderson Cancer Center showed that chemoradiation leads to durable control of pelvic symptoms in 80% and avoidance of colostomy in 90%.[27] At M. D. Anderson, patients with surgically incurable metastatic rectal cancer are treated with either standard fractionation radiotherapy or with hypofractionated radiation (35 Gy in 14 fractions/3 weeks, or 30 Gy in 6 fractions/3 weeks) with concurrent fluoropyrimidine-based chemotherapy.

Management of Recurrent Rectal Cancer

Rectal cancer patients treated with surgery and chemoradiation have local recurrence rates of 5 to 30% depending on their initial T and N stages.[20] For patients with an isolated local recurrence, surgery plays the most important role in treatment. Patients who have not received prior radiotherapy to the pelvis can be treated with preoperative or postoperative radiotherapy (50.4 to 54 Gy in 1.8- to 2-Gy daily fractions) with concurrent 5-FU. Even in patients who have received prior radiotherapy, chemoradiation has been used to treat local recurrences. In a series from the University of Kentucky Medical Center, patients were treated with concurrent 5-FU and radiotherapy at a dose of either 30 Gy in 1.2-Gy twice-daily fractions or 30.6 Gy in 1.8-Gy daily fractions, followed by a boost dose to a limited volume.[28] Among 103 patients who received reirradiation, 33 experienced grade 3 or higher toxicity, and 22 developed late complications; the 5-year survival rate was 19%. Thus, reirradiation with concurrent 5-FU appears to be well tolerated with acceptable long-term toxicity in patients with recurrent rectal cancer.

Intraoperative Radiation Therapy

Intraoperative radiation therapy (IORT) allows delivery of high-dose radiotherapy to the tumor bed while sparing surrounding normal tissues. IORT has been used for locally advanced and recurrent rectal cancers. Studies from MGH and the Mayo Clinic suggest that IORT (10 to 20 Gy, in combination with 45 to 55 Gy external beam radiation therapy) improves local control in patients with locally advanced rectal cancer.[29,30] In the MGH series, patients with residual tumor or positive or close (< 5 mm) margins were given IORT. The 5-year local control rate was 89% in those undergoing complete resection and 65% in those with residual disease. Studies from MGH and the Mayo Clinic also indicate that IORT may improve local control in locally recurrent rectal cancers, although the local control rate is only 35% even with IORT.[31,32] The most important toxicities of IORT in these studies were pelvic neuropathy, soft tissue or sacral injury, and ureteral strictures. While IORT has not been evaluated in phase III trials, carefully selected patients with locally advanced or recurrent rectal cancer may benefit from IORT.

Adjuvant Therapy after Local Excision

Local excision can be an alternative to radical surgery in selected patients with limited rectal cancer. In patients undergoing local excision, T stage, grade, and lymphovascular invasion are associated with the risk of lymph node involvement.[33] Patients with T2 lesions, poorly differentiated histology, or lymphovascular invasion also have higher rates of local failure.[34] In patients undergoing local excision, adjuvant chemoradiation is therefore indicated for those with ≥T2 tumors, and for those with T1 tumors with high-grade histology or lymphovascular invasion. Adjuvant chemoradiation is also indicated if the margins of resection are close.

The Radiation Therapy Oncology Group (RTOG) conducted a phase II trial of local excision in patients with a clinically mobile rectal tumor located less than 10 cm from the anal verge.[35] Patients with stage ≥ T2, tumor size > 3 cm, grade 3, margins < 3 mm, lymphovascular invasion, or elevated carcinoembryonic antigen level were treated with adjuvant radiotherapy (50 to 65 Gy) with concurrent 5-FU. Patients who had none of these adverse features received no adjuvant therapy. The rate of local failure was 12% for the entire population and 14% for those treated with chemoradiation. Thus, high rates of local control are achievable with this combination of local excision and adjuvant chemoradiation in carefully selected patients.

Radiotherapy Technique

The radiotherapy volume should encompass the primary rectal tumor and draining lymph nodes, including the mesorectal, presacral, and internal iliac nodes. In general, patients are given an initial course of radiation to the pelvis (45 Gy), followed by a boost (5.4 to 9 Gy) to the rectal tumor and surrounding margin. A multifield approach helps spare normal tissue, such as small bowel. Bowel exclusion techniques can be used to move bowel out of the irradiated volume, thereby reducing toxicity. A three-field prone technique with an open tabletop ("belly board") has been shown to reduce the median dose to the small bowel, the volume of small bowel in the field, and the incidence of small bowel obstruction.[36,37] Prone positioning with a three-field or four-field technique without an open tabletop device also can exclude bowel from the field. The rectal tumor should be defined with the help of rectal contrast and/or computed tomographic (CT) imaging. Typically, the superior border of the field is placed at the L5/S1 interspace, and the inferior border is placed at least 3 cm below the inferior extent of the tumor for preoperative treatments, and at least 3 cm below the anastomosis for postoperative treatments. For patients treated after an abdominoperineal resection, the inferior border should be placed at least 1.5 cm below the perineal scar. The lateral borders are placed 1.5 to 2 cm lateral to the widest bony margin of the pelvis sidewalls, and the posterior border is placed 1 to 1.5 cm posterior to the sacral margin. The anterior border should be placed such that the internal iliac nodes are included. Traditionally, the external iliac nodes were also included if the tumor invaded the cervix, vagina, prostate, or bladder, but the risk of external iliac nodal recurrence is low in patients with T4 tumors who do not receive radiotherapy to the external iliac region.[38] The risk of inguinal nodal recurrence is also low ($< 5\%$) for tumors extending to the anal canal.[39] Since treatment of the inguinal nodes increases the volume of radiation and thereby increases the risk of severe skin reactions, scrotal edema, and diarrhea, elective groin irradiation is not routinely recommended for patients whose tumor extends to the anal canal. Nevertheless, clinically involved inguinal nodes should be included in the radiation field.

References

1. Anonymous. Prolongation of the disease-free interval in surgically treated rectal carcinoma. Gastrointestinal Tumor Study Group. N Engl J Med 1985;312:1465–72.

2. Douglass HO Jr, Moertel CG, Mayer RJ, et al. Survival after postoperative combination treatment of rectal cancer. N Engl J Med 1986;315:1294–5.

3. Krook JE, Moertel CG, Gunderson LL, et al. Effective surgical adjuvant therapy for high-risk rectal carcinoma. N Engl J Med 1991;324:709–15.

4. Fisher B, Wolmark N, Rockette H, et al. Postoperative adjuvant chemotherapy or radiation therapy for rectal cancer: results from NSABP protocol R-01. J Natl Cancer Inst 1988;80:21–9.

5. Wolmark N, Wieand HS, Hyams DM, et al. Randomized trial of postoperative adjuvant chemotherapy with or without radiotherapy for carcinoma of the rectum: National Surgical Adjuvant Breast and Bowel Project Protocol R-02. J Natl Cancer Inst 2000;92:388–96.

6. O'Connell MJ, Martenson JA, Wieand HS, et al. Improving adjuvant therapy for rectal cancer by combining pro-tracted-infusion fluorouracil with radiation therapy after curative surgery. N Engl J Med 1994;331:502–7.

7. Tepper JE, O'Connell M, Niedzwiecki D, et al. Adjuvant therapy in rectal cancer: analysis of stage, sex, and local control—final report of intergroup 0114. J Clin Oncol 2002;20:1744–50.

8. Tepper JE, O'Connell MJ, Petroni GR, et al. Adjuvant postoperative fluorouracil-modulated chemotherapy combined with pelvic radiation therapy for rectal cancer: initial results of intergroup 0114. J Clin Oncol 1997;15:2030–9.

9. Smalley SR, Benedetti J, Williamson S, et al. Intergroup 0144—phase III trial of 5-FU based chemotherapy regimens plus radiotherapy (XRT) in postoperative adjuvant rectal cancer. Bolus 5-FU vs prolonged venous infusion (PVI) before and after XRT + PVI vs bolus 5-FU + leucovorin (LV) + levamisole (LEV) before and after XRT + bolus 5-FU +LV. Proc Am Soc Clin Oncol 2003;22:251.

10. Twelves C, Wong A, Nowacki MP, et al. Capecitabine as adjuvant treatment for stage III colon cancer. N Engl J Med 2005;352:2696–704.

11. Dunst J, Reese T, Sutter T, et al. Phase I trial evaluating the concurrent combination of radiotherapy and capecitabine in rectal cancer. J Clin Oncol 2002;20:3983–91.

12. Lin EH, Skibber J, Delclos M, et al. A phase II study of capecitabine and radiotherapy plus consomitant boost in patients with locally advanced rectal cancer: preliminary safety analysis. Proc Am Soc Clin Oncol 2003;22:287.

13. Andre T, Boni C, Mounedji-Boudiaf L, et al. Oxaliplatin, fluorouracil, and leucovorin as adjuvant treatment for colon cancer. N Engl J Med 2004;350:2343–51.

14. Gerard JP, Chapet O, Nemoz C, et al. Preoperative concurrent chemoradiotherapy in locally advanced rectal cancer with high-dose radiation and oxaliplatin-containing regimen: the Lyon R0-04 phase II trial. J Clin Oncol 2003; 21:1119–24.

15. Rodel C, Grabenbauer GG, Papadopoulos T, et al. Phase I/II trial of capecitabine, oxaliplatin, and radiation for rectal cancer. J Clin Oncol 2003;21:3098–104.

16. Sauer R, Becker H, Hohenberger W, et al. Preoperative versus postoperative chemoradiotherapy for rectal cancer. N Engl J Med 2004;351:1731–40.

17. Kwok H, Bissett IP, Hill GL. Preoperative staging of rectal cancer. Int J Colorectal Dis 2000;15:9–20.

18. Anonymous: improved survival with preoperative radiotherapy in resectable rectal cancer. Swedish Rectal Cancer Trial [published erratum appears in N Engl J Med 1997 22;336: 1539]. N Engl J Med 1997;336:980–7.

19. Kapiteijn E, Marijnen CA, Nagtegaal ID, et al. Preoperative radiotherapy combined with total mesorectal excision for resectable rectal cancer. N Engl J Med 2001;345:638–46.

20. Gunderson LL, Sargent DJ, Tepper JE, et al. Impact of T and N stage and treatment on survival and relapse in adjuvant rectal cancer: a pooled analysis. J Clin Oncol 2004; 08:173.

21. Willett CG, Badizadegan K, Ancukiewicz M, et al. Prognostic factors in stage T3N0 rectal cancer: do all patients require postoperative pelvic irradiation and chemotherapy? Dis Col Rectum 1999;42:167–73.

22. Marijnen CA, Nagtegaal ID, Kapiteijn E, et al. Radiotherapy does not compensate for positive resection margins in rectal cancer patients: report of a multicenter randomized trial. Int J Radiat Oncol Biol Phys 2003;55: 1311–20.

23. Tepper JE, O'Connell MJ, Niedzwiecki D, et al. Impact of number of nodes retrieved on outcome in patients with rectal cancer. J Clin Oncol 2001;19:157–63.

24. Benson AB 3rd, Schrag D, Somerfield MR, et al. American Society of Clinical Oncology recommendations on adjuvant chemotherapy for stage II colon cancer. J Clin Oncol 2004;22:3408–19.

25. Bosset JF, Calais G, Mineur L, et al. Preoperative radiation (Preop RT) in rectal cancer: effect and timing of additional chemotherapy (CT) 5-year results of the EORTC 22921 trial. J Clin Oncol 2005;23:247S.

26. Abdalla EK, Vauthey JN, Ellis LM, et al. Recurrence and outcomes following hepatic resection, radiofrequency ablation, and combined resection/ablation for colorectal liver metastases. Ann Surg, 239:818–25; discussion 825–7.

27. Crane CH, Janjan NA, Abbruzzese JL, et al. Effective pelvic symptom control using initial chemoradiation without colostomy in metastatic rectal cancer. Int J Radiat Oncol Biol Phys 2001;49:107–16.

28. Mohiuddin M, Marks G, Marks J. Long-term results of reirradiation for patients with recurrent rectal carcinoma. Cancer 2002;95:1144–50.

29. Nakfoor BM, Willett CG, Shellito PC, et al. The impact of 5-fluorouracil and intraoperative electron beam radiation therapy on the outcome of patients with locally advanced primary rectal and rectosigmoid cancer. Ann Surg 1998; 228:194–200.

30. Gunderson LL, Nelson H, Martenson JA, et al. Locally advanced primary colorectal cancer: intraoperative electron and external beam irradiation +/- 5-FU. Int J Radiat Oncol Biol Phys 1997;37:601–14.

31. Lindel K, Willett CG, Shellito PC, et al. Intraoperative radiation therapy for locally advanced recurrent rectal or rectosigmoid cancer. Radiother Oncol 2001;58:83–7.

32. Haddock MG, Gunderson LL, Nelson H, et al. Intraoperative irradiation for locally recurrent colorectal cancer in previously irradiated patients. Int J Radiat Oncol Biol Phys 2001;49:1267–74.

33. Minsky BD, Rich T, Recht A, et al. Selection criteria for local excision with or without adjuvant radiation therapy for rectal cancer. Cancer 1989;63:1421–9.

34. Chakravarti A, Compton CC, Shellito PC, et al. Long-term follow-up of patients with rectal cancer managed by local excision with and without adjuvant irradiation. Ann Surg 1999;230:49–54.

35. Russell AH, Harris J, Rosenberg PJ, et al. Anal sphincter conservation for patients with adenocarcinoma of the distal rectum: long-term results of radiation therapy oncology group protocol 89-02. Int J Radiat Oncol Biol Phys 2000; 46:313–22.

36. Mak AC, Rich TA, Schultheiss TE, et al. Late complications of postoperative radiation therapy for cancer of the rectum and rectosigmoid. Int J Radiat Oncol Biol Phys 1994;28: 597–603.

37. Koelbl O, Richter S, Flentje M. Influence of patient positioning on dose-volume histogram and normal tissue complication probability for small bowel and bladder in patients receiving pelvic irradiation: a prospective study using a 3D planning system and a radiobiological model. Int J Radiat Oncol Biol Phys 1999;45:1193–8.

38. Sanfilippo NJ, Crane CH, Skibber J, et al. T4 rectal cancer treated with preoperative chemoradiation to the posterior pelvis followed by multivisceral resection: patterns of failure and limitations of treatment. Int J Radiat Oncol Biol Phys 2001;51:176–83.

39. Taylor N, Crane C, Skibber J, et al. Elective groin irradiation is not indicated for patients with adenocarcinoma of the rectum extending to the anal canal. Int J Radiat Oncol Biol Phys 2001;51:741–7.

CHAPTER 34

SURGICAL TREATMENT OF LOCALLY ADVANCED AND RECURRENT RECTAL CANCER

NESTOR F. ESNAOLA, MD, MPH

Despite recent advances in surgical technique and adjuvant therapy for rectal cancer, up to one-third of patients will recur after curative resection. Multiple studies have shown higher rates of recurrence in patients who present with low to mid rectal cancers, transmural extension, or nodal involvement. Although definitive external beam radiation therapy (EBRT) can provide short-term palliation in the majority of patients, its effects are short lived, and long-term cure is achieved in less than 5% of patients. In patients with primary locally advanced rectal cancer (tumors extending to or invading adjacent pelvic structures), the incidence of local failure is 54 to 67% after surgery alone.[1]

Most rectal cancer recurrences occur within 2 years after resection. Among patients who recur, approximately one-third will have isolated pelvic recurrences, and one-third of these will in turn be amenable to re-resection. Attempted curative surgery often requires multivisceral resections, en bloc bone resections, and creation of multiple stomas. These procedures are associated with significant postoperative morbidity and can have a significant impact on a patient's post-treatment quality of life. With careful selection, however, 25 to 30% 5-year survival rates can be achieved after complete, negative-margin resection.

Locally advanced or recurrent rectal cancers represent a challenge to the surgeon due to their bulky, extensive nature and the anatomic confines of the pelvis, which often preclude wide margin resection. Resection is often technically difficult and results in significant morbidity. Furthermore, many patients prove to be unresectable at exploration or ultimately succumb to distant metastases after "curative" resection. Therefore, management of these complex patients requires careful selection, detailed preoperative staging, and a thoughtful, stepwise treatment plan centered on multimodality therapy.

Preoperative Evaluation

PATIENT CHARACTERISTICS AND SELECTION

Certain signs and symptoms at presentation are suggestive of local pelvic invasion and can help guide the initial clinical evaluation. Patients with large, bulky rectal tumors often complain of intestinal cramping, obstipation, or diarrhea due to intermittent, partial large-bowel obstruction. Tenesmus and/or fecal incontinence should alert the clinician to potential involvement of the levator muscles or infiltration of the sphincter complex. Anterior invasion with infiltration of the genitourinary tract can present as dysuria, hematuria, pneumaturia, or urinary tract dysfunction (Figure 1). In women, new vaginal bleeding or discharge often indicate the presence of an emerging rectovaginal fistula. Posterior or lateral invasion by tumor often present as unilateral or bilateral lower extremity swelling secondary to venous obstruction or pain radiating down the back of the leg due to sciatic nerve involvement. These symptoms are particularly ominous and suggestive of lateral pelvic side wall involvement, which is almost uniformly unresectable.

On physical exam, careful attention should be paid to the supraclavicular and inguinal nodal basins. Suspected inguinal node involvement should be confirmed by ultrasonography and fine-needle aspiration, particularly

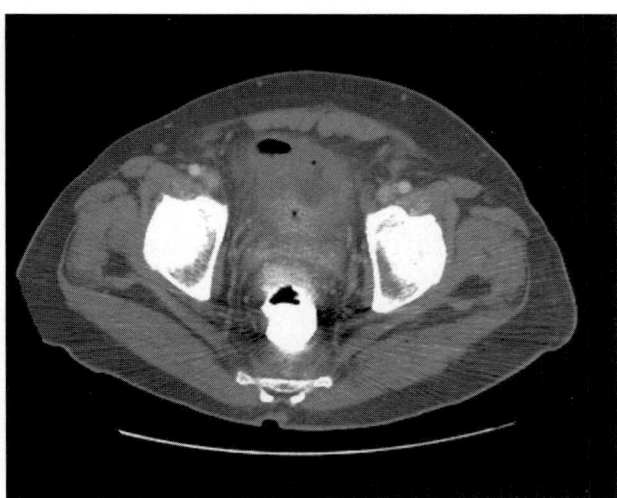

Figure 1 Pelvic computed tomography of a patient with locally advanced rectal cancer who presented with dysuria and pneumaturia. There is a large, necrotic rectal mass with surrounding fat stranding. The urinary bladder is thickened and contains air.

because it is often associated with disseminated disease and poor prognosis after resection.[2] New gynecologic complaints in women require a full pelvic examination, including a bimanual exam to assess the rectovaginal septum. Digital rectal exam and proctoscopy are required to assess the degree of luminal narrowing, the location of the tumor (ie, anterior, lateral, posterior), and potential involvement of the bony pelvis. Although tethering to adjacent pelvic structures often represents invasion in patients with primary locally advanced tumors, it can represent scarring from previous surgery or radiation in patients with recurrent tumors and should be interpreted with caution.

IMAGING AND STAGING

Accurate and detailed anatomic information is required to identify patients for neoadjuvant therapy or intraoperative radiotherapy and properly plan wide en bloc resections to ensure negative margins. Although endorectal ultrasound has proven to be a valuable tool in the staging of patients with mobile, T1 to T3 rectal tumors, its accuracy in patients with bulky T4 tumors is limited due to difficulty with probe placement and poor visualization of the endopelvic fascia. Computed tomography (CT) can provide useful information about local extent of disease and distant metastases. Although CT can also help predict the need for hysterectomy and sacrectomy, it cannot distinguish between tumor and inflammation/fibrosis on pelvic sidewalls and tends to overestimate urinary tract involvement.[3] The presence of unilateral of bilateral hydronephrosis on a CT in patients

with recurrent cancers is almost uniformly associated with unresectable pelvic disease due to lateral pelvic sidewall involvement or carcinomatosis. This radiologic finding is associated with survival equivalent to metastatic disease, and should be considered as a contraindication to exploration and attempted resection.[4]

Magnetic resonance imaging (MRI) has an inherently high soft tissue contrast resolution and a high sensitivity and specificity rate for detecting tumor infiltration into adjacent pelvic structures. Sagittal views are particularly useful for detecting anterior tumor invasion into the genitourinary tract (eg, bladder trigone, seminal vesicles, prostate) in male patients (Figure 2). MRI results should be interpreted with caution in patients following radiation because areas with residual viable tumor can often mimic fibrosis on T2 weighted images. Because colorectal cancer is known to be fluorodeoxyglucose (FDG) avid, FDG-positron emission tomography (FDG-PET) has been used to distinguish between nonglucose avid scar and viable tumor. Moore and colleagues reported a positive predictive value of 76% and negative predictive value of 92% in detecting pelvic recurrence in previously irradiated rectal cancer patients, although they noted a higher false-positive rate when scans were performed within 6 to 12 month of radiation therapy, likely due to persistent radiation-induced inflammation.[5] Given the limitations of MRI and FDG-PET in predicting

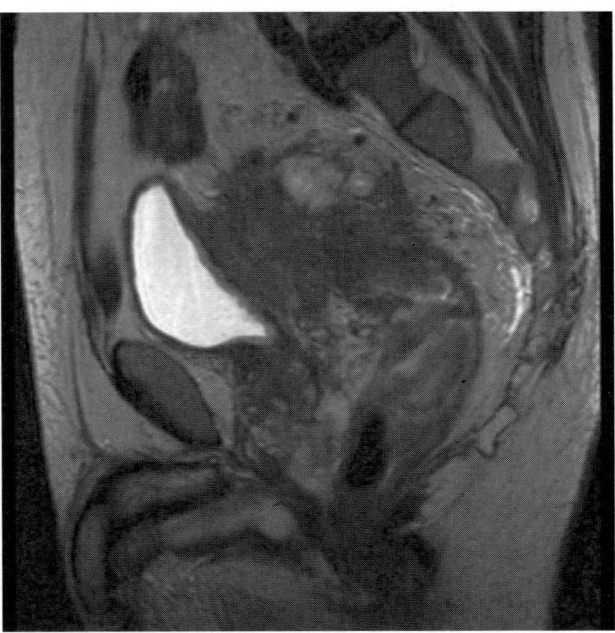

Figure 2 Sagittal T2-weighted magnetic resonance image of a patient with locally advanced rectal cancer. There is anterior invasion of the genitourinary tract by the tumor with involvement of the trigone and seminal vesicles.

the extent of viable, residual tumor after neoadjuvant therapy, resection of the original tumor area is still warranted to ensure complete resection with negative margins.

Neoadjuvant Therapy

In rectal cancer patients with stage II or III disease, postoperative chemoradiation improves local control and survival compared to surgery without radiation and is considered the standard of care in the United States.[6] Janjan and colleagues reported their results using preoperative chemoradiation in 117 rectal cancer patients with T3 and/or N1 disease. Tumor downstaging occurred in 62% of cases, resulting in sphincter-sparing procedures in 59% of cases. The pathologic complete response rate (pCR) was 27%, and response to preoperative therapy was associated with improved disease-free survival (DFS) and overall survival (OS) on multivariate analysis.[7] More recently, the German Rectal Cancer Study Group randomized patients with T3, T4, or node-positive rectal cancer to preoperative versus postoperative chemoradiation consisting of fluorouracil (FU) and 50.4 Gy in 28 fractions. Preoperative treatment resulted in higher rates of sphincter preservation (39% versus 19%), improved local control (6% versus 13%), and lower treatment-related toxicity, but did not improve OS.[8]

Given the importance of complete resection with negative margins and the significant risk of local and systemic recurrence after "curative" resection in patients with locally advanced and recurrent rectal cancer, strong consideration should be given to using neoadjuvant therapy whenever possible. Recent studies have evaluated the role of FU-based neoadjuvant chemoradiation (with and without adjuvant chemotherapy) in patients with fixed or tethered T4 primaries or recurrent tumors.[9,10] The pCR rate in these studies ranged from 16 to 25%, and the DFS and OS rate among the complete responders was 97 to 100%. In both studies, postchemoradiation stage was the most powerful independent predictor of recurrence and survival.

Although it is clear that neoadjuvant therapy downsizes a significant portion of patients, thus increasing rates of resection and sphincter preservation, preoperative clinical assessment of complete responses is limited. In a study from Duke University, the positive predictive value of examination, proctoscopy, and CT after neoadjuvant chemoradiation was only 60%.[11] In a study from the University of Texas M. D. Anderson Cancer Center, 17% of patients with pathologic T0-2 tumors after chemoradiation had evidence of residual nodal disease in the mesorectum at resection.[12] These data

suggest that the surgical strategy at the time of attempted curative resection should ultimately be based on the stage of the tumor at presentation, rather than post-treatment stage following neoadjuvant therapy.

Operative Considerations

SURGICAL STRATEGY

The main objective of surgery in patients with locally advanced or recurrent rectal cancer is complete resection with negative margins (so-called R0 resection). Preoperative evaluation can help identify patients who will require en bloc resection of adjacent pelvic structures, while neoadjuvant therapy can help facilitate surgery and sterilize potential margins. The role of total mesorectal excision (wide anatomic resection of the rectum and its surrounding lymphatics, or mesorectum) in reducing local recurrence and improving survival is well established. This is the procedure of choice in cases of local recurrence after previous local excision, and small, anastomotic recurrences following previous low anterior resection. In patients with tumors within 5 to 7 cm of the anal verge and in previously irradiated patients, strong consideration should be given to creating a temporary diverting loop ileostomy at the time of resection to minimize the risk of a postoperative anastomotic leak. In patients with low-lying primary tumors and/or sphincter involvement, and patients who recur after low anterior resection, abdominoperineal resection is often required for complete resection. It is important to avoid performing a total mesorectal excision down to the pelvic floor in these cases in order to avoid dissecting down onto the tumor, thus compromising the radial margin. Instead, the levator muscles can be transected above and lateral to the tumor, which is often best performed through the perineum. For low-lying tumors grossly involving the levators, a paravesical approach can be used to provide better exposure and access for resection (Figure 3).[13] The dissection is begun laterally, and the ipsilateral ureter and bladder are mobilized and rotated medially off the symphysis pubis to the level of the prostate and urethral hiatus. The lateral ligament of the rectum can be divided to provide better access to the levators. Once the tumor is exposed, the levators can then be transected lateral to the tumor.

INVOLVEMENT OF ADJACENT VISCERA

The need for en bloc resection of adjacent pelvic organs is usually established by preoperative evaluation and

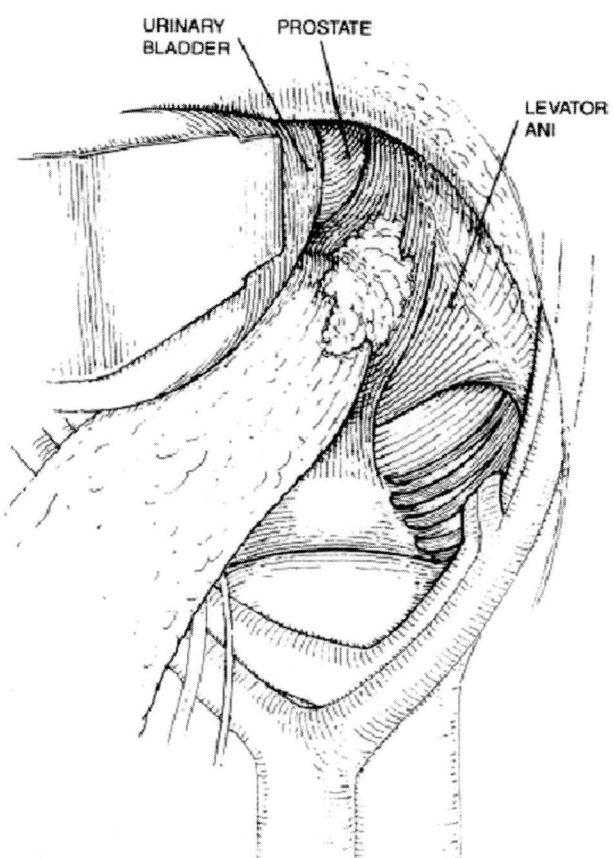

Figure 3 Paravesical approach to low-lying rectal tumor involving the levator ani. The ipsilateral ureter and urinary bladder have been mobilized medially to the level of the prostate and urethral hiatus to better expose the tumor.[13]

imaging. Is difficult to differentiate between a benign adhesion and malignant invasion intraoperatively, and up to half of such adherences will demonstrate tumor involvement on final pathology. For this reason, it is safest to proceed with partial or complete en bloc resection of any adherent organs when discovered incidentally.

The most commonly resected structures in female patients with tumors with anterior invasion are the ovaries, uterus, and vagina. In patients with isolated involvement of the posterior vaginal wall, a "posterior exenteration" involving en bloc resection of the rectum, ovaries, uterus, and posterior vaginal wall can be performed with subsequent reconstruction of the vaginal canal using a rectus abdominis pedicle flap.

Early participation by an experienced urologic team is imperative to determine the full extent of involvement of the urinary tract and the best means of resection and reconstruction. Isolated, unilateral involvement of the ureter can be managed by simple resection and psoas

hitch procedure. Assessment of bladder involvement is based on preoperative imaging and intraoperative evaluation. In a study by Balbay and colleagues, the sensitivity of imaging and palpation were 69% and 70%, respectively. In contrast, the joint sensitivity of preoperative imaging and intraoperative palpation for bladder involvement was 90%.[14] In the absence of extensive bladder involvement or invasion of the trigone, bladder-sparing procedures (eg, partial cystectomy, prostatectomy) should be considered. Although the rate of urinary complications was not diminished after bladder-sparing procedures in Balbay's study, gastro-intestinal complications after total cystectomy and permanent urinary diversion (eg, small bowel obstruction, enteric fistulas) were avoided. Furthermore, 3-year local control and OS rates were similar in both groups. The presence of positive margins after en bloc bladder resection for locally advanced rectal cancer has a significant impact on subsequent survival. In a report by Talamonti and colleagues, patients with negative resection margins had a median survival of 34 months and a 5-year survival rate of 51.8%. In contrast, the median survival for six patients who had positive margins was 11 months, with no survivors at 5 years.[15] Therefore, intraoperative assessment of margins during bladder-sparing procedures is required, and total cystectomy should be performed if necessary.

ABDOMINOSACRAL RESECTION

In patients with posterior extension of the tumor involving the sacrum, abdominoperineal or total pelvic exenteration combined with en bloc resection of the sacrum may be necessary. These are formidable procedures, and early, preoperative involvement of an experienced orthopedic or neurosurgical team should be sought. A thorough preoperative assessment of lower extremity neuromuscular function should be performed and carefully documented. Upper sacral (S1-S2) involvement must be ruled out by preoperative imaging, as transection at this level will result in loss of plantar flexion and foot-drop.

Abdominosacral resections are most often performed in two phases, as recently described by Temple and colleagues.[16] The abdominal phase is performed in the lithotomy position. After laparotomy, a thorough abdominal exploration is performed to rule out extra-pelvic or locally unresectable disease. If the there is extensive involvement of the pelvic or lower periaortic nodes, the procedure should be terminated. Otherwise, the ureters should be mobilized medially to avoid inadvertent damage during sacral transection. The internal iliac and middle sacral artery and veins are identified and ligated to enhance subsequent hemostasis.

The rectum is transected and mobilized down to the level of the sacrum in the standard fashion. Any necessary rectus abdominis myocutaneous flaps are mobilized and advanced into the pelvis for later access. Any necessary urinary conduits or end colostomies should be created and brought out through the anterior abdominal wall, which is then closed.

The patient is then turned onto the prone jack-knife position for the perineal phase of the procedure (Figure 4). A midline incision is made over the sacrum, and the gluteal muscles are transected and mobilized to expose the lateral edges of the sacrum. The sciatic nerve and piriformis are identified bilaterally and laminectomies are performed above the level of the planned transection. This allows for ligation of the dural sac and identification and preservation of the proximal nerve roots under direct vision. The sacrum is divided using an osteotome or oscillating saw, and the sacrum, tumor, and involved pelvic organs are removed en bloc. The defect may need to be packed temporarily to facilitate hemostasis. Once the specimen has been oriented and discussed with the pathologists, any close margins should be evaluated by frozen section to determine the need for further resection or intraoperative radiation therapy.

RECONSTRUCTION OF THE PELVIC SPACE

Patients with locally advanced and recurrent rectal cancers treated with neoadjuvant chemoradiation are at higher risk for perineal wound infection and dehiscence after surgery. Furthermore, the extensive nature of these resections often makes primary closure unsafe or technically impossible. These problems can often be avoided by using vascularized tissue flaps to reconstruct the resulting pelvic defect.[18] Although the greater omentum can be used to obliterate some of the pelvic dead space after low anterior or abdominoperineal resection, it is often damaged by previous abdominal procedures and is inadequate after more extensive resections. Gluteal myocutaneous rotation flaps can be used to reconstruct large posterior defects and have low complication rates. However, because they require intact gluteal vessels they often cannot be use in the setting of previous sacral radiation. Rectus abdominis myocutaneous flaps based on the inferior epigastric vessels are an excellent alternative in this setting (Figure 5). These flaps provide the surgeon with a large cutaneous island based on perforating vessels from the underlying muscle, and are particularly useful in reconstructing the posterior vaginal wall after posterior exenteration. As noted earlier, these flaps should be harvested and mobilized into the pelvis during the abdominal phase of an abdominosacral

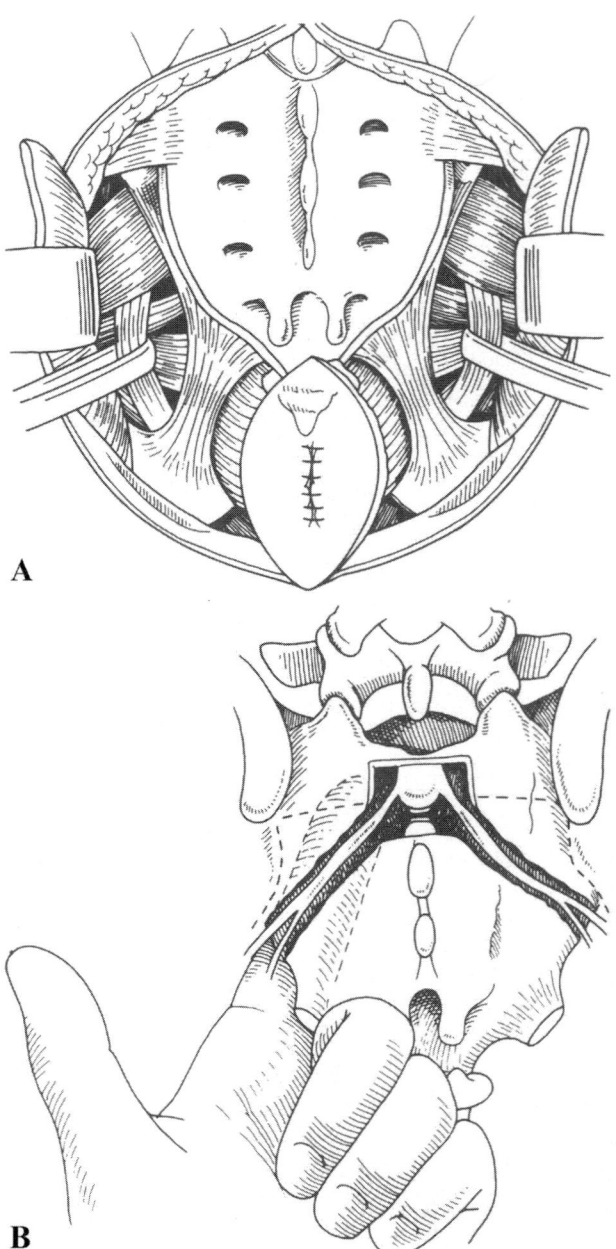

A

B

Figure 4 Perineal phase of abdominosacral resection, performed in the prone jack-knife position. *A*, A posterior sacral incision is made from L5 to the perineum and flaps are raised to the level of the periosteum. The gluteus maximus and medius are dissected from their sacral origins and the sciatic nerves are identified on both sides. *B*, After breaking through the endopelvic fascia to the anterior surface of the sacrum, laminectomies are performed above the level of the planned transection to allow for identification and preservation of the proximal nerve roots. The sacrum is divided using an osteotome, and the sacrum, tumor, and involved organs are removed en bloc.[17]

resection prior to turning the patient onto the prone position. Mobilization may be difficult after previous laparotomy or ostomies. In patients undergoing total

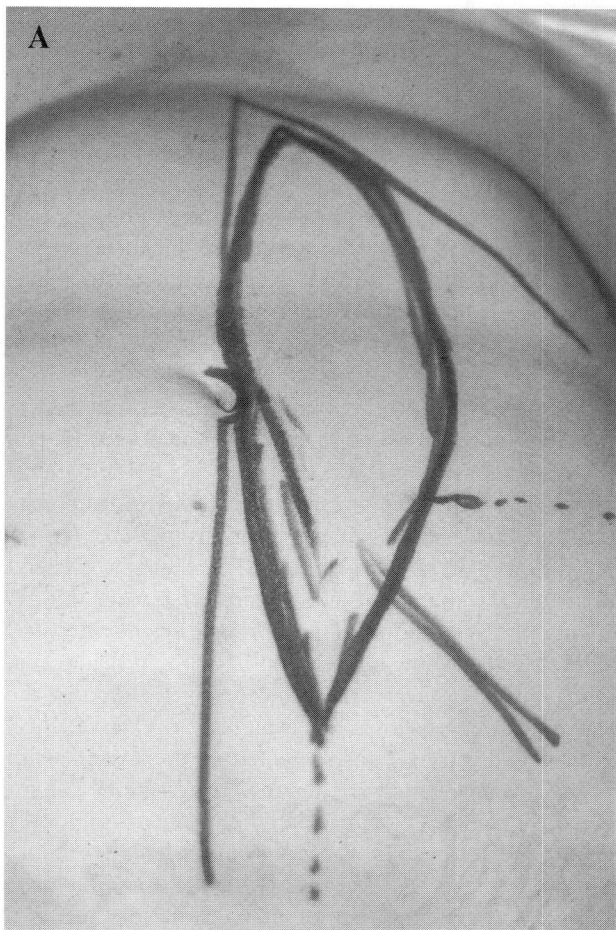

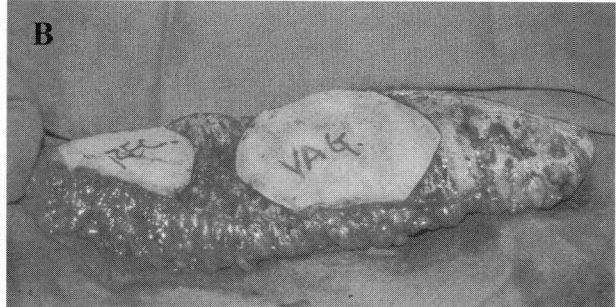

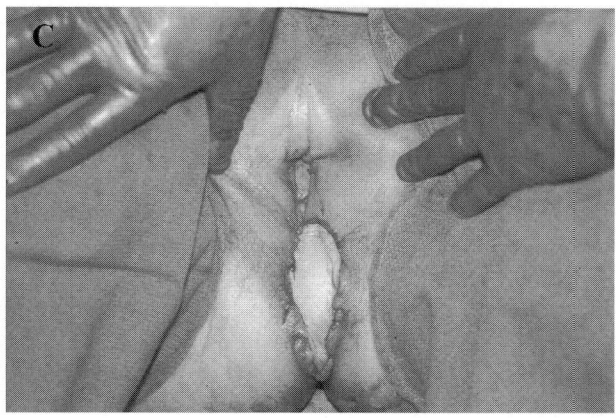

Figure 5 Use of vertical rectus abdominis myocutaneous flap to reconstruct posterior vaginal wall and perineal defects after posterior exenteration. Courtesy of David W. Chang, MD, Department of Plastic Surgery, The University of Texas M. D. Anderson Cancer Center.

pelvic exenteration, the rectus flap should be harvested from the same side as urinary conduit to avoid prolapse of the end colostomy. Other options for pelvic reconstruction include composite thigh flaps (eg, gracilis and/or sartorius myocutaneous flaps) and free flaps (eg, tensor fascia lata or latissimus dorsi). Free flap reconstruction can be extremely difficult due to limited access to recipient vessels in the pelvis. However, it may be the best last resort given the high complication rates and poor results associated with composite thigh flaps.

IORT and Brachytherapy

Approximately one-third of patients with locally advanced or recurrent rectal cancer recur locally despite neoadjuvant therapy and aggressive en bloc resection. Due to the fact that small bowel toxicity prevents the use of additional EBRT, the use of intraoperative radiation therapy (IORT) has been explored in this setting.[19] IORT

allows for the displacement of dose-limiting structures (by packing or shielding during treatment) while allowing for the administration of high, biologically equivalent doses of radiation. The dose of IORT given is often based on the margin status at the time of resection: 10 Gy is usually administered after an R1 resection (ie, microscopically positive margins) and 15 to 20 Gy after an R2 resection (ie, grossly positive margins). It is estimated that a dose of IORT is biologically equivalent to 2 to 3 times the same dose of EBRT. Thus, patients who received 45 Gy during neoadjuvant chemoradiation, followed by 10 Gy of IORT after resection would effectively receive a total dose 65 to 75 Gy of radiation.

IORT can be delivered using electrons (intraoperative electron radiation therapy [IOERT]) or high-dose-rate brachytherapy (HDR-IORT). IOERT takes less time (approximately 5 to 10 minutes) and has greater tissue penetration, allowing for treatment of areas of residual tumor thicker than 0.5 to 1 cm. Unfortunately, delivery of IOERT requires a linear accelerator. Due to shielding requirements, this often requires a dedicated operating room (OR) for IORT or intraoperative transfer of the patient to the radiation oncology department. Finally, IORT applicators are often awkward and difficult to position within the deep or posterior pelvis.

HDR-IORT delivers photon radiation (usually from a mobile Ir^{192} source) via hollow catheters usually embedded in flexible pads of Silicone Rubber at 1 cm intervals. These Harrison-Anderson-Mick applicators allow for the treatment of larger, more complex treatment areas, such as the pelvic sidewalls. Once the applicator has been placed and secured intraoperatively, adjacent organs and sensitive structures can be packed and shielded prior to advancing the source into the afterloading catheters. In centers without dedicated ORs, afterloading catheters embedded in absorbable mesh can be used instead, and tissue flaps can be used to displace and shield adjacent organs. These patients can then be treated postoperatively in the radiation oncology department, after which time the catheters can be removed. HDR-IORT takes longer than IOERT (usually 30 to 45 minutes) and can only be used to treat tumor beds less than 0.5 to 1 cm due to inherent dose inhomogeneity.

A theoretical disadvantage of IORT is that a large dose of radiation is given over a short period of time, limiting the repair of sublethal damage within normal tissues seen during EBRT. The dose limiting structures during pelvic IORT are the peripheral nerves and ureters. Up to one-third of patients who receive IORT will develop peripheral neuropathy, which most commonly presents as pelvic pain, numbness, or weakness. The symptoms are rarely severe and resolve in the majority of cases. Ureteral stenosis is less common, and can often be avoided with use of ureteral stents. The risk of peripheral nerve or ureteral damage is related to the length of nerve or ureter treated and doses above 12.5 Gy and 15 Gy, respectively.

Results of Therapy

LOCAL CONTROL, DISTANT FAILURE, AND SURVIVAL

The literature on multimodality therapy for locally advanced or recurrent rectal cancer consists largely of nonrandomized, phase II studies that rely on comparisons to historical controls. These studies often combine patients from both disease groups, and vary greatly with respect to treatments delivered (eg, radiation versus chemoradiation, timing of (neo)adjuvant therapy, extent of resection, use of IORT, etc.). Nonetheless, closer inspection of the data yields several conclusions about the role of multimodality therapy in these patients.

Postoperative radiation ensures better selection based on margin status, but results in unacceptably high rates of incomplete resection and local failure. Preoperative radiation can be used to "downsize" tumors, and results in higher rates of resection and sphincter preservation. Combined chemoradiation results in higher response rates and better DFS and OS rates compared to radiation alone. Local control, however, continues to be a problem, particularly in the setting of incomplete resections.

Multimodality therapy combining chemoradiation, attempted curative resection, and IORT increases the rate of complete resection, local control, and DFS of patients with locally advanced or recurrent rectal cancers. The bulk of these studies have come from three major institutions: the Mayo Clinic, Massachusetts General Hospital, and Memorial Sloan-Kettering Cancer Center. Representative results of multimodality therapy (ie, IORT, EBRT with or without 5-FU, and maximal surgical resection) from two large series reported by the Mayo Clinic are shown in Table 1.[20,21] Overall, local control and survival rates are better in patients with locally advanced tumors. Incomplete resection is associated with lower OS, particularly in patients with locally advanced disease. In both groups, distant failure remained a persistent problem, highlighting the need for adjuvant systemic chemotherapy in these patients.

Several studies have documented worse prognosis in patients who recur locally after resection and radiation therapy compared to patients who recur after resection alone. In one study, patients who recurred locally after preoperative radiation and total mesorectal excision had higher rates of distant disease at presentation, underwent resection less often, and received radiotherapy for their recurrence less often than their counterparts.[22] The use of aggressive multimodality therapy (surgical resection and IOERT with or without EBRT) in previously irradiated patients with locally recurrent rectal cancer was recently explored.[23] The median IOERT dose was 20 Gy, and 73% of patients received additional EBRT (median dose 25.2 Gy). Local control within the IOERT field was 72%, and local control at 2 years was 81% in patients who received ≥ 30 Gy EBRT compared to 54% in patients who received ≤ 30Gy or no EBRT ($p = .16$). Almost all patients who developed neuropathy or ureteral stenosis received IOERT doses ≥ 20Gy. Only 6% of patients received adjuvant systemic therapy. Not surprisingly, 76% of patients went on to develop distant disease and the overall 5-year survival rate for the entire group was only 12%. Patients who recur locally after previous resection and radiation may have more biologically

Table 1 Selected Results of Multimodality Therapy in Patients with Locally Advanced or Recurrent Rectal Cancer

	Extent of Resection	Local Failure (3 yr)	Distant Failure (3 yr)	Overall Survival (3 yr)
Locally Advanced Rectal Cancer (20)	R0, R1	9%	37%	69%
	R2	27%	66%	28%
Locally Recurrent Rectal Cancer (21)	R0, R1	16%	64%	41%
	R2	32%	64%	36%

R0 = negative margin resection; R1 = microscopically positive margin resection; R2 = grossly positive margin resection.

aggressive disease and should routinely be referred for adjuvant systemic therapy.

QUALITY OF LIFE AFTER TREATMENT

Aggressive surgical resection and multimodality therapy are often associated with significant morbidity and toxicity and can have a significant impact of patients' quality of life after treatment. The impact of multimodality therapy on anorectal function and quality of life was recently examined in a group of 18 patients with locally advanced or recurrent rectal cancer using questionnaires.[24] Thirty percent of patients after "high" low anterior resection reported unfavorable (poor or fair) symptoms or problems approximately 2 years after treatment compared to 88% of patients after "very low" low anterior resection or coloanal anastomosis. Over half of patients were dissatisfied with their quality of life due to restriction in their social activity, sexual function, or travel.

More recently, post-treatment pain and quality of life were studied prospectively in a group of 45 patients with locally recurrent rectal cancer using the Brief Pain Inventory and Functional Assessment of Cancer Therapy-Colorectal questionnaires.[25] Surprisingly, resected patients reported significant levels of mild to moderate pain and impaired quality of life up to 3 years after surgery, despite apparently adequate pain management. Pain at presentation, total pelvic exenteration, and sacrectomy were associated with higher rates of post-treatment pain. Clinicians faced with patients with locally recurrent disease and pelvic pain at presentation should proceed with extreme caution, given that neither cure nor palliation is likely in these patients.

Summary

Patients with locally advanced or recurrent rectal cancers present a special challenge to the surgeon. These tumors are locally extensive by nature, and attempts at curative resection with negative margins are often limited by anatomic constraints. Resection and multimodality therapy are associated with significant morbidity and have a significant impact on patients' post-treatment quality of life. Careful patient selection and preoperative counseling is necessary to identify patients who are more likely to benefit from aggressive therapy. Detailed preoperative imaging plays a central role in treatment planning and is necessary to rule out locally unresectable or metastatic disease at presentation. All potentially resectable patients should receive neoadjuvant chemoradiation in an effort to "downsize" their tumors and improve their chances of sphincter preservation and negative margin resection. An aggressive, well-coordinated surgical strategy (often requiring close collaboration between multiple surgical subspecialties) should be outlined at the outset of therapy and designed to minimize morbidity while optimizing oncologic outcome. Furthermore, resections should be performed in institutions with IOERT or HDR-IORT capabilities, given the high rates of local failure after neoadjuvant chemoradiation and resection alone. A significant proportion of patients with locally advanced or recurrent rectal cancer succumb to distant disease despite optimal surgical and multimodality therapy, emphasizing the importance adjuvant systemic therapy after resection. Finally, enrollment of patients in clinical trials evaluating novel neoadjuvant chemoradiation strategies and new chemotherapeutic and biologic agents should be strongly encouraged.

References

1. Rich T, Gunderson LL, Lew R, et al. Patterns of recurrence of rectal cancer after potentially curative surgery. Cancer 1983;52:1317–29.

2. Tocchi A, Lepre L, Costa G, et al. Rectal cancer and inguinal metastases: prognostic role and therapeutic indications. Dis Colon Rectum 1999;42:1464–6.

3. Farouk R, Nelson H, Radice E, et al. Accuracy of computed tomography in determining resectability for locally advanced primary or recurrent colorectal cancers. Am J Surg 1998;175:283–7.

4. Cheng C, Rodriguez-Bigas MA, Petrelli N. Is there a role for curative surgery for pelvic recurrence from rectal carcinoma in the presence of hydronephrosis? Am J Surg 2001;182:274–7.

5. Moore HG, Akhurst T, Larson SM, et al. A case-controlled study of 18-fluorodeoxyglucose positron emission tomography in the detection of pelvic recurrence in previously

irradiated rectal cancer patients. J Am Coll Surg 2003;197: 22–8.

6. NIH consensus conference. Adjuvant therapy for patients with colon and rectal cancer. JAMA 1990;264:1444–50.

7. Janjan NA, Crane C, Feig BW, et al. Improved overall survival among responders to preoperative chemoradiation for locally advanced rectal cancer. Am J Clin Oncol 2001; 24:107–12.

8. Sauer R, Becker H, Hohenberger W, et al. Preoperative versus postoperative chemoradiotherapy for rectal cancer. N Engl J Med 2004;351:1731–40.

9. Mohiuddin M, Hayne M, Regine WF, et al. Prognostic significance of postchemoradiation stage following preoperative chemotherapy and radiation for advanced/ recurrent rectal cancers. Int J Radiat Oncol Biol Phys 2000;48:1075–80.

10. Chan AK, Wong A, Jenken D, et al. Posttreatment TNM staging is a prognostic indicator of survival and recurrence in tethered or fixed rectal carcinoma after preoperative chemotherapy and radiotherapy. Int J Radiat Oncol Biol Phys 2005;61:665–77.

11. Onaitis MW, Noone RB, Fields R, et al. Complete response to neoadjuvant chemoradiation for rectal cancer does not influence survival. Ann Surg Oncol 2001;8:801–6.

12. Bedrosian I, Rodriguez-Bigas MA, Feig B, et al. Predicting the node-negative mesorectum after preoperative chemoradiation for locally advanced rectal carcinoma. J Gastrointest Surg 2004;8:56–62; discussion 62–3.

13. Enker WE, Kafka NJ, Martz J. Planes of sharp pelvic dissection for primary, locally advanced, or recurrent rectal cancer. Semin Surg Oncol 2000;18:199–206.

14. Balbay MD, Slaton JW, Trane N, et al. Rationale for bladder-sparing surgery in patients with locally advanced colorectal carcinoma. Cancer 1999;86:2212–6.

15. Talamonti MS, Shumate CR, Carlson GW, et al. Locally advanced carcinoma of the colon and rectum involving the urinary bladder. Surg Gynecol Obstet 1993;177:481–7.

16. Temple WJ, Saettler EB. Locally recurrent rectal cancer: role of composite resection of extensive pelvic tumors with strategies for minimizing risk of recurrence. J Surg Oncol 2000;73:47–58.

17. Wanebo HJ, Turk PS. Abdominosacral resection for recurrent cancer of the rectum. In: Bauer JJ, editor. Colorectal surgery illustrated. St. Louis: Mosby; 1993. p. 245–7.

18. Miles WK, Chang DW, Kroll SS, et al. Reconstruction of large sacral defects following total sacrectomy. Plast Reconstr Surg 2000;105:2387–94.

19. Hu KS, Harrison LB. Results and complications of surgery combined with intra-operative radiation therapy for the treatment of locally advanced or recurrent cancers in the pelvis. Semin Surg Oncol 2000;18:269–78.

20. Gunderson LL, Nelson H, Martenson JA, et al. Locally advanced primary colorectal cancer: intraoperative electron and external beam irradiation +/- 5-FU. Int J Radiat Oncol Biol Phys 1997;37:601–14.

21. Gunderson LL, Nelson H, Martenson JA, et al. Intraoperative electron and external beam irradiation with or without 5-fluorouracil and maximum surgical resection for previously unirradiated, locally recurrent colorectal cancer. Dis Colon Rectum 1996;39:1379–95.

22. van den Brink M, Stiggelbout AM, van den Hout WB, et al. Clinical nature and prognosis of locally recurrent rectal cancer after total mesorectal excision with or without preoperative radiotherapy. J Clin Oncol 2004;22:3958–64.

23. Haddock MG, Gunderson LL, Nelson H, et al. Intraoperative irradiation for locally recurrent colorectal cancer in previously irradiated patients. Int J Radiat Oncol Biol Phys 2001;49:1267–74.

24. Shibata D, Guillem JG, Lanouette N, et al. Functional and quality-of-life outcomes in patients with rectal cancer after combined modality therapy, intraoperative radiation therapy, and sphincter preservation. Dis Colon Rectum 2000;43:752–8.

25. Esnaola NF, Cantor SB, Johnson ML, et al. Pain and quality of life after treatment in patients with locally recurrent rectal cancer. J Clin Oncol 2002;20:4361–7.

CHAPTER 35

SURGERY AND CHEMORADIATION FOR ANAL CANCER

MIGUEL A. RODRIGUEZ-BIGAS, MD

CATHY ENG, MD

CHRISTOPHER H. CRANE, MD

Chemoradiation and Surgery for Anal Squamous Cancer

In order to treat tumors in the anal region, it is imperative to know the exact location of the lesion. The treatment of perianal squamous cancer is primarily surgical, whereas chemoradiation is appropriate for invasive squamous cell carcinoma (SCC) of the anal canal, with surgical therapy used for persistent or recurrent disease after chemoradiation.

Anatomy

The perianal skin starts at the anal verge (the junction of the anal canal and the hair-bearing skin) and extends approximately 5 to 6 cm from the anal verge.[1] The anal canal has been subdivided into the surgical anal canal and the anatomic anal canal.[2] The former extends from the anorectal junction where the puborectalis muscle encompasses the rectum to the anal verge. The latter extends from the dentate line to the anal verge. The dentate line is the midpoint of the anal canal and is usually about 2 cm proximal to the anal verge.[2]

Due to the nature of its epithelium, the anal canal can give rise to a variety of neoplasms. Below the dentate line there is squamous epithelium. Above the dentate line the epithelium is columnar. In the anal transition zone, defined as the area 6 to 12 mm proximal to the dentate line, columnar, basal, cuboidal, transitional, and squa-mous epithelium can be encountered.[2] Squamous cell carcinoma of the anal canal is a broad term that includes epidermoid, basaloid (cloacogenic), and transitional cell carcinomas. However, the treatment of these neoplasms is the same with chemoradiation as the primary initial therapeutic modality.

Epidemiology and Etiology

Squamous cell cancer of the anus is not a common neoplasm. In 2005, there will be 3,990 new cases of carcinoma of the anus diagnosed in the United States compared to 145,290 new colorectal adenocarcinoma cases.[3] SCC is slightly more common in women than in men, but there has been an increase in incidence in males under the age of 40 years.[4]

Human papilloma virus (HPV) infection has been associated with condyloma acuminata, high-grade intrae-pithelial neoplasia, and invasive squamous cell carcinoma of the anus.[5] HPV 16 is the most common subtype causing invasive cancer.[6] Cervical dysplasia, receptive anal intercourse, greater than 10 sexual partners, human immunodeficiency virus (HIV) infection, immunosup-pression, cigarette smoking, and sexually transmitted diseases all have been implicated as factors increasing the risk of affected individuals to develop SCC of the anus.[5]

Similar to cervical intraepithelial dysplasia in invasive cervical cancer, it appears that anal intraepithelial neoplasia (AIN) is the precursor of anal squamous cell cancer.[7] AIN can involve both the anal canal and the perianal skin. It is a multifocal process associated with HPV infection.[8] Because of confusion in terminology, it has been recommended that only the terms low-grade intraepithelial dysplasia and high-grade intraepithelial dysplasia be used when referring to AIN.[9] The former should be used for AIN grade I or low-grade dysplasia, and the latter for AIN grade II, AIN grade III, carcinoma in situ, Bowen's disease, and severe dysplasia.[9]

Clinical Presentation

Because it is frequently associated with coexistent benign pathology, it is common for the diagnosis of SCC of the anus to be delayed. The most common presenting symptom is a mass that has increased in size over a period of time, but other symptoms such as pruritus, perianal pain, bleeding, tenesmus, and incontinence can occur.[10] At times these cancers present as perianal abscesses or fistulae, fissures, erythematous or white plaques skin lesions, and on occasion, are diagnosed in a hemorrhoidectomy specimen. Perianal SCC rarely metastasizes to distant organs. However, regional metastasis to

inguinal lymph nodes has been reported in up to 25% of cases.[11] Anal canal cancers are locally aggressive. They can extend to invade adjacent organs and structures. Regional lymph node metastases occur in up to 45% of patients with SCC of the anal canal.[11] Even though the main pattern of recurrence in SCC of the anal canal is locoregional, distant metastases do occur, primarily to the liver and lungs. The risk of lymph node metastases appears to increase according to the T stage. The T staging in anal cancer is based on size of the primary tumor and invasion to adjacent structures (Table 1).[12]

These patients should be evaluated in a multidisciplinary fashion by a surgeon, radiation oncologist, and medical oncologist. These clinicians should communicate frequently so as to be one step ahead of any potential complication during treatment and to address persistent or recurrent disease in a timely fashion.

Anal Intraepithelial Lesions

Anal intraepithelial lesions represent a unique problem in diagnosis and management because of the multifocality. It is important to assess the local extent of the disease.

Table 1 AJCC Staging of Perianal and Anal Canal Cancer

Perianal Skin

Primary Tumor (T)	Lymph Nodes (N)	Distant Metastasis (M)	Staging (TNM)
TX tumor can not be assessed	NX Regional nodes cannot be assessed	MX Distant metastasis cannot be assessed	Stage 0 TisN0M0
T0 no evidence of tumor	N1 No regional node metastasis	M0 No distant metastasis	Stage 1 T1N0M0
Tis Carcinoma in situ	N2 Regional lymph node metastasis	M1 Distant metastasis	Stage II T2N0M0
			T3N0M0
T1 Tumor ≤ 2 cm in greatest dimension			Stage III T4N0M0
			Any TN1M0
T2 Tumor > 2 cm but ≤ 5 cm in greatest dimension			Stage IV Any T Any N M1
T3 Tumor > 5 cm in greatest dimension			
T4 Tumor invades deep extradermal structures			

Anal Canal

Primary tumor (T)	Lymph Nodes (N)	Distant Metastasis (M)	Staging (TNM)
Tx tumor can not be assessed	Nx Regional nodes can not be assessed	MX Distant metastasis cannot be assessed	Stage 0 TisN0M0
T0 no evidence of tumor	N0 No regional node metastasis	M0 No distant metastasis	Stage I T1N0M0
Tis Carcinoma in situ	N1 Metastasis in perirectal lymph lymph node(s)	M1 Distant metastasis	Stage II T2N0M0
			T3N0M0
T1 Tumor ≤ 2 cm in greatest dimension	N2 Metastasis in unilateral internal iliac and/or inguinal lymph node(s)	Stage IIIA T1,2,or 3N1M0	
T2 Tumor > 2 cm but ≤ 5 cm in greatest dimension	N3 Metastasis in perirectal and inguinal lymph nodes and/or bilateral internal iliac and or inguinal lymph node(s)		T4N0M0
			Stage IIIB T4N1M0
			Any T N2M0
			Any T N3M0
T3 Tumor > 5 cm in greatest dimension			Stage IV Any T Any N M1
T4 Tumor invades deep extradermal structures (vagina, urethra, bladder			

AJCC = American Joint Committee on Cancer; TNM = tumor node metastasis.
Adapted from Green FL et al.[12]

The extent of the disease can be assessed by the application of 3% acetic acid to the anal mucosa and the perianal skin. The affected areas will turn white.[7] This method can guide the clinician to areas of suspicion, but it is not very specific.

The natural history of AIN is not well known. Two studies, one a survey of practicing colorectal surgeons, and the other a single institution retrospective study, have reported that approximately 5% of AIN grade III (Bowen's disease) undergo progression to an invasive malignancy over a period of about 20 years.[13,14] Because of the slow progression and the extensive resection that at times is required to eliminate AIN, we observe patients with close follow-up. Biopsies are performed in suspicious areas. If an invasive carcinoma is diagnosed then it is treated. Other therapies for AIN that have been tried with varying success include topical 5-fluorouracil (5-FU) cream, topical imiquimod, photodynamic therapy, cryotherapy, and argon laser tissue coagulation.[7]

Perianal Squamous Cell Cancer (Anal Margin)

In general, the approach to SCC of the perianal skin is surgical. However, in selected situations chemoradiation followed by wide excision or even abdominoperineal resection is required for persistent or locally recurrent disease. The clinical presentation varies from a simple small mass to an obstructing mass in the anal canal (Figure 1). Thus, the treatment varies according to the size of the lesion. In general, for tumors up to 5 cm (T1 and T2), most surgeons would perform a wide local excision with a negative margin. Primary closure should be attempted, but in some cases, careful preoperative planning is warranted because there may be a need for a skin graft or advancement flaps. Radiation therapy alone for smaller lesion has been undertaken with good results.[11] Some authors recommend elective inguinal node irradiation in patients with T2 tumors.[15] In larger tumors (> 5 cm), or tumors that invade adjacent structures, consideration should be given to chemoradiation (5-FU-based, usually combined with cisplatin or mitomycin-C).[15] In these larger tumors, including the inguinal nodal basins bilaterally in the radiation field is recommended. If there is persistent disease after combined therapy, surgical resection should be considered. Again, careful consideration should be given preoperatively to the reconstruction because the resulting defects are quite large. At times a radical procedure such as an abdominoperineal resection is warranted, especially when there is fecal incontinence or persistent or recurrent tumor invading the sphincters. Table 2 illustrates the results of selected series of patients treated

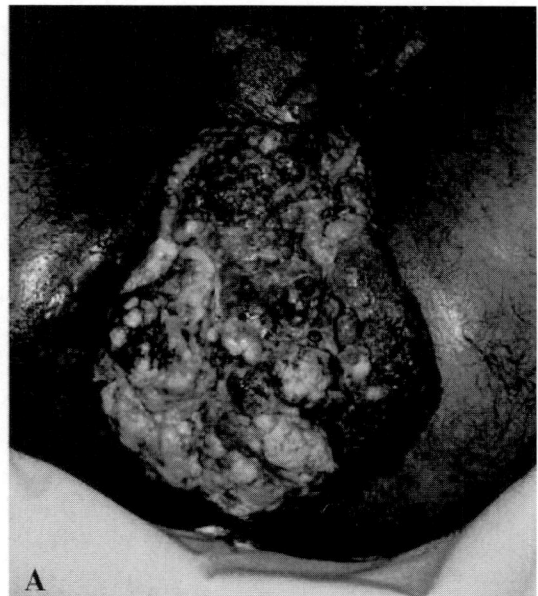

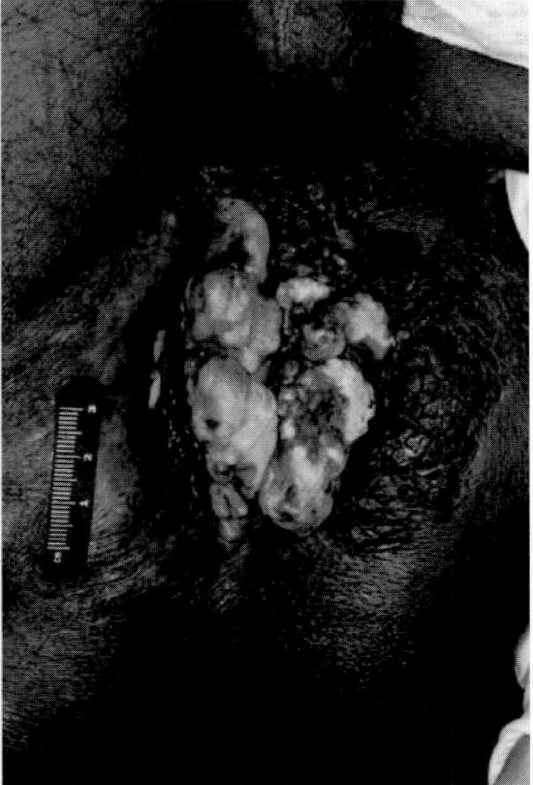

Figure 1 *A*, Primary invasive perianal squamous cell carcinoma. *B*, After treatment with 55 Gy and Capecitabine.

for anal margin or perianal squamous cell carcinoma. Figures 1a, 1b, and 2 show illustrative cases of primary and recurrent perianal SCC.

Table 2 Selected Series on Treatment for Anal Margin or Perianal Skin Squamous Cell Carcinomas

Author and year	Number of Patients	Treatment	Follow-Up (Median Months)	5-Year Local Survival Rate (%)	Recurrence Rate (%)
Greenall MJ et al, 1985[35]	31	LE	NS	68	46
Jensen SL et al, 1988[36]	58	LE	120	53*	41
Peiffert D et al,1997[37]	31	RT	54 (mean)	67	23
Pintor MP et al, 1989[38]	49	LE, APR, RT	NS	65	NS
Mendenhall WM et al, 1996[15]	10	RT, Chemo/RT	60	100	100

APR = abdominoperineal resection; LE = local excision; NS = not stated; RT = radiation therapy.
* 15-year actuarial survival.

Anal Canal SCC

In situ SCC of the anal canal can be treated with local excision alone. As previously mentioned, the treatment of choice for invasive SCC of the anal canal is chemoradiation with surgical therapy as salvage for persistent or recurrent disease. However, there are still proponents of radiation therapy alone for small ≤ 1 cm tumors.[16]

After chemoradiation for anal canal SCC, the expected local control ranges between 61 and 85%, whereas the overall 5-year survival is expected to be between 58 and 92%.[17] However, persistent disease will be diagnosed in up to 15% of patients after chemoradiation and an additional 10 to 30% will develop recurrent disease.[11] Prognosis depends on staging with approximately 50% of T3/T4 primary tumors developing local failure after chemoradiation.[18] Nodal metastases risk increases as the T stage of the primary tumor increases. Most synchronous nodal metastases will be controlled with chemoradiation.

Chemoradiation

In the mid-1970s, Nigro and colleagues reported on three patients who were treated with preoperative chemoradiation utilizing a total of 30 Gy of external beam irradiation and concurrent 5-FU and mitomycin-C, followed by abdominoperineal resection with a complete pathologic response in the specimen.[19] These results were corroborated in multiple centers by different investigators in non-randomized studies with reported 5-year survival rates of 65% to 85% and sphincter preservation rates of 80 to 90% in these patients.[20]

Once chemoradiation was established as the primary treatment for SCC of the anal canal, it was important to determine whether concurrent chemotherapy was indeed necessary. To address this, two prospective randomized trials were conducted in the UK. In the first trial, the United Kingdom Coordinating Committee on Cancer Research (UKCCCR) conducted a study of 585 patients randomized to receive either 45 Gy of external beam radiation alone, or combined modality therapy with 45 Gy of radiation with concurrent 5-FU and mitomycin-C.[21] In a smaller second study conducted by the European Organization for Research and Treatment of Cancer (EORTC), the randomization was similar to the UKCCCR except that the patients in the EORTC study had locally advanced anal cancer and did receive a boost of dose radiation of 15 to 20 Gy if there was incomplete response or persistent disease after multimodality therapy.[22] In both of these studies, patients receiving combined modality therapy had statistically better

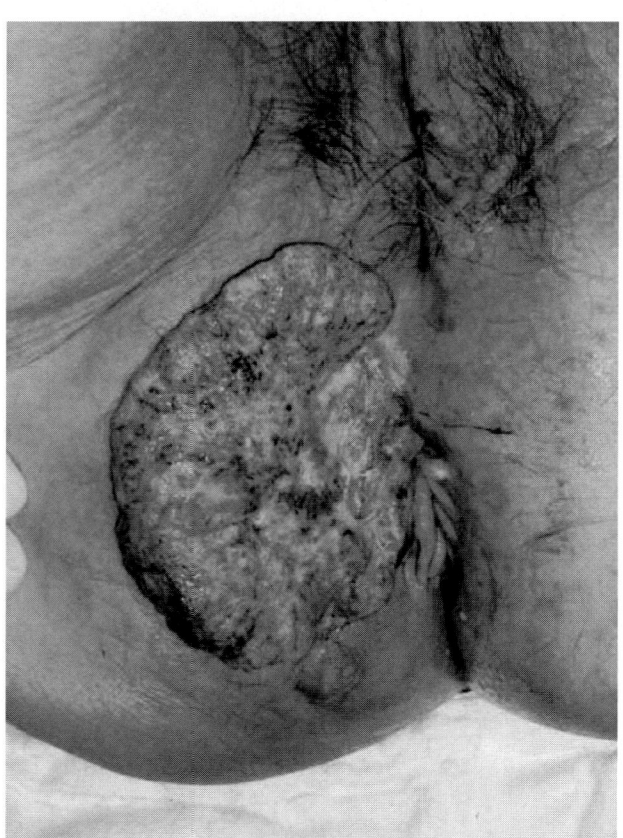

Figure 2 Recurrent perianal squamous cell carcinoma. Note the tumor nodule adjacent to the recurrence.

locoregional control, but there was no statistical improvement in overall survival (OS) rate (Table 3). It must be noted that there was late toxicity, including severe fibrosis, anal, skin, and rectal stenosis, in both of the studies.

The Eastern Cooperative Group (ECOG) and the Radiation Therapy Oncology Group (RTOG) evaluated the role of mitomycin-C in combined modality therapy. In their study, 291 evaluable patients were randomized to receive either 45 Gy radiation + continuous infusion 5-FU with or without mitomycin-C.[23] After 4 to 6 weeks, all patients underwent full-thickness biopsy to assess treatment response. Patients with partial response received an additional boost of 9 Gy of radiation with a cycle of 5-FU and cisplatin while those with complete response did not receive any further therapy.[23] If repeat full thickness biopsies after the salvage therapy revealed less than a complete response, patients underwent abdominoperineal resection. The results of this trial revealed that even though there was no statistically significant improvement in OS rate, patients who received mitomycin-C had a statistically significant improvement in disease-free survival (DFS) rate and colostomy-free survival (CFS) rate (see Table 3).[23] In addition, patients receiving mitomycin-C had higher complete response rate than who did not receive mitomycin-C (92% versus 85%).[23] However, there was a significantly higher Grade 4 and 5 toxicity in the mitomycin-C arm of the study (23% versus 7%).[23]

Patients receiving chemoradiation with 5-FU and mitomycin-C-based chemotherapy have approximately an 84% (81 to 87%) complete response rate, 73% (64 to 86%) local control rate, and 77% (66 to 92%) 5-year survival rate.[18] Approximately half of patients with T3/T4 tumors will require salvage radical surgery.[18] Additionally, about 25% of these patients with a complete response to chemoradiation will require salvage

radical surgery.[18] There is room for improvement, especially in locally advanced tumors.

Cisplatin has been utilized both in conjunction with 5-FU during radiation and in a neoadjuvant fashion prior to definitive chemoradiation. In 35 consecutive patients treated with two cycles of continuous infusion 5-FU $\times$ 96 hours and bolus cisplatin on day 1 with concomitant radiation, a 94% complete response rate was reported.[24] At a median follow-up of 37 months (range 6 to 57), 33 patients (94%) were disease free and 30 patients (86%) were colostomy free. Another prospective nonrandomized study was reported of 80 patients with locally advanced (tumor $>$ 4 cm, N+) anal canal cancers. All were treated with neoadjuvant 5-FU and cisplatin (two cycles), followed by definitive chemoradiation with 5-FU and cisplatin and 45 Gy of external beam irradiation followed by a 15 to 20 Gy boost.[25] After completing treatment, there was a 93% complete response rate. At a median follow-up of 29 months (range 15 to 50), the actuarial 3-year DFS rate and CFS rate was 73%. A similar Phase II pilot study was conducted by the Cancer and Leukemia Group B (CALGB), except that the chemotherapy during the radiation was 5-FU and mitomycin-C and if persistent disease was present, a 9 Gy boost with concomitant 5-FU and cisplatin was administered.[26] Forty-five patients were enrolled in this Phase II study. The complete response rates were 18% after induction chemotherapy and 82% after combined modality therapy. Twenty-two of 44 (50%) patients followed-up for 4 years were disease free and colostomy free. Overall, there were 30 (68%) patients alive, of whom 27 were disease free. In this Phase II pilot study, the most common Grade 3 and 4 toxicities were neutropenia, thrombocytopenia, anemia, stomatitis, and nausea.[26]

The recently reported intergroup trial led by RTOG (98-11) accrued over 550 patients with Stage II and III

Table 3 Selected Prospective Randomized Trials in Invasive Squamous Cell Carcinoma of the Anal Canal

Investigators	Patients	Median Follow-Up (Months)	Regimen	Locoregional Failure Rate %	Overall Survival Rate %	Colostomy Free Survival Rate %
UKCCCR[21]	279	42 (28–62)	45 Gy radiation	59*	58*	
	283		45 Gy radiation + 5-FU + mitomycin-C	36#	65 (NS)	
EORTC [22]	52	42 (9–88)	45 Gy radiation	50**	57**	40**
	51		45 Gy radiation + 5-FU + mitomycin-C	32##	52 (NS)	70###
ECOG/RTOG[23]	145	36 (8.5–74)	45-50.4 Gy + 5-FU	49***	64***	59***
	146		45-50.4Gy + 5-FU + mitomycin-C	27####	78 (NS)	71#####

*3-year; **5-year; ***4-year estimated failure rate and overall survival.
# $p < .0001$; ## $p = .02$; ### $p = .002$; #### $p = .0003$; ##### $p = .014$.
5-FU = 5-fluorouracil; ECOG/RTOG = Eastern Cooperative Group/ Radiation Therapy Oncology Group; EORTC = European Organization for Research and Treatment of Cancer; NS = not significant; UKCCCR = United Kingdom Coordinating Committee on Cancer Research.

anal canal cancer. Patients were randomized to 5-FU and mitomycin-C with concurrent radiation (45 Gy initially and a boost to 55 Gy for T2, 59 Gy for T3/T4 tumors) versus the neoadjuvant approach with two cycles of 5-FU and cisplatin followed by 5-FU and cisplatin with the same concurrent radiation doses. In this trial, neither the estimated overall survival nor the estimated disease-free survival was statistically different between arms.[27] The former was 69% p = (0.24) whereas the latter was 56% for the mitomycin–C arm and 48% for the cisplatin arm (p = 0.28). There was no significant difference in colostomy free survival 10% mitomycin arm versus 20% cisplatin arm (p = 0.12). Grade 3 and 4 hematologic toxicity rates were higher in the mitomycin C arm compared to the cisplatin arm 67% versus 47% respectively (p = 0.0004) while there was no difference between arms in non-hematologic grade 3 and 4 toxicity rates. The authors concluded that 5-FU/cisplatin followed by 5-FU/cisplatin/radiation failed to improve

disease free survival compared to 5-FU mitomycin C/radiation.[27]

At the University of Texas M. D. Anderson Cancer Center, we have been utilizing continuous infusion 5-FU (250 mg/m^2/day, cisplatin (4 mg/m^2/day), 5 days a week on all days of radiation with 55 Gy of radiation to the primary tumor and lymph node basins. In 92 patients evaluated retrospectively, at a median follow-up of 44 months the 5-years actuarial survival rate was 77%, the DFS rate was 55%, and the CFS rate was 82%.[28] Locoregional failure and distant metastases occurred in 17% and 9% of the patients, respectively. We rarely introduce a break during radiation treatment, which likely has contributed to these favorable results. This is possible because of aggressive skin care, optimization of nausea, diarrhea, and pain management and the most critical factor: the radiation technique (Figures 3 to 5),[28] which is designed to spare the small bowel and genitalia from the high doses of radiation. Based on this analysis,

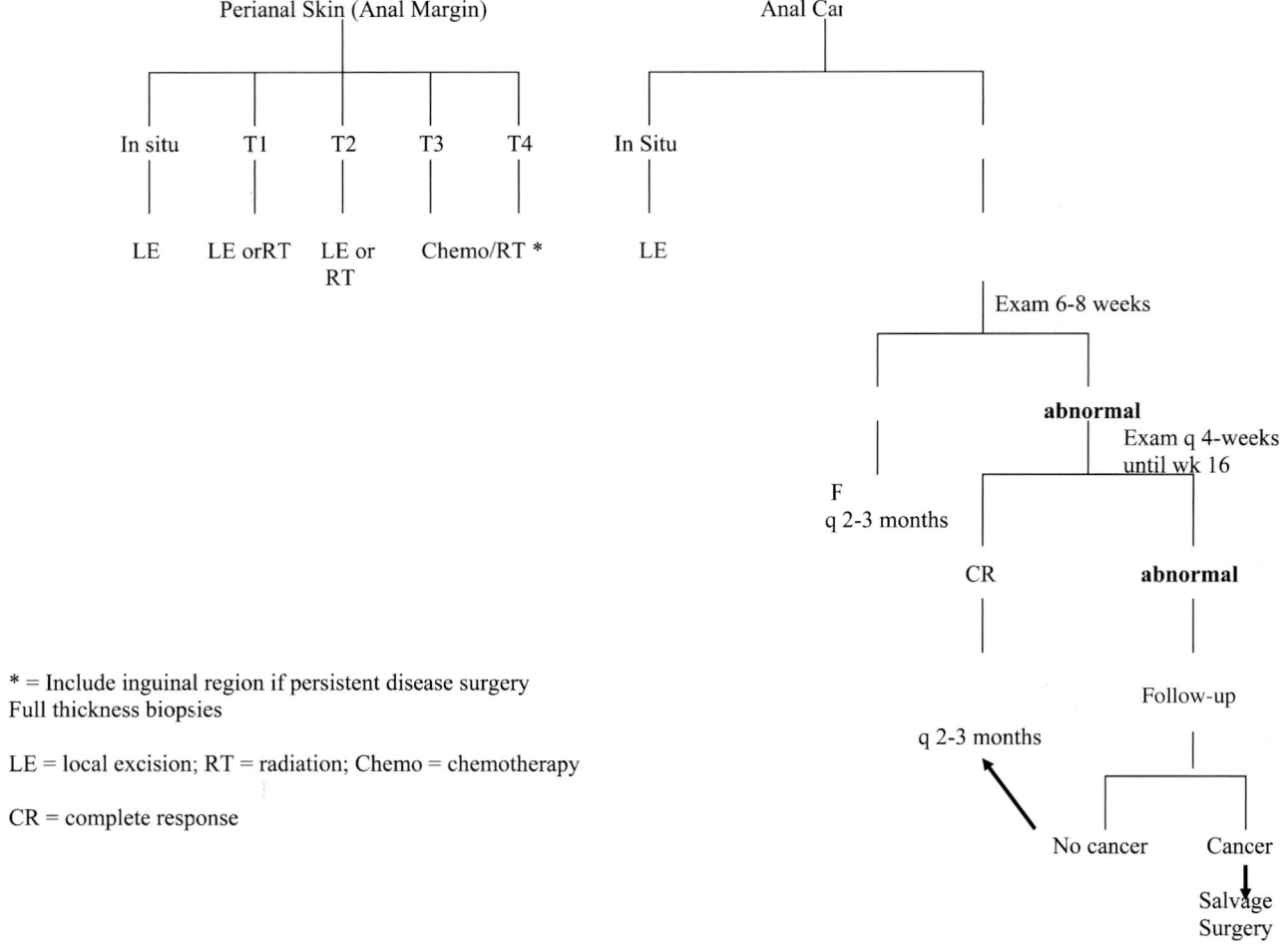

* = Include inguinal region if persistent disease surgery
Full thickness biopsies

LE = local excision; RT = radiation; Chemo = chemotherapy

CR = complete response

Figure 3 Management of squamous cell anal cancer.

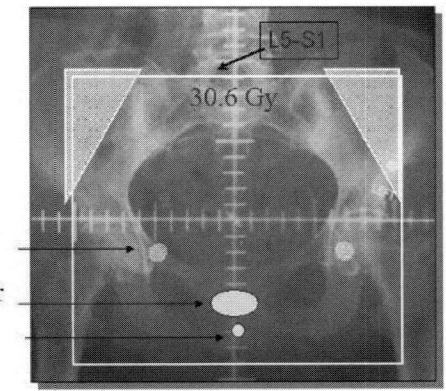

Figure 4 Recommended radiation technique: Initial Fields (Dose: 30.6 Gy at 1.8 Gy per day). All patients will initially be treated with either opposed anterior and posterior fields encompassing the pelvic, anus, perineum, and inguinal lymph nodes. Either prone or supine positioning is acceptable. The superior border of the AP/PA fields is placed at the top of the L5 vertebral body and the inferior border is placed at least 2.5 cm below the most inferior portion of the primary tumor or anal verge (whichever is lower). The lateral borders of the anterior and posterior fields are placed 1 cm lateral to the bony acetabulum to encompass the medial inguinal lymph nodes.

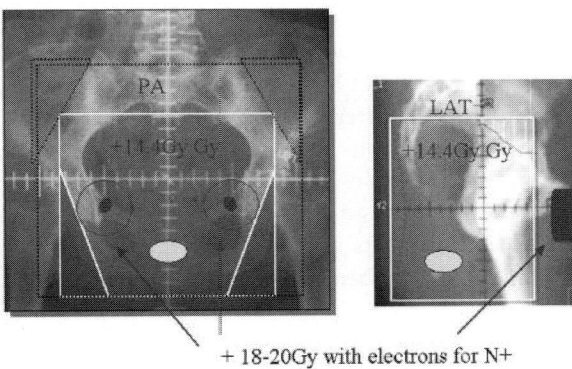

Figure 5 Reduced pelvic field (Dose: 14.4 Gy in 8 fractions for a total pelvic dose of 45 Gy at 1.8 Gy/day). A three-field technique (posterior field and right and left wedged lateral fields) is recommended for this reduction. The superior border of the posterior field is reduced to level of the greater sciatic notch (the inferior border of the sacroiliac joints) and the lateral borders will be placed 1.5 to 2.0 cm lateral to the pelvic brim. The femoral heads must be blocked in the PA field. The inferior border shall be unchanged from the initial fields. In the lateral fields, the superior and inferior borders will be the same as the posterior field, the posterior border will be placed 1 cm behind the sacrum and the anterior border will be placed 1 to 2 cm behind the pubic symphysis. The fields must cover all gross disease and increased if necessary for unusually large tumors. Because the inguinal lymph nodes will be treated only in the initial fields (30.6 Gy), a boost technique will be required to a higher dose if the inguinal lymph nodes ≥ 1 cm at presentation. In that case, the goal is to treat inguinal nodes to a total dose of 55 Gy. This can usually be accomplished using electron supplementation from anterior electron fields.

limitations of local failure in T3/T4 patients and distant failure in N2/N3 patients were identified. To address this, we have increased the total radiation dose to 59 Gy for T3/T4 patients. Presently we have a Phase II trial evaluating capecitabine and oxaliplatin with concurrent radiation in patients with Stage II and III anal cancer.

Importantly, we examine our patients 8 weeks after chemoradiation so that persistent disease can be identified for a salvage operation. If there is suspected persistent disease clinically, we follow our patients every 4 to 6 weeks up to 16 weeks post therapy prior to performing biopsies. Biopsies performed sooner can be falsely positive for active disease and depending on the location, biopsy of irradiated tissue can result in fistula, ulceration, or infection. If the area in question is responding clinically, the patients are closely observed with a very low threshold to perform biopsies. Hallmark signs of active disease are an enlarging mass, pain in the anal canal, bleeding, and ulceration of the mucosa during this critical follow-up period. If there is persistent cancer on biopsies, then these patients proceed to radical surgery.

Persistent or recurrent SCC of the anal canal

Persistent disease after multimodality treatment for anal canal SCC has been defined by most as disease diagnosed within 6 months of completion of multimodality chemoradiation therapy. SCC diagnosed 6 months after a complete clinical response following chemoradiation is considered recurrent disease. Although further radiation with chemotherapy has been utilized as conservative salvage therapy for recurrent or persistent SCC of the anal canal, radical surgery is the procedure of choice. In a retrospective study conducted at the Veterans Administration Hospitals, 53% of the patients treated with salvage abdominoperineal resection were alive versus 19% of those treated with radiation alone or combined chemoradiation.[29]

Radical surgery for persistent or recurrent disease commonly entails an abdominoperineal resection or an exenterative procedure.[1] In general, the most common pattern of failure after surgical treatment is locoregional. In females, the posterior vaginal wall has been reported to be the site of recurrent disease in over 50% of patients whose primary treatment was abdominoperineal resection and thus, an en bloc posterior vaginectomy has been advocated in female patients at the time of abdominoperineal resection.[30] In males, the most common site of failure is the pelvis and perineum. It is important to note that recurrent SCC is infiltrative, and at times, negative margins of resections are not obtained. Needless to say, an involved margin of resection implies a dire prognosis and all attempts should be made to obtain complete clearance at the margins of resection. If available, intraoperative radiation can be utilized, but the surgeon should not rely on this modality to address the unfortunate situation of an involved margin. In multivariate analysis, a positive resection margin has been reported to be the strongest predictor of survival after salvage surgery for anal cancer.[31] If in the preoperative period it is concluded that negative margins will not be achieved by radical surgery, then the salvage procedure should not be performed. The morbidity and potential interference with quality of life outweigh the benefits, if any, of an incomplete resection.

Results after salvage surgery for persistent or recurrent disease vary, but in general the overall 5-year survival rate is approximately 40 to 50% and the local recurrence rate is approximately 60% (Table 4). The most common major morbidity after salvage abdominoperineal resection is related to the perineal wound. Nonhealing perineal wounds and wound infections occur in up to 60% of the patients.[30,32] In our experience, myocutaneous flaps, such as rectus abdominis and gracilis or posterior thigh, are extremely useful to obliterate the pelvic space and reconstruct the vagina and perineum. We therefore include our plastic surgery colleagues in the planning of the salvage procedure for the reconstruction. At times when musculocutaneous flaps are not available, the omentum may be used to obliterate the resulting pelvic defect. Figure 6 illustrates an algorithm for the management of these patients.

Management of Inguinal Lymph Node Metastases

The incidence of inguinal lymph node involvement is related to the tumor size and histology.[15] In anal carcinoma, the incidence of lymph node metastasis has

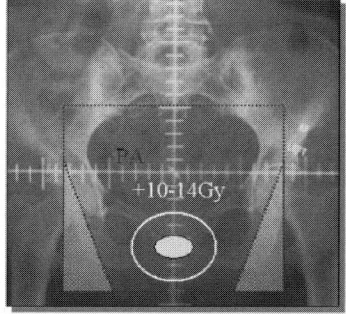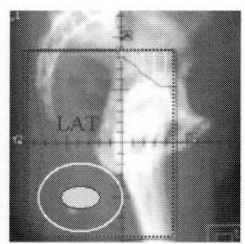

Figure 6 Primary tumor boost (10 Gy in 5 fractions for T_2 tumors and 14 Gy in 7 fractions for T_3-T_4 tumors). The boost will be delivered with the same field arrangement as the second phase of treatment (using 3 fields). A 2.5 cm margin in the posterior and the lateral fields should be placed around all initially involved gross tumor (including pelvic lymphadenopathy > 1 cm).

been reported to be between 15 and 63%.[5] For the most accurate staging, suspicious lymph nodes or abnormally enlarged lymph nodes should be evaluated by fine-needle aspiration (FNA) or image-guided biopsy. However, any lymph node greater than 1 cm in size on CT scan should be presumed to be positive and boosted with additional doses of radiation regardless of the FNA results. Rarely is an open biopsy indicated. The use of sentinel lymph node techniques have been reported,[33] but because chemoradiation is extremely effective for microscopic and small gross lymph node metastases, the accurate nodal staging is not essential, particularly if it adds increased morbidity risks.

Retrospective reports indicate that radiation alone or in combination with chemotherapy will control inguinal lymph node metastases in approximately 65 to 90% of the patients.[34] Therefore, (chemo)radiation is the treatment of choice for metastatic squamous cell cancer of the anus metastatic to the inguinal nodes. In patients who have persistent disease, consideration should be given for

Table 4 Selected Series of Salvage Surgery after Conservative Therapy for Anal Squamous Cell Carcinoma

Author	Year	Patients	Salvage Surgery	Follow-Up Months (Media)	Overall Survival Rate % 3-year	Overall Survival Rate % 5-year	Overall Recurrence Rate (%)	Local Recurrence Rate (%)
Ellerhorn JD et al[32]	1994	38	APR	47		44	61	66*
Pocard M et al[39]	1998	21	APR	40		33	61	NS
van der Wal BC et al[40]	2001	17	APR/PPE	53		47 (44 DFS)	62	62**
Smith AJ et al[41]	2001	22	APR	19 ***	72			81
Nilsson PJ et al[42]	2002	35	APR	33	52		42	93
Renehan AG et al[31]	2005	73	APR/TPE/LE		55	40		
Ghouti L et al[43]	2005	36	APR	67		69	64	70

*Pelvic recurrence; **5/13 patients with recurrence, 5 patients pelvis or groin and 3 patients pelvis and distant; ***Follow-up from salvage APR to death;^ anal margin and anal canal.
APR = abdominoperineal resection; LE = local excision; PPE = posterior pelvic exenteration; TPE = total pelvic exenteration.

inguinal lymph node dissection. Metachronous inguinal lymph node metastases should be initially managed by combined modality therapy in patients who have not reached the maximum radiation tissue tolerance, with surgery reserved for persistent disease. In patients with metachronous metastatic disease, the 5-year survival rate after therapeutic lymph node dissection has been reported to be over 50%.[35] However, the surgical morbidity of a groin dissection in radiated tissue should not be taken lightly.

Chemoradiation in HIV patients

HIV-positive patients whose CD4 count is greater than 200/μL and who do not have signs or symptoms of any other HIV-related diseases should be treated with full dose chemoradiation for their anal cancers.[18] The treating physician should understand that these patients may require dose reductions during therapy, thus they need to be followed closely during therapy. Patients whose CD4 counts are less than 200/μL or who have evidence of any other HIV-related disease should not be treated with full dose chemoradiation at the start of treatment.[18] The clinician needs to be alert for toxicities in these patients because any toxicity from treatment in immunocompromised patients can result in death. It is important that the patients continue to take their antiretroviral medications while on treatment. Multimodality treatment in these individuals remains challenging.

References

1. Skibber J, Rodriguez-Bigas MA, Gordon PH. Surgical considerations in anal cancer. Surg Oncol Clin N Am 2004; 13:321–38.

2. Dujovny N, Quiros RM, Saclarides TJ. Anorectal anatomy and embryology. Surg Oncol Clin N Am 2004;13:277–93.

3. Jemal A, Murray T, Ward E, et al. Cancer statistics, 2005. CA Cancer J Clin 2005;55:10–30.

4. Cress RD, Holly EA. Incidence of anal cancer in California: increased incidence among men in San Francisco, 1973–1999. Prev Med 2003;36:555–60.

5. Rousseau DL Jr, Petrelli NJ, Kahlenberg MS. Overview of anal cancer for the surgeon. Surg Oncol Clin N Am 2004; 13:249–62.

6. Frisch M, Glimelius B, van den Brule AJ, et al. Sexually transmitted infection as a cause of anal cancer. N Engl J Med 1997;337:1350–8.

7. Abbasakoor F, Boulos PB. Anal intraepithelial neoplasia. Br J Surg 2005;92:277–90.

8. Scholefield JH, Sonnex C, Talbot IC, et al. Anal and cervical intraepithelial neoplasia: possible parallel. Lancet 1989;2: 765–9.

9. Welton ML, Sharkey FE, Kahlenberg MS. The etiology and epidemiology of anal cancer. Surg Oncol Clin N Am 2004; 13:263–75.

10. Beahrs OH, Wilson SM. Carcinoma of the anus. Ann Surg 1976;184:422–8.

11. Fuchshuber PR, Rodriguez-Bigas M, Weber T, Petrelli NJ. Anal canal and perianal epidermoid cancers. J Am Coll Surg 1997;185:494–505.

12. Green FL, Page DL, Fleming ID, et al, editors. AJCC Cancer Staging Handbook. 6th ed. New York: Springer-Verlag, Inc., 2002. p. 139–44.

13. Marfing TE, Abel ME, Gallagher DM. Perianal Bowen's disease and associated malignancies. Results of a survey. Dis Colon Rectum 1987;30:782–5.

14. Marchesa P, Fazio VW, Oliart S, et al. Perianal Bowen's disease: a clinicopathologic study of 47 patients. Dis Colon Rectum 1997;40:1286–93.

15. Mendenhall WM, Zlotecki RA, Vauthey JN, Copeland EM 3rd. Squamous cell carcinoma of the anal margin. Oncology (Williston Park). 1996;10:1843–8; discussion 1848, 1853–44.

16. Ortholan C, Ramaioli A, Peiffert D, et al. Anal canal carcinoma: early-stage tumors < or =10 mm (T1 or Tis): therapeutic options and original pattern of local failure after radiotherapy. Int J Radiat Oncol Biol Phys 2005;62: 479–85.

17. Ryan DP, Mayer RJ. Anal carcinoma: histology, staging, epidemiology, treatment. Curr Opin Oncol 2000;12:345–52.

18. Eng C, Abbruzzese J, Minsky BD. Chemotherapy and radiation of anal canal cancer: the first approach. Surg Oncol Clin N Am 2004;13:309–20, viii.

19. Nigro ND, Vaitkevicius VK, Considine B Jr. Combined therapy for cancer of the anal canal: a preliminary report. Dis Colon Rectum 1974;17:354–6.

20. Shank B, Enker WE, Flam MS. Neoplasms of the anus. In: Kufe DW, Pollock RE, Weichselbaum RC, et al, editors. Holland-Frei Cancer Medicine, 6th ed. Hamilton: B.C. Decker; 2003:1667–74.

21. Epidermoid anal cancer. results from the UKCCCR randomised trial of radiotherapy alone versus radiotherapy, 5-fluorouracil, and mitomycin. UKCCCR Anal Cancer Trial Working Party. UK Co-ordinating Committee on Cancer Research. Lancet 1996;348:1049–54.

22. Bartelink H, Roelofsen F, Eschwege F, et al. Concomitant radiotherapy and chemotherapy is superior to radiotherapy alone in the treatment of locally advanced anal cancer: results of a phase III randomized trial of the European Organization for Research and Treatment of Cancer

Radiotherapy and Gastrointestinal Cooperative Groups. J Clin Oncol 1997;15:2040–9.

23. Flam M, John M, Pajak TF, et al. Role of mitomycin in combination with fluorouracil and radiotherapy, and of salvage chemoradiation in the definitive nonsurgical treatment of epidermoid carcinoma of the anal canal: results of a phase III randomized intergroup study. J Clin Oncol 1996;14:2527–39.

24. Doci R, Zucali R, La Monica G, et al. Primary chemoradiation therapy with fluorouracil and cisplatin for cancer of the anus: results in 35 consecutive patients. J Clin Oncol 1996;14:3121–5.

25. Peiffert D, Giovannini M, Ducreux M, et al. High-dose radiation therapy and neoadjuvant plus concomitant chemotherapy with 5-fluorouracil and cisplatin in patients with locally advanced squamous-cell anal canal cancer: final results of a phase II study. Ann Oncol 2001;12:397–404.

26. Meropol NJ, Niedzwiecki D, Shank B, et al. Combined-modality therapy of poor prognosis anal canal carcinoma: a phase II study of the Cancer and Leukemia Group B. Gastrointestinal Cancers Symposium. Am Soc Clin Oncol 2005;a238.

27. Ajani JA, Winter KA, Gunderson LL, et al. Intergroup RTOG 98-11: A phase III randomized study of 5-fluorouracil (5-FU), mitomycin, and radiotherapy versus 5-fluorouracil, cisplatin and radiotherapy in carcinoma of the anal canal. J Clin Oncol, 2006 ASCO Annual Meeting Proc (Post-Meeting Edition) 2006;24(18S):4009.

28. Hung A, Crane C, Delclos M, et al. Cisplatin-based combined modality therapy for anal carcinoma: a wider therapeutic index. Cancer 2003;97:1195–202.

29. Longo WE, Vernava AM 3rd, Wade TP, et al. Recurrent squamous cell carcinoma of the anal canal. Predictors of initial treatment failure and results of salvage therapy. Ann Surg 1994;220:40–9.

30. Singh R, Nime F, Mittelman A. Malignant epithelial tumors of the anal canal. Cancer 1981;48:411–5.

31. Renehan AG, Saunders MP, Schofield PF, O'Dwyer ST. Patterns of local disease failure and outcome after salvage surgery in patients with anal cancer. Br J Surg 2005;92:605–14.

32. Ellerhorn JD, Enker WE, Quan SH. Salvage abdominoperineal resection following combined chemotherapy and radiotherapy for epidermoid carcinoma of the anus. Ann Surg Oncol 1994;1:105–10.

33. Peley G, Farkas E, Sinkovics I, et al. Inguinal sentinel lymph node biopsy for staging anal cancer. Scand J Surg 2002;91:336–8.

34. Shank B, Cunningham JD, Kelsen DP. Cancer of the anal region. In: DeVita DT, Hellman S, Rosenberg SA, editors. Cancer: principles and practices of oncology. Philadelphia: Lippincott-Raven; 1997. p. 1234–51.

35. Greenall MJ, Quan SH, Stearns MW, et al. Epidermoid cancer of the anal margin. Pathologic features, treatment, and clinical results. Am J Surg 1985;149:95–101.

36. Jensen SL, Hagen K, Harling H, et al. Long-term prognosis after radical treatment for squamous-cell carcinoma of the anal canal and anal margin. Dis Colon Rectum 1988;31:273–8.

37. Peiffert D, Bey P, Pernot M, et al. Conservative treatment by irradiation of epidermoid carcinomas of the anal margin. Int J Radiat Oncol Biol Phys 1997;39:57–66.

38. Pintor MP, Northover JM, Nicholls RJ. Squamous cell carcinoma of the anus at one hospital from 1948 to 1984. Br J Surg 1989;76:806–10.

39. Pocard M, Tiret E, Nugent K, et al. Results of salvage abdominoperineal resection for anal cancer after radiotherapy. Dis Colon Rectum 1998;41:1488–93.

40. van der Wal BC, Cleffken BI, Gulec B, et al. Results of salvage abdominoperineal resection for recurrent anal carcinoma following combined chemoradiation therapy. J Gastrointest Surg 2001;5:383–7.

41. Smith AJ, Whelan P, Cummings BJ, Stern HS. Management of persistent or locally recurrent epidermoid cancer of the anal canal with abdominoperineal resection. Acta Oncol 2001;40:34–6.

42. Nilsson PJ, Svensson C, Goldman S, Glimelius B. Salvage abdominoperineal resection in anal epidermoid cancer. Br J Surg 2002;89:1425–9.

43. Ghouti L, Houvenaeghel G, Moutardier V, et al. Salvage abdominoperineal resection after failure of conservative treatment in anal epidermoid cancer. Dis Colon Rectum 2005;48:16–22.

CHAPTER 36

MANAGEMENT OF DIFFERENTIATED THYROID CANCER

STEVEN I. SHERMAN, MD

It was estimated that nearly 26,000 individuals would be diagnosed in 2005 with carcinoma of the thyroid gland and that about 1,600 patients would die as a consequence of complications of these diseases or their treat-ments.[1] Now the eighth most commonly diagnosed malignancy in women, the age-adjusted incidence of thyroid carcinoma has risen faster than that of any other cancer, and the age-adjusted mortality is also among the most rapidly increasing.[2] Histologically, 80% and 14%, respec-tively, are either papillary or follicular carci-nomas, differentiated carcinomas that derive from the thyroid hormone producing follicular epithelial cells. Another 4% are medullary carcinoma, a neuroen-docrine malignancy, and the remaining 2% are the highly aggressive anaplastic car-cinoma. Rates of disease recur-rence and cancer-specific mortality are increased in patients with metastases, especially those with extra-cervical spread. In the Surveillance, Epidemiology, and End Results (SEER) report of 15,700 patients, the overall 10-year age- and gender-corrected survival rates were 98% for papillary, 92% for follicular, 80% for medullary, and 13% for anaplastic carcinoma.[3] Older age at diagnosis and wider spread of disease are associated with a worse prognosis, independent of the type of can-cer. Although differentiated carcinomas have a 2:1 female predominance, male gender confers a slightly worse prognosis.

Because of a lack of randomized compara-tive trials, decisions regarding the selection of treatments for these diseases are based largely on retrospective analyses and consensus recommendations.[4] Therapy routinely involves multiple modalities, including surgery and thyroid hormone, radioiodine (for differentiated tumors), and external radiation and chemotherapy for selected patients with advanced disease. However, the poor response to treatment for metastatic thyroid cancer has recently triggered a spate of clinical trials of newer thera-peutic strategies.

Diagnostic Evaluation of the Solitary Thyroid Nodule

The most common clinical presentation of a patient with thyroid carcinoma is with a solitary thyroid nodule (Table 1).[5] Ultrasonography, however, reveals clinically unsuspected nodules in up to 30% of individuals without palpable lesions, and multiple nodules are frequent. Sonographic criteria that increase the likelihood of malignancy include the presence of microcalcifications, hypoechogenicity, and increased intranodular vascular-ity.[6] In the setting of an unsuppressed serum thyroid-stimulating hor-mone (TSH) concentration, thyroid ultrasound followed by cytologic examina-tion of a fine-needle aspirate (FNA) of solitary nod-ules at least 1 cm in size is the most appropriate diagnostic procedure; in the setting of multiple nodules, those with suspicious sonographic appearances should be preferentially aspi-rated.[7] Papillary, medullary, and anaplastic carcinomas can be readily diagnosed on the basis of cytologic criteria; however, the dis-tinction between follicular carcinoma and benign follicular adenoma requires histologic demonstration of either invasion through the tumor capsule or vascular invasion. Fol-licular adenomas and carcinomas are therefore grouped together cytologically as indeterminate or suspi-cious follicular neoplasms. Up

Table 1 Differential Diagnosis of a Thyroid Nodule

Benign
    Macrofollicular colloid adenoma
    Adenomatoid hyperplasia
    Microfollicular adenoma
    Hurthle cell adenoma
    Hashimoto's thyroiditis
    Graves' disease
    Infection
    Cyst
    Infiltrative and granulomatous disease
Malignant
    Differentiated carcinoma (papillary, follicular, Hurthle cell)
    Medullary carcinoma
    Anaplastic carcinoma
    Thyroid lymphoma
    Metastatic carcinoma (breast, renal cell, lung, melanoma, colon, gastric)
Extrathyroidal Disease
    Parathyroid adenoma, cyst, or carcinoma
    Esophageal diverticulum
    Lipoma
    Aberrant subclavian artery

to 25% of aspira-tions are inadequate or nondiagnostic, largely because of aspiration of cystic, hemorrhagic, or hypocellular colloid nodules.[8] The false-positive and false-negative rates for nodules characterized as "malig-nant" and "benign," respectively, are less than 5%.[9] For suspicious follicular lesions, the overall rate of carcinoma is approximately 20%, with higher rates associated with larger nodule size, older age, and male gender.[10–12] Intraopera-tive frozen section evaluation adds little to the evaluation of follicular neoplasms, but may occasionally be helpful to confirm the diagnosis of cytologically suspected papillary carci-noma.[13,14] For nod-ules in which FNA yields inad-equate diagnostic material, repeat aspiration, particularly with ultrasono-graphy guidance, can augment the accuracy of the procedure.[15]

By radionuclide scanning, malignant thyroid lesions are usually hypofunctioning or "cold," but this finding is both nonspecific and nondiag-nostic. In contrast, a "hot" hyperfunctioning nodule-causing thyrotoxicosis is highly likely to be a benign follicular adenoma. Thus, only patients with a suppressed TSH should undergo radioiodine scanning to determine the function of significant nodules, and FNA should only be performed for nonfunctioning lesions. Other imaging procedures, such as com-puted tomography (CT), magnetic reso-nance imaging (MRI), and positron emission tomogra-phy (PET) have no role in the routine diagnostic evaluation of thyroid nodules.

Pathogenesis

The only well-established risk factor for differentiated thyroid cancer is radia-tion exposure, especially during infancy.[16] Exter-nal radiation, delivered therapeutically decades ago for benign conditions, such as thymic and tonsillar enlargement, and currently for malig-nant diseases, such as Hodgkin's lymphoma and before bone marrow transplantation, is associated with an excess relative risk for thyroid malignancy of 3 to 9 per Gy. Exposure to inter-nal sources of radiation after the Chernobyl nuclear accident led to a 3- to 75-fold increase in the incidence of papillary carcinoma, the highest risks seen in younger children.[17] Although nuclear weapon testing and other sources of radiation fallout have affected large areas of the US, follow-up studies have yet to identify definite evidence of increased rates of thyroid cancer.[18,19]

Differentiated carcinoma is a component of several inherited syndromes, including familial adenomatous polyposis, Gardner syndrome, Cowden disease, Turcot syndrome, and Carney complex. Familial nonmedullary carcinoma, described in families with at least two first-degree relatives with the disease, has been reported in 5% of all papillary carcinoma patients, and may portend a more-aggressive disease course.[20–23]

Pathologic Features

Papillary carcinomas are characterized by the presence of papillae con-sisting of a well-defined fibrovascular core sur-rounded by one or two layers of tumor cells. Follicles and colloid are typically absent. Nuclei tend to be large, oval, and appear crowded and overlapping on micro-scopic sections. The nuclei contain hypodense powdery chromatin, cytoplasmic pseudoinclusions caused by a redun-dant nuclear membrane, and nuclear grooves. Indi-vidually, these features are not pathognomonic of papillary carcinoma, but in combination they define the disease. About one-half of papillary car-cinomas contain calcified psammoma bodies, which are the scarred and calcified remnants of tumor papillae that presumably infarcted.

Of the several histologic subtypes, the follic-ular variant accounts for approximately 10% of all papillary carcinomas.[24] The cells are orga-nized into follicles rather than papillae, but cyto-logically they display the typical nuclear fea-tures of papillary carcinomas. Rates of recurrence and survival with the follicular vari-ant are very similar to those of patients with common-type papillary carcinomas. In contrast, the tall-cell variant of papillary carcinoma is a more aggres-sive tumor, characterized by tumor cells with eosinophilic cytoplasm that are twice as tall as they are wide.[25] The primary tumors tend to be large, are often invasive, and frequently have both local and distant metastases at the time of diagnosis. The 5-year survival rate is 75 to 85%.

Follicular carcinomas are distinguished from benign follicular lesions on the basis of invasive-ness. These tumors are commonly encapsulated, and invasion can commonly be demonstrated in one or more foci along the capsule or across vas-cular endothelial walls. Semiquantitative assess-ment of the magnitude of invasion can separate follicular carcinomas into mini-mally invasive and widely invasive lesions; a minimally inva-sive follicular carcinoma has only scattered foci of capsular or vascular invasion. Cytologic fea-tures do not reliably distinguish benign from malignant follicular lesions.

Hurthle cell neoplasms are formed by cells containing numerous mitochondria, which impart a granular, eosinophilic appearance to their cytoplasm.[26] Most have a follicular archi-tecture and are diagnosed as adenomas or carci-nomas by the same criteria applied to other fol-licular neoplasms. A Hurthle-cell variant of papillary carcinoma is much less common and tends to be more aggressive than typical papil-lary carcinomas.

Insular carcinomas are often placed in the category of poorly differentiated thyroid carci-nomas, which implies a status between that of differentiated and anaplastic carcinomas. Insu-lar carcinomas generally concentrate radioio-dine and are therefore treated as differentiated cancers. They are formed by small cells with variable mitotic activity, arranged in nests, with foci of necrosis.

Clinicopathologic Staging

Although multiple clinicopathologic staging schemes exist for differentiated thyroid carcinoma, the sixth edition of the TNM (tumor, node, metastasis) staging approach (Table 2) is generally recommended for use; however, evidence for a superior value for predicting death caused by thyroid can-cer has only been reported for the previous fifth edition.[27] Both TNM versions classify patients with distant metastases but who are under the age of 45 years as being at "low risk" for death, one of several significant caveats to clinical use of these schemes. The importance of histologic features such as tumor size and extrathyroidal invasion underscore the need for pathologists to report these data uniformly on thyroidectomy specimens.[28,29]

Primary Surgical Management

Total thyroidectomy is the preferred initial surgical procedure for most patients with differentiated thyroid carcinoma, as supported by these arguments: (1) foci of papillary carcinoma are found in both thyroid lobes in 60 to 85% of patients; (2) 5 to 10% of recurrences of papillary carcinoma after unilateral surgery occur in the contralateral lobe, with subsequent high risk of disease-related death; and (3) the efficacy of therapy with radioiodine and the specificity of serum thyroglobulin levels as a tumor marker are max-imized by resection of as much thyroid tissue as possible.[30–32] In contrast, the major argument put forth to support a unilateral procedure is the risk for more complications following bilateral surgery, including hypoparathyroidism and recurrent laryngeal nerve paralysis. In a retrospective analysis of the outcomes of 1,685 low-risk patients, the 20-year recurrence rate after lobectomy was 22%, compared with 8% for patients treated with total thy-roidectomy.[33] Other retrospective studies (although not all) reported similar results of reduced recurrence.[34–36] Most recently, analysis of a multicenter prospective thyroid cancer registry database has demonstrated improved survival associated with total or near-total thyroidectomy in patients with stages II to IV.[37]

In the absence of prospective trials, consensus recommendations have generally recommended that a near-total or total thyroidectomy should be performed if the primary papillary carcinoma or Hurthle cell carci-noma is at least 1 cm in diameter, if there is extrathyroidal exten-sion of tumor, or if there are metastases.[4,38] This operation should also be performed in patients with a history of exposure to ionizing radiation of the head and neck.[39] In selected patients whose papillary tumor is < 1 cm in diameter and confined to one lobe of the gland, a unilateral lobectomy may be sufficient. For patients with a cytologically suspicious follicular neoplasm, unilateral lobec-tomy and isthmusectomy should be performed; a complete thyroidectomy is done if there is a diagnosis of malignancy.

Although microscopic regional nodal metas-tasis of papillary carcinoma occurs in up to 80% of patients, only about 35% have cervical or mediastinal node metastasis grossly detectable at the time of surgery, most commonly found in lateral cervical compartments.[40–42] Lymph node metastasis is only a minor risk factor for mortality, although bulky nodes or a large number of involved nodes may be more significant.[43,44] Whereas resection of bilateral central, level VI nodes has been associated with improved survival, a meta-analysis of nine studies demonstrated no rela-tionship between the lateral lymph node status at pre-sentation and survival.[40,45] However, incomplete resection of metastatic lateral nodes may portend an increased risk of tumor recur-rence.[46–48] Thus, routine central compartment (level VI) neck dis-

Table 2 TNM Classification, Version 6

T: tumor status	
T1	< 2 cm
T2	2–4 cm
T3	> 4 cm, or minimal extraglandular invasion
T4	extraglandular invasion
T4a	gross invasion
T4b	prevertebral, carotid, or mediastinal invasion
Tx	tumor status cannot be determined
N: regional node status	
N0	no nodes involved
N1a	cervical level VI nodes positive
N1b	unilateral, contralateral, or bilateral levels II-V or VII nodes positive
Nx	node status cannot be determined
M: distant metastasis status	
M0	no distant metastasis
M1	distant metastasis present
Mx	distant metastases cannot be determined

Stage Assignments	< 45 years old	≥ 45 years old
Stage I	Any T, any N, M0	T1, N0, M0
Stage II	Any T, any N, M1	T2, N0, M0
Stage III		T3-4, N0, M0
		Any T, N1a, M0
Stage IV		A: T4a, any N, M0
		Any T, N1b, M0
		B: T4b, any N, M0
		C: Any T, any N, M1

TNM = tumor node metastases.
Adapted from Greene et al.[27]

section should be performed at the time of thyroidectomy and compartment-oriented modified radical lateral dissections if node involvement is identified.

In the presence of invasion of aerodigestive tract structures, similar survival rates are achieved from either complete surgical resection or shave excision leaving only micro-scopic residual disease.[49] In the presence of frank cartilage destruction or intraluminal involvement of the aerodigestive tract structures, a shave excision cannot be performed without leaving gross tumor behind, leading to a 50% death rate within 4 years. Surgery in patients with extensively invasive thyroid carcinoma should therefore aim to remove all gross tumor, attempting to retain as much airway, vocal, and digestive function as possible. However, only if the tumor is unresectable or the patient does not agree to a radical resection should gross tumor be left behind in the neck.

Postoperative Adjuvant Therapy

RADIOIODINE

Adjuvant ablation of residual thyroid tissue following primary surgery has two ratio-nales: (1) to destroy any residual microscopic foci of disease, and (2) to increase the speci-ficity and negative predictive value of subsequent serum thyroglobulin measurements and ^{131}I scanning for detection of recurrent or metastatic disease by eliminating residual nor-mal tissue. Conflicting data have been reported from multiple retrospective studies of the efficacy of radioiodine. In a recent meta analysis, only 1 of the 7 included studies reported improved survival following adjuvant radioiodine, and improved locoregional disease-free survival (DFS) in 3.[34,50] In the more recent multicenter thyroid cancer registry, improved survival was associated with postoperative radioiodine use in stages II to IV disease patients after adjustment for extent of thyroidectomy, and in stage III to IV patients when also adjusted for thyroid hormone suppression therapy.[37] For patients with residual disease following optimal surgery, including extracervical metastases, radioiodine therapy is also recommended. In contrast, ablation may be withheld for patients with small solitary primary tumors without evidence of extrathyroidal invasion or metastasis, particularly those under age 45 at diagnosis.

The efficacy of radioiodine depends on patient preparation, tumor-specific characteristics, sites of disease, and administered radioio-dine activity. Iodide uptake by thyroid tissue is stimulated by TSH and is suppressed by increased endogenous iodide stores. Following thyroidectomy, the patient's thyroid hormone lev-els must decline sufficiently to allow the TSH concentration to rise to above 25 to 30 mU/L.[51] This period of hormone withdrawal typically lasts 4 to 5 weeks. To minimize the resulting symptoms of hypothyr-oidism, the shorter-acting hormone liothyronine (T3) can be given at doses of 25 μg two times per day until 2 weeks prior to radioiodine dosing. Lower doses are administered to elderly patients and those with ischemic heart disease. An alternative to thyroid hormone with-drawal may be use of thyrotropin alfa, which in a recent, small randomized study appeared equivalent to thyroid hormone withdrawal for stimulating radioiodine uptake and successful ablation.[52] Patients should avoid foods with high iodine content for at least 2 weeks prior to the scanning.[53] For similar reasons, radioio-dine uptake can be iatrogenically suppressed for 1 to 3 months after administration of iodinated intravenous contrast for radiographic procedures. Urinary iodine content can be measured to confirm excessive iodine intake if suspected.

Whole-body radioiodine scans for localization of uptake prior to ablation or therapy are fre-quently performed 24 to 72 hours after administration of a diagnostic activity of 2 to 5 mCi of [131]I. Most patients demonstrate significant uptake of radioiodine within the thyroid bed following thy-roidectomy, presumably from normal residual thyroid. Greater sensitivity for the detection of residual or metastatic tumor can be attained with the use of higher amounts of [131]I. But larger radioisotope activities can lead to "stunning," in which reduced uptake of the subsequent ablative or therapeutic dose occurs as a consequence of radiation delivered by the diagnostic dose.[54,55] Use of ^{123}I, with a lower radiation dose to thyroid tissue, may prevent stunning of therapeutic uptake after a diagnostic scan without loss of diagnostic accuracy.[56] However, the exact utility of scanning before therapy in the absence of known metastatic disease is undefined, and therefore scanning before ablation may be considered optional for such patients.[57] An alternative approach is to use a low activity of ^{123}I to measure radioiodine uptake in the thyroid bed before treatment, without requiring greater activities necessary for imaging.

With postoperative radioiodine uptake in the thyroid bed, or if no pretherapy scanning or uptake has been performed, an empirically selected activity of 131I is administered for adjuvant ablation, typi-cally 30 to 100 mCi. In general, higher efficacy rates have been reported with larger administered activities. Assuming that the 24-hour radioiodine uptake is less than 5%, this lower activity has a similar efficacy of successful abla-tion and could be considered for patients with dis-ease entirely confined to the thyroid gland.[58,59] Nonetheless, there is scant information about long-term outcomes, and considerably more study is required before such low doses can be generally recommended. When substantial yet unsuspected locore-gional disease or excessive thyroid remnants are detected, strong consideration is given to addi-tional surgery before radioiodine admin-istration.

A post-treatment scan is performed several days after administration of the radioiodine dose, but the diag-nostic utility of such scans immediately after ablative treatments is maximal in patients whose thyroid bed activity was previ-ously ablated.[54]

Thyroid Hormone

Patients require life-long thyroid hormone treatment to treat postsurgical hypothyroidism and to minimize TSH stimula-tion to tumor growth. With TSH-suppressive thy-roid hormone therapy, both overall survival (OS) and DFS may be improved two- to threefold, particularly in TNM or National Thyroid Cancer Treatment Cooperative Study (NTCTCS) stages III and IV patients.[37,60,61] Lesser degrees of suppression may also improve OS in stage I and II patients. However, potential morbidity from overly aggressive thyroid hormone suppression therapy includes acceleration of osteoporo-sis, provocation of atrial fibrillation, and possibly cardiac hypertrophy and dysfunction and impaired quality of life.[62–65] The clinician must balance the risk for disease recurrence or progression with the risk for thyrotoxic complica-tions in determining the degree of TSH-suppres-sive therapy. At least during the initial years of follow-up, patients at lower risk for thyroid can-cer morbidity and mortality should have their TSH levels maintained between 0.1 and 0.5 mU/L, whereas patients at higher risk should have TSH levels suppressed to less than 0.1 mU/L. Patients who remain disease-free for 5 to 10 years may potentially have their degree of TSH suppression reduced by lowering their doses of thyroid hormone; other mitigating factors, such as concurrent cardiac disease, may also dictate a need for reduced hormone dosing.

External Beam Radiation

External-beam radiotherapy (EBRT) may be an effective adju-vant therapy to prevent locoregional recurrence in older patients with locally invasive papillary car-cinoma. A review of 282 patients found that postoperative EBRT did not significantly affect the locoregional control of disease-specific sur-vival rates. However, in a subgroup of 155 patients with papillary histology and microscopic residual disease (evidence of disease at or within 2 mm of the resection margin, or tumor that was shaved off cervical structures), EBRT produced a significant improvement in 10-year rates of locoregional control (93% versus 78%) and disease-specific survival (100% versus 95%).[66] Increased freedom from locoregional and distant relapse has been reported in patients older than age 40 years with extrathyroidal extension and lymph node involvement from papillary carcinoma when treated with adjuvant EBRT in addition to total thyroidectomy, two courses of ^{131}I, and TSH suppression.[67] In neither study was a benefit of adjuvant EBRT demonstrated for patients with follicular carcinoma. Adjuvant EBRT is likely of little benefit to those younger than age 45 years, and esophageal and tracheal side effects may be poorly tolerated by the elderly patient (> 65 years). EBRT, 40 to 50 Gy to the thyroid bed, is recommended in the setting of gross extrathy-roidal invasion with presumed microscopic resid-ual disease as well as following incomplete resection near aerodigestive structures.

Long-Term Follow-Up: Diagnostic Imaging and Serum Thyroglobulin Monitoring

The follow-up paradigm for differentiated thyroid carcinomas has undergone significant changes in the past several years, in part due to the improved utility of cervical ultrasound and serum thyroglobulin measure-ments. Whereas patients following initial radioiodine ablation previously underwent routine periodic radio-iodine scanning, this procedure is now being used more selectively.[68]

Ultrasonography of the thyroid bed and cervi-cal node compartments can accurately identify locoregional metastases and recurrence measur-ing several millimeters in diameter and facilitate confirmatory FNA of such lesions.[47,69] Neither CT nor MRI is as sensitive for detect-ing such small lesions, although these techniques are more readily standardized and less operator dependent. Routine chest radiographs are of limited sensitiv-ity and probably can be avoided in low-risk patients.

The synthesis and secretion of thyroglobulin (Tg) is a differentiated characteristic of thyroid follicular cells. In the long-term follow-up of patients, measurement of the serum Tg concentration aids the detection of residual, recurrent, or metastatic disease, particularly given the rough correlation between tumor size and Tg level. After thyroid resection and ablation, serum Tg concentrations should approach the limits of assay detectability but may take several years to decline to an undetectable nadir following primary ther-apy.[70] An important factor in the interpretation of Tg concentrations is the concurrent level of TSH, given the dependence on TSH for Tg production. The sensitivity for detection of residual cancer is enhanced by eleva-tion of the serum TSH during thyroid hormone withdrawal or by the use of recombinant TSH (thyro-tropin alfa).[71] The sensitivity of detecting disease by measurement of Tg following TSH stimulation is 85 to 95% but may be as low as 50% during TSH suppression or with dedifferen-tiated tumors.[72] The utility of stimulated Tg measurements in the absence of scanning combined with cervical ultrasound has the greatest accuracy in low-risk patients, but radioiodine scanning remains valuable for follow-up in high-risk patients.[73,74]

In immunometric assays, reported Tg concen-trations can be falsely lowered by autoantibodies that bind Tg and prevent antigen interaction with assay's antibodies. For the 25% of the thyroid cancer population with anti-Tg autoantibodies, serum Tg levels must be interpreted with caution. The persistence of anti-Tg autoantibodies follow-ing thyroidectomy and radioiodine ablation may in itself indicate the presence of residual thyroid tissue and an increased risk for recurrence, although antibody persistence has been reported for up to 18 years after resection of a gland affected by Hashimoto's thyroiditis.[75,76]

Therapy of Metastatic Disease: Surgery

Function-preserving compartmental node dissection is pre-ferred, if possible, for patients with nodes > 1 cm in diameter. In the setting of disease invading aerodigestive structures, grossly complete surgical excision can improve survival, but may require more extensive procedures such as tracheal resection and anastamosis or pharyngectomy. Palliative procedures can be employed when curative resection is not feasible and can include tracheal stents, tracheotomy, and laser ablation in addition to partial excision. For extracervical metastases, sur-gical resection can lead to improved survival in selected patients.[77] In one report, nearly 30% of patients who underwent complete resection of their skeletal, pulmonary, or intra-abdominal metastases remained disease free after an average follow-up of 8 years.[78] Among patients with one or more brain metastases, surgical removal significantly improved med-ian survival from 4 to 22 months.[79] Symptom palliation can also result from surgical treatment, particularly for lesions causing pain or spinal cord compression.

Radioiodine

[131]I treatment of regional nodal metastases yields a complete response in 80% of patients when at least 8,000 to 10,000 cGy is delivered, but it can be suboptimal in patients with bulky disease.[80] Patients with resid-ual

postoperative disease in the thyroid bed or in the regional lymph nodes are treated with high activities of [131]I. Efficacy has been reported with 150 mCi as an average dose, either as a result of empiric therapy or as determined by dosimetry.

Patients treated for iodine-concentrating pul-monary metastases, which occur in approxi-mately 5% of cases of differentiated cancer, have a 5-year survival rate of 60 to 80% as compared with a 5-year survival rate of 30% for those whose tumors do not take up iodine.[81] Long-term survival is highest in those patients with pul-monary metastases seen on [131I] scanning but not seen on chest radiography or CT. Nevertheless, only a minority of patients with such micronodu-lar disease have a complete remission. Patients with macronodular pul-monary metastases seen on chest radiography but not detected by ^{131}I scanning have the worst prognosis, and only rarely respond to large doses of [131]I. Radioiodine activities of 150 to 175 mCi are rec-ommended for empiric treatment of pulmonary metastases. Advocates of dosimetry suggest treatment of distant metastases with the maximum tolerable doses, that is, that dose which delivers no more than 200 cGy to the red marrow and 80 to 120 mCi whole-body retention.[82] Such activities may exceed 300 to 400 mCi but are calculated to allow the greatest degree of tumor kill without dose-limiting toxicity. Skele-tal metastases often do not concentrate ^{131}I; complete resolution of disease occurs in fewer than 10% of treated patients and partial remis-sion in only 35%.[83] Patients with follicular car-cinoma may be more likely to respond. Empiric doses of 200 mCi are generally suggested for distant metastases outside the lungs. Following surgical debulking, radioiodine therapy can also be administered to patients with iodine-concentrat-ing intracerebral metastases.[79]

Acute and chronic complications of ^{131}I can limit the usefulness of this treatment. In the short-term, radiation thyroiditis, painless neck edema, sialoadenitis, and tumor hemorrhage or edema occur in 10 to 20% of patients, particu-larly when higher doses are given. The radiopro-tectant amifostine may prevent symptomatic reduction in long-term salivary gland function as a result of [131]I. Over the long-term, ^{131}I therapy may be associated with development of secondary malignancies, such as acute myelocytic leukemia, usually occurring between 2 and 10 years after therapy. The risk is considerably lower when the total blood dose per treatment is less than 2 Gy and when repeat treatments are given no more frequently than annually. Increased prevalence of cancers of the bladder, salivary gland, colon, and female breast has also been reported in patients, but with little agree-ment on the degree of absolute risk.[84,85] Oligospermia and transient ovarian failure also occur, but subsequent infertility is rare, except after high doses. Patients who receive repeated high radiation doses to the lung parenchyma from radioiodine treatment of diffuse pulmonary metastases rarely develop pulmonary fibrosis.

As production of Tg and incorporation of radioiodine represent distinct differentiated functions of follicular cells, metastatic disease can be suspected by the presence of a detectable serum Tg in the absence of radioiodine uptake. Such "false-negative" results occur in up to 15% of diagnostic radioiodine scans in patients with detect-able Tg levels following thyroid ablation. Because a high frequency of post-therapy scans demonstrate foci of radioiodine uptake com-bined with a subsequent decrease in the serum Tg level, it has been proposed that patients with elevated serum Tg and negative diagnostic radioiodine scans should receive empiric ^{131}I therapy with 100 to 300 mCi.[86] However, the underlying risk for disease-related morbidity or mortality in patients with scan-negative, Tg -positive disease is not well defined, particularly for patients without evidence of tumor mass by other imaging modalities. At present, there is no evidence that either partial reductions in serum Tg levels or elimination of radioiodine uptake visible only on post-therapy scans is associated with improved patient outcome, and Tg levels often decline over a period of years after the last radioiodine treatment.[87] The potential risks of repeated high-dose empiric therapy must be considered as well. Diagnostic imaging should be performed to identify foci of disease that could be surgically resected or treated by other means, such as cervical ultrasonography, CT, or MRI.[88,89] PET imaging following injection of fluoro-D-glucose can be particularly useful in localizing disease in patients with Tg levels greater than 10 ng/mL and negative radioiodine imaging. Given the propensity of follicular thyroid carcinoma to metastasize to bone, skeletal imaging with [99m]technetium pyrophosphate may also be of value. In the absence of surgically resectable disease, only patients with evidence of progres-sive metastases, patients with rising Tg levels greater than 10 ng/mL, or those who are at high risk for dis-ease-related mortality might receive a therapeu-tic trial of radioiodine before embarking on other systemic treat-ment modalities. However, for younger patients with stable or minimally elevated Tg lev-els and no radio-graphic evidence of disease, evi-dence of benefit is insufficient to warrant empiric radioiodine.

Biologic Modifiers of Radioiodine Responsiveness

Poor uptake and diminished retention of radioiodine are associated with tumor dedifferentiation and poor response to treatment. Certain histologic subtypes, such as Hurthle cell carcinoma and the tall-cell variant of papillary carcinoma, concentrate ^{131}I less effec-tively. Older patients and women may also be less likely to have adequate uptake in metastases. Restoration of respon-siveness to radioiodine therapy has therefore been a major goal of investigation during the past several years. Because lithium can increase iodine retention by thyroid tissue, it has been suggested that lithium administration can augment radiation dose in tumors with low iodine retention.[90] Whether these findings will result in improved eradication of metastases remains to be determined.

Loss of iodide uptake may be related to decreased expression of the sodium-iodide sym-porter in the tumor cells, which has been partially attributed to epigenetic alterations affecting gene expression. On the basis of the hypothesis that hypermethylation and/or histone deace-tylation affecting the promoter region of thyroid-specific transcription factors or the sodium-iodine symporter genes leads to decreased expression and loss of iodide uptake, it could be presumed that hypomethylation might restore iodide uptake. In vitro, increased iodide uptake has been demonstrated in dedifferentiated thyroid cancer cell lines treated with the demethylating agent 5-azacytidine or the histone deacetylase inhibitor, depsi-peptide.[91,92]

External-Beam Radiation

Patients with unresectable gross locally invasive or metastatic disease in the neck may also benefit from the addition of EBRT, as can patients with painful skeletal metastases. When surgical resection is not feasible, palliative radiation should be offered to patients with bone lesions that either cause pain or pose a risk for pathologic fracture. Radiation doses of 50 Gy in 25 fractions may be given for solitary lesions, but reduced doses should be administered for vertebral foci.[93]

Chemotherapy

Although 10 to 15% of patients with differentiated thyroid cancer die from their disease, and an even higher proportion suffer morbidity from recurrence, little progress has been made since the original reports of partial responses to doxoru-bicin in approximately one-third of patients. The best responses occur in patients with pulmonary metastases and high performance status, in whom dox-orubicin probably yields no greater than a 30% response rate for progressive differentiated cancers unresponsive to radioiodine. The recommended dose is 60 to 75 mg/m^2 every 3 weeks, administered as a contin-uous intravenous infusion for 48 to 72 hours to mini-

mize the risk of cardiac toxicity. Cumulative doses of up to 600 mg/m^2 can be administered in responsive patients. Other single chemothera-peutic agents that have been attempted include paclitaxel, bleomycin, cisplatin, car-boplatin, methotrexate, melphalan, mitoxantrone, etopo-side, and aclaru-bicin, without suggestion of improved response rates. In one comparative trial, the combination of doxorubicin (60 mg/m^2) and cisplatin (40 mg/m^2) induced complete or partial response in 16%, whereas doxorubicin alone yielded a 31% response rate.[94] Toxicities, including pancytopenia and gastroin-testinal side effects, are markedly more common and severe, however, during these combination therapies without clear evidence of greater ben-efit. More recently, multiple phase II studies have been initiated with therapies targeted at cellular mechanisms active in thyroid carcinoma, including small molecule tyrosine kinase inhibitors, proteasome inhibitors, and epigenetic modi-fiers. Given the marked increase in availability of such trials, it can now be recommended that patients with metastatic thyroid carcinoma unresponsive to radio-iodine should be considered for participation in clinical trials as an alternative to the currently available typical chemotherapeutic agents such as doxorubicin.

References

1. Jemal A, Murray T, Ward E, et al. Cancer statistics, 2005. CA Cancer J Clin 2005;55:10–30.

2. SEER Cancer Statistics Review, 1975–2001. National Cancer Institute, 2004. http://seer.cancer.gov/csr/1975_2001/ (accessed September 5, 2005).

3. Gilliland FD, Hunt WC, Morris DM, Key CR. Prognostic factors for thyroid carcinoma: a population-based study of 15,698 cases from the Surveillance, Epidemiology and End Results (SEER) program 1973–1991. Cancer 1997;79:564–73.

4. Sherman SI, Angelos P, Ball DW, et al. Thyroid carcinoma. J Natl Compr Canc Netw 2005;3:404–57.

5. Mandel SJ. A 64-year-old woman with a thyroid nodule. Jama 2004;292:2632–42.

6. Papini E, Guglielmi R, Bianchini A, et al. Risk of malignancy in nonpalpable thyroid nodules: predictive value of ultrasound and color-Doppler features. J Clin Endocrinol Metab 2002;87:1941–6.

7. Ravetto C, Colombo L, Dottorini ME. Usefulness of fine-needle aspiration in the diagnosis of thyroid carcinoma: a retrospective study in 37,895 patients. Cancer 2000;90:357–63.

8. Cochand-Priollet B, Guillausseau PJ, Chagnon S, et al. The diagnostic value of fine-needle aspiration biopsy under ultrasonography in nonfunctional thyroid nodules: a

prospective study comparing cytologic and histologic findings. Am J Med 1994;97:152–7.

9. Gharib H. Fine-needle aspiration biopsy of thyroid nodules: advantages, limitations, and effect. Mayo Clin Proc 1994;69:44–9.

10. Tyler DS, Winchester DJ, Caraway NP, et al. Indeterminate fine-needle aspiration biopsy of the thyroid. Identification of subgroups at high risk for invasive carcinoma. Surgery 1994;116:1054–60.

11. Tuttle RM, Lemar H, Burch HB. Clinical features associated with an increased risk of thyroid malignancy in patients with follicular neoplasia by fine-needle aspiration. Thyroid 1998;8:377–83.

12. Baloch ZW, Fleisher S, LiVolsi VA, Gupta PK. Diagnosis of "follicular neoplasm": a gray zone in thyroid fine-needle aspiration cytology. Diagn Cytopathol 2002;26:41–4.

13. Udelsman R, Westra WH, Donovan PI, et al. Randomized prospective evaluation of frozen-section analysis for follicular neoplasms of the thyroid. Ann Surg 2001;233:716–22.

14. Roach JC, Heller KS, Dubner S, Sznyter LA. The value of frozen section examinations in determining the extent of thyroid surgery in patients with indeterminate fine-needle aspiration cytology. Arch Otolaryngol Head Neck Surg 2002;128:263–7.

15. Cramer H. Fine-needle aspiration cytology of the thyroid: an appraisal. Cancer 2000;90:325–9.

16. Rubino C, Cailleux AF, De Vathaire F, Schlumberger M. Thyroid cancer after radiation exposure. Eur J Cancer 2002;38:645–7.

17. Pacini F, Vorontsova T, Demidchik EP, et al. Post-Chernobyl thyroid carcinoma in Belarus children and adolescents: comparison with naturally occurring thyroid carcinoma in Italy and France. J Clin Endocrinol Metab 1997;82:3563–9.

18. Gilbert ES, Tarone R, Bouville A, Ron E. Thyroid cancer rates and ^{131}I doses from Nevada atmospheric nuclear bomb tests. J Natl Cancer Inst 1998;90:1654–60.

19. Burke JP, Hay ID, Dignan F, et al. Long-term trends in thyroid carcinoma: a population-based study in Olmsted County, Minnesota, 1935–1999. Mayo Clin Proc 2005;80:753–8.

20. Maxwell EL, Hall FT, Freeman JL. Familial non-medullary thyroid cancer: a matched-case control study. Laryngoscope 2004;114:2182–6.

21. Hemminki K, Eng C, Chen B. Familial Risks for Non-Medullary Thyroid Cancer. J Clin Endocrinol Metab 2005.

22. Musholt TJ, Musholt PB, Petrich T, et al. Familial papillary thyroid carcinoma: genetics, criteria for diagnosis, clinical features, and surgical treatment. World J Surg 2000;24:1409–17.

23. Alsanea O, Wada N, Ain K, et al. Is familial non-medullary thyroid carcinoma more aggressive than sporadic thyroid cancer? A multicenter series. Surgery 2000;128:1043–50.

24. Tielens ET, Sherman SI, Hruban RH, Ladenson PW. Follicular variant of papillary thyroid carcinoma. A clinicopathologic study. Cancer 1994;73:424–31.

25. Machens A, Holzhausen HJ, Lautenschlager C, Dralle H. The tall-cell variant of papillary thyroid carcinoma: a multivariate analysis of clinical risk factors. Langenbecks Arch Surg 2004;389:278–82.

26. Lopez-Penabad L, Chiu AC, Hoff AO, et al. Prognostic factors in patients with Hurthle cell neoplasms of the thyroid. Cancer 2003;97:1186–94.

27. Greene FL, Page DL, Fleming ID, et al, editors. AJCC Cancer Staging Manual. 6th ed. New York: Springer-Verlag; 2002.

28. Sherman SI. Toward a standard clinicopathologic staging approach for differentiated thyroid carcinoma. Semin Surg Oncol 1999;16:12–5.

29. Association of Directors of Anatomic and Surgical Pathology. Recommended reporting format for thyroid carcinoma. Am J Clin Pathol 2000;114:684–6.

30. Machens A, Hinze R, Lautenschlager C, et al. Prophylactic completion thyroidectomy for differentiated thyroid carcinoma: prediction of extrathyroidal soft tissue infiltrates. Thyroid 2001;11:381–4.

31. Katoh R, Sasaki J, Kurihara H, et al. Multiple thyroid involvement (intraglandular metastasis) in papillary thyroid carcinoma. A clinicopathologic study of 105 consecutive patients. Cancer 1992;70:1585–90.

32. Silverberg SG, Hutter RVP, Foote Jr FW. Fatal carcinoma of the thyroid: Histology, metastases, and causes of death. Cancer 1970;25:792–802.

33. Hay ID, Grant CS, Bergstralh EJ, et al. Unilateral total lobectomy: is it sufficient surgical treatment for patients with AMES low-risk papillary thyroid carcinoma? Surgery 1998;124:958–64; discussion 64–6.

34. Mazzaferri EL, Jhiang SM. Long-term impact of initial surgical and medical therapy on papillary and follicular thyroid cancer. Am J Med 1994;97:418–28.

35. DeGroot LJ, Kaplan EL, Straus FH. Does the method of management of papillary thyroid carcinoma make a difference in outcome? World J Surg 1994;18:123–30.

36. Samaan NA, Schultz PN, Hickey RC, et al. The results of various modalities of treatment of well differentiated thyroid carcinoma: a retrospective review of 1,599 patients. J Clin Endocrinol Metab 1992;75:714–20.

37. Jonklaas J, Sarlis NJ, Litofsky D, et al. Outcomes of patients with differentiated thyroid carcinoma following initial therapy. [In press].

38. Thyroid Carcinoma Task Force. AACE/AAES medical/surgical guidelines for clinical practice: Management of thyroid carcinoma. Endocr Pract 2001;7:203–20.

39. Rubino C, Cailleux AF, Abbas M, et al. Characteristics of follicular cell-derived thyroid carcinomas occurring after external radiation exposure: results of a case control study nested in a cohort. Thyroid 2002;12:299–304.

40. Tisell LE, Nilsson B, Molne J, et al. Improved survival of patients with papillary thyroid cancer after surgical microdissection. World J Surg 1996;20:854–9.

41. Machens A, Holzhausen HJ, Lautenschlager C, et al. Enhancement of lymph node metastasis and distant metastasis of thyroid carcinoma. Cancer 2003;98:712–9.

42. Kupferman ME, Patterson M, Mandel SJ, et al. Patterns of lateral neck metastasis in papillary thyroid carcinoma. Arch Otolaryngol Head Neck Surg 2004;130:857–60.

43. Sugitani I, Kasai N, Fujimoto Y, Yanagisawa A. A novel classification system for patients with PTC: addition of the new variables of large (3 cm or greater) nodal metastases and reclassification during the follow-up period. Surgery 2004;135:139–48.

44. Leboulleux S, Rubino C, Baudin E, et al. Prognostic factors for persistent or recurrent disease of papillary thyroid carcinoma with neck lymph node metastases and/or tumor extension beyond the thyroid capsule at initial diagnosis. J Clin Endocrinol Metab 2005.

45. Grebe SK, Hay ID. Thyroid cancer nodal metastases: biologic significance and therapeutic considerations. Surg Oncol Clin N Am 1996;5:43–63.

46. Kouvaraki MA, Lee JE, Shapiro SE, et al. Preventable reoperations for persistent and recurrent papillary thyroid carcinoma. Surgery 2004;136:1183–91.

47. Kouvaraki MA, Shapiro SE, Fornage BD, et al. Role of preoperative ultrasonography in the surgical management of patients with thyroid cancer. Surgery 2003;134:946–54.

48. Gemsenjager E, Perren A, Seifert B, et al. Lymph node surgery in papillary thyroid carcinoma. J Am Coll Surg 2003;197:182–90.

49. Gillenwater AM, Goepfert H. Surgical management of laryngotracheal and esophageal involvement by locally advanced thyroid cancer. Semin Surg Oncol 1999;16:19–29.

50. Sawka AM, Thephamongkhol K, Brouwers M, et al. Clinical review 170: a systematic review and metaanalysis of the effectiveness of radioactive iodine remnant ablation for well-differentiated thyroid cancer. J Clin Endocrinol Metab 2004;89:3668–76.

51. Sanchez R, Espinosa-de-los-Monteros AL, Mendoza V, et al. Adequate thyroid-stimulating hormone levels after levothyroxine discontinuation in the follow-up of patients with well-differentiated thyroid carcinoma. Arch Med Res 2002;33:478–81.

52. Pacini F, Ladenson PW, Schlumberger M, et al. Radioiodine ablation of thyroid remnants after preparation with recombinant human thyrotropin in differentiated thyroid carcinoma: results of an international, randomized, controlled study. [In press].

53. Lakshmanan M, Schaffer A, Robbins J, et al. A simplified low iodine diet in I-131 scanning and therapy of thyroid cancer. Clin Nucl Med 1988;13:866–8.

54. Sherman SI, Tielens ET, Sostre S, et al. Clinical utility of posttreatment radioiodine scans in the management of patients with thyroid carcinoma. J Clin Endocrinol Metab 1994;78:629–34.

55. Muratet JP, Daver A, Minier JF, Larra F. Influence of scanning doses of iodine-131 on subsequent first ablative treatment outcome in patients operated on for differentiated thyroid carcinoma. J Nucl Med 1998;39:1546–50.

56. Mandel SJ, Shankar LK, Benard F, et al. Superiority of iodine-123 compared with iodine-131 scanning for thyroid remnants in patients with differentiated thyroid cancer. Clin Nucl Med 2001;26:6–9.

57. Cailleux AF, Baudin E, Travagli JP, et al. Is diagnostic iodine-131 scanning useful after total thyroid ablation for differentiated thyroid cancer? J Clin Endocrinol Metab 2000;85:175–8.

58. Logue JP, Tsang RW, Brierley JD, Simpson WJ. Radioiodine ablation of residual tissue in thyroid cancer: relationship between administered activity, neck uptake and outcome. Br J Radiol 1994;67:1127–31.

59. Bal CS, Kumar A, Pant GS. Radioiodine dose for remnant ablation in differentiated thyroid carcinoma: a randomized clinical trial in 509 patients. J Clin Endocrinol Metab 2004;89:1666–73.

60. McGriff NJ, Csako G, Gourgiotis L, et al. Effects of thyroid hormone suppression therapy on adverse clinical outcomes in thyroid cancer. Ann Med 2002;34:554–64.

61. Pujol P, Daures J-P, Nsakala N, et al. Degree of thyrotropin suppression as a prognostic determinant in differentiated thyroid cancer. J Clin Endocrinol Metab 1996;81:4318–23.

62. Stall GM, Harris S, Sokoll LJ, Dawson-Hughes B. Accelerated bone loss in hypothyroid patients overtreated with L-thyroxine. Ann Intern Med 1990;113:265–9.

63. Bauer DC, Ettinger B, Nevitt MC, et al. Risk for fracture in women with low serum levels of thyroid-stimulating hormone. Ann Intern Med 2001;134:561–8.

64. Sawin CT, Geller A, Wolf PA, et al. Low serum thyrotropin concentrations as a risk factor for atrial fibrillation in older persons. N Engl J Med 1994;331:1249–52.

65. Biondi B, Fazio S, Palmieri EA, et al. Effects of chronic subclinical hyperthyroidism from levothyroxine on cardiac morphology and function. Cardiologia 1999;44:443–9.

66. Tsang RW, Brierley JD, Simpson WJ, et al. The effects of surgery, radioiodine, and external radiation therapy on the clinical outcome of patients with differentiated thyroid carcinoma. Cancer 1998;82:375–88.

67. Farahati J, Geling M, Mader U, et al. Changing trends of incidence and prognosis of thyroid carcinoma in lower

Franconia, Germany, from 1981–1995. Thyroid 2004;14: 141–7.

68. Grigsby PW, Baglan K, Siegel BA. Surveillance of patients to detect recurrent thyroid carcinoma. Cancer 1999;85: 945–51.

69. Krishnamurthy S, Bedi DG, Caraway NP. Ultrasound-guided fine-needle aspiration biopsy of the thyroid bed. Cancer (Cytopathology) 2001;93:199–205.

70. Ozata M, Suzuki S, Miyamoto T, et al. Serum thyroglobulin in the follow-up of patients treated with differentiated thyroid cancer. J Clin Endocrinol Metab 1994;79:98–105.

71. Mazzaferri EL, Robbins RJ, Spencer CA, et al. A consensus report of the role of serum thyroglobulin as a monitoring method for low-risk patients with papillary thyroid carcinoma. J Clin Endocrinol Metab 2003;88:1433–41.

72. Haugen BR, Pacini F, Reiners C, et al. A comparison of recombinant human thyrotropin and thyroid hormone withdrawal for the detection of thyroid remnant or cancer. J Clin Endocrinol Metab 1999;84:3877–85.

73. Pacini F, Molinaro E, Castagna MG, et al. Recombinant human thyrotropin-stimulated serum thyroglobulin combined with neck ultrasonography has the highest sensitivity in monitoring differentiated thyroid carcinoma. J Clin Endocrinol Metab 2003;88:3668–73.

74. Robbins RJ, Chon JT, Fleisher M, et al. Is the serum thyroglobulin response to recombinant human thyrotropin sufficient, by itself, to monitor for residual thyroid carcinoma? J Clin Endocrinol Metab 2002;87:3242–7.

75. Spencer CA, Takeuchi M, Kazarosyan M, et al. Serum thyroglobulin autoantibodies: prevalence, influence on serum thyroglobulin measurement, and prognostic significance in patients with differentiated thyroid carcinoma. J Clin Endocrinol Metab 1998;83:1121–7.

76. Chiovato L, Latrofa F, Braverman LE, et al. Disappearance of humoral thyroid autoimmunity after complete removal of thyroid antigens. Ann Intern Med 2003;139(5 Pt 1):346–51.

77. Pak H, Gourgiotis L, Chang WI, et al. Role of metastasectomy in the management of thyroid carcinoma: the NIH experience. J Surg Oncol 2003;82:10–8.

78. Niederle B, Roka R, Schemper M, et al. Surgical treatment of distant metastases in differentiated thyroid cancer: indication and results. Surgery 1986;100:1088–97.

79. Chiu AC, Delpassand ES, Sherman SI. Prognosis and treatment of brain metastases in thyroid carcinoma. J Clin Endocrinol Metab 1997;82:3637–42.

80. Maxon HR, Englaro EE, Thomas SR, et al. Radioiodine-131 therapy for well-differentiated thyroid cancer —a quantitative radiation dosimetric approach: outcome and validation in 85 patients. J Nucl Med 1992;33:1132–6.

81. Ronga G, Filesi M, Montesano T, et al. Lung metastases from differentiated thyroid carcinoma. A 40 years' experience. Q J Nucl Med Mol Imaging 2004;48:12–9.

82. Furhang EE, Larson SM, Buranapong P, Humm JL. Thyroid cancer dosimetry using clearance fitting. J Nucl Med 1999;40:131–6.

83. Maxon HR, Smith HS. Radioiodine-131 in the diagnosis and treatment of metastatic well differentiated thyroid cancer. Endocrinol Metab Clin North Am 1990;19:685–718.

84. Rubino C, de Vathaire F, Dottorini ME, et al. Second primary malignancies in thyroid cancer patients. Br J Cancer 2003;89:1638–44.

85. Chen AY, Levy L, Goepfert H, et al. The development of breast carcinoma in women with thyroid carcinoma. Cancer 2001;92:225–31.

86. Schlumberger M, Mancusi F, Baudin E, Pacini F. 131I therapy for elevated thyroglobulin levels. Thyroid 1997;7: 273–6.

87. Fatourechi V, Hay ID, Javedan H, et al. Lack of impact of radioiodine therapy in tg-positive, diagnostic whole-body scan-negative patients with follicular cell-derived thyroid cancer. J Clin Endocrinol Metab 2002;87:1521–6.

88. Schluter B, Bohuslavizki KH, Beyer W, et al. Impact of FDG PET on patients with differentiated thyroid cancer who present with elevated thyroglobulin and negative 131I scan. J Nucl Med 2001;42:71–6.

89. Frilling A, Gorges R, Tecklenborg K, et al. Value of preoperative diagnostic modalities in patients with recurrent thyroid carcinoma. Surgery 2000;128:1067–74.

90. Koong SS, Reynolds JC, Movius EG, et al. Lithium as a potential adjuvant to 131I therapy of metastatic, well differentiated thyroid carcinoma. J Clin Endocrinol Metab 1999;84:912–6.

91. Kitazono M, Robey R, Zhan Z, et al. Low concentrations of the histone deacetylase inhibitor, depsipeptide (FR901228), increase expression of the Na(+)/I(-) symporter and iodine accumulation in poorly differentiated thyroid carcinoma cells. J Clin Endocrinol Metab 2001;86:3430–5.

92. Venkataraman GM, Yatin M, Marcinek R, Ain KB. Restoration of iodide uptake in dedifferentiated thyroid carcinoma: relationship to human Na+/I-symporter gene methylation status. J Clin Endocrinol Metab 1999;84:2449–57.

93. Brierley JD, Tsang RW. External-beam radiation therapy in the treatment of differentiated thyroid cancer. Semin Surg Oncol 1999;16:42–9.

94. Shimaoka K, Schoenfeld DA, DeWys WD, et al. A randomized trial of doxorubicin versus doxorubicin plus cisplatin in patients with advanced thyroid carcinoma. Cancer 1985;56:2155–60.

CHAPTER 37

Surgical Treatment of Medullary Thyroid Cancer

Emily Reiff, BS

Electron Kebebew, MD

Medullary thyroid cancer (MTC) accounts for only 3 to 7% of all thyroid cancer cases, but for 14% of thyroid cancer deaths.[1] Its biochemical, genetic, and clinical profile is distinct from other thyroid cancers of follicular cell origin. MTC arises from the parafollicular or C-cells (calcitonin secreting) of the thyroid gland, which originate from the neuroectoderm. The C-cells are infrequent and dispersed throughout the normal thyroid gland. Most of the C-cells are located in the upper one-third of each thyroid lobe where MTC most commonly develops. Approximately 25% of MTC cases are hereditary and 75% are sporadic. A germline mutation in the *RET* proto-oncogene is responsible for hereditary MTC and has been effectively used for screening at-risk family members.[2] Multiple endocrine neoplasia (MEN) types 2A and 2B and isolated familial medullary thyroid cancer compose the hereditary forms of MTC. Genetic screening has resulted in improved patient outcome because of earlier diagnosis of MTC and prophylactic thyroidectomy. Data from international cooperative consortiums have led to the recognition of important RET genotype-phenotype associations that should be considered in determining the best treatment options for patients who have germline RET mutations.[2–4]

The surgical approach to patients with MTC is unique and must be individualized for each patient in order to result in cure. In this chapter, we review the appropriate preoperative evaluation and the best surgical treatment of patients with MTC, including the optimal timing for prophylactic surgical treatment in hereditary cases, extent of resection and technique of thyroidectomy, and lymph node dissection.

Clinical Features

Most patients with sporadic MTC or index cases of hereditary MTC present in the fourth decade of life. Patients with MEN 2B usually present early with aggressive MTC within the first two decades of life. The frequency of MTC is equal among both sexes, unlike other thyroid neoplasms, which occur in a high proportion of women. Patients with sporadic MTC or index cases of hereditary MTC commonly present with a thyroid mass with or without enlarged cervical lymph nodes or one or more enlarged cervical lymph nodes.

Approximately 10% of patients with MTC who present with a neck mass will have hoarseness, respiratory difficulty, and dysphasia. These symptoms often indicate locally invasive tumors involving the recurrent laryngeal nerve, trachea, or esophagus because this tumor commonly occurs in the upper posterior one-third of the thyroid lobe. Distant metastasis from MTC occur in approximately 12% of all cases and is frequently to the liver, lung, and bone.[5] Rarely, patients with MTC will present with flushing and diarrhea from heavy tumor burden or distant metastases that secrete vasoactive hormones such as serotonin.

Regional lymph node metastases are common in patients with MTC. Although MTC is a relatively slow-growing tumor, lymph node metastasis to the cervical and upper mediastinal lymph nodes occurs early and frequently (Table 1).[5–8] Cervical lymph nodes in the central neck compartment (Level VI) are most frequently involved followed by the ipsilateral lateral neck compartment (levels II, III, IV) and contralateral lateral nodes,

Table 1 Patterns of cervical lymph node metastasis in patients with MTC

| | | Overall | | Central neck | | Lateral neck | | | |
| | | | | | | Ipsilateral | | Contralateral | |
tumor size (cm)	Number of patients	N1 total	(%)	total	(%)	Number of patients	(%)	Number of patients	(%)
0–1.9^	64	25	39%	25	39%	23	40%	5	8%
2.0–3.9^	85	48	56%	48	56%	42	49%	20	24%
> 4.0^	44	36	82%	36	82%	30	68%	18	41%
total^	193	109	56%	109	56%	95	49%	43	22%
total lymph node metastasis^^	1296	690	63%						

^Data from references.[6,28]
^^Data from references.[5,6,8,28,29]

MTC= medullary thyroid cancer.

and less commonly level VII lymph nodes (Figure 1, see Table 1).

Hereditary MTC has an autosomal pattern of inheritance. MEN 2A is characterized by MTC (100%), pheochromocytoma (30 to 50%), and hyperparathyroidism (20%). Approximately 9% of MEN 2A families will have cutaneous lichens amyloidosis, which occur exclusively in the intrascapular region. Patients with MEN 2B have MTC (100%), pheochromocytoma (70%), and characteristic physical features such as a marfinoid body habitus, ganglioneuromatosis, mucosal neuromas, prominent corneal nerves, and skeletal abnormalities. In familial MTC, patients have only MTC and no other components of MEN 2. Hirschsprung's disease may be associated with familial MTC and MEN 2A.

Diagnosis

In patients who present with a neck mass, fine-needle aspiration (FNA) biopsy and cytologic examination is cost-effective and accurate for establishing a diagnosis of MTC. If the cytologic features are equivocal, immunohistochemical staining for calcitonin, amyloid, and carcinoembryonic antigen are helpful and discriminate MTC from other thyroid cancers of follicular cell origin. All patients diagnosed with MTC should have preoperative measurement of serum basal or stimulated calcitonin and carcinoembryonic antigen levels. A preoperative ultrasound of the neck should also be done to evaluate the thyroid gland for multicentric and bilateral thyroid nodules and to detect any enlarged central and lateral cervical lymph nodes.

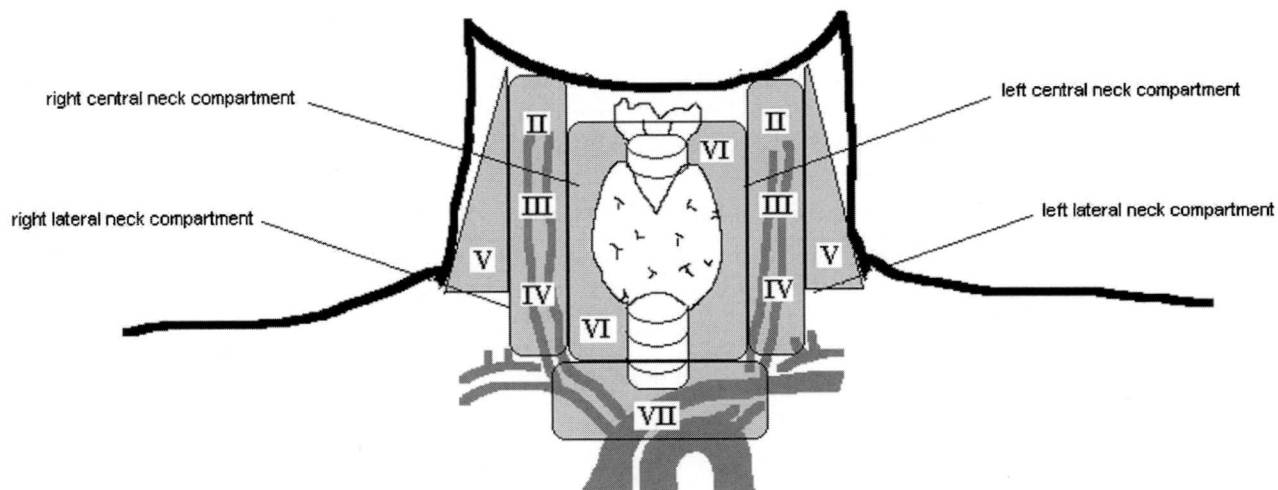

Figure 1 Cervical and mediastinal lymph node compartments. The level VI central neck lymph nodes are the primary site of lymphatic drainage for the thyroid gland, followed by the lateral neck jugular vein lymph node compartments (level II, III, IV) and the posterior triangle (level V). The level VII mediastinal lymph nodes may be involved with MTC either by direct extension or in the perithymic lymph nodes. The level I submandibular and submental lymph nodes are rarely involved with MTC.

A comprehensive history and physical examination is integral in making the diagnosis and determining the familial nature of MTC. Patients should be questioned specifically about local symptoms and symptoms that can occur from vasoactive hormone secretion secondary to widely metastatic MTC, such as diarrhea and flushing. A thorough family history is important and should include questions regarding a family history of thyroid cancer, pheochromocytoma, hyperparathyroidism, or a history of unexplained sudden death in any first degree family members (suggesting an undiagnosed pheochromocytoma). During the physical examination, the extent of the thyroid mass should be carefully determined, as should the presence of enlarged lymph nodes, phenotypic features of MEN 2B, and cutaneous lichen amyloidosis. In all patients with MTC, preoperative 24-hour urinary catecholamine and metabolite levels should be measured to rule out pheochromocytoma. Operating on a patient with an undiagnosed and untreated pheochromocytoma can be catastrophic. Therefore, the pheochromocytoma should be removed before thyroidectomy. The preoperative serum calcium level should also be measured to exclude a diagnosis of hyperparathyroidism. Because the penetrance of hyperparathyroidism and pheochromocytoma in MEN 2A is variable, some patients may have either disorder even if no one in the kindred has hyperparathyroidism or pheochromocytoma disguised as familial MTC.

Genetic Screening and Genotype-Phenotype Associations

In 99% of hereditary MTC cases, a germline RET proto-oncogene mutation is identified in exon 10, 11, 13, 14, 15, or 16 by direct deoxyribonucleic acid (DNA) sequence analysis.[2] All patients with MTC should have a blood test for the presence of germline RET proto-oncogene mutations because 9% of apparently sporadic cases may turn out to be the index case in a kindred with a de novo mutation. Family members of patients found to have hereditary MTC should also be screened. Genetic screening has replaced biochemical screening consisting of basal or stimulated calcitonin measurements for several reasons: 1) it is more accurate and cost effective, 2) it results in earlier diagnosis and higher surgical cure rates, and 3) existing genotype-phenotype associations can help with the risk assessment both of what components of MEN 2 the patient might develop and the onset and aggressiveness of MTC.

Because national and international cooperative efforts have improved the collective experience with and data on germline RET proto-oncogene mutations, genotype-phenotype associations for hereditary MTC have emerged and should be considered when evaluating patients diagnosed with hereditary MTC.[2,4,9] The different codons in which RET proto-oncogene mutations may occur have been stratified into three risk groups based on the earliest age of MTC onset in patients who had prophylactic thyroidectomy and the risk of lymph node metastasis (Table 2). These three risk categories are the basis for the guidelines on the appropriate age for prophylactic thyroidectomy and the need for cervical lymph node dissection. The level 3 group of RET proto-oncogene mutations in codons 883, 918, and 922 has the highest risk of early and aggressive MTC. The level 2 group of RET proto-oncogene mutations in codons 611, 618, 620, 630, and 634 is also at high risk for early development of MTC, as early as 1 year old for codon 634. The level 1 RET proto-oncogene mutations in codons 609, 768, 790, 791, 804, and 891 have the lowest risk for aggressive MTC. The most common RET mutation is in codon 634, which accounts for about two-thirds of hereditary MTC cases. Patients with codon 634 mutations of Cysteine-to-Arginine substitutions

Table 2 Risk Stratification for MTC Aggressiveness and Associated Phenotypes Based on RET Genotype^

Risk level	Codon Mutations	Lowest age reported to have MTC	Earliest age reported to have MTC lymph node metastasis	Genotype-Phenotype Correlation
High (level 3)	883, 918, 922	9 months	10 years	MEN 2B (918, 922) FMTC (883)
Intermediate (level 2)	611, 618, 620, 630, 634	1 years	16 years	630 only in MEN 2A 634 accounts for two-thirds of all MEN 2A cases 634 associated with a higher risk of pheochromocytoma, hyperparathyroidism, and cutaneous lichens amyloidosis
Low (level 1)	609, 768, 790, 791, 804, 891	6 years	34 years	768, 804, 891 in FMTC 790, 791 in MEN 2A

^Data from references.[2–4,23,25,30]
FMTC = familial medullary thyroid cancer; MTC = medullary thyroid cancer; MEN = multiple endocrine neoplasia.

have the highest risk for developing primary hyperparathyroidism, pheochromocytoma, and cutaneous lichen amyloidosis.[10] Approximately 95% of MEN 2B cases are due to mutations in codon 918.

Treatment

The best treatment approach for MTC is based on several unique features of MTC: 1) MTC is more aggressive than differentiated thyroid cancer of follicular cell origin, 2) radioiodine ablation is ineffective in patients with MTC because the c-cells do not trap iodine, 3) MTC is commonly bilateral and multicentric, especially in hereditary cases, 4) cervical lymph node metastasis is present in up to 80% of MTC cases, and 5) persistent or recurrent MTC occurs in over 50% of patients who present with clinically evident tumors even after apparent curative surgical resection.

SURGICAL TREATMENT FOR MTC

Surgical resection is the only effective treatment for MTC. Patients with MTC or at risk for developing MTC can be classified into three groups. Group 1 consists of patients with a thyroid mass and or lymph node involvement that shows MTC on FNA biopsy. This commonly occurs in patients with sporadic MTC or hereditary MTC index cases. Group 2 consists of patients who have positive germline RET proto-oncogene mutations without clinically evident disease but a thyroid nodule or nodules are found by ultrasound testing or have an elevated basal or stimulated preoperative calcitonin level. Group 3 consists of patients who have a positive germline RET proto-oncogene mutation but no clinical, imaging, or biochemical evidence of disease. It is important to consider which of these groups a patient may belong in and to select the appropriate surgical treatment accordingly.

Patients who belong in Group 1 should have a total or near total thyroidectomy, bilateral central (level VI), and ipsilateral functional modified radical neck node (levels II, III, IV and V) dissection. The rationale for this approach is that MTC is multicentric and bilateral.[11-13] The presence of cervical lymph node metastasis also cannot be accurately determined intraoperatively.[6] Furthermore, cervical lymph node metastasis occurs in up to 80% of patients with a primary tumor ≥ 1cm and frequently involves the central and ipsilateral neck nodes (see Table 1).[5,6,13] Finally, total thyroidectomy and bilateral central neck node clearance is associated with a lower risk of persistent or recurrent MTC than less extensive operations.

Patients who belong in Group 2 should also have a total or near total thyroidectomy and at least a bilateral central neck node dissection, especially if the primary tumor is > 1 cm in size by ultrasound. If any of the central neck nodes are positive for MTC, an ipsilateral lateral (Levels II, III, IV, V) neck node dissection should be performed.

For the Group 3 patients who are diagnosed by genetic testing as carriers of the RET germline mutations, the type of surgical procedure and the best time to perform it should be based on the specific codon mutation. Those who have high risk level 3 RET codon mutations (883, 918, 922) should undergo immediate total or near total thyroidectomy or before age 1 year. Those who have level 2 risk RET codon mutations (609, 611, 618, 620, 630, 634) should have a total or near total thyroidectomy before the age of 5. The best age for prophylactic thyroidectomy in patients with level 1 RET codon mutations (768, 790, 791, 804, 891) is controversial because of limited data and the variable age of MTC onset observed. Some experts recommend prophylactic thyroidectomy before age 5 or 10 years, whereas others recommend waiting until the stimulated calcitonin level becomes elevated. We recommend total or near total thyroidectomy before age 5 because thyroidectomy is a safe operation when performed by skilled surgeons, lymph node metastasis may occur early even if the MTC is microscopic, and the aggressiveness of MTC in this group is variable.

Total thyroidectomy for MTC should include a complete extracapsular removal of both thyroid lobes, the isthmus, and the pyramidal lobe. At times, it may be necessary to perform a near-total thyroidectomy to avoid injury to the recurrent laryngeal nerve by leaving a small (1 to 5%) thyroid remnant in the posterolateral portion. Every effort should be made to preserve the function of the recurrent laryngeal nerve unless it is documented not to function by preoperative direct laryngoscopy. For the bilateral central neck node dissection, all lymphatic and fibrofatty tissue from the hyoid bone down to the perithymic region and from carotid sheath to the carotid sheath should be removed (see Figure 1). For a modified functional radical neck dissection, the dissection is extended laterally to remove the level II, III, and IV jugular lymph nodes and level V posterior triangle nodes. Fibrofatty and lymphatic tissue from the angle of the mandible and anterior margin of the trapezius muscle down to the innominate vessels and to the anterior surface of the scalene muscle are removed. The phrenic nerve, spinal accessory, internal jugular vein, sternocleidomastoid muscle, cervical sensory nerves, and brachial plexus should be preserved in the functional modified radical neck dissection.

The best approach for managing the parathyroid glands in patients with MTC is controversial. Some surgeons routinely perform parathyroidectomy with autotransplantation. The rationale for this is that some surgeons do not believe that an adequate total thyroidectomy and central neck lymph node clearance can be done without devascularizing the parathyroid glands. In our experience, however, the parathyroid glands can usually be left in-situ without preventing complete removal of cervical nodes and minimizing the risk of hypoparathyroidism. If the viability of the parathyroid gland(s) is questionable, the gland or glands can be autotransplanted into the forearm of patients with MEN 2A and to the sternocleidomastoid muscle of patients with sporadic MTC, familial MTC, and MEN 2B because they are not at risk of developing hyperparathyroidism.

NONSURGICAL TREATMENT FOR MTC

Several cytotoxic chemotherapy agents (dacarbazine, 5-fluorouracil, epirubicin, cyclophosphamide, doxorubicin, streptozocin, interferon α 2) have been evaluated in patients with metastatic MTC without observing any significant tumor response.[1] Somatostatin analog (octreotide) therapy may reduce calcitonin and carcinoembryonic antigen levels in patients with metastatic MTC and may improve symptoms such as flushing and diarrhea.[14] Long-term octreotide therapy, however, requires continued dose-escalation. Most studies in patients with metastatic MTC have not documented any significant tumor response to octreotide therapy. Patients with metastatic MTC to the liver who have flushing and diarrhea may benefit from radiofrequency ablation for tumor debulking and symptomatic relief.[15] In patients with advanced and progressing metastatic MTC, referral to experimental clinical trials that are evaluating radionuclide therapy with octreotide, 131-I labeled anticarcinoembryonic antigen monoclonal antibody, and tyrosine-kinase inhibitors and anti-angiogenesis agents should be considered.[16,17]

The efficacy of external beam radiatiotherapy (EBRT) in patients with MTC is unclear.[18] Some investigators have suggested improved local control, but no difference in survival has been observed. Because EBRT can be associated with significant side effects and at best results in improved local control and not complete tumor response, the routine use of postoperative radiotherapy is not warranted. The group of patients most likely to benefit from postoperative EBRT are those with gross extrathyroidal invasion of tumor or those that have positive microscopic tumor margins. It should be considered for patients who have unresectable locoregional MTC as determined by a skilled surgeon and in patients with symptomatic bone metastasis that cannot be resected.

Follow-up Monitoring

Serum calcitonin is an accurate marker for MTC and undetectable levels indicate biochemical cure. All patients treated for MTC should have postoperative basal or stimulated serum calcitonin levels measured annually. Postoperative detectable or elevated (hypercalcitoninemia) serum calcitonin levels most commonly indicate persistent or recurrent MTC, often before any disease can be localized by imaging studies. Some patients may have elevated postoperative serum calcitonin levels because of delayed clearance. If so, they should have calcitonin levels measured again in 3 to 6 months. Although calcium- or pentagastrin-stimulated calcitonin levels are more accurate than basal calcitonin levels for indicating persistent or recurrent disease, pentagastrin is neither widely available nor routinely used in the US.

Patients who have elevated or detectable serum calcitonin levels should have an ultrasound of the neck, a magnetic resonance image of the mediastinum to detect locoregional disease, and a computed tomography scan of the chest and abdomen to detect distant disease or a bone scan if the patient has symptoms suggesting bone metastasis. If these imaging studies are negative, octreotide and positron emission tomography scanning may be helpful for locating regional or distant sites of disease.[16,19] If none of these localizing studies show any evidence of disease, selective venous catheterization with stimulated calcitonin measurement may be useful for detecting MTC.[20] Because MTC liver metastases can be as small as millet seeds, some investigators have used diagnostic laparoscopy and biopsy to detect liver metastasis.[21]

Prognosis

The survival of patients with MTC is intermediate to that of patients with differentiated thyroid cancer of follicular cell origin and anaplastic thyroid cancer; the overall survival rate is 75% at 10 years follow-up.[22] There is, however, great variability in the aggressiveness of MTC.[5] Some patients may survive several decades with known metastatic MTC or hypercalcitoninemia, whereas others will have rapidly progressive tumors and die within months of presentation. Only early diagnosis and at least a total thyroidectomy with bilateral central neck node dissection gives the patient the best chance of biochemical cure and disease-free survival. In contemporary series, patients diagnosed with hereditary MTC by screening have a nearly 100% survival rate and over a 95% biochemical cure rate after prophylactic total thyroidectomy and removal of the cervical lymph nodes.[11,12,23–25]

Several clinical, pathologic, biochemical, and molecular variables predict the risk of persistent or recurrent MTC and prognosis in patients with MTC. These include older age, systemic symptoms such as flushing or diarrhea at diagnosis, large primary tumor size, lymph node involvement (2 or more cervical compartments, lymph node > 1cm in size, 10 or more positive lymph node metastases), presence of distant metastasis, serum basal calcitonin > 10,000 pg/mL, elevated carcinoembryonic antigen level, decreased or absent amyloid staining, and tumors with DNA aneuploidy. The most important and independent prognostic factors that predict survival in patients with MTC are the TNM (tumor, nodes, metastasis) stage and patient age at diagnosis.[5]

Persistent and Recurrent MTC

Over half of the patients who present with clinically evident MTC have persistent or recurrent MTC, manifested by elevated postoperative basal or stimulated serum calcitonin levels. When evaluating patients who have persistent or recurrent MTC based on elevated postoperative calcitonin levels, the prior surgical treatment(s) and the results of localizing studies need to be considered carefully. Patients who had less than total thyroidectomy and less than at least a bilateral central neck node dissection usually have residual disease in the neck and should undergo cervical reexploration and removal of all remaining thyroid tissue. If there is no evidence of distant metastasis to the liver, lung, and bone, a bilateral modified functional radical neck dissection should be considered. If the patient had an appropriate initial surgical treatment, the elevated calcitonin commonly indicates occult MTC in the neck, mediastinum, or at distant sites.

The best treatment remains uncertain for patients with hypercalcitoninemia after appropriate initial surgical treatment who have no radiographic or clinical evidence of MTC. Such patients may enjoy long-term survival without the need for another surgical intervention. Several investigators have shown that reoperation with removal of the remaining cervical and mediastinal fibrofatty and lymphatic tissues in patients with persistent or recurrent MTC may result in biochemical cure (normalization of basal or stimulated calcitonin) in 10 to 38% of patients.[26,27] Such an approach may be reasonable to consider in patients with either: 1) increasing calcitonin levels, or 2) postoperative hypercalcitoninemia and a positive localizing study for locoregional residual MTC but without distant metastasis, or for palliation of aggressive locoregional MTC in patients with widely metastatic MTC.

Summary

Significant advances in our understanding of MTC have resulted in significantly improved patient outcome. All patients diagnosed with MTC should undergo genetic screening. Patients who have clinically evident MTC should have at least a total or near total thyroidectomy and bilateral central neck node dissection. If the central neck lymph nodes are involved or the primary tumor is 1 cm, these patients should have an ipsilateral modified functional radical neck dissection. Patients who are RET germline mutation carriers should have prophylactic total thyroidectomy and the timing of the operation should be based on the codon involved. All patients with MTC require lifelong follow-up consisting of serum basal or stimulated calcitonin levels measured annually or more frequently if clinically indicated.

References

1. Kebebew E, Clark OH. Medullary thyroid cancer. Curr Treat Options Oncol 2000;1:359–67.

2. Brandi ML, et al. Guidelines for diagnosis and therapy of MEN type 1 and type 2. J Clin Endocrinol Metab 2001;86: 5658–71.

3. Eng C, et al. The relationship between specific RET proto-oncogene mutations and disease phenotype in multiple endocrine neoplasia type 2. International RET mutation consortium analysis. Jama 1996;276:1575–9.

4. Machens A, et al. Early malignant progression of hereditary medullary thyroid cancer. N Engl J Med 2003;349: 1517–25.

5. Modigliani E, et al. Prognostic factors for survival and for biochemical cure in medullary thyroid carcinoma: results in 899 patients. The GETC Study Group. Groupe d'etude des tumeurs a calcitonine. Clin Endocrinol (Oxf) 1998;48: 265–73.

6. Moley JF, DeBenedetti MK. Patterns of nodal metastases in palpable medullary thyroid carcinoma: recommendations for extent of node dissection. Ann Surg 1999;229:880–7; discussion 887–8.

7. Weber T, et al. Impact of modified radical neck dissection on biochemical cure in medullary thyroid carcinomas. Surgery 2001;130:1044–9.

8. Scollo C, et al. Rationale for central and bilateral lymph node dissection in sporadic and hereditary medullary thyroid cancer. J Clin Endocrinol Metab 2003;88:2070–5.

9. Yip L, et al. Multiple endocrine neoplasia type 2: evaluation of the genotype-phenotype relationship. Arch Surg 2003; 138:409–16; discussion 416.

10. Gertner ME, Kebebew E. Multiple endocrine neoplasia type 2. Curr Treat Options Oncol 2004;5:315–25.

11. Kebebew E, et al. Medullary thyroid carcinoma: clinical characteristics, treatment, prognostic factors, and a comparison of staging systems. Cancer 2000;88:1139–48.

12. Yen TW, et al. Medullary thyroid carcinoma: results of a standardized surgical approach in a contemporary series of 80 consecutive patients. Surgery 2003;134:890–9; discussion 899–901.

13. Machens A, et al. Enhancement of lymph node metastasis and distant metastasis of thyroid carcinoma. Cancer 2003; 98:712–9.

14. Lupoli GA, et al. The role of somatostatin analogs in the management of medullary thyroid carcinoma. J Endocrinol Invest 2003;26(8 Suppl):72–4.

15. Siperstein AE, et al. Laparoscopic thermal ablation of hepatic neuroendocrine tumor metastases. Surgery 1997; 122:1147–54; discussion 1154–5.

16. Kaltsas G, et al. Recent advances in radiological and radionuclide imaging and therapy of neuroendocrine tumours. Eur J Endocrinol 2004;151:15–27.

17. Cuccuru G, et al. Cellular effects and antitumor activity of RET inhibitor RPI-1 on MEN2A-associated medullary thyroid carcinoma. J Natl Cancer Inst 2004;96:1006–14.

18. Brierley JD, Tsang RW. External radiation therapy in the treatment of thyroid malignancy. Endocrinol Metab Clin North Am 1996;25:141–57.

19. McDougall IR, Davidson J, Segall GM. Positron emission tomography of the thyroid, with an emphasis on thyroid cancer. Nucl Med Commun 2001;22:485–92.

20. Abdelmoumene N, et al. Selective venous sampling catheterisation for localisation of persisting medullary thyroid carcinoma. Br J Cancer 1994;69:1141–4.

21. Tung WS, Vesely TM, Moley JF. Laparoscopic detection of hepatic metastases in patients with residual or recurrent medullary thyroid cancer. Surgery 1995;118:1024–9; discussion 1029–30.

22. Hundahl SA, et al. A National Cancer Data Base report on 53,856 cases of thyroid carcinoma treated in the U.S., 1985–1995. Cancer 1998;83:2638–48.

23. Dralle H, et al. Prophylactic thyroidectomy in 75 children and adolescents with hereditary medullary thyroid carcinoma: German and Austrian experience. World J Surg 1998;22:744–50; discussion 750–1.

24. Machens A, et al. Improved prediction of calcitonin normalization in medullary thyroid carcinoma patients by quantitative lymph node analysis. Cancer 2000;88:1909–15.

25. Wells SA Jr, et al. Predictive DNA testing and prophylactic thyroidectomy in patients at risk for multiple endocrine neoplasia type 2A. Ann Surg 1994;220:237–47; discussion 247–50.

26. Moley JF, Dilley WG, DeBenedetti MK. Improved results of cervical reoperation for medullary thyroid carcinoma. Ann Surg 1997;225:734–40; discussion 740–3.

27. Kebebew E, et al. Long-term results of reoperation and localizing studies in patients with persistent or recurrent medullary thyroid cancer. Arch Surg 2000;135:895–901.

28. Machens A, et al. Pattern of nodal metastasis for primary and reoperative thyroid cancer. World J Surg 2002;26:22–8.

29. Beressi N, et al. Sporadic medullary microcarcinoma of the thyroid: a retrospective analysis of eighty cases. Thyroid 1998;8:1039–44.

30. Gimm O, et al. Timing and extent of surgery in patients with familial medullary thyroid carcinoma/multiple endocrine neoplasia 2A-related RET mutations not affecting codon 634. World J Surg 2004;28:1312–6.

CHAPTER 38

SURGICAL MANAGEMENT OF LOCALLY ADVANCED THYROID CANCER

MICHAEL E. KUPFERMAN, MD

RANDAL S. WEBER, MD

Although well-differentiated thyroid carcinoma is a curable disease with a favorable long-term prognosis, locally invasive tumors pose therapeutic challenges that contribute to significant morbidity and mortality in patients. Extrathyroidal involvement portends for recurrence and poor prognosis, and up to 50% of all cancer-related deaths results from uncontrolled local disease.[1] Eighty percent of patients with differentiated thyroid cancer have local recurrence at the time of death. Involvement of the neck musculature and upper-aerodigestive tract with thyroid cancers occurs in approximately 5 to 15% of all patients, and complete tumor extirpation is absolutely required to prevent the dreaded sequelae of massive hemoptysis, airway compromise, and pharyngoesophageal obstruction.[2] The management of invasive thyroid cancer is complex, requiring a thorough understanding of tumor behavior, expertise in complex resections and reconstructions of the visceral organs of the neck, and the need for anatomic and functional preservation of structures vital to voice and swallowing. This chapter will review the evaluation and management of invasive thyroid cancer.

Pathology

Papillary thyroid carcinoma (PTC) is the most common form of thyroid cancer and accounts for the majority of invasive lesions in most published series. Despite its indolent behavior, PTC has a predilection for local and regional metastases. In a review of patients treated at the

Mayo Clinic, McCaffrey and colleagues found that 89% of invasive thyroid cancers were PTC.[3] Variants of PTC, including tall cell and insular carcinomas, display more aggressive behaviors and should prompt the surgeon to evaluate for extraglandular spread. As opposed to PTC, which has a rate of extrathyroidal extension approximating 15%, these histological variants display extrathyroidal extension in 35 to 50% of cases.[4]

While follicular carcinoma is known to spread distantly to the lung, brain and bone, its propensity for involvement of cervicovisceral structures is variable. Tumors with follicular histology accounted for 5 to 40% of invasive thyroid cancers, and 20% of patients with follicular thyroid carcinoma (FTC) presented with widely invasive lesions.[3,5,6] Hürthle cell carcinoma, a variant of FTC, is a particularly aggressive subtype with a propensity for regional metastasis and local recurrences.[7] Both sporadic and familial forms of medullary thyroid carcinoma (MTC) have a high propensity for laryngotracheal invasion. In one series from Germany, 44% of patients treated at a single institution for invasive thyroid cancer had MTC.[8]

Anaplastic thyroid carcinoma (ATC) is the most aggressive histological subtype of thyroid carcinoma and is often not responsive to standard therapeutic modalities. The overall 1-year survival rate for ATC remains about 10% and has not improved with the advent of multimodality treatment approaches. A recent review of 134 cases of ATC identified locally invasive disease in 98% of patients.[9] Although most patients are treated with chemotherapy and radiation therapy, some do undergo extensive extirpations for this disease, often requiring the surgical removal of adjacent structures.

Presenting Signs and Symptoms

With the exception of strap muscle involvement, invasion of surrounding structures by thyroid cancer will result in symptoms that should alert the surgeon to the presence of a locally aggressive lesion. However, evidence of local extension is often identified intra-operatively, and the surgeon must be comfortable with surgical management of cervical viscera to provide the patient with a thorough oncological resection.

RECURRENT LARYNGEAL NERVE

The recurrent laryngeal nerve is the structure most commonly involved by thyroid cancer, after taking into account strap muscle invasion.[10] Patients may present with hoarseness or early vocal fatigue, although young patients may accommodate to long-standing paralyses with contralateral vocal cord hyperfunction. Nasopharyngolaryngoscopy should be performed on all patients prior to surgery to assess vocal cord function and may reveal vocal cord weakness or frank paralysis with concomitant vocal cord atrophy. Vocal fold fasiculations and tremor in the setting of recurrent thyroid cancer is also an ominous sign of neuronal involvement. If laryngeal dysfunction is noted preopera-tively, the surgeon should document this with video stroboscopy. Laryngeal electromyography has a limited role under these circumstances. Preoperative counseling should include discussions regarding the need to resect the recurrent laryngeal nerve and potential procedures for future vocal rehabilitation. In the setting of recurrent disease with a preexisting vocal cord paralysis, injury to the remaining functioning nerve will result in emergent airway obstruction and necessitate the placement of a tracheotomy.

TRACHEA

Despite its anatomic proximity to the thyroid gland, the trachea is rarely involved with aggressive thyroid cancer. Symptoms related to tracheal invasion may be subtle, such as chronic cough, globus sensation, or wheezing. Hemoptysis, dysphagia, stridor, or dyspnea are suggestive of a more invasive lesion and may require immediate surgical management of the airway.[11] In certain patients, office bronchoscopy may be performed after topically anesthetizing the vocal cords to evaluate the status of the tracheal lumen.

ESOPHAGUS

Posterior extension of thyroid carcinoma to involve the hypopharynx and cervical esophagus is rare and may be difficult to distinguish from extrinsic tumor compres-sion. Patients may complain only of dysphagia, but with more aggressive disease, hematemesis and esophageal obstruction may ensue. In most instances, the tumor will invade the muscular wall; however, transmural\intra-luminal extension is rare.[12]

LARYNX

Invasion into the laryngeal skeleton usually occurs via direct extension through the laryngeal cartilages or via the paraglottic space at the posterior free margin of the thyroid cartilage. Tumor may then progress superiorly to enter the supraglottis or inferiorly into the pyriform sinus or glottis.[3] Complaints of hoarseness or globus sensation are suggestive of laryngeal framework invasion. Subtle findings on physical examination include sub-mucosal fullness, rotation of the hemilarynx, and restriction of vocal cord mobility. In more advanced disease, thyroid cancer will directly invade the laryngeal lumen and result in airway obstruction necessitating immediate surgical intervention.

INTERNAL JUGULAR VEIN\CAROTID ARTERY

It is uncommon for vascular invasion with thyroid cancer to incur physical symptoms unless gross invasion of the internal or common carotid arteries has occurred. Mental status changes and neurological insults suggest complete carotid encasement, stenosis, or thrombosis. Tumor emboli from direct invasion of the carotid or vertebral system are exceedingly rare.

Diagnostic Studies

All patients suspected of having an invasive thyroid cancer should undergo diagnostic imaging to evaluate the extent of disease. While ultrasound is useful in evaluating the extent of nodal disease, it has limited utility in evaluating for soft tissue involvement. Therefore, patients suspected of having extensive soft tissue disease should have anatomic imaging with either computerized tomography (CT) with iodinated contrast or magnetic resonance imaging (MRI). CT has the advantage of identifying bony or cartilaginous invasion of the laryngotracheal comple, and is superior to MRI for the identification of metastatic lymphadenopathy. On the other hand, MRI provides superior soft tissue and luminal characterization than CT (Figure 1). Additionally, the administration of radioactive iodine

A

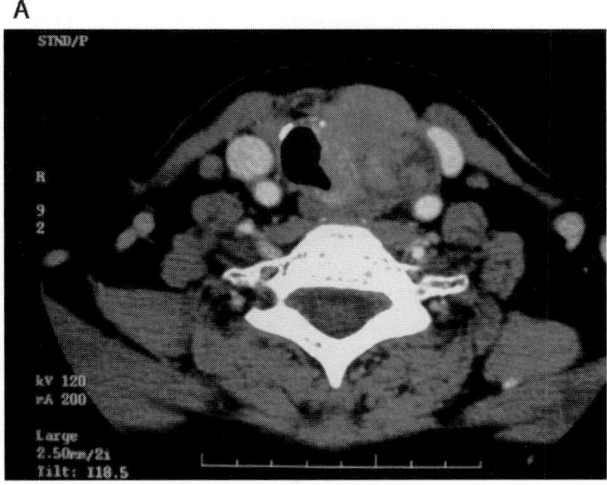

B

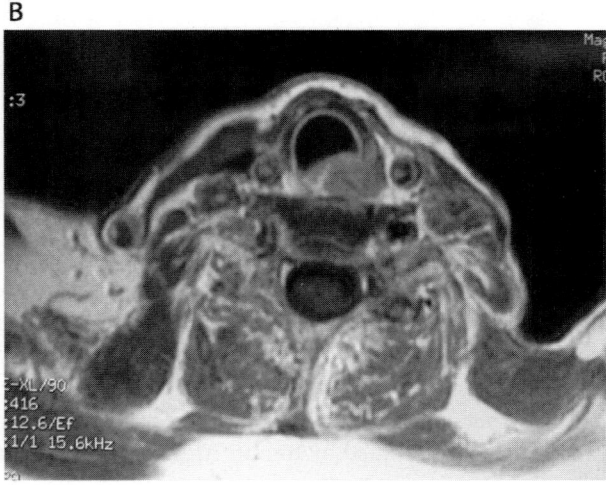

Figure 1 *A,* Computed tomography scan of the neck with iodinated contrast in a patient with a large thyroid cancer with aggressive local invasion of the left trachea. Tracheal ring destruction is evident. *B,* Magnetic resonance image of the same patient demonstrating intraluminal involvement. Although the tumor encroaches upon the esophagus, only the serosa is involved.

must be delayed by 6 weeks after the administration of iodinated contrast agents. Determining the appropriate study is usually based on the surgeon's preference and the experience of the head and neck radiologist.

Any suspected recurrences or soft tissue deposits should be assessed histopathologically using fine-needle aspiration, which may be performed with ultrasound guidance to increase the diagnostic yield. Suspected intraluminal lesions should be biopsied in the operating room under general anesthesia, particularly if there is concern for impending airway compromise.

Esophagoscopy or barium swallow should be performed when there is concern that tumor has spread to the esophagus. These studies have greater sensitivity for esophageal involvement than axial imaging and can direct the surgeon as to whether the esophagus will need to be addressed intraoperatively. Thorough evaluation of the larynx and trachea with a direct laryngoscopy and bronchoscopy prior to definitive resection should be performed when airway involvement is likely.

Operative Management

One of the more controversial areas in the management of locally invasive thyroid cancers is the issue of extent of resection. Historically, authors have stated that total excision of all tumor-bearing tissues to microscopically negative margins is required for the appropriate treatment of aggressive thyroid cancers. More recently, the use of partial, or "shave" resections have been advocated to minimize the morbidity of ablative surgery, with residual microscopic disease addressed with radioactive iodine ablation or external beam radiation. No survival benefit has been demonstrated for total tumor resection compared to "shave resection" in various retrospective reviews, and thus debate persists.[3,13] For differentiated thyroid cancer, minimal margins are adequate in contrast to other solid tumor of the head and neck. There is still no clear consensus on the extent of resection for patients with tumor invading the aerodigestive tract; thus, the surgeon must rely on his or her clinical acumen and experience to make these decisions. A guiding principle is the knowledge the patients with recurrent disease can be expected to have a prolonged life expectancy, so any treatment morbidity will have a significant impact on quality of life.

RECURRENT LARYNGEAL NERVE

Despite its intimate relationship with the thyroid gland and the paratracheal nodes, the recurrent laryngeal nerve is rarely invaded by tumor. In most situations, the surgeon can clear the recurrent laryngeal nerve (RLN) of tumor by carefully skeletonizing the nerve in a superior and inferior direction. However, when the tumor or metastatic lymph nodes actually encase the nerve circumferentially, there may be no option other than to sacrifice the nerve. Extreme care must be taken with dissection on the contralateral side in avoiding injury to the other RLN—bilateral vocal cord paralysis is a feared complication of thyroid surgery and can rapidly lead to acute airway distress upon extubation. The unfortunate patient who does require bilateral RLN divisions need to be trachetomized prophylactically to avoid upper airway obstruction.

Postoperatively, the paralyzed vocal cord will initially be in a medialized position with a gradual lateralization of the cord and an ensuing diminution in voice quality. Surgical rehabilitation with a medialization thyroplasty, in conjunction with an arytenoid adduction can restore adequate voice quality.

STRAP MUSCLE

Numerous facial bands and blood vessels connect the thyroid gland to the overlying sternothyroid and sternohyoid musculature, making them a common structure involved in locally advanced thyroid cancer. With further extension, the thyrohyoid and omohyoid muscles may be invaded by tumor. Although they play a role in deglutition and vocal pitch, the strap muscles can be resected with impunity without untoward patient morbidity. Preoperative imaging may suggest local extension into these structures, but often the decision to include the strap muscles in the resection specimen is made intraoperatively. Involvement of the sternocleidomastoid muscle usually occurs in the setting of lateral neck lymphatic metastases with extracapsular spread and should be resected in the course of a modified radical neck dissection.

LARYNX

Difficult management decisions arise when thyroid cancer extends superiorly to enter the laryngeal skeleton, either directly though the cricothyroid membrane or into the paraglottic space. It is imperative to determine the extent of cricoid involvement because this will dictate the extent of resection and the need for complex reconstruction. Some advocate a shave resection for anterior invasion of the cricoid, but there is higher risk of recurrence when this is performed.[14] Up to one-third of the cricoid can be resected without the need for grafting—the defect can be reconstructed using a local muscle or myoperiosteal flap. Resection of the anterior one-third to one-half of the cartilage can be performed, with a rib cartilage graft interpositioned into the defect to prevent postoperative stenosis. Costal perichondrium should be kept intact and placed intraluminally to provide a bed for remucosalization.[15] More invasive subglottic extension necessitates a total laryngectomy for oncologic control, although some authors advocate a cricotracheal resection and primary anastomosis under these circumstances. As is done for subglottic stenosis, a thin portion of cricoid cartilage, upon which the arytenoids sit, may be preserved and sutured directly to the remnant trachea. The experience of the surgeon should dictate the reconstruction offered to the patient.

When the thyroid cartilage is the site of a small focus of invasion and no paraglottic or preepiglottic space invasion has occurred, resection of the cartilage to the inner perichondrium can be curative. Ipsilateral laryngeal involvement can be managed with conservative procedures such as the vertical hemilaryngectomy if the surgeon is assured of the ability to obtain negative margins. Preoperative imaging and intraoperative laryngoscopy are critical for accurate assessment of the extent of laryngeal resection necessary. When thyroid cancer invades the anterior commissure or both hemilarynges, a total laryngectomy is indicated for complete tumor eradication.

TRACHEA

In most circumstances, tracheal invasion is identified during the preoperative evaluation. However, previously unrecognized foci of tracheal invasion may be seen during the course of surgical resection. Invasion of the trachea with thyroid cancer occurs via the intercartilagenous spaces or directly through the cartilaginous rings Figure 2). In both instances, full thickness resection of the tracheal wall is necessary for complete tumor extirpation (Figure 3). Shave resection is an option when the tumor is adherent but has not invaded the tracheal cartilage or lumen. Some surgeons advocate a "shave resection" of the perichondrium fascia and tracheal rings, but this technique does not allow for pathologic evaluation of the specimen margins. We therefore recommend complete tumor resection under these circumstances.

Early invasion of the trachea with thyroid carcinoma can be managed with a window resection of the involved tracheal cartilage and intercartilagenous space. To minimize postoperative tracheomalacia and stenosis, a regional myofascial flap can be effectively rotated into the defect for repair. Placement of a temporary tracheostomy may be necessary to maintain an adequate airway in the perioperative setting. Larger anterior wall defects that involve up to six tracheal rings should be reconstructed with rib cartilage grafting, ensuring that that the grafted perichondrium is placed intraluminally to prevent postoperative granulation. Some authors advocate the use of a temporary tracheal stent with or without free mucosal grafts to ensure the success of the reconstruction without excessive granulation and cicatrix formation.

When greater than 50% of the tracheal circumference or more than 6 tracheal rings are invaded by tumor, total resection of the involved segment with primary anastomosis must be performed (Figure 4). Meticulous surgical technique, using interrupted submucosal sutures, is necessary to prevent postoperative granulation tissue and scar formation, which will render the reconstruction

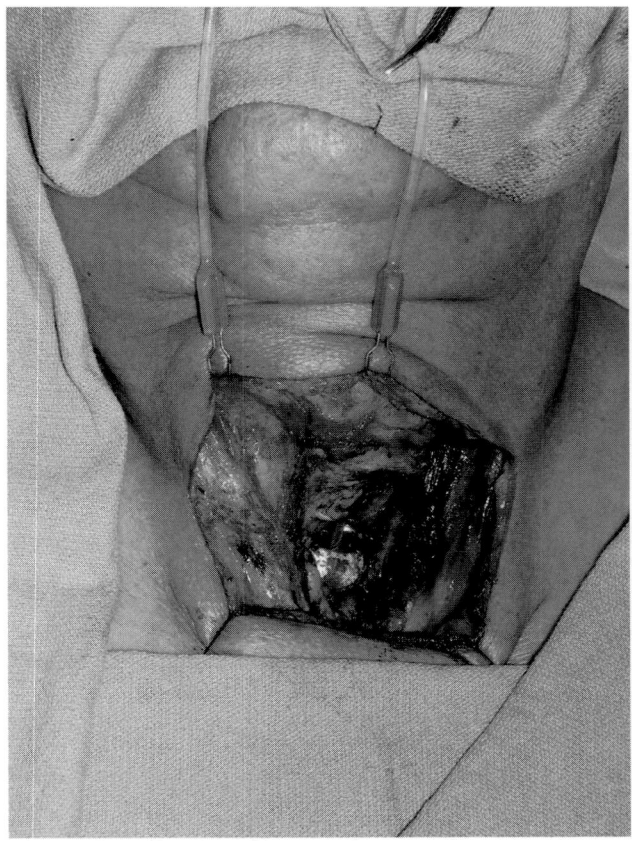

A

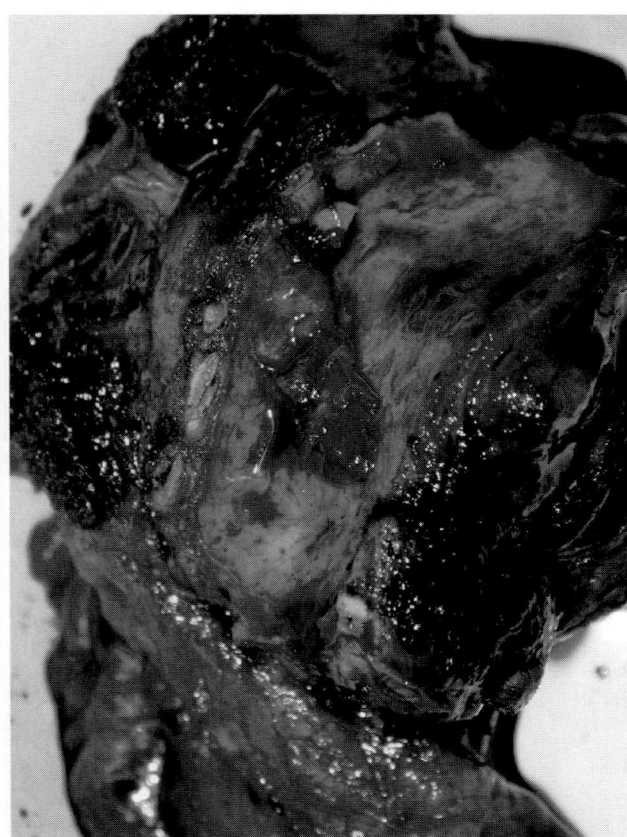

B

Figure 2 *A*, Intraoperative view of a partial tracheal resection for invasive thyroid carcinoma. *B*, The resected surgical specimen, demonstrating intraluminal invasion.

nonfunctional. Close collaboration with the anesthesiology team is critical for maintenance of the airway during reconstruction. Closure can be facilitated by inferior dissection of the anterior tracheal wall down to the carina, and an additional 5 cm of lengthening can be obtained with a suprahyoid release at the expense of increased postoperative aspiration. Tracheal resection can usually be performed without the need for a tracheostomy tube. The decision to extubate the patient at the end of the procedure should take into consideration the skills and experience of the surgical and anesthesiology teams. Postoperatively, the patient needs to be monitored closely for signs of aspiration, infection, obstruction, and fistula formation.

Alternatively, there has been recent interest in the use of vascularized free tissue transfer in the reconstruction of large circumferential tracheal defects, particularly in the reoperative setting when scarring and previous resections may limit the ability to perform an end-to-end-anastomosis.[16] The pliable radial forearm-free flap can be tubed around a flexible tracheal stent or may be used as an epithelial lining for an external tracheal scaffold (Figure 5). Disadvantages of this approach include absence of a mucosal lining, pooling of secretions, mucus plugging, and the risk of infection. The long-term outcome of this reconstructive approach remains to be seen.

Occasionally, patients with thyroid cancer may present with airway disease that is unresectable. The primary approach to treating these patients is to establish the airway and bypass the obstructing lesion, with subsequent palliative endotracheal resection using either cold or laser techniques. Repeated endoscopic ablative procedures are often necessary for comfort measures and can temporarily relieve the chronic dyspnea and obstruction. The addition of tracheal stenting or a Montgomery T-tube can provide further symptom control to this group of patients.

PHARYNX AND ESOPHAGUS

Pharyngeal invasion rarely occurs without concomitant laryngeal and esophageal invasion, but when encoun-

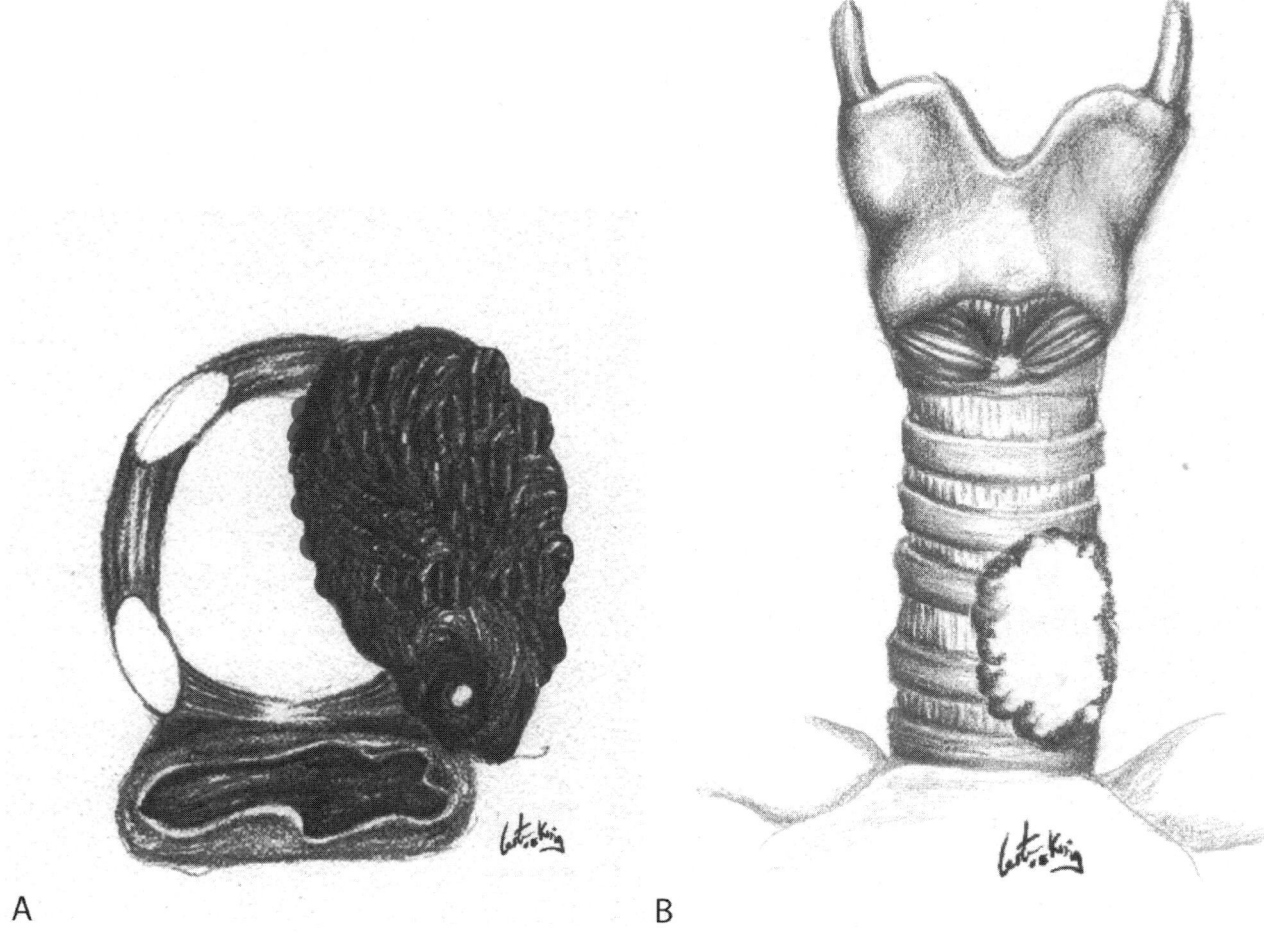

A   B

Figure 3 *A*, Artist's rendering of an invasive thyroid carcinoma, extending into the trachea and involvement of the recurrent laryngeal nerve. *B*, Defect of the trachea after resection for invasive thyroid carcinoma.

tered, the tumor can be approached with a lateral pharyngotomy and primary resection. However, laryngopharyngectomy is often required for total gross tumor resection.

When thyroid cancer invades the esophagus, extensive resection and reconstruction is often necessary. Cervical esophagectomy is a morbid procedure necessitating reconstruction with a tubed radial forearm or jejunal-free tissue transfer for small defects. However, in most situations, only the muscular wall is invaded, allowing for preservation of the mucosa and submucosa.[2] The defect can then be reinforced with a pedicled muscle flap interposed between the esophagus and the trachea and carotid sheath. When the distal anastomosis extends below the thoracic inlet, total esophagectomy with gastric pull-up will be required for adequate local control. These procedures pose high risks of morbidity and mortality to the patient, and consideration of the patient's general medical fitness and overall survival must be taken into

account. Regardless of the treatment plan, ensuring adequate nutritional intake with placement of an enteral feeding tube, either via gastrostomy or jejunostomy, should not be neglected.

Adjuvant Therapies

Patients with locally advanced thyroid cancer should receive additional therapy to control microscopic disease, prevent locoregional recurrences, and reduce the risk of distant metastases. Options include radioactive iodine therapy and external beam radiation. Certainly, all patients with iodine-avid invasive thyroid cancers should be treated with I^{131} and suppressive exogenous thyroxine.[17] Although no prospective studies have been undertaken, external beam radiation is felt to be beneficial for patients with extrathyroidal extension of tumor because they have a high risk of recurrence in the thyroid bed. Further, patients who have microscopic disease on final

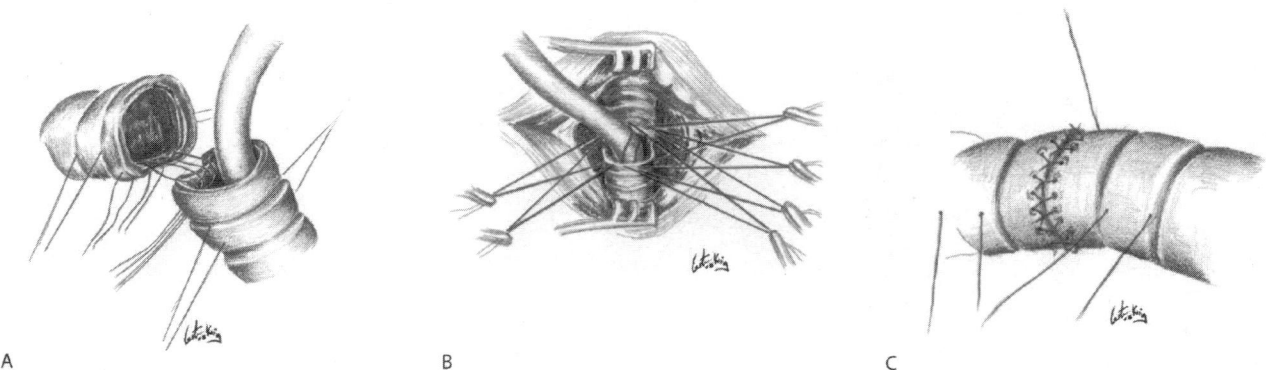

A   B   C

Figure 4 Reconstruction of the trachea after a full-thickness resection of multiple tracheal rings. *A,* The posterior wall of the trachea is closed using interrupted sutures. *B,* The lateral tracheal walls are closed using submucosally placed absorbable sutures with the knots tied extra-luminally. *C,* Completed tracheal reconstruction.

pathologic may also benefit from external beam radiation.[18]

Prognosis

A lack of uniformity in reporting results in the literature makes it difficult to provide concrete survival statistics for patients with locally aggressive thyroid cancer. Nonetheless, it is clear that invasion of the aerodigestive tract portend for a high rate of local recurrence, distant metastasis, and poor survival. Among patients in whom complete resection is possible, a 5-year survival benefit between 60 to 80% is possible.[3,5,19–21] This decreases when gross tumor extirpation is not possible.

Conclusions

The management of locally invasive thyroid cancer is complex, with little agreement in the literature over the extent of treatment necessary. This is primarily due to the lack of well-designed prospective studies and the rarity of disease occurrence. Despite the infrequent incidence of locally aggressive thyroid cancers, careful attention to presenting signs and symptoms should alert the surgeon to the presence of upper aerodigestive tract involvement. Thorough evaluation with imaging and endoscopy is warranted to determine the extent of disease and helps guide the surgeon in determining the extent of resection needed. The primary goals of treatment should be (1) complete tumor eradication and (2) minimization of patient morbidity. Adjuvant therapies, including radioactive iodine and external beam radiation, should be included in all management strategies to maximize local control and minimize distant metastasis.

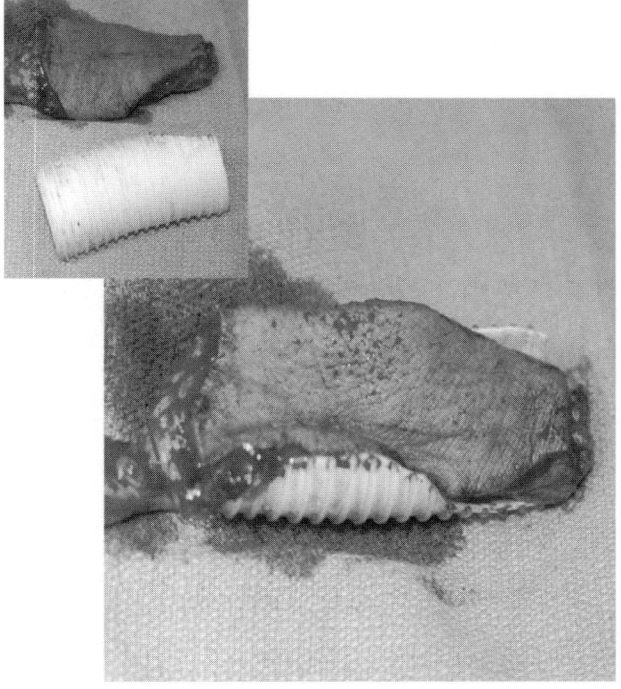

Figure 5 Radial forearm free flap reconstruction of a large anterior tracheal wall defect with a polytetrafluoroethylene scaffold (Courtesy of Dr. Peirong Yu).

References

1. Tollefsen HR, Decosse JJ, Hutter RV. Papillary carcinoma of the thyroid. A clinical and pathological study of 70 fatal cases. Cancer 1964;17:1035–44.

2. Hammoud ZT, Mathisen DJ. Surgical management of thyroid carcinoma invading the trachea. Chest Surg Clin N Am 2003;13:359–67.

3. McCaffrey TV, Bergstralh EJ, Hay ID. Locally invasive papillary thyroid carcinoma: 1940–1990. Head Neck 1994; 16:165–72.

4. McConahey WM, Hay ID, Woolner LB, et al. Papillary thyroid cancer treated at the Mayo Clinic, 1946 through 1970: initial manifestations, pathologic findings, therapy, and outcome. Mayo Clin Proc 1986;61:978–96.

5. Kowalski LP, Filho JG. Results of the treatment of locally invasive thyroid carcinoma. Head Neck 2002;24:340–4.

6. D'Avanzo A, Treseler P, Ituarte PH, et al. Follicular thyroid carcinoma: histology and prognosis. Cancer 2004;100:1123–9.

7. Lopez-Penabad L, Chiu AC, Hoff AO, et al. Prognostic factors in patients with Hurthle cell neoplasms of the thyroid. Cancer 2003;97:1186–94.

8. Machens A, Hinze R, Dralle H. Surgery on the cervicovisceral axis for invasive thyroid cancer. Langenbecks Arch Surg 2001;386:318–23.

9. McIver B, Hay ID, Giuffrida DF, et al. Anaplastic thyroid carcinoma: a 50-year experience at a single institution. Surgery 2001;130:1028–34.

10. Breaux GP Jr, Guillamondegui OM. Treatment of locally invasive carcinoma of the thyroid: how radical? Am J Surg 1980;140:514–7.

11. Grillo HC, Suen HC, Mathisen DJ, Wain JC. Resectional management of thyroid carcinoma invading the airway. Ann Thorac Surg 1992;54:3–9; discussion 9–10.

12. Gillenwater AM, Goepfert H. Surgical management of laryngotracheal and esophageal involvement by locally advanced thyroid cancer. Semin Surg Oncol 1999;16:19–29.

13. Czaja JM, McCaffrey TV. The surgical management of laryngotracheal invasion by well-differentiated papillary thyroid carcinoma. Arch Otolaryngol Head Neck Surg 1997;123:484–90.

14. Park CS, Suh KW, Min JS. Cartilage-shaving procedure for the control of tracheal cartilage invasion by thyroid carcinoma. Head Neck 1993;15:289–91.

15. Friedman M. Surgical management of thyroid carcinoma with laryngotracheal invasion. Otolaryngol Clin North Am 1990;23:495–507.

16. Beldholm BR, Wilson MK, Gallagher RM, et al. Reconstruction of the trachea with a tubed radial forearm free flap. J Thorac Cardiovasc Surg 2003;126:545–50.

17. Tsang RW, Brierley JD, Simpson WJ, et al. The effects of surgery, radioiodine, and external radiation therapy on the clinical outcome of patients with differentiated thyroid carcinoma. Cancer 1998;82:375–88.

18. Brierley JD, Tsang RW. External-beam radiation therapy in the treatment of differentiated thyroid cancer. Semin Surg Oncol 1999;16:42–9.

19. Bayles SW, Kingdom TT, Carlson GW. Management of thyroid carcinoma invading the aerodigestive tract. Laryngoscope 1998;108:1402–7.

20. Kasperbauer JL. Locally advanced thyroid carcinoma. Ann Otol Rhinol Laryngol 2004;113:749–53.

21. Ballantyne AJ. Resections of the upper aerodigestive tract for locally invasive thyroid cancer. Am J Surg 1994;168:636–9.

CHAPTER 39

EVALUATION AND MANAGEMENT OF ANAPLASTIC THYROID CARCINOMA

CHRISTOPHER KLEM, MD

DANIELLE D. ELLIOTT, MD

ERICH M. STURGIS, MD, MPH

Anaplastic thyroid carcinoma (ATC) is the least common and most lethal thyroid malignancy. It typically presents as a rapidly enlarging central and/or lower neck mass, often with symptoms of airway obstruction or dysphagia. Even with aggressive treatment, patients rarely live longer than 12 months after the time of diagnosis. Because of the rarity, aggressiveness, and overall poor prognosis of ATC, correct pathologic diagnosis is critical, but little progress has been made in the successful treatment and management of this disease.

Epidemiology

ATC is extremely rare, with approximately 500 new cases diagnosed annually in the US.[1–3] For reasons that are not readily apparent, the number of cases has been decreasing in recent decades.[4] Although this disease represents less than 2% of all primary thyroid malignancies, it is responsible for 25 to 50% of the 1,490 deaths attributed annually to thyroid cancer.[5,6] This is primarily a disease of the elderly; almost all patients are older than 50 years of age, and most are older than 70 years of age (mean, 71.3 ± 12.7 years).[1,2,7] There is a 2.0 to 2.5:1.0 female-to-male preponderance of the disease, a lower female preponderance than in differentiated thyroid malignancies.[1,2,7] Most patients are white and approximately 5% are African-American.[7]

A multi-institutional prospective cohort study of more than 5,000 patients with thyroid cancer treated in 1996 included 96 patients with ATC and 5,310 patients with differentiated thyroid carcinoma. Of patients with ATC, 9.4% had a history of head and neck radiation therapy compared with less than 5% of patients with differentiated thyroid cancer.[1] In addition, one-quarter of the patients with ATC had a history of an enlarged thyroid compared with less than 15% of those with differentiated thyroid carcinoma. Of those with ATC, 11.5% had a history of a nonthyroid malignancy, but only 7% of the patients with differentiated thyroid cancer had such a history. No dramatic differences were noted in the frequency of family history of thyroid carcinoma or personal history of Graves' disease or thyroiditis. A matched pair analysis from Serbia of 110 patients with ATC and 110 hospital-based control patients without ATC matched for age, sex, time of hospitalization, and place of residence revealed that ATC was significantly associated with a history of goiter, residence in endemic goiter areas, and a previous nonthyroid malignancy.[8] In addition, the data suggested an association with diabetes mellitus and a low education level. Only two patients (both with ATC) reported a history of radiation exposure. Other studies have also reported the association between ATC and the presence of a long-standing goiter.[1,9–11] In summary, ATC is an extremely rare disease that generally occurs in the elderly, but a history of radiation exposure, a goiterous thyroid, and a prior nonthyroid malignancy are associative risk factors.

Pathologic Characteristics

On gross examination, ATC is characterized by a diffusely infiltrative, firm tumor mass that usually obliterates most of the normal thyroid parenchyma. The cut surface is typically tan-white, firm, and homogeneous with areas of hemorrhage and necrosis (Figure 1a). ATCs commonly demonstrate significant extraglandular extension with invasion of adjacent structures, including the skin, the strap muscles, the laryngotracheal complex, and the esophagus (see Figure 1a). These gross findings may aid in the diagnosis, but they are seen with decreasing frequency by surgical pathologists because most disease is inoperable at the time of presentation. As a result, pathologic examination is usually based on material obtained during fine-needle aspiration (FNA) biopsy, core biopsy, or open biopsy.

The histologic diagnosis of ATC is always considered in the setting of a poorly differentiated malignant thyroid

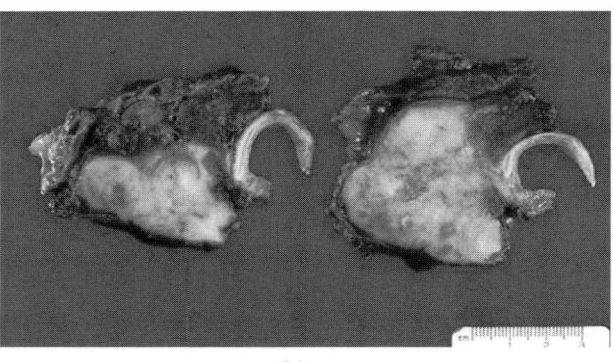

(a)

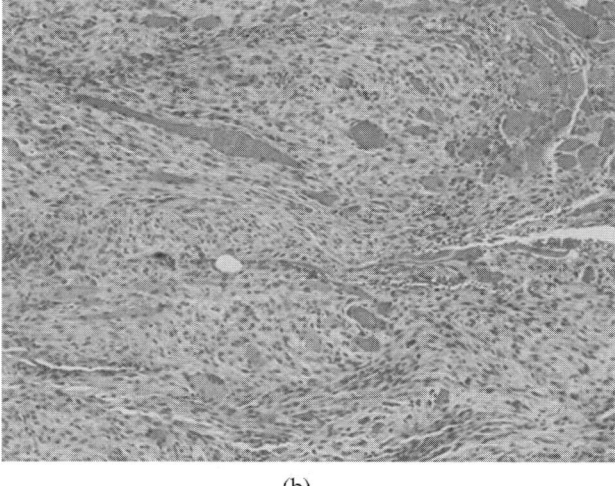

(b)

Figure 1 Pathologic characteristics of anaplastic thyroid carcinoma. A, Photograph shows anaplastic thyroid carcinoma invading adjacent strap muscles and tracheal cartilage. B, Photomicrograph of anaplastic thyroid carcinoma shows spindle cells infiltrating skeletal muscle.

tumor. However, the broad histologic differential diagnosis combined with often limited biopsy material does pose some difficulty. There are three major histologic subtypes of ATC that may be found alone or in combination. While these subtypes have little clinical relevance, each requires its own differential diagnosis.[10] ATCs of all histologic subtypes are usually markedly atypical epithelial tumors with high mitotic activity, nuclear pleomorphism, and areas of vascular invasion and necrosis.[9,12] The spindle cell variant may be indistinguishable from sarcoma on light microscopy, mimicking a spindle cell sarcoma such as fibrosarcoma, leiomyosarcoma, or malignant fibrous histiocytoma (Figure 1b). Scattered areas or even large portions may be paucicellular with fibrosis and marked collagen deposition mimicking benign fibrosing processes such as Riedel's thyroiditis.[13] The giant cell variant is composed of sheets of epithelial and/or spindled cells infiltrated by histiocytic giant cells and tumor giant cells. This variant tends to show more marked nuclear atypia and resembles pleomorphic sarcomas such as malignant fibrous histiocytoma. The squamoid variant, as its name implies, has epithelial differentiation that may mimic squamous cell carcinoma (SCC). This subtype must be distinguished from the rare primary SCC of the thyroid, papillary thyroid carcinoma with squamous metaplasia, and SCCs from adjacent sites that secondarily involve the thyroid gland since such entities can often be successfully treated with surgery.

The histologic distinction between ATC (undifferentiated thyroid carcinoma) and poorly differentiated thyroid carcinomas such as insular carcinomas and tall cell or solid variants of papillary thyroid carcinoma is important because these tumors portend longer survival and are amendable to surgical treatment. This differentiation can be made with careful histologic examination by identifying classic areas of differentiated thyroid carcinoma or follicular differentiation.[10,14] Metastases to the thyroid are infrequent but should also be excluded from the differential diagnosis. Metastatic tumors may clinically present similarly to ATC, with a rapidly growing thyroid mass or an enlarging goiter. Lung, breast, and kidney adenocarcinomas are sources of the most common metastases to the thyroid found at autopsy and in clinical series.[15] Despite similarities in the clinical presentation, histologic evaluation with supporting immunohistochemical studies and a thorough clinical history will lead to the correct diagnosis.

Immunohistochemical analysis can help differentiate ATC from other poorly differentiated malignancies. Demonstration of epithelial differentiation is critical in excluding other entities, particularly sarcoma. While expression of most markers is variable between and within individual tumors, up to 80% of ATCs will show some form of epithelial expression with the use of antibodies to various keratins or epithelial membrane antigen.[9,16–19] ATC may also stain positive for thyroglobulin, indicating a thyroid epithelial origin; however, a negative result does not exclude the diagnosis.[16] The often uniform expression of thyroid transcription factor-1 seen in differentiated thyroid carcinomas is absent in ATC.[20] Most immunostaining patterns in ATC are patchy and variable and thus lead to diagnostic difficulty on small biopsy samples. Electron microscopy, though not routinely used, may be helpful in establishing a diagnosis of ATC with the identification of ultrastructural epithelial cell features such as desmosomes and tight junctions.[12] All of these ancillary techniques are helpful in establishing a diagnosis of ATC, but ultimately, the diagnosis is one of exclusion and requires correlation with clinical findings.

As discussed above, the presence of a long-standing goiter is an apparent risk factor for the development of ATC.[1,8–11] In addition, many series have reported the presence of a preexisting differentiated thyroid carcinoma in cases of ATC, with rates between 23 and 90%.[21–24] Such areas of differentiated thyroid carcinoma serve to aid in the diagnosis of and provide evidence for a presumed malignant transformation from a differentiated thyroid carcinoma.[9] Some investigators have identified molecular events thought to play a role in the anaplastic transformation of differentiated thyroid carcinoma and normal follicular epithelium. Mutations in tumor suppressor genes such as *p53* and *PTEN* have been identified in ATC but not in coexisting differentiated thyroid carcinoma.[11,24,25] Other researchers have found loss of heterozygosity at multiple loci, including microsatellite markers in ATC, but not in differentiated thyroid carcinomas.[26,27] In addition, various growth factor receptors known to participate in thyroid tumorigenesis are overexpressed in ATC. Recent reports of overexpression of epidermal growth factor receptor and platelet-derived growth factor receptor in ATC show that they hold great promise for therapeutic intervention.[28–30] It is hoped that such an understanding of the molecular pathogenesis of ATC will ultimately lead to easier diagnosis and better targeted, more effective, and less toxic therapies.

Clinical Presentation

Most patients with ATC present with a rapidly enlarging central and/or lower neck mass (Figure 2), and approximately 25% of them have a history of a preexisting goiterous mass.[1,2,6,9,31–33] Common associated symptoms include dysphagia, hoarseness or voice change, neck pain,

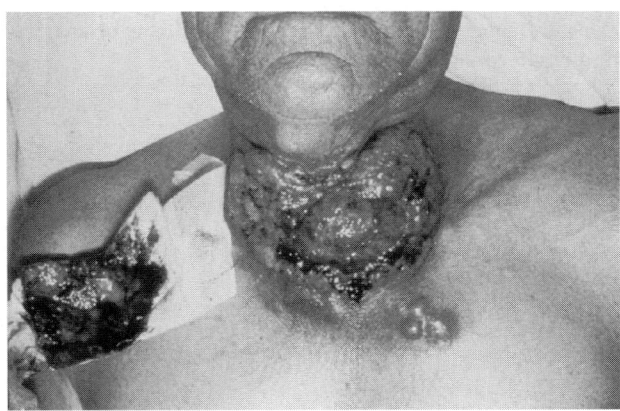

Figure 2 Photograph of an elderly man with locally advanced anaplastic thyroid carcinoma and dermal metastases.

stridor, and weight loss (Table 1).[1–3,9,32,33] Hemoptysis, which implies airway involvement, is a grave but uncommon presenting symptom.

Physical examination typically reveals a large, fixed thyroid mass usually larger than 5 cm.[1–3,4,33] Approximately 50% of patients have palpable cervical lymphadenopathy at the time of presentation (see Table 1).[1,2,4,6,7,31,34] Approximately 33% of patients have unilateral or bilateral vocal cord paralysis and direct invasion into the trachea or esophagus occurs in approximately 25% of patients.[1–4,9,33] Airway obstruction from bilateral vocal fold paralysis and/or airway involvement is common at presentation, and subsequent airway obstruction and aspiration pneumonia are leading causes of death.[6] Distant metastatic disease is present in 50% of patients at the time of diagnosis, most commonly to the lungs (90%), bones (15%), and brain (15%) (see Table 1).[4,6,7,10,31,32]

Evaluation

The diagnostic evaluation of ATC centers on correct pathologic diagnosis, understanding the extent of local disease and the critical structures involved, and detecting distant metastatic spread. FNA biopsy is typically sufficient to diagnose the disease, though open biopsy is occasionally necessary and can often be performed at the time of a tracheotomy. When cytopathologic differentiation from poorly differentiated variants of papillary and follicular carcinomas is in question, a core-needle biopsy may more effectively permit a histopathologic diagnosis. As mentioned above, immunohistochemical testing and careful histologic examination can often be used to differentiate ATC from other poorly differentiated malignancies.

Table 1 Demographics and presenting symptoms of anaplastic thyroid carcinoma patients.

Demographics and Presenting Symptoms	No. of Patients (%)
Sex	
Female	345 (66.9)
Male	171 (33.1)
Ethnicity	
White	437 (85.0)
Asian/Pacific Islander	49 (9.5)
African-American	26 (5.1)
Native-American	2 (0.4)
Extent of disease	
Local	39 (8.6)
Regional	194 (42.6)
Distant	222 (48.8)
Local symptoms	
Thyroid mass	74 (77.1)
Hoarseness/voice change	39 (40.6)
Dysphagia	38 (40.0)
Stridor	23 (24.0)
Regional symptoms	
Lymph node mass	52 (54.2)
Neck pain	25 (26.0)
Systemic or distant symptoms	
Weight loss	20 (20.8)
Bone pain	6 (6.3)
Pathologic fracture	1 (1.0)
Other	22 (23.2)

Demographics of 516 patients with anaplastic thyroid carcinoma from Surveillance Epidemiology and End Results (SEER) registries from 1973 to 2000[7] and presenting symptoms of 96 patients with anaplastic thyroid carcinoma from a prospective cohort of over 5,000 patients in the US with newly diagnosed thyroic cancer in 1996.[1]

Prior to treatment of ATC, radiographic imaging is essential. If an ATC is suspected, a computed tomography (CT) scan with contrast or magnetic resonance imaging (MRI) with gadolinium can be used to evaluate the involvement by the tumor of any surrounding critical structures, including the larynx, trachea, esophagus, deep cervical muscles, and carotid artery (Figure 3). When an advanced, aggressive thyroid cancer is being imaged, CT typically provides superior imaging of the thyroid and surrounding structures over MRI. The need to adequately assess local extension of aggressive thyroid malignancies supersedes the concerns about iodine administration in patients with thyroid cancer. Sonography allows adequate imaging of early thyroid cancers and nodal disease, but is usually inadequate for evaluating the extent of extraglandular extension common in ATCs. In addition, a CT scan of the chest can be obtained at the time of head and neck CT imaging and should be included in the work-up of all patients with ATC to evaluate for distant metastatic disease. The precise role of positron emission tomography (PET) in the evaluation and follow-up of patients with ATC is not

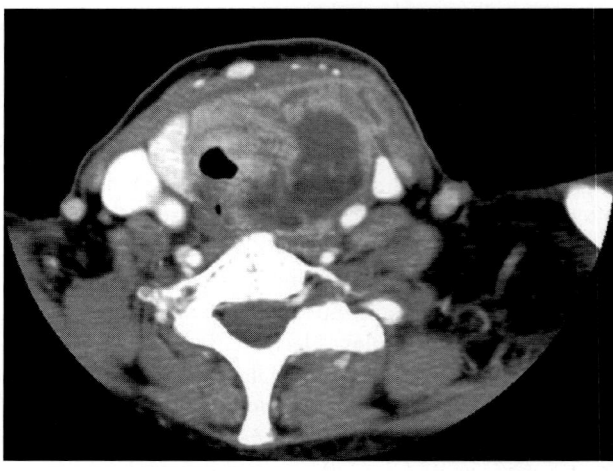

Figure 3 Anaplastic thyroid carcinoma of the left thyroid lobe with CT scan evidence of strap muscle invasion, early esophageal and tracheal involvement, and pending invasion of the carotid artery and prevertebral fascia.

well defined. Case reports have documented the ability of PET to detect the disease, but there are no comparative data for more traditional imaging modalities.[35–37]

Staging

The sixth edition of the American Joint Committee on Cancer's cancer staging manual includes changes to staging system of thyroid cancer to account for the significant differences in outcome between the different histologic subtypes.[38] All ATCs are considered T4 tumors. The T4 category for anaplastic carcinomas is subcategorized into T4a (intrathyroidal anaplastic carcinoma–surgically resectable) and T4b (extrathyroidal anaplastic carcinoma–surgically unresectable) (Table 2). In addition, regardless of the patient's age at presentation and the presence of nodal or distant metastases, all ATCs are considered stage IV. According to Surveillance Epidemiology and End Results (SEER) registry data from 1973 to 2000, only a small minority of patients presented with disease only at the primary site (see Table 1).[7]

Treatment

The management of ATC presents a dilemma for both physicians and patients because of the rapid progression of the disease and virtually universal poor outcome. In addition, the literature on this disease consists of primarily small, retrospective case series without controls, and the level of evidence supporting particular treatments is poor. Treatment options are based primarily on the extent of the primary tumor and

Table 2 National Cancer Institute and TNM Staging of Anaplastic Thyroid Carcinoma

National Cancer Institute stage	T stage	N stage	M stage
IV			
A	T4a–intrathyroidal, surgically resectable	Any	0
B	T4b–extrathyroidal, unresectable	Any	0
C	Any	Any	1

TMN = tumor, nodes, metastasis.
Adapted from Greene FL et al.[38]

presence of distant metastatic disease and include surgery, radiation therapy, and chemotherapy, but rarely will one of these modalities be successful alone. In highly selected cases, combination therapy with surgery and adjuvant postoperative chemoradiation therapy or a combination of chemotherapy and radiation therapy may provide improved local control, palliation, and possibly survival.

Initial therapeutic priorities must include the safety of the patient's airway and nutritional support; many surgeons recommend placement of a tracheotomy and enteral feeding tube soon after diagnosis, before disease progression creates an emergent situation. However, the role of prophylactic tracheotomy is unclear because of the lack of evidence of a prognostic benefit despite clear detriments to the patient's quality of life. In a review of 67 patients with ATC, Pierie and colleagues found that the placement of a tracheotomy or enteral feeding tube had no effect on survival.[32] Holting and colleagues reported on 32 patients with anaplastic thyroid cancer whose treatment included a tracheotomy.[39] In that study, the mean survival time was 2 months compared with 5 months for 45 patients who did not undergo a tracheotomy. In addition, many patients with tracheotomies experienced local wound complications that delayed or prevented postoperative radiation therapy, and the authors point out the likelihood that patients who had tracheotomies had more aggressive tumors and delays in treatment.[39] At a minimum, discussion of these issues should be undertaken with the patient soon after diagnosis, but it should be kept in mind that tracheotomy brings with it significant local problems and quality-of-life changes of its own, particularly in patients with an aggressive mass growing immediately adjacent to the tracheotomy, which can cause significant bleeding and hemorrhagic aspiration.

Surgery

Ruling out distant metastatic disease is imperative before surgical resection can be considered, but complete surgical resection of ATC is rarely feasible because the disease is often locally advanced at the time of diagnosis.

Few data exist to support surgery as the sole method of treatment, but much controversy exists over the role and extent of surgery. All studies of the benefit of surgical treatment of ATC have been confounded by selection bias because typically the smaller, more confined ATCs will be operated on and the most advanced will be treated nonsurgically, often in a palliative fashion. In addition, many ATCs treated surgically are pathologically diagnosed postoperatively as a smaller component of a differentiated tumor for which the surgery was initially planned and consequently are much more likely to be cured.[3] Multiple retrospective studies suggest a survival benefit in patients who undergo surgery, but these results should be interpreted cautiously because of significant biases in the reported retrospective experiences.[31,32,40,41]

Haigh and colleagues reviewed 33 cases of ATC treated over 25 years.[31] Of the 26 patients who underwent surgical treatment, 4 were considered macroscopically free of disease and 4 had minimal residual disease after total thyroidectomy and resection of tumor adherent to adjacent structures. Of those 8 patients, 4 were alive 5 years after surgery and postoperative radiation therapy and chemotherapy. A significant survival benefit was found for patients treated with total or near-total resection followed by chemoradiation therapy compared with that in patients treated with either palliative resection plus chemoradiation therapy or chemoradiation therapy alone (43 months versus 3 months, $p = .002$). The authors note that a strategy of aggressive surgical management with organ preservation was used throughout the study period: sacrifice of structures with radical en-bloc resections of the larynx or esophagus was not performed, nor were recurrent laryngeal nerves resected unless vocal cord paresis was documented preoperatively or tumor invasion of the nerve was found intraoperatively. Inherent bias in surgical selection could easily explain the survival of those four patients. In addition, various chemotherapeutic agents and radiation doses and schedules were used during the study period, making conclusions regarding effective alternative therapies difficult.[31]

Pierie and colleagues reported retrospectively on 67 patients with ATC treated between 1969 and 1999.[32]

Surgery was performed on 44 patients; 12 underwent complete resections. The respective survival rates at 6 months, 1 year, and 3 years were 92%, 92%, and 83% after complete resection and 22%, 4%, and 0% after no surgery ($p < .0001$). Improved outcome was also seen in patients who received radiation doses higher than 45 Gy. It must be noted, however, that 10 patients had incidentally found ATC and that 8 of the 12 completely resected carcinomas were incidentally found. These incidental ATCs behaved in a more indolent fashion than those in patients who initially presented with the disease.[32]

In a 50-year review of 134 patients with ATC treated at a single institution, McIver and colleagues found no significant differences in the median survival between those treated with surgery (3.5 months) and those treated with radiation (2.3 months).[6] Both groups had longer survival than did those undergoing only palliative care (3 weeks), and all 13 patients who survived longer than 1 year had undergone surgical resection (8 complete, 3 with minimal residual tumor, and 2 with gross residual tumor). In another review, Besic and colleagues found the survival at 1 year to be 25% for the 26 patients whose primary treatment was surgery, 21% for the 53 patients treated with radiation and chemotherapy, and 0% for the 83 patients treated with palliative intent.[42] In a retrospective population-based cohort from the SEER database of 516 patients with ATC treated between 1973 and 2000, Kebebew and colleagues found surgical resection to have a significant positive effect on survival, but on multivariate analysis, only age (< 60 years), SEER extent of disease, and combined surgery and radiation therapy were associated with significantly improved survival.[7]

Some have suggested that debulking surgery may play a role in the initial treatment of local ATC in the absence of distant metastases. In one study from Japan, Sugino and colleagues reviewed the cases of 40 patients treated over a 10-year period.[41] Of the 26 patients who initially presented with localized ATC, 15 underwent surgical debulking as part of their initial therapy. Debulking surgery was indicated if reduction of more than 90% of the tumor was resected. The 1-year survival of the 15 patients who underwent debulking surgery was significantly improved over that of the 11 patients who did not undergo surgery (60% versus 21%, $p = .01$). Three patients who underwent surgical debulking survived more than 2 years. No survival advantage was found for either radiation therapy or chemotherapy.[41] However, in the study by Haigh and colleagues discussed above, the median survival of 3 months after debulking surgery plus chemotherapy and radiation therapy was not significantly different than that for chemoradiation therapy alone ($p = .063$).[31] In the series reported by Pierie and

colleagues, the 6- and 12-month survival rates were better for those undergoing debulking surgery (53% and 35% versus 22% and 4%; $p = .008$), but no patients survived at 3 years.[32]

While it would seem that patients who undergo surgery for ATC have improved longer survival than those who undergo nonsurgical treatment, the gains are minimal and the locally aggressive behavior of the disease puts such patients at significant risk for perioperative morbidity and mortality. Most surgeons believe that the risks of surgery outweigh the potential benefits of longer survival in most patients with ATC.

Despite its inclusion in some of the retrospective series discussed above, ATC found incidentally in patients who undergo surgery for presumed differentiated thyroid carcinoma is a different disease. In fact, the overall survival (OS) rates may approach those of patients with other poorly differentiated thyroid carcinoma histologies.[32,41] However, because of the proclivity of ATC for local recurrence and distant metastases, aggressive multimodality therapy, including postoperative radiation therapy, chemotherapy, or chemoradiation therapy is recommended for patients with incidental disease.[41]

Radiation Therapy

ATC has not been traditionally thought to be particularly radiosensitive, but multiple studies have shown a benefit in local disease control with radiation therapy, either alone or as an adjunct to surgery and/or chemotherapy. Levendag and colleagues retrospectively reviewed the cases of 51 patients with ATC to investigate the potential role of definitive external beam radiation therapy (EBRT) with or without chemotherapy.[43] Those patients treated with less than 30 Gy had less than a 1-month median survival duration, whereas those treated with doses more than 30 Gy had a median survival duration of 3.3 months and a 1-year survival rate of 10%. For patients without residual disease at the end of radiation therapy, an actuarial median survival of 8 months was observed. In patients with local residual disease after therapy, the median survival was 1.6 months, and 100% had died within 8 months. This analysis supported the conclusion that local control is imperative for achieving improved short-term survival rates and that radiation can improve local control.[43]

Because ATCs are rapidly growing tumors with short doubling times, accelerated radiation therapy should decrease cell repopulation and reduce the opportunity for tumor cells to repopulate during the course of treatment. Hyperfractionation of radiation therapy theoretically allows higher total doses of radiation to be delivered with less toxicity. In a study of hyperfractionated radiation therapy to a total dose of 60.8 Gy in 32 fractions without adjuvant treatment, Mitchell and colleagues treated 17 patients with ATC.[44] Three patients experienced a complete clinical response and seven patients experienced a partial response. However, most patients experienced grades 3 and 4 toxicities, including severe esophagitis, dysphagia, and tracheoesophageal fistula, and five patients died before the toxicity had fully resolved.[44]

Other studies have also shown a survival advantage with hyperfractionated radiation therapy over conventional radiation therapy. Heron and colleagues retrospectively reviewed the cases of 32 patients with anaplastic thyroid cancer, 9 of whom had been treated with daily radiation therapy and 23 of whom had undergone twice-daily radiation therapy with concurrent chemotherapy.[45] Twelve of the patients underwent surgical resection prior to radiation therapy (4 in the daily radiation therapy group and 8 in the twice-daily radiation therapy group). Overall 2-year survival rates were 44% for the daily radiation therapy group and 52% for the twice-daily radiation therapy group. In this study, the authors included poorly differentiated histologic subtypes, (which tend to be more treatable), with the true anaplastic tumors; this may explain the better survival rates obtained in this series than the historical rates reported for ATC. Among 516 patients in the SEER database, EBRT was associated with significantly improved survival, but these results were not seen after multivariate adjustment.[7]

Therefore, as a single modality of local therapy, radiation will cure exceedingly few patients with ATC, and although hyperfractionation offers some advantages, the most appropriate schedule and dose remain to be determined.

Chemotherapy

ATC often presents with or proceeds to distant metastatic disease, so systemic therapy is considered vital to successful treatment. However, this tumor is notoriously chemo resistant, and none of the currently available chemotherapeutic agents have been effective when used alone in preventing disease progression. Doxorubicin has long been considered the mainstay of chemotherapy in ATC but is ineffective as monotherapy, with a response rate of less than 25%. Other agents, used alone, have been even less effective.[46–48] After preclinical studies demonstrated significant antineoplastic activity of paclitaxel, Ain and colleagues used it in a phase II trial to treat ATC in patients with persistent metastatic disease despite surgery and/or radiation therapy.[49] Twenty patients were

treated with a 96-hour infusion of paclitaxel every 3 weeks for one to six cycles. The authors found a 53% response rate, with one complete response and nine partial responses (including one off protocol); however, no survival benefit was demonstrated.[49] Combination chemotherapy used alone has been shown to have little benefit over single-agent treatment, though newer combinations continue to be tried and a better understanding of multidrug resistance is emerging.

Multimodality Treatment

Because surgery, radiation therapy, and chemotherapy are ineffective alone, successful treatment of ATC must involve multiple methods. Retrospective studies have shown a benefit in locoregional control and occasionally in survival with aggressive combination therapy, but such studies have been hampered by numerous biases, heterogeneous treatments, and limited power, all common limitations of retrospective series of rare diseases.[5,40,42,50]

In a prospective study of locally advanced thyroid cancer, Kim and Leeper prospectively treated 19 patients with ATC with a combination regimen of low-dose doxorubicin (10 mg/m^2 once-weekly) before hyperfractionated radiation therapy (160 cGy per treatment twice daily for 3 days per week to a total dose of 5,760 cGy in 40 days).[51] The complete tumor response rate was 84%, and the local control rate at 2 years was 68%, a significant improvement over historic controls. The median survival rate of 1 year was also longer than that in control patients. Although no patient had obvious metastatic disease when treatment was initiated, most eventually developed distant metastases and died of the disease.[51]

In one of the largest prospective studies of ATC, Tennvall and colleagues used a combined regimen consisting of hyperfractionated radiation therapy, doxorubicin, and when feasible, debulking surgery in 55 consecutive patients.[52] The authors found improved local control in all 33 patients treated with surgery compared with historical controls. Nine patients (16%) survived for more than 1 year, and five patients (9%) were free of disease at 2 years, but no significant difference was observed in the distant metastases rate. It is notable that patients with incidentally found ATCs were not included in this study.[52]

De Crevoisier and colleagues prospectively treated 30 patients with a combination of surgery, chemotherapy, and hyperfractionated radiation therapy.[40] Complete macroscopic resection was performed as the initial modality when feasible (n = 17). Chemotherapy was given immediately after surgery and consisted of a combination of doxorubicin and cisplatin every 4 weeks.

Hyperfractionated radiation therapy was started 15 days after the second cycle of chemotherapy finished and consisted of two daily fractions of 1.25 Gy, to a total dose of 40 Gy. Survival rates at 1 and 3 years were 46% and 27%, respectively, and the median survival time was 10 months. Significant poor prognostic factors omit were tracheal extension and the inability to achieve macroscopically complete resection.[40]

In several retrospective series, complete surgical resection resulted in the longest survival times and, in rare cases, cures.[5,31–33,42] Multimodality therapy did not clearly improve survival duration, though adjuvant radiation therapy and chemotherapy seemed to provide some benefit. However, these single-institutional retrospective series of cases, collected over a long time involve inherent biases and differences in surgical technique, radiotherapeutic schema, and chemotherapeutic agents. In a study of 516 ATC patients in the population-based SEER registry from 1973 to 2000, Kebebew and colleagues found, in multivariate analysis, that surgery combined with EBRT was associated with significantly better outcomes, though survival of this group was only approximately 10% at 4 years.[7]

Taken together, the prospective and retrospective data suggest that aggressive multimodality treatment, including surgical resection, offers some modest benefits but that treatment morbidities are significant, the prognosis is dismal, and careful selection, frank patient counseling, and multidisciplinary evaluations are critical.

Future Directions

Despite advances in surgical techniques, chemotherapeutic agents, and radiation therapy schema, the prognosis for ATC remains dismal. Because patients with the disease have a median survival time of less than 6 months, even with aggressive treatment, innovative treatments for this aggressive malignancy are being actively investigated.

Yu and colleagues reported on the treatment of aggressive thyroid cancer with an oncolytic herpes virus in an animal model.[53] These viruses are promising therapeutic agents when they are genetically modified to attenuate their toxicity to normal tissues while maintaining lytic activity against malignant tumors. Intratumoral injection of the virus resulted in significantly decreased tumor volume with no associated morbidity.[53] In two patients with end-stage ATC, Barzon and colleagues have demonstrated necrosis of tumor masses injected with a retroviral vector carrying the human interleukin-2 gene and the suicide gene thymidine kinase of herpes simplex virus type 1, followed by ganciclovir administration.[54]

The results of two recent studies exemplify the shift toward targeted molecular therapy in the treatment of ATC. Schiff and colleagues found that epidermal growth factor receptor is consistently overexpressed in ATC cell lines in vitro and in vivo and in human tissue arrays.[29] They found that gefitinib, an epidermal growth factor receptor inhibitor, effectively blocked activation of the receptor, inhibited anaplastic cellular proliferation, and induced apoptosis in vitro. Gefitinib also had significant antitumor activity against anaplastic thyroid cancer in a mouse thyroid cancer tumor model.[29] And in preclinical study of AEE788, a dual inhibitor of epidermal growth factor receptor and vascular endothelial growth factor receptor tyrosine kinases, Kim and colleagues demonstrated that AEE788 inhibited proliferation and induced apoptosis of ATC cell lines in vitro.[30] In a mouse model, administration of AEE788, alone and in combination with paclitaxel, inhibited the growth of ATC xenografts by 44% and 69%, respectively. The group treated with AEE788 plus paclitaxel also showed a 6- to 8-fold increase in tumor cell apoptosis compared with the control group.[30]

Ultimately, the understanding of the molecular pathogenesis of ATC will lead to targeted, more effective, and less toxic therapies.

Conclusions

In conclusion, ATC is a rare disease with an extremely poor prognosis. Successful treatment is uncommon, but rarely nonmutilating surgery will be possible and may be attempted with aggressive adjuvant chemoradiation therapy. For small ATCs that are incidentally found postoperatively on histopathologic review of a thyroid specimen, aggressive adjuvant chemoradiation should also be seriously considered. However, for most patients, complete surgical resection will not be possible, and such patients should be offered experimental nonsurgical treatment. Frank discussions of palliative options should be included in treatment planning.

References

1. Hundahl SA, Cady B, Cunningham MP, et al. Initial results from a prospective cohort study of 5583 cases of thyroid carcinoma treated in the United States during 1996. Cancer 2000;89:202–17.

2. Hundahl SA, Fleming ID, Fremgen AM, Menck HR. A National Cancer Data Base report on 53,856 cases of thyroid carcinoma treated in the U.S., 1985–1995. Cancer 1998;83:2638–48.

3. Ain KB. Anaplastic thyroid carcinoma: a therapeutic challenge. Semin Surg Oncol 1999;16:64–9.

4. Pasieka JL. Anaplastic thyroid cancer. Curr Opin Oncol 2003;15:78–83.

5. Jemal A, Taylor M, Ward E, et al. Cancer statistics, 2005. CA Cancer J Clin 2005;55:10–30.

6. McIver MB, Hay ID, Giuffrida DF. Anaplastic thyroid carcinoma: a 50-year experience at a single institution. Surgery 2001;130:1028–34.

7. Kebebew E, Greenspan FS, Clark OH, et al. Anaplastic thyroid carcinoma, treatment outcome and prognostic factors. Cancer 2005;103:1330–5.

8. Zivaljevic V, Vlajinac H, Jankovic R, et al. Case-control study of anaplastic thyroid cancer. Tumori 2004;90:9–12.

9. Venkatesh YS, Ordonez NG, Schultz PN, et al. Anaplastic carcinoma of the thyroid. A clinicopathologic study of 121 cases. Cancer 1990;66:321–30.

10. Carcangiu ML, Steeper T, Zampi G, Rosai J. Anaplastic thyroid carcinoma: a study of 70 cases. Am J Clin Path 1985;83:135–58.

11. Lam KY, Lo CY, Chan KW, Wan KY. Insular and anaplastic carcinoma of the thyroid: a 45-year comparative study at a single institution and a review of the significance of p53 and p21. Ann Surg 2000;231:329–38.

12. Austin JR, El-Naggar AK, Goepfert H. Thyroid cancers II: medullary, anaplastic, lymphoma, sarcoma, squamous cell. Otolaryngol Clin North Am 1996;29:611–27.

13. Canos JC, Serrano A, Matias-Guiu X. Paucicellular variant of anaplastic thyroid carcinoma: report of two cases. Endocr Pathol 2001;12:157–61.

14. Breau RL, Suen JY. Lymphoma and anaplastic carcinoma of the thyroid. In: Randolph GW, editor. Surgery of the thyroid and parathyroid glands. Philadelphia: Saunders; 2003. p. 245–52.

15. Nakhjavani MK, Gharib H, Goellner JR, van Heerden JA. Metastasis to the thyroid gland. A report of 43 cases. Cancer 1997;79:574–8.

16. Ratnatnga N, Ramadasa S. Immunohistochemical staining for thyroglobulin in poorly differentiated carcinoma of the thyroid. Ceylon Med J 1993;38:113–6.

17. Kobayashi S, Yamadori I, Ohmori M, et al. Anaplastic carcinoma of the thyroid with osteoclast-like giant cells. An ultrastructural and immunohistochemical study. Acta Pathol Jpn 1987;37:807–15.

18. Hurlimann J, Gardiol D, Scazziga B. Immunohistology of anaplastic thyroid carcinoma. A study of 43 cases. Histopathology 1987;11:567–80.

19. Ordonez NG, El-Naggar AK, Hickey RC, Samaan NA. Anaplastic thyroid carcinoma. Immunocytochemical study of 32 cases. Am J Clin Pathol., 1991;96:15–24.

20. Miettinen M, Franssila KO. Variable expression of keratins and nearly uniform lack of thyroid transcription factor 1 in thyroid anaplastic carcinoma. Hum Pathol 2000;31:1139–45.

21. Wiseman SM, Loree TR, Rigual NR. Anaplastic transformation of thyroid cancer: review of clinical, pathologic, and molecular evidence provides new insights into disease biology and future therapy. Head Neck 2003;25:662–70.

22. Wiseman SM, Loree TR, Hicks WL, et al. Anaplastic thyroid cancer evolved from papillary carcinoma: demonstration of anaplastic transformation by means of the inter-simple sequence repeat polymerase chain reaction. Arch Otolaryngol Head Neck Surg 2003;129:96–100.

23. Segev DL, Umbricht C, Zeiger MA. Molecular pathogenesis of thyroid cancer. Surg Oncol 2003;47:709–22.

24. Hunt JL, Tometsko M, LiVolsi VA, et al. Molecular evidence of anaplastic transformation in coexisting well-differentiated and anaplastic carcinomas of the thyroid. Am J Surg Pathol 2003;27:1559–64.

25. Moretti F, Farsetti A, Soddu S, et al. p53 re-expression inhibits proliferation and restores differentiation of human thyroid anaplastic carcinoma cells. Oncogene 1997;14:729–40.

26. Kitamura Y, Shimizu K, Tanaka S, et al. Allelotyping of anaplastic thyroid carcinoma: frequent allelic losses on 1q, 9p, 11, 17, 19p, and 22q. Genes Chromosomes Cancer 2000;27:244–51.

27. Kadota M, Tamaki Y, Sekimoto M, et al. Loss of heterozygosity on chromosome 16p and 18q in anaplastic thyroid carcinoma. Oncol Rep 2003;10:35–8.

28. Elliott DD, El-Naggar AK. Growth factor receptor expression in anaplastic thyroid carcinoma, implications for a therapeutic approach. Modern Pathol 2005;18:90A.

29. Schiff BA, McMurphy AB, Jasser SA, et al. Epidermal growth factor receptor (EGFR) is overexpressed in anaplastic thyroid cancer, and the EGFR inhibitor gefitinib inhibits the growth of anaplastic thyroid cancer. Clin Cancer Res 2004;10:8594–602.

30. Kim S, Schiff BA, Orhan GY, et al. Targeted molecular therapy of anaplastic thyroid carcinoma with AEE788. Mol Cancer Ther 2005;4:632–40.

31. Haigh PI, Ituarte PH, Wu HS, et al. Completely resected anaplastic thyroid carcinoma combined with adjuvant chemotherapy and irradiation is associated with prolonged survival. Cancer 2001;91:2335–42.

32. Pierie JP, Muzikansky A, Gaz RD, et al. The effect of surgery and radiation therapy on outcome of anaplastic thyroid carcinoma. Ann Surg Oncol 2002;9:57–64.

33. Tan RK, Finley RK, Driscoll D, et al. Anaplastic carcinoma of the thyroid: a 24-year experience. Head Neck 1995;17:41–8.

34. Ain KB. Anaplastic thyroid carcinoma: behavior, biology, and therapeutic approaches. Thyroid 1998;8:715–26.

35. Poppe K, Lahoute T, Everaert H, et al. Images in thyroidology. The utility of multimodality imaging in anaplastic thyroid carcinoma. Thyroid 2004;14:981–2.

36. Zettinig G, Leitha T, Niederle B, et al. FDG positron emission tomographic, radioiodine, and MIBI imaging in a patient with poorly differentiated insular thyroid carcinoma. Clin Nucl Med 2001;26:599–601.

37. Jadvar H, Fischman AJ. Evaluation of rare tumors with [F-18] fluorodeoxyglucose positron emission tomography. Clin Pos Imag 1999;2:153–8.

38. Greene FL, Page DL, Fleming ID, et al, editors. Thyroid. In: AJCC Cancer Staging Manual, 6th ed. New York: Springer-Verlag; 2002. p. 77–88.

39. Holting T, Meybier H, Buhr H. Stellenwert der tracheotomie in der behandlung des respiratorischen notfalls beim anaplastischer schilddrusenkarzinom. [Status of tracheotomy in treatment of the respiratory emergency in anaplastic thyroid cancer]. Wien Klin Wochenschr 1990; 102:264–6.

40. De Crevoisier R, Baudin E, Bachelot A, et al. Combined treatment of anaplastic thyroid carcinoma with surgery, chemotherapy, and hyperfractionated accelerated external radiation therapy. Int J Radiat Oncol Biol Phys 2004;60: 1137–43.

41. Sugino K, Ito K, Mimura T, et al. The important role of operations in the management of anaplastic thyroid carcinoma. Surgery 2002;131:245–8.

42. Besic N, Auerrsperg M, Us-Krasovec M, et al. Effect of primary treatment on survival in anaplastic thyroid carcinoma. Eur J Surg Oncol 2001;27:260–4.

43. Levendag PC, DePorre PM, van Putten WL. Anaplastic carcinoma of the thyroid gland treated by radiation therapy. Int J Radiat Oncol Biol Phys 1993;26:125–8.

44. Mitchell G, Huddart R, Harmer C. Phase II evaluation of high dose accelerated radiation therapy for anaplastic thyroid carcinoma. Radiother Oncol 1999;50:33–8.

45. Heron DE, Karimpour S, Grigsby PW. Anaplastic thyroid carcinoma: comparison of conventional radiation therapy and hyperfractionation chemoradiation therapy in two groups. Am J Clin Oncol 2002;25:442–6.

46. Poster DS, Bruno S, Penta J, et al. Current status of chemotherapy in the treatment of advanced carcinoma of the thyroid gland. Cancer Clin Trials 1981;4:301–7.

47. Shimoaoka K. Adjunctive management of thyroid cancer: chemotherapy. J Surg Oncol 1980;15:283–6.

48. DeBesi P, Busnardo B, Toso S, et al. Combined chemotherapy with bleomycin, adriamycin, and platinum in advanced thyroid cancer. J Endocrinol Invest 1991;14: 475–80.

49. Ain KB, Egorin MJ, DeSimone PA. Treatment of anaplastic thyroid carcinoma with paclitaxel: phase 2 trial using ninety-six hour infusion. Collaborative anaplastic thyroid cancer health intervention trials (CATCHIT) group. Thyroid 2000;10:587–94.

50. Nilsson O, Lindeberg J, Zedenius J, et al. Anaplastic giant cell carcinoma of the thyroid gland: treatment and survival over a 25-year period. World J Surg 1998;22: 725–30.

51. Kim JH, Leeper RD. Treatment of locally advanced thyroid carcinoma with combination doxorubicin and radiation therapy. Cancer 1987;60:2372–5.

52. Tennvall J, Lundell G, Wahlberg P. Anaplastic thyroid carcinoma: three protocols combining doxorubicin, hyperfractionated radiation therapy and surgery. Br J Cancer 2002;86:1848–53.

53. Yu Z, Eisenberg DP, Singh B, et al. Treatment of aggressive thyroid cancer with an oncolytic herpes virus. Int J Cancer 2004;112:525–32.

54. Barzon L, Pacenti M, Taccaliti A, et al. A pilot study of combined suicide/cytokine gene therapy in two patients with end-stage anaplastic thyroid carcinoma. J Clin Endocrinol Metab 2005;90:2831–4.

CHAPTER 40

PRIMARY HYPERPARATHYROIDISM

REBECCA S. SIPPEL, MD

HERBERT CHEN, MD

The parathyroid gland was first discovered during the dissection of an Indian rhinoceros in 1850. Ivar Sandstrom later described the gross and histologic appearance of the glands in several animals and humans. The connection between an enlarged parathyroid and bone disease was identified in the early twentieth century, and subsequently Felix Mandl performed the first successful parathyroidectomy in 1925.

Almost all patients have at least four parathyroid glands, two upper parathyroids derived from the IV branchial pouch and two lower parathyroids derived from the III branchial pouch. A normal parathyroid gland weighs between 30 and 50 mg, with the lower glands typically slightly larger than the superior glands. Approximately 10 to 20% of patients have a supernumerary gland. The most common location for a supernumerary gland is within the thymus. The blood supply of the parathyroid glands is almost always derived from the inferior thyroid artery.

Primary hyperparathyroidism (HPT) has an incidence of 25 to 100 per 100,000 in the general population and up to 1,500 per 100,000 in the elderly. The incidence increases with age and is most common in postmenopausal women. Primary HPT is caused by a single adenoma in approximately 80% of patients. Fifteen percent of patients have multigland disease and 3 to 5% have double adenomas. Less than 1% of patients will have parathyroid carcinoma as the cause of their HPT.

Historically, patients with HPT were diagnosed as they developed symptoms of bone disease or kidney stones. However, since the development of serum chemistry autoanalyzers in the early 1970s, hypercalcemia identified on routine laboratory analysis has become the most common presentation of primary HPT. Because these patients do not present with classic renal and skeletal abnormalities, they are frequently labeled as being "asymptomatic," which is a misnomer. Over 80% of patients with HPT will have subjective, identifiable symptoms that are associated with HPT.[1] The symptoms of HPT are varied and are often difficult to appreciate due to their lack of specificity. The many manifestations of HPT are listed in Figure 1. The most common early symptoms are vague and consist of weakness, fatigue, nausea, anorexia, and constipation. Skeletal and renal manifestations occur later and are much more likely to bring the patient to medical attention.

The laboratory diagnosis of HPT consists of an elevated calcium level in conjunction with an inappropriately high normal or elevated parathyroid hormone (PTH) level. Other associated laboratory abnormalities include hypophosphatemia (50%), hypomagnesemia (5 to 10%), and an elevated alkaline phosphatase (a marker for bone disease). A chloride to phosphate ratio greater than 30 is thought to be highly suggestive of HPT. Urinary calcium levels are either normal or elevated. A low urinary calcium level (< 100 mg/24 hrs) is suggestive of familial hypocaluric hypercalcemia (which should not be treated with parathyroidectomy). Bone mineral density testing, while not diagnostic in HPT, can help to determine the effects of HPT on bone loss and assess the need for operative treatment.

Rarely a patient presents with an acute hyperparathyroid crisis and a markedly elevated calcium level. The symptoms of hyperparathyroid crisis include the rapid onset of nausea, vomiting, weight loss, fatigue, weakness, and confusion. The first goal in the treatment of hyperparathyroid crisis is to increase the excretion of calcium. This is done first by rehydrating the patient with normal saline, followed by diuresis with a loop diuretic. The second goal of treatment is to inhibit bone resorption

Manifestations of Primary Hyperparathyroidism

- **Renal**
  - Nephrocalcinosis, nephrolithiasis, calciuria, polyuria, overflow incontinence

- **Bone**
  - Osteitis fibrosa cystica, osteopenia/osteoporosis, bone pain, pathological fractures

- **Gastrointestinal**
  - Nausea, vomiting, anorexia, constipation, abdominal pain, pancreatitis

- **Psychiatric**
  - Depression, anxiety, psychosis

- **Neuromuscular**
  - Fatigue, myalgias, muscle weakness

- **Cardiovascular**
  - Hypertension

Figure 1 Clinical manifestations of primary hyperparathyroidism.

with bisphosphonates. Bisphosphonates inhibit osteoclast function and start working within 3 to 6 days with their effects lasting weeks. In most cases prompt parathyroidectomy after hydration is preferred over bisphosphonates due to the prolonged postoperative hypocalcemia that can occur after the use of bisphosphonates.

Primary HPT can be part of several genetic syndromes, most notably the multiple endocrine neoplasia (MEN) syndromes. Nearly 100% of patients with MENI will develop primary HPT, which is due to parathyroid gland hyperplasia. Primary HPT is less frequently seen in MEN IIA, occurring in approximately 25% of cases.

Indications for Surgery

Surgery provides the only cure for primary hyperparathyroidism. In experienced hands the cure rate of parathyroidectomy is > 95% with a complication rate of < 3%. The guidelines for surgical intervention continue to expand as our understanding of the disease and the potential benefits of earlier treatment in apparently "asymptomatic" patients become realized. The advantages of intervention in a symptomatic patient are clear. Any symptomatic patient should be considered for

Table 1 NIH Consensus Guidelines 2002: Indications for Surgery in the Asymptomatic Patient

- Age < 50
- Serum calcium 1.0 mg/dL > the normal range
- Reduction in creatinine clearance by > 30%
- 24-hr urinary calcium excretion > 400 mg
- Reduction in bone mass marked by a t-score < -2.5 at any site (lumbar spine, hip, or forearm)
- Medical surveillance is neither desired nor possible

surgical intervention. Patients who do not present with classical symptoms are frequently labeled as asymptomatic. The original NIH consensus guidelines for the management of these asymptomatic patients with primary HPT were established back in 1990, and then revised in 2002.[2] The recommendations of the 2002 consensus conference are listed in Table 1.

Labeling patients without overt bone or renal manifestations as asymptomatic is inappropriate. Several studies in recent years have examined these "asymptomatic" patients trying to decipher the myriad symptoms and the potential benefits of surgical treatment. Studies have shown a significant increase in bone mineral densities, an improvement in subtle neurocognitive symptoms, a reduction in fatigue, a decrease in premature cardiovascular death, and an improved quality of life.[1,3–9] Because of the potential benefits of treatment and the minimal risks of surgery, many advocate offering surgical treatment to nearly all patients. The many benefits of parathyroidectomy are listed in Table 2.

The role of nonoperative management in primary HPT has been examined by several studies. They have shown that approximately 25% of patients will have progression of their disease to the point of requiring surgery.[2] If nonoperative management is chosen, then patients must be monitored on a regular basis. They should be observed for the development of symptoms and should have serum calcium measurements every 6 months and serum creatinine and bone mineral densities (three sites: lumbar spine, hip, forearm) annually. Calcimimetic agents, such as cinacalcet, are now available clinically for the treatment of intractable HPT. These drugs reduce circulating PTH levels by increasing the

Table 2 Benefits of Parathyroidectomy

- Improvement in renal function
- Improvement in bone mineral density
- Resolution of neuropsychiatric symptoms
- Reduction of fatigue
- Decrease in cardiovascular morbidity
- Improved survival
- Improved quality of life
- Decreased cost over surveillance after 5 years

sensitivity of the calcium sensing receptor (CaR) to extracellular calcium. The indications for the use of this new class of drugs are still evolving. Clinical trials clearly support their efficacy in secondary HPT as well as in the treatment of parathyroid carcinoma, and some data suggest they may play a role in the treatment of primary HPT as well.[10,11]

Bilateral Neck Exploration

The standard surgical approach to hyperparathyroidism is a bilateral neck exploration. This technique has proven over time to be highly successful with cure rates of 95% in experienced hands. The long-term complication rate of a bilateral neck exploration is low (< 3%), but the incidence of transient hypocalcemia can be as high as 40%. This technique is dependent upon the successful identification of all four parathyroid glands and requires surgeon expertise in the recognition of the parathyroid glands in their normal and ectopic locations. No preoperative localization is necessary and no special intraoperative adjuncts are required. In the past, each parathyroid gland was biopsied to confirm that all glands were identified. However, due to the risk of devascularization, biopsies of normal appearing glands are no longer recommended.

BILATERAL NECK EXPLORATION OPERATIVE TECHNIQUE

Positioning/Set-up

The patient is positioned on the operating room (OR) table in a beach chair position with their arms tucked at their side. An intravenous (IV) bag or inflatable pressure bag is placed under the shoulders to assist in exposure of the neck.

Operative Approach

A 2 to 4 cm incision is made two fingerbreadths above the sternal notch. The strap muscles are separated down their midline and the thyroid is exposed. The thyroid is then retracted medially enabling the search for parathyroid tissue.

The variations seen in the locations of the parathyroid glands are based mostly on their embryogenesis. Understanding where they descended from can help guide the search for an aberrant gland. The inferior glands descend with the thymus and can be found anywhere from the larynx to the mediastinum. Inferior glands are most frequently located just posterior to the inferior lobe of the thyroid gland and anterior and medial to the recurrent laryngeal nerve (RLN). They can be displaced inferiorly and located within the thymus or

anterior mediastinum, or located more posterior within the tracheoesophageal groove. Eighty percent of all inferior glands are located within 2 cm of the inferior pole of the thyroid. If no inferior gland is identified, then resection of the thymic tissue on that side should be performed because up to 15% of lower glands are located within thymus or between the thyroid and thymus. If you are still unable to identify a lower gland, the carotid sheath on that side should be opened to the level of the bifurcation. A final option is to obtain an intraoperative ultrasound of the thyroid looking for an intrathyroidal parathyroid adenoma, which occurs in 1 to 4% of cases. A blind thyroid lobectomy should not be performed.

The superior glands are typically located posterior to the upper pole of the thyroid near the point that the RLN enters the larynx. The gland is most commonly located posterior and lateral to the recurrent laryngeal nerve. If no superior gland is seen, then the tracheoesophageal groove should be explored, taking care to avoid injuring the RLN. Next the retropharyngeal space should be explored.

Frozen section can be used to determine that the resected tissue is indeed parathyroid tissue. However, pathology cannot reliably distinguish between an adenoma and hyperplasia (Figure 2). Because the incidence of multiple gland disease is as high as 20%, it is essential to make every effort to identify all four parathyroid glands. The goal of the first exploration is to clear the neck of any disease. However, if after a thorough exploration no abnormal parathyroid tissue is identified, it is important for the surgeon to meticulously document which parathyroids were identified and what areas were explored in the search for the missing gland. Normal appearing parathyroid glands should never be removed. Median sternotomy and mediastinal exploration, in the absence of definitive preoperative localization to the mediastinum, should never be pursued at the initial exploration.

If four gland disease is present then the treatment options are a subtotal (3 1/2 gland) parathyroidectomy or a total parathyroidectomy with autotransplantation to the forearm.

Minimally Invasive Parathyroidectomy

Because the majority of patients with primary HPT have only a single abnormal gland (80 to 85%), attempts have been made to minimize the extent of surgery in those patients with a single adenoma. Minimally invasive parathyroidectomy (MIP) consists of identifying a single abnormal gland and removing it without the identification of the remaining normal parathyroid glands. MIP consists not just of one procedure, but a variety of techniques that have been used either alone or in combination. The central component of each of these techniques is accurate

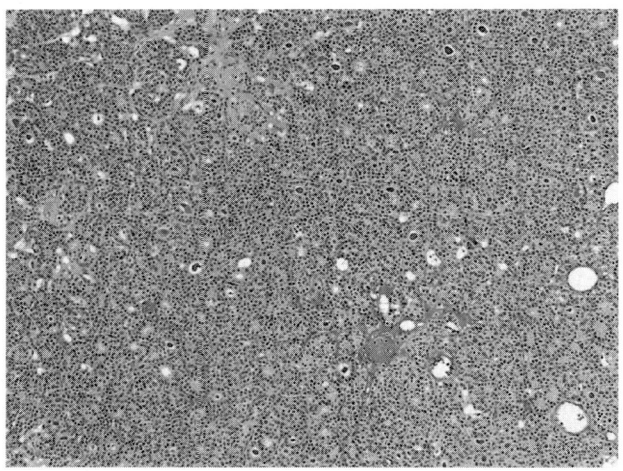

Figure 2 Parathyroid adenoma demonstrating increased cellularity (200X magnification).

preoperative localization. A second component, not adopted by all, but we believe to be essential part of a successful MIP technique, is intraoperative PTH testing. The use of intraoperative PTH testing allows determination of biochemical cure at the time of surgery. Intraoperative PTH testing has been shown to improve the cure rate of MIP, and it expands the population of patients who are candidates for MIP.[12,13] Other adjuncts such as intraoperative gamma detection, video assistance, and the use of local anesthesia have been adopted by some.

The cure rate of a bilateral exploration is approximately 95%. There have been several large case series and one randomized prospective clinical trial that have shown that the cure rate of MIP (defined as normocalcemia 6 months postoperatively) appears to be equal if not better than a conventional exploration.[14–17] While cure rates appear similar, there is limited long-tem data available about recurrence rates. Some are concerned that biochemically silent adenomas may be missed due to the limited incision and then become activated at a later date, leading to a higher recurrence rate. Preliminary data do not support this concept.

There are several advantages of MIP over a bilateral neck exploration (Table 3). The incidence of symptomatic postoperative hypocalcemia has been shown to be reduced from 25% in a bilateral exploration to 7% with MIP.[17] The ability to perform a MIP under local anesthesia is another major advantage because the risks of general anesthesia can be avoided. This is especially important in the elderly population who are at higher risk for general anesthestic complications. In addition, using local anesthesia allows assessment of recurrent laryngeal nerve function by having the patient talk during the surgical procedure. A smaller incision size leads to improved cosmesis and potentially less postoperative pain. MIP has been shown to reduce OR

Table 3 Advantages and Disadvantages of Minimally Invasive Parathyroidectomy

Advantages of MIP	Disadvantages of MIP
• Ability to perform under local anesthesia	• Requires special adjuncts (intraoperative PTH testing, gamma probe)
• Improved cosmesis	• Requires accurate preoperative localization
• Decreased operating room time	• Requires surgeon expertise in the technique
• Ability to perform surgery as an outpatient	
• Decreased incidence of transient hypocalcemia	
• Possible cost savings	

MIP = minimally invasive parathyroidectomy; PTH = parathyroid hormone.

time by up to 50%.[15] Because only one side of the neck is explored, the risk of hypocalcemia is reduced and most patients can safely be discharged on the same day, leading to a reduction in hospital length of stay and overall cost savings.[14,18]

PREOPERATIVE LOCALIZATION

When performing a bilateral exploration, no preoperative localization is necessary. However, if a MIP is going to be considered then accurate preoperative localization is an essential component. The most commonly performed and most accurate localization test is a Tc-99m sestamibi scan (Figure 3). The sensitivity of the test is very institution specific as it is greatly altered by the quality of the equipment used and the skill of the interpreter. The sensitivity of Tc-99m sestamibi with SPECT (single photon emission computed tomography) imaging is around 80 to 90%. The advantages of Tc-99m sestamibi are its availability, the ability to obtain three-dimensional anatomic information, and the ability to evaluate ectopic locations such as the mediastinum at the same time. Thallium pertechnetate/Tc-99m sestamibi subtraction scanning is an alternative nuclear imaging modality that has been used with some success. This study appears to be very institution specific with a sensitivity around 75%.[19]

Ultrasound is another commonly used imaging modality. It is noninvasive and inexpensive; however, it is very operator dependent and is unable to image things located either deep in the neck or outside of the neck. Ultrasound is frequently used as an adjunct to confirm a finding on another imaging modality. When combined with Tc-99m sestamibi, the combined sensitivity is > 90%.[20]

Other imaging tests including computed tomography and magnetic resonance imaging are more expensive and less sensitive at localizing a parathyroid within the anterior neck, but can be useful in identifying abnorm-

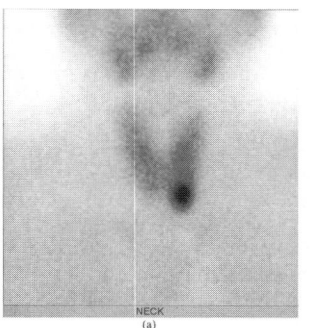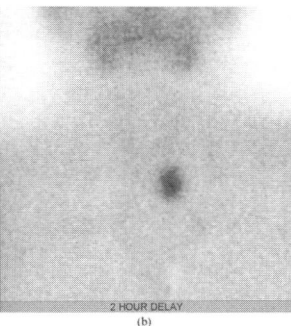

Figure 3 A Tc-99m sestamibi scan demonstrating a parathyroid adenoma. *A*, Early 10-minute images show uptake in a left lower parathyroid adenoma as well as the thyroid gland. *B*, Delayed 2-hour images reveal washout of the tracer from the thyroid gland with persistent uptake in the parathyroid adenoma.

alities deep within the neck or mediastinum. More invasive localization tools, such as arteriography and venography, should be reserved for patients with symptomatic disease and a failed prior exploration.

INTRAOPERATIVE PTH TESTING

While the majority of patients with primary HPT have a single abnormal gland, up to 20% of patients will have either multiple adenomas or hyperplasia of all four glands. The sensitivity of Tc-99m sestamibi is good for single adenomas but is substantially poorer when trying to identify hyperplasia. Therefore a method other than visual inspection is needed to confirm the adequacy of resection. PTH has a half-life of 2 to 4 minutes. Hence, within 5 to 10 minutes of resecting an abnormal gland, over one-half of the PTH in the bloodstream will have been cleared. By testing PTH levels preoperatively and then again after resection of the abnormal gland you can determine if there are additional hyperfunctioning glands present. The definition we use to define a cure is a fall in intraoperative PTH of > 50% 5 minutes after resection of a parathyroid gland.

The intraoperative assay is also being used to replace frozen section in the identification of parathyroid tissue. Fine-needle aspiration samples or small biopsies of presumed parathyroid tissue can be placed in saline and an intraoperative PTH sample can be run to confirm that the tissue is indeed parathyroid tissue.

INTRAOPERATIVE GAMMA PROBE

Intraoperative gamma probe localization uses the same principles as a Tc-99m sestamibi scan. It relies on the fact that there is variable sestamibi uptake in the thyroid compared to abnormal parathyroid tissue. Patients typically receive a preoperative injection of 10 mCi of Tc-99m sestamibi 1 to 4 hours prior to being taken back

to the OR. A gamma probe is used intraoperatively to guide incision placement as well as to direct the dissection, allowing the surgeon to focus in on the location of the abnormal parathyroid tissue. The gamma probe is then used to confirm that the tissue resected is indeed parathyroid tissue. Counts > 20% of background are considered diagnostic for parathyroid tissue.[21] The benefits of the intraoperative gamma probe have been debated. The greatest benefit appears to be in reducing operative time when the parathyroid adenoma is located in an ectopic position or when the sestamibi scan has a false positive due to a thyroid nodule. In these cases, the radioprobe can direct the intraoperative exploration to a location of the abnormal gland. In our experience, the gamma probe has been useful in the majority of patients, and it reduces operative time and minimizes the extent of dissection.[21] Furthermore, the technology can be used for patients with primary, secondary, or tertiary HPT.[22]

MIP TECHNIQUE

There are many variations in how MIP is performed based on institutional resources and surgeon preference. Below is a description of our current technique of MIP, which includes the use of radioguidance as well as intraoperative PTH testing.

Preoperative Preparation

Prior to being considered for a MIP, a patient must have undergone preoperative imaging that revealed a single abnormal gland. One to two hours prior to surgery the patient is given an IV injection of 10 mCi of Tc-99m sestamibi, which is used intraoperatively to help localize the parathyroid tissue.

Positioning/Set-up

The patient is positioned the same as with a conventional exploration. An additional large bore peripheral IV is placed to be used for intraoperative PTH testing. If local anesthesia is to be used, a superficial cervical block is performed at this time with 1% lidocaine. Sedation with either midazolam or propofol may be used to aid in patient comfort.[23]

Operative Approach

Prior to making an incision, a baseline PTH level is drawn from the patient's peripheral IV line by anesthesia. If a peripheral site for blood draws is not available, the internal jugular vein can be used. An 11 mm collimated gamma probe (Neoprobe 2000, Ethicon Endo-Surgery, Cincinnati, Ohio) is then used to localize the area of highest radioactivity. Because both the thyroid and the parathyroid take up Tc-99m sestamibi, the background level is set over the thyroid isthmus. The spot in the neck with the highest counts above background is marked and used to guide placement of our incision. Our standard incision is 2 cm in length and is placed favoring the side of the abnormal gland. The strap muscles are divided down the middle and the thyroid is exposed. The gamma probe is then used to focus our dissection to the area of highest uptake. The abnormal parathyroid is identified and its vascular pedicle is ligated. The adenoma is then resected and ex-vivo counts of the tissue are obtained by placing the gland atop the gamma probe. Ex-vivo counts > 20% of background are consistent with parathyroid tissue. After confirming that parathyroid tissue was removed, the intraoperative PTH assay is then used to determine the adequacy of the resection. Because the half-life of PTH is 2 to 4 minutes, intraoperative PTH levels are obtained 5 and 10 minutes after resection of the abnormal gland. Our criterion is a 50% drop from our baseline PTH level (baseline obtained in the OR) as the definition of an adequate resection. If there is not a 50% drop in PTH levels, then the ipsilateral parathyroid gland is visualized and, if abnormal, resected. Intraoperative PTH levels are again used to confirm that there is not any additional disease. If the ipsilateral gland is normal or the PTH does not fall after resection of the second gland a bilateral exploration is performed. All four parathyroid glands are identified and any abnormal parathyroid tissue is resected.

Management of Recurrent Disease

Cure after parathyroidectomy is typically defined as normocalcemia at least 6 months postoperatively. Biochemical HPT within 6 months of surgery is termed persistent disease. Persistent disease is typically do to failure to identify the causative adenoma, a missed second adenoma, or inadequately resected hyperplasia. If the patient develops HPT more than 6 months after surgery then it is referred to as recurrent disease. Recurrent disease is most commonly due to growth of hyperplastic tissue left at the original surgery.

The key to minimizing the risks of parathyroid surgery is to avoid reoperative surgery by performing an adequate operation at the first exploration. Reoperative surgery carries greater risks and the indications for operative intervention must be clear. Localization studies, while optional for an initial exploration, are mandatory prior to pursuing a re-exploration. Two concordant imaging localizing studies should be sought prior to offering any patient a re-exploration. If noninvasive studies are nonlocalizing or discordant, then invasive localization procedures, such as selective arteriography and venous sampling, are justified prior to pursuing reoperative neck surgery.

References

1. Perrier ND. Asymptomatic hyperparathyroidism: a medical misnomer? Review. Surgery 2005;137:127–31.

2. Bilezikian JP, Potts JT Jr, Fuleihan G, et al. Summary statement from a workshop on asymptomatic primary hyperparathyroidism: a perspective for the 21st century. Review. J Clin Endocrinol Metab 2002;87:5353–61.

3. Vestergaard P, Mosekilde L. Cohort study on effects of parathyroid surgery on multiple outcomes in primary hyperparathyroidism. BMJ 003, 327:530–4.

4. Vestergaard P, Mollerup CL, Frokjaer VG, et al. Cardiovascular events before and after surgery for primary hyperparathyroidism. World J Surg 2003;27:216–22.

5. Hedback G, Oden A. Increased risk of death from primary hyperparathyroidism—an update. Eur J Clin Invest 1998; 28:271–6.

6. Nilsson IL, Aberg J, Rastad J, Lind L. Circadian cardiac autonomic nerve dysfunction in primary hyperparathyroidism improves after parathyroidectomy. Surgery 2003;34: 1013–9; discussion 1019.

7. Nilsson IL, Yin L, Lundgren E, Rastad J, Ekbom A. Clinical presentation of primary hyperparathyroidism in Europe—nationwide cohort analysis on mortality from nonmalignant causes. J Bone Miner Res 2002;7 Suppl 2:N68–74.

8. Pasieka JL, Parsons LL, Demeure MJ, et al. Patient-based surgical outcome tool demonstrating alleviation of symptoms following parathyroidectomy in patients with primary hyperparathyroidism. World J Surg 2002;26:942–9.

9. Quiros RM, Alef MJ, Wilhelm SM, et al. Health-related quality of life in hyperparathyroidism measurably improves after parathyroidectomy. Surgery 2003;134:675–81; discussion 681–3.

10. Barman Balfour JA, Scott LJ. Cinacalcet hydrochloride. Review. Drugs 2005;65:271–81.

11. Peacock M, Bilezikian JP, Klassen PS, et al. Cinacalcet hydrochloride maintains long-term normocalcemia in patients with primary hyperparathyroidism. J Clin Endocrinol Metab 2005;90:135–41.

12. Chen H, Pruhs Z, Starling J, Mack E. Intraoperative parathyroid hormone testing improves cure rates in patients undergoing minimally invasive parathyroidectomy. Surgery 2005;138:583–7; discussion 587–90.

13. Chen H, Mack E, Starling J. A comprehensive evaluation of peri-operative adjuncts during minimally invasive parathyroidectomy: which is most reliable? Ann Surg 2005;242: 375–80; discussion 380–3.

14. Udelsman R, Donovan PI, Sokoll LJ. One hundred consecutive minimally invasive parathyroid explorations. Ann Surg 2000;232:331–9.

15. Udelsman R. Six hundred fifty-six consecutive explorations for primary hyperparathyroidism. Ann Surg 2002;235:665–70; discussion 670–2.

16. Irvin GL 3rd, Solorzano CC, Carneiro DM. Quick intraoperative parathyroid hormone assay: surgical adjunct to allow limited parathyroidectomy, improve success rate, and predict outcome. World J Surg 2004;28:1287–92.

17. Bergenfelz A, Lindblom P, Tibblin S, Westerdahl J. Unilateral versus bilateral neck exploration for primary hyperparathyroidism: a prospective randomized controlled trial. Ann Surg 2002;236:543–51.

18. Chen H, Sokoll LJ, Udelsman R. Outpatient minimally invasive parathyroidectomy: a combination of sestamibi-SPECT localization, cervical block anesthesia, and intraoperative parathyroid hormone assay. Surgery 1999;126: 1016–21; discussion 1021–2.

19. Sippel RS, Bianco J, Wilson M, et al. Can thallium-pertechnetate subtraction scanning play a role in the preoperative imaging for minimally invasive parathyroidectomy? Clin Nucl Med 2004;29:21–6.

20. Sosa JA, Udelsman R. New directions in the treatment of patients with primary hyperparathyroidism. Review. Curr Probl Surg 2003;40:812–49.

21. Chen H. Radioguided parathyroid surgery. Review. Adv Surg 2004;38:377–92.

22. Chen H, Mack E, Starling JR. Radioguided parathyroidectomy is equally effective for both adenomatous and hyperplastic glands. Ann Surg 2003;238:332–7; discussion 337–8.

23. Sippel RS, Becker YT, Odorico JS, et al. Does propofol anesthesia affect intraoperative parathyroid hormone levels? A randomized, prospective trial. Surgery 2004;136: 1138–42.

CHAPTER 41

PARATHYROID CARCINOMA

MOUHAMMED AMIR HABRA, MD

RENA VASSILOPOULOU-SELLIN, MD

GARY L. CLAYMAN, MD, DDS

Parathyroid carcinoma is a rare neoplasm accounting for 0.4 to 5% of all cases of primary hyperparathyroidism. The estimated prevalence of parathyroid carcinoma is around 0.005% of all cancers.[1–6] This carcinoma was first described in 1904 in a patient with nonfunctioning parathyroid carcinoma.[7] Twenty-nine years later, the first functioning parathyroid carcinoma was reported.[8]

Recently, there has been a growing number of clinical reports and case series describing the clinical course, genetics, and role of different therapeutic modalities in the treatment of this rare disorder. There are also rare reports of familial parathyroid carcinoma, but there are not enough data on this disorder that could be used as the basis for screening family members for this rare disorder.[9] There is also an increased incidence of parathyroid carcinoma in patients with hyperparathyroidism-jaw tumor syndrome, but the exact etiology of parathyroid carcinoma is still undetermined in most cases.[10,11] Head and neck irradiation does not seem to be a major risk factor for parathyroid carcinoma despite the few reports describing it as occurring within an adenoma, hyperplastic gland, or even normal glands after radiation exposure.[12–14] Parathyroid carcinoma has also been described in patients with end-stage renal disease and multiple endocrine neoplasia type 1, thereby raising the possibility that benign hyperplastic parathyroid glands may transform into malignant tumors, though this has not been confirmed.[13,15]

Clinical Presentation

The mean age of diagnosis is 47 years, which is at least 10 years younger than the mean age of diagnosis in primary hyperparathyroidism resulting from benign adenoma.[16] No firm relationship to sex and ethnicity has been established; most reported studies involve few patients, but it is believed that parathyroid carcinoma has a similar incidence in both sexes.[2,16] Rare cases of nonfunctioning parathyroid carcinoma have been described, and its clinical course is similar to that in patients with functioning tumors.[17]

Parathyroid carcinoma can be asymptomatic and incidentally discovered by the finding of hypercalcemia on routine blood tests; it can also present as life-threatening hypercalcemia. The classical presentation consists of hypercalcemia, hypophosphatemia, elevated alkaline phosphatase, and a remarkably elevated level of intact parathyroid hormone (PTH). These findings can overlap with the presentation of benign parathyroid adenoma or hyperplasia, though severe hypercalcemia (serum calcium > 13.5 mg/dL) and elevated PTH should raise the suspicion of parathyroid carcinoma. The presence of a large neck mass (Figure 1), often palpable on physical exam, in a patient with PTH-mediated hypercalcemia is also suggestive of parathyroid carcinoma.[16] The presence of skeletal or renal manifestations of hyperparathyroidism is somewhat more common in patients with functioning parathyroid cancer compared with patients with benign disease.

Pathology

The finding of an indurated mass invading the surrounding structures of the neck at the time of surgery is highly predictive of parathyroid carcinoma. The tumor may invade the strap musculature, ipsilateral thyroid lobe, the esophagus, trachea, and/or recurrent laryngeal nerve.[18] Parathyroid carcinomas tend to occur more in the inferior parathyroid glands[16,19]; lymphatic invasion is found in 11% of cases.[16]

Macroscopically, parathyroid carcinomas tend to be larger (often greater than 3 cm), lobulated, and firm;

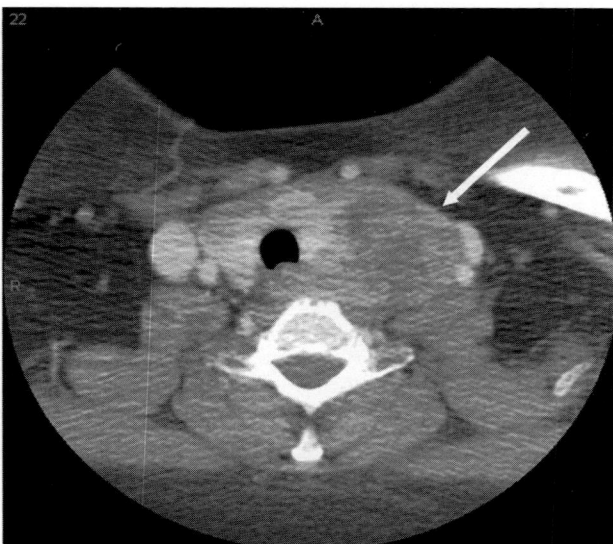

Figure 1 Computed tomography scan of the neck showing a heterogeneous left-sided neck mass (white arrow) that proved to be a parathyroid carcinoma.

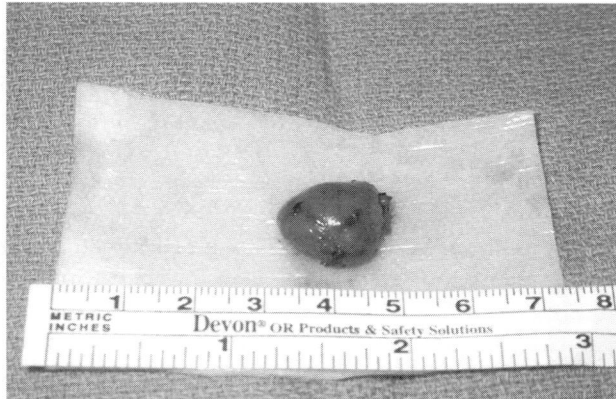

Figure 3 Gross appearance of parathyroid adenoma. This benign adenoma appears as a small, brownish tumor.

However, they are not universally found. In our recent series of 27 patients treated at The University of Texas M. D. Anderson Cancer Center during a 22-year period, these criteria were found in less than half of all cases of parathyroid carcinoma.[16]

Molecular Oncogenesis

Because the classic pathologic features are not always present in parathyroid carcinoma, studies have been conducted to try to find a common abnormality to help physicians properly diagnose the condition. In a limited number of cases, several genetic abnormalities have been associated with parathyroid carcinoma. For example, the loss of a region on chromosome 13 that contains the coding regions for retinoblastoma has been reported in multiple studies.[21–23] Other abnormalities include *p53* mutation,[24] loss of *BRCA2*,[21] downregulation of the

additionally, they have a dense fibrous capsule and appear to have a grayish color (Figure 2). This is in contrast to parathyroid adenomas, which tend to be oval, soft, smaller, and brownish red to tan (Figure 3). Despite these differences, in many cases, it is hard to distinguish the two entities on the basis of gross appearance alone.

The current pathologic diagnostic criteria for parathyroid carcinoma were described in 1973 by Schantz and Castelman[20] and are as follows: (1) uniform sheets of cells arranged in a lobulated fashion with intervening fibrous trabeculae, (2) capsular and/or vascular invasion, and (3) the presence of mitotic figures (Figure 4).

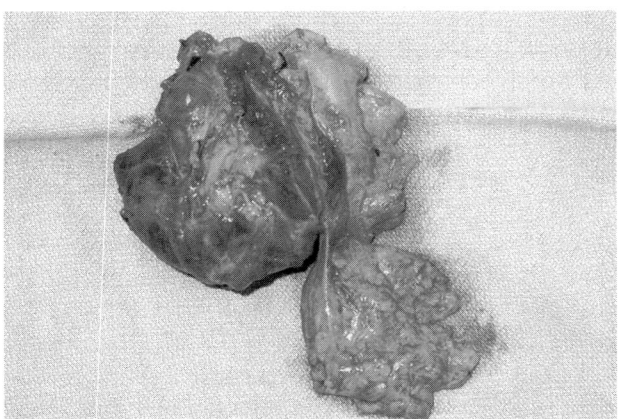

Figure 2 Gross appearance of parathyroid carcinoma. The tumor is large, invading the surrounding structures.

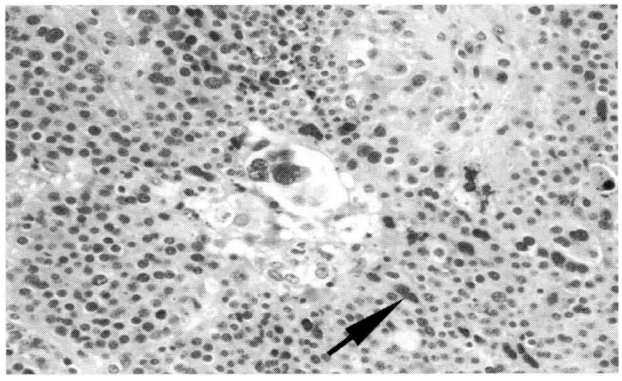

Figure 4 Microscopic appearance of parathyroid carcinoma. The cells show pleomorphic nuclei. A large nucleus with irregular shape is shown (black arrow).

expression of the calcium-sensing receptor with loss of heterozygosity of the chromosome 1q region containing the *HRPT2* gene and chromosome 11q containing the menin gene.[25] Pericentromeric inversion of chromosome 11, which activates the *PRAD1/cyclin D1* gene, is considered important in the pathogenesis of parathyroid neoplasms[26,27] and can be found in some cases of parathyroid carcinoma.[26] *HRPT2* is a recently described tumor suppressor gene that is associated with the hyperparathyroidism-jaw tumor syndrome and encodes parafibromin, a protein of unclear function.[28] In one study, somatic mutations of this gene were seen in cases of sporadic parathyroid carcinoma,[10,11] and germline mutations were seen in 3 of 15 patients.[10]

Staging

There are no accepted staging criteria for parathyroid carcinoma; the commonly used tumor-node-metastasis staging system is not applicable to this disease for two reasons. First, parathyroid carcinoma infrequently metastasizes to regional lymph nodes, and second, tumor size does not seem to carry a major prognostic value in parathyroid carcinomas. We have used staging criteria based on the extent of the disease at diagnosis in a series of patients treated at M. D. Anderson Cancer Center. We divided the patients into the following three groups: group 1, localized disease histologically defined as carcinoma but confined to the parathyroid gland; group 2, locally invasive disease defined as microscopic or macroscopic disease and extending outside the parathyroid gland and invading the surrounding tissues (adipose tissue, striated muscle, thyroid, and esophagus); and group 3, metastatic disease defined as tumor spread to distant organs[16] (Figure 5).

Management

Hypercalcemia is the leading cause of morbidity and mortality in patients with parathyroid carcinoma.[16] This morbidity and mortality is generally due to PTH secretion and hypercalcemia rather than to the tumor burden itself. Thus, treatment goals include controlling hypercalcemia by various modalities as well as attempting to cure the disease when feasible with surgery and radiation therapy.

MANAGEMENT OF HYPERCALCEMIA

We have tried to control and correct hypercalcemia, especially in patients with unresectable disease or with

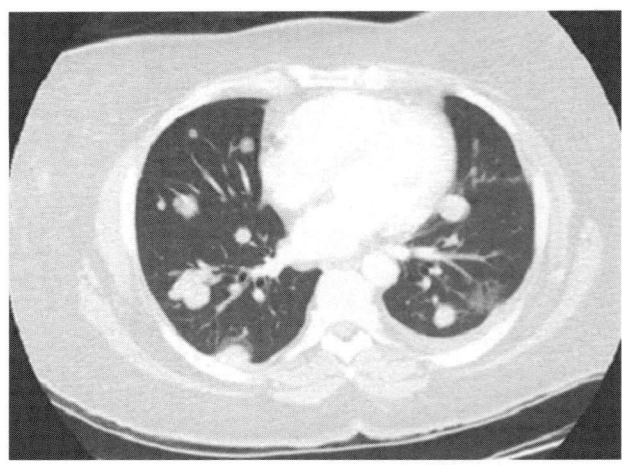

Figure 5 Computed tomography scan of the chest showing multiple lung metastases in a patient with parathyroid carcinoma.

persistent PTH-mediated hypercalcemia and negative results on localization tests. Various modalities can be used to achieve this goal. The general principle is to begin by maintaining adequate hydration either orally on a permanent basis or intravenously in the case of a hypercalcemic emergency. Usually, intravenous saline therapy reduces the calcium level by expanding the extracellular space and increasing the renal excretion of calcium. This increase in renal excretion is caused by an increase in glomerular filtration and sodium delivery, which reduce passive calcium resorption. Many patients with severe hypercalcemia and hypovolemia may require at least 4 to 6 liters of fluids in the first day of treatment. Loop diuretics are often used after a patient achieves a reasonable level of rehydration because they increase calcium excretion by inhibiting calcium resorption into the loop of Henle.

Along with hydration and loop diuretics, other agents should be used to inhibit the bone resorption caused by the high levels of PTH. Multiple agents have been used for this over the years, including plicamyin, intravenous bisphosphonates, calcitonin, and gallium nitrate. Plicamyin, though proven effective, has been associated with serious side effects, which has led to ceased production of the agent. Calcitonin, in a dose of 4 to 8 units per kg administered subcutaneously every 6 to 8 hours, has been used with a good safety profile. Though the effects of calcitonin are usually seen within a few hours after its first administration, the drug is generally a weak agent with short-term benefit because of the development of tachyphylaxis.[29] Bisphosphonates (pamidronate and zoledronic acid) have been the mainstay of medical therapy because they inhibit the activity of the osteoclasts. They are generally nontoxic and available for intravenous infusion. Pamidronate acid is usually given intravenously in doses ranging from 30 to 90 mg over 1 to 2 hours. Zoledronic acid is more potent than pamidronate and requires a shorter period of administration. It is usually given in a dose of 4 mg administered intravenously over at least 15 minutes. The duration of response to these agents is variable and can last for few weeks in some patients. Calcimimetic agents have also been studied in patients with parathyroid carcinoma.[30] Oral cinacalcet is the first calcimimetic agent approved by the US Food and Drug Administration for the management of hypercalcemia in patients with parathyroid carcinoma. Calcimimetic agents bind to the calcium-sensing receptor and increase its sensitivity to circulating calcium, thereby reducing PTH secretion.[31] Gallium nitrate also inhibits osteoclastic activity and reduces the serum calcium level. It has potential nephrotoxic side effects and requires continuous infusion over a few days, which makes it less preferable as a first-line choice of treatment in patients with hypercalcemia. In some cases of severe hypercalcemia and cases not responding properly to other treatments, patients may require hemodialysis.

SURGICAL MANAGEMENT

Surgery is the mainstay of therapy to achieve disease control and a potential cure of parathyroid carcinoma. In many cases, the diagnosis of parathyroid carcinoma cannot be made preoperatively in the absence of regional or distant metastases. Comprehensive resection of the tumor and the surrounding tissues should be attempted in patients with preoperative suspicion of parathyroid carcinoma on the basis of clinical and/or radiographic evidence of soft tissue invasion. Patients often require resection of the parathyroid tumor, as well as thyroid lobectomy, resection of the strap musculature, and the paratracheal fibrolymphatic compartment and its adjacent soft tissues, as required. Simultaneously, an attempt should be made to preserve a normally functioning recurrent laryngeal nerve unless it is circumferentially involved by tumor.

A comprehensive lymphadenectomy is not indicated except in the local area of the primary malignancy because parathyroid carcinoma is not commonly associated with cervical lymphadenopathy. Therefore, dissection of cervical lymphatic levels I, II, or V is rarely indicated in these patients. Large neoplasms may include contents of neck levels III or IV depending on the location of the primary tumor. If dissection is performed, the carotid artery should be identified and spared.

Because significant reduction of PTH should be sought and observed, intraoperative analysis of intact PTH is recommended, especially in patients who have not previously undergone surgery. In patients with extensive soft tissue extension, normal values of intact PTH may not be observed intraoperatively, and the decrease in PTH may not be as rapid as in benign parathyroid disorders (15 to 30 minutes). In some cases, the malignant potential of parathyroid tumors is not appreciated until patients present with local relapse or distant metastases years after surgery.[16]

ADJUVANT RADIATION THERAPY

Patients with parathyroid carcinoma have a significant risk of locoregional disease progression or recurrence when treated with surgery alone. Whether adjuvant radiation therapy should become the standard of care in patients with parathyroid carcinoma is currently a subject of extensive discussion. In selected cases, adjuvant radiation therapy appears to effectively decrease the local relapse rate. Radiation therapy has been reported to improve the disease-free interval, especially in high-risk patients.[32] In the most recent series of patients studied at M. D. Anderson, the local relapse rate appeared lower when adjuvant radiation therapy (50 to 60 Gy) was administered within 2 months after initial surgery, independent of the type of surgery and disease stage.[16] One would expect that patients with cancer confined to the gland (localized) would be less likely to have a recurrence, yet in our experience, of the 8 patients with cancer confined to the gland who did not receive adjuvant radiation therapy, 5 (62.5%) had a recurrence, including 1 patient who was treated with comprehensive resection. Likewise, one would expect that patients with locally invasive cancers would be more likely to experience a recurrence. Yet only 6 (33%) of 18 patients with locally invasive cancer in our series experienced a recurrence, 3 after complete resection and 3 after comprehensive resection. It should be noted that only 1 (17%) of 6 patients who received adjuvant radiation therapy in this group had a recurrence, independent of the extent of surgery.[16] While the small number of patients in our series precludes quantitative analyses, we believe that adjuvant radiation therapy may play an important role in the local control of parathyroid carcinomas. Other reports have confirmed this observation and have even found a survival benefit to radiation therapy, though the number of treated patients in these studies was also too small to provide strong statistical analysis.[33]

Survival

Parathyroid carcinoma is a disease with an often indolent but progressive course. Some reports indicate that the surgical margin status and the institution at which the initial surgery is performed can determine the risk of postoperative disease progression.[33] Our experience suggests that younger males (< 45 years) presenting with higher calcium values (> 13mg/dL) tend to have more aggressive disease. In our series, the 5-year survival rate was 85%, which is consistent with that of previous reports, but the 10-year survival rate of 77% is somewhat higher than that shown by other studies.[16,17,34] It is thought that improvements in supportive medical care in general and in the control of hypercalcemia more specifically are behind the improved survival of these patients.

References

1. Fujimoto Y, Obara T, Ito Y, et al. Surgical treatment of ten cases of parathyroid carcinoma: importance of an initial en bloc tumor resection. World J Surg 1984;8:392–400.

2. Shane E. Clinical review 122: parathyroid carcinoma. J Clin Endocrinol Metab 2001;86:485–93.

3. Wang CA, Gaz RD. Natural history of parathyroid carcinoma. Diagnosis, treatment, and results. Am J Surg 1985;149:522–7.

4. van Heerden JA, Weiland LH, ReMine WH, et al. Cancer of the parathyroid glands. Arch Surg 1979;114:475–80.

5. Dotzenrath C, Goretzki PE, Sarbia M, et al. Parathyroid carcinoma: problems in diagnosis and the need for radical surgery even in recurrent disease. Eur J Surg Oncol 2001; 27:383–9.

6. Hundahl SA, Fleming ID, Fremgen AM, Menck HR. Two hundred eighty-six cases of parathyroid carcinoma treated in the U.S. between 1985–1995: a National Cancer Data Base Report. The American College of Surgeons Commission on Cancer and the American Cancer Society. Cancer 1999;86:538–44.

7. De Quervain F. Parastruma maligna aberrata. Deutsche Zeitschrift Fuer Chirurgie 1904;100:334–52.

8. Saniton P, Millot J. Malegne dun adenoma parathyroidiene eosinophile, Aucours dune de Recklinghausen. Annales Anatomie pathologique 1933;10:813.

9. Frayha RA, Nassar VH, Dagher F, Salti IS. Familial parathyroid carcinoma. J Med Liban 1972;25:299–309.

10. Shattuck TM, Valimaki S, Obara T, et al. Somatic and germ-line mutations of the HRPT2 gene in sporadic parathyroid carcinoma. N Engl J Med 2003;349:1722–9.

11. Howell VM, Haven CJ, Kahnoski K, et al. HRPT2 mutations are associated with malignancy in sporadic parathyroid tumours. J Med Genet 2003;40:657–63.

12. Christmas TJ, Chapple CR, Noble JG, et al. Hyperparathyroidism after neck irradiation. Br J Surg 1988;75:873–4.

13. Ireland JP, Fleming SJ, Levison DA, et al. Parathyroid carcinoma associated with chronic renal failure and previous radiotherapy to the neck. J Clin Pathol 1985;38: 1114–8.

14. Obara T, Fujimoto Y, Kanaji Y, et al. Flow cytometric DNA analysis of parathyroid tumors. Implication of aneuploidy for pathologic and biologic classification. Cancer 1990;66: 1555–62.

15. Dionisi S, Minisola S, Pepe J, et al. Concurrent parathyroid adenomas and carcinoma in the setting of multiple endocrine neoplasia type 1: presentation as hypercalcemic crisis. Mayo Clin Proc 2002;77:866–9.

16. Busaidy NL, Jimenez C, Habra MA, et al. Parathyroid carcinoma: a 22-year experience. Head Neck 2004;26:716–26.

17. Anderson BJ, Samaan NA, Vassilopoulou-Sellin R, et al. Parathyroid carcinoma: features and difficulties in diagnosis and management. Surgery 1983;94:906–15.

18. Koea JB, Shaw JH. Parathyroid cancer: biology and management. Surg Oncol 1999;8:155–65.

19. Cohn K, Silverman M, Corrado J, Sedgewick C. Parathyroid carcinoma: the Lahey Clinic experience. Surgery 1985;98:1095–100.

20. Schantz A, Castleman B. Parathyroid carcinoma. A study of 70 cases. Cancer 1973;31:600–5.

21. Pearce SH, Trump D, Wooding C, et al. Loss of heterozygosity studies at the retinoblastoma and breast cancer susceptibility (BRCA2) loci in pituitary, parathyroid, pancreatic and carcinoid tumours. Clin Endocrinol (Oxf) 1996;45:195–200.

22. Cryns VL, Thor A, Xu HJ, et al. Loss of the retinoblastoma tumor-suppressor gene in parathyroid carcinoma. N Engl J Med 1994;330:757–61.

23. Subramaniam P, Wilkinson S, Shepherd JJ. Inactivation of retinoblastoma gene in malignant parathyroid growths: a candidate genetic trigger? Aust N Z J Surg 1995;65:714–6.

24. Cryns VL, Rubio MP, Thor AD, et al. p53 abnormalities in human parathyroid carcinoma. J Clin Endocrinol Metab 1994;78:1320–4.

25. Haven CJ, van Puijenbroek M, Karperien M, et al. Differential expression of the calcium sensing receptor and combined loss of chromosomes 1q and 11q in parathyroid carcinoma. J Pathol 2004;202:86–94.

26. Hsi ED, Zukerberg LR, Yang WI, Arnold A. Cyclin D1/PRAD1 expression in parathyroid adenomas: an immunohistochemical study. J Clin Endocrinol Metab 1996;81: 1736–9.

27. Hemmer S, Wasenius VM, Haglund C, et al. Deletion of 11q23 and cyclin D1 overexpression are frequent aberra-

tions in parathyroid adenomas. Am J Pathol 2001;158: 1355–62.

28. Carpten JD, Robbins CM, Villablanca A, et al. HRPT2, encoding parafibromin, is mutated in hyperparathyroid-ism-jaw tumor syndrome. Nat Genet 2002;32:676–80.

29. Ljunghall S. Use of clodronate and calcitonin in hypercal-cemia due to malignancy. Recent Results Cancer Res 1989; 116:40–5.

30. Collins MT, Skarulis MC, Bilezikian JP, et al. Treatment of hypercalcemia secondary to parathyroid carcinoma with a novel calcimimetic agent. J Clin Endocrinol Metab 1998;83: 1083–8.

31. Nemeth EF, Heaton WH, Miller M, et al. Pharmacodynamics of the type II calcimimetic compound cinacalcet HCl. J Pharmacol Exp Ther 2004;308:627–35.

32. Chow E, Tsang RW, Brierley JD, Filice S. Parathyroid carcinoma—the Princess Margaret Hospital experience. Int J Radiat Oncol Biol Phys 1998;41:569–72.

33. Munson ND, Foote RL, Northcutt RC, et al. Parathyroid carcinoma: is there a role for adjuvant radiation therapy? Cancer 2003;98:2378–84.

34. Hakaim AG, Esselstyn CB Jr. Parathyroid carcinoma: 50-year experience at The Cleveland Clinic Foundation. Cleve Clin J Med 1993;60:331–5.

Chapter 42

Management and Treatment of Solitary Adrenal Nodules

Johanna R. Askegard-Giesmann, MD

David R. Farley, MD

Efficient evaluation and effective treatment of an adrenal nodule must be based on the truisms of modern medicine:

Adrenal Nodules

1. are *common*, and become more so as humans age.
2. are *usually* harmless, *infrequently* hormonally active, and *rarely* cancerous.
3. that go undetected, and happen to be those rare functional or malignant adrenal nodules, may have *lethal* consequences.

Any management algorithm must acknowledge the above facts regarding adrenal nodules and scrutinize unsuspecting patients efficiently, safely, and cost-effectively. This chapter will attempt to offer a best practice for physicians to evaluate patients with adrenal nodules and offer five real patient scenarios to work through. This treatise is based on the *assumptions* that we have:

1. an imaging study that highlights an adrenal mass, and
2. a *thorough* history and physical examination is accurately performed.

Additionally, we *assume* that astute physicians agree that removing hormonally active adrenal masses (secreting cortisol, catecholamines, aldosterone, and/or sex hormones) and those likely to be cancer is logical; both types of neoplasms (either functioning or suspicious for

cancer) mandate careful workup, while the "extremes" of adrenal nodules—obviously benign tumors or frankly metastatic disease—typically require little further evaluation.

The National Institutes of Health (NIH) Consensus Conference on "Management of the Clinically Inapparent Adrenal Mass" (hereafter referred to as "incidentaloma" or "adrenaloma")[1] held in February of 2002 offered ten "Take Home Points" for physicians in practice.[2]

1. Patients with an incidentaloma ($\geq$ 1 cm) should have a 1-mg dexamethasone suppression test and measurement of plasma-free metanephrines.
2. Patients with hypertension should also undergo measurement of serum potassium and plasma aldosterone concentration-plasma renin activity ratio.
3. Homogeneous adrenal masses with a low attenuation value (< 10 Hounsfield units) on unenhanced computed tomography (CT) are probably benign.
4. Surgery should be considered in all patients with functional adrenal cortical tumors that are clinically apparent.
5. All patients with biochemical evidence of pheochromocytoma should undergo operative resection (following alpha blockade).
6. Surgical versus nonsurgical management remains controversial in patients with subclinical, hyperfunctioning adrenal cortical adenomas.
7. Although data are retrospective and nonstandardized, patients with tumors > 6 cm are usually

treated surgically, while those with tumors < 4 cm are generally monitored.

8. Patients with incidentalomas are best treated by a multidisciplinary team approach.
9. Laparoscopic and open adrenalectomy are both acceptable surgical options, and the choice must be based on tumor characteristics and operative expertise.
10. Incidentalomas stable in size over 6 months without evidence of hormonal hypersecretion over 4 years do not mandate further follow-up.

Based on the simplistic truisms and assumptions that begin this chapter, and the take-home points recommended by the NIH, we offer a simplistic algorithm for evaluating and caring for patients with incidental adrenal masses, defined as an adrenal tumor ≥ 1 cm in diameter *without* clinical evidence of function (Figure 1). Using this algorithm coupled with careful scrutiny of the adrenal images and efficient evaluation based on a multidisciplinary approach, let us evaluate several patient scenarios involving incidentally discovered adrenal nodules at the Mayo Clinic:

Scenario 1: An abdominal CT scan shows a 1.5-cm adrenal mass in a 68-year-old man with abdominal pain.

Scenario 2: An abdominal X-ray identifies a calcified adrenal gland in a fit, elderly woman.

Scenario 3: Magnetic resonance imaging (MRI) highlights a 7-cm adrenal mass in a patient with hypertension.

Scenario 4: Positron emission tomography (PET) suggests a right-sided adrenal hot spot in a 42-year-old woman with breast cancer.

Scenario 5: A chest CT scan shows a 2-cm adrenal mass in a middle-aged man with a smoking history.

Five different initial images and five separate studies either based on physician concern for underlying disease or as part of a general evaluation: specifically, what can these images tell us about the adrenal nodule? How should we proceed with our multidisciplinary team to evaluate and care for these patients based on the recommendations of the NIH Consensus Conference? And, what does evidence-based literature suggest about each patient's management and eventual outcome?

SCENARIO 1

This CT scan (Figure 2) was obtained in a 68-year-old man for vague abdominal pain. He is otherwise fit without evidence of malignancy, hypertension, or adrenal hypersecretion. There is no family history of endocrinopathy.

LITERATURE BACKGROUND

The scenario is not unusual: at least 2 to 4% of abdominal CT scans will identify an adrenal nodule.[3] CT scans are based on tissue density with Hounsfield units (HUs) ranging from -1,000 (air) to +1,000 (bone) with water being zero. The radiologic literature is secure:[4,5] adrenal nodules with tissue density less than water (ie, ≤ 0 HU) represent benign lesions; myelolipomas, lipomas, or simple cysts do not mandate resection or further work-up. Adrenalomas with densities between zero and 10 HU are overwhelmingly benign, but size, shape, and border characteristics take on more importance as CT density increases. Homogeneous, smaller (< 4 cm), low density (≤ 10 HU) masses with discrete borders in fit patients are benign tumors nearly 100% of the time. Heterogeneous, larger (> 6 cm), dense masses with ill-defined borders on CT are worrisome for malignancy (primary adrenal or metastatic) or bleeding. Adrenal nodules with elevated HU (> 30) are especially concerning for either adrenal malignancies (adrenal cortical carcinoma [ACC] or metastatic from lung, breast, kidney, or brain primaries), pheochromocytoma, or recent hemorrhage.[6]

Multidisciplinary Assessment of Patient 1

RADIOLOGY INTERPRETATION

This CT scan shows a 1.5-cm homogeneous right adrenal mass with relatively discrete borders. HU values on the noncontrast component of the CT approximated 8. CT criteria would suggest this mass is overwhelmingly likely to be a benign adrenal tumor. Liver, pancreas, kidneys, and left adrenal gland appear normal.

ENDOCRINOLOGY ASSESSMENT

Although seemingly benign in appearance, *functioning* adrenal nodules will cause patient health issues. Among 2,000+ adrenalomas, 82% were found to be nonfunctioning adenomas, 5% caused subclinical Cushing syndrome, 5% were pheochromocytomas, and 1% were aldosteronomas.[7] Adrenal cortical carcinoma (4.7%) and metastatic disease (2.5%) represented 7% of this study group. Therefore, ruling out (or in!) endocrine function (catecholamines and cortisol) by assessing urinary metanephrines and free catecholamines, and a 1-mg overnight dexamethasone suppression test will be necessary in this 68-year-old patient. Recent favor for plasma-free metanephrines to rule out pheochromocytoma has been evident,[8] but we continue to favor the combined urine studies (metanephrines, nor/epinephrine, and dopamine) that offer slightly better accuracy and lower rates of false positivity.[9] Potassium, aldosterone,

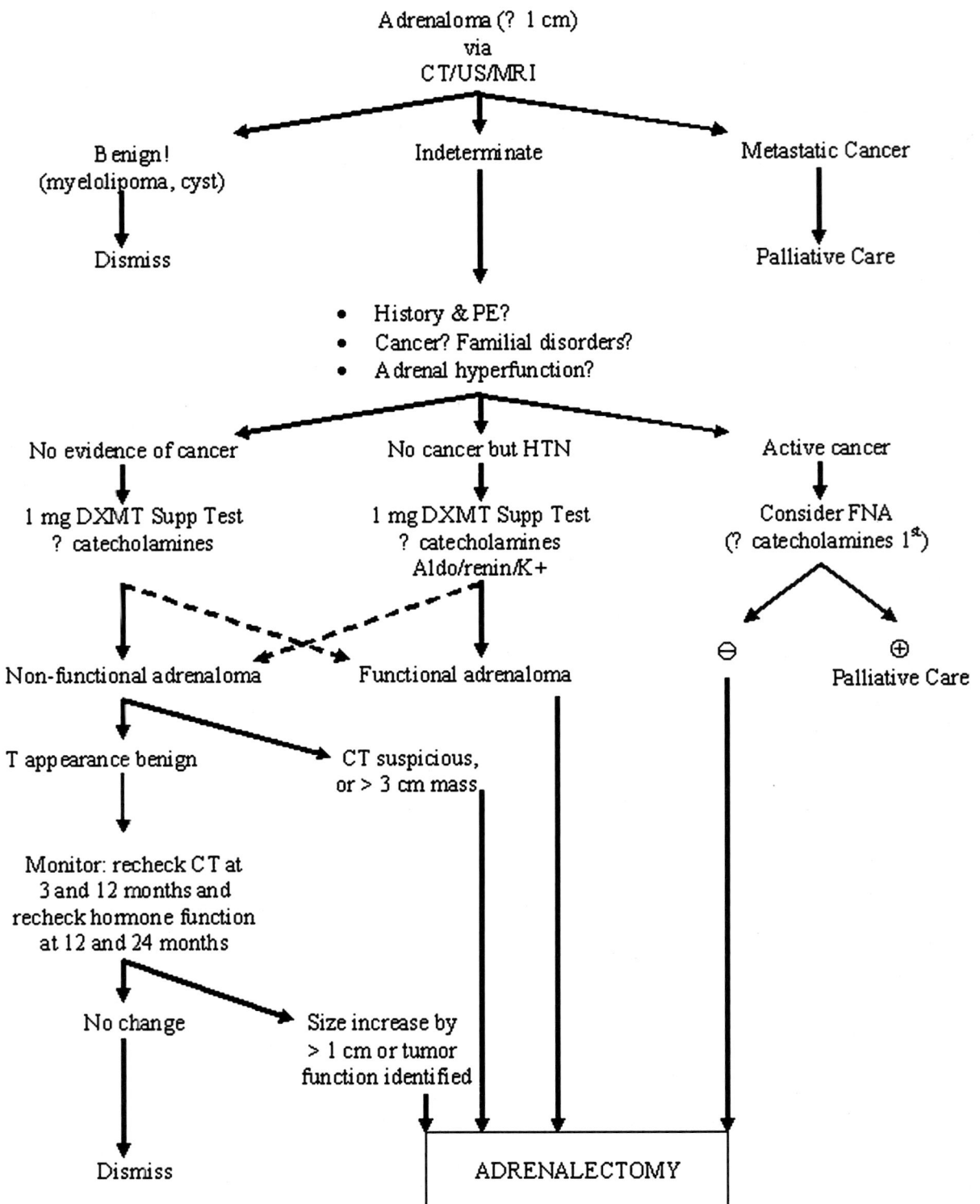

Figure 1 Management algorithm for incidentaloma.

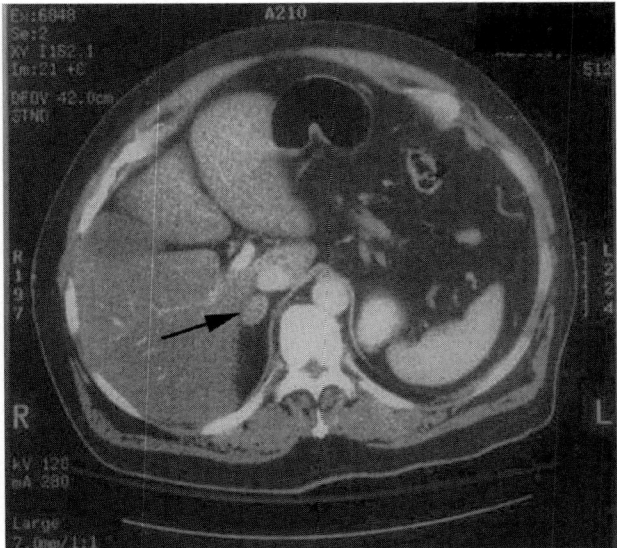

Figure 2 Contrast enhanced computed tomography scan with 1.5-cm right adrenal mass (arrow) posterior to the inferior vena cava.

and renin levels are unnecessary to obtain in this normotensive patient. Reassuring the patient of likely benignancy (> 95% for this 1.5-cm tumor) and nonfunctioning status (> 82%) seems likely, but awaiting the results of hormone function studies is mandatory.

SURGICAL VIEW

Surgical consultation for a functioning adrenal mass or one likely to be malignant is always warranted. Given the benign image shown and presumably negative functional tests, consultation is currently premature in this gentleman. If a functional neoplasm is identified, consultation and subsequent resection would then be indicated (Table 1).

Table 1.

DATA	Patient 1	Normal Levels
Serum		
cortisol	7 μg/dL	
		AM: 5–25; PM: 2–14
1-mg dexamethasone test	2.0 μg/dL	
Urine		Normal=suppression to < 5
norepinephrine	41 μg/24h	
epinephrine	10 μg/24h	15–80
dopamine	128 μg/24h	0–20
metanephrines	0.9 mg/24h	65–400
		< 1.3

OUTCOME

Functional studies were normal in this patient. With no need for surgical consultation, the endocrinologist repeated the CT scan in 3 months and again in 12 months. No change in size was noted. Functional studies at 12 and 24 months were negative and this patient was reassured of benignancy and dismissed from further follow-up. The NIH recommendations would include reassessing adrenal function at 36 and 48 months, but our own data would suggest *this* patient requires no additional evaluation.[10]

SCENARIO 2

A healthy, elderly woman undergoing a general medical exam has a plain, abdominal X-ray (Figure 3) performed (constipation). The history and physical examination are normal. She has no family history of endocrinopathies.

LITERATURE BACKGROUND

Plain X-rays rarely identify adrenal masses, but this exam appears to do just that. The possibility of pancreatic, splenic, gastric, or hepatic abnormalities as the source of this "adrenal mass" must be considered: we have now seen nearly a dozen patients with erroneously labeled "adrenal" neoplasms that operative intervention found to be something other than adrenal tissue.[11]

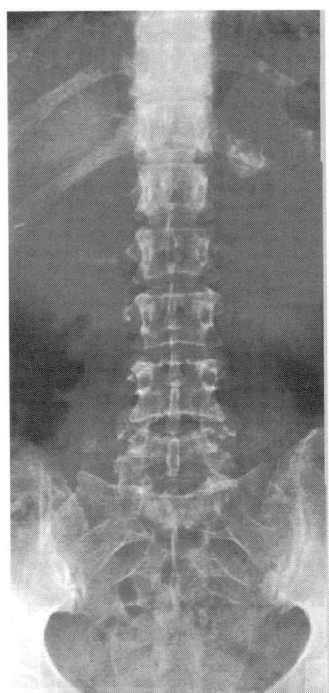

Figure 3 Plain abdominal X-ray with calcification noted in area of left adrenal gland.

While calcium within an adrenal gland brings to mind long ago bleeds, tuberculosis, histoplasmosis, or perhaps a hamartomatous lesion, it is important for us to recall that as patients age, adrenal nodules become more common. Inherently more common in women than in men, autopsy studies (25 studies pooled to include more than 85,000 cadavers) suggest the incidence of adrenal masses is 5.9% with a range from 1 to 32%.[12] Clinical series suggest that the incidence of adrenal nodules increases with age: < 30 years old = 0.2% and > 70 years = 6.9%.[13–15]

Multidisciplinary Assessment of Patient 2

RADIOLOGY INTERPRETATION

The abdominal plain film shows a calcified right adrenal gland, likely benign but indeterminate. Normal, nonspecific bowel gas pattern. Suggest abdominal CT to further evaluate both adrenal glands.

ENDOCRINOLOGIST ASSESSMENT

Given this patient is currently healthy and well, one must query this woman about a history of previous trauma, infection, anticoagulant use, or surgical procedures. Following radiologic advice, obtaining either an abdominal CT (our preference) or an MRI exam seems prudent, although the likelihood of any underlying concerning pathology is low in this setting. Consideration for ruling out hormone production (dexamethasone suppression and catecholamine assessment) will likely reassure both patient and endocrinologist that this "mass" is of no clinical importance.

SURGICAL VIEW

While likely to agree the mass is harmless, the meticulous surgeon must similarly question whether the lesion is indeed adrenal in nature. A CT or MRI will help make sure the calcified mass is adrenal and not in fact, a pancreatic, splenic, hepatic, or gastric abnormality. Nevertheless, this mass is unlikely to lead to any surgical intervention (Table 2).

OUTCOME

A CT scan (Figure 4) shows benign adrenal features bilaterally and functional studies were normal. This patient was reassured of a benign adrenal process void of hormonal secretion and no further work-up or follow-up was mandated.

SCENARIO 3

A family practitioner struggling to control hypertension in a middle-aged CEO erroneously opts early on for an abdominal image (Figure 5: MRI!), serendipitously finding a right-sided adrenal mass. The patient is overweight, smokes, requires antihypertensive medications to keep blood pressures below 140s/90s, and denies familial endocrine problems. With long-standing hypertension (HTN), the physician interprets the findings as essential HTN and elects to repeat the abdominal MRI for each of the next 5 years (!) watching the mass grow in size to 5 cm in diameter.

LITERATURE BACKGROUND

Millions of Americans have HTN, and not infrequently abdominal images are obtained long before appropriate serologic and urine studies are evaluated. While primary hyperaldosteronism is the number one cause of secondary hypertension in nonsmokers,[16] MRI is uniquely

Table 2.

DATA	Patient 2	Normal Levels
Serum		
cortisol	AM: 15 µg/dL	AM: 5–25; PM: 2–14
1-mg dexamethasone test	3.0 µg/dL	Normal=suppression to < 5
Urine		
norepinephrine	60 µg/24h	15–80
epinephrine	13 µg/24h	0–20
dopamine	227 µg/24h	65–400
metanephrines	0.8 mg/24h	< 1.3

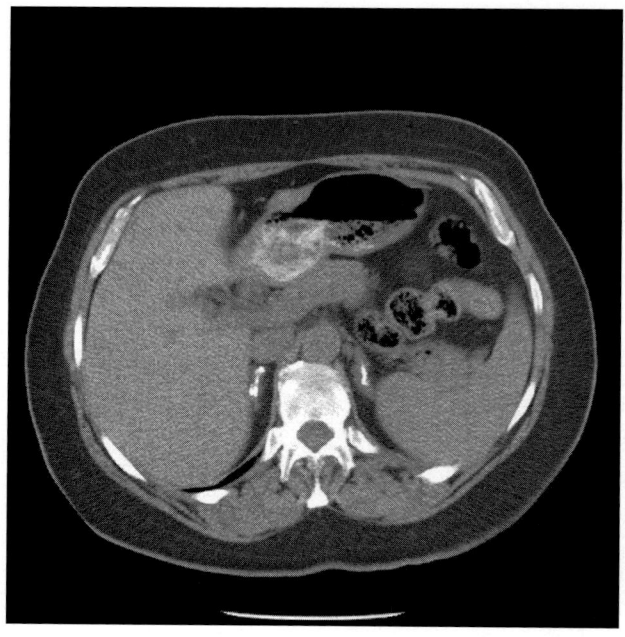

Figure 4 Computed tomography showing benign adrenal calcifications without any obvious "mass."

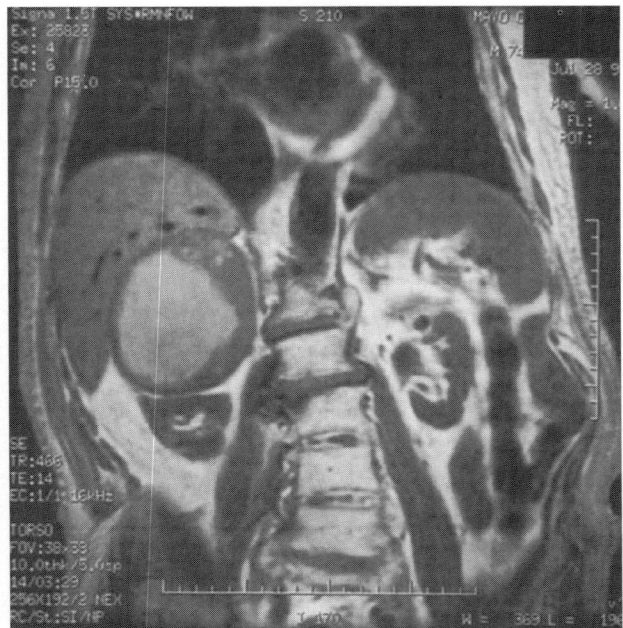

Figure 5 Magnetic resonance imaging identifies a right-sided adrenal mass consistent with adrenal cortical carcinoma or a large pheochromocytoma.

adept at evaluating catecholamine-secreting tumors, and this image (see Figure 5) is characteristic for a pheochromocytoma.[17] Round or oval adrenal masses with cortical thinning suggest a medullary process, and areas of necrosis are common within pheochromocytomas. Given 50% of patients with pheochromocytoma have sustained hypertension, and 45% have intermittent HTN with "spells" of palpitations, sweating, or headaches, this patient presents within the confines of a common presentation.[18] Only 5% of catecholamine secreting tumors are truly asymptomatic. While MRI or CT are clearly effective in identifying such volatile adrenal masses, physicians should spend extra time with the radiologist to rule out abnormalities of the contralateral gland (~10% occurrence) as well as nodal, liver, or locally invasive characteristics.

Multidisciplinary Assessment of Patient 3

RADIOLOGY INTERPRETATION

This MRI depicts a right-sided adrenal tumor consistent with pheochromocytoma or less likely an ACC. No evidence of local invasion or liver metastases. Normal-appearing left adrenal gland.

ENDOCRINOLOGY ASSESSMENT

Questions for the patient regarding his family history of endocrinopathies (thyroid, parathyroid, adrenal, or

pancreas abnormalities), heart disease, and stroke seem prudent. Laboratory analysis to rule in hormone excess (ideally obtained 5 years earlier!) must certainly involve urinary and serum analysis for catecholamines and cortisol. Although unlikely with larger masses (most aldosteronomas are < 2 cm in diameter),[19] all hypertensive patients should have preoperative evaluation of potassium, aldosterone, and renin levels. With confirmation of catecholamine production (checked *before* ordering a $2,000 MRI), Mayo patients undergo 5 to 10 days of alpha blockade, salt loading and hydration, and typically 3 days of beta blockade in preparation for surgical resection. Our preference is for initial oral phenoxybenzamine (titrating intake to nasal congestion and orthostatic hypotension) and subsequent propranolol to prepare the patient fully over 7 to 10 days in hopes of minimizing intraoperative blood pressure changes.

SURGICAL VIEW

Larger adrenal masses (unless cysts, lipomas, myelolipomas, or obvious metastases) in otherwise healthy people mandate surgical resection. However, before adrenalectomy is offered in this patient with a pheochromocytoma, careful analysis of familial endocrinopathies, potential thyroid nodules, (+/- ultrasound exam), serum calcitonin and calcium (to rule out MEN 2 syndromes), and completing 7+ days of alpha blockade and ~3 days of beta blockade is mandatory (Table 3).

OUTCOME

Urine-free catecholamines and metanephrines were elevated. Alpha blockade using phenoxybenzamine and subsequent beta blockade with propranolol along with volume restoration were secured. Laparoscopic right adrenalectomy was technically straightforward, but several hypertensive spells intraoperatively (Figure 6) mandated surgical patience, intravenous nitroprusside

Table 3.

DATA	Patient 3	Normal Levels
Serum		
cortisol	AM: 11 µg/dL	
		AM: 5–25; PM: 2–14
1-mg dexamethasone test	2.5 µg/dL	
calcitonin	9 pg/mL	Normal=suppression to < 5
calcium	9.3 mg/dL	< 16
Urine		8.9–10.1
norepinephrine	111 µg/24h	
epinephrine	42 µg/24h	15–80
dopamine	444 µg/24h	0–20
metanephrines	1.6 mg/24h	65–400
Neck US	normal thyroid	< 1.3
		--

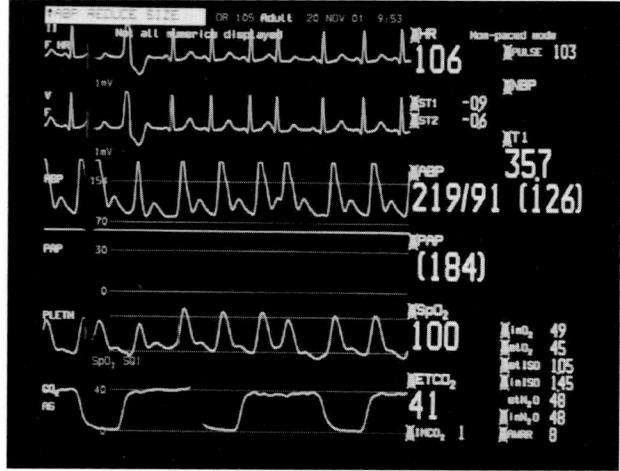

Figure 6 Intraoperative hypertensive episode.

and esmolol administration, and early ligation of the right adrenal vein. Postoperatively, the patient was dismissed in 2 days and fares well today. Like most patients with a pheochromocytoma, he is now normotensive following surgical resection.

SCENARIO 4

This PET scan (Figure 7) in a 42-year-woman lights up a hypermetabolic spot in the region of the right adrenal gland. Three years previously, the patient underwent breast conservation therapy for a T2 N1 M0 left breast ductal adenocarcinoma followed by adjuvant radiation and chemotherapy. Seemingly fit and well (no hypertension), this "routine follow-up" study is concerning for

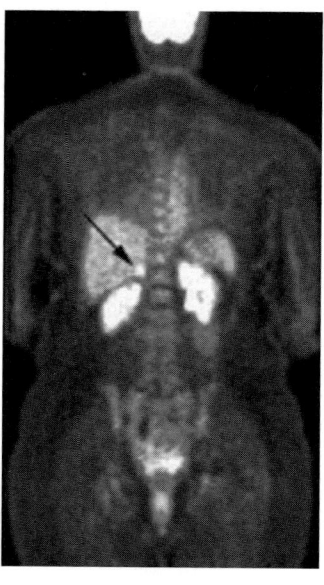

Figure 7 Positron emission tomography scan with adrenal hot spot.

metastatic disease in the right adrenal gland and nowhere else.

LITERATURE BACKGROUND

Although expensive (~$3,330), imperfect, and lacking years of data analysis and clinical confirmation, PET identifies high metabolic activity that most consistently points to malignancy. PET scanning for adrenal nodules is in its infancy, but early studies show that PET scans can characterize adrenal lesions (ie, malignant versus benign) with a sensitivity as high as 100%, a specificity of 94%, and an accuracy of 96%.[20,21]

Adrenalectomy for metastatic disease is an uncommon indication, but surgical literature does offer numerous case reports of laparoscopic or open adrenalectomy for evidence of solitary adrenal metastasis in the face of controlled primary disease.[22,23]

Fine-needle aspiration (FNA) of adrenal masses is unusual but finds a role in patients unfit for either general anesthesia or surgical intervention or in patients with high suspicion for metastatic disease. A skilled cytopathologist may facilitate immediate palliative treatment (institution of radiation or chemotherapy) in those patients with metastatic disease that are unlikely to benefit from surgical intervention. Prior to any FNA of the adrenal gland (or other tumors potentially capable of secreting catecholamines), evaluation of an underlying pheochromocytoma is imperative. Serious consequences of needle biopsy in unprotected (no alpha or beta blockade) patients with pheochromocytomas have been reported.[24]

Multidisciplinary Assessment of Patient 4

RADIOLOGY INTERPRETATION

The PET scan identifies a solitary, hypermetabolic focus in the right adrenal gland. In the face of known breast cancer, consider metastatic disease; primary adrenal cancer or benign adrenal neoplasms are less likely. Obtaining a CT abdominal study with and without contrast (checking for washout) may prove useful.

ENDOCRINOLOGY ASSESSMENT

Differentiating primary ACC versus metastatic breast cancer versus a benign incidentaloma is of crucial importance with great ramifications to this patient and her multidisciplinary team. Depending on prior evaluation, numerous studies seem reasonable in this woman: mammography, chest X-ray, bone scan, a battery of blood tests (liver function tests, hemoglobin, creatinine, etc.), and CT of the brain, chest, abdomen, and pelvis. Abdominal CT (Figure 8) was performed and considera-

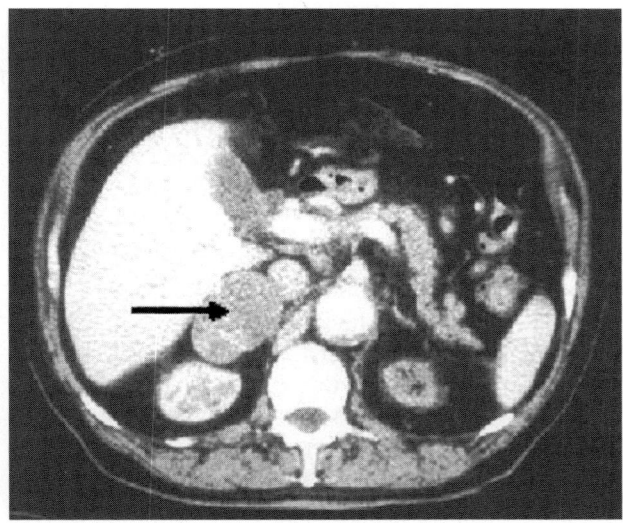

Figure 8 Computed tomography scan of metastatic cancer to adrenal gland.

Table 4.

DATA	Patient 4	Normal Levels
Serum		
cortisol	7 µg/dL	
		AM: 5–25; PM: 2–14
1-mg dexamethasone test	2.0 µg/dL	
Urine		Normal=suppression to < 5
norepinephrine	21 µg/24h	
epinephrine	9 µg/24h	15–80
dopamine	89 µg/24h	0–20
metanephrines	0.6 mg/24h	65–400
FNA	indeterminate cells	< 1.3
		--

tion given for percutaneous biopsy of the right adrenal mass (HU=28). Prior to such intervention, serum metanephrines (or urinary studies) *must* be obtained to avoid placing a needle into a patient with an undetected (and pharmacologically unprotected) pheochromocytoma. Should the catecholamine studies prove negative, FNA to secure a diagnosis of likely metastatic breast cancer is reasonable. Should the laboratory studies identify a pheochromocytoma, FNA is contraindicated and continued preparation for elective resection would progress. If the catecholamine work-up is negative, *and* the FNA is indeterminate, completing the assessment for cortisol production is a given prior to likely adrenalectomy.

SURGICAL VIEW

In the pre-PET era, patients with an underlying, and potentially active, malignancy harboring an adrenal mass on CT still had a reasonable chance of having a benign adrenal neoplasm: metastatic disease was found in "only" 35 to 75%.[25–29] PET scanning will likely refine these numbers, and a positive PET scan is extremely worrisome in this woman. Removing metastatic disease is rarely useful to patients, and the CT and PET images do suggest some form of malignancy. Assuming catecholamine analysis is negative, FNA is appropriate. Should the FNA be indeterminate or show benign cells, resection would be offered in this patient with a 5-cm solitary adrenal mass. If metastatic breast cancer is identified, chemotherapy would be recommended. Cells suspicious for ACC would force open adrenalectomy, potentially preceded by laparoscopic evaluation (Table 4).

OUTCOME

We remained worried about metastatic disease in this woman, and following careful assessment for endocrine function (none found), this patient underwent FNA of the right adrenal gland. Cells obtained were indeterminate. Following careful scrutiny of the chest, abdomen, and pelvis CT and reassessing the PET scan to be sure we had not missed evidence of other metastatic sites, we offered laparoscopy. At the time of operation, no evidence for metastatic liver or peritoneal disease was found, and a laparoscopic right adrenalectomy was performed. Pathologic analysis revealed metastatic breast cancer.

SCENARIO 5

A 55-year-old male smoker with fatigue underwent CT imaging following normal upper and lower endoscopic evaluations for a presumed underlying malignancy (Figure 9). In retrospect, the patient was hypertensive on physical examination (presumed at the time to be "white coat hypertension"). In follow-up with his internist, the hypertension was in fact difficult to control and required three medications.

LITERATURE BACKGROUND

Current studies suggest that primary hyperaldosteronism is now the most common surgically treatable cause of hypertension.[16] While the diagnosis of primary hyperaldosteronism is relatively straightforward, elevated serum aldo levels (> 15 ng/dL), low renin levels, with a aldo/renin ratio of > 20, clarifying the etiology (unilateral: left or right? Or bilateral?) may be more difficult. Mayo Clinic data would suggest that in young patients (< 40 years) with a secure serologic diagnosis and a unilateral adrenal mass > 1 cm in diameter, the source is apparent and unilateral adrenalectomy is indicated.[30] All others with evidence of hyperaldosteronism need adrenal venous (AV) sampling.

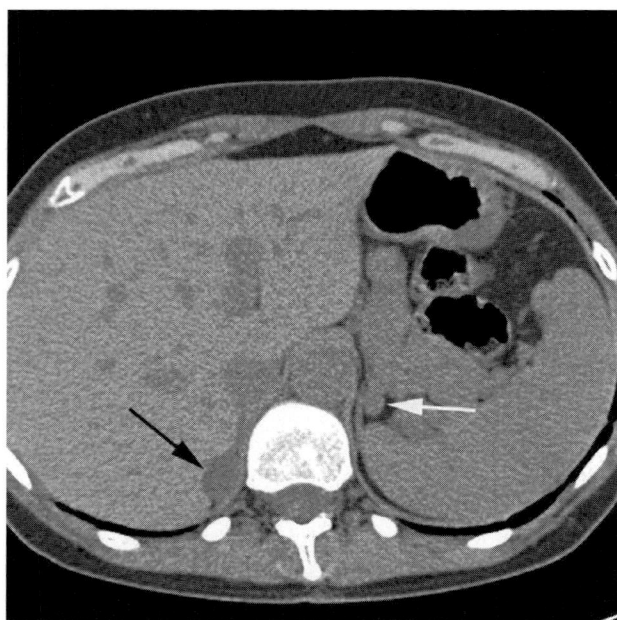

Figure 9 Computed tomography shows a right adrenal mass (Hounsfield unit=7) (black arrow). A 7-mm nodule is additionally identified projecting from the left adrenal gland (white arrow).

Multidisciplinary Assessment of Patient 5

RADIOLOGY INTERPRETATION

This abdominal CT scan identifies a right-sided adrenal nodule measuring 1.8 cm in size. The left adrenal gland harbors less impressive nodularity. Kidneys, liver, pancreas, and gallbladder appear normal.

ENDOCRINOLOGY ASSESSMENT

Poorly controlled hypertension requires careful scrutiny. Combined with an adrenaloma, most would agree with the NIH take-home points and check for adrenal functionality highlighting analysis for aldosterone, renin, and potassium. Assessment for cortisol and catecholamine function must similarly occur. Contemplation for AV sampling is wise given the sensitivity and specificity of CT or MRI is far from perfect, and with realization that patients > 40 years of age may have up to a 10% chance of harboring adrenal nodules.[30]

SURGICAL VIEW

While the endocrinologist will likely fixate initially over whether operative or nonoperative management will be best for this patient, the surgeon's concern must address right from left: which side contains the aldosteronoma? Primary hyperaldosteronism is often caused by very small tumors (range: 5 to 20 mm) with mean size usually far less than 2 cm in diameter.[31] Assuming clinical findings confirm primary hyperaldosteronism, we favor AV sampling in patients older than age 40 (Figure 10) (Table 5).

OUTCOME

With confirmation of primary hyperaldosteronism, (hypokalemia, elevated aldo levels, and aldo/renin ration of > 20) this patient underwent AV sampling despite suspicion of a right-sided aldosteronoma on CT. Expensive and invasive, this patient demonstrates the exact reason for obtaining AV sampling: supranormal aldosterone levels emanate from the *left* side, opposite the side of the visualized nodule. Nearly 25% of patients will have operative management changed on the basis of AV sampling.[31] With a secure diagnosis, a straightforward, laparoscopic, LEFT adrenalectomy was performed. As with many patients with long-standing hypertension from hyperaldosteronism, postoperative hypertension was improved but not corrected; Eukalemia was restored.

We agree a multidisciplinary approach to incidentalomas is warranted and will expedite the evaluation and improve the overall care of patients. Importantly, careful radiologic assessment shortens the need for extending work-ups with most adrenal masses. As seen from the patients above, nodules from 1 to 6 cm in size and *not* classical for any known diagnosis, require meticulous and

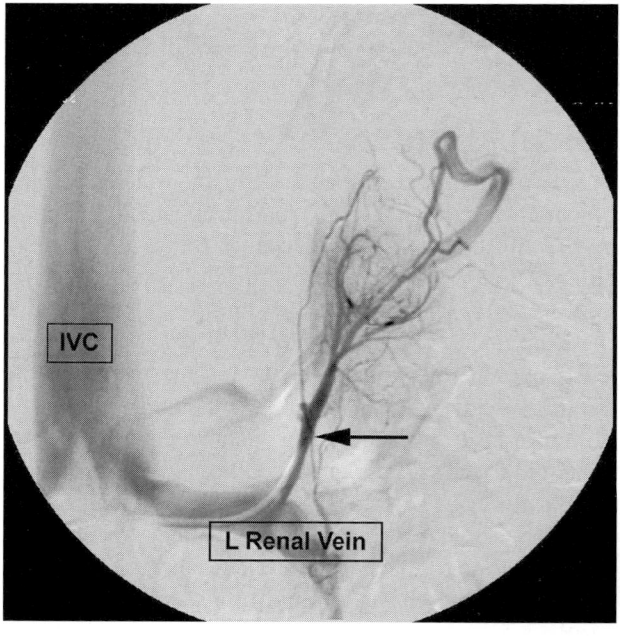

Figure 10 Fluoroscopic image taken during adrenal venous sampling (left adrenal vein).

Table 5.

DATA	Patient 5	Normal Levels	
Serum			
cortisol	17 µg/dL		
		AM: 5–25; PM: 2–14	
1-mg dexamethasone test	4.0 µg/dL		
potassium	3.2 mEq/L	Normal=suppression to < 5	
rennin	1.1 ng/mL/h	3.6–4.8	
		Na+ deplete upright=2.9–10.8	
aldosterone	32 ng/dL	Na+ replete upright=≤ 0.6–3.0	
Urine		1–21	
norepinephrine	22 µg/24h		
epinephrine	7 µg/24h	15–80	
dopamine	82 µg/24h	0–20	
metanephrines	0.5 mg/24h	65–400	
		< 1.3	

Adrenal Venous Sampling	R Adrenal Vein	L Adrenal Vein	IVC
aldosterone ng/dL cortisol µg/d/L	296	7248	63
	1500	970	37
Right Adrenal Vein Ratio:	aldo/cortisol =	296/1500 = 0.2	
Left Adrenal Vein Ratio:	aldo/cortisol =	7248/970 = 7.5	
Left to Right	aldo/cortisol=	7.5/0.2 = 37.5 to 1.0	

logical assessment: benign adrenal cysts, lipomas, or hemorrhage identified accurately shortens the evaluation to zero. With larger, malignant-appearing masses or evidence of metastatic disease picked up via CT or MRI, rapid evaluation and prompt surgical treatment or transition to palliative care of metastatic disease is expedited.

Surgical Management

While the surgical management of adrenal masses harbors pitfalls, nuances, and pearls of technique, logistically the decisions are relative simplistic:

1. Surgical candidates must be able to tolerate general anesthesia.
2. Functioning adrenal masses mandate resection.
3. Tumors larger than 6 cm (unless myelolipomas) require resection.
4. Nonfunctioning tumors < 3 to 4 cm should be observed.
5. Endoscopic adrenalectomy is the gold standard of surgical care.
6. Open adrenalectomy is used for larger (> 8 cm) and/or malignant tumors.

When the multidisciplinary approach identifies a functioning adrenaloma or a neoplasm suspicious for malignancy, operative preparation is undertaken and laparoscopic removal planned. Endoscopic resection from pooled studies suggest that smaller adrenalomas can be safely removed (Table 6). While malignant tumors have been removed laparoscopically, our preference

Table 6.

	Pheo	Aldo	Uni	Bilateral	Malignant?	Overall
			Hypercortisolism			
Patients	255	192	148	110	153	2550
OR Time (min)	160	173	124	282	171	156
Blood loss (mL)	129	219	NA	171	192	104
Conversion (%)	2	1	2	4	7	4
Complications (%)	18	8	NA	13	12	10
Hospital days	3.5	3.7	NA	3.7	3.1	3.3

OR = operating room; NA = not available.

remains open en bloc resection for larger (> 8 cm) masses or any primary cancer.

Summary

Although adrenal nodules in fit, asymptomatic patients are usually benign and harmless, identifying the nearly 1 in 5 that are either functioning (11%) or malignant (7%) pressures multidisciplinary team members into evaluating their patients meticulously. Combining CT or MRI characteristics and ruling out catecholamine, cortisol, or aldosterone secretion, most adrenal nodules are benign and nonfunctioning and can be observed. Larger masses (> 6 cm), or functioning tumors should be removed. Laparoscopic (for smaller, benign tumors) and open (for ACC or tumors > 8 cm) adrenalectomy are usually well tolerated by patients.

References

1. Linos DA, Stylopoulos N, Raptis SA. Adrenaloma: a call for more aggressive management. World J Surg 1996;20:788–92; discussion 792–3.

2. Grumbach MM, Biller BM, Braunstein GD, et al. Management of the clinically inapparent adrenal mass ("incidentaloma"). Ann Intern Med 2003;138:424–9.

3. Korobkin M, Francis IR, Kloos RT, Dunnick NR. The incidental adrenal mass. Radiol Clin North Am 1996;34:1037–54.

4. Glazer HS, Weyman PJ, Sagel SS, et al. Nonfunctioning adrenal masses: incidental discovery on computed tomography. Am J Roentgenol 1982;139:81–5.

5. Mitnick JS, Bosniak MA, Megibow AJ, Naidich DP. Non-functioning adrenal adenomas discovered incidentally on computed tomography. Radiology 1983;148:495–9.

6. Shuman WP, Moss AA. The adrenal glands. In: Moss AA, Gamsu G, Genant HK, editors. Computed tomography of the body with magnetic resonance imaging; Vol 3. 2nd ed Philadelphia: Saunders; 1992. p. 1021–57.

7. Young WF Jr. Management approaches to adrenal incidentalomas. A view from Rochester, Minnesota. Endocrinol Metab Clin North Am 2000;29:159–85.

8. Lenders JW, Pacak K, Walther MM, et al. Biochemical diagnosis of pheochromocytoma: which test is best? JAMA 2002;287:1427–34.

9. Kudva YC, Sawka AM, Young WF Jr. Clinical review 164: the laboratory diagnosis of adrenal pheochromocytoma: the Mayo Clinic experience. J Clin Endocrinol Metab 2003;88:4533–9.

10. Barry MK, van Heerden JA, Farley DR, et al. Can adrenal incidentalomas be safely observed? World J Surg 1998;22:599–604.

11. Teh SW, Grant CS, van Heerden JA, et al. "Adrenal" masses that are not adrenal. Contemporary Surg 2001;57:550–5.

12. Thompson GB, Young WF Jr. Adrenal incidentaloma. Curr Opin Oncol 2003;15:84–90.

13. Commons RR, Callaway CP. Adenomas of the adrenal cortex. Arch Intern Med 1948;81:37.

14. Devenyi I. Possibility of normokalaemic primary aldosteronism as reflected in the frequency of adrenal cortical adenomas. J Clin Pathol 1967;20:49–51.

15. Kokko JP, Brown TC, Berman MM. Adrenal adenoma and hypertension. Lancet 1967;1:468–70.

16. Lim PO, Rodgers P, Cardale K, et al. Potentially high prevalence of primary aldosteronism in a primary-care population. Lancet 1999;353:40.

17. Egglin TK, Hahn PF, Stark DD. MRI of the adrenal glands. Semin Roentgenol 1988;23:280–7.

18. Farley DR, van Heerden JA. Pheochromocytoma. In: McIntyre RC Jr, Stiegmann GV, Eiseman B, editors. Surgical decision making; 5th ed. Philadelphia: Saunders; 2004. p. 312–3.

19. Al Fehaily M, Duh QY. Clinical manifestation of aldosteronoma. Surg Clin North Am 2004;84:887–905.

20. Yun M, Kim W, Alnafisi N, et al. 18F-FDG PET in characterizing adrenal lesions detected on CT or MRI. J Nucl Med 2001;42:1795–9.

21. Frilling A, Tecklenborg K, Weber F, et al. Importance of adrenal incidentaloma in patients with a history of malignancy. Surgery 2004;136:1289–96.

22. Sarela AI, Murphy I, Coit DG, Conlon KC. Metastasis to the adrenal gland: the emerging role of laparoscopic surgery. Ann Surg Oncol 2003;10:1191–6.

23. Feliciotti F, Paganini AM, Guerrieri M, et al. Laparoscopic anterior adrenalectomy for the treatment of adrenal metastases. Surg Laparosc Endosc Percutan Tech 2003;13:328–33.

24. Mansmann G, Lau J, Balk E, et al. The clinically inapparent adrenal mass: update in diagnosis and management. Endocr Rev 2004;25:309–40.

25. Abrams HL, Spiro R, Goldstein N. Metastases in carcinoma; analysis of 1000 autopsied cases. Cancer 1950;3:74–85.

26. Lumb G, Mackenzie DH. The incidence of metastases in adrenal glands and ovaries removed for carcinoma of the breast. Cancer 1959;12:521–6.

27. Belldegrun A, Hussain S, Seltzer SE, et al. Incidentally discovered mass of the adrenal gland. Surg Gynecol Obstet 1986;163:203–8.

28. Gillams A, Roberts CM, Shaw P, et al. The value of CT scanning and percutaneous fine needle aspiration of adrenal masses in biopsy-proven lung cancer. Clin Radiol 1992;46:18–22.

29. Lenert JT, Barnett CC Jr, Kudelka AP, et al. Evaluation and surgical resection of adrenal masses in patients with a history of extra-adrenal malignancy. Surgery 2001;130: 1060–7.

30. Young WF Jr. Primary aldosteronism: management issues. Ann NY Acad Sci 2002;970:61–76.

31. Assalia A, Gagner M. Laparoscopic adrenalectomy. Br J Surg 2004;91:1259–74.

CHAPTER 43

ADRENAL CORTICAL CARCINOMA

ALAN PB. DACKIW, MD, PhD

Adrenal cortical carcinoma is an uncommon endocrine neoplasm with a worldwide incidence of approximately two per million population. There is a bimodal age distribution with an increased incidence in children less than 5 years of age and in individuals in the fourth and fifth decades of life.[1] Among 1891 cases reported in the English-language literature, adrenal cortical carcinomas were slightly more common in women (58.6%) than in men (41.4%).[2] The adrenal cortex is responsible for synthesizing and secreting several different classes of hormones, which include glucocorticoids, mineralocorticoids, and sex steroids. These hormones which consist mainly of cortisol, aldosterone, dehydroepiandrosterone (DHEA) and their biologically active metabolites, play essential roles in regulating multiple processes throughout the body including glucose metabolism, fluid-electrolyte balance, inflammation, wound healing, and sexual development. Tumors may be functional or nonfunctional, depending on whether they produce cortisol, aldosterone, androgens, or estrogens. More than 50% of patients with adrenal cortical cancers have clinical evidence of excess hormone production. The etiology of adrenal cortical carcinoma is unknown, although recent studies documenting chromosomal abnormalities and alterations in growth factor production have provided insight into possible mechanisms of molecular pathogenesis. Epidemiologic studies have suggested an increased risk of adrenal cortical cancer in association with cigarette smoking in men and with the use of oral contraceptives in women.[3] Complete surgical resection is currently the only potentially curative therapy for localized adrenal cortical carcinoma. Locally recurrent or isolated distant metastatic disease may also be amenable to surgical resection in carefully selected patients. Response rates to cytotoxic systemic che-

motherapy and the adrenolytic agent mitotane have been modest.

Clinical Presentation and Diagnostic Evaluation

The clinical presentation of adrenal cortical neoplasms will vary depending on tumor size and the hormonal secretory status of the tumor. Patients with large tumors will often present with abdominal pain and pressure due to mass effect and may report other symptoms including weight loss, malaise, dyspnea, hematuria, and varicocele. Excessive hormone production and secretion is observed in over 50% of patients. These functional tumors most commonly secrete cortisol (30%), androgens (20%), estrogen (10%), and aldosterone (2%), while 35% of patients will secrete a mixed pattern of hormones.[4]. A large proportion of nonfunctional adrenal cortical tumors are incidental or serendipitous findings unrelated to the clinical presentation of the patient and appropriately termed incidentalomas and more recently as clinically inapparent adrenal masses. Incidentalomas are relatively common occurring in up to 4% of individuals undergoing abdominal CT and in up to 7% of individuals at autopsy.[5] Most commonly, these tumors are smaller than 6 cm and represent benign nonfunctional adrenal cortical adenomas.

Once a clinical diagnosis of an adrenal tumor is suspected based on the patient history or radiologic findings, it is important to determine if the neoplasm is functional or nonfunctional, benign or malignant, and in the case of malignant tumors, if the adrenal neoplasm is a primary lesion or a secondary metastatic focus. To determine the hormonal secretory status of an adrenal tumor, a careful history and physical examination looking for clinical features suggestive of Cushing's syndrome, hypertension, and virilization should be performed. An office biochemical evaluation that initially involves a random afternoon plasma sample to measure circulating cortisol and electrolyte levels and a 24-hour urine collection to measure vanillylmandelic acid (VMA), metanephrine, normetanephrine, dopamine, and catecholamine concentrations should be obtained. The patient is administered oral dexamethasone (1 mg) at 10 pm the same evening and instructed to return to the clinic the following morning at 8 am to determine serum cortisol concentration and in the afternoon to return their timed 24-hour urine collection specimen. If the patients serum cortisol level is not suppressed below 5 ug/dL, a second 24-hour urine collection is performed to measure cortisol, 17-hydroxysteroid, and 17-ketosteroids. Hypokalemia is suggestive of aldosterone excess, elevated cortisol levels that cannot be suppressed with dexamethasone suggest a cortisol excess, abnormal urine 17-ketosteroids suggest a masculinizing or feminizing tumor, and elevated urine catecholamine and metanephrine concentration raise suspicion of a pheochromocytoma.[6]

The size of a unilateral adrenal tumor as measured on computed tomography (CT) or magnetic resonance imaging (MRI) remains the single best indicator of malignancy. It is estimated that an adrenal mass larger than 6 cm in diameter may have a 35 to 98% likelihood of being an adrenal cortical carcinoma.[7] In contrast, large adrenal adenomas (> 6 cm) are uncommon, although the exact frequency is unknown. Although malignancy cannot be ruled out in tumors between 3 and 5 cm in diameter, specific radiologic features can be important.[6,7] CT characteristics of malignancy include tumor inhomogeneity, irregular shape, and irregular margins. MRI characteristics of malignancy include signal intensity on T2 weighed images, with adenomas being of low signal intensity compared to liver (adrenal mass/liver ratio ≤ 1.4), adrenal cortical carcinomas and metastasis being moderately bright (adrenal mass/liver ratio 1.2 to 2.8), and pheochromocytomas being very bright (adrenal mass/liver ratio ≥ 3.0).[8] Unfortunately, the use of signal intensity ratios to differentiate benign from malignant neoplasms may be unreliable because these ratios overlap in up to 40% of cases. Percutaneous biopsies of the adrenal mass should be avoided unless metastatic disease is suspected. Lung cancer is the most common primary tumor to metastasize to the adrenal gland, while cancer of the breast, stomach, prostate, kidney, colon, and melanoma can metastasize to the adrenals. Patient symptoms, previous history of cancer, physical examination findings, radiologic or biochemical tests will often suggest the origin of the underlying

malignancy; however, occult primary malignancies can occur.

Perioperative Management

In patients with corticosteroid producing tumors, careful attention must be given to ensure adequate corticosteroid coverage and replacement during the perioperative and postoperative period, as suppression of the contralateral gland can be expected. Perioperative steroids should also be considered in patients with nonfunctional tumors to compensate for any steroidal production by the tumor. The dose and duration of replacement must be individualized and can vary depending on the tumor. For example patients presenting with Cushing's syndrome may take longer to regain adequate steroid production in the contralateral adrenal gland. Steroid replacement during the perioperative time period should resemble that administered to patients receiving long-term exogenous steroids prior to surgery. For example, 100 mg of hydrocortisone intravenously on call to the operating room and continued every 8 hours until a tapering regimen is commenced. Mineralocorticoid replacement should also be considered in patients with total adrenal ablation. While corticosteroids exhibit mineralocorticoid effects, this compensatory response may not be sufficient and patients may need to be administered synthetic adrenocorticoid fludrocortisone acetate. The dosing regimen will need to be individualized based on the patient's weight gain and serum electrolytes; however, an initial dose of 0.1 mg three times a week can be given and adjusted up to a dose of 0.1 mg/day. All patients with aldosterone-producing adrenal tumors must have their blood pressure controlled and their potassium levels monitored before surgery. Administration of spironolactone, an aldosterone antagonist, for 3 to 4 weeks prior to surgery has been the mainstay of medical treatment. While several doses have been reported in the literature ranging from 25 to 400 mg per day, it is associated with considerable side effects at higher doses (> 100 mg per day). These side effects include gastrointestinal symptoms, impotence, fatigue, and gynectomastia. It is advisable to limit doses below 50 mg per day especially in men. Spironolactone can be used in combination with other antihypertensive medications, including angiotensin-converting enzyme inhibitors and calcium-channel blockers.[9]

Staging

The Sullivan modification[10] of the MacFarlane system[11] for staging adrenal cortical carcinoma is the most widely used staging system. In contrast to most modern staging systems for solid tumors, this system groups patients with evidence of adjacent, direct organ invasion and positive lymph nodes with those who have distant metastatic disease. Icard and colleagues[4] and Lee and colleagues[12] have suggested modifications to this system that would classify patients with locally advanced tumors in stage III and only patients with distant metastatic disease in stage IV (Table 1). These modifications to the traditional staging systems of MacFarlane and Sullivan more accurately reflect the natural history of the disease and correlate more closely with cancer staging systems used for other solid tumors and are reflected in the most recent American Joint Committee on Cancer (AJCC) tumor, node, metastasis (TNM) classification.

Treatment

SURGERY

Complete surgical resection is the only potentially curative treatment for adrenal cortical carcinoma. The strongest predictor of outcome in this disease is the ability to perform a complete margin negative resection. A number of series have demonstrated that the 5-year actuarial survival ranges from 32 to 48% for patients who undergo complete resection (Table 2) [reviewed in 6,8]. Neither extended resection nor the presence of tumor thrombus in the inferior vena cava (IVC) or renal vein predicted a poor prognosis in patients who underwent complete resection. Venovenous bypass or cardiac bypass techniques may be necessary in patients with tumor extension to the IVC. In contrast, patients who undergo incomplete resection of adrenal cortical carcinomas (less than total resection of the primary tumor or resection of the primary tumor in the setting of unresectable metastatic disease) have a uniformly poor prognosis

with a median survival of less than 1 year (Table 3) [reviewed in 6,8]. Therefore, resection should generally be performed only if preoperative imaging studies indicate that a complete margin-negative resection is possible. In a report from Memorial Sloan-Kettering Cancer Center, pathologic prognostic factors were analyzed in 46 patients who underwent a complete, potentially curative resection for localized adrenal cortical carcinoma.[13] Predictors of short survival were tumor diameter. 12 cm, six or more mitotic figures per 10 high-power fields, and the presence of histologic evidence of intratumoral hemorrhage. All seven patients whose tumor specimens exhibited all three of these risk factors were dead within slightly over 2 years from the time of complete resection of their primary tumor. The six patients whose tumors exhibited no pathologic risk factors had a 5-year survival of 83%; this survival decreased to 42% for tumors with one risk factor and to 33% for tumors with two risk factors. Therefore, pathologic variables predicted aggressive biologic behavior in a small subset of patients who underwent a complete margin-negative resection. For most patients, however, the technical aspects of tumor resection remain critical for completion of a margin-negative resection, the most important predictor of survival. We recommend a transabdominal approach through a subcostal or midline incision for any suspected or proven adrenal cortical malignancy. This facilitates the maximal exposure necessary for complete resection, minimizes the chance for tumor spillage, and allows vascular control of the IVC, aorta, and renal vessels when necessary. The surgeon performing operative procedures for adrenal cortical carcinoma should be prepared for the en bloc resection of contiguous structures including the liver, IVC, kidney, spleen, and pancreas. Areas of technical difficulty during resection of large adrenal tumors are

Table 1 Staging Systems for Adrenal Cortical Carcinoma

Stage	Macfarlane (1958)[11]	Sullivan (1978)[10]	Icard (1992)[4]	Lee (1995)[12]
I	T_1 ($\leq$ 5 cm), N_0, M_0	T_1 ($\leq$ 5 cm), N_0, M_0	T_1 ($\leq$ 5 cm), N_0, M_0	T_1 ($\leq$ 5 cm), N_0, M_0
II	T_2 (>5 cm), N_0, M_0	T_2 (>5 cm), N_0, M_0	T_2 (> 5 cm), N_0, M_0	T_2 (> 5 cm), N_0, M_0
III	T_3 (local invasion without involvement of adjacent organs) or mobile positive lymph nodes, M_0	T_3 (local invasion), N_0, M_0 or T_{1-2}, N_1 (positive lymph nodes), M_0	T_3 (local invasion) and/or N1 (positive regional lymph nodes), M_0	$T_{3/T4}$ (local invasion as demonstrated by histologic evidence of adjacent organ invasion, direct tumor extension to IVC, and/or tumor thrombus within IVC or renal vein) and/or N1 (positive regional lymph nodes), M_0
IV	T_4 (invasion of adjacent organs) or fixed positive lymph nodes or M_1 (distant metastases)	T_4 (local invasion), N_0, M_0; or T_3, N_1, M_0; or T_{1-4}, N_{0-1}, M_1 (distant metastases)	T_{1-4}, N_{0-1}, M_1 (distant metastases)	T_{1-4}, N_{0-1}, M_1 (distant metastases)

Table 2 Survival of Patients Who Underwent a Potentially Curative Resection for Adrenal Cortical Carcinoma

First Author	Institution	Year	N	Margin Analysis	Median Follow-up (months)	Overall Survival (months)	5-Year actuarial Survival (%)
Harrison	MSKCC	1999	46	No	20	28†	36
Crucitti	Italy	1996	91	No	--	28	48
Lee	MDA	1995	16	Yes	43	46†	46
Zografos	Roswell Park	1994	15	No	--	13†	38
Icard	France	1992	127	No	--	--	42
Icard	France	1992	31	No	--	44‡	45
Pommier	MSK	1992	53	No	28	28‡	47
Gröndal	Sweden	1990	22	No	--	--	--
Henley	Mayo Clinic	1983	31	No	--	--	32

Table 3 Patient Survival Following Incomplete Resection* of Adrenal Cortical Carcinoma

Series	Institution	Year	N	Median Survival (months)
Crucitti	Italy	1996	33	16+
Lee	MDA	1995	7	8.5
Zografos	Roswell Park	1994	28	2
Icard	France	1992	28	< 12
Icard	France	1992	10	< 4
Gröndal	Sweden	1990	12	10
Henley	Mayo Clinic	1983	14	< 6

*Patients with incomplete resections included those who underwent incomplete resection of the primary tumor and those who underwent complete resection of the primary tumor in the presence of unresectable distant metastatic disease.
MDA, M. D. Anderson Cancer Center
+ mean survival

predictable on the basis of fundamental anatomic considerations. For example, a locally invasive right adrenal cortical carcinoma commonly invades the posterior segment of the right hepatic lobe and the IVC (Figure 1). Positive resection margins can be expected if blunt dissection is used to separate a locally invasive tumor from these structures. Complete mobilization of the liver combined with proximal and distal control of the IVC should therefore be performed routinely at the time of right adrenalectomy. Large right adrenal tumors may require a thoracoabdominal approach to adequately contend with tumor-induced compression of the liver, which may otherwise prevent the successful hepatic mobilization necessary for vascular control of the suprahepatic IVC. Incomplete resection of a large left adrenal cortical carcinoma is usually due to tumor extension along the mesenteric plexus at the origin of the celiac axis (Figure 2). Tumor encasement of the celiac axis, aorta, or proximal superior mesenteric artery represents clear evidence of a locally unresectable tumor. These vital tumor–vessel relations should be apparent before operation on contrast-enhanced CT images. Intraoperative assessment of the relation of a large left adrenal tumor to the celiac axis or proximal superior mesenteric artery is extremely difficult, may be associated

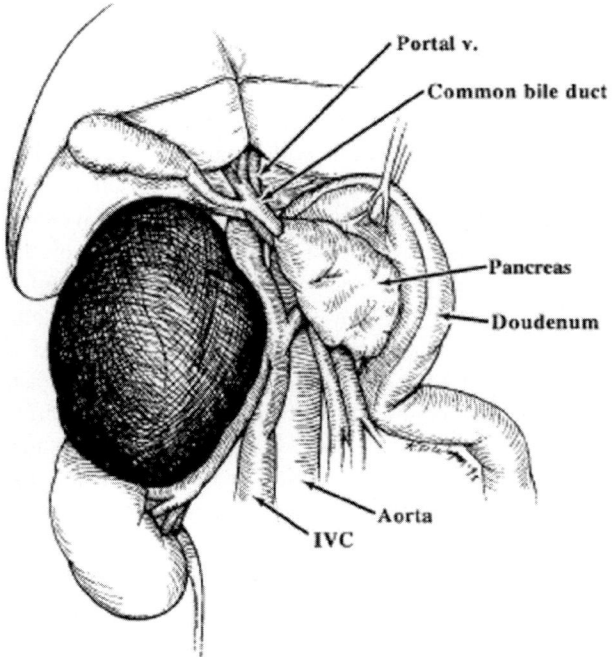

Figure 1 Large right adrenal carcinoma demonstrating the frequent finding of tumor invasion of the liver (posterior segment of the right hepatic lobe) and the inferior vena cava. v = vein. Reprinted with permission from Dackiw et al.[6]

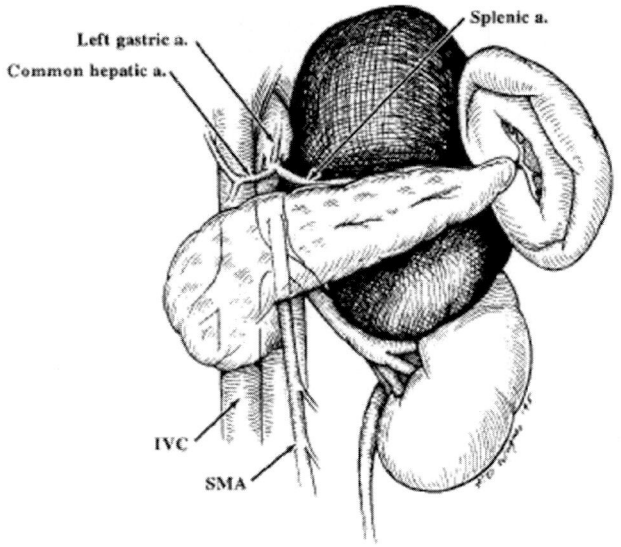

Figure 2 Large left adrenal carcinoma demonstrating the intimate relation between the tumor and the origin of the celiac axis and the superior mesenteric artery. a = artery. Reprinted with permission from Dackiw et al.[6]

with iatrogenic arterial injury, and when incorrect is likely responsible for the high incidence of incomplete tumor resection.[6] Laparoscopic adrenalectomy should be reserved for resection of presumed benign cortical tumors, aldosteronomas, pheochromocytomas, and for the rare patient who requires adrenalectomy for metastatic disease. If the differential diagnosis of a cortical neoplasm includes adrenal cortical carcinoma, the patient requires the best oncologic operation the surgeon can perform to achieve a wide margin resection. For most surgeons that would be an open transabdominal procedure. Preresection biopsies should be avoided. Locoregional recurrence may occur irrespective of the technique used for adrenalectomy; however, an open transabdominal operation should be performed if one suspects malignancy on the basis of tumor size and if pheochromocytoma has been excluded. In contrast, laparoscopic resection should be considered for palliative removal of metastatic disease to the adrenal gland.. Thus, for a malignant adrenal cortical mass, radical surgical excision with en bloc resection of any locally invaded structures offers the patient the greatest potential for cure (see Table 2), especially in children and adult patients with stage I and II tumors (see Table 1). In patients with stage III and IV disease, the role of surgery remains more controversial, as several of the studies outlined in Table 3 clearly indicate no overall improvement in patient survival, especially in patients presenting with metastatic disease where death usually occurs within 1 year. The presence of IVC extension should not be considered

metastatic disease but local tumor extension, which warrants a more aggressive surgical procedure that should include an attempt at removing the intravascular extension.

Laparoscopic adrenalectomy via a transperitoneal or retroperitoneal approach has become the preferred treatment for presumed benign adrenal cortical nonfunctional and functional tumors. While patients undergoing laparoscopic resection demonstrate reduced hospital stay, lower morbidity, and a faster recovery, several factors including tumor size, malignancy, and surgeon experience limit the use of minimally invasive surgery in the management of adrenal cortical carcinoma. If a preoperative diagnosis of adrenal cortical carcinoma is suspected, the surgeon must select an operative approach that will maximize the likelihood of achieving a margin negative resection.

In summary, for adrenal cortical carcinomas less than 10 cm, a transabdominal approach through a subcostal incision to remove the suspected adrenal cortical malignancy is recommended. This approach allows adequate exposure to the tumor mass and common sites of metastasis including the liver, omentum, periaortic nodes, and the peritoneum, and allows for vascular control of the IVC, aorta, and renal vessels when necessary. Local tumor invasion is common and may require the en-bloc excision of contiguous structures including the kidney, liver, IVC, spleen, pancreas, and regional lymph nodes. Extreme care should be taken not to violate the tumor to minimize tumor spillage and the chance of local tumor recurrence. Limited hepatic resection for metastasis and excision of omental or peritoneal implants are justified and may provide the patient with some symptom relief due to hormone excess. For larger lesions greater than 10 cm, a thoracoabdominal approach will often provide better access to the tumor and in the case of right adrenal tumors, allow for better hepatic mobilization and control of the supra-hepatic IVC if necessary. For lesions with intracaval extension, cardiac bypass is required if the lesions extend above the subhepatic vena cava and into the right atrium. Prior knowledge of the superior extent of the lesion is needed to prevent a tumor embolus at the time of clamping of the IVC, which may result in hemodynamic instability or neovascularization and growth in the lung. These patients should have bypass techniques used early in the operation prior to tumor manipulation.

Postoperative follow-up should include a physical examination, biochemical assessment if the tumor was functional, CT scan, and chest radiograph every 4 months following a potentially curative resection for primary tumor. Bone metastasis are often symptomatic and should be suspected in patients with elevated alkaline phosphatase levels. In patients that remain disease free, the duration of radiologic surveillance remains unclear. Continued CT scanning beyond 5 years after diagnosis due to unpredictable biological behavior of these tumors is recommended. In patients presenting with an isolated tumor recurrence amenable to reoperation, surgery should be recommended and the tumor resected (see below). In patients presenting with recurrence in multiple sites, systemic therapy may prolong overall survival.

MULTI-DISCIPLINARY THERAPY

Studies have demonstrated a beneficial role for mitotane (ortho, para-DDD or 1,1-dichloro-2-[o-chlorophenyl]-2-[p-chlorophenyl] ethane) as adjuvant therapy in the treatment of adrenal cortical carcinoma as indicated in Table 4. Mitotane acts via several different mechanisms including reducing corticoid biosynthesis by preventing cholesterol side chain cleavage and 11-β hydroxylation and by inducing structural damage to mitochondria in the zona reticularis and zona fasciculata leading to necrosis of both normal and tumor tissue.[14] These actions appear to be dose dependant with doses < 3 g per day leading to marked suppression of adrenal steroid secretion and doses > 3 g per day producing an adrenolytic effect. Typically, initial daily dosing begins with the administration of 1.5 to 2.0 g divided into three or four doses. The daily dosage is gradually increased to 8 to 12 g a day to achieve a target serum level above 15 μg/l[15] This threshold is based on previous studies that demonstrated a correlation between plasma serum levels and survival, with the best response seen in patients with serum levels more than 14 μg/mL.[15] Typically, serum levels reach a plateau after approximately 8 to 10 weeks of treatment and persist for 6 to 9 weeks following discontinuation of the drug due to extensive storage in adipose tissue. Glucocorticoid replacement should commence simultaneously (nonfunctional tumors) or within 2 to 4 weeks (functional tumors) after commencing

mitotane due to the suppressive effects on healthy adrenal tissue. A dose of 20 to 40 mg hydrocortisone is recommended, with two-thirds of the dose administered in the morning and the remainder administered in the afternoon with the exception of perioperative phase when higher doses may be required. Mineralocorticoid replacement with fludrocortisone may also be indicated depending on serum electrolyte measurements. Once mitotane treatment has been terminated, no attempt at tapering the corticosteroid replacement dose should be attempted for at least 1 month.

In general, mitotane treatment is associated with frequent serious side effects that appear to be dose dependent. The most common side effects include gastrointestinal symptoms such as nausea, vomiting, anorexia, and diarrhea, which occur in > 80% of patients. Neuropsychiatric symptoms including ataxia, dysarthria, confusion, lethargy, and somnolence occur in < 25% of patients, while skin rashes have also been reported in approximately 10% of patients. Other infrequent side effects include hepatotoxicity and hypercholesterolemia. All side effects can be reversed or reduced by reducing the dose of mitotane or by interrupting therapy, although, as previously mentioned, serum levels can remain elevated for a substantial time period.

Anecdotal reports and retrospective studies involving small series of patients have yielded conflicting results concerning the efficacy of mitotane either as adjuvant therapy or for the treatment of locally unresectable or metastatic disease (see Table 4). In the study by Luton and colleagues[16] mitotane therapy had no significant effect on survival but was effective in controlling hormone secretion in 75% of patients with adrenal cortical carcinoma. Further, In a report by Vassilopoulou-Sellin and colleagues,[17] no improvement in survival was observed in 8 patients treated with mitotane treatment; in fact only 1 of the 8 patients that received mitotane remained disease free 2 years after

Table 4 Adrenal Cortical Carcinoma Response to Mitotane Therapy

Study	Institution	Year	N	Result/Conclusion
Kasperlik-Zaluska et al.[18]	Poland	1995	36	Suggested benefit with adjuvant mitotane treatment
Haak et al.[15]	Netherlands	1994	62	Response rate 21% (6/29)
Vassilopoulou-Sellin et al.[17]	MDACC	1993	13	No effect on survival
Pommier et al.	MSKCC	1992	29	PR 24%
Luton et al.[16]	France	1990	37	PR 22%, no effect on survival
Venkatesh et al.	MDACC	1989	72	Stable disease or PR 29%
Karakousis et al.	Roswell Park	1985	10	Stable disease or response 40% (n=4)
van Slooten et al.	Netherlands	1984	34	Serum level >14 μg/ml associated with improved survival
Henley et al.	Mayo Clinic	1983	24	PR 4% (n=1)

PR = partial response.

diagnosis. These observations were in marked contrast to other studies that demonstrated improved survival[15,18] including cases of complete remission up to 4 years. Although there are currently no prospective studies available, the collective findings from both anecdotal and retrospective studies suggest a putative role for mitotane in the treatment of adrenal cortical cancer. The challenge involves attempting to translate information from this body of literature into clinical practice, which is further complicated by several factors, including (1) differing endpoints studied in the various studies, which makes direct comparisons difficult, ie, survival versus hormone production; (2) nonprotocol-based therapy, which often involves using differing treatment regimens of mitotane often in combination with various other cytotoxic agents that are administered at different times following the surgery; (3) failure to measure serum levels of mitotane, which appear to correlate with treatment response.[6,9]

Chemotherapeutic agents have been shown to be of some benefit in patients who do not respond to mitotane, experience intolerable side effects while administered mitotane, or in patients who present with unresectable tumors or recurrent tumors (Table 5). Cisplatin-based therapy in combination with other cytotoxic agents has been most commonly reported to be effective in several small patient series. For example, cisplatin administered in a dose of 100 mg/m^2 on day 1 and etoposide (VP16) in a daily dose of 100 mg/m^2 on days 1 to 3 resulted in three complete and three partial response rates in 18 patients, for an overall response rate of 33%.[19] Similar response rates were observed in patients treated with combination 5-fluorouracil, doxorubicin, and cisplatin.[20]

The heterogeneous response to classic cytotoxic chemotherapy can in part be explained by the expression of the *multidrug resistance 1* (*mdr1*) gene and its protein product p-glycoprotein that is frequently expressed on the surface of malignant adrenal cells. P-glycoprotein is an ATP-binding cassette that is able to actively transport chemotherapeutic agents out of the cell, thereby conferring chemotherapy resistance. Interestingly, mitotane has been shown to act as a P-glycoprotein antagonist in vitro,[21] suggesting that mitotane therapy may enhance the tumorolytic effect of classical cytotoxic chemotherapeutic agents. This approach has been evaluated by Berruti and colleagues,[22] who treated 28 patients with advanced inoperable disease with combination etoposide, doxorubicin, and cisplatin (EDP). The EDP schedule (etoposide 100 mg/m^2 on days 5 to 7; doxorubicin 20 mg/m^2 on days 1 and 8; cisplatin 40 mg/m2 on days 2 and 9) was repeated every 4 weeks and repeated for a maximum of six cycles. Mitotane was started at 1 g per day and escalated to 4 g per day or the maximum dose tolerated, which usually was less than 4 g due to the side effects of this combination. Complete response was achieved in 2 patients and a partial response in 13 for an overall response rate of 53.5%. The median time to disease progression in responding patients was 24 months. These results are encouraging and support the concept of combining classical cytotoxic agents with mitotane.

Additional pharmacologic agents are available for inhibiting the endogenous production of steroids, especially in patients who have failed surgery and mitotane. Ketoconazole is an imidazole antifungal agent that is able to suppress androgen and corticosteroid production but does not inhibit tumor growth. Ketoconazole treatment results in long-term hormonal suppression and can be administered preoperatively to patients with Cushing's disease and adrenal cortical carcinoma.[23] The maximal daily dose is 200 mg four times daily and requires routine measurements of liver transaminases to monitor for liver toxicity. Therapy should be temporarily disrupted in patients that exhibit elevated liver enzymes. Metyrapone is another pharmacologic agent that is able to inhibit adrenal cortisol production when the combination of mitotane and ketoconazole fail.[24] Doses range from 750 to 5,000 mg

Table 5 Adrenal Cortical Carcinoma Response to Chemotherapy

Study	Institution	Year	N	Regimen	Response
Abraham et al.	NCI	1999	28	M E D V	CR 1, PR 4
Berruti et al.	Italy	1998	28	M E D P	CR 2, PR 13
Zidan et al.	Israel	1996	1	E P*	PR 1
Bukowski et al.	SWOG	1993	37	M P	PR 11
Berruti et al.[22]	Italy	1992	2	E D P	PR 2
Schlumberger et al.	France	1991	13	D P 5-FU	CR1, PR 2
Hesketh et al.	Boston Univ.	1987	4	E P B	CR 1, PR 1
Johnson et al.	Vanderbilt	1986	2	E C	PR 2

B = bleomycin; CR = complete resection; D = doxorubicin; E = etoposide; 5-FU = 5-fluorouracil; M = mitotane; NCI = National Cancer Institute; P = cisplatin; PR = partial response; SWOG = Southwest Oncology Group; V = vincristine.
*Mitotane failure.

per day and result in the suppression of normal adrenal tissue, making it essential to provide patients with hydrocortisone replacement. A randomized trial examining the adjuvant use of mitotane and other chemotherapeutic agents appears warranted.

Follow-up and Reoperation

Postoperative follow-up generally includes physical examination, biochemical assessment if the tumor was originally functional, CT scanning, and chest radiography every 4 months following potentially curative resection of the primary tumor. Bone metastases are usually symptomatic and may be suspected on the basis of elevation of the alkaline phosphatase level. In patients with recurrence, systemic therapy for progressive, multisite, recurrent disease may prolong survival, but the potential for long-term survival exists only in patients with isolated recurrence amenable to reoperation.

Two large series of patients who underwent reoperation for recurrent adrenal cortical carcinoma have been reported.[25,26] The Italian registry report included 140 patients from 21 institutions who underwent potentially curative resection of a primary adrenal cortical carcinoma.[25] Disease recurred in 52 (37%) of the 140 patients: at distant sites (liver, lungs, bone) in 25 patients, locally in 13 patients, and at distant and local sites in 14 patients. The mean disease-free interval was 22 months. Twenty of the 52 (38%) patients underwent reoperation for recurrent disease. These 20 patients had a 5-year survival of 50% compared with 8% in the 32 patients whose recurrent disease was not amenable to surgical resection. The long survival of these 20 patients was likely due to favorable tumor biology and aggressive therapy. Similar results were recently reported from Memorial Sloan-Kettering Cancer Center.[26] Following resection of local or distant recurrences, complete resection was associated with a median survival of 74 months (5-year survival 57%) and incomplete resection was associated with a median survival of 16 months (5-year survival 0%). Although the number of patients in these studies is small, these data do support the use of careful clinical and radiographic follow-up in patients after their initial adrenalectomy in the hope of discovering recurrent disease that would be amenable to reoperation. For patients who enjoy a long disease-free interval, the recommended duration of continued radiographic surveillance is unclear. Because of the unpredictable biologic behavior of adrenalcortical carcinoma, continuing CT scans beyond 5 years after diagnosis is not unreasonable.

Summary

Adrenal cortical carcinoma is a rare endocrine tumor with a worldwide incidence of approximately two pre million population for which complete surgical resection is the only potentially curative treatment. Accurate preoperative biochemical and radiographic evaluation of the patient who presents with an adrenal mass will optimize patient management and facilitate a complete margin-negative resection of the primary tumor; the most powerful prognostic variable for long-term survival. Response to mitotane or chemotherapy is modest in patients with advanced disease.

References

1. Norton JA. Adrenal tumors. In: DeVita V, Hellman S, Rosenberg S, editors. Cancer: principles and practice of oncology. 5th ed. Philadelphia: Lippincott-Raven Publishers; 1997. p. 1659.

2. Wooten MD, King DK. Adrenal cortical carcinoma. Epidemiology and treatment with mitotane and a review of the literature. Cancer., 1993;72:3145.

3. Hsing AW, Nam JM, Co Chien HT, et al. Risk factors for adrenal cancer: an exploratory study. Int J Cancer 1996;65:432.

4. Icard P, Chapuis Y, Andreassian B, et al. Adrenal cortical carcinoma in surgically treated patients: a retrospective study on 156 cases by the French association of endocrine surgery. Surgery 1992;112:972–9; discussion 979–80.

5. Lee JE, Evans DB, Hickey RC, et al. Unknown primary cancer presenting as an adrenal mass: frequency and implications for diagnostic evaluation of adrenal incidentalomas. Surgery 1998;124:1115–22.

6. Dackiw AP, Lee JE, Gagel RF, Evans DB. Adrenal cortical carcinoma. World J Surg 2001;25:914–26.

7. Ross NS, Aron DC. Hormonal evaluation of the patient with an incidentally discovered adrenal mass. N Engl J Med 1990;323:1401–5.

8. Doppman JL, Reinig JW, Dwyer AJ, et al. Differentiation of adrenal masses by magnetic resonance imaging. Surgery 1987;102:1018–26.

9. Boushey RP, Dackiw AP. Adrenal cortical carcinoma. Curr Treat Options Oncol 2001;2:355–64.

10. Sullivan M, Boileau M, Hodges CV. Adrenal cortical carcinoma. J Urol 1978;120:660.

11. Macfarlane DA. Cancer of the adrenal cortex: the natural history, prognosis and treatment in a study of fifty-five cases. Ann R Coll Surg Engl 1958;23:155.

12. Lee JE, Berger DH, El-Naggar AK, et al. Surgical management, DNA content, and patient survival in adrenal cortical carcinoma. Surgery 1995;118:1090.

13. Harrison LE, Gaudin PB, Brennan MF. Pathologic features of prognostic significance for adrenocortical carcinoma after curative resection. Arch Surg 1999;134:181.

14. Kopf D, Goretzki PE, Lehnert H. Clinical management of malignant adrenal tumors. J Cancer Res Clin Oncol 2001; 127:143–55.

15. Haak HR, Hermans J, van de Velde CJ, et al. Optimal treatment of adrenal cortical carcinoma with mitotane: results in a consecutive series of 96 patients. Br J Cancer 1994;69:947–51.

16. Luton JP, Cerdas S, Billaud L, et al. Clinical features of adrenal cortical carcinoma, prognostic factors, and the effect of mitotane therapy. N Engl J Med 1990;322:1195–201.

17. Vassilopoulou-Sellin R, Guinee VF, Klein MJ, et al. Impact of adjuvant mitotane on the clinical course of patients with adrenal cortical cancer. Cancer 1993;71:3119–23.

18. Kasperlik-Zaluska AA, Migdalska BM, Zgliczynski S, et al. Adrenal cortical carcinoma. A clinical study and treatment results of 52 patients. Cancer 1995;75:2587–91.

19. Bonacci R, Gigliotti A, Baudin E, et al. Cytotoxic therapy with etoposide and cisplatin in advanced adrenal cortical carcinoma. Reseau comete inserm. Br J Cancer 1998;78: 546–9.

20. Schlumberger M, Gicquel C, Lumbroso J, et al. Malignant pheochromocytoma: clinical, biological, histologic and therapeutic data in a series of 20 patients with distant metastases. J Endocrinol Invest 1992;15:631–42.

21. Bates SE, Shieh CY, Mickley LA, et al. Mitotane enhances cytotoxicity of chemotherapy in cell lines expressing a multidrug resistance gene (mdr-1/p-glycoprotein) which is also expressed by adrenal cortical carcinomas. J Clin Endocrinol Metab 1991;73:18–29.

22. Berruti A, Terzolo M, Paccotti P, et al. Favorable response of metastatic adrenal cortical carcinoma to etoposide, adriamycin and cisplatin (EAP) chemotherapy. Report of two cases. Tumori 1992;78:345–8.

23. Engelhardt D, Weber MM. Therapy of Cushing's syndrome with steroid biosynthesis inhibitors. J Steroid Biochem Mol Biol 1994;49:261–7.

24. Thoren M, Adamson U, Sjoberg HE. Aminoglutethimide and metyrapone in the management of Cushing's syndrome. Acta Endocrinol (Copenh) 1985;109:451–7.

25. Bellantone R, Ferrante A, Boscherini M, et al. Role of reoperation in recurrence of adrenal cortical carcinoma: results from 188 cases collected in the Italian national registry for adrenal cortical carcinoma. Surgery 1997;122: 1212.

26. Schulick RD, Brennan MF. Long-term survival after complete resection and repeat resection in patients with adrenocortical carcinoma. Ann Surg Oncol 1999;6:719–26.

CHAPTER 44

MANAGEMENT OF ADRENAL MEDULLARY NEOPLASMS

WILLIAM F. YOUNG, JR., MD, MSc

CLIVE S. GRANT, MD

Catecholamine-secreting tumors that arise from chromaffin cells of the adrenal medulla are termed pheochromocytomas. Although catecholamine-secreting tumors are rare (annual incidence of 2 to 8 cases per million people),[1] it is important to suspect, confirm, localize, and resect these tumors because (a) the associated hypertension is curable with surgical removal of the tumor, (b) there is the risk of a lethal paroxysm, and (c) approximately 10% of the adrenal medullary neoplasms are malignant. These tumors occur with equal frequency in men and women, primarily in the third, fourth, and fifth decades. Patients harboring pheochromocytomas may be asymptomatic. However, symptoms usually are present and are due to the pharmacologic effects of excess circulating catecholamines. The resulting hypertension may be sustained or paroxysmal. Episodic symptoms may occur in "spells," or paroxysms, that can be extremely variable in presentation but typically include forceful heartbeat, pallor, tremor, headache, and diaphoresis. Spells may be either spontaneous or precipitated by postural change, anxiety, medications (eg, metoclopramide, anesthetic agents), exercise, medical procedures (eg, colonoscopy), or maneuvers that increase intra-abdominal pressure. Although the types of spells experienced across all patients with pheochromocytoma are highly variable, spells tend to be stereotypical for each patient. However, a key point for all clinicians is that most patients with spells do not have a pheochromocytoma,[2] and that most patients with "classic pheochromocytoma spells" do not have pheochromocytoma.

Additional clinical signs of pheochromocytoma include hypertension, hypertensive retinopathy, orthostatic hypotension, constipation (megacolon may be the presenting symptom), hyperglycemia, diabetes mellitus,

hypercalcemia, and erythrocytosis. Some of the cosecreted hormones that may dominate the clinical presentation include adrenocorticotropin (Cushing's syndrome), parathyroid hormone-related peptide (hypercalcemia), vasoactive intestinal peptide (watery diarrhea), and growth hormone-releasing hormone (acromegaly). Cardiomyopathy, myocardial infarction with normal coronary arteries, and congestive heart failure are the symptomatic presentations that are perhaps most frequently unrecognized by clinicians to be caused by pheochromocytoma. Many physical examination findings are associated with genetic syndromes that predispose to pheochromocytoma; these findings include retinal angiomas, marfanoid body habitus, café au lait spots, axillary freckling, subcutaneous neurofibromas, and mucosal neuromas on the eyelids and tongue.

The surgical experience with pheochromocytomas at the Mayo Clinic during the era of laparoscopic adrenalectomy started in October 1995. A total of 131 pheochromocytomas were operated from October 1995 through April 2004, from which considerable data can be gleaned (Table 1). Pheochromocytomas are localized to the adrenal glands, with a mean size of 4.5 to 4.9 cm[3] (Figure 1). Paragangliomas are found where there is chromaffin tissue: along the para-aortic sympathetic chain, within Zuckerkandl's organs (at the origin of the inferior mesenteric artery), in the wall of the urinary bladder, and along the sympathetic chain in the neck or mediastinum.[4]

Syndromic Pheochromocytoma

Approximately 10 to 20% of patients with catecholamine-secreting tumors have associated germline muta-

Table 1 Surgically resected adrenal pheochromocytomas at Mayo Clinic (131 patients), October 1995 through April 2004

Category	Frequency	%
Male/Female	58/73	44/56
Age, yrs, average (min-max)	55 (16–86)	
Associated condition:	17	13
MEN-2A	6	5
MEN-2B	4	3
VHL	4	3
Neurofibromatosis	3	2

Imaging	True Pos/False Neg/Not Done	%TP/%TN
CT	118/2/10	98/2
MRI	52/1/76	98/2
MIBG	20/1/109	95/5

Surgical technique	Frequency	%
Anterior	35	27
Laparoscopic	86	66
Hand-assisted	1	1
Lap converted to open	7	5
Posterior	1	1

Adrenalectomy	Frequency	%
Right	70	54
Left	53	41
Bilateral	7	5

Intraoperative BP		Peak, Minimum
Systolic, Avg Max, Min	192, 83	310, 31

Intraoperative BP meds		%
used: Yes, No	90, 40	69, 31
α-Adrenergic blockade		
Phenoxybenzamine	120	92
Other medications	3	2
None	8	6

Tumor size, avg; range	4.9 cm	0.7–16 cm
Presented as adrenal incidentaloma: Yes, No	49, 81	38%, 62%

BP = blood pressure; CT = computed tomography; MEN = multiple endocrine neoplasia; MIBG = metaiodobenzylguanidine; MRI = magnetic resonance imaging; VHL = von Hippel-Lindau disease.

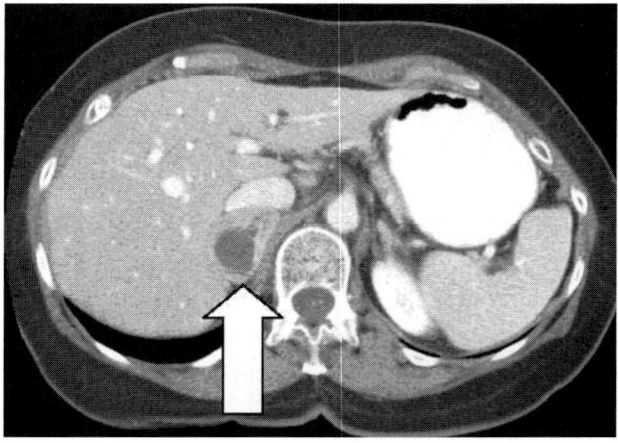

Figure 1 A computed tomographic (CT) scan of the abdomen with intravenous contrast agent of a 66-year-old woman with spells of heart pounding, anxiety, and tremor. The 24-hour urine studies were abnormal: total metanephrine, 2,500 μg (normal < 1,300). The CT image shows a 4.0 × 2.5 cm enhancing right adrenal mass with central cystic degeneration consistent with pheochromocytoma (arrow). After α-and β-adrenergic blockade, a 4.8 × 3.4 × 2.1 cm pheochromocytoma was removed laparoscopically. Postoperatively, the 24-hour urinary metanephrines have been checked annually for 6 years and remain normal.

tions (inherited mutations present in all cells of the body) in genes known to cause genetic disease.[5] The familial neurocristopathic syndromes associated with adrenal pheochromocytoma include multiple endocrine neoplasia (MEN) type 2A (pheochromocytoma, medullary thyroid carcinoma (MTC), and hyperparathyroidism) and type 2B (MEN-2B) (pheochromocytoma, medullary thyroid carcinoma, mucosal neuromas, thickened corneal nerves, intestinal ganglioneuromatosis, and marfanoid body habitus); neurofibromatosis type 1 (NF1); von Hippel-Lindau disease (VHL) (pheochromocytoma, retinal angiomas, cerebellar hemangioblastoma, renal and pancreatic cysts, and renal cell carcinoma); familial pheochromocytoma (specific mutations yet to be identified); and familial paraganglioma. Another syndrome associated with catecholamine-secreting tumors that does not appear to be inherited is Carney's triad (gastric leiomyosarcoma, pulmonary chondroma, and extra-adrenal pheochromocytoma).[6] Bilateral adrenal pheochromocytoma has also been reported in children with Beckwith-Wiedemann syndrome.[7]

Familial paraganglioma is an autosomal dominant syndrome characterized by paragangliomas that are located most often in the head and neck, but they also have been found in the thorax, abdomen, adrenal medulla, pelvis, and urinary bladder. The occurrence of catecholamine hypersecretion in familial paraganglioma depends on tumor location; approximately 5% of head and neck paragangliomas and 50% of abdominal paragangliomas are hormone-producing tumors.[4] Familial paraganglioma is caused by mutations in the succinate dehydrogenase (SDH; succinate:ubiquinone oxidoreductase) subunit genes *SDHB, SDHC, SDHD*, which compose portions of mitochondrial complex II.[8] *SDHB* mutations have been associated with increased risk of malignant paraganglioma.[8,9] Patients with the *SDHB* mutation are also at increased risk for renal cell carcinoma and papillary thyroid cancer.[8]

Diagnostic Investigation

CASE FINDING

Pheochromocytoma should be suspected in patients who have hypertension accompanied by one or more of the following: hyperadrenergic spells (eg, self-limited episodes of nonexertional palpitations, diaphoresis, headache, tremor, and pallor); resistant hypertension; a familial syndrome that predisposes to catecholamine-secreting tumors (eg, MEN-2); an incidentally discovered adrenal mass; or a history of gastric stromal tumor or pulmonary chondromas (Carney's triad). The diagnosis must be confirmed biochemically by the presence of increased concentrations of catecholamines and/or metanephrines in the urine or plasma.

At Mayo Clinic, the single most reliable screening method for identifying catecholamine-secreting tumors is measuring metanephrines in a 24-hour urine collection.[10] If clinical suspicion is high, then urinary catecholamines (epinephrine, norepinephrine, and dopamine) are measured in addition to the 24-hour urine metanephrines. Fractionated plasma-free metanephrines, which are products of intrapheochromocytoma catecholamine metabolism, are also obtained in high clinical suspicion cases.[11,12] The index of suspicion should be high for the following scenarios: resistant hypertension; spells; a family history of pheochromocytoma; a genetic syndrome that predisposes to pheochromocytoma (eg, MEN-2); a past history of resected pheochromocytoma

and present history of recurrent hypertension or spells; or an incidentally discovered adrenal mass that has imaging characteristics consistent with pheochromocytoma (eg, marked enhancement with intravenous contrast medium on computed tomography [CT], high signal intensity on T2-weighted magnetic resonance imaging [MRI], cystic and hemorrhagic changes, and larger size [eg, > 4 cm], or bilaterality). In addition, measuring fractionated plasma-free metanephrines is a good first-line test for children since obtaining a complete 24-hour urine collection is difficult.

LOCALIZATION

Localization studies should not be initiated until biochemical studies have confirmed the diagnosis of a catecholamine-secreting tumor. Computer-assisted imaging of the adrenal glands and abdomen with MRI or CT should be the first localization test (sensitivity, > 95%; specificity, > 65%)[13] (Figure 2). In the Mayo Clinic experience, the true positive rate for either CT or MRI for pheochromocytomas has been 98% (see Table 1). Approximately 90% of catecholamine-secreting tumors are found in the adrenal glands and 98% are found in the abdomen.[14] If the results of abdominal imaging are negative, scintigraphic localization with ^{123}I-metaiodobenzylguanidine (^{123}I-MIBG) is indicated (Figure 3). This radiopharmaceutical agent accumulates preferentially in catecholamine-producing tumors; however, this procedure is not as sensitive as initially hoped (sensitivity, 80%; specificity, 99%).[15] In a study of 282 patients

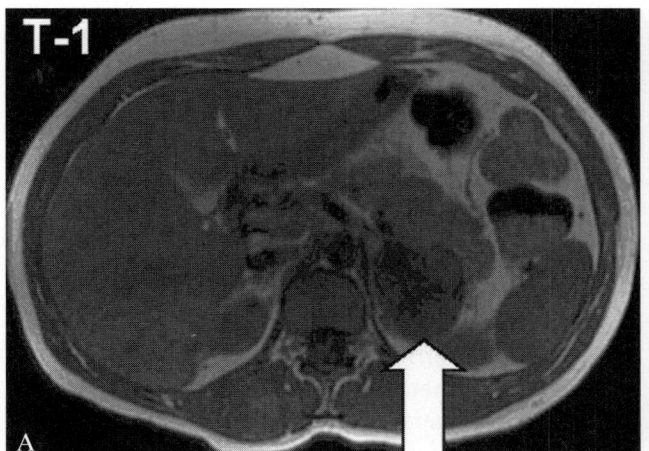 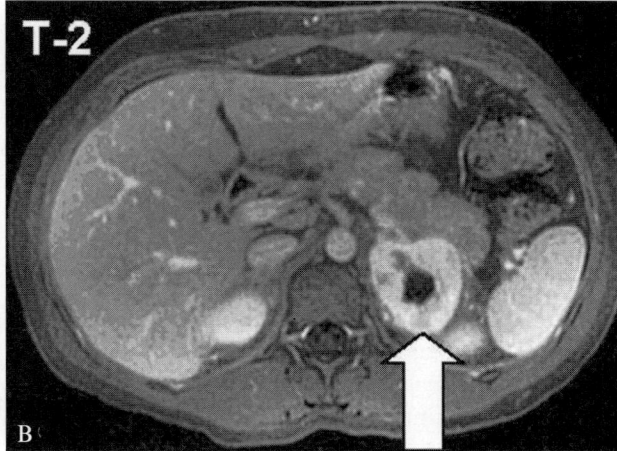

Figure 2 Magnetic resonance images of the abdomen of a 22-year-old woman with a 1-year history of hypertension. She also had been troubled by spells of palpitations, diaphoresis, and lightheadedness for the last 6 months. The fractionated plasma-free metanephrines were abnormal: metanephrine, 0.31 nmol/L (normal < 0.5) and normetanephrine, 14.6 nmol/L (normal < 0.9). The 24-hour urine test for fractionated metanephrines was also markedly abnormal: metanephrine, 86 μg (normal < 400); normetanephrine, 4,256 μg (normal < 900). The images show a 4.8 × 4.2 × 6.4 cm left adrenal mass consistent with pheochromocytoma (arrows) that has increased signal intensity on T2-weighted images. *A*, T1-weighted image. *B*, T2-weighted image (note area of central necrosis). Following α- and β-adrenergic blockade, a 8.0 × 5.0 × 4.8 cm pheochromocytoma was removed laparoscopically. Postoperatively, the fractioned plasma-free metanephrines normalized.

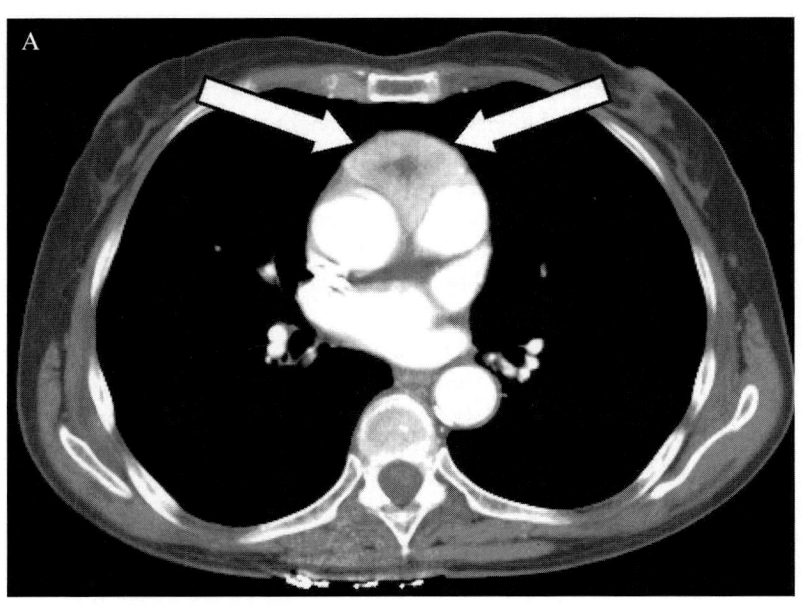

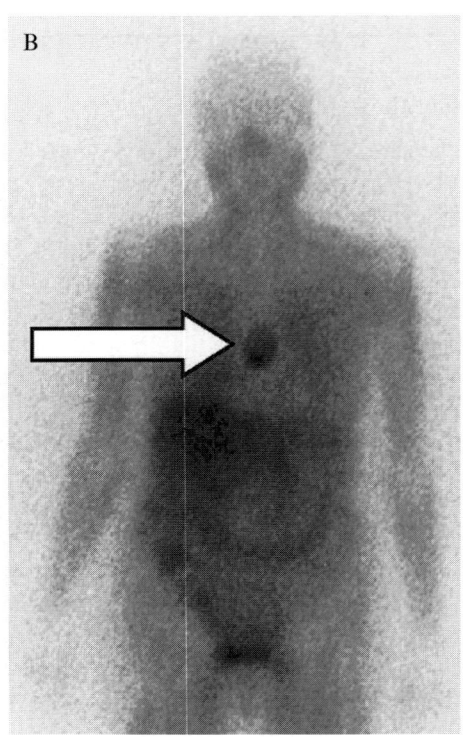

Figure 3 Computed tomography (CT) and ^{123}I-metaiodobenzylguanidine (^{123}I-MIBG) imaging from a 79-year-old woman. Her primary symptom was excessive diaphoresis and she was recently diagnosed with hypertension. A catecholamine-secreting neoplasm was appropriately suspected and confirmed with a 24-hour urine test for fractionated metanephrines and catecholamines: metanephrine, 330 µg (normal < 400); normetanephrine, 17,157 µg (normal < 900); norepinephrine, 2,106 µg (normal < 170); epinephrine, 7 µg (normal < 35); and dopamine, 1,108 µg (normal < 700). MRI of the abdomen was normal. **A**, Chest CT image showing a 5.5 × 4.5 × 4.0 cm mixed attenuation mass (arrow) in the anterior mediastinum. **B**, ^{123}I-MIBG whole body scan showing a large intense area of uptake in midline anterior mediastinum near the base of the heart (arrow) that corresponds to the mass seen on the CT image; no other abnormal uptake is seen.

with catecholamine-secreting tumors that were surgically confirmed, the overall sensitivity was 89% for CT, 98% for MRI, and 81% for ^{131}I-MIBG.[16] If a typical (< 10 cm) unilateral adrenal pheochromocytoma is found on CT or MRI, ^{123}I-MIBG scintigraphy is superfluous and the results may confuse the clinician.[17,18] ^{123}I-MIBG scintigraphy is preferred over ^{131}I-MIBG because of more avid tumor uptake, shorter scan times, and the ability to perform single photon emission computed tomography. However, if a paraganglioma is identified on CT or MRI, then ^{123}I-MIBG scintigraphy is indicated because the patient has increased risk of having additional paragangliomas and malignant disease. Performing preoperative ^{123}I-MIBG scintigraphy in patients with large (> 10 cm) adrenal pheochromocytomas may be indicated to identify metastatic disease; however, finding metastatic disease preoperatively does not usually change the initial surgical treatment plan.

Localizing procedures that can also be used, but are rarely required, include computer-assisted imaging of the chest, neck, and head. Other localizing studies, such as somatostatin receptor imaging with In-pentetreotide,

may also be considered. Although positron emission tomography (PET) scanning with ^{18}F-fluorodeoxyglucose (FDG) or ^{11}C-hydroxyephedrine or 6-[^{18}F]fluorodopamine can identify paragangliomas,[19] these expensive techniques probably should be reserved for identifying sites of metastatic disease in patients with negative ^{123}I-MIBG scintigraphic results (Figure 4).

Treatment

The treatment of choice for pheochromocytoma is complete surgical resection. Careful preoperative pharmacologic preparation is crucial for successful treatment. Most catecholamine-secreting tumors are benign and can be totally excised. Tumor excision usually cures hypertension in patients who lack a family history of essential hypertension.

PREOPERATIVE MANAGEMENT

Some form of preoperative pharmacologic preparation is indicated for all patients with catecholamine-secreting neoplasms. However, no randomized controlled trials

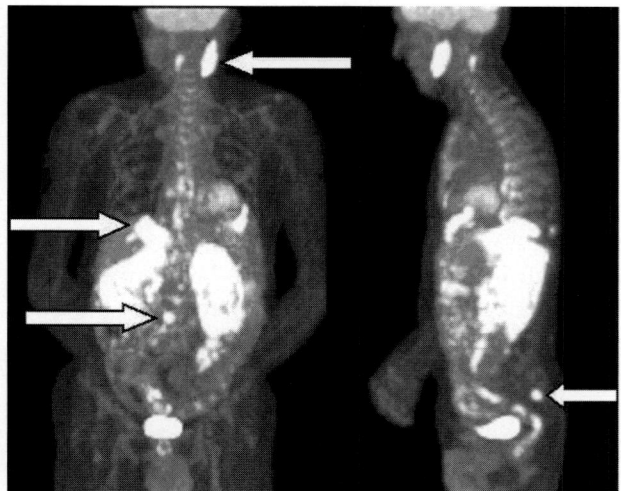

Figure 4 F-18 flurodeoxyglucose (FDG) positron emission tomography (PET) scan from a 63-year-old man who had a right periadrenal paraganglioma resected 31 years previously. The patient developed recurrent signs and symptoms of a catecholamine-secreting tumor, and because of invasion of the liver and inferior vena cava, the recurrent paraganglioma proved unresectable. The fractionated plasma-free metanephrines were abnormal: metanephrine, < 0.2 nmol/L (normal < 0.5); normetanephrine, 20.5 nmol/L (normal < 0.9). ^{123}I-metaiodobenzylguanidine scintigraphy showed uptake limited to the right supra-renal region. The FDG-PET scan shows soft tissue hypermetabolism in the large right supra-renal mass (arrow) and bony and nodal metastatic disease involving the right sacrum (arrow), third lumbar vertebral body (arrow), left mandible (arrow), and anterior mediastinum.

have compared the different approaches. Combined α- and β-adrenergic blockade is one approach to control blood pressure and prevent intraoperative hypertensive crises.[20] α-Adrenergic blockade should be started at least 7 to 10 days preoperatively to normalize blood pressure and expand the contracted blood volume. Target blood pressure is less than 120/80 mm Hg (seated), with systolic blood pressure greater than 90 mm Hg (standing); both targets should be modified on the basis of the patient's age and comorbid disease. On the second or third day of α-adrenergic blockade, patients are encouraged to start a diet high in sodium content because of the catecholamine-induced volume contraction and the orthostasis associated with α-adrenergic blockade. After adequate α-adrenergic blockade has been achieved, β-adrenergic blockade is initiated, which typically occurs 2 to 3 days preoperatively.

α-Adrenergic Blockade

Phenoxybenzamine is the preferred drug for preoperative preparation to control blood pressure and arrhythmia, and we have utilized this drug in nearly all pheochro-mocytoma patients. It is an irreversible, long-acting, nonspecific α-adrenergic blocking agent. The initial dosage is 10 mg 1 or 2 times daily, and it is increased by 10 to 20 mg every 2 to 3 days as needed to control blood pressure and prevent spells. The final target dosage of phenoxybenzamine is typically 20 to 100 mg daily. The patient should be warned about the orthostasis, nasal stuffiness, and fatigue that occur in almost all patients. With their more favorable side-effect profile, prazosin, terazosin, or doxazosin, selective α₁-adrenergic blocking agents, are preferable to phenoxybenzamine when long-term pharmacologic treatment is indicated (eg, for metastatic pheochromocytoma). However, treatment with these agents is not routinely used preoperatively because of incomplete α-adrenergic blockade.

β-Adrenergic Blockade

The β-adrenergic antagonist should be administered only after α-adrenergic blockade is effective, because with β-adrenergic blockade alone, hypertension may be more severe from the unopposed α-adrenergic stimulation. Preoperative β-adrenergic blockade is indicated to control the tachycardia associated with both the high concentrations of circulating catecholamines and the α-adrenergic blockade. The clinician should exercise caution if the patient is asthmatic or has congestive heart failure. Chronic catecholamine excess can produce a myocardiopathy; this may become evident with the initiation of β-adrenergic blockade, resulting in acute pulmonary edema. Therefore, when the β-adrenergic blocker is administered, it should be used cautiously and at a low dose. For example, a patient is usually given 10 mg of propranolol every 6 hours to start; on the second day of treatment, the β-adrenergic blockade (assuming the patient tolerates the drug), propranolol is converted to a single long-acting dose. The dose is then increased as necessary to control the tachycardia (goal heart rate is 60 to 80 beats per minute).

Catecholamine Synthesis Inhibitor

α-Methyl paratyrosine (metyrosine) should be used with caution and only when other agents have been ineffective or when significant tumor manipulation is anticipated. Although some centers have used this agent preoperatively, most reserve it primarily for patients who cannot be treated with the typical combined α- and β-adrenergic blockade protocol because of cardiopulmonary reasons. Metyrosine inhibits catecholamine synthesis by blocking the enzyme tyrosine hydroxylase. Metyrosine's side effects can be disabling, and they include sedation, depression, diarrhea, anxiety, nightmares, crystalluria and urolithiasis, galactorrhea, and extrapyramidal signs.

Calcium Channel Blockers–

Calcium channel blockers, which block norepinephrine-mediated calcium transport into vascular smooth muscle, have been used successfully at several medical centers to preoperatively prepare patients with pheochromocytoma.[21–23] Nicardipine is the most commonly used calcium channel blocker in this setting. It is given orally to control blood pressure preoperatively and is given as an intravenous infusion intraoperatively. When calcium channel blockers are used as the primary mode of antihypertensive therapy, they appear to be just as effective as α- and β-adrenergic blockade.[21–23]

ACUTE HYPERTENSIVE CRISES

Acute hypertensive crises may occur before or during an operation, and they should be treated intravenously with sodium nitroprusside, phentolamine, or nicardipine. Sodium nitroprusside is an ideal vasodilator for intraoperative management of hypertensive episodes because of its rapid onset of action and short duration of effect. It is administered as an intravenous infusion at 0.5 μg/kg to 5.0 μg/kg per minute; the maximal dose should not exceed 800 μg per minute. Phentolamine is available in lyophilized form in 5 mg vials; the initial infused dose should be 1 mg, followed by repeat 5 mg boluses or a continuous infusion. Nicardipine can be started at an infusion rate of 2.5 mg per hour and titrated for blood pressure control (maximum dose is 15 mg per hour).

ANESTHESIA AND SURGERY

Surgical resection of a catecholamine-secreting tumor is a high-risk surgical procedure, and an experienced surgeon/anesthesiologist team is required. The last oral doses of α- and β-adrenergic blockers can be administered orally early in the morning on the day of the operation. Fentanyl, ketamine, and morphine should be avoided because they can potentially stimulate catecholamine release from a pheochromocytoma.[24] Also, parasympathetic nervous system blockade with atropine should be avoided because of the associated tachycardia. Anesthesia may be induced with intravenous injection of propofol, etomidate, or barbiturates in combination with synthetic opioids.[24] Most anesthetic gases can be used, but halothane and desflurane should be avoided.[24] Cardiovascular and hemodynamic variables must be monitored closely. In our experience over the past 10 years, nitroprusside has been used only rarely, replaced by intermittent small doses of esmolol (Brevibloc). Whereas dopamine previously was the preferred agent to treat hypotension, short bolus administration of ephedrine or phenylephrine have more commonly been used. Continuous measurement of intra-arterial pressure

and heart rhythm is required. If the patient has congestive heart failure or decreased cardiac reserve, monitoring of pulmonary capillary wedge pressure is indicated. Surgical survival rates are 98 to 100%. Four perioperative deaths occurred in a series of 165 patients operated on in Paris, France, from 1975 to 1997.[25] No perioperative deaths occurred in our series of 131 patients, and adverse perioperative complications occurred in 4%, equally divided between problems directly related to the adrenalectomy and those unrelated specifically to the procedure. The preoperative and perioperative treatment approach outlined here is the same for adults and children.[26,27]

In the past, an anterior midline abdominal surgical approach was generally used for resecting adrenal pheochromocytoma. However, the laparoscopic approach to the adrenal gland is currently the procedure of choice for patients with solitary intra-adrenal pheochromocytomas less than 8 to 10 cm in diameter.[28] Our average length of hospitalization for patients who underwent laparoscopic adrenalectomy for pheochromocytoma has been 2.8 days, comparable to 2 reported series of 39 and 80 patients with mean hospitalization times of 1.7[29] and 2.3[30] days, respectively. If the pheochromocytoma is in the adrenal gland, the entire gland should be removed.

Laparoscopic adrenalectomy for pheochromocytoma should be converted to open adrenalectomy for difficult dissection, invasion, adhesions, or surgeon inexperience.[31] If the tumor is malignant, as much of the tumor should be removed as possible. If a bilateral adrenalectomy is planned preoperatively, the patient should receive glucocorticoid stress coverage while awaiting transfer to the operating room. Glucocorticoid coverage should be initiated in the operating room if unexpected bilateral adrenalectomy is necessary. Cortical-sparing bilateral adrenalectomies have been used to treat patients with MEN-2 and VHL disease.[32–34] However, with MEN-2 patients, there is a concern of leaving residual adrenal medullary tissue behind, and thus increase the risk of recurrent pheochromocytoma. An anterior midline abdominal surgical approach is indicated for abdominal paragangliomas. Paragangliomas of the neck, chest, and urinary bladder require specialized approaches. "Unresectable" cardiac pheochromocytomas may require cardiac transplantation.[35]

Hypotension may occur after surgical resection of the pheochromocytoma, and it should be treated with fluids and small, intermittent doses of intravenous pressor agents. Postoperative hypotension is less frequent in patients who have had adequate preoperative α-adrenergic blockade. If both adrenal glands were manipulated during surgery, adrenocortical insufficiency should be considered as a potential cause of postoperative hypotension. Because hypoglycemia can occur in the immediate postoperative period, blood glucose levels should be monitored, and fluid given intravenously should contain 5% dextrose.

Blood pressure is usually normal by the time of hospital discharge. Some patients remain hypertensive for up to 4 to 8 weeks postoperatively. Long-standing, persistent hypertension does occur and may be related to inadvertent ligation of a polar renal artery, resetting of baroreceptors, hemodynamic changes, structural changes of the blood vessels, altered sensitivity of the vessels to pressor substances, functional or structural renal changes, or coincident primary hypertension.

LONG-TERM POSTOPERATIVE FOLLOW-UP

Approximately 1 to 2 weeks after surgery, catecholamines and metanephrines should be measured by collecting a 24-hour urine. If the levels are normal, the resection of the pheochromocytoma should be considered complete. The survival rate after removal of a benign pheochromocytoma is nearly that of age- and sex-matched normal controls. Increased levels of catecholamines and metanephrines detected postoperatively are consistent with residual tumor, either a second primary lesion or occult metastases. If bilateral adrenalectomy was performed, life-long glucocorticoid and mineralocorticoid replacement therapy is prescribed. Twenty-four hour urinary excretion of catecholamines and fractionated metanephrines or fractionated plasma metanephrines should be checked annually for life. Annual biochemical testing assesses for metastatic disease, tumor recurrence in the adrenal bed, or delayed appearance of multiple primary tumors. Recurrence rates are highest for patients with familial disease, right-sided adrenal pheochromocytoma, or a paraganglioma.[36] Only 2 patients have suffered recurrence in our recent experience, 1 with malignancy and the other with contralateral pheochromocytoma in a MEN-2B patient. Follow-up CT or MRI is not needed unless the metanephrine and/or catecholamine levels become elevated or the original tumor was associated with minimal catecholamine excess.

Consider genetic testing for patients with 1 or more of the following: a family history of pheochromocytoma, paraganglioma, or any sign that suggests a genetic cause (eg, retinal angiomas, axillary freckling, café au lait spots, cerebellar tumor, MTC, hyperparathyroidism).[37] In addition, all first-degree relatives of a patient with pheochromocytoma or paraganglioma should have biochemical testing (eg, 24-hr urine for fractionated metanephrines and catecholamines). If mutation testing in a patient is positive, first-degree relatives should have stepwise (eg, parents first) germline screening.

Malignant Pheochromocytoma

Distinguishing between benign and malignant catecholamine-secreting tumors is difficult on the basis of clinical, biochemical, or histopathologic characteristics. In the future, analyses of circulating biomarkers may be able to distinguish malignant from benign pheochromocytomas.[38] Malignancy is rare in patients with an adrenal familial syndrome, but is common in those with familial paraganglioma caused by mutations in *SDHB*. Patients with *SDHB* mutations are more likely to develop malignant disease and nonparaganglioma neoplasms (eg, renal cell carcinoma).[8,9] Although the 5-year survival rate for patients with malignant pheochromocytoma is less than 50%, the prognosis is variable: approximately 50% of patients have an indolent form of the disease, with a life expectancy of more than 20 years, and the other 50% of patients have rapidly progressive disease, with death occurring within 1 to 3 years. Metastatic sites include local tissue invasion, liver, bone, lung, and lymph nodes. Metastatic lesions should be resected if possible. Skeletal metastatic lesions that are painful or threaten structural function can be treated with external radiotherapy or cyroablation therapy. External radiotherapy can also be used to treat unresectable soft tissue lesions.

Local tumor irradiation with therapeutic doses of ^{131}I-MIBG has produced partial and temporary responses in approximately one-third of patients.[39–42] Thrombotic therapy for large unresectable liver metastases and radiofrequency ablation for small liver metastases are options to be considered. In selected cases, long-acting octreotide has been beneficial. If the tumor is considered aggressive and the patient's quality of life is affected, combination chemotherapy may be considered. In a nonrandomized, single-arm trial, the efficacy of chemotherapy (CVD protocol: cyclophosphamide 750 mg/m^2 body surface area on day 1; vincristine, 1.4 mg/m^2 on day 1; and dacarbazine 600 mg/m^2 on days 1 and 2 and every 21 days) was studied in 14 patients with malignant pheochromocytoma.[43] The combination CVD protocol produced a complete and partial response rate of 57% (median duration, 21 months; range, 7 to > 34). Complete and partial biochemical responses were seen in 79% of patients (median duration, > 22 months; range, 6 to > 35). All responding patients had objective improvement in performance status and blood pressure. Management of a patient who has malignant pheochromocytoma can be frustrating because curative options are limited. Clearly, innovative prospective protocols are needed to seek new treatment options for this neoplasm.[44]

References

1. Stenstrom G, Svardsudd K. Phaechromocytoma in Sweden, 1958–81. An analysis of the National Cancer Registry Data. Acta Med Scand 1986;220:225–32.

2. Young WF Jr, Maddox DE. Spells: in search of a cause. Mayo Clin Proc 1995;70:757–65.

3. Kinney MA, Warner ME, vanHeerden JA, et al. Perianesthetic risks and outcomes of pheochromocytoma and paraganglioma resection. Anesth Analg 2000;91:1118–23.

4. Erickson D, Kudva YC, Ebersold MJ, et al. Benign paragangliomas: clinical presentation and treatment outcomes in 236 patients. J Clin Endocrinol Metab 2001;86:5210–6.

5. Neumann HP, Bausch B, McWhinney SR, et al. Germ-line mutations in nonsyndromeic pheochromocytoma. N Engl J Med 2002;346:1459–66.

6. Carney JA. Gastric stromal sarcoma, pulmonary chondroma, and extra-adrenal paraganglioma (Carney Triad): natural history, adrenocortical component, and possible familial occurrence. Mayo Clin Proc 1999;74:543–52.

7. Baldisserotto M, Peletti AB, Angelo de Araujo M, et al. Beckwith-Wiedemann syndrome and bilateral adrenal pheochromocytoma: sonography and MRI findings. Pediatr Radiol 2005;35:1132–4.

8. Neumann HP, Pawlu C, Peczkowska M, et al. Distinct clinical features of paraganglioma syndromes associated with SDHB and SDHD gene mutations. JAMA 2004;292:943–51.

9. Gimenez-Roqueplo AP, Favier J, Rustin P, et al. Mutations in SDHB gene are associated with extra-adrenal and/or malignant phaeochromocytomas. Cancer Res 2003;63:5615–21.

10. Kudva YC, Sawka AM, Young WF Jr. Clinical review 164: the laboratory diagnosis of adrenal pheochromocytoma: the Mayo Clinic experience. J Clin Endocrinol Metab 2003;88:4533–9.

11. Lenders JW, Pacak K, Walther MM, et al. Biochemical diagnosis of pheochromocytoma: which test is best? JAMA 2002;287:1427–34.

12. Sawka AM, Prebtani AP, Thabane L, et al. A systematic review of the literature examining the diagnostic efficacy of measurement of fractionated plasma free metanephrines in the biochemical diagnosis of pheochromocytoma. BMC Endorc Disord 2004;4:2.

13. Jackson JA, Kleerekoper M, Mendlovic D. Endocrine grand rounds: a 51-year-old man with accelerated hypertension, hypercalcemia, and right adrenal and paratracheal masses. Endocrinologist 1993;3:5.

14. van Gils APG, Falke THM, van Erkel AR, et al. MR imaging and MIBG scintigraphy of pheochromocytomas and extraadrenal functioning paragangliomas. Radiographics 1991;11:37–57.

15. Shapiro B, Gross MD, Fig L, et al. Localization of functioning sympathoadrenal lesions. In: Biglieri EG, Melby JC, editors. Endocrine hypertension. New York: Raven Press; 1990. p. 235–55.

16. Jalil ND, Pattou FN, Combemale F, et al. Effectiveness and limits of preoperative imaging studies for the localisation of pheochromocytomas and paragangliomas: a review of 282 cases. French Association of Surgery (AFC), and the French Association of Endocrine Surgeons (AFCE). Eur J Surg 1998;164:23–8.

17. Miskulin J, Shulkin BL, Doherty GM, et al. Is preoperative iodine 123 meta-iodobenzylguanidine scintigraphy routinely necessary before initial adrenalectomy for pheochromocytoma? Surgery 2003;134:918–22.

18. Taieb D, Sebag F, Hubbard JG, et al. Does iodine-131 meta-iodobenzylguanidine (MIBG) scintigraphy have an impact on the management of sporadic and familial phaeochromocytoma? Clin Endocrinol (Oxf) 2004;61:102–8.

19. Pacak K, Eisenhofer G, Carrasquillo JA, et al. Diagnostic localization of pheochromocytoma: the coming of age of positron emission tomography. Ann N Y Acad Sci 2002;970:170–6.

20. Young WF Jr. Pheochromocytoma: 1926–1993. Trends Endocrinol Metab 1993;4:122–7.

21. Bravo EL. Pheochromocytoma: an approach to antihypertensive management. Ann N Y Acad Sci 2002;970:1–10.

22. Combemale F, Carnaille B, Tavernier B, et al. Exclusive use of calcium channel blockers and cardioselective beta-blockers in the pre- and per-operative management of pheochromocytomas. 70 cases. Ann Chir 1998;52:341–45.

23. Lebuffe G, Dosseh ED, Tek G, et al. The effect of calcium channel blockers on outcome following the surgical treatment of phaeochromocytomas and paragangliomas. Anaesthesia 2005;60:439–44.

24. Memtsoudis SG, Swamidoss C, Psoma M. Anesthesia for adrenal surgery. In: Linos D, van Heerden JA, editors. Adrenal glands: diagnostic aspects and surgical therapy. New York: Springer-Verlag; 2005. p. 287–97.

25. Plouin PF, Duclos JM, Soppelsa F, et al. Factors associated with perioperative morbidity and mortality in patients with pheochromocytoma: analysis of 165 operations at a single center. J Clin Endocrinol Metab 2001;86:1480–6.

26. Hack HA. The perioperative management of children with phaeochromocytoma. Paediatr Anaesth 2000;10:463–76.

27. Reddy VS, O'Neill JA Jr, Holcomb GW III, et al. Twenty-five-year surgical experience with pheochromocytoma in children. Am Surg 2000;66:1085–91.

28. Grant C. Pheochromocytoma. In: Clark OH, Duh Q-Y, Kebebew E, editors. Textbook of endocrine surgery, 2nd ed. Philadelphia: W. B. Saunders; 2005. p. 621–33.

29. Cheah WK, Clark OH, Horn JK, et al. Laparoscopic adrenalectomy for pheochromocytoma. World J Surg 2002; 26:1048–51.

30. Kercher KW, Novitsky YW, Park A, et al. Laparoscopic curative resection of pheochromocytomas. Ann Surg 2005; 241:919–26.

31. Shen WT, Sturgeon C, Clark OH, et al. Should pheochromocytoma size influence surgical approach? A comparison of 90 malignant and 60 benign pheochromocytomas. Surgery 2004;136:1129–37.

32. Lee JE, Curley SA, Gagel RF, et al. Cortical-sparing adrenalectomy for patients with bilateral pheochromocytoma. Surgery 1996;120:1064–71.

33. Walther MM, Keiser HR, Choyke PL, et al. Management of hereditary pheochromocytoma in von Hippel-Lindau kindreds with partial adrenalectomy. J Urol 1999;161: 395–8.

34. Diner EK, Franks ME, Behari A, et al. Partial adrenalectomy: the National Cancer Institute experience. Urology 2005;66:19–23.

35. Jeevanandam V, Oz MC, Shapiro B, et al. Surgical management of cardiac pheochromocytoma. Resection versus transplantation. Ann Surg 1995;221:415–9.

36. Amar L, Servais A, Gimeniz-Roqueplo AP, et al. Year of diagnosis, features at presentation, and risk of recurrence in patients with pheochromocytoma or secreting paraganglioma. J Clin Endocrinol Metab 2005;90:2110–6.

37. Pawlu C, Bausch B, Reisch N, Neumann HP. Genetic testing for pheochromocytoma-associated syndromes. Ann Endocrinol (Paris) 2005;66:178–85.

38. Brouwers FM, Petricoin EF III, Ksinantova L, et al. Low molecular weight proteomic information distinguishes metastatic from benign pheochromocytoma. Endocr Relat Cancer 2005;12:263–72.

39. Sisson JC. Radiopharmaceutical treatment of pheochromocytomas. Ann N Y Acad Sci 2002;970:54–60.

40. Safford SD, Coleman RE, Gockerman JP, et al. Iodine-131 metaiodobenzylguanidine is an effective treatment for malignant pheochromocytoma and paraganglioma. Surgery 2003;134:956–62.

41. Rose B, Matthay KK, Price D, et al. High-dose 131I-metaiodobenzylguanidine therapy for 12 patients with malignant pheochromocytoma. Cancer 2003;98:239–48.

42. Loh KC, Fitzgerald PA, Matthay KK, et al. The treatment of malignant pheochromocytoma with iodine-131 metaiodobenzylguanidine (131I-MIBG): a comprehensive review of 116 reported patients. J Endocrinol Invest 1997;20:648–58.

43. Averbuch SD, Steakley CS, Young RC, et al. Malignant pheochromocytoma: effective treatment with a combination of cyclophosphamide, vincristine, and dacarbazine. Ann Intern Med 1988;109:267–73.

44. Eisenhofer G, Bornstein SR, Brouwers FM, et al. Malignant pheochromocytoma: current status and initiatives for future progress. Endocr Relat Cancer 2004;11:423–36.

CHAPTER 45

SURGICAL TREATMENT AND MANAGEMENT OF GASTRINOMA

JONATHAN C. HUNDLEY, MD

PAUL G. GAUGER, MD

Introduction

Gastrinomas are neuroendocrine tumors that produce gastrin, resulting in hypergastrinemia. This in turn is manifested by complications of excessive gastric acid secretion, such as peptic ulcer disease or diarrhea. Gastrinomas are commonly located in the region of the duodenum or pancreas. The diagnosis of gastrinoma is often termed the Zollinger-Ellison syndrome (ZES), which was first described in 1955, even before the identification of (or the ability to measure) the hormone gastrin, which mediates the disease.[1]

Gastrinomas are the most common type of functional, potentially malignant pancreatic endocrine tumor. They are 0.5 to 1.5 times as frequent as nonfunctioning pancreatic endocrine tumors, 2 to 4 times more common than VIPomas, and 8 to 15 times more common than glucagonomas or somatostatinomas.[2] Gastrinomas are still rare, however, with an incidence of only 1 to 3 per million people per year.[3]

Gastrinomas occur in patients in either sporadic or familial patterns. Sporadic gastrinomas are not inherited. Familial gastrinomas develop in patients who have multiple endocrine neoplasia type 1 (MEN-1), also known as Wermer's syndrome. Sporadic and familial gastrinoma are two separate entities that require somewhat different surgical and management strategies. Much of the following information refers to management of sporadic gastrinoma, although information referable to MEN-1 patients is indicated separately.

Pathology and Pathogenesis

On histology, gastrinomas contain sheets of small, uniform and usually well-differentiated cells with few mitoses and fine granular eosinophilic cytoplasm (Figure 1). Gastrinomas are neuroendocrine neoplasms and fall under the category of amine precursor uptake and decarboxylation tumors (APUDomas). Gastrinomas were first described as "islet cell tumors,"[1] but this is a misnomer since they do not develop from pancreatic islet cells directly. Gastrinomas probably develop from pluripotent neuroendocrine stem cells located within the duct epithelium of the exocrine pancreas and duodenum.[4,5] Distinction between benign and malignant tumors usually cannot be made by histologic examination alone. Metastasis or gross invasion of normal tissues remains the only reliable histologic criterion for the diagnosis of malignancy in these tumors. Gastrinomas metastasize primarily to regional lymph nodes and

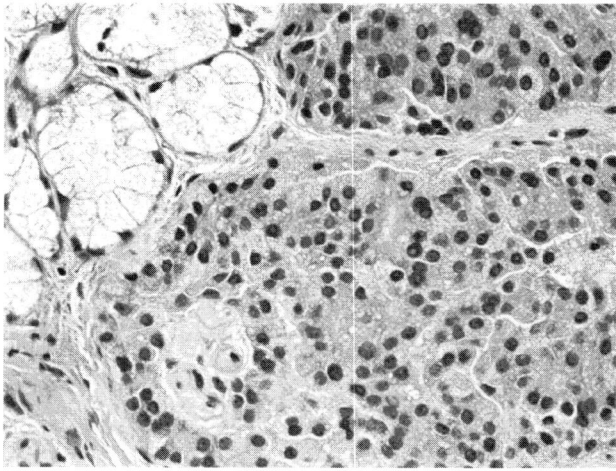

Figure 1 Typical histology of a gastrinoma demonstrates sheets of small, uniform, well-differentiated cells with few mitoses and fine granular eosinophilic cytoplasm.

the liver, although metastases to bony structures such as the pelvis, scapula, and ribs has been reported in up to 31% of patients with liver metastases.[6] In much of the literature, approximately one-third of patients have presented with liver metastases, one-third with localized disease, and one-third with an occult primary tumor.

Before the standard inclusion of duodenotomy during surgical exploration for ZES, pancreatic gastrinomas were thought to be 3 times more frequent than duodenal gastrinomas. Since the increased awareness of the role of duodenotomy, the incidence of duodenal gastrinomas has been recognized to be much higher than previously appreciated.[7] In a recent study of 212 consecutive patients with ZES, approximately 40% had pancreatic gastrinomas, 40% duodenal gastrinomas, and 20% a gastrinoma in some other location.[8] Depending on the patient series and the specific surgical strategies employed, duodenal gastrinomas may be 3 to 10 times more common than pancreatic gastrinomas.[9]

Sixty to 90% of gastrinomas occur in the "gastrinoma triangle," whose apices are the junction of the pancreatic body and neck, the junction of the second and third parts of the duodenum, and the junction of the cystic duct and common bile duct. In the duodenum, the frequency of gastrinomas decreases from proximally to distally, with over half of duodenal gastrinomas found in the first portion of the duodenum. Rarely, they are found in the first portion of the jejunum. The distribution of gastrinomas in the pancreas was previously thought to occur in the head, body, and tail in a 4:1:4 distribution, but more recent studies support a more balanced distribution in the pancreas.[10,11] Gastrinomas have been reported in many other sites including the stomach, gallbladder, biliary tree, liver, ovary, omentum, mesentery, spleen, heart, and renal capsule. Gastrinomas have been found in lymph nodes draining the pancreas and duodenum and resected for apparent cure with no accompanying primary tumor identified, raising the question of whether gastrinomas can arise in lymph nodes or whether these all represent metastases from occult primary tumors.[9,12]

In recent years, researchers have realized that duodenal gastrinomas are biologically and clinically distinct from pancreatic gastrinomas. Pancreatic gastrinomas are usually larger and more commonly associated with liver metastases. Duodenal gastrinomas are usually small (< 1 cm), may be multiple, are more likely to metastasize to lymph nodes (40–70%), and are less likely to metastasize to the liver (< 5%).[9] Duodenal gastrinomas therefore appear to have a better prognosis than pancreatic gastrinomas.

All initial symptoms in ZES are due to gastric acid hypersecretion that results directly from hypergastrinemia. Gastric acid hypersecretion directly causes peptic ulcer disease and severe GERD and indirectly causes diarrhea by damaging the small bowel mucosa, inactivating lipase, and causing the precipitation of bile acids.[13]

Symptoms, signs, and diagnosis of ZES

The most common initial symptoms of ZES are abdominal pain, diarrhea, heartburn, nausea, vomiting, and gastrointestinal bleeding. Clinical conditions that are suspicious for ZES (Table 1) include severe or complicated peptic ulcer disease (PUD), multiple ulcers, ulcers in unusual locations (eg, jejunum), and PUD associated with diarrhea. At diagnosis, the majority of patients have been previously diagnosed with chronic idiopathic PUD, although other potential misdiagnoses include GERD, chronic idiopathic diarrhea, Crohn's disease, irritable bowel syndrome, and celiac sprue.[14] If a duodenal ulcer is present, it is often clinically and endoscopically indistinguishable from typical peptic ulcer disease.

The diagnosis of gastrinoma is elusive and is usually delayed several years beyond the onset of symptoms. The diagnosis requires proving the existence of autonomous gastrin secretion that does not respond to normal physiologic mechanisms. Figure 2 provides an algorithm that will effectively aid in diagnosis or exclusion of ZES in the majority of patients using three tests: a fasting serum gastrin level, a fasting gastric acid analysis (pH and basal acid output), and a provocative secretin test.

The initial screening test is a fasting serum gastrin level. If the gastrin level is < 100 pg/mL, ZES is ruled out

Table 1 Clinical and Laboratory Conditions Suspicious for ZES

1. Duodenal ulcer with one or more of the following:
   - diarrhea
   - no *Helicobacter pylori* infection
   - refractory to medical or surgical management
   - known pancreatic tumor
   - nephrolithiasis, hypercalcemia, or other endocrinopathy (suspicion of MEN-1)
   - perforation
   - clinically significant bleeding
   - prominent gastric folds on UGI or endoscopy
   - gastric acid hypersecretion
   - gastric carcinoid tumor
   - elevated serum chromogranin level
2. GERD associated with the following:
   - diarrhea
   - severe or resistant symptoms
3. Chronic secretory diarrhea
4. Family History of nephrolithiasis, endocrinopathies, peptic ulcer disease, or MEN-1

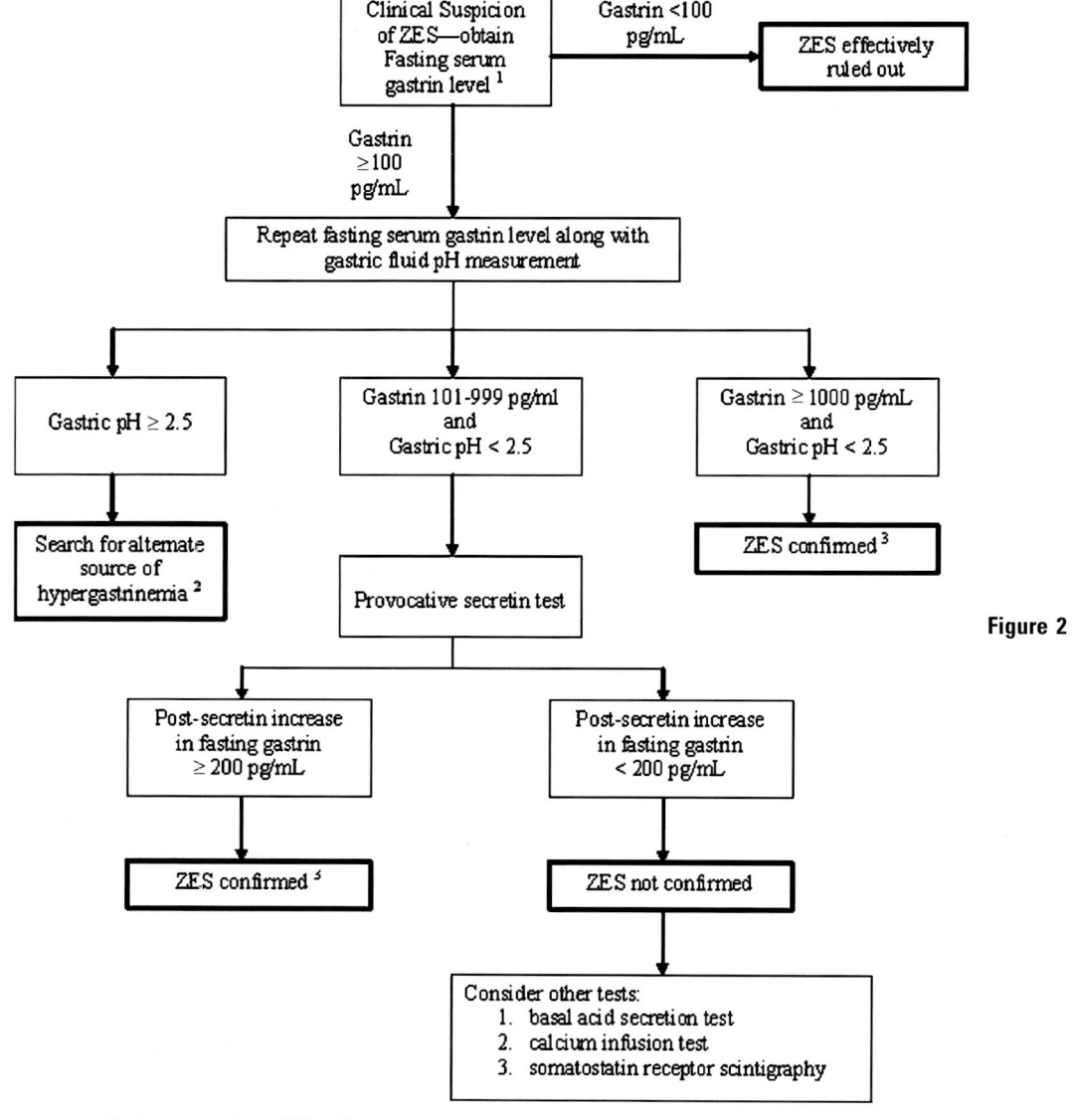

Figure 2

1. Patient must be off H+-K+ ATPase inhibitor for 5 days and off histamine H2-receptor antagonists for 30 hours.
2. See Table 2
3. If retained gastric antrum syndrome is not a possibility, no further confirmatory tests are required.

with no further work-up required. If the gastrin level is ≥ 100 pg/mL, further work-up is necessary to distinguish between ZES and other causes of hypergastrinemia (Table 2). Such testing includes fasting serum gastrin level, which is repeated along with measurement of gastric fluid pH. It should be noted that current therapy with proton pump inhibitor (PPI) medication at the time of measurement can elevate fasting gastrin levels significantly. The patient's PPI should be stopped for 5 days before remeasurement of basal gastrin levels. If symptoms make this 5-day period difficult for patients to

tolerate, H_2 blockers may be used during this time without significant interference with the gastrin measurement if they are also stopped at least a day before testing. ZES is effectively ruled out with a gastric pH ≥ 2.5. Retained gastric antrum syndrome (RGAS) occurs in patients who undergo antrectomy with a Billroth II reconstruction, in which part of the antrum is left attached to the excluded duodenal stump. RGAS is associated with a high serum gastrin level and a low gastric pH, and is therefore very difficult to distinguish from ZES. RGAS can be cured by surgical resection of the

Table 2 Causes of Hypergastrinemia

1. Associated with gastric acid hypersecretion
   - *Helicobacter pylori* infection
   - gastric outlet obstruction
   - antral G-cell hyperfunction/hyperplasia
   - chronic renal failure
   - retained gastric antrum syndrome
   - short-bowel syndrome
   - Zollinger-Ellison syndrome
2. Associated with gastric acid hyposecretion/achlorhydria
   - pernicious anemia
   - atrophic gastritis
   - H+-K+ ATPase inhibitors
   - chronic renal failure
   - *Helicobacter pylori* infection
   - post-gastric acid reducing surgery

excluded antral segment . If RGAS has been ruled out, the presence of a fasting serum gastrin level $\geq$ 1,000 pg/mL associated with a gastric pH $<$ 2.5 confirms the diagnosis of ZES—unfortunately, only one-third of patients with ZES have a gastrin level $\geq$ 1,000 pg/mL (which can make secure diagnosis in the remainder more challenging).

Two-thirds of patients with ZES have only moderate hypergastrinemia (gastrin level 100–999 pg/mL) and a gastric pH $<$ 2.5. The provocative secretin test is used to differentiate between ZES and other syndromes in this setting. Fasting serum gastrin levels are measured before and after administration of secretin (2 units/kg IV bolus). A postsecretin increase in gastrin of $\geq$ 200 pg/mL confirms the diagnosis of ZES (the only false positives are patients with achlorhydria, but these patients do not have low gastric pH). Secretin may often be difficult to obtain, and a calcium infusion test (using calcium as a secretagogue instead of secretin) may be performed. Overall, the experience with administration and interpretation of this test is less well defined than with secretin. If ZES is strongly suspected in a patient with a negative secretin test, further work-up can include a basal acid secretion test, calcium infusion test, and somatostatin receptor scintigraphy (SRS).[14,15]

After the diagnosis of ZES has been established, all patients should undergo screening for MEN-1, including a thorough family history, and then biochemical screening such as calcium and parathyroid hormone, prolactin, pancreatic peptide, and other serum or imaging tests guided by specific clinical suspicion.

Localization of Gastrinoma

Once the diagnosis of ZES is confirmed, attempts at accurate localization in preparation for surgical resection are very important. Imaging also provides the opportu-

nity to detect those patients with advanced stages of disease, such as those with established liver metastases. Functional imaging with somatostatin receptor scintigraphy (SRS) has recently replaced CT scanning and MRI as the first localization study that should be obtained.[16] Gastrinomas often express somatostatin receptors that bind [111]I octreotide and are then visualized using SPECT (single photon emission computed tomography) imaging. SRS images the entire body and detects distant metastases and primary gastrinomas in unusual intra-abdominal locations. SRS is more sensitive than all conventional imaging combined for localization of extrahepatic gastrinomas, liver metastases, and primary tumors.[16] It is also the most sensitive modality for detecting bony metastases. However, SRS misses 50% of small duodenal gastrinomas and provides no information on tumor size or exact location of the tumor.[9] Because of these limitations, functional imaging with SRS alone is inadequate and should be combined with either MRI or a CT scan for anatomic correlation in patients being evaluated for surgical resection.

Endoscopic ultrasound (EUS) has high sensitivity for pancreatic gastrinomas and allows for cytologic confirmation of tumor if a biopsy is performed. EUS has therefore been recommended by many authors for routine preoperative tumor localization and staging in ZES.[9,17,18] Conversely, EUS has low sensitivity for duodenal gastrinomas, does not provide information regarding metastases, is operator-dependent, and cytologic confirmation of tumor is usually not required in patients with confirmed ZES.

In a recent review, Norton and Jensen concluded the following about the application of localization procedures: (1) SRS and CT scan with intravenous contrast are the recommended routine initial studies in patients with biochemically diagnosed ZES; (2) routine preoperative EUS is not warranted; and (3) if SRS and CT scan are both negative, angiography with secretin stimulation and hepatic vein gastrin sampling or EUS may be helpful.[9] However, we continue to utilize EUS early in localization testing.

Medical Management of Gastric Acid Hypersecretion

The natural history of gastrinoma has been changed by the development of H$^+$-K$^+$ ATPase inhibitor drugs (proton pump inhibitors, or PPIs). Whereas in the past, patients were often affected by the end result of gastric acid hypersecretion (ie, upper gastrointestinal hemorrhage), these events are much less common in the current era. The natural history of gastrinoma is now often ultimately determined by the neoplastic aspects of the disease (the potential for the tumor to behave in a malignant fashion). PPIs have replaced histamine H2-receptor antagonists as the standard of care in the medical management of gastric acid hypersecretion in ZES. The use of PPIs such as omeprazole, pantoprazole, and lansoprazole provides for control of gastric acid hypersecretion in almost all patients with ZES. Unlike use of PPIs in simple PUD or GERD, in which efficacy of medical management is determined by cessation of symptoms, measurement of therapeutic response may be very helpful. It has been suggested that basal acid secretion of < 10 mEq/hr for the hour before the next dose of antisecretory drug is the goal (< 5 mEq/hr in patients with previous acid-reducing surgery). For the best titration of therapy, this should be determined initially and at least once a year thereafter.[19,20] Most authors recommend a starting dose of the equivalent of 60 mg of omeprazole daily, although some patients will require more than 200 mg per day (divided in 2 doses). After a maintenance dose is established, attempts should be made to reduce the dose to 20 mg once or twice a day.[19] Octreotide, a somatostatin analogue, may be helpful in patients with gastric acid hypersecretion that is not controlled with PPIs, which is exceedingly rare.

Surgical Management of Gastric Acid Hypersecretion

Prior to the advent of PPI's, total gastrectomy or vagotomy with antrectomy was frequently performed to control gastric acid hypersecretion. Acid hypersecretion can now be controlled in all patients by PPIs, making these operations necessary only in patients who are medically noncompliant. Routine parietal cell vagotomy at the time of surgical exploration for cure is a reasonable proposition owing to the following observations: (1) two-thirds of patients with ZES are not cured long term and require PPIs; (2) many patients are noncompliant with PPIs owing to the considerable expense; and (3) PPIs frequently cause achlorhydria, which may lead to vitamin B_{12} and iron malabsorption.[9]

Surgical Resection of Gastrinoma

In patients with newly diagnosed sporadic ZES who do not have distant metastatic disease, routine abdominal exploration with attempt at resection of gastrinoma is indicated. Table 3 details the important steps of an adequate operative exploration for ZES. An important component of this exploration is complete inspection and palpation of the duodenum and entire pancreas. Aside from duodenotomy and palpation, two additional intraoperative procedures can potentially help to localize gastrinomas. These include endoscopic transillumination of the duodenum, and intraoperative ultrasound (IOUS).[21,22]

Duodenotomy has been shown to increase the long-term cure rate.[23] We perform routine duodenotomy during all gastrinoma explorations in which an obvious pancreatic gastrinoma (ie, not just a positive peripancreatic lymph node) is not found. An anterior longitudinal duodenotomy approximately 6 cm in length in

Table 3 Abdominal Gastrinoma Exploration

1. Initial thorough examination of the abdomen including the peritoneum, liver, bowel, ovaries, and mesenteries
   - bilateral subcostal incision for most patients
   - midline incision for thin patients with a narrow subcostal angle
2. Mobilize the splenic and hepatic flexures of the colon
3. Open the lesser sac
   - divide the gastrocolic ligament close to the transverse colon to expose the body and tail of the pancreas
     - alternately, the omentum can be retracted superiorly and detached from the transverse colon, leaving it attached to the stomach
   - perform a Kocher maneuver to expose the body and neck of the pancreas as well as the posterior aspect of the duodenum
   - division of the hepatoduodenal and hepatogastric ligaments may be necessary
4. Mobilize the pancreas
   - incise the peritoneum along the inferior border of the pancreas until the pancreas is elevated out of the retroperitoneum
   - incision of the lateral peritoneal attachments of the spleen or division of the gastrolienal ligament may be necessary
   - bimanual palpation and intraoperative ultrasonography (IOUS) of the pancreas
5. Perform a lateral duodenotomy for palpation of duodenal mucosa
6. Multiple lymph node biopsies
   - paraduodenal
   - pancreatic capsule "nodule"
   - transverse mesocolon
7. Optional intraoperative maneuvers
   - endoscopy with transillumination of the duodenum
   - consider routine parietal cell vagotomy

the second part of the duodenum allows for digital palpation of the mucosa from the antrum to the proximal jejunum if the mucosa is then everted over a fingertip on the serosal surface, inspected, and palpated meticulously. Very small tumors (< 5 mm in diameter) may be locally excised with a partial thickness of mucosa, tumor, and submucosa, after which the mucosal defect is closed in 2 layers with interrupted sutures. Larger tumors are more likely to be locally invasive and are removed by a full thickness elliptical excision of duodenal wall. With sufficient foresight, these larger tumors can be palpated externally and incorporated into the original duodenotomy if possible. The duodenotomy is then closed using a full-thickness running absorbable suture and a second layer of interrupted silk sutures.[21,24]

Most gastrinomas in the pancreatic head are amenable to enucleation. Distal pancreatectomy, often with splenectomy, is indicated in patients with invasive, malignant pancreatic body or tail tumors and tumors abutting the pancreatic ducts or vessels. Pancreaticoduodenectomy (Whipple procedure) is warranted in patients (1) with a large pancreatic head or duodenal tumor not amenable to enucleation; (2) with multiple duodenal tumors where multiple enucleations are impractical or unsafe; (3) with multiple involved lymph nodes with a duodenal or pancreatic head tumor; or (4) if the patient is not cured after removal of a duodenal or pancreatic head gastrinoma as assessed by intraoperative secretin stimulation or other methods.[9]

A postoperative fasting serum gastrin level (before discharge) should be obtained. Others advocate for not only this test, but also a secretin-stimulated gastrin level, as both of these tests correlate significantly with a long-term cure.[25]

Metastatic Gastrinoma

Approximately ≤ 25% of patients with liver metastases have localized disease that is amenable to surgical resection. Norton and colleagues reported a 5-year survival of 85% and a 5-year cure rate of 29% in 17 patients with localized gastrinoma within the liver who underwent hepatic resection.[26] This study and others support aggressive resection of hepatic gastrinoma when localized disease can be completely removed. There may also be an evolving role for techniques such as radio-frequency ablation in controlling hepatic metastases not amenable to resection.

Patients with widely metastatic disease require lifelong medical management. The role of debulking operations is controversial. In general and because effective medications are available to control the effects of gastrin hypersecretion, patients should not be subjected to an operation unless the tumor can be completely resected for potential cure. Palliative surgical debulking may be performed in those rare patients refractory to medical management. It is important that radiographically diffuse liver lesions that suggest metastatic disease that would preclude curative resection be confirmed histologically with a CT or ultrasound-guided biopsy to further inform the decision making.

Long-acting octreotide may help control hormone secretion and has been shown to slow tumor growth in 50% of patients with metastatic gastrinoma.[27,28] Interferon-alpha has shown some efficacy in slowing tumor growth in a minority of patients, but no decrease in the overall tumor burden has been achieved.[29] Combining octreotide and interferon-alpha in patients refractory to either agent alone may be beneficial.[30,31] Patients refractory to octreotide and interferon-alpha are candidates for hepatic arterial embolization, radiofrequency ablation, or cryosurgery. Streptozotocin-based chemotherapy can be used when significant extrahepatic disease is present.[32]

Prognosis

Gastrinomas demonstrate two general growth patterns: an aggressive variant in 25% of ZES patients and a nonaggressive variant in the remaining 75%.[8,9,33] The aggressive form is more common in women and those without MEN-1. Typically seen are higher serum gastrin levels, large pancreatic tumors, and more frequent liver metastases, all of which contribute to a 10-year survival rate of 30% compared with 96% in patients with the nonaggressive tumor variant.[9,33]

Yu and colleagues reported a series of 212 consecutive patients with ZES (143 of whom underwent laparotomy) followed over nearly 20 years at the NIH with important long-term survival data and analysis.[8] The 10-year survival probabilities for patients who never developed liver metastases, developed liver metastases during observation, or had liver metastases present at the time of initial evaluation after were 96%, 85%, and 26%, respectively.[8] This underscores the main conclusion of many long-term ZES analyses: The single most important prognostic factor is the presence or absence of liver metastases.[8,9,33] More specifically, the most important factor is the presence of unresectable hepatic metastases. Norton and colleagues reported an 85% 5-year survival rate and a 29% 5-year cure rate in 17 patients who underwent resection for localized hepatic gastrinoma.[26] This survival rate is less than that seen in extrahepatic gastrinoma (95%) but far better than that seen in unresectable liver metastases (30%).

Bony metastases and ectopic ACTH production by the gastrinoma are poor prognostic signs—even in patients with already established liver metastases.[8] Other poor prognostic factors, such as primary pancreatic tumor size > 2 cm, local invasion, and poor tumor differentiation, likely impact survival mainly by predicting which tumors will metastasize to the liver.

Norton and colleagues analyzed data from 151 consecutive patients with ZES who underwent 180 exploratory operations.[15] Gastrinomas were found in 93% of patients. The immediate postoperative biochemical cure rate in sporadic gastrinoma was 51%, and was 49% at 5 years.[15] The immediate postoperative biochemical cure rate in MEN-1 gastrinoma was 16%, and was only 6% at 5 years.[15]

MEN-1 and Gastrinoma

MEN-1 is an autosomal dominant inherited syndrome characterized by multiglandular hyperparathyroidism, pancreatic and duodenal neuroendocrine tumors (such as gastrinomas), and anterior pituitary adenomas. Secondary manifestations include adrenal tumors, thyroid tumors, and bronchial and thymic carcinoid tumors. Nonfunctional pancreatic endocrine tumors are the most common tumors overall. Gastrinomas are the most common functional gastrointestinal neuroendocrine tumors, present in approximately half of patients with the syndrome. MEN-1 is found in 10 to 38% of all patients with ZES.[34] Compared with sporadic ZES, gastrinoma in MEN-1 patients is characterized by less frequent diarrhea; otherwise, ZES-related signs/symptoms are similar.[2]

Before 1990, it was not fully appreciated that the majority of gastrinomas in patients with MEN-1 and ZES were located in the duodenum. Most of these patients (60–100%) have multiple small submucosal duodenal gastrinomas and, in addition, usually possess pancreatic microadenomas or larger tumors detected on conventional imaging studies or SRS.[2,9] In many, if not most, of these patients, these larger pancreatic tumors are not gastrinomas.[2] EUS may be helpful in identifying the exact location of the pancreatic tumors in these patients as well as metastatic lymph nodes. Therefore, EUS should be considered routinely in preoperative evaluation of patients with MEN-1 and ZES despite the fact that the test is of little value in imaging the duodenal tumors.[9]

Compared with patients with sporadic ZES, patients with MEN-1 and ZES are more likely to have the nonaggressive form of ZES.[2] They are therefore less likely to present with liver metastases and have a significantly better long-term survival than patients without MEN-1. Gastrinomas in MEN-1 are invariably multiple and small, making complete resection of all gastrinoma tumors challenging.[30] Because of the high incidence of multiple, small duodenal gastrinomas, the surgical cure rate in these patients is very low (0–10%) without pancreaticoduode-

nectomy.[9,15] However, some centers have reported significantly higher cure rates.[35] Because of the excellent long-term survival and low surgical cure rate, it is difficult to argue for any type of aggressive surgical resection in the majority of patients with MEN-1 and ZES, although this remains controversial since most patients so treated are realizing good long-term prognoses.[2,9]

Many experts who consider surgical exploration in patients with MEN-1 and ZES agree that surgical exploration in patients with MEN-1 and ZES should be performed routinely only in patients with tumors that are ≥ 2 cm, since patients with tumors < 2 cm have an excellent long-term prognosis.[9] However, we emply a strategy of early imaging and surgery in these patients.[35,36] Although duodenotomy is included to address ZES when present, the overall operative strategy in MEN-1 patients is often predicated on management of the imaged pancreatic endocrine tumors in an attempt to prevent lymph node and liver metastases related to these tumors (although this could potentially occur related to the gastrinoma as well). Parathyroidectomy in MEN-1 patients with hyperparathyroidism should precede operative exploration for gastrinoma because gastric acid hypersecretion often improves when parathyroidectomy achieves eucalcemia.

Summary

Gastrinoma and its resultant syndrome affect a diverse group of patients who may develop the condition on a sporadic or familial (MEN-1) basis. Although there are some differences in the course of disease among these patients, some common management principles are shared. Diagnosis often depends on basal and stimulated gastrin levels and gastric acid analysis. Preoperative localization often utilizes somatostatin receptor scintigraphy, cross-sectional imaging, and endoscopic ultrasound. Symptoms may be well controlled with proton pump inhibitor medicines. Especially with sporadic patients, the malignant potential of the disease is difficult to predict. Operative treatment often involves enucleation of pancreatic tumors, resection of duodenal tumors via duodenotomy, and resection of regional lymph nodes. Long-term survival is often determined by the development of liver metastases. When possible, limited metastatic disease should be addressed surgically in order to mitigate against this influence.

References

1. Zollinger RM, Ellison EH. Primary peptic ulcerations of the jejunum associated with islet cell tumors of the pancreas. Ann Surg 1955;142:709–23.

2. Jensen RT. Management of the Zollinger-Ellison syndrome in patients with multiple endocrine neoplasia type 1. J Intern Med 1998;243:477–88.

3. Meko JB, Norton JA. Management of patients with Zollinger-Ellison syndrome. Annu Rev Med 1995;46:395–411.

4. Kloppel G, Heitz PU. Pancreatic endocrine tumors. Pathol Res Pract 1988;183:155–68.

5. Andrew A, Kramer B, Rawdon BB. Gut and pancreatic amine precursor uptake and decarboxylation cells are not neural crest derivatives. Gastroenterology 1983;84:429–31.

6. Gibril F, Schumann M, Pace A, Jensen RT. Multiple endocrine neoplasia type 1 and Zollinger-Ellison syndrome: a prospective study of 107 cases and comparison with 1009 cases from the literature. Medicine (Baltimore) 2004;83:43–83.

7. Sugg SL, Norton JA, Fraker DL, et al. A prospective study of intraoperative methods to diagnose and resect duodenal gastrinomas. Ann Surg 1993;218:138–44.

8. Yu F, Venzon DJ, Serrano J, et al. Prospective study of the clinical course, prognostic factors, causes of death, and survival in patients with long-standing Zollinger-Ellison syndrome. J Clin Oncol 1999;17:615–30.

9. Norton JA, Jensen RT. Resolved and unresolved controversies in the surgical management of patients Zollinger-Ellison syndrome. Ann Surg 2004;240:757–73.

10. Zollinger RM, Ellison EC, Fabri PJ, et al. Primary peptic ulcerations of the jejunum associated with islet cell tumors. Twenty-five year appraisal. Ann Surg 1980;192:422–30.

11. Soga J, Yakuwa Y. The gastrinoma/Zollinger-Ellison syndrome: statistical evaluation of a Japanese series of 359 cases. J Hepatol Bil Pancreatic Surg 1998;5:77–85.

12. Perrier ND, Batts KP, Thompson GB, et al. An immunohistochemical survey for neuroendocrine cells in regional pancreatic lymph nodes: a plausible explanation for primary nodal gastrinomas? Surgery 1995;118:957–65.

13. Jensen RT, Gardner JD, Raufman JP, et al. Zollinger-Ellison syndrome: current concepts and management. Ann Intern Med 1983;98:59–75.

14. Roy PK, Venzon DJ, Feigenbaum KM, et al. Gastric secretion in Zollinger-Ellison syndrome. Correlation with clinical expression, tumor extent and role in diagnosis—a prospective NIH study of 235 patients and a review of 984 cases in the literature. Medicine (Baltimore) 2001;80:189–222.

15. Norton JA, Fraker DL, Alexander HR, et al. Surgery to cure the Zollinger-Ellison syndrome. N Engl J Med 1999;341:635–44.

16. Gibril F, Reynolds JC, Doppman JL, et al. Somatostatin receptor scintigraphy: its sensitivity compared with that of other imaging methods in detecting primary and metastatic gastrinomas. A prospective study. Ann Intern Med 1996;125:26–34.

17. Proye C, Malvaux P, Pattou F, et al. Noninvasive imaging of insulinomas and gastrinomas with endoscopic ultrasonography and somatostatin receptor scintigraphy. Surgery 1998;124:1134–43.

18. Thompson NW, Czako PF, Fritts LL, et al. Role of endoscopic ultrasonography in the localization of insulinomas and gastrinomas. Surgery 1994;116:1131–8.

19. Termanini B, Gibril F, Stewart CA, et al. A prospective study of the effectiveness of low dose omeprazole as initial therapy in Zollinger-Ellison syndrome. Aliment Pharmacol Ther 1996;10:61–71.

20. Metz DC, Soffer E, Forsmark CE, et al. Maintenance oral pantoprazole therapy is effective for patients with Zollinger-Ellison syndrome and idiopathic hypersecretion. Am J Gastroenterol 2003;98:301–7.

21. Thompson NW, Pasieka J, Fukuuchi A. Duodenal gastrinomas, duodenotomy, and duodenal exploration in the surgical management of Zollinger-Ellison syndrome. World J Surg 1993;17:455–62.

22. Lowney J, Doherty GM. Surgery for endocrine tumors of the pancreas. In: Doherty GM, Skogseid B, editors. Surgical endocrinology. Philadelphia: Lippincott Williams & Wilkins; 2001. p. 381–92.

23. Norton JA, Alexander HR, Fraker DL, et al. Does the use of routine duodenotomy (DUODX) affect rate of cure, development of liver metastases, or survival in patients with Zollinger-Ellison syndrome? Ann Surg 2004;239:617–25.

24. Thompson NW, Vinik AI, Eckhauser FE. Microgastrinomas of the duodenum. A cause of failed operations for the Zollinger-Ellison syndrome. Ann Surg 1989;209:396–404.

25. Alexander HR, Bartlett DL, Venzon DJ, et al. Analysis of factors associated with long-term (five or more years) cure in patients undergoing operation for Zollinger-Ellison syndrome. Surgery 1998;124:1160–6.

26. Norton JA, Doherty GM, Fraker DL, et al. Surgical treatment of localized gastrinoma within the liver: a prospective study. Surgery 1998;124:1145–52.

27. Cadiot G, Vuagnat A, Doukhan I, et al. Prognostic factors in patients with Zollinger-Ellison syndrome and multiple endocrine neoplasia type 1. Groupe d'Etude des Neoplasies Endocriniennes Multiples (GENEM and groupe de Recherche et d'Etude du Syndrome de Zollinger-Ellison (GRESZE). Gastroenterology 1999;116:286–93.

28. Shojamanesh H, Gibril F, Louie A, et al. Prospective study of the antitumor efficacy of long-term octreotide treatment in patients with progressive metastatic gastinoma. Cancer 2002;94:331–43.

29. Eriksson B. Systemic therapy for neuroendocrine tumors of the pancreas. In: Doherty GM, Skogseid B, editors. Surgical endocrinology. Philadelphia: Lippincott Williams & Wilkins; 2001. p. 393–404.

30. Pipeleers-Marchal M, Somers G, Willems G, et al. Gastrinomas in the duodenums of patients with multiple endocrine neoplasia type 1 and the Zollinger-Ellison syndrome. N Engl J Med 1990;322:723–7.

31. Fjallskog ML, Sundin A, Westlin JE, et al. Treatment of malignant endocrine pancreatic tumors with a combination of alpha-interferon and somatostatin analogs. Med Oncol 2002;19:35–42.

32. Brentjens R, Saltz L. Islet cell tumors of the pancreas: the medical oncologist's perspective. Surg Clin North Am 2001;81:527–42.

33. Weber HC, Venzon DJ, Lin JT, et al. Determinants of metastatic rate and survival in patients with Zollinger-Ellison syndrome: a prospective long-term study. Gastroenterology 1995;108:1637–49.

34. Mignon M, Cadiot G. Diagnostic and therapeutic criteria in patients with Zollinger-Ellison syndrome and multiple endocrine neoplasia type 1. J Intern Med 1998;243:489–94.

35. Thompson N. Current concepts in the surgical management of multiple endocrine neoplasia type 1 pancreatic-duodenal disease. Results in the treatment of 40 patients with Zollinger-Ellison syndrome, hypoglycaemia or both. J Intern Med 1998;243:495–500.

36. Gauger PG, Thompson NW. Early surgical intervention and strategy in patients with multiple endocrine neoplasia type 1. Best Pract Res Clin Endocrinol Metab 2001;15:213–23.

CHAPTER 46

SURGICAL TREATMENT AND MANAGEMENT OF INSULINOMAS

GEOFFREY B. THOMPSON, MD

CLIVE S. GRANT, MD

DAVID R. FARLEY, MD

Historical Background

With the discovery of insulin by Banting and Best in 1922,[1] it was only 5 short years before a malignant tumor composed of insulin-secreting cells was recognized by Drs. W. J. Mayo and R. Wilder at Mayo Clinic in 1927.[2] In 1929, Graham in Toronto performed the first curative operation for benign insulinoma.[3] Dr. Alan O. Whipple, in 1935, described his classic clinical triad, which remains today the first-line criteria for diagnosing an insulinoma.[4] In 1944, the first successful total pancreatectomy was performed in the United States by Dr. James Priestley at Mayo Clinic for an occult insulinoma.[5] Since 1927, over 450 operations for endogenous hyperinsulinism have been successfully completed at Mayo Clinic and serve as the basis for this chapter on insulinoma.[6,7,8]

Classification of Hyperinsulinemic Hypoglycemia in Adults

Far and away, insulinoma comprises the most common cause of endogenous hyperinsulinism in adults. Other causes include insulin and sulfonylurea factitial hypoglycemia, the rare insulin autoimmune hypoglycemia, and noninsulinoma pancreatogenous hypoglycemia syndrome (NIPHS).[9,10]

Demographics

Insulinomas have comprised over one-half of all islet cell tumors seen at Mayo Clinic in recent decades. They are by far the most common functioning islet cell tumors, with 4 cases reported per 1,000,000-person years. Fifty-eight percent of the insulinomas occur in women, with a median age of 47 years and a range of 8 to 85 years. One hundred percent of these tumors are intrapancreatic, and these are equally distributed throughout the gland. Ninety percent are solitary, and 90% are less than 2 cm in greatest diameter. Six percent are malignant, and 5% are seen in association with the multiple endocrine neoplasia type 1 (MEN-1) syndrome. Approximately 3% of patients with sporadic insulinomas have multiple tumors.[6–10]

Clinical Presentation and Diagnosis

Classically, patients with insulinoma present with symptoms during fasting and exercise, but symptoms can also occur during the postprandial period within 1 to 5 hours after consuming a meal. This is especially true in patients with NIPHS.[10] The presenting symptoms can be autonomic in nature, a reflection of catecholamine excess in response to hypoglycemia (ie, sweating, palpitations, anxiety) or, more specifically, neuroglycopenic. It is the neuroglycopenic symptoms that are the hallmark in patients with insulinoma. Typically, symptoms arise when the serum glucose level falls below 55 mg/dL, and central nervous system (CNS) dysfunction becomes apparent at levels less than 50 mg/dL. Over 85% of our patients with insulinoma present with a combination of visual disturbances, palpitations, sweating, and profound weakness; 80% demonstrate confusion and/or abnormal behavior; 53%, amnesia or coma; and 12% present with a seizure disorder.[7,9]

Table 1 Diagnostic Criteria: 72-Hour Fast*

• Glucose	$\leq$ 45 mg/dL
• Insulin (ICMA)	$\geq$ 3 μu/mL
• C-peptide (ICMA)	$\geq$ 200 pmol/L
• Proinsulin (ICMA)	$\geq$ 5 pmol/L
• Sulfonylureas screen (1st and 2nd generation)	Negative
• β-hydroxybutyrate	< 2.7 mmol/L
• Δ glucose with 1 mg IV glucagon	$\geq$ 25 mg/dL @ 30′
• Glycated hemoglobin	< 4.1 %

*Plasma values at end of fast with neuroglycopenic symptoms present.

The confirmation of hypoglycemia requires satisfaction of Whipple's triad. This includes the demonstration of a serum glucose level $\leq$ 50 mg/dL, associated neuroglycopenic symptoms, and the relief of symptoms with the administration of glucose-containing substances. It is best to document Whipple's triad during a spontaneous "hypoglycemic" episode. Failing to do so requires the need for dynamic testing (72-hour fast).[9] It is important to remember that capillary glucose levels are not definitive, and only serum glucose levels can accurately measure *low levels* of glucose in the bloodstream. Once Whipple's triad has been documented, one needs to establish the role of the β-cell polypeptides in order to confirm the hyperinsulinemic nature of the hypoglycemia. In patients who have already satisfied Whipple's triad with neuroglycopenic symptoms and a serum glucose level $\leq$ 50 mg/dL, it is necessary only to lower serum glucose levels to 55 mg/dL (with or without symptoms) in order to obtain diagnostic β-cell polypeptide levels. The criteria for endogenous hyperinsulinemic hypoglycemia are outlined in Table 1. In the presence of neuroglycopenic symptoms with serum glucose levels less than 50 mg/dL, concomitant demonstration of insulin levels $\geq$ 3 μIU/mL by ICMA assay is essential. In addition, C-peptide levels $\geq$ 200 pmol/L by ICMA assay are confirmatory of the *endogenous* nature of the hyperinsulinism. Proinsulin levels $\geq$ 5 pmol/L by

ICMA assay are also supportive of this diagnosis. Insulin surrogates are available that can be rapidly determined during a hypoglycemic event. β-hydroxybutyrate levels $\leq$ 2.7 mmol/L, in the presence of hypoglycemia, is highly indicative of a hyperinsulinemic state owing to the antiketogenic effect of insulin on ketones. Insulin has an antiglycogenolytic effect as well; therefore, one would expect to see a rise in serum glucose after administration of glucagon. A $\geq$ 25 mg/dL rise in serum glucose during the first 30 minutes after administration of 1 mg of glucagon is again supportive of a hyperinsulinemic state.

To ensure the diagnosis of insulinoma, one should also check for (negative) insulin antibodies, primarily today to rule out autoimmune hypoglycemia. In the past, measurement of beef and pork insulin antibody levels were imperative to rule out factitial insulin-induced hypoglycemia. Today, with the widespread use of recombinant human insulin, C-peptide levels have taken over that role. One also needs to screen for sulfonylureas and meglitinides to rule out factitial drug-induced hypoglycemia. The mixed meal test is sometimes helpful in patients suspected of having NIPHS. The C-peptide suppression test is rarely indicated in the diagnostic schema.[11] With a formal 72-hour fast, one-third of our patients with proven insulinoma were able to terminate their fast in less than 12 hours, 65% in less than 24 hours, 93% in less than 48 hours, and 99% in less than 72 hours; thus, the selection of the 72-hour cutoff. Table 2 reviews the spectrum of hyperinsulinemic hypoglycemia in adults comparing and contrasting the lab values of the various conditions that have been described.[7,9,12]

Localization

With heightened awareness of NIPHS in our clinical practice, preoperative localization has become increasingly necessary. Once the diagnosis of endogenous hyperinsulinism has been confirmed, then, and only then, are localization studies obtained. The utilization of

Table 2 Hyperinsulinemic Hypoglycemia in Adults (Differential Diagnosis)

Diagnostic Interpretation	Symptoms or Signs	Glucose (mg/dL)	Insulin (μU/mL)	C-Peptide (pmol/L)	Proinsulin (pmol/L)	B-Hydroxybutyrate (mmol/L)	Glucose Response to Glucagon (mg/dL)	Sulfonylurea/ Meglitinide in Serum	Insulin Antibodies
Normal	No	40–60	< 3	< 200	< 5	> 2.7	< 25	No	Neg
Insulinoma/ NIPHS	Yes	$\leq$ 45	$\geq$ 3	$\geq$ 200	$\geq$ 5	$\leq$ 2.7	> 25	No	Neg
Insulin factitious	Yes	$\leq$ 45	> 3	< 200	< 5	$\leq$ 2.7	> 25	No	Neg/Pos
Sulfonylurea factitious	Yes	$\leq$ 45	$\geq$ 3	$\leq$ 200	$\geq$ 5	$\leq$ 2.7	$\geq$ 25	Yes	Neg
IAS*	Yes	$\leq$ 45	>> 3	>> 200	>> 5	< 2.7	> 25	No	Pos
Insulin-like factor†	Yes	$\leq$ 45	< 3	< 200	< 5	$\leq$ 2.7	$\geq$ 25	No	Neg

*insulin autoimmune hypoglycemia
†rare sarcomas (never occult)

localizing studies to make the diagnosis of insulinoma is fraught with hazard and can lead to disastrous consequences in the setting of a false-positive study.

Transabdominal ultrasonography (Figure 1) is very much observer-dependent and has a reported sensitivity of approximately 65%.[13] The advantage of this modality is that it is noninvasive and, in experienced hands, has a high positive predictive value.

With succeeding generations of spiral computed tomography (CT) scanners (Figures 2 and 3) and the use of triple-phase contrast, the sensitivity of this form of cross-sectional imaging has improved. Sensitivities in the range of 55 to 85% have been reported with a positive predictive value of 88%.[6,14]

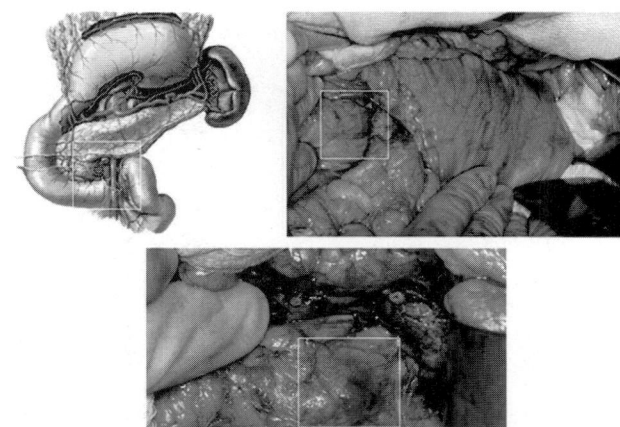

Figure 3 Corresponding gross photographs to spiral CTs in Figure 2.

Endoscopic ultrasonography (EUS)[15,16] has become increasingly popular for examining the pancreas for both large and small neoplasms (Figure 4). It has reported sensitivities from 80 to 93% with a positive predictive value of 82%. EUS has the advantage of being able to perform fine-needle aspiration if the imaging criteria are indeterminate. It appears best suited for nonpedunculated tumors and tumors confined to areas away from the pancreatic tail.

Between 1982 and 2004, 247 patients have been operated on at Mayo Clinic utilizing a combined approach of careful palpation and intraoperative ultrasonography.[6] The sensitivity of this method is 98%, with a positive predictive value of 97%. During this time period, we have had, however, 4 false-negative results and 5 false-positive results. Ultrasonography, in any form, has the ability not only to identify the tumor and its size, but

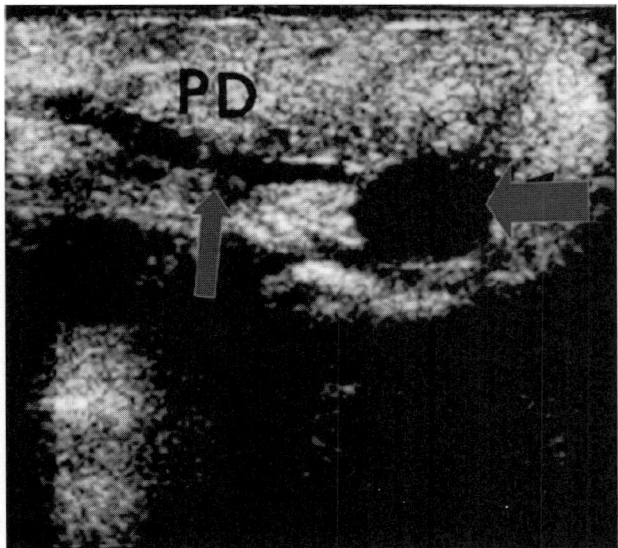

Figure 1 Transabdominal ultrasound demonstrating hypoechoic insulinoma adjacent to the pancreatic duct.

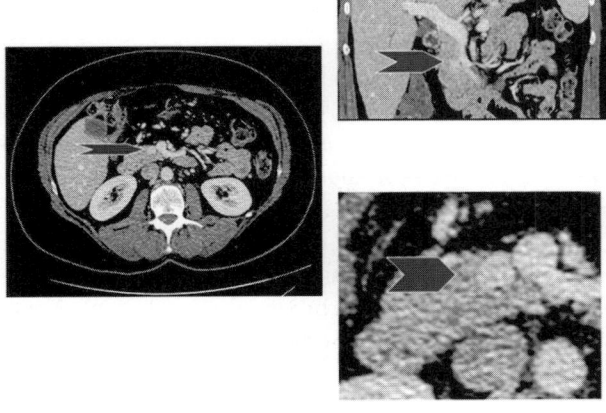

Figure 2 Late arterial, early venous phase of spiral CT demonstrating vascular blush in the pancreatic uncinate adjacent to superior mesenteric vein.

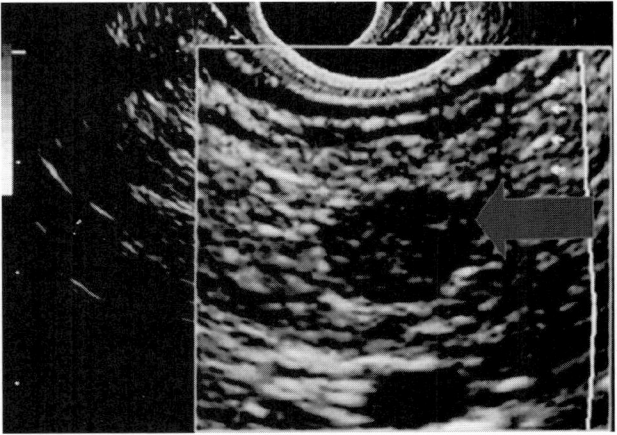

Figure 4 Endoscopic ultrasound demonstrating a hypoechoic insulinoma in the body of the pancreas.

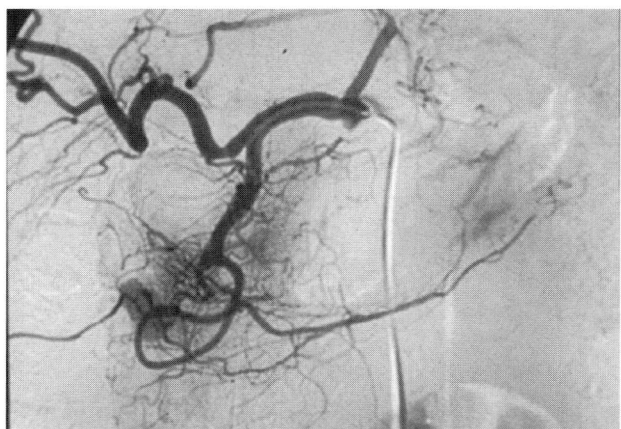

Figure 5 Selective gastroduodenal arteriogram demonstrating a vascular tumor blush in the pancreatic head.

also to delineate its location with regard to major vessels, the pancreatic duct, and the biliary tree. With the application of color flow Doppler, the characteristic vascular enhancement of an islet cell tumor can be differentiated from other processes, such as an intrapancreatic lymph node.

Introduced in the 1970s, angiography (Figure 5) was the earliest localizing study[17] for localization of insulinomas. A characteristic vascular blush can be seen in approximately 60% of arteriograms with a positive predictive value of 80%.

More recently, the selective arterial calcium stimulation test has been introduced for the regionalization of insulinomas based on the arterial distribution of the pancreas (Figure 6). This modality has reported sensitivities as high as 100% with a positive predictive value of 90%. This test has become particularly useful in patients

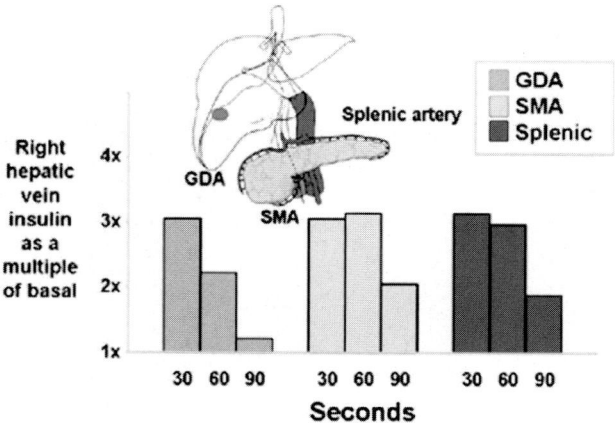

Figure 6 Results of selective arterial calcium stimulation test in patient with NIPHS. Note positive gradients in all 3 arterial distributions.

with radiographically occult insulinomas, in reoperative cases, and in patients with profound postprandial hypoglycemia when NIPHS is suspected. A catheter is placed via the femoral vein and wedged into the right hepatic vein for continuous insulin measurements. A femoral artery catheter is introduced and is utilized to selectively cannulate the splenic artery, gastroduodenal artery, superior mesenteric artery, and, in cases of suspected hepatic metastases, the hepatic arteries. Calcium is a known secretagogue for insulin in the presence of abnormal β cells. Rapid injection of calcium into the selectively cannulated arteries, followed by hepatic vein insulin measurements, can establish abnormal gradients within the pancreas. A 2-fold or greater step-up in hepatic vein insulin levels (as a multiple of basal) predicts abnormal β-cell function in that particular arterial distribution. A step-up in the splenic artery suggests an abnormality in the body or tail of the pancreas; the gastroduodenal artery, the head, and, to a lesser extent, the uncinate process of the pancreas; and the superior mesenteric artery, the uncinate, and, to a lesser degree, the head of the pancreas. A step-up in multiple arterial distributions suggests nesidioblastosis or multiple adenomas.[10,18,19]

Noninsulinoma Pancreatogenous Hypoglycemia Syndrome[10,20]

To date, we have seen over 40 cases of NIPHS at Mayo Clinic. This syndrome is characterized by profound postprandial hyperinsulinemic hypoglycemia, is more commonly seen in males, and all patients have a negative formal 72-hour fast. Conventional preoperative localizing studies are true-negatives, but all of these patients have a positive selective arterial calcium stimulation test, most often in multiple arterial distributions. Effective palliation has been achieved by gradient-guided partial pancreatectomy, and pathologic specimens have uniformly demonstrated islet hypertrophy and nesidioblastosis (Figure 7; Table 3). Because of the often diffuse nature of this process, cure rates are not as high (80%—early results) as with sporadic insulinomas, and long-term data are still pending.

More recently, we have cared for 25 patients who have developed hyperinsulinemic hypoglycemia of the NIPHS variety following gastric bypass surgery for medically complicated obesity. These patients have also benefited from gradient-guided partial pancreatectomy. It is thought that the rapid delivery of nutrients into the distal ileum following Roux-en-Y gastric bypass results in elevated glucagon-like peptide 1 levels (GLP-1), which serves as an incretin, stimulating β-cell proliferation, and

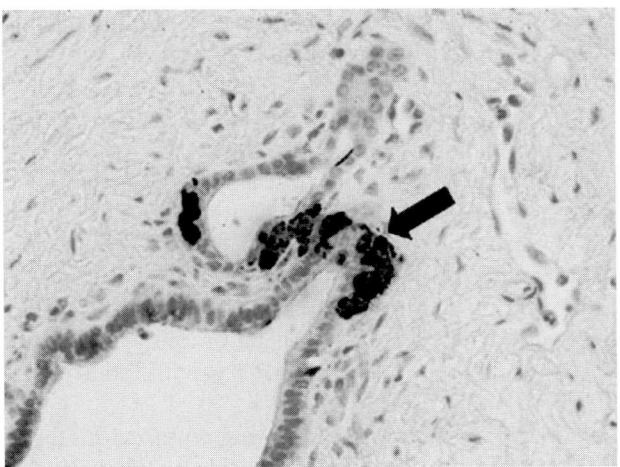

Figure 7 Immunostain for insulin demonstrating β cells budding off an exocrine duct (nesidioblastosis).

inhibiting β-cell apoptosis, thus resulting in inappropriately high insulin levels.[21]

In our last 247 patients, 95% had sporadic disease (3% with multiple tumors), and 5% had the MEN-1 syndrome. Twenty-two (9%) of the sporadic cases had NIPHS.[6]

Insulinoma in MEN-1

Endogenous hyperinsulinism represents the second most common functioning syndrome of duodenopancreatic origin in the MEN-1 syndrome, following gastrinomas. However, in MEN-1 patients under the age of 25, hyperinsulinism is the most common functional syndrome related to the presence of a pancreatic islet cell tumor. Although patients with hyperinsulinism in MEN-1 often have multiple tumors throughout the pancreas, frequently it is only 1 or 2 of these tumors that are responsible for the excess secretion of insulin. Cure rates are not as high with surgical intervention as with sporadic cases, but palliation is quite satisfactory with an extended distal pancreatectomy (with or without splenic preservation).[22] In addition, other tumors within the pancreatic head are enucleated, and if gastrin levels

Table 3 Noninsulinoma Pancreatogenous Hypoglycemia Syndrome

- Postprandial hyperinsulinemic hypoglycemia
- More common in males
- Negative 72-hour fast
- Negative perioperative radiologic localization studies
- Positive selective arterial calcium stimulation test
- Relief of symptoms by gradient-guided partial pancreatectomy
- Islet hypertrophy and nesidioblastosis

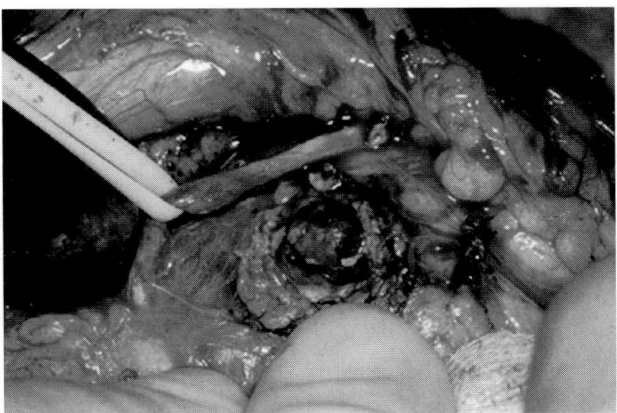

Figure 8 Enucleation of islet cell tumor in the head of the pancreas just deep to the gastroduodenal artery.

are elevated, a duodenotomy with excision of duodenal carcinoid tumors is also performed along with a regional lymphadenectomy.

Procedures Performed

Fifty-eight percent of our patients have been treated with enucleation, 35% by distal pancreatectomy with or without splenic preservation, and in only 3% of patients have Whipple procedures been required for large tumors involving the head of the pancreas or smaller tumors nestled alongside major ductal structures. Twelve percent of our operations were reoperative in nature, related to failures elsewhere.[6] To date, only a small proportion of insulinomas have been managed laparoscopically at our institution, most often for benign tumors in the pancreatic tail.[23] These tumors were amenable to limited distal pancreatectomy or enucleation with splenic preservation. Several series have examined the role of minimally invasive pancreatic surgery for insulinoma.[24,25] Certainly, in select patients, the procedure can be carried out expeditiously, resulting in less pain and quicker recovery, but to date, fistula rates appear to be higher with the laparoscopic approach.

In days gone by, it was customary to perform a blind distal pancreatectomy in patients with a suspected insulinoma but no visible or palpable tumor at the time of operation. This procedure is to be condemned, since insulinomas are equally distributed throughout the gland, and most occult insulinomas end up being found in the head and uncinate. Blind distal pancreatectomy only complicates future reoperations and increases the risk of diabetes and its inherent complications.[26] If gradient-guided information from selective arterial calcium stimulation testing is unavailable at the time of operation, the abdomen should be closed and the patient sent for calcium stimulation testing before any further surgery is performed.

Operative Technique

STANDARD OPEN TECHNIQUE

The peritoneal cavity is explored through a transverse epigastric or long midline incision. After ruling out obvious metastatic disease, primarily on the surface of the liver, peritoneum, and regional lymph nodes, the gastrocolic omentum is taken down from left to right off the transverse colon to allow entry into the lesser sac. The hepatic flexure of the colon is mobilized and the duodenum is widely kocherized out to and including the ligament of Treitz, thereby fully exposing the head, neck, and uncinate of the pancreas. The superior mesenteric vein is identified, and the vascular plane along the inferior border of the body of the pancreas is incised to mobilize the body and proximal tail of the pancreas. With bimanual and bidigital palpation, most insulinomas can be detected. Should the insulinoma not be readily apparent at this point, the lateral peritoneal attachments to the spleen are incised using electrocautery, and the spleen and remaining tail of the pancreas are mobilized into the wound. Once thorough palpation is completed, intraoperative ultrasonography is performed, and in the case of a sporadic insulinoma, over 98% of lesions can be demonstrated with these two modalities.

Most insulinomas, because of their benign and well-encapsulated nature, are amenable to enucleation after incising the overlying pancreatic capsule and exposing the underlying insulinoma. It is often helpful to perform the enucleation using a carotid endarterectomy spatula. Small vessels are coapted with bipolar cautery. Sutures and clips are best avoided if possible. Once the superficial portion of the insulinoma is free, placing a stay suture in a figure-of-eight fashion through the adenoma often facilitates completion of the enucleation by providing slight countertraction. When the insulinoma is right on the main pancreatic duct within the body and tail of the gland, a spleen-preserving distal pancreatectomy is advisable, rather than risk major ductal injury. For tumors in the head of the gland in close proximity to the bile and pancreatic ducts, a Whipple procedure, although generally frowned on and rarely indicated, can be performed safely rather than taking the chance of missing a major bile or pancreatic ductal injury.

Helpful hints for performing a pancreatojejunostomy in the setting of a soft, normal pancreas include using as few absorbable sutures as possible, thereby minimizing necrosis. The routine use of fibrin glue and intravenous octreotide to prevent pancreatic leak is of unproven benefit.

Whether enucleation or resection is undertaken, close-suction drainage is imperative and should be maintained until the patient is eating without signs of a pancreatic leak. Following enucleation procedures, we will frequently administer 75 to 150 IU of secretin intravenously to check for major ductal disruption. Intraoperative ultrasonography can also be beneficial at this point as secretin causes dilatation of the pancreatic duct, making it possible to visualize its entire course with the ultrasound probe.

Intraoperative glucose monitoring is utilized routinely at our institution. Patients are brought to the operating room off all glucose containing fluids for 2 hours prior to surgery. Frequent plasma glucose levels are determined, and patients are maintained at levels > 60 mg/dL using incremental doses of 50% dextrose administered intravenously. Following removal of the tumor, plasma glucose levels are checked at 5-minute intervals with the aid of a radial arterial line, until rebound hyperglycemia is demonstrated. Typically, after successful removal of an insulinoma, blood glucose levels rebound by 20 mg or more during the first 30 minutes. False-negative and false-positive results, however, do occur, and surgical judgment should be the final determinant (not the plasma glucose level) for assessing the completeness of resection. Patients generally develop rebound hyperglycemia within a few hours following surgery, if not sooner. Depending on the extent of the pancreatic resection, glucose levels as high as 300 mg/dL can be seen within the first 24 to 48 hours. We typically do not treat levels under 250 mg/dL. Plasma glucose levels will generally return to normal within 7 to 10 days. Long-term follow-up of patients undergoing insulinoma surgery have shown a 7% risk of developing diabetes mellitus.[7]

Apparent ductal injury following enucleation can be managed in a number of ways. Minor side branch injuries can be treated with simple ligation with absorbable suture and closed-suction drainage. Major pancreatic ductal injury involving the body and tail of the pancreas is best treated with distal pancreatectomy. Major ductal injury in the head of the gland can be treated with closure of the hole with fine interrupted absorbable sutures and closed-suction drainage, while others close this type of injury over a small silastic stent brought out through the papilla to decrease back pressure. One other option is to drain the site of injury into a defunctionalized Roux limb. Finally, if all else fails, a Whipple procedure can be considered, but in general, it should be a procedure of last resort.

LAPAROSCOPIC APPROACH

The pancreas can be approached laparoscopically through 5 or 6 ports placed along the upper abdomen. Positioning is dependent on preoperative knowledge of the whereabouts of the tumor. For tumors that are in the body and tail of the pancreas, the lesion can be approached through a lateral decubitus or semidecubitus position. For lesions more proximal in the pancreas, supine positioning is preferable. The use of ultrasonic dissectors and laparoscopic ultrasound facilitate such operative procedures.

Outcomes

Between 1982 and 2005, 247 patients underwent surgery for endogenous hyperinsulinism at our institution with 0% mortality. Although most patients had no perioperative complications, 18% experienced complications, primarily pancreatic in nature; most of these were low-output fistulas that were managed with closed-suction drainage. In our group of 247 patients, 2% (5 patients) developed recurrent disease. Two of our MEN-1 patients developed new insulinomas, 2 of our nesidioblastosis patients have experienced symptomatic recurrence, as has 1 of our sporadic patients with multiple insulinomas. In only 1 case of suspected insulinoma was no tumor found.[6]

Survival after diagnosis and treatment of insulinoma is no different when compared with an age- and sex-matched controlled population. Survival after diagnosis of a malignant insulinoma is significantly different with a 5-year survival of 45% and a 10-year survival of less than 30%.[7] Malignant insulinomas are managed like any malignant islet cell carcinoma with formal pancreatic resection and lymphadenectomy. Hepatic metastases can be managed with a number of modalities, including arterial chemoembolization, hepatic resection, and radio-frequency ablation.[27] Chemotherapy (streptozotocin, doxorubicin, and 5-fluorouracil) has been shown to offer effective palliation in select patients.[28] Frequent meals, continuous intravenous glucose infusion, calcium channel blockers, and diazoxide have also been utilized with limited palliative effect. Because of the absence of specific somatostatin receptors within insulinomas, somatostatin analogues are generally ineffective.

The recurrence rates for insulinoma following initial curative surgery is less than 10% in non-MEN-1 patients and over 20% in the MEN-1 group.[7]

Summary

Patients with neuroglycopenia and a positive 72-hour fast or positive end-of-fast study during a spontaneous episode of hypoglycemia are referred for transabdominal US and spiral CT. Although EUS is being utilized at many centers with increasing frequency, we favor its use to follow-up on equivocal cross-sectional imaging. With a positive imaging study, patients are taken to the operating room with intraoperative ultrasonography. Enucleation or resection is performed depending on the size and location of the tumor, and its proximity to ductal and vascular structures. From our experience, we can predict, in this subgroup of patients, a 100% cure rate for sporadic insulinoma. The only recurrences that we have had in this particular group have been in the MEN-1 subcategory. In the one-third of patients with negative preoperative imaging, we will generally refer those patients today for selective arterial calcium stimulation testing, and if positive, the patient is taken to the operating room.

If one were to take a patient with nonfamilial disease to the operating room with a negative preoperative imaging study, visible pathology would either be palpable or visible to the surgeon or radiologist performing intraoperative ultrasound in 98% of the patients. One could then select to close the other 2% and move on to a calcium stimulation test. Today, however, patients are quite aware of what is available and will often opt for selective arterial calcium stimulation testing prior to operation.

In patients with postprandial neuroglycopenia and Whipple's triad, but a negative 72-hour fast, a similar imaging battery is performed. In less than 1% of these patients will an insulinoma be found. These patients will almost certainly have NIPHS that can be confirmed by selective arterial calcium stimulation testing. With a positive selective arterial stimulation test, the patient is taken to the operating room with intraoperative ultrasound to rule out the possibility of an insulinoma and a gradient-guided resection is performed.

With advances in minimally invasive techniques and robotic surgery, we will likely see an increasing number of operations performed utilizing this advanced technology in the future.

References

1. Banting FG, Best CH. The internal secretion of the pancreas. J Lab Clin Med 1922;7:251–66.

2. Wilder RM, Allan FN, Power MH, Robertson HE. Carcinoma of the islets of the pancreas: hyperinsulinism and hypoglycemia. JAMA 1927;89:348–55.

3. Howland G, Campbell WR, Maltby EJ, Robinson WL. Dysinsulinism: convulsions and coma due to islet cell tumor of the pancreas with operation and cure. JAMA 1929;93:674–9.

4. Whipple AO, Franz VK. Adenoma of the islet cells with hyperinsulinism. Am Surg 1935;101:1299–335.

5. Laroche GP, Ferris DO, Priestley JT. Hyperinsulinism. Arch Surg 1968;96:765–72.

6. Grant CS. Insulinoma. In: Tytgat GN, editor. Best practice & research: clinical gastroenterology. United Kingdom: Elsevier Science. [In press].

7. Service FJ, McMahon MM, O'Brien PC, Ballard DJ. Functioning insulinoma—incidence, recurrence, and long-term survival of patients: a 60-year study. Mayo Clin Proc 1991;66:711–9.

8. Thompson GB, Service FJ. Insulinoma. In: Saclarides T, Millikan KW, Godellas CV, editors. Surgical oncology: an algorithmic approach. New York: Springer-Verlag; 2003. p. 104–13.

9. Service FJ. Hypoglycemic disorders. N Engl J Med 1995; 332:1144–52.

10. Service F, Natt N, Thompson G, et al. Noninsulinoma pancreatogenous hypoglycemia: a novel syndrome of hyperinsulinemic hypoglycemia in adults independent of mutations in Kir6.2 and SUR1 genes. J Clin Endocrinol Metab 1999;84:1582–9.

11. Service FJ, O'Brien PC, Kao PC, Young WF Jr. C-peptide suppression test: effects of gender, age, and body mass index; implications for the diagnosis of insulinoma. J Clin Endocrinol Metab 1992;74:204–10.

12. O'Brien T, O'Brien PC, Service FJ. Insulin surrogates in insulinoma. J Clin Endocrinol Metab 1993;77:448–51.

13. Grant CS, van Heerden JA, Charboneau JW, et al. Insulinoma: the value of intraoperative ultrasonography. Arch Surg 1988;123:843–8.

14. Fidler JL, Fletcher JG, Reading CC, et al. Preoperative detection of pancreatic insulinomas in multiphasic helical CT. Am J Roentgenol 2003;181:775–80.

15. Roche T, Lightdale CJ, Botet JF. Localization of pancreatic endocrine tumors by endoscopic ultrasonography. N Engl J Med 1992;326:1721–6.

16. Zimmer T, Stolzel U, Bader M, et al. Endoscopic ultrasonography and somatostatin receptor scintigraphy in the preoperative localization of insulinomas and gastrinomas. Gut 1996;39:562–8.

17. Fulton RE, Sheedy PT, McIlrath DC. Preoperative angiographic localization of insulin-producing tumors of the pancreas. AJR 1975;123:367–77.

18. Doppman JL, Chang R, Fraker DL. Localization of insulinomas to regions of the pancreas by intra-arterial stimulation with calcium. An Intern Med 1995;123:269–73.

19. Doppman JL, Miller DL, Chang R, et al. Insulinomas: localization with selective intra-arterial injection of calcium. Radiology 1991;178:237–41.

20. Thompson GB, Service FJ, Andrews JC, et al. Noninsulinoma pancreatogenous hypoglycemia syndrome: an update in 10 surgically treated patients. Surgery 2000; 128:937–5.

21. Service GJ, Thompson GB, Service FJ, et al. Hyperinsulinemic hypoglycemia with nesidioblastosis after gastric-bypass surgery. N Engl J Med 2005;353:249–54.

22. O'Riordain DS, O'Brien T, van Heerden JA, et al. Surgical management of insulinoma associated with multiple endocrine neoplasia type I. World J Surg 1994;18:488–94.

23. Jaroszewski DE, Schlinkert RT, Thompson GB, Schlinkert DK. Laparoscopic localization and resection of insulinomas. Arch Surg 2004;139:270–4.

24. Lo C-Y, Chan W-F, Lo C-M, et al. Surgical treatment of pancreatic insulinomas in the era of laparoscopy. Surg Endosc 2004;18:297–302.

25. Mabrut JY, Fernando-Cruz L, Azagra JS, et al. Laparoscopic pancreatic resection: results of a multicenter European study of 127 patients. Surgery 2005;137:597–605.

26. Thompson GB, Service FJ, Carney JA, et al. Reoperative insulinomas, 1927 to 1992: an institutional experience. Surgery 1993;114:1196–206.

27. Siperstein AE, Rogers SJ, Hanson PD, Gitomirsky A. Laparoscopic thermal ablation of hepatic neuroendocrine tumor metastases. Surgery 1997;122:1147–55.

28. Moertel CG, Lefkopoulo M, Lipsitz S. Streptozocin-doxorubicin, streptozocin-fluorouracil, or chlorozotocin in the treatment of advanced islet-cell carcinoma. N Engl J Med 1992;326:519–23.

CHAPTER 47

RARE FUNCTIONING NEUROENDOCRINE TUMORS OF THE PANCREAS

ELIJAH DIXON, MD, MSC (EPI)

JANICE L. PASIEKA, MD

Introduction

In 1902 Nicholls was the first to describe an islet cell tumor of the pancreas, yet it took the discovery of insulin in 1922 to open up a new field in oncological diseases, that of functioning islet cell tumors of the pancreas. Endocrinopathies from functioning islet cell or neuroendocrine tumors of the pancreas was first appreciated when in 1926 Charles Mayo operated on a physician with metastatic insulinoma. Although the tumor was unresectable, extracts from the biopsied liver metastases caused hypoglycemia when injected into rabbits, reproducing the hypoglycemic symptoms that the patient suffered from.[1] With a better understanding of the physiology of the endocrine pancreas, endocrinopathies from the overproduction of other hormones secreted by these islet cell tumors have since been described during the latter part of the twentieth century (Table 1). These rare tumors occur in approximately 1 out of 100,000 people and are much less common than pancreatic adenocarcinoma by a ratio of 125:1. With the exception of insulinomas, the majority of islet cell tumors or neuroendocrine tumors of the pancreas (NETPs) are malignant. Neuroendocrine tumors may be further classified as functional or nonfunctional. Functional tumors are characterized by a recognized clinical endocrinopathy that results from excessive hormone production. Nonfunctioning neuroendocrine tumors of the pancreas histologically are similar to functioning neuroendocrine tumors of the pancreas; however, they do not produce a clinical syndrome. The potential reasons for the lack of a syndrome include inadequate

secretion of hormone, secretion of a hormone in an inactive form, or the hormone released results in a yet to be described clinical syndrome. Up to 40% of NETPs are nonfunctioning.

Although NETPs generally behave less aggressively than pancreatic adenocarcinoma, they do spread to the liver more frequently than any other malignancy, with the exception of colorectal cancers.[2] Excluding insulinomas, at the time of diagnosis, 50 to 60% of NETPs have already spread to the liver.[3] It is, however, the clinical endocrinopathy produced by these tumors that are potentially life threatening.

Embryology and Histology

Islet cells have a rich blood supply. They are interspersed between acinar cells of the pancreas. Pancreatic endocrine cells make up 1 to 2% of the pancreatic mass. Alpha cells secrete glucagon and comprise 20% of the islet cells, beta cells produce insulin (70% of islet cell mass), and delta cells secrete mainly somatostatin (5–10% islet cell mass). Within the islets of Langerhans, beta cells are located at the center, a mantle zone 3 cells thick contains alpha, delta, and clear cells. This relationship facilitates paracrine communication between the cells. The origin of NETPs has been debated; originally they were felt to arise from the islets of Langerhans; more recently, evidence suggests they likely arise from pluripotent cells in the ductal epithelium.[4] The neuroendocrine cell lineage is suggested by silver staining of the cytoplasm. The typical histologic appearance of an NETP is one of

Table 1: Characteristics of NETPs

	Glucagonoma	VIPoma	PPoma	Somatostatinoma
First Described	1942	1954	1980	1980
Mean Age	53	42/7*		55
Male:Female	1:1.3	1:1		1:1.2
Malignant	60–100%	> 70%	> 60%	40–75%
5-Year Survival	50–60%	50–70%	30–50%	40%
Mean Size	> 4cm	> 3 cm	Large, or hyperplasia	5 cm
% MEN-1	1–20%	5–10%	20–40%	45–50%
Location				
Head	22%	< 10%	NC	68%
Body	32%	< 10%	NC	4%
Tail	54%	> 75%	NC	26%
Diffuse	4%	4%	NC	2%
Combination	< 5%	< 5%	< 5%	< 5%
Extra-pancreatic	0.7%	< 10%	< 5%	0

NC = not characterized, too few cases.
*Neurogenic extrapancreatic VIPomas.

uniform cytology with scant mitoses. Microscopically, NETPs are composed of small, uniform, cuboidal cells with an eosinophilic or aminophilic finely granular cytoplasm that may be arranged into trabeculae, festoons, or solid nests (Figure 1A). Electron microscopy shows nanosecretory granules in the cytoplasm. The bland histologic appearance of NETPs can be confused with acinar exocrine carcinoma of the pancreas, pacreatoblastoma, microadenomas of the pancreas, and solid pseudopapillary tumors.[5]

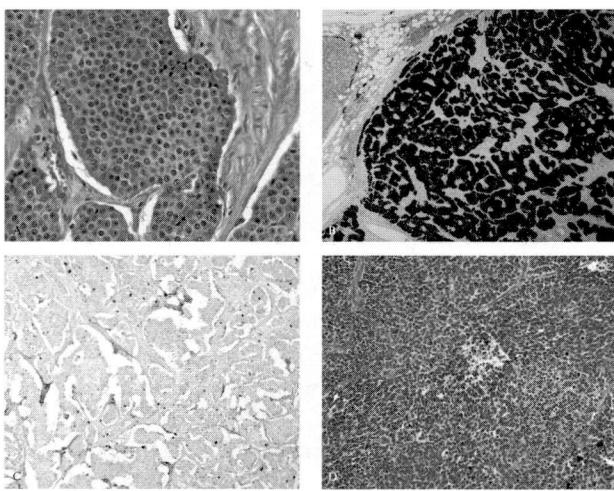

Figure 1 Histological appearance of NETPs. *A*, Well-differentiated demonstrating small, uniform, cuboidal cells with an eosinophilic or aminophilic finely granular cytoplasm that may be arranged into trabeculae, festoons, or solid nests. *B*, Immunohistochemical staining of synaptophysin uniformly distributed throughout the tumor. *C, Ki67* index with 10% of these cells staining positive. *D*, Poorly differentiated NEPTs.

Pathological Classification

Several authors have recently devised a variety of classification systems for neuroendocrine tumors to help better predict prognosis. Schindl and colleagues stratified NETPs into either: benign, uncertain, or malignant.[6] These groups were defined by tumor risk factors that included size, local invasion, angioinvasion, cellular atypia, gross invasion, and metastases.[6] Tumors less than or equal to 20 mm in size with no evidence of the other risk factors are categorized as benign. Tumors greater than 20 mm in size with evidence of local infiltration, angioinvasion, and atypia, but without gross invasion or metastases are classified as "uncertain." Malignant tumors have the presence of all the risk factors. Utilizing this classification, the 5-year estimated cumulative survival for benign, uncertain, and malignant were 100%, 100%, and 52%, respectively. More recently, the World Health Organization (WHO) published a classification that takes into account the differentiation of the tumor histologically[7,8] (Table 2). Well-differentiated endocrine tumors express markers of neuroendocrine differentiation both diffusely and intensely, in particular, chromogranin A and synpatophysin (Figure 1B). These lesions have a low proliferative index measured by the percentage of cells staining for *Ki67* (Figure 1C). In

Table 2 WHO Classification of Neuroendocrine Tumors

WHO Classification of Neuroendocrine Tumors
Well-differentiated endocrine tumor
Well-differentiated endocrine carcinoma
Poorly differentiated endocrine carcinoma
Mixed endocrine/exocrine tumors
Tumor-like lesions

contrast, poorly differentiated endocrine carcinomas express cytosol neuroendocrine markers together with synaptophysin, with rare expression of chromogranin A. These lesions have greater than 16% of the cells expressing and commonly demonstrate central necrosis (Figure 1D). The difference between a well-differentiated endocrine tumor and a well-differentiated endocrine carcinoma is the demonstration of local invasion or metastasis. Both of these classifications illustrate the spectrum of disease that NETPs display, from an indolent benign behavior to an aggressive tumor with a poor prognosis.

Risk Factors

An increased risk for developing NETPs (odds ratio = 2) has been reported in a recent European study,[8] the common features that were identified were exposure to organic solvents and rust-preventing paints that contains lead. In a large Swedish study, socioeconomic status may have impact on the development of these tumors, with an odds ratio of 3.0 among professionals.[9] There are several hereditary conditions that are associated with the development of NETPs. The most common is multiple endocrine neoplasia type 1(MEN-1). MEN-1 is characterized by the development of hyperparathyroidism (98%), multiple pancreatic islet cell tumors (50%), pituitary adenomas (30%), adrenal cortical lesions (20%), and carcinoid tumors. MEN-1 is known to be caused by the loss of the tumor suppressor MENIN gene located on chromosome 11. Other hereditary conditions that have a greater incidence of NETPs are von Hippel-Lindau (VHL) and neurofibromatosis type 1 (NF-1). VHL disease is an autosomal dominant disorder characterized by hemangioblastomas of the central nervous system, renal cell carcinoma, pheochromocytoma, pancreatic tumors, and endolymphatic sac tumors. The pancreatic tumors are varied and include true cyst (91%), serous cystadenoma (12%), NETPs (12%), or combination of each of these.[10] The chromosomal abnormality in VHL is found on chromosome 3. NF-1 has a unique association of somatostatinomas, usually arising in the periampullar region of the duodenum. These duodenal tumors do not appear to cause the typical somatostatinoma syndrome seen with the pancreatic lesions.

Functioning Neuroendocrine Tumors of the Pancreas

Functioning NETPs are characterized by the clinical syndrome resulting from excess hormone production. Many times the endocrinopathy can produces life-threatening and sometimes debilitating symptoms.

Diagnosis and treatment of these tumors is, therefore, twofold. Firstly, to alleviate the excessive hormone production and counteract the symptoms, while at the same time addressing the malignant potential of these tumors. NETPs are classified into different subtypes based on function and clinical symptoms. The most common functioning NETP is an insulinoma causing hypoglycemia, followed by a gastrinoma causing Zollinger-Ellison syndrome. The majority of NETPs have immunohistochemical staining of more than one hormone or peptide. It is not uncommon for the clinical syndrome to evolve or change over time, depending on the predominate hormone produced. This change in the clinical syndrome over time is most commonly seen in poorly differentiated metastatic NETs.

Glucagon secreting tumors (Glucagonoma)

In 1922, Murlin postulated a glucose agonist he termed glucagon by observing a temporary rise in blood sugar level before hypoglycemia caused by pancreatic extracts. Glucagon was separated from impure insulin 25 years later and is known now to originate from the alpha cells of the islets. Glucagonomas are the third most common NETP. These tumors produce a syndrome that has been variously termed glucagonoma syndrome, hyperglycemic cutaneous syndrome, diabetes dermatitis syndrome, and catabolic syndrome.[11] Becker and colleagues[12] were the first to describe the characteristic syndrome in 1942. In an extensive review of the literature by Soga and Yakuwa, they found over 70% of the of 407 glucagonomas were greater than 2 cm in size.[11] The characteristic clinical presentation has been termed the "4D syndrome," diabetes, dermatitis, deep vein thrombosis, and depression.[5] The characteristic rash of a glucagonoma is termed "necrolytic migratory erythema," and was first described in 1973.[13] The rash occurs in 70% of patients at diagnosis, and they typically present with erythematous plaques on the face, abdomen, groin, lower extremities, and rarely the mucous membranes[5] (Figure 2). The central areas are clear and the borders become blistered and encrusted. Patients often complain of pain and pruritus at the site of the rash. The rash is believed to be the result of decreased levels of amino acids, since the majority of patients with glucagonomas will present with hypoaminoacidemia. Biopsy of the rash will lead to the diagnosis, as it is characterized by pallor and spongiosis of the upper stratum, necrotic keratinocytes, and a perivascular infiltrated are commonly seen. Complete surgical resection of the tumor will result in a rapid resolution of the rash within days to weeks of surgery. Almost half of these patients will present with throm-

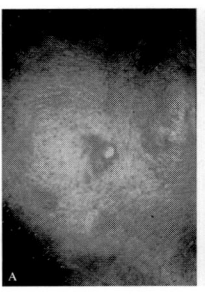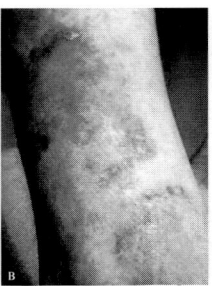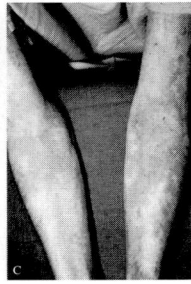

Figure 2 Necrolytic migratory erythema presents with erythematous plaques on the extremities of a patient with a glucagonoma.

boembolic disease. The cause of the thromboembolic disease is unknown, yet leads to a lifelong need for anticoagulation. Other findings include anemia, weight loss, hypoaminoaciduria, and other neuropsychiatric symptoms (see Table 1; Table 3). In contrast to insulinomas, the majority of these tumors are malignant. Untreated, these patients die of sepsis secondary to malnutrition or complication from thromboembolic disease. Aggressive surgical intervention is the only hope of curtailing the devastating symptoms.

Vasoactive Intestinal Peptide-Producing Tumors (VIPomas)

VIPomas are very rare tumors, occurring in 1 in 10,000,000 people per year.[5] The characteristic syndrome was first described in 1957[14] by Priest, followed in 1958 by a case report of 2 patients with watery diarrhea, hypokalemia, and an noninsulin secreting islet cell tumor of the pancreas.[15] In their paper that bears the name of the clinical syndrome, Verner and Morrison found an additional 9 patients with similar clinical characteristics and nonbeta cell islet tumors in the pancreas. It was not until 1970 that the hormone responsible for the syndrome, vasoactive intestinal polypeptide (VIP) was discovered.[16,17] Other names for this syndrome include VIPoma, pancreatic cholera, and watery diarrhea hypokalemia achlorhydria (WDHA) syndrome. VIP is known to bind to a receptor in the intestinal lumen, which activates adenylate cyclase and cyclic AMP (adenosine monophosphate). This results in the secretion of sodium, chloride, potassium, and water into the small bowel, along with an increase in bowel motility.[5] This leads to secretory diarrhea, hypokalemia, and dehydration. Other effects include the inhibition of gastric acid secretion, vasodilatation, bone resorption, and glycogenolysis.[5] This may result in hypochlorhydria, flushing, hypercalcemia, and hyperglycemia. Water loss can be significant, with 70% of patients having stool volumes of greater than 3 liters per day.[5] The diagnosis is suspected clinically when patients present with a secretory diarrhea that persists with fasting. Examination of the stool reveals a high sodium load, and a low osmol gap. The extreme nature of the diarrhea syndrome makes the rate of preoperative diagnosis relatively high, at 67% compared with only 50% of other functioning NETPs.[17] Extrapancreatic VIPomas have been reported in neurogenic tumors such as ganglioneuroblastomas, gang-

Table 3

	Hormone	Syndrome	Extrapancreatic
Glucagonoma	Glucagon	Diabetes	Necrolytic Migratory Erythema DVT Depression
VIPoma	VIP	Diarrhea Hypokalemia Achlorhydria Dehydration	Neurogenic tumors
Somatostatinoma	Somatostatin	Diabetes Cholelithiasis Steatorrhea	Duodenal (NF-1)
PPoma	Pancreatic Polypeptide	Asymptomatic ? Diarrhea	Islet Hyperplasia
Carcinoid	5-HPT Serotonin	Flushing Diarrhea Valvular Heart Disease Carcinoid syndrome	
PTHrPoma	PTHrP	Hypercalcemia Hypophosphatemia Undetectable PTH	
ACTH	ACTH	Cushing's syndrome	

lioneuromas, and neuroblastomas, as well as the colon and bronchus.[5] Extrapancreatic VIPomas tend to occur in the pediatric population with a mean age 7 years versus 42 years for the pancreatic VIPomas. In a review by Soga and Yakuwa of 241 patients, pancreatic VIPomas had a significantly greater rate of metastases compared with the neurogenic group (56% vs 29%)[17] (see Tables 1 and 3).

Somatostatinoma

Somatostatin is a hormone that normally acts in a paracrine fashion to inhibit the secretion of insulin, glucagon, gastrin, and growth hormone. It also inhibits the CCK-mediated secretion of pancreatic enzymes, intestinal absorption, and gastric acid secretion.[5] In 1977 the first case of a somatostatinoma was reported, and in a review done by Sugo in 1999, only 173 cases had been reported in the world literature.[18] Somatostatinomas are equally distributed between the pancreas and duodenum. The site of origin does appear to dictate a slightly different clinical presentation. The classic inhibitory symptoms consisting of diabetes mellitus, cholelithiasis, and steatorrhea are seen in approximately 20% of pancreatic primaries and in only 3% of duodenal lesions[5,19] (see Table 3). Most patients present with a variety of gastrointestinal symptoms, including hypochlorhydria, abdominal pain, postprandial fullness, steatorrhea, and diarrhea. Patients with duodenal somatostatinomas may present with obstruction of the biliary tract because of their close approximation to the ampulla, despite the fact that the majority of these lesions are under 2 cm in size[5] (Figure 3). In contrast to the duodenal lesions, pancreatic somatostatinomas are most commonly found in the head of the pancreas, 86% are greater than 2 cm, and over half will present with distant metastases. Sixty-five percent of all the Somatostatinomas in the literature demonstrate invasiveness, 70% of the pancreatic and 56% of the duodenal lesions.[19] Von Recklinghausen's disease (NF-1) is associated with the duodenal lesions (43%), yet rarely seen in association with the pancreatic lesions (1%). Somatostatinomas are associated with MEN-1 7% of the time.

Similar to all NETPs, the calculated 5-year survival rates are dependent on the presence of metastases or not. Overall, Kaplan-Meier estimated of the 5-year survival in 90 reported cases in the world literature was 75%, 60% in those patients with metastases and 100% in those without.[18]

Pancreatic Polypeptide (PPomas)

In 1976 Larsson and colleagues were the first to describe a syndrome caused by pancreatic polypeptide (PP) hormone production.[20] These patients presented with a secretory diarrhea similar to that seen in VIPomas. However, it is possible that another hormone may have been responsible for these symptoms. When injected into animals, PP rarely causes any symptoms and, therefore, PPomas have traditionally been classified as nonfunctioning NETPs. Islet cell hyperplasia that stains predominately for PP is seen adjacent to many of the islet cell tumors, resulting in elevated levels of PP in up to 80% of patients with other NETPs. This has allowed for utilization of PP as a screening tool in patients known to be predisposed to NETPs such as MEN-1 and VHL patients.[21] More recently, there has been an increased number of case reports of diarrhea associated with either a PPomas or PP islet cell hyperplasia[20,22] (Figure 4). In an extensive review in the literature, 58 cases of PPomas were reviewed by Soga and Yakuwa.[18] A total of 54 of these cases were from NETPs, and 4 were a result of islet cell hyperplasia. Almost half (48%) of the cases secreted multihormones, including gastrin, ACTH, and glucagon.

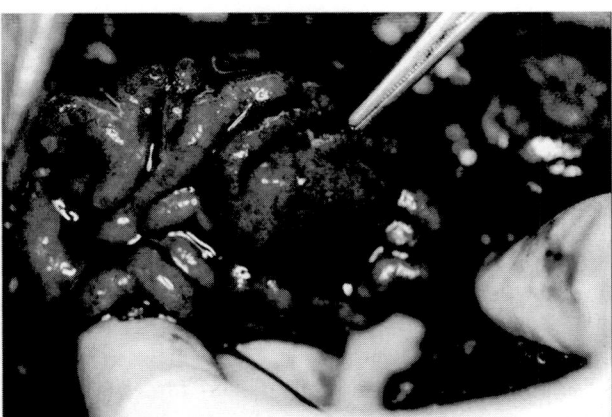

Figure 3 Duodenal somatostatinoma in a patient with NF-1, duodenal resection with preservation of the ampulla of Vater.

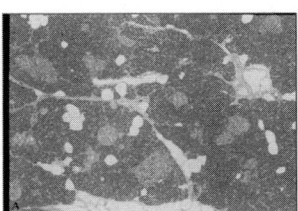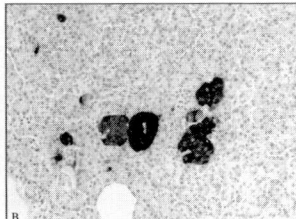

Figure 4 PP hyperplasia in a woman presenting with secretory diarrhea. *A*, Demonstrates islet cell hyperplasia, and *B*, demonstrates immunohistochemical staining intensely for PP. Distal pancreatectomy resulted in a reduction of serum PP and resolution of her secretory diarrhea.

Presenting symptoms ranged from asymptomatic to abdominal pain, diarrhea, and weight loss (see Tables 1 and 3).

Pancreatic Carcinoids

Only 40 cases of pancreatic carcinoid tumors, otherwise known as pancreatic serotoninoma, or serotonin-producing tumor of the pancreas, have been described.[23] These tumors usually present late, with 88% being malignant. They can produce the typical "carcinoid syndrome," characterized by facial flushing, diarrhea, abdominal pain, and valvular heart diseae.[23] Prognosis is generally poor because of the late stage of presentation. Being a "foregut" carcinoid, they lack the decarboxylating enzyme that converts 5-hydroxythyrophan (5-HPT) to serotonin. Therefore, one would not expect high levels of urinary 5-HIAA (5-hydroxyindoleacetic acid) in the early stages of this disease, but would find elevated levels of 5-HPT in the urine. Elevation of urinary 5-HIAA usually occurs when there is a significant tumor burden. Measurement of urinary 5-HIAA chromogranin A (CgA) and/or the demonstration of elevated serotonin levels in the tumor and/or the serum are key to making the diagnosis (see Table 3).

Ectopic Hypercalcemia Syndrome (Pancreatic PTHrPoma)

Pancreatic neuroendocrine tumors can produce parathyroid hormone-related peptide (PTHrP), which has similar activity to that of parathyroid hormone (PTH).[24] The diagnosis is often initially confused with primary hyperparathyroidism when the patient presents with elevated calcium and low phosphate levels in the serum. The clue to the diagnosis is the rapid onset of symptoms, including muscle weakness, bony pain, and fatigue, along with significantly elevated calcium levels usually greater than 3.5 mmol/L and undetectable PTH levels in the serum (see Table 3). PTHrP has molecular heterogeneity and, therefore, is not detected by the standard PTH assay. Aggressive resuscitation and lowering of the serum calcium levels are required prior to surgical intervention. Following complete resection, following serum calcium levels provides an excellent tumor marker for recurrence. Bisphosphonates can and should be utilized both preoperatively and as palliative therapy in persistent disease. The majority of these tumors are malignant, usually presenting with liver metastases. Patients usually die from complications of resistant hypercalcemia, not from the tumor itself.

ACTH-Secreting NETPs

Twenty-six percent of the cases of Cushing's syndrome owing to ectopic ACTH production reported in the literature are from NETPs.[25] Pancreatic ACTH tumors are second only to bronchogenic tumors is ectopic production of this hormone. This syndrome is more common in men than women and usually occurs in patients over the age of 50. The diagnosis of ectopic ACTH-dependant Cushing's is suspected in patients with a rapid onset of the manifestations of Cushing's syndrome (see Table 3). The diagnosis is confirmed by an elevated 24-hour urinary cortisol, elevated ACTH, and a nonsuppression high-does dexamethasone suppression test. Most patients present with distant metastases and, therefore, surgical cure is unlikely. Utilization of ketoconazole, an antifungal agent that inhibits the synthesis cortisol through P-450 enzyme inhibition, has been used in a limited number of patients with mixed results. Therefore, recent studies have addressed the suppression of ACTH from the tumor with a somatostatin analogue instead with good results.

Other hormones that have been described in isolated case reports include prostatic acid phosphotase,[26] calcitonin, and growth hormone.

Mixed Endocrine/Exocrine (Adenocarcinoid)

These very rare tumors have dual features of both a neuroendocrine tumor and an adenocarcinoma. These tumors co-express mucin and neurosecretory granules.[27] They very rarely have a humoral syndrome associated with them, and more typically present as a mass lesion. These tumors behave much more aggressively than NETPs, and in this regard are more closely related to the typical adenocarcinoma of the pancreas.[27]

Preoperative Imaging

Vast improvements in the quality of both anatomic and functional imaging have improved the preoperative detection of NETPs. Abdominal ultrasound (US) has the advantage of low cost, wide availability, lack of radiation exposure, and noninvasiveness. Most NETPs appear as hypoechoic, well-circumscribed masses within the pancreas, in contrast, the liver metastases appear as hyperechoic lesions. Abdominal ultrasound is highly operator-dependent, with sensitivity between 66 and 80%.[28] Endoscopic ultrasound (EUS) utilizes the same tumor properties and is an excellent modality to detect small pancreatic tumors. It is most sensitive for tumors of the head of the pancreas or the duodenum. Lesions in the tail are not seen as well because of the lack of proximity to the luminal gastrointestinal tract. EUS has the advantage of being able to obtain a biopsy to aid in preoperative diagnosis and planning. Although it is also operator-dependent, lesions of the pancreas can generally be identified with this modality with a sensitivity of 93%[19] (Figure 5).

The hypervascular nature of NETPs often makes them visible on contrast-enhanced imaging. A biphasic computerize tomography (CT) scan with both arterial and venous phases has a sensitivity, depending on the size, between 40 and 100%[28] (Figure 6). With improvements in magnetic resonance imaging (MRI), as well as its ability to demonstrate high contrast between small NETPs and normal pancreas, MRI has become an invaluable modality to image NETPs. NETPs demonstrate low signal intensity on T1 weighted images and high signal intensity on T2 weighted images. Contrast

enhancement using gadolinium has also improved the sensitivity of the modality (Figure 7). Similar to CT imaging, the sensitivity of this modality is size-dependent, with lesions less than 1 cm rarely being detected, lesions 1 to 2 cm in diameter being detected 50% of the time, and all lesions greater than 3 cm being detected.[29] Despite the recent advantages in both CT and MRI, both of these modalities can underestimate the tumor burden in up to 50% of patients.

The expression of somatostatin receptors on over 85 to 90% of NETPs allows for the utilization of somatostatin receptor scintigraphy for detection of occult tumors (Figure 8). With the exception of insulinoma, the sensitivity for octreotide scintigraphy is 80%.[30,31] In a study by Scherubl and colleagues, up to 40% of liver metastases were detected using scintigraphy

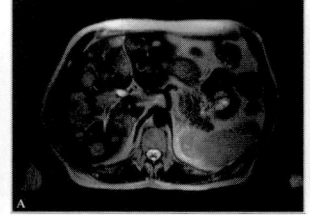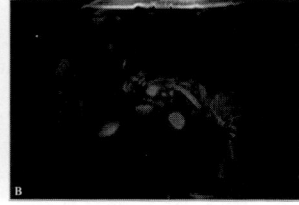

Figure 7 *A*, MRI scan of liver metastases from an NETP. Gadolinium enhancement demonstrates high signal intensity on T2 weighted images. *B*, T1 image of the primary in the tail of the pancreas.

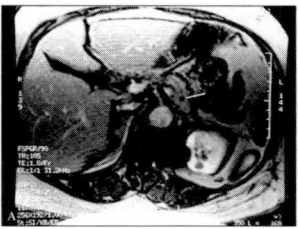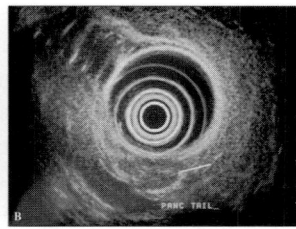

Figure 5 *A*, MRI demonstrating small NETPs in the tail of the pancreas. *B*, Endoscopic ultrasound demonstrating this small hypoechoic and well-circumscribed lesion.

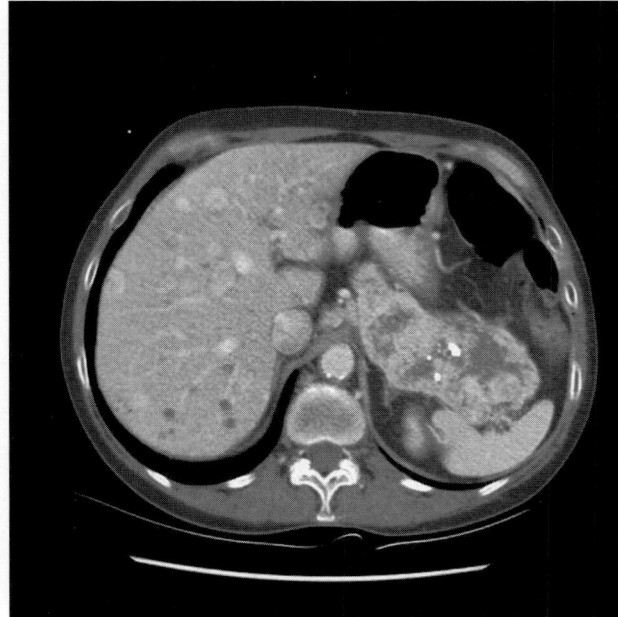

Figure 6 A CT scan of a large NETP in the tail of the pancreas.

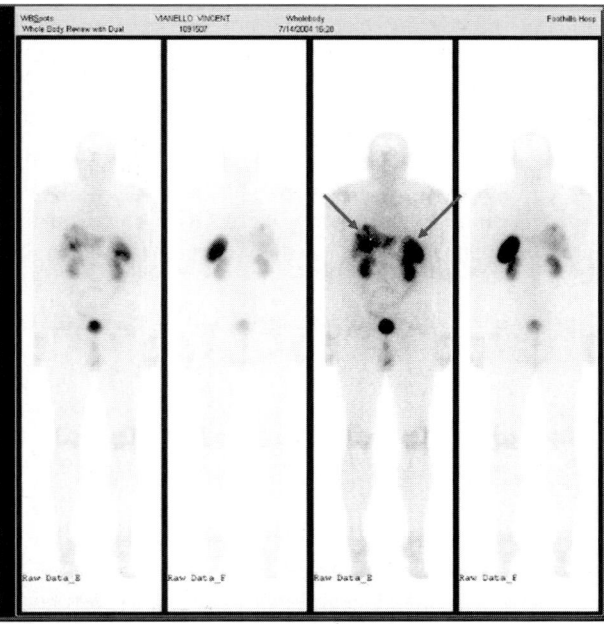

Figure 8 Somatostatin receptor scintigraphy. ^{111}In-octreotide scan detecting both the primary tumor in the tail of the pancreas and several liver metastases.

when CT, MRI, and US failed to demonstrate the lesions.[32] SPECT imaging improves the sensitivity further when compared with traditional planar imaging. Metaiodobenzylguanidine (mIBG) is incorporated into the secretory granules in neuroendocrine tumors approximately 70% of the time. This additional functional modality can provide additional information in some of the NETPs, and should be considered in patients with octreotide scan-negative tumors or for assessment of radionuclide therapy. Recently, the combination of functional and anatomical imaging has allowed for the identification of these unique tumors with CT-PET (positive emission tomography) (Figure 9). Unfortunately FDG-PET has not been advantageous for imaging NETPs, likely because of their low proliferation. The development of alternative compounds such as [11]C 5-HTP may enhance the detection rate of these tumors in the future. In a recent comparison of conventional imaging, 5-HTP PET proved better than CT and somatostatin scintigraphy for tumor visualization in NETPs and carcinoid tumors.[33]

Preoperative Management

Patients will generally either present with symptoms related to a functioning NETP, local symptoms related to the tumor, or a lesion found incidentally. Because of the rarity of these tumors, the average delay in diagnosis can sometimes be years. A very thorough history and physical can at times provide the clues and should direct the clinician in ordering specific tumor markers for NETPs (see Table 3). These include the specific hormone causing the endocrinopathies, such as glucagon, somatostatin, VIP, and ACTH, as well as nonspecific markers of NETPs, such as PP and CgA. Imaging should include either a biphasic CT scan and/or contrast-enhanced MRI. If the lesion has features of a NET on imaging (hypervascular, discrete), then functional imaging

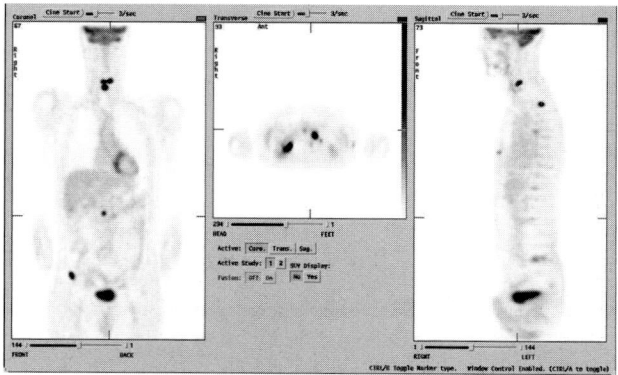

Figure 9 PET/CT scan of NETPs.

including both octreotide and mIBG studies should be done. EUS with or without fine-needle aspiration biopsy may be completed if it is available.

Preoperative fluid and electrolyte resuscitation is needed in patients with syndromes related to VIP, PTHrP, or somatostatin secretion. As well, patients with a glucagon-secreting tumor may benefit from a course of preoperative hyperalimentation because of their catabolic state. All patients should receive deep venous thrombosis prophylaxis in the form of unfractionated or low-molecular weight heparin, which will need to be continued indefinitely in patients with unresectable glucagonomas. Our practice is to also include perioperative antibiotics, subcutaneous injection of 100 ug of octreotide followed with an intraoperative infusion of octreotide at 10 ug/hr throughout the course of the operation.

Surgical Management

GENERAL PRINCIPLES

The key determinants of a successful outcome following surgical extirpation include a thorough understanding of endocrine surgical diseases and prior training and expertise in both pancreatic and endocrine surgery. A multidisciplinary approach to these patients is necessary. Intraoperative ultrasonography may be required to aid in localization, although the majority of these tumors are large and seen preoperatively on imaging. Exploration can be accomplished through either a midline incision or a bilateral subcostal incision, depending on body habitus and the presence or absence of hepatic disease. If hepatic lesions are expected, then the bilateral subcostal incision is preferred. Celiotomy is performed, with a careful examination for metastatic disease.

Combinations of maneuvers are utilized to completely expose the pancreas. These include mobilization of the right colon and extended kocherization of the duodenum and head of the pancreas over to the aorta so that the superior mesenteric artery can be felt as a cord running anterior to the fingers of the surgeon's left hand. Small branches from the pancreas into the superior mesenteric vein (SMV) are divided in order to allow the surgeon to palpate the entire uncinate process (Figure 10). Division of the gastrocolic ligament and mobilization and exposure of the caudal aspect of the pancreas is performed along its entirety, the mesentery of the right colon and small bowel is mobilized off of the second and third portions of the duodenum, and the gastrocolic trunk of the superior mesenteric vein is sometimes divided to expose the SMV-portal vein confluence at the neck of the pancreas. Caudal mobilization of the gland is

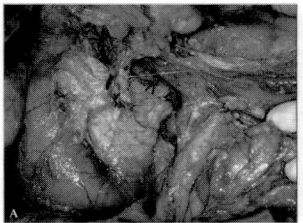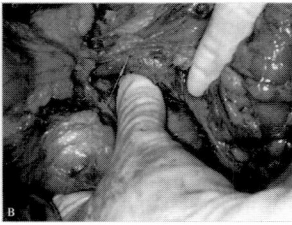

Figure 10 *A,* Kocherization of the duodenum and head of the pancreas so that the superior mesenteric vein (SMV) is exposed. *B,* Small branches into the SMV are divided in order to allow the surgeon to palpate the entire uncinate process between their thumb and index finger.

performed to facilitate bimanual palpation of the gland; this involves division of the splenocolic ligaments (Figure 11).

The NETPs, with the exception of insulinomas and gastrinomas, as a group have many similarities. They are often large at presentation and frequently liver metastases are identified. Therefore, the only chance of cure for these patients is surgical resection. This most often involves either a distal pancreatectomy or pancreatico-duodenectomy, depending on the location of the tumor.[5] Anatomic resection as opposed to enucleation is preferred in this setting because of the high rate of malignancy. Even in the setting of disseminated disease, because of the endocrinopathy, aggressive resection and/or debulking is warranted to minimize symptoms and to provide palliation. The methods used to achieve this must be individualized. Anatomic resection of the pancreas is preferable to enucleation if an R0 (complete) resection can be achieved, since long-term cure is possible. This principle holds with regards to liver metastases; if an R0 state can be achieved, then resection is preferable to ablative therapies.[34,35] Pape and collegues reported in a recent series, however, that up to 50% of patients with R0 resection of NETPs reoccur in long-term follow-up.[36] Adjuvant therapy may, therefore, prove in the future to be important in the treatment of these tumors. At the present time, there is no adjuvant therapy following complete resection.

When less than complete resection is possible, cytoreduction by debulking the tumor burden may be achieved by anatomic resection and/or ablative therapies in the pancreas and liver, respectively. There is mounting evidence that incomplete resection or debulking of metastatic neuroendocrine disease results in improved survival.[37,38] Another important caveat in these patients relates to palliative therapy such as radionuclide therapy. If these tumors have significant uptake on functional imaging, then debulking may maximize the dose effect of palliative radionuclide therapy. If long-term somatostatin analogue therapy is contemplated, a cholecystectomy should be performed at the time of surgery to prevent future development of cholelithiasis caused by this drug.

Systemic Therapy

SOMATOSTATIN ANALOGUES (SA)

The presence of somatostatin receptors on the cell surface of many NETPs is useful both for diagnosis and therapy. Tumors that have the greatest number of receptors generally respond the best to SA therapy. The development of long-acting analogues given monthly intramuscularly has simplified treatment for many patients. Symptomatic along with biochemical response to therapy occurs in between 60 and 90% of patients.[5,39] The median duration of response to treatment is 12 months, at which time tachyphylaxis often develops. The cause of tachyphylaxis is unknown. Somatostatin analogues not only inhibit hormone release, both also play a role in inhibiting angioneogensis. Between 5 and 15% of patients will have a reduction in tumor burden.[5] The future developments of subtype-specific analogues have demonstrated promise for the future.[39] Targeting somatostatin receptor subtype 3, which is involved in angiogenesis, may provide a better tumor response while continuing to provide excellent palliation. At the present time, this drug is under investigation. The side effects of SA include nausea, vomiting, cholelithiasis, diarrhea, steatorrhea, and pain at the injection site.

INTERFERON (IFN)-ALPHA

IFN acts through both direct antiproliferative effects as well as inhibition of tumor angiogenesis mediated by suppression of VEGF gene expression in NETPs.[24] In trials of neuroendocrine patients, INF has shown a 50% biochemical response for a median duration of 20 months.[5,39] A significant tumor response (> 50% reduction) is, however, modest, occurring in only 10 to 15% of patients, whereas tumor stabilization is reported

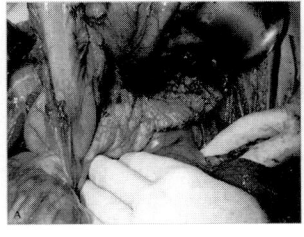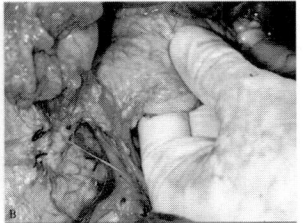

Figure 11 *A,* Mobilization of the body and tail of the pancreas along the inferior aspect of the pancreas allows for *B,* bimanual palpation of the gland.

to in 40 to 60%.[5] Interferon 3 to 5 million units subcutaneously 3 times weekly is tolerated in most patients. Side effects include flu-like symptoms, arthralgias, and depression. The majority of these symptoms can be counteracted with NSAIDs. The combination of SA and IFN has shown promise when given in combination together, with tumor stabilization reported in 67% of patients.[39]

CHEMOTHERAPY

There are limited data regarding chemotherapy for NETPs, most studies are small, with a mix of carcinoid tumors and other NETs. Response rates vary between studies (30–70%).[39–41] Chemotherapy is generally reserved for patients with symptoms that are unresponsive to SA or IFN. Single-agent therapy has lower response rates (20%).[5] Generally, streptozocin is given with either doxorubicin or 5-flourouracil (5-FU), with response rates of 69% and 45%, respectively, and median survival is 2.2 years versus 1.4 years, respectively.[40] Unfortunately many of these responses are short lived (median 6 months), and many patients experience toxicity from the streptozocin, including renal failure, myelosuppression, and nausea.[5] Some authors reserve the use of chemotherapy for the poorly differentiated tumors, as they appear to have a better response rate than the well-differentiated NETs. At the present time, chemotherapy should be give under a study protocol if we are to learn the value and role for these patients in the future.

RADIOLABELED THERAPY

Radionuclide therapy is not a new concept in the treatment of endocrine tumors. It has been utilized since the 1940s for the treatment of thyroid carcinoma. The success of such therapy is dependent on a high target-to-background uptake ratio of the radioisotope and on the amount time that the radionuclide is retained within the tumor cells. mIBG is a guanethidine derivative, structurally similar to norepinephrine. mIBG localizes to adrenal-medullary tumors as well as many NETs. mIBG is transported into NETs by vesicular monoamine transport proteins. It has been shown that up to 70% of NETs and 12 to 35% of MTC will concentrate [131]I mIBG. Therapeutic doses of [131]I mIBG have been utilized in the treatment of metastases of pheochromocytomas, NETPs, and carcinoid tumors, demonstrating a modest tumor and biochemical response while providing symptomatic control.[42–44]

Octreotide is an 8-amino acid analogue of somatostatin. In a large series from Rotterdam, the percentage of tumor uptake with ^{111}In-octreotide was reported as high as 96% of carcinoid tumors, 71% of MTC, 61% of insulinomas, and 100% of the gastrinomas studied.[45] To date, several series have reported promising beneficial effects of ^{111}In-octreotide on clinical symptoms, hormone production, and tumor growth in NETs.[42]

With limited numbers of patients with these NETPs, it is difficult to know if a glucagonoma would respond differently to this type of therapy versus a VIPoma. When faced with disseminated disease that is resistant to the systemic therapies mentioned above, candidates with either mIBG or octreotide-avid tumors should be considered for radionuclide therapy (Figure 12). Although the numbers are small, our experience and those of others has been that radionuclide therapy can provide palliative benefit and improve one's perceived quality of life in patients with functioning disseminated NETPs, and there may prove to be a survival benefit in some patients.[42–44] At the present time, research is ongoing with the development of different ligands for these compounds in order to deliver a better therapeutic effect.

Summary

NETPs are a rare diverse group of tumors that require a multidisciplinary approach to their treatment. Clinical endocrinopathies will dictate the preoperative treatment. Correction of fluid and electrolyte abnormalities sometimes requires direct intervention with somatostatin analogues, bisphosphate, and ketoconazole. Surgical intervention remains the primary treatment not only for complete resection, but also for palliative cytoreduc-

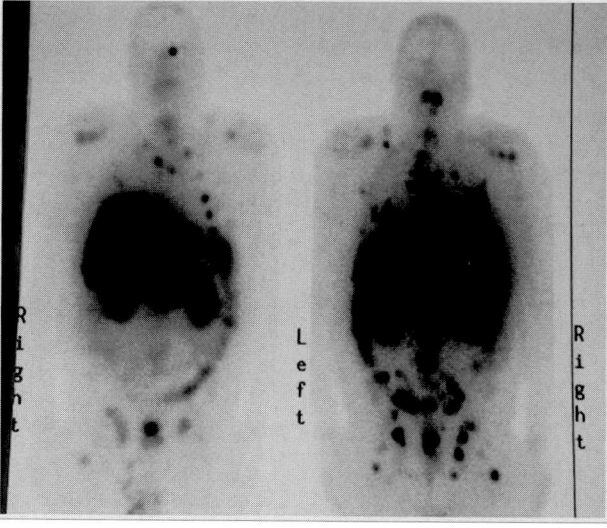

Figure 12 Disseminated glucagonoma treated with ^{111}In-octreotide therapy. Symptomatic improvement of his bone pain and diarrhea occurred for 7 months before progression and ultimate death.

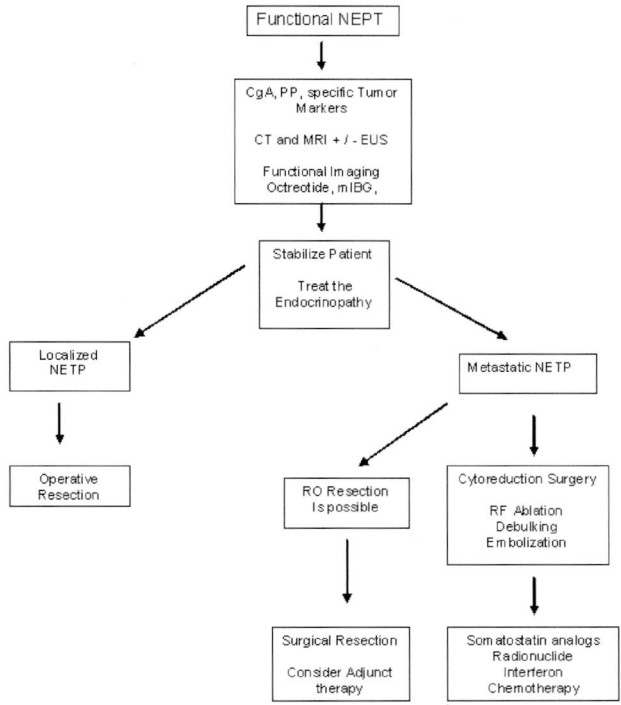

Figure 13 An algorithm of the work-up on functional neuroendocrine tumors of the pancreas (NETPs).

tion of metastatic disease. Even with complete resection, almost half of these tumors will recur and, therefore, in the future, adjuvant therapy may prove to be crucial. At the present time, palliative therapies include hormonal therapy, biotherapy, radionuclide therapy, and chemotherapy (Figure 13).

References

1. Welbourn RB, Friesen SR, Johnston IDA, Sellwood RA. History of endocrine surgery. New York: Praeger Publishers; 1990.

2. Chen H, Hardacre JM, Uzar A, et al. Isolated liver metastases from neuroendocrine tumors: does resection prolong survival? J Am Coll Surg 1998;187:88–93.

3. Kloppel G, Solcia E, Capella C, Heitz PU. Classification of neuroendocrine tumours. Ital J Gastroenterol Hepatol 1999;31 Suppl 2:111–6.

4. Pour PM, Schmied B. The link between exocrine pancreatic cancer and the endocrine pancreas. Int J Pancreatol 1999; 25:77–87.

5. Mansour JC, Chen H. Pancreatic endocrine tumors. J Surg Res 2004;120:139–61.

6. Schindl M, Kaczirek K, Kaserer K, Niederle B. Is the new classification of neuroendocrine pancreatic tumors of clinical help? World J Surg 2000;24:1312–8.

7. Solcia E, Kloppel G, Sobin LH. Typing of endocrine tumors. World Health Organization international histological classification of endocrine tumors. 2nd ed. New York: Springer; 2000.

8. Kaerlev L, Teglbjaerg PS, Sabroe S, et al. Occupational risk factors for small bowel carcinoid tumor: a European population-based case-control study. J Occup Environ Med 2002;44:516–22.

9. Hemminki K, Li X. Familial carcinoid tumors and subsequent cancers: a nation-wide epidemiologic study from Sweden. Int J Cancer 2001;94:444–8.

10. Hammel PR, Vilgrain V, Terris B, et al. Pancreatic involvement in von Hippel-Lindau disease. The Groupe Francophone d'Etude de la Maladie de von Hippel-Lindau. Gastroenterology 2000;119:1087–95.

11. Soga J, Yakuwa Y. Glucagonomas/diabetico-dermatogenic syndrome (DDS): a statistical evaluation of 407 reported cases. J Hepatobiliary Pancreat Surg 1998;5:312–9.

12. Becker SW, Kahn D, Rothman T. Cutaneous manifestations of internal malignant tumors. Arch Dermatol Syph 1942;45:1069–80.

13. Wilkinson DS. Necrolytic migratory erythema with carcinoma of the pancreas. Trans St Johns Hosp Dermatol Soc 1973;59:244–50.

14. Priest WM, Alexander MK. Islet cell tumour of the pancreas with peptic ulceration, diarrhoea, and hypokalaemia. Lancet 1957;273:1145–7.

15. Verner JV, Morrison AB. Islet cell tumor and a syndrome of refractory watery diarrhea and hypokalemia. Am J Med 1958;25:374–80.

16. Welbourn R. His, 1990.

17. Soga J, Yakuwa Y. Vipoma/diarrheogenic syndrome: a statistical evaluation of 241 reported cases. J Exp Clin Cancer Res 1998;17:389–400.

18. Soga J, Yakuwa Y. Somatostatinoma/inhibitory syndrome: a statistical evaluation of 173 reported cases as compared to other pancreatic endocrinomas. J Exp Clin Cancer Res 1999;18:13–22.

19. Proye C, Malvaux P, Pattou F, et al. Noninvasive imaging of insulinomas and gastrinomas with endoscopic ultrasonography and somatostatin receptor scintigraphy. Surgery 1998;124:1134–4.

20. Larsson LI, Schwartz T, Lundqvist G, et al. Occurrence of human pancreatic polypeptide in pancreatic endocrine tumors. Possible implication in the watery diarrhea syndrome. Am J Pathol 1976;85:675–84.

21. Adrian TE, Uttenthal LO, Williams SJ, Bloom SR. Secretion of pancreatic polypeptide in patients with pancreatic endocrine tumors. N Engl J Med 1986;315:287–91.

22. Pasieka JL, Hershfield N. Pancreatic polypeptide hyperplasia causing watery diarrhea syndrome: a case report. Can J Surg 1999;42:55–8.

23. Mao C, el Attar A, Domenico DR, et al. Carcinoid tumors of the pancreas. Status report based on two cases and review of the world's literature. Int J Pancreatol 1998;23: 153–64.

24. Rosewicz S, Detjen K, Scholz A, von Marschall Z. Interferon-alpha: regulatory effects on cell cycle and angiogenesis. Neuroendocrinology 2004;80 Suppl 1:85–93.

25. Becker M, Aron DC. Ectopic ACTH syndrome and CRH-mediated Cushing's syndrome. Endocrinol Metab Clin North Am 1994;23:585–606.

26. Kaneko Y, Motoi N, Matsui A, et al. Neuroendocrine tumors of the liver and pancreas associated with elevated serum prostatic acid phosphatase. Intern Med 1995;34: 886–91.

27. Jordan PH Jr. A personal experience with pancreatic and duodenal neuroendocrine tumors. J Am Coll Surg 1999; 189:470–82.

28. Angeli E, Vanzulli A, Castrucci M, et al. Value of abdominal sonography and MR imaging at 0.5 T in preoperative detection of pancreatic insulinoma: a comparison with dynamic CT and angiography. Abdom Imaging 1997;22:295–303.

29. Boukhman MP, Karam JM, Shaver J, et al. Localization of insulinomas. Arch Surg 1999;134:818–3.

30. Gibril F, Reynolds JC, Chen CC, et al. Specificity of somatostatin receptor scintigraphy: a prospective study and effects of false-positive localizations on management in patients with gastrinomas. J Nucl Med 1999;40:539–53.

31. Gibril F, Reynolds JC, Doppman JL, et al. Somatostatin receptor scintigraphy: its sensitivity compared with that of other imaging methods in detecting primary and metastatic gastrinomas. A prospective study. Ann Intern Med 1996; 125:26–34.

32. Scherubl H, Bader M, Fett U, et al. Somatostatin-receptor imaging of neuroendocrine gastroenteropancreatic tumors. Gastroenterology 1993;105:1705–9.

33. Sundin A, Eriksson B, Bergstrom M, et al. PET in the diagnosis of neuroendocrine tumors. Ann N Y Acad Sci 2004;1014:246–57.

34. Strasberg SM, Linehan D. Radiofrequency ablation of liver tumors. Curr Probl Surg 2003;40:459–98.

35. Galandi D, Antes G. Radiofrequency thermal ablation versus other interventions for hepatocellular carcinoma. Cochrane Database Syst Rev 2002;(3):CD003046.

36. Pape UF, Bohmig M, Berndt U, et al. Survival and clinical outcome of patients with neuroendocrine tumors of the gastroenteropancreatic tract in a german referral center. Ann N Y Acad Sci 2004;1014:222–33.

37. Chamberlain RS, Canes D, Brown KT, et al. Hepatic neuroendocrine metastases: does intervention alter outcomes? J Am Coll Surg 2000;190:432–45.

38. Sarmiento JM, Heywood G, Rubin J, et al. Surgical treatment of neuroendocrine metastases to the liver: a plea for resection to increase survival. J Am Coll Surg 2003;197: 29–37.

39. Oberg K. Diagnosis and treatment of carcinoid tumors. Expert Rev Anticancer Ther 2003;3:863–77.

40. Brentjens R, Saltz L. Islet cell tumors of the pancreas: the medical oncologist's perspective. Surg Clin North Am 2001;81:527–42.

41. Eriksson B, Oberg K. Neuroendocrine tumours of the pancreas. Br J Surg 2000;87:129–31.

42. Pasieka JL, McEwan AJ, Rorstad O. The palliative role of ^{131}I-MIBG and ^{111}In-octreotide therapy in patients with metastatic progressive neuroendocrine neoplasms. Surgery 2004;136:1218–26.

43. Sywak MS, Pasieka JL, McEwan A, et al. ^{131}I-meta-iodobenzylguanidine in the management of metastatic midgut carcinoid tumors. World J Surg 2004;28:1157–62.

44. Taal BG, Hoefnagel CA, Valdes Olmos RA, Boot H. Combined diagnostic imaging with ^{131}I-metaiodobenzyl-guanidine and ^{111}In-pentetreotide in carcinoid tumours. Eur J Cancer 1996;32A:1924–32.

45. Krenning EP, Kwekkeboom DJ, Bakker WH, et al. Somatostatin receptor scintigraphy with [^{111}In-DTPA-D-Phe1]- and [^{123}I-Tyr3]-octreotide: the Rotterdam experience with more than 1000 patients. Eur J Nucl Med 1993; 20:716–31.

CHAPTER 48

MANAGEMENT OF NONFUNCTIONAL ISLET CELL CARCINOMAS OF THE PANCREAS

JAMES C. YAO, MD

SANJAY GUPTA, MD

JEAN-NICOLAS VAUTHEY, MD

DOUGLAS B. EVANS, MD

Introduction

Islet cell carcinomas, sometimes referred to as pancreatic endocrine tumors or low-grade neuroendocrine tumors of the pancreas, are rare tumors that arise from neuroendocrine cells of the pancreas. According to the SEER 11 database, the incidence of islet cell carcinomas was 0.3 per 100,000 persons in 1999.[1] Because the nonfunctional variants of islet cell carcinoma are not associated with syndromes that produce bioactive amines and peptides, they often present insidiously. Although this cancer is sometimes diagnosed incidentally after laboratory abnormalities are detected, it frequently is not diagnosed until advanced. Occasionally, however, islet cell carcinomas present in a dramatic fashion. For example, tumors located in the head of the pancreas can present with biliary obstruction, and those located in the tail can cause splenic vein obstruction and present with massive upper gastrointestinal bleeding resulting from gastric varices.

Whereas most islet cell carcinomas occur sporadically, some can arise in the setting of multiple endocrine neoplasia type 1 or tuberous sclerosis. The tumors associated with these syndromes can be multifocal.

Pathology

The diagnosis of islet cell carcinoma is based on pathology. Microscopically, these neuroendocrine tumors of epithelial origin are well differentiated. The tumors cells are typically small and uniform in appearance, with round to oval regular nuclei.[2] Immunohistochemical markers, including synaptophysin, chromogranin, and CD56, are frequently used to diagnose islet cell carcinoma. Although staining for neuron-specific enolase is also usually positive, this marker is less specific and may be present in other tumors, such as solid-cystic tumors of the pancreas.[2] Islet cell carcinomas can also show positive staining for the epithelial maker cytokeratin. Additionally, although nonfunctional tumors generally do not produce elevated plasma hormone levels, specific peptides and amines related to cellular products, such as insulin, glucagon, pancreatic polypeptide, and vasoactive intestinal peptide, may be detected in their cancer cells by immunohistochemical analysis.

Low-grade tumors should have no more than 2 mitoses per 10 high power fields and a Ki-67 labeling index of less than 2%. Tumors with more than 2 mitoses per 10 high power fields are considered intermediate grade and therefore more aggressive. Poorly differentiated tumors with many mitoses and frequent central necrosis are considered high-grade neuroendocrine carcinomas. Their clinical and biologic behaviors are highly aggressive and similar to those of small cell carcinoma of the lung. Occasionally, it is not possible to classify tumor grade on the basis of a small specimen obtained by fine-needle aspiration. In such cases, a core needle biopsy is appropriate, if it can be performed safely.

Diagnostic Testing

The goal of diagnostic testing in patients with islet cell carcinoma is to establish the location and extent of the disease. In this regard, plasma markers can help in the long-term follow-up of patients. Nonfunctional islet cell carcinomas also frequently present as neuroendocrine carcinomas of unknown primary origin. In these cases, the identification of a primary pancreatic tumor is of particular clinical significance, as islet cell carcinomas are more likely to respond to streptozocin-based chemotherapy than are carcinoid tumors of the bowel.[3]

In addition to a routine history, a physical examination, and laboratory studies, we also recommend assessing tumor markers and performing detailed anatomic and functional imaging studies. Chromogranin A, neuron-specific enolase, and pancreatic polypeptide are all tumor markers that can be detected in the blood.

For precise imaging of the primary tumor and determination of its resectability, our current practice is to initially perform high-resolution multidetector, multiphasic computed tomography (CT) with a 2.5 mm slice thickness. Because islet cell carcinomas are often hypervascular, it is necessary to perform imaging at the peak of the arterial phase of the contrast enhancement. The detailed images thus obtained allow for the precise definition of the tumor location in relation to the superior mesenteric artery, the superior mesenteric vein (SMV), and the celiac axis. Magnetic resonance imaging (MRI) can also be helpful, especially in patients unable to receive iodinated contrast agents. In fact, a recent study comparing the relative effectiveness of CT, MRI, and somatostatin receptor scintigraphy for detecting liver metastases in patients with neuroendocrine tumors showed that MRI detected the greatest number of liver lesions. T2-weighted imaging may detect the most lesions when a contrast agent cannot be given. However, the optimal imaging method will likely depend on the specific clinical scenario and on the equipment, technique, and expertise of the individual institution.

Nuclear imaging is also frequently used in the diagnosis of neuroendocrine tumors. Diethylenetriaminepentaacetic acid-D-Phe10-[octreotide] (OctreoScan, St. Louis, MO), a ^{111}In-labeled somatostatin analogue, shares the receptor-binding profile of octreotide, and thus is a good agent for the imaging of tumors positive for somatostatin receptors 2 and 5.[4] The overall sensitivity of OctreoScan appears to be 80 to 90%.[4]

OctreoScan may also be effective in detecting occult lesions not apparent by conventional radiologic imaging techniques.[5,6]

An additional method for identifying the anatomic location of islet cell carcinomas is esophagogastroduodenoscopy with endoscopic ultrasonography. A visual inspection with this technique can identify invasion of the duodenum. The ultrasonography not only allows inspection of the tumor's relationship to the superior mesenteric artery and SMV, but also facilitates the identification of the lymph nodes. If warranted, tissue diagnosis can be achieved by CT-guided percutaneous needle biopsy or endoscopic ultrasound (EUS)-guided biopsy.

Management of Locoregional Disease

In general, complete surgical resection, when technically possible, is the treatment of choice for patients with low- or intermediate-grade nonfunctional islet cell carcinoma of the pancreas. In a retrospective series of 163 patients with nonfunctional islet cell carcinoma treated at The University of Texas M. D. Anderson Cancer Center, patients with localized resectable disease had longer overall survival durations than did those with locally advanced disease (median survival durations, 7.1 years versus 5.2 years, $P = 0.04$).[7] We thus advocate surgery to achieve complete margin-negative resection whenever possible. Occasionally, this may require the resection of the SMV or the SMV and portal vein confluence, with graft reconstruction. In patients with arterial encasement, successful resection may require upper abdominal exenteration. Because of the morbidity and mortality associated with this procedure, however, it is rarely performed.

In patients with bulky tumors that are considered borderline for resectability, we frequently initiate induction systemic therapy with the aim of reducing the tumor bulk, thereby allowing some of the tumors to become resectable. During this treatment, we can assess whether a tumor has a favorable biology that makes it suitable for resection, thus sparing those patients with rapidly progressive or occult metastatic disease from unnecessary surgical morbidity.

We generally do not advocate immediate resection of high-grade neuroendocrine carcinoma of the pancreas. As with small cell carcinoma of the lung, these tumors are aggressive, are fast growing, and rapidly metastasize. In addition, the systemic relapse rate is high after resection of the local disease. Therefore, we frequently treat affected patients with systemic chemotherapy before resection.

The resection of primary islet cell carcinomas in patients with known metastatic disease is more controversial, and randomized data in this area are lacking. In general, we recommend complete resection of the primary tumor if all metastases can also be resected. Resection can also be considered in patients with relatively indolent systemic disease that is clearly symptomatic from the primary tumor. A common example of this is recurrent variceal bleeding from the tail of the pancreas caused by islet cells obstructing the splenic vein. A partial pancreatectomy and splenectomy can help control the variceal bleeding.

Management of Advanced Disease

SYSTEMIC CHEMOTHERAPY

There is considerable controversy over the role of systemic chemotherapy in the management of advanced islet cell carcinoma. However, several agents have already shown single-agent activity when used in chemotherapy trials. Chemotherapy agents with known activity in islet cell carcinoma include streptozocin, doxorubincin, and dacarbazine.

The activity of streptozocin in islet cell carcinoma was first reported in 1973 by Broder and Carter.[8] They treated 52 patients who had islet cell carcinoma with streptozocin and observed a response rate of 50%. Similarly, Moertel and colleagues treated 42 patients who had islet cell carcinoma with single-agent streptozocin in 1 arm of a randomized trial;[9] they observed a response rate of 36%. Doxorubicin similarly induced responses in 4 of 20 patients (20%) in a single-arm phase II trial.[10] Dacarbazine was also studied in a phase II trial that included 42 patients with islet cell carcinoma, and a 33% response rate was observed.[11] Chlorozotocin likewise demonstrated clinical activity in 2 single-agent clinical trials,[12,13] but this drug is not currently commercially available. Finally, temozolomide, a new orally administered imidazole tetrazinone, appears promising in the management of islet cell carcinoma.[13]

The combinations of 5-fluorouracil plus streptozocin and 5-fluorouracil plus doxorubicin have achieved response rates ranging from 27 to 69%.[9,14–17] However, in a retrospective study of 16 patients with islet cell carcinoma who received streptozocin and doxorubicin at Memorial Sloan-Kettering Cancer Center, only 1 response (6%) was observed.[18] Similarly, a retrospective review of 16 patients treated with streptozocin and doxorubicin at the Dana Faber Cancer Institute found only 1 objective response (6%).[19] Studies of triplet chemotherapy consisting of all 3 drugs have found response rates of 40% and 55% in 2 small series.[20,21] At

M. D. Anderson, we recently reviewed the records of 84 consecutive patients with islet cell carcinoma treated with fluorouracil, doxorubicin, and streptozocin (Table 1).[3] Using the criteria proposed by the Response Evaluation Criteria in Solid Tumors Committee (RECIST), we observed a response rate of 39%. The 2-year progression-free survival rate was 41%, and the 2-year overall survival rate was 74%.

BIOLOGIC THERAPY

Although octreotide is effective in reducing the hormonal output of functional islet cell carcinomas, its role in nonfunctional islet cell carcinoma is less well defined. Although there have been anecdotal reports of tumor shrinkage in patients with neuroendocrine carcinoma, a large series showed that octreotide caused tumor shrinkage in only 2 to 3% of patients.[22] The stabilization of growing neuroendocrine tumors with octreotide has also been shown.[23,24] However, definitive randomized trials are lacking.

Interferon also shows antitumor activity in pancreatic endocrine tumors. However, most clinical trials in patients with neuroendocrine carcinoma have included a mix of islet cell carcinomas and carcinoid tumors, so its effectiveness as a chemotherapeutic agent specifically for islet cell carcinomas is unknown.

HEPATIC ARTERY EMBOLIZATION OR CHEMOEMBOLIZATION

Although we believe that systemic chemotherapy has a major role in the management of nonfunctional islet cell carcinoma, most patients eventually become resistant to the therapy. Among patients with advanced disease, liver is the most common site of metastasis.

Although systemic chemotherapy has a major role in the management of nonfunctional islet cell carcinoma, most cases eventually become resistant to therapy. Liver is one of the most common sites of metastasis. Liver metastases from islet cell tumors derive more than 80% of their blood supply primarily from the hepatic artery.

Table 1 Chemotherapy Regimens for Islet Cell Carcinoma

5-fluorouracil, streptozocin, and doxorubicin – 28-day cycle
  5-fluorouracil 400 mg/m^2/day IV bolus days 1–5
  Streptozocin 400 mg/m^2/day IV days 1–5
  Doxorubicin 40 mg/m^2 on day 1 only
5-fluorouracil, and streptozocin – 42-day cycle
  5-fluorouracil 400 mg/m^2/day IV bolus days 1–5
  Streptozocin 500 mg/m^2/day IV days 1–5
Streptozocin and doxorubicin – 42-day cycle
  Streptozocin 500 mg/m^2/day IV days 1–4
  Doxorubicin 50 mg/m^2 on days 1 and 22

This feature, combined with the fact that the liver has a dual vascular supply, provides a good rationale for inducing tumor ischemia and necrosis by occluding the hepatic arterial supply to the tumor. Early studies of vascular occlusion involved surgical ligation of the common hepatic artery or embolization of the common hepatic artery. Despite early successes, responses were usually short lived because of collateral formation. Hence peripheral hepatic artery embolization (HAE) with gelfoam or polyvinyl alcohol particles using percutaneous interventional radiologic techniques has become the preferred method. Because hepatic metastases derive most of their blood supply from the hepatic artery, regional delivery of chemotherapy offers pharmacokinetic advantages over systemic administration. This has prompted many investigators to use hepatic arterial chemoembolization (HACE), which combines embolization and intra-arterial delivery of chemotherapy. Such an approach creates ischemia, slows the transit, and increases the contact time between the chemotherapy and the tumor cells. Several reports have documented that such an approach can palliate symptoms and reduce the tumor burden in many patients with hepatic metastases from neuroendocrine tumors.

Most trials of HAE and HACE have included a mix of carcinoid and islet cell carcinoma. Small studies using blend bland hepatic artery embolization have reported tumor responses of 17 to 87%.[25–27] Those using chemoembolization or intra-arterial chemotherapy in addition to embolization have reported tumor response rates from 8 to 60%.[28–34] At the current time there are no data from randomized trials to evaluate whether chemoemboliz/tion is superior to particulate embolization alone. Our experience (unpublished data) suggests that patients with islet cell tumors with metastases to liver seem to benefit from the addition of intra-arterial chemotherapy to embolization. Patients treated with HACE had a prolonged overall survival (31.5 vs 18.2 months) and improved response (50% vs 25%) compared with patients treated with HAE, although the differences did not reach statistical significance.

HEPATIC RESECTION

Because of the relatively indolent nature of low-grade neuroendocrine carcinomas, some investigators have advocated the resection of limited liver metastases. Most studies on this topic have included both carcinoid tumors and islet cell carcinomas. However, islet cell carcinomas may be more aggressive than carcinoid tumors. In 1 series, for example, 31 patients with low-grade neuroendocrine carcinomas underwent resection of their liver metastases;[35] patients with islet cell carcinomas had inferior survival durations (median,

< 2 years) compared with the survival durations of patients with carcinoid tumors (median, > 5 years).

As mentioned earlier, our approach to liver metastases in patients with islet cell carcinoma is to resect solitary metastases. In patients with more numerous but potentially resectable liver lesions, we typically analyze the biology of the disease before making a decision about liver surgery. Systemic chemotherapy can be given before the decision is made, and surgery can be ruled out in patients with aggressive tumors destined to spread or recur quickly after a major resection.

EMERGING NOVEL THERAPEUTIC APPROACHES

Although islet cell carcinoma is generally thought to be fairly resistant to many cytotoxic chemotherapeutic agents, substantial clinical activity has been observed with streptozocin-based therapy. Regarding future therapy, a number of novel therapeutic strategies are under development. For example, peptide receptor radiotherapy will take advantage of the presence of somatostatin receptors on low-grade neuroendocrine carcinomas. Compounds using indium-111, yttrium-90, and lutetium-177 attached to somatostatin analogues have been designed, and some have been studied in clinical trials. Only limited clinical activity has been observed with the indium- and yttrium-based compounds. Lutetium-177 octreotide is currently in development and has been shown to improve the quality of life of patients with gastroenteropancreatic tumors.[36]

The introduction of novel molecularly targeted therapeutics into clinical use has generated renewed interest and research activity in the treatment of neuroendocrine carcinomas. For example, because low-grade neuroendocrine carcinomas are vascular tumors, therapeutic strategies targeting vascular endothelial growth factor (VEGF) signaling are under development. At M. D. Anderson, we conducted a phase II study comparing low-dose peginterferon alfa-2b and bevacizumab, which is a humanized monoclonal antibody targeting VEGF-A. All patients also received octreotide. A significant improvement in the progression-free survival rate at week 18 was observed in the bevacizumab arm (96% vs 68%, $P = 0.02$).[37] In a separate multicenter trial, investigators studied the effects of SU11248, an inhibitor of VEGF and platelet-derived growth factor receptor tyrosine kinases, in patients with carcinoid tumors and islet cell carcinomas; they found a higher response rate in the patients with islet cell carcinomas.[38] These studies showed that strategies targeting VEGF signaling are promising. However, larger confirmatory trials are needed.

In conclusion, continued development of novel targeted therapeutic strategies and improvements in our understanding of the molecular biology of cancer are needed to further advance the treatment of islet cell carcinoma.

References

1. Talamonti M, Stuart K, Yao JC. Neuroendocrine tumors of the gastrointestinal tract: how aggressive should we be? In: Perry M (ed): American society of clinical oncology 2004 education book. Alexandria: American Society of Clinical Oncology, 2004, 206–15.

2. Capella C, Heitz PU, Hofler H, et al. Revised classification of neuroendocrine tumors of the lung, pancreas and gut. Digestion 1994;55:11–23.

3. Kouvaraki MA, Ajani JA, Hoff P, et al. Fluorouracil, doxorubicin, and streptozocin in the treatment of patients with locally advanced and metastatic pancreatic endocrine carcinomas. J Clin Oncol 2004;22:4762–71.

4. Krenning EP, Kooij PPM, Bakker WH, et al. Radiotherapy with a radiolabeled somatostatin analogue, [111 In-DTPA-D-Phe 1]-octreotide. Ann NY Acad Sci 1994;733:496–506.

5. Westlin JE, Janson ET, Arnberg H, et al. Somatostatin receptor scintigraphy of carcinoid tumours using the [111 In-DTPA-D-Phe 1]-octreotide. Acta Oncol 1993;32:783–6.

6. Shi W, Johnston CF, Buchanan KD, et al. Localization of neuroendocrine tumours with [111 In] DTPA-octreotide scintigraphy (Octreoscan): a comparative study with CT and MRs imaging. QJM 1998;91:295–301.

7. Solorzano CC, Lee JE, Pisters PW, et al. Nonfunctioning islet cell carcinoma of the pancreas: survival results in a contemporary series of 163 patients. Surgery 2001;130:1078–85.

8. Broder LE, Carter SK. Pancreatic islet cell carcinoma. II. Results of therapy with streptozotocin in 52 patients. Ann Intern Med 1973;79:108–18.

9. Moertel CG, Hanley JA, Johnson LA. Streptozocin alone compared with streptozocin plus fluorouracil in the treatment of advanced islet-cell carcinoma. N Engl J Med 1980;303:1189–94.

10. Moertel CG, Lavin PT, Hahn RG. Phase II trial of doxorubicin therapy for advanced islet cell carcinoma. Cancer Treat Rep 1982;66:1567–9.

11. Ramanathan RK, Cnaan A, Hahn RG, et al. Phase II trial of dacarbazine (DTIC) in advanced pancreatic islet cell carcinoma. Study of the Eastern Cooperative Oncology Group-E6282. Ann Oncol 2001;12:1139–43.

12. Bukowski RM, McCracken JD, Balcerzak SP, Fabian CJ. Phase II study of chlorozotocin in islet cell carcinoma. A Southwest Oncology Group study. Cancer Chemother Pharmacol 1983;11:48–50.

13. Fine R, Fogelman D, Schreibman S. Effective treatment of neuroendocrine tumors with temozolomide and capecitabine. J Clin Oncol 2005;23:361s.

14. Chernicoff D, Bukowski RM, Groppe CW Jr. Hewlett JS. Combination chemotherapy for islet cell carcinoma and metastatic carcinoid tumors with 5-fluorouracil and streptozotocin. Cancer Treat Rep 1979;63:795–6.

15. Moertel CG, Lefkopoulo M, Lipsitz S, et al. Streptozocin-doxorubicin, streptozocin-fluorouracil or chlorozotocin in the treatment of advanced islet-cell carcinoma.[comment]. N Engl J Med 1992;326:519–23.

16. Eriksson B, Oberg K. An update of the medical treatment of malignant endocrine pancreatic tumors. Acta Oncol 1993;32:203–8.

17. Eriksson B, Skogseid B, Lundqvist G, et al. Medical treatment and long-term survival in a prospective study of 84 patients with endocrine pancreatic tumors. Cancer 1990;65:1883–90.

18. Cheng PN, Saltz LB. Failure to confirm major objective antitumor activity for streptozocin and doxorubicin in the treatment of patients with advanced islet cell carcinoma. Cancer 1999;86:944–8.

19. McCollum AD, Kulke MH, Ryan DP, et al. Lack of efficacy of streptozocin and doxorubicin in patients with advanced pancreatic endocrine tumors. Am J Clin Oncol 2004;27:485–8.

20. von Schrenck T, Howard JM, Doppman JL, et al. Prospective study of chemotherapy in patients with metastatic gastrinoma. Gastroenterology 1988;94:1326–34.

21. Rivera E, Ajani JA. Doxorubicin, streptozocin, and 5-fluorouracil chemotherapy for patients with metastatic islet-cell carcinoma. Am J Clin Oncol 1998;21:36–8.

22. Schnirer II, Yao JC, Ajani JA. Carcinoid: a comprehensive review. Acta Oncol 2003;42:672–92.

23. Arnold R, Trautmann ME, Creutzfeldt W, et al. Somatostatin analogue octreotide and inhibition of tumour growth in metastatic endocrine gastroenteropancreatic tumours. Gut 1996;38:430–8.

24. Saltz L, Trochanowski B, Buckley M, et al. Octreotide as an antineoplastic agent in the treatment of functional and nonfunctional neuroendocrine tumors. Cancer 1993;72:244–8.

25. Carrasco CH, Charnsangavej C, Ajani J, et al. The carcinoid syndrome: palliation by hepatic artery embolization. AJR Am J Roentgenol 1986;147:149–54.

26. Nobin A, Mansson B, Lunderquist A. Evaluation of temporary liver dearterialization and embolization in patients with metastatic carcinoid tumour. Acta Oncol 1989;28:419–24.

27. Eriksson BK, Larsson EG, Skogseid BM, et al. Liver embolizations of patients with malignant neuroendocrine gastrointestinal tumors. Cancer 1998;83:2293–301.

28. Ruszniewski P, Rougier P, Roche A, et al. Hepatic arterial chemoembolization in patients with liver metastases of endocrine tumors. A prospective phase II study in 24 patients. Cancer 1993;71:2624–30.

29. Therasse E, Breittmayer F, Roche A, et al. Transcatheter chemoembolization of progressive carcinoid liver metastasis. Radiology 1993;189:541–7.

30. Perry LJ, Stuart K, Stokes KR, Clouse ME. Hepatic arterial chemoembolization for metastatic neuroendocrine tumors. Surgery 1994;116:1111–7.

31. Diaco DS, Hajarizadeh H, Mueller CR, et al. Treatment of metastatic carcinoid tumors using multimodality therapy of octreotide acetate, intra-arterial chemotherapy, and hepatic arterial chemoembolization. Am J Surg 1995;169: 523–8.

32. Drougas JG, Anthony LB, Blair TK, et al. Hepatic artery chemoembolization for management of patients with advanced metastatic carcinoid tumors. Am J Surg 1998; 175:408–12.

33. Diamandidou E, Ajani JA, Yang DJ, et al. Two-phase study of hepatic artery vascular occlusion with microencapsulated cisplatin in patients with liver metastases from neuroendocrine tumors. AJR Am J Roentgenol 1998;170: 339–44.

34. Kim YH, Ajani JA, Carrasco CH, et al. Selective hepatic arterial chemoembolization for liver metastases in patients with carcinoid tumor or islet cell carcinoma. Cancer Invest 1999;17:474–78.

35. Nave H, Mossinger E, Feist H, et al. Surgery as primary treatment in patients with liver metastases from carcinoid tumors: a retrospective, unicentric study over 13 years. Surgery 2001;129:170–5.

36. Teunissen JJ, Kwekkeboom DJ, Krenning EP. Quality of life in patients with gastroenteropancreatic tumors treated with [177Lu-DOTA0,TYR3]octreotate. J Clin Oncol 2004;22: 2724–9.

37. Yao JC, Ng C, Hoff PM, et al. Improved progression free survival (PFS), and rapid, sustained decrease in tumor perfusion among patients with advanced carcinoid treated with bevacizumab. J Clin Oncol 2005;23:309s.

38. Kulke MH, Lenz HJ, Meropol NJ, et al. A phase 2 study to evaluate the efficacy and safety of SU11248 in patients (pts) with unresectable neuroendocrine tumors (NETs). J Clin Oncol 2005;23:310s.

CHAPTER 49

THE SURGICAL TREATMENT OF MEN-1

MARIA A. KOUVARAKI, MD

NANCY D. PERRIER, MD

THEREASA A. RICH, MS

JEFFREY E. LEE, MD

DOUGLAS B. EVANS, MD

Introduction

Multiple endocrine neoplasia type 1(MEN-1) is a hereditary disease transmitted in an autosomal dominant pattern with more than 95% penetrance of at least 1 clinical manifestation by age 40. Its prevalence is estimated to be between 2 and 20 per 100,000 individuals. MEN-1 was first described in 1954 by Wermer as "adenomatosis of endocrine glands," affecting several members of a family in 2 consecutive generations. Wermer was the first to propose a genetic basis for the disease. Affected individuals inherit a mutated *MEN1* allele, and inactivation of the remaining *MEN1* allele through a spontaneous somatic mutation results in tumor development in specific tissues. More than 350 germline mutations have been reported in this gene, which are distributed throughout exons 2 through 10 as well as in splice sites within the noncoding introns.

Patients with MEN-1 develop various combinations of functioning and nonfunctioning tumors of the parathyroid glands (90–97%), pancreatic islet cells and duodenum (30–80%), and the anterior pituitary gland (20–65%). A wide spectrum of tumors including adrenal tumors (5–41%), foregut carcinoid tumors (2–8%), thyroid neoplasms (8–27%), meningiomas (8%), ependymoma (1%), malignant melanoma (0.5%), and testicular teratoma (0.5%) are also seen in MEN-1 patients. Lipomas, facial angiofibromas, and collagenomas are common. Endocrine tumors associated with MEN-1 usually become clinically evident in late adolescence or young adulthood.

The most common clinical manifestations of MEN-1 are caused by functional effects of hormone hypersecretion, such as hypercalcemia (hyperparathyroidism [HPT]), ulcer diathesis (hypergastrinemia), or hypoglycemia (insulinoma). Primary hyperparathyroidism (PHPT) is usually the first clinical manifestation of the syndrome, typically appearing between the ages of 20 and 25 years, but sometimes as late as the fifth decade of life. HPT may occur in up to 97% of affected individuals. In addition, HPT is present in most asymptomatic gene carriers and is often synchronously diagnosed in MEN-1 patients who present with other clinical manifestations of the disease. Pancreatic islet cell neoplasms are the second most common manifestation of MEN-1, and these tumors, when functioning, may secrete various hormones, including gastrin, insulin, glucagon, somatostatin, and pancreatic polypeptide (PP). Among the functioning tumors, gastrinomas are the most common and account for up to 60% of functioning pancreatic tumors in MEN-1. Insulinomas are the next most frequent functional pancreatic tumor, accounting for 10 to 33% of all MEN-1-associated hormonally active pancreatic tumors. Insulinomas are more common in patients of younger age (< 40 years), whereas gastrinomas and somatostatinomas typically occur in older patients (> 40 years).

Complications from hypercalcemia and peptic ulcer disease rarely cause death in patients with MEN-1 syndrome today, owing to the development of proton pump inhibitors. Progressive metastatic neuroendocrine pancreatic carcinoma now represents the greatest health risk to patients with MEN-1 and is currently the major cause of disease-specific mortality in these patients. Up to 50% of MEN-1 patients with malignant pancreatic neoplasms will develop liver metastasis. In addition, most MEN-1-related carcinoids (thymic and bronchial) are malignant and represent the second leading cause of MEN-1-related death. This chapter reviews the available data necessary to develop an appropriate surgical strategy for patients with MEN-1-associated neoplasms.

Genetic Testing and Counseling Issues in MEN-1

Genetic testing for MEN-1 is currently available through several commercial laboratories in the United States and can be an extremely useful tool in identifying individuals affected with MEN-1. Genetic testing should be preceded by thorough counseling regarding the benefits, risks, limitations, and alternatives to genetic testing (Table 1), as well as the natural history and medical management of MEN-1. The genetic counselor reviews cancer genetics and autosomal dominant inheritance; likelihood of a positive result; cost; insurance and employment discrimination issues; and reproductive, familial, and psychosocial implications.

Although consensus guidelines for MEN-1 genetic testing are still being developed, compelling reasons to consider genetic testing include but are not limited to (1) confirmation of a clinical diagnosis, (2) confirmation or reduction of suspicion of MEN-1 in individuals with an atypical presentation of MEN-1, and (3) discrimination between affected and unaffected relatives of a known mutation carrier to determine necessity of clinical screening.

Sequencing of the coding exons (exons 2 through 9) identifies mutations in 75 to 90% of patients with a clinical diagnosis of MEN-1 (involvement of 2 or more principle endocrine glands: parathyroid, pituitary, and pancreas). Detection rates vary depending on the techniques used and the experience of individual laboratories. Detection rates are also lower for simplex cases (single occurrence of MEN-1 in a family) than familial cases, which may, in part, be due to somatic mosaicism in some simplex cases. Therefore, a significant proportion of individuals with clinical evidence of MEN-1 will not have an identifiable mutation, and, importantly, a negative genetic test does *not* necessarily rule out a diagnosis of MEN-1. Genetic testing of at-risk relatives in these cases is not useful for discriminating affected from unaffected individuals. Recommendations for appropriate clinical follow-up are controversial. Occasionally, genetic testing may reveal a variant of uncertain significance, which would require testing additional affected and unaffected family members to aid in distinguishing benign polymorphisms from disease-causing mutations.

For those families in which a mutation is identified, presymptomatic genetic testing can identify affected individuals before the disease is clinically manifested as well as identify unaffected individuals in which MEN-1 screening is not necessary. Genetic testing of at-risk relatives should be performed by the same laboratory that identified the mutation in the family's index case. The benefits of earlier diagnosis and screening must be considered in light of the lack of consensus on prophylactic intervention and the inability to predict the clinical pattern of future disease. Genetic testing of asymptomatic minors raises particular concern in that minors, in general, are not able to give true informed consent for genetic testing. We currently recommend

Table 1 Benefits, Risks, and Limitations of Genetic Testing for MEN-1

Benefits	Risks	Limitations
• Confirmation of diagnosis	• Potential risk for health insurance/ employment discrimination	• Detection rate significantly less than 100%
		• No genotype-phenotype correlations
• Early screening for tumors	• Psychological (anxiety, depression, fear, blame, guilt, reproductive anxiety etc)	• Inability to predict disease course
		• Lack of proven mechanisms for cure/prevention
• Risk assessment for relatives	• Laboratory error in reporting results	• Potential for uncertain result (variants of uncertain significance)
• Exclude diagnosis for at-risk members of an affected family	• Financial cost (if not covered by insurance)	
• Psychological counseling (reduce anxiety of the uncertain)		

that at-risk relatives consider presymptomatic genetic analysis at an age when MEN-1 manifestations typically first appear (ie, late adolescence or early adulthood) or when the patient develops the maturity to participate in the informed consent process.[1] In lieu of genetic testing, at-risk relatives should be clinically screened for associated individual neoplasms.

Clinical Screening in MEN-1

Screening in the Affected Patient with MEN-1

Continued tumor surveillance for MEN-1-related neoplasms is recommended for all MEN-1 patients. It is reasonable for asymptomatic at-risk MEN-1 patients (confirmed to be affected through genetic testing) to undergo a complete physical examination and routine biochemical screening (serum levels of prolactin, calcium, phosphorus, intact parathyroid hormone, PP, chromogranin A (CgA), gastrin, and glucagon) and imaging studies (computed tomography [CT] of chest and abdomen) at an interval appropriate for the patient's age and kindred-associated risk. Currently, no specific guidelines exist for the frequency of abdominal imaging in patients with MEN-1. In patients at high risk for the development of islet cell tumors (by family history), we currently recommend abdominal imaging (CT or magnetic resonance imaging [MRI]) every 1 to 2 years beginning at age 20 or earlier if islet cell carcinoma has been diagnosed at an earlier age within the patient's family. The frequency of abdominal imaging is also based on the aggressiveness of the tumor in the individual kindred. We currently perform endoscopic ultrasound (EUS) for pancreatic endocrine tumors (PETs) only in MEN-1 patients in whom a tumor is seen on screening CT or MRI. CT and MRI are noninvasive and clearly the tests of choice for pancreatic imaging in at-risk MEN-1 patients.

Patients who have been surgically treated for an MEN-1-associated PET should undergo postoperative abdominal imaging at approximately 6 months after resection to create a baseline for further follow-up imaging. Long-term surveillance of these patients, according to National Comprehensive Cancer Network guidelines, should include physical examination and assessment of biochemical tumor markers every 6 months for the first 3 years and annually after year 4.[2] At The University of Texas M. D. Anderson Cancer Center, we advocate abdominal CT or MRI and chest CT every 12 to 24 months based on risk factor assessment to include the patient's personal and family history.

Screening in the Healthy Relative at Risk for MEN-1

The frequency of diagnostic evaluations and the exact tests that should be performed in relatives at risk for MEN-1 (based on the presence of an established family history without genetic confirmation in the proband or the patient in question) are not clearly defined. Diagnostic screening of kindred members with MEN-1 syndrome leads to earlier tumor detection by approximately 2 decades. The aim of screening (both patients who are known to be affected and those relatives at risk for MEN-1) is to detect abnormalities at a presymptomatic stage, and thus to reduce morbidity and mortality resulting from identifying MEN-1-related malignancies at an advanced stage. We advocate yearly biochemical screening, including serum levels of prolactin, calcium, intact parathyroid hormone, fasting glucose, gastrin, PP, and CgA. In addition to biochemical screening, we recommend radiographic screening for PETs and carcinoid tumors to include CT or MRI of the abdomen and CT of the chest; the use and frequency of such imaging in patients of unknown MEN-1 status within an affected kindred are controversial, and clear recommendations are not available.

MEN-1-Related Neoplasms

1. PARATHYROID TUMORS

Natural History and Presentation

Asymmetric benign hyperplasia of all 4 parathyroid glands causing hypercalcemia owing to PHPT is the most prevalent (90–97%) and usually the first manifestation in MEN-1 patients, typically appearing between the ages of 20 and 25 years. MEN-1-associated HPT is often asymptomatic. However, when symptoms occur, they are similar to those seen in sporadic PHPT and include nephrolithiasis, fatigue, muscles weakness, bone mass abnormalities, and depression (along with other neuro-cognitive symptoms). PHPT in MEN-1 exhibits some differences from sporadic PHPT with respect to the age of onset (earlier in MEN-1), female to male ratio (1:1 in MEN-1 vs 3:1 in sporadic), parathyroid pathology (multiglandular disease vs singular adenoma in sporadic), and rates of recurrent HPT (higher in MEN-1, owing to the multigland involvement and the greater complexity of surgical treatment).

Treatment

Surgery is the only effective treatment for PHPT in patients with MEN-1. The timing and the extent of surgery remain controversial. Early parathyroidectomy in asymptomatic patients with elevated PTH levels and hypercalcemia who meet the NIH criteria may minimize lifetime exposure to HPT and thereby preserve bone mass.[3] In addition, surgery should not be delayed in patients with asymptomatic PHPT and concurrent Zollinger-Ellison syndrome (ZES). However, because of the high recurrence rate of MEN-1-associated HPT, the morbidity from neck reoperation, and the risk for postoperative permanent hypoparathyroidism, as well as the excellent medical management of hypergastrinemia in patients with ZES, the timing of parathyroid surgery in asymptomatic patients remains controversial. Careful assessment of end organ function, especially bone mineral density evaluation, is critically important in the decision to proceed with the initial operation as well as reoperation. In the asymptomatic patient with a mild elevation in serum calcium (less than 1 mg/dL above the upper limit of normal) the need for parathyroidectomy should be based on the findings from serial bone mineral density evaluations. Surgical options include subtotal parathyroidectomy (leaving 50 mg of the most normal gland in situ) and cryopreservation (Figure 1), or total parathyroidectomy, cryopreservation, and parathyroid autotransplantation in the nondominant forearm (Figure 2). In addition, transcervical thymectomy should always be performed at the initial operation because MEN-1 patients have a high incidence of supernumerary glands (which exist in ectopic locations) and are at risk to develop thymic carcinoid tumors.

The 2005 NCCN (National Comprehensive Cancer Network) guidelines suggest that MEN-1 patients with biochemical confirmation of PHPT should either undergo subtotal parathyroidectomy with cryopreservation and bilateral upper thymectomy, or total parathyroidectomy, cryopreservation, parathyroid autotransplantation in the nondominant forearm, and bilateral upper thymectomy. We currently recommend subtotal parathyroidectomy as the initial operation in patients with primary HPT in the setting of MEN-1.[4] We would not perform a forearm autograft at the initial operation, assuming a portion of 1 gland is clearly viable in situ. This avoids the complication of autograft hyperfunction and also avoids the need to determine whether recurrent HPT is secondary to the autograft in the forearm or the remaining parathyroid in the neck. If recurrent HPT develops after an initial subtotal parathyroidectomy, completion total parathyroidectomy is performed by removing the remaining parathyroid in the neck. At that time, forearm autografting is mandatory. The decision to proceed with reoperative completion total parathyroidectomy should be made with the knowledge that some autografts may take months to years to function, and

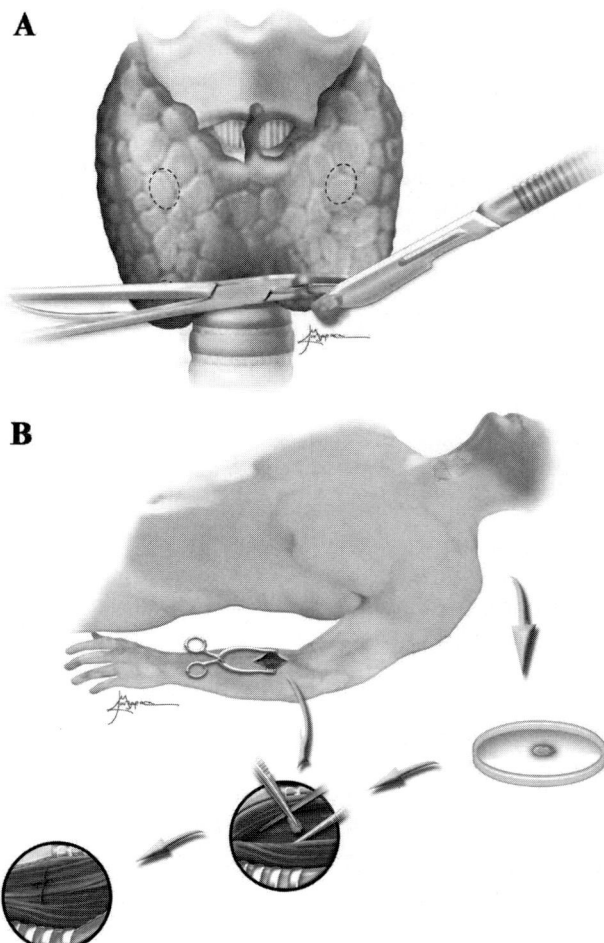

Figure 1 *A*, Illustrates a subtotal parathyroidectomy performed though a standard Kocher incision. After 3-gland removal, the lateralmost part of the fourth gland is divided with a scalpel across a large or medium size hemoclip, leaving in situ the gland's remnant along with its vascular pedicle. We prefer to preserve the most normal appearing parathyroid gland. If all of them are equally enlarged, we prefer to preserve a viable remnant of the inferior gland. *B*, One can see a parathyroid autotransplantation in the branchioradialis muscle of the nondominant arm, after the performance of a 4-gland paratyroidectomy. One of the parathyroids is immediately autotransplanted in the nondominant forearm and the rest is cryopreserved. A small 1–1.5 cm incision is performed longitudinally on the anterior surface of the forearm. A pouch is then created in the bracheoradialis muscle using a curved mosquito clamp. A small portion of parathyroid is minced in a Petri dish and then placed with forceps into a single muscle pouch. The pouch is closed with a prolene suture and a small metallic clip.

some may not function at all, resulting in permanent hypoparathyroidism and the need for long-term administration of calcium and vitamin D.

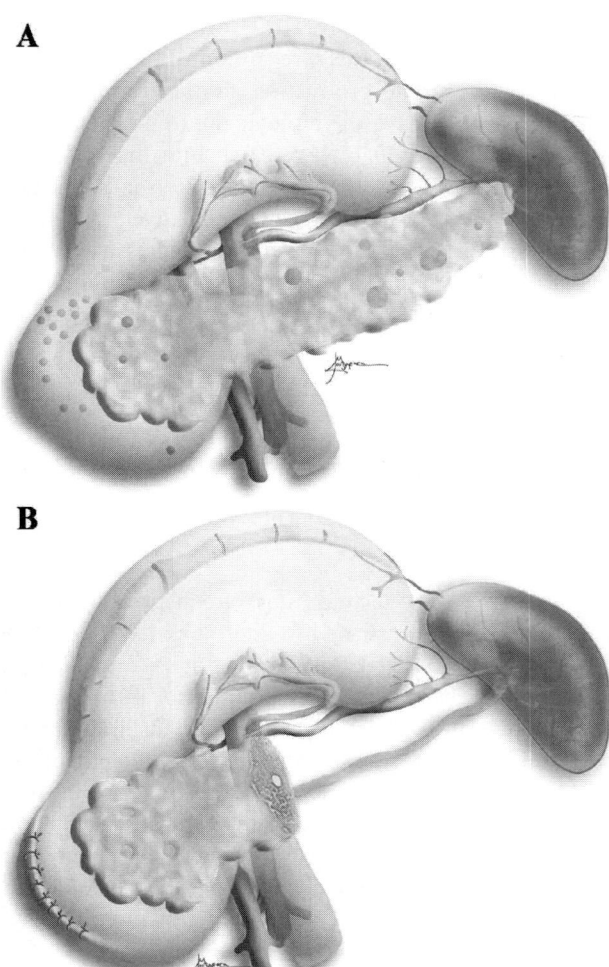

Figure 2 Illustration of selected aspects of the operative procedure for islet cell neoplasms in the setting of MEN-1 as described by Thompson, which consists of distal subtotal pancreatectomy, enucleation of islet cell neoplasms in the pancreatic head, and peripancreatic and portal lymphadenectomy (owing to the high frequency of regional lymph node metastases). *A*, One can see the possible distribution of multifocal small tumors extending to the surface of the pancreas, and within the duodenum. *B*, The distal pancreas has been separated from the splenic vessels and removed. The spleen is preserved whenever possible and the authors prefer to preserve the splenic artery and vein rather than attempt splenic preservation on just the short gastric vessels.

2. PANCREATIC ENDOCRINE TUMORS

The Natural History of Pancreatic Tumors in MEN-1

Pancreatic endocrine tumors in MEN-1 are often indolent, making natural history assessment difficult. Most patients with MEN-1 syndrome will develop islet cell hyperplasia or a discrete pancreatic neoplasm during their lifetime. Approximately 50% of MEN-1-associated pancreatic neoplasms are functional and produce clinical symptoms because of the hypersecretion of one or more pancreatic hormones such as gastrin and/or insulin. Nonfunctioning pancreatic neuroendocrine tumors are defined as those without clinical evidence of peptide hypersecretion. However, most clinically nonfunctioning pancreatic tumors are associated with some degree of elevation of one or more pancreatic hormones, such as PP. Patients with nonfunctioning tumors usually come to medical attention because of symptoms related to local tumor growth or metastases. Although immunohistochemical studies have been used to better characterize the cell of origin of various endocrine tumors of the pancreas in MEN-1 patients, the clinical syndrome caused by hormone hypersecretion is not necessarily associated with the immunohistochemical expression.

Gastrinoma

Gastrinoma is the most common functioning islet cell tumor associated with MEN-1. MEN-1-associated gastrinomas often occur within the gastrinoma triangle (pancreatic head and the first and second portions of the duodenum), and in contrast to sporadic gastrinomas, they can also occur in the body and tail of the pancreas and more distal duodenum.[5] Most of the duodenal tumors are small (often only 2–3 mm in diameter or less), multicentric, and located within the submucosal layer of the duodenum. Duodenal gastrinomas frequently coexist with other functioning and nonfunctioning neuroendocrine tumors located throughout the pancreas. Despite their small size, these tumors metastasize frequently (minimum of 40%) to the peripancreatic and periduodenal lymph nodes; however, liver metastases are much less common.[5–7] Interestingly, liver metastases from sporadic gastrinomas located in the duodenum (in contrast to the pancreas) are rare; however, less is known about the natural history of MEN-1-associated pancreatic and duodenal gastrinomas than their sporadic counterpart.[8]

In patients with sporadic gastrinoma, liver metastases may be more frequent in patients whose primary tumors are of increased size (> 3 cm), but it is not known whether such data can be applied to patients with MEN-1-associated gastrinoma.[8] Few studies (involving small numbers of patients) have attempted to correlate the size of the primary tumor with the incidence of synchronous or metachronous liver metastasis.[8] It is reasonable to assume that studies that correlate the size of the primary tumor with the presence of synchronous liver metastases overestimate the size of the primary tumor as there is no way to determine how long the metastases were present. In contrast, the report by Lowney and colleagues does not support a correlation between the size of the primary tumor and the risk of metastasis.[9] Clearly, the number of patients with MEN-1-related gastrinoma (or other neuroendocrine pancreatic tumors) are too small and their follow-up too brief to assess accurately a possible relationship between tumor size and malignant potential, especially with respect to the development of distant metastases to liver, lung, or bone. However, it is reasonable to assume that all MEN-1-associated PETs have malignant potential, and, therefore, a delay in diagnosis of the primary tumor in the pancreas would incur some level of increased risk for distant metastases.

We recently reviewed our experience with MEN-1-related PETs and found that patients with localized tumors at the time of diagnosis had a longer survival compared with those with synchronous distant metastatic disease (median, 19.5 years vs 3 years; $p < 0.0001$), a finding that was confirmed on multivariate analysis.[10] Patients who underwent surgical resection of their PETs had a longer survival than those who did not undergo PET resection (median, 22 years vs 5 years, $p = 0.0043$). Surgical resection of PETs was independently associated with improved survival in our multivariate analysis when including only patients with localized disease at diagnosis. Our data suggested that early surgical intervention for MEN-1-related PETs may delay PET recurrence and prevent or delay the development of distant metastatic disease. In addition, we showed that patients who underwent formal pancreatic resection as the first surgical procedure were free of disease significantly longer than those patients who underwent enucleation alone. This reflects the clinical observation that pancreatic disease in MEN-1 is a multifocal disease and enucleation alone will result in the need for reoperation.

Lymph node metastases do not appear to be a consistent marker of distant organ metastasis as occurs with other solid tumors, nor do they predict early mortality in patients with MEN-1.[8] Obviously, lymph node metastases can be detected only if lymph nodes are removed by the surgeon and histologically examined by the pathologist. Furthermore, published studies have probably underestimated the frequency of lymph node metastases because of the absence of uniform criteria for histologic sectioning of lymph nodes. Despite probable under-reporting, lymph node metastases are common in patients with MEN-1-related PETs, occurring in at least 39 to 55% of patients, and are thought to be even more common in patients with duodenal gastrinomas.[9,11,12] The uncertain biologic significance of lymph node metastases combined with inconsistencies in lymph node assessment justify the use of liver metastases (or other distant metastases) as the proper end point for studies examining the malignant potential of neuroendocrine

tumors in patients with MEN-1. However, currently, it is best to assume that all PETs, regardless of the presence or absence of hormone production or the immunohistochemical profile, have the biologic ability to metastasize to distant organs. Ongoing research into the molecular profiling of PETs may alter this conclusion in the future. Some investigators have suggested that liver metastases from gastrinomas tend to have a less aggressive natural history in MEN-1 patients compared with patients with sporadic gastrinomas.[13] However, Gibril and colleagues[14] suggested that there is a subset of MEN-1 patients with gastrinomas in which tumors exhibit aggressive growth. In summary, the results of these studies suggest that the natural history of MEN-1-associated PETs (nonfunctioning and gastrin-producing) remains poorly defined and unpredictable.

Insulinoma

Insulinoma is the second most frequent functioning pancreatic tumor, occurring in approximately 10 to 20% of patients with MEN-1. Insulinomas arise from the beta cells of the pancreas and may be multifocal throughout the pancreas. In contrast to gastrinomas, insulinomas are not found in the duodenum and are rarely malignant (9–20%).[15] However, within specific kindreds, insulin- and proinsulin-producing tumors can be highly malignant. When distant metastases occur, they are typically present in the liver. In approximately 10% of MEN-1-associated tumors, insulinoma may coexist with gastrinoma.[16]

Glucagonoma

Glucagonoma arises from alpha cells of the pancreatic islets and occurs in fewer than 3% of MEN-1 patients.[17] Notably, glucagonoma hypersecretion in patients with MEN-1 only rarely produces a clinical syndrome with the characteristic necrolytic migrating erythema, diabetes, weight loss, and normochromic, normocytic anemia. In most MEN-1 patients, glucagonoma-producing tumors are asymptomatic, especially when tumor size is small (< 3 cm), complicating the diagnosis. As such, a small glucagonoma is usually diagnosed as a clinically occult tumor found during the routine screening of an MEN-1 patient with abdominal imaging. Glucagonomas are located most frequently within the pancreatic tail and body, and when symptomatic, these tumors tend to be large, and the majority are malignant (50–80%).[17]

VIPomas

VIPomas arise from VIP secreting delta cells of the pancreas and are rare in patients with MEN-1. These tumors are almost exclusively located within the body and tail of the pancreas (90%) and are associated with significant malignant potential (66%).

Somatostatinomas

Somatostatinomas also arise from delta cells but are exceedingly rare in patients with MEN-1. Somatostatinomas may metastasize to the liver; however, the exact incidence of liver metastases is unknown because of the rarity of these neoplasms.

Pancreatic Polypeptidomas

Pancreatic polypeptidomas (PPomas) are commonly considered within the group of nonfunctioning PETs because hypersecretion of PP does not lead to a recognized clinical syndrome. PPomas are located most frequently in the pancreatic head but can be found anywhere within the pancreas. These tumors arise from F cells (or PP cells or delta 2 [D2 cells]). Pancreatic polypeptidomas may metastasize to the liver, and it has been suggested that large tumor size is a predictor of metastasis. By definition, nonfunctioning PETs are not associated with an elevated level of peptide hormone. MEN-1-related nonfunctioning PETs are almost exclusively malignant (80–100%) and are associated with both lymph node and liver metastasis.

Surgical Management of Pancreatic Tumors in MEN-1

The surgical management of pancreatic neuroendocrine tumors in patients with MEN-1 remains controversial because MEN-1-associated pancreatic tumors have unique characteristics when compared with pancreatic tumors of sporadic etiology. First, MEN-1-associated pancreatic tumors are almost always multifocal, and second, they are usually distributed throughout the pancreatic parenchyma, with or without a hormone-excess syndrome. Unlike the situation with medullary thyroid cancer in multiple endocrine neoplasia type 2 (MEN-2) where total thyroidectomy is performed as a prophylactic procedure, total pancreatectomy would result in insulin dependence and pancreatic exocrine insufficiency, both of which may result in significant patient morbidity. Therefore, the timing and proper extent of pancreatic resection remain controversial. Also, in contrast to MEN-2, the relationship between genotype and phenotype in MEN-1 is still unclear.[18,19] Therefore, genotype cannot be used to guide the timing and extent of pancreatic resection (as occurs in the timing of thyroidectomy in MEN-2). Currently, clinical features of MEN-1 such as patient age, sites of tumor involvement, and tempo of disease progression vary extensively among patients with MEN-1 and even among affected members within the same family who have the same genetic mutation.

Gastrinoma

MEN-1 patients with clinical evidence of hyperparathyroidism and gastrinoma have been reported to show a reduction in fasting gastrin levels and basal acid output after parathyroidectomy. Parathyroidectomy is accepted as the initial surgical procedure for these patients. In contrast, the role of surgery in the management of MEN-1 patients with ZES remains controversial. As gastrin levels rarely decline to normal after surgery, and control of acid hypersecretion without surgery is now possible with the introduction of Na+-K+-ATPase inhibitors (eg, omeprazole). However, correction of hypercalcemia or medical control of increased acid production because of hypergastrinemia obviously does not address the malignant potential of gastrin-producing neoplasms in the pancreas or duodenum. Thus, the long-term survival of MEN-1 patients with gastrinoma is dependent on the biologic behavior of the tumor and the effectiveness of surgical therapy to prevent the development of metastatic disease.

Skogseid and colleagues[20] and Thompson[21] advocated early surgical intervention for all MEN-1-associated gastrinomas to include a distal pancreatectomy with enucleation (after ultrasound localization) of any tumor within the pancreatic head.[20,21] Duodenotomy is considered essential for all MEN-1 patients with elevated gastrin levels, as small duodenal gastrinomas are frequently present (87%) and cannot be found without opening the duodenum. These authors also recommend a peripancreatic and portal lymph node dissection to include those lymph nodes in the porta hepatis and along the common hepatic artery.[21] Bartsch and colleagues[18] and Lairmore and colleagues[22] also advocate early surgery for all MEN-1 patients with hypergastrinemia. According to these authors, pancreaticoduodenectomy may be the procedure of choice for MEN-1-related gastrinomas,[18] as well as for very large PETs within the head and uncinate process of the pancreas, especially when regional lymph node metastases are present.[22]

In contrast, Norton and colleagues and Jensen have advocated a much less aggressive approach for the management for MEN-1-associated gastrinomas.[23,24] They suggest surgical resection of tumors only if 2.5 cm in size or larger.[6,25,26] The rationale for this strategy is that major pancreatic operations are associated with significant morbidity and possible mortality, and, therefore, pancreatic resection should not be performed unless there is a clinically significant risk for the development of distant metastases (which they feel is based on tumor size).[8,25] These authors recommend enucleation for gastrinomas located within the head of the pancreas and segmental pancreatic resection or enucleation for tumors located within the body or the tail.[6] Mignon and

Cadiot[16] suggested that surgery is not curative for MEN-1 patients with hypergastrinemia. Although pancreatic tumors larger than 3 cm may be associated with synchronous or metachronous liver metastases, these authors do not feel that surgery is likely to prevent the development of liver metastasis.[16] The report from the Group d'Etude des Neoplasies Endocriniennes Multiples de Type 1 in France agreed with this conservative strategy.[27]

Published reports on the surgical management of MEN-1-related gastrinoma appear in Table 2. Indolent tumor growth, long survival duration, and the uncommon nature of this disease make for a natural history that is difficult to document accurately. As such, in the absence of accurate natural history data, consensus on treatment recommendations is not easily achieved.

Insulinoma

There is general consensus that patients with insulinoma syndrome should be managed with surgery. Mignon and colleagues[28] suggested that in MEN-1-associated insulinoma, removal of the functionally dominant islet cell areas is essential, but near total or total pancreatectomy should be avoided.[28] Bartsch and colleagues[18] and Lairmore and colleagues[22] also suggested that all MEN-1 patients with hyperinsulinism should be treated with surgery.[18] A combination of enucleation and/or distal pancreatectomy can be performed in patients with insulinoma. Table 3 summarizes the surgical approaches used to treat insulinomas in MEN-1 patients in 12 reported series. Given the difficulty of extrapolating treatment recommendations from such small numbers of patients, it appears that a logical surgical approach is

Table 2 Surgical Management of MEN-1-Associated Gastrinoma (Zollinger-Ellison Syndrome [ZES]) Reproduced with permission from Kouvaraki et al.[35]

Author, Year	MEN-1 and ZES	Surgery	PD or TP	Duo-denotomy	DP ± Enucleation	Enucleation or NAR	Biochemical Cure (%)	m–LM (%)	DOD(%)	Follow-up
	No. of patients									
Kloppel, 1986	NA	2	1 (PD)	NA	0	1	2/2 (100%)*	NA	NA	NA
Van Heerden, 1986	25	10	1 (PD)†	NA	4	5	0/10	NA	0/10	Mean: 79.75 m
Sheppard, 1989	22	7	0	2	6	1	0/7	NA	NA	Range: 3–84 m
Samaan, 1989	6	4	1 (TP)	2	2	1‡	1/4 (25%)	1/4 (25%)	0/4	NA
Thompson, 1989	NA	6	0	6	6	0	1/6 (17%) 5/6 (83%)*	0/6	0/6	Mean: 7 y (5–144 m)
Pipeleers-Marichall 1990	NA	7	2 (PD)‡	2	4	1‡	4/7 (57%)*	NA	NA	NA
Grama,1992	19	14	NA	5	NA	NA	0/14	2/19 (11%)	4/19 (21%)	Range: 7–14 y
Thomson, 1992	11	11	0	11	10¶	1‡	3/11 (27%) 10/11 (91%)*	0/11	0/11	Range: 3 m–14 y
Cherner, 1992	1	1	0	0	1	0	0/1	0/1	0/1	16 m
Thomson, 1993	NA	3	0	3	3	0	0/3	0/3	0/3	NA
Melvin, 1993	19	17	NA	NA	NA	NA	1/17 (6%)	NA	4/19 (21%)	Mean: 14 y (1–39 y)
Mignon, 1993	36	33	3 (PD)	9	21	9	1/33 (3%)	7/33 (21%)	2/33 (6%)	Median: 95 m (17–278 m)
Thompson, 1998	43	38	NA	38	38	0	33% 67%*	1/38	0/38	Up to 19 y
Cadiot, 1999	NA	48	5 (PD) 1 (TP)	NA	32	4	NA	8/48 (17%)	3/48 (6%)	Median: 102 m (12–366 m)
Lowney, 1998	NA	12	NA	NA	NA	NA	NA	0/12	0/12	NA
Norton, 1999	NA	28	NA	NA	NA	NA	0/28	NA	NA	Median: 5 ± 7 y
Bartsch, 2000	21	8	3 (PD)§	7	3	2	87%	0/8	NA	Median: 53 m (1–198 m)
Lairmore, 2000	NA	2	0	2	NA	1	NA	0/2	0/2	Range: 1.5 y–6.8 y
Total	*203*	*251*	*17*	*87*	*130*	*25*	*Range: 0–87%*	*0–25%*	*0–6%*	*Range: 3 m–21 y*

DOD = dead of disease; DP = distal pancreatectomy; m-LM = metachronous liver metastases; NA = not applicable; NAR = nonanatomic resection; PD = pancreaticoduodenectomy; ZES = Zollinger-Ellison syndrome.
*Eugastrinemic
†Reoperation after recurrence (prior simple enucleation of duodenal tumor)
‡Excision of the tumor from duodenum
‡1 patient has both PD and distal pancreatectomy
¶3 patients had reoperation after recurrence (prior simple enucleation of duodenal tumor)
§2 patients had reoperations after recurrence

Table 3 Surgical Management of MEN-1-Associated Insulinoma Reproduced with permission from Kouvaraki et al.[35]

Author, Year	No. of patients							Follow-up
	Surgery	PD or TP	DP	Enucleation or NAR	Cure	m-LM	DOD	
Kloppel, 1986	2	0	0	2	2/2 (100%)	0/2	0/2	NA
Tisell, 1988,1989	3	2 (TP)	1	0	2/3 (67%)	NA	0/3	Range: 3.5–9+ y
Sheppard, 1989	2	0	1	1	100%	NA	0/2	Range: 3–84 m
Samaan, 1989	2	0	2	0	100%	0/2	0/2	Range: 18 m–7 y
Demeure, 1991	6	0	5	1*	5/6 (84%)[†]	NA	0/6	NA (up to 15 y)
Grama, 1992	7	0	NA	NA	4/7 (57%)	1/7	0/7	Range: 7–14 y
O' Riordain, 1994	18	1 (TP)	12	5	16/18	0/18	4/18 (22%)	Median:10.3 y (1.7–18.8 y)
Chung-Yau Lo, 1998	3	0	2	1‡	2/3 (67%)[†]	0/3	0/3	Mean: 26 m (6–57 m)
Thompson, 1998	7	0	7	0	100%	0/7	0/7	Up to 18 y
Lowney, 1998	10	NA	NA	NA	NA	1/10 (10%)	1/10 (10%)	NA
Bartsch, 2000	6‡	1¶	2	3	100%	0/6	0/6	Median: 41 m (1–181 m)
Lairmore, 2000	3	1	NA	NA	NA	NA	1/3 (33%)§	Range: 1.5 y–6.8 y
Total	*69*	*5*	*32*	*13*	*Range: 57–100%*	*0–10%*		*Range: 3 m–21 y*

DOD = dead of disease; DP = distal pancreatectomy; m-LM = metachronous liver metastases; NA = not available; NAR = nonanatomic resection; PD = pancreaticoduodenectomy; TP = total pancreatectomy.
*Reoperation: total pancreatectomy: no reccurence
[†]100% cure after reoperation
‡ Reoperation: distal pancreatectomy: no recurrence
‡2 patients had gastrinoma and insulinoma
¶The patient underwent PD because of concomitant gastrinoma
§One perioperative death

distal subtotal pancreatectomy and enucleation of ultrasound-visible disease in the pancreatic head and uncinate process.

VIPoma, Glucagonoma

Clinical studies have suggested that VIPomas and glucagonomas represent a relatively small percentage of MEN-1-associated pancreatic tumors. Two of the 3 surgically treated MEN-1 patients with reported glucagonomas (Table 4) underwent distal pancreatectomy with enucleation of synchronous tumors within the head or the uncinate process of the pancreas. Tisell and Ahlman[29] reported a patient with metastatic disease secondary to glucagonoma who underwent debulking surgery; this patient died 4 years after surgery. Of the 5 reported patients who were operated on for VIPomas, only 2 underwent distal pancreatectomy with a cure rate of 100%. The limited number of surgically treated patients with VIPoma reported to date precludes any definite conclusions unique to the management of these specific tumors.

Pancreatic Polypeptidomas and Nonfunctioning Tumors

Nonfunctioning tumors of the pancreas, including PPomas, represent as many as 71% of surgically treated MEN-1-associated pancreatic tumors (see Table 4). Several surgical strategies have been proposed for the management of clinically nonfunctioning neuroendo-

crine pancreatic tumors in MEN-1 patients. The most aggressive approach is advocated by Skogseid and colleagues[20] who suggest that pancreatic imaging is ineffective for the early detection of MEN-1-associated pancreatic tumors. They obtain annual biochemical markers from the age of 15 years, and surgery is recommended if peptide levels increase, even in the absence of radiographic evidence of a pancreatic neoplasm. All patients with elevations in at least 2 pancreatic peptides were found at surgery to have a grossly visible pancreatic or duodenal tumor, with an average size of 1.3 cm.[20] According to these investigators, the appropriate surgical approach includes intraoperative ultrasonography, duodenotomy (if Zollinger-Ellison syndrome diagnosed), subtotal distal pancreatectomy, and enucleation of any tumor within the pancreatic head or uncinate process.

Thompson[21] advocates surgery in all MEN-1 patients with a nonfunctioning PET greater than 1 cm found on endoscopic ultrasound (EUS). The operation now commonly referred to as the "Thompson procedure" includes distal pancreatectomy (at the level of the superior mesenteric vein), enucleation of any identified lesions in the pancreatic head or uncinate process, and regional lymphadenectomy.[21] In the absence of gastrin hypersecretion, duodenal exploration is not performed.

Norton and colleagues suggested surgical resection for nonfunctioning PETs that are 2 to 3 cm or larger.[26] The rationale for this strategy is based on their experience in

Table 4 Surgical Management of MEN-1-Associated Nonfunctioning and Other Rare PETs Reproduced with permission from Kouvaraki et al.[35]

Author, Year	Surgery	PD or TP	Duodenotomy	DP	Enucleation or NAR	Biochemical Cure (%)	M-LM	DOD	Follow-up
Kloppel, 1986	4 (NPET)*	0	NA	4	0	0/4	NA	1/4	NA
	1 (VIP)	1 (PD)	NA	0	0	NA	NA	NA	NA
Tisell, 1988,1989	1 (SOM/GLU)	1	0	0	0	0/1	0/1	1/1 (100%)	NA
Sheppard, 1989	1 (VIP)	0	0	1	0	100%	NA	NA	17 m
Samaan, 1989	2 (GLU)	0	0	2	0	1/2	0/2	1/2	NA
Grama, 1992	7	NA	NA	NA	NA	NA	1/7	4/7	Range: 7–14 y
Thompson, 1998	3 (NPET)	0	3	3	0	NA	0/3	0/3	Up to 19 y
Lowney, 1999	19 (NPET)*	NA	NA	NA	NA	16/19†	0/19	0/19	NA
	2 (VIP)	NA	NA	NA	NA	NA	0/2	0/2	Up to 21 y
Bartsch, 2000	3 (NPT)	0	0	3	0	3/3 (100%)‡	0/3	0/3	Median: 78 m (1–198 m)
	1 (VIP)	0	0	1	0	0/1	1/1 (100%)	0/1	Median: 78 m (1–198 m)
Lairmore, 2000	15 (NPET)*	NA	NA	NA	NA	NA	NA	NA	Range: 1.5–6.8 y
	1 (VIP)	NA	NA	NA	NA	NA	NA	NA	Range: 1.5–6.8 y
Total	62	2§	3§	14§	0§	21§	2§	7§	Range: 17 m–19 y

DOD = dead of disease; DP = distal pancreatectomy; GLU = glucagonoma; m-LM = metachronous liver metastases; NA = not available; NAR = nonanatomic resection; NPET = nonfunctioning pancreatic endocrine tumors; PD = pancreaticoduodenectomy; SOM = somatostatinoma; VIP = VIPoma.
*PPomas included with nonfunctioning tumors
†2/19 patients recurred
‡Imaging studies were positive in 2 patients
§Insufficient information to total

patients with sporadic gastrinoma in which primary tumor size appeared to correlate with metastatic potential.[8] Mignon and Cadiot also suggested surgery for nonfunctioning PETs larger than 3 cm.[16]

Bartsch and colleagues. suggested that patients with nonfunctioning PETs should undergo surgery if tumor size is larger than 1 cm.[18] Pancreaticoduodenectomy may be necessary for very large tumors that are located within the head and uncinate process of the pancreas in close proximity to the pancreatic duct or tumors with synchronous metastatic disease in regional lymph nodes.[18]

Consensus Statement on the Management of MEN-1 Patients with Pancreatic Neuroendocrine Tumors

Brandi and colleagues recently published a consensus statement on the management of MEN-1 patients and confirmed that surgery should be considered the main treatment for insulinoma.[30] For MEN-1-related gastrinoma, these authors were less enthusiastic about surgery because of the finding that few patients have a normal serum level of gastrin after operation. Their consensus statement reflects the difficulty in developing treatment recommendations, especially with regard to major abdominal surgery, when there are limited data on

which to base recommendations. It is reasonable to conclude that patients with MEN-1-related neuroendocrine carcinoma of the pancreas should be managed at a center experienced with the global management of this disease and, specifically, the operative management of complex pancreatic tumors. Both an in-depth knowledge of the disease and the technical aspects of pancreatic surgery are necessary components of a favorable outcome.

NCCN Treatment Guidelines for Patients with MEN-1-Related Pancreatic Neuroendocrine Tumors

Since 2003 the National Comprehensive Cancer Network has also provided treatment guidelines for patients with MEN-1-related neuroendocrine tumors. The current publication (2005) suggests that patients with radiographically occult presumed sporadic gastrinoma (no primary tumor has been found by preoperative imaging studies) may be observed or referred for surgery.[2] Surgery for most forms of functioning and nonfunctioning tumors should include distal pancreatectomy, duodenotomy, enucleation of any palpable or ultrasound-visible tumors in the pancreatic head, and regional lymphadenectomy (Thompson procedure).[2] For tumors in the pancreatic head that cannot be enucleated (size > 5 cm or invasive) and VIPomas, pancreaticoduodenectomy and periduodenal node dissection is required.[2]

Authors Recommendations for the Surgical Management of MEN-1-Associated PETs

Tables 2 through 4 illustrate the small number of surgically treated patients with MEN-1-associated PETs. From an endocrine perspective, patients with Zollinger-Ellison Syndrome (gastrinoma) and insulinoma syndrome should receive surgical treatment. Although the results with surgery for Zollinger-Ellison Syndrome in patients with MEN-1 have been suboptimal with respect to rendering patients eugastrinemic, advances in surgical technique, the routine use of intraoperative ultrasound, and the appreciation that the duodenum harbors small tumors in the majority of patients provide an optimistic outlook for surgery performed by experienced pancreatic surgeons. Even if postoperative-stimulated gastrin levels remain abnormal, control of gastric acid production may be improved by a reduction in tumor burden. In addition, PETs may be a unique neoplasm in oncology and one in which overall tumor burden may be related to metastatic potential. Although this concept is foreign to the management of other solid tumors, patients with sporadic and familial PETs may receive a survival advantage by maintaining a tumor volume as low as possible, even if all gross or microscopic disease cannot be removed.

With regard to patients with tumors other than gastrinomas or insulinomas, oncologic concerns become even more compelling. In such patients, it seems most appropriate to operate when disease is confirmed on imaging studies (CT or MRI). We concur that the operation described by Thompson appears to be the most appropriate approach, because it removes all visible tumor while decreasing the overall islet cell mass and, therefore, the volume of at-risk pancreas (see Figure 2). This clearly represents a compromise procedure by leaving islet cell mass in the pancreatic head and, therefore, the risk of metachronous neoplasms while preventing the complications of insulin-dependent diabetes associated with total pancreatectomy. This operation attempts to delay the need for total pancreatectomy (assuming patients may develop metachronous neoplasms in the remaining pancreas and, therefore, the need for completion total pancreatectomy), and thereby avoid the long-term complications of type 1 diabetes, especially in young patients. Very long-term follow-up will be necessary to determine the wisdom of this approach. In patients with large tumors within the head of the pancreas that are not amenable to enucleation, pancreatoduodenectomy is an appropriate alternative. Total pancreatectomy, as the initial operative procedure, is rarely recommended to cure nonfunctioning MEN-1-associated PETs because of the resulting endocrine and exocrine insufficiency.

Treatment of Metastatic Pancreatic Endocrine Tumors

Medical treatment of patients with advanced neuroendocrine carcinoma of the pancreas attempts to control symptoms of hormonal excess and prevent tumor growth and metastasis. In patients with gastrinoma, acid hypersecretion is now effectively controlled with H+/K+-ATPase inhibitors (omeprazole) in almost all patients. In contrast, medical management of insulinoma is rarely effective and indicated only in patients with a high surgical risk or those who have previously failed surgical treatment.[31] Diazoxide or somatostatin analogues may be used for this purpose. For VIPomas or metastatic carcinoid tumors, regiments such as corticosteroids, indomethacin, and lithium carbonate have been used in symptomatic patients.[32] Octreotide may also control watery diarrhea in most patients with VIPomas.

Controlled trials of chemotherapy and radiation have not been performed in MEN-1 patients with malignant PETs because of the small number of patients available for study. Therefore, empiric treatment based on our larger experience with sporadic disease is usually the basis for therapy. A multimodality approach with somatostatin analogue, systemic triple chemotherapy consisting of Adriamycin, 5-fluorouracil (5-FU), streptozotocin, and biotherapy with interferon-alpha represent common alternatives. In addition, hepatic artery embolization has been proposed by several investigators.[33]

Octreotide is a human somatostatin analogue that inhibits the secretion of different peptide hormones from neuroendocrine tumors, which express somatostatin receptors. These receptors mediate the antiproliferative and antisecretory action of somatostatin. Octreotide analogues are effective in controlling hormone-related symptoms in patients with gastrinoma, but their efficacy with respect to tumor response (tumor size) remains controversial. Burgess and colleagues[34] reported rapid symptomatic improvement and biochemical response in MEN-1 patients with gastrinomas; gastrin levels decreased by at least 25% of the pretreatment level.[34] These investigators also reported that the size of hepatic metastases in patients with metastatic disease was reduced by up to 15% after treatment with octreotide.[34] Other investigators also found objective biochemical or tumor response to octreotide. Octreotide has been used as palliative therapy for metastatic insulinoma, but it is not generally recommended, as insulinomas usually do not possess somatostatin receptors, and thus octreotide only rarely improves hypoglycemic symptoms. Octreotide has a well-established role in the systemic management of unresectable or metastatic VIPomas and hormonally active metastatic carcinoid tumors.[34]

Systemic chemotherapy has been evaluated in sporadic PETs, with variable rates of tumor response, and these data are used as a basis for the treatment of MEN-1 patients with metastatic neuroendocrine carcinoma. The most commonly used chemotherapeutic agents include streptozocin, 5-FU, doxorubicin, chlorozotocin, and dacarbazine. Streptozocin-based combination chemotherapy (usually with 5-FU and doxorubicin) has a response rate of up to 63% in patients with sporadic disease. Previous data from our institution suggest that the response rate is probably closer to 35 to 40%.[35] Grama and colleagues[36] reported a biochemical response of 25% in MEN-1 patients treated with this regimen.[36] Response to streptozocin-based combination chemotherapy may be associated with the histologic type of PET. It has been suggested that malignant insulinoma and VIPoma have superior response rates to streptozotocin and 5-FU than do gastrinomas and nonfunctioning PETs. Interferon-alpha alone or in combination with somatostatin has been used in the treatment of patients with sporadic metastatic PETs, and has therefore been proposed for patients with MEN-1-associated malignant PETs. For gastrinomas, the administration of human leukocyte interferon may be beneficial.[37]

Selective hepatic artery embolization of metastatic tumors can control hormonal symptoms and reduce tumor burden. The metastatic lesions in the liver are typically hypervascular with a blood supply derived from the hepatic artery. However, there are currently no specific guidelines concerning the optimal timing of embolization. It is not clear whether liver embolization should be attempted early in the course of the disease or after response or failure of systemic therapy. The indolent and often variable nature of disease progression in patients with metastatic PETs makes for a very heterogeneous population that is difficult to study. It is very difficult to determine the impact of various treatment interventions versus the frequently witnessed variations in tumor progression. For example, one cannot often differentiate the impact of therapy from stable disease unrelated to treatment response. Patient management is therefore often based on the judgment of an experienced clinician combined with knowledge of the overall tumor burden and tempo of disease progression. Finally, the role of radiotherapy is largely limited to the palliative management of metastases to bone, skin, or brain.

NCCN Treatment Guidelines for MEN-1 Patients with Distant Metastases

In patients with distant metastatic disease from PETs, NCCN guidelines suggest surgical excision of resectable metastases that are confined to the liver or lung. For unresectable or extrahepatic metastatic disease, one can consider observation with tumor markers and cross-sectional imaging every 3 to 6 months, or chemotherapy in the settings of a clinical trial. According to the guidelines, if progression occurs or the patient is symptomatic from hormonal excess or from tumor burden, then one should consider short- or long-acting octreotide. If metastases are confined to the liver, hepatic arterial chemoembolization or systemic chemotherapy to include doxorubicin plus streptozocin or chemotherapeutic agents in the setting of a clinical trial should be considered. If distant metastatic sites are in bone, radiotherapy should be considered, and for lung metastases, systemic chemotherapy represents the best alternative.

3. CARCINOID TUMORS

Carcinoid tumors occur in 2 to 8% of MEN-1 patients. They are usually foregut in origin, located mainly in the thymus, bronchus, or stomach. Most bronchial and thymic carcinoids are malignant and therefore represent the second leading cause of MEN-1-related death after malignant PETs. There are no currently diagnostic or treatment guidelines for MEN-1-related carcinoid tumors. Therefore, the diagnosis and management of these tumors is based on our experience with sporadic disease.

Thymic Carcinoids

MEN-1-related thymic carcinoids are rare (0–6%), aggressive, and occur more often in men. Thymic carcinoids are usually diagnosed after age 45, and the diagnosis is usually delayed because patients are generally asymptomatic.[38] When symptoms do occur, they are due to tumor compression and include dysarthria, dyspnea, cough, and chest and neck discomfort.[38,39] Most MEN-1-associated thymic carcinoids are malignant (up to 50% have hepatic metastases at the time of diagnosis) and frequently are the cause of disease-specific mortality. Prophylactic transcervical thymectomy during neck exploration for parathyroidectomy is recommended in MEN-1 patients to both remove a supernumerary ectopic parathyroid and reduce the volume of thymic tissue, and thereby possibly prevent the development of a thymic carcinoid tumor.[40] The treatment of choice for an established thymic carcinoid tumor is surgical excision, which may prevent local disease progression and facilitate the use of adjuvant therapy.[38] Adjuvant therapy includes radiotherapy, chemotherapy, and interferon-alpha.[38] Brandi and colleagues[30] recommended CT imaging every 3 years to screen at-risk MEN-1 patients for thymic carcinoids; however, in kindreds with a history of thymic carcinoids, more frequent screening with chest CT or magnetic resonance imaging (MRI) may be reasonable.[30]

Bronchial Carcinoids

MEN-1-associated bronchial carcinoids are also rare neoplasms occurring in only 8% of MEN-1 patients, and in contrast to thymic carcinoids, bronchial tumors are more prevalent in women. Bronchial carcinoids may rarely secrete ACTH or GHRH, and may also produce the atypical carcinoid syndrome, or foregut carcinoid syndrome, as a result of histamine secretion. Foregut carcinoid tumors rarely secrete serotonin because of a lack of the enzyme aromatic amino acid decarboxylase. Dominant symptoms include flushing and headache. Flushing with foregut tumors tends to be prolonged, purple in color, and distributed predominantly in the face and neck. Bronchospasm, cutaneous edema, and hypotension may also be present. In contrast, with midgut carcinoids, cutaneous flushing is usually short in duration and pink-red in color. Carcinoid symptoms can be precipitated by a particular "trigger" agent, such as alcohol, cheese, coffee, chocolate, red wine, or exercise. Like sporadic bronchial carcinoids, 66% of MEN-1-associated bronchial carcinoid tumors are centrally located in the pulmonary lobes, and the remaining tumors may be peripheral. Pulmonary carcinoids in MEN-1 patients are usually classified as low-grade typical or intermediate-grade atypical carcinoid. Metastases to regional lymph nodes or to the liver have only rarely been reported. High-grade large cell and small cell neuroendocrine carcinoma have not been described in MEN-1 patients. Bronchial carcinoid tumors seen on imaging studies may be confused with bronchogenic carcinomas of the lung. Surgical excision is the preferred treatment, and radiation therapy is used for patients with regional lymph node metastases.

Gastric Carcinoids

Type II gastric carcinoids arise from histamine-secreting enterochromaffin-like (ECL) cells in up to 30% of MEN-1 patients with ZES owing to prolonged exposure to high levels of serum gastrin.[7] Type I gastric carcinoids are due to secondary hypergastrinemia in the setting of achlorhydria, chronic atrophic gastritis, and pernicious anemia, and type III gastric carcinoids are sporadic in origin and not associated with hypergastrinemia. Type III gastric carci-

noids are thought to have a much greater malignant potential than types I and II, which rarely metastasize to distant sites. MEN-1-associated carcinoid tumors are multifocal in up to 92% of patients and are usually very small (80% are less than 2 cm).[41] They are distributed throughout the fundus or corpus of the stomach and are accompanied by diffuse argyrophilic cell hyperplasia of ECL cells or dysplasia in the entire oxyntic mucosa, which is not atrophic. The natural history of gastric carcinoids in MEN-1 patients is not well studied because they are so uncommon. Recently, it has been found that gastric carcinoid tumors express vesicular monoamine transporter type 2, which is used as a histologic marker to distinguish carcinoids and their metastases from PETs. Upper endoscopy with biopsy will accurately assess the size, number, and extent of carcinoid tumors in the stomach. Although the precise malignant potential is unknown, distant metastases from type II gastric carcinoid tumors are very rare. Therefore, when possible, type II gastric carcinoids should be removed endoscopically, especially if such lesions are small and relatively few in number. Importantly, if one can reduce the serum gastrin level by removing the tumors in the pancreas and duodenum, the stimulus for carcinoid production should be lost, thereby preventing the further development of type II gastric carcinoids.

4. MISCELLANEOUS ENDOCRINE TUMORS

Other less common endocrine neoplasms in MEN-1 include adrenocortical tumors (including pheochromocytomas) and thyroid neoplasms.

Adrenal Tumors

Adrenal tumors are found in up to 45% of MEN-1 patients and arise more often in the cortex (up to 35%) and rarely in the adrenal medulla (up to 3%).[36,42] Unlike other heritable causes of pheochromocytomas, which vastly cause bilateral tumors, adrenal tumors in MEN-1 patients may often be unilateral.[43,44] The majority of adrenocortical tumors are nonfunctional. However, some of these tumors may be functional, causing Cushing's syndrome and primary hyperaldosteronism.[42-44] Most adrenocortical tumors are benign, although adrenocortical carcinomas have been reported.[43,44] There is controversy concerning the potential role of the *MEN1* gene in adrenocortical lesions. Skogseid and colleagues[43] demonstrated loss of heterozygosity (LOH) at 11q13 in adrenocortical carcinoma from patients with MEN-1, but not in benign cortical nodules.[43] Other studies suggested direct involvement the *MEN1* gene in adrenocortical proliferation, and thus in the pathogenesis of these tumors.[42] Because adrenal tumors occur in association with PETs, it has been also proposed that growth factors released by PETs in MEN-1 patients may be related to the adrenocortical tumor formation. However, hormonal hypersecretion by PET does not seem to be the primary cause adrenocortical tumor development.

The occurrence of pheochromocytoma in patients with MEN-1 is rare (up to 3%).[44] Pheochromocytomas in MEN-1 are usually unilateral, and only one case of malignancy has been reported. Germline *MEN1* mutations have been detected in these tumors, and LOH of the wild-type allele around the *menin* locus, implicating inactivation of *MEN1* has been associated with adrenomedullary tumorigenesis.[44]

The vast majority of adrenal tumors in MEN-1 are nonfunctioning cortical adenomas and usually have an indolent course that can be followed annually with CT or MRI. A hormonally active cortical adenoma or pheochromocytoma should be ruled-out in all MEN-1 patients with an adrenal mass. The biochemical evaluation should include an overnight 1 mg dexamethasone suppression test to exclude Cushing's syndrome. In addition, the current NCCN guidelines recommend measurements of 24-hour free urine cortisol, serum ACTH, cortisol, and electrolytes.[2] Plasma-free metanephrines levels can be measured to exclude pheochromocytoma. Any hormonally active adrenal neoplasm, regardless of size, should be resected. For hormonally inactive adrenal neoplasms, resection should be considered for (1) tumors larger than 4 cm, (2) tumors of any size that demonstrate malignant characteristics (heterogeneous density, irregular borders) on radiographic imagining, or (3) tumors that enlarge during follow-up.[45] A laparoscopic approach is appropriate for patients with MEN-1 whose disease is limited to one adrenal gland and does not demonstrate any malignant characteristics.

Thyroid Neoplasms

Follicular thyroid neoplasms, colloid goiters, and thyroid carcinomas, have been found in up to 27% of MEN-1 patients.[46] However, studies have failed to identify LOH of the *MEN1* gene in these thyroid lesions, suggesting that thyroid neoplasms found in these patients are unrelated to MEN-1.[46] It has been suggested that the higher incidence of thyroid tumors in MEN-1 patients when compared to the general population, may be associated with the frequent neck exploration for hyperparathyroidism.

5. MISCELLANEOUS NONENDOCRINE TUMORS

A wide spectrum of other non-endocrine mesenchymal tumors such as cutaneous or visceral lipomas (in up to 34%), facial angiofibromas and collagenomas (up to 88%), leiomyomata, and "café au lait" macules have also been reported in patients with MEN-1. The causal relationship between angiofibromas, collagenomas, lipomas, and leiomyomas with MEN-1 syndrome has only recently been confirmed by studies showing loss of heterozygosity of the *MEN1* in these tumors.[47] Other rare nonendocrine tumors observed in MEN-1 patients include malignant melanomas and testicular teratomas.

References

1. Shapiro SE, Cote GC, Lee JE, et al. The role of genetics in the surgical management of familial endocrinopathy syndromes. J Am Coll Surg 2003;197:818–31.

2. Clark OH, Ajani J, Benson AB III, et al. NCCN oncology practice guidelines v.1.2005. National Comprehensive Cancer Network 2005.

3. Proceedings of the NIDDK workshop program. Asymptomatic primary hyperparathyroidism: A perspective for the 21st century. Bethesda, Maryland, USA. April 8–9, 2002. J Bone Miner Res 2002;17Suppl 2:N1–162.

4. Lambert LA, Shapiro SE, Lee JE, et al. Surgical treatment of hyperparathyroidism in patients with multiple endocrine neoplasia type 1. Arch Surg 2005;140:374–82.

5. Pipeleers-Marichal M, Somers G, Willems G, et al. Gastrinomas in the duodenums of patients with multiple endocrine neoplasia type 1 and the Zollinger-Ellison syndrome [see comments]. N Engl J Med 1990;322:723–7.

6. Norton JA, Fraker DL, Alexander HR, et al. Surgery to cure the Zollinger-Ellison syndrome [see comments]. N Engl J Med 1999;341:635–44.

7. Gibril F, Schumann M, Pace A, Jensen RT. Multiple endocrine neoplasia type 1 and Zollinger-Ellison syndrome: a prospective study of 107 cases and comparison with 1009 cases from the literature. Medicine (Baltimore) 2004;83:43–83.

8. Weber HC, Venzon DJ, Lin JT, et al. Determinants of metastatic rate and survival in patients with Zollinger-Ellison syndrome: a prospective long-term study. Gastroenterology 1995;108:1637–49.

9. Lowney JK, Frisella MM, Lairmore TC, Doherty GM. Pancreatic islet cell tumor metastasis in multiple endocrine neoplasia type 1: correlation with primary tumor size. Surgery 1998;124:1043–9.

10. Kouvaraki MA, Shapiro SE, Cote GJ, et al. Management of pancreatic endocrine tumors in multiple endocrine neoplasia type 1. World J Surg 2006;30:643–53.

11. Thompson NW. Surgical treatment of the endocrine pancreas and Zollinger-Ellison syndrome in the MEN 1 syndrome. Henry Ford Hosp Med J 1992;40:195–8.

12. Donow C, Pipeleers-Marichal M, Schroder S, et al. Surgical pathology of gastrinoma. Site, size, multicentricity, associa-

tion with multiple endocrine neoplasia type 1, and malignancy. Cancer 1991;68:1329–34.

13. Cadiot G, Vuagnat A, Doukhan I, et al. Prognostic factors in patients with Zollinger-Ellison syndrome and multiple endocrine neoplasia type 1. Groupe d'Etude des Neoplasies Endocriniennes Multiples (GENEM and Groupe de Recherche et d'Etude du Syndrome de Zollinger-Ellison (GRESZE). Gastroenterology 1999;116:286–93.

14. Gibril F, Venzon DJ, Ojeaburu JV, et al. Prospective study of the natural history of gastrinoma in patients with MEN1: definition of an aggressive and a nonaggressive form. J Clin Endocrinol Metab 2001;86:5282–93.

15. Demeure MJ, Klonoff DC, Karam JH, et al. Insulinomas associated with multiple endocrine neoplasia type I: the need for a different surgical approach. Surgery 1991;110: 998–1005.

16. Mignon M, Cadiot G. Diagnostic and therapeutic criteria in patients with Zollinger-Ellison syndrome and multiple endocrine neoplasia type 1. J Intern Med 1998;243:489–94.

17. Thakker RV. Multiple endocrine neoplasia type 1. Endocrinol Metab Clin North Am 2000;29:541–67.

18. Bartsch DK, Langer P, Wild A, et al. Pancreaticoduodenal endocrine tumors in multiple endocrine neoplasia type 1: surgery or surveillance? Surgery 2000;128:958–66.

19. Kouvaraki MA, Lee JE, Shapiro SE, et al. Genotype-phenotype analysis in multiple endocrine neoplasia type 1. Arch Surg 2002;137:641–7.

20. Skogseid B, Oberg K, Eriksson B, et al. Surgery for asymptomatic pancreatic lesion in multiple endocrine neoplasia type I. World J Surg 1996;20:872–7.

21. Thompson NW. Current concepts in the surgical management of multiple endocrine neoplasia type 1 pancreatic-duodenal disease. Results in the treatment of 40 patients with Zollinger-Ellison syndrome, hypoglycaemia or both. J Intern Med 1998;243:495–500.

22. Lairmore TC, Chen VY, DeBenedetti MK, et al. Duodenopancreatic resections in patients with multiple endocrine neoplasia type 1. Ann Surg 2000;231:909–18.

23. Norton JA, Doppman JL, Jensen RT. Curative resection in Zollinger-Ellison syndrome. Results of a 10-year prospective study. Ann Surg 1992;215:8–18.

24. Jensen RT. Management of the Zollinger-Ellison syndrome in patients with multiple endocrine neoplasia type 1. J Intern Med 1998;243:477–88.

25. Doherty GM, Olson JA, Frisella MM, et al. Lethality of multiple endocrine neoplasia type I. World J Surg 1998;22: 581–7.

26. Norton JA, Alexander HR, Fraker DL, et al. Comparison of surgical results in patients with advanced and limited disease with multiple endocrine neoplasia type 1 and Zollinger-Ellison syndrome. Ann Surg 2001;234:495–506.

27. Chanson P, Cadiot G, Murat A. Management of patients and subjects at risk for multiple endocrine neoplasia type 1: MEN 1. GENEM 1. Groupe d'Etude des Neoplasies Endocriniennes Multiples de Type 1. Horm Res 1997;47:211–20.

28. Mignon M, Ruszniewski P, Podevin P, et al. Current approach to the management of gastrinoma and insulinoma in adults with multiple endocrine neoplasia type I. World J Surg 1993;17:489–97.

29. Tisell LE, Ahlman H. Treatment of the pancreatic disease of multiple endocrine neoplasia type 1 (MEN 1). Acta Oncol 1989;28:415–7.

30. Brandi ML, Gagel RF, Angeli A, et al. Guidelines for diagnosis and therapy of MEN type 1 and type 2. J Clin Endocrinol Metab 2001;86:5658–71.

31. Veldhuis JD, Norton JA, Wells SA Jr. et al. Surgical versus medical management of multiple endocrine neoplasia (MEN) type I. J Clin Endocrinol Metab 1997;82:357–64.

32. Pannett AA, Thakker RV. Multiple endocrine neoplasia type 1. Endocr Relat Cancer 1999;6:449–73.

33. Eriksson BK, Larsson EG, Skogseid BM, et al. Liver embolizations of patients with malignant neuroendocrine gastrointestinal tumors. Cancer 1998;83:2293–301.

34. Burgess JR, Greenaway TM, Parameswaran V, Shepherd JJ. Octreotide improves biochemical, radiologic, and symptomatic indices of gastroenteropancreatic neoplasia in patients with multiple endocrine neoplasia type 1 (MEN-1). Implications for an integrated model of MEN-1 tumorigenesis. Cancer 1999;86:2154–9.

35. Kouvaraki M, Shapiro SE, Lee JE, Evans DB. Multiple endocrine neoplasia type 1. In: Von Hoff DD, Evans DB, Hruban RH, editors. Pancreatic cancer. 1st edition. Sudbury, MA: Jones and Bartlett Publishers; 2005. p. 631–54.

36. Grama D, Skogseid B, Wilander E, et al. Pancreatic tumors in multiple endocrine neoplasia type 1: clinical presentation and surgical treatment. World J Surg 1992;16:611–9.

37. Thakker RV. Multiple endocrine neoplasia—syndromes of the twentieth century. J Clin Endocrinol Metab 1998;83: 2617–20.

38. Gibril F, Chen YJ, Schrump DS, et al. Prospective study of thymic carcinoids in patients with multiple endocrine neoplasia type 1. J Clin Endocrinol Metab 2003;88:1066–81.

39. Teh BT, McArdle J, Chan SP, et al. Clinicopathologic studies of thymic carcinoids in multiple endocrine neoplasia type 1. Medicine (Baltimore) 1997;76:21–9.

40. Burgess JR, Greenaway TM, Shepherd JJ. Expression of the MEN-1 gene in a large kindred with multiple endocrine neoplasia type 1. J Intern Med 1998;243:465–70.

41. Rindi G, Bordi C, Rappel S, et al. Gastric carcinoids and neuroendocrine carcinomas: pathogenesis, pathology, and behavior. World J Surg 1996;20:168–72.

42. Beckers A, Abs R, Willems PJ, et al. Aldosterone-secreting adrenal adenoma as part of multiple endocrine neoplasia

type 1 (MEN1): loss of heterozygosity for polymorphic chromosome 11 deoxyribonucleic acid markers, including the MEN1 locus. J Clin Endocrinol Metab 1992;75:564–70.

43. Skogseid B, Larsson C, Lindgren PG, et al. Clinical and genetic features of adrenocortical lesions in multiple endocrine neoplasia type 1. J Clin Endocrinol Metab 1992;75:76–81.

44. Langer P, Cupisti K, Bartsch DK, et al. Adrenal involvement in multiple endocrine neoplasia type 1. World J Surg 2002;26:891–6.

45. Clark OH, Ajani J, Benson AB III, et al. NCCN oncology practice guidelines v.1.2003. National Comprehensive Cancer Network; 2003.

46. Desai D, McPherson LA, Higgins JP, Weigel RJ. Genetic analysis of a papillary thyroid carcinoma in a patient with MEN1. Ann Surg Oncol 2001;8:342–6.

47. Pack S, Turner ML, Zhuang Z, et al. Cutaneous tumors in patients with multiple endocrine neoplasia type 1 show allelic deletion of the MEN1 gene. J Invest Dermatol 1998; 110:438–40.

CHAPTER 50

SURGICAL TREATMENT OF MULTIPLE ENDOCRINE NEOPLASIA TYPE 2 (MEN-2)

MARIA A. KOUVARAKI, MD, PhD

NANCY D. PERRIER, MD

SUZANNE E. SHAPIRO, MS

JEFFREY E. LEE, MD

DOUGLAS B. EVANS, MD

Introduction

Multiple endocrine neoplasia type 2 (MEN-2) is a genetic syndrome caused by germline mutations in the *RET* proto-oncogene, is transmitted in an autosomal dominant pattern, and affects approximately 1 in 30,000 individuals.[1–3] MEN-2 is divided into 3 clinical subtypes depending on the presence or absence of tissue-specific tumors, phenotypic characteristics, and the number of affected family members (Table 1). MEN-2A, or Sipple's syndrome, is the most common subtype (occurs in approximately 80–90% of patients with hereditary medullary thyroid cancer [MTC]) and is characterized by MTC (> 95% of affected individuals), pheochromocytoma (50%), and primary hyperparathyroidism (HPT; 20%).[4] Sipple[5] first reported the association of MTC with pheochromocytoma in 1961; however, the term "multiple endocrine neoplasia type 2" was first used by Steiner and colleagues,[6] who associated the presence of primary HPT with the syndrome.[6] Two rare subtypes of MEN-2A have been described, one with Hirschsprung's disease (HSCR) and the other with cutaneous lichen amyloidosis (CLA).[7–9] HSCR is due to the absence of autonomic ganglia in the terminal hindgut, which results in colonic dilatation, obstipation, constipation, and obstruction in neonates. CLA is a pruritic lichenoid skin lesion, usually located on the upper back. Each of these rare subtypes has been associated only with specific *RET* mutations in MEN-2A patients.

MEN-2B is far less common than MEN-2A, accounting for approximately 5% of MEN-2 cases. It is characterized by aggressive MTC (100%); pheochromocytoma (50%); marfanoid habitus; the presence of distinctive mucosal neuromas on the tongue, lips, and subconjunctival areas; and diffuse ganglioneuromas of the gastrointestinal tract.[4,10] HPT is not known to develop in patients with MEN-2B. The MEN-2B phenotype may be recognized during early childhood by the characteristic neuromas on the lips and tongue. MTC in the setting of MEN-2B develops during infancy and has a more aggressive course compared with MTC in other MEN-2 clinical subtypes. The majority of cases of MEN-2B are the result of spontaneous new *RET* mutations, which are not inherited from either parent; therefore, most patients with MEN-2B lack a family history of the disease and would not be identified as

Table 1 Classification of Hereditary MTC

Subtype	MTC	Pheochromocytoma	HPT	Number of affected family members
MEN-2A*	Yes	Yes (50%)	Yes (20%)	Any
MEN-2B†	Yes	Yes (50%)	No	Any
FMTC	Yes	No	No	≥ 4
Unclassified	Yes	No	No	≤ 3

FMTC = familial medullary thyroid carcinoma; HPT = hyperparathyroidism; MEN = multiple endocrine neoplasia; MTC = medullary thyroid carcinoma.
*Diagnosis of pheochromocytoma and/or HPT is required.
†Characteristic mucosa neuromas on the tongue, lips, subconjunctival areas, and gastrointestinal tract are required.

candidates for early screening and prophylactic thyroidectomy. As such, these MEN-2B patients often experience a delay in diagnosis until signs of mucosal neuromas and/or palpable thyroid tumors are appreciated by their parents, pediatrician, or dentist.

Familial MTC (FMTC), the third clinical subtype of inherited MTC, accounts for 5 to 15% of hereditary MTC cases. It is defined as the presence of MTC in kindreds with 4 or more affected members and with objective evidence of the absence of adrenal and parathyroid gland involvement.[11] FMTC represents a less aggressive form of hereditary MTC, and it has a corresponding older age at onset—often between 20 and 40 years—compared with MEN-2A and MEN-2B.[12]

Prognosis is related to the development of MTC, as metastatic MTC is the leading cause of disease-specific mortality in MEN-2 patients. In contrast to MEN-1, where prophylactic total pancreatectomy (to avoid the development of pancreatic neuroendocrine tumors) is not routinely performed, prophylactic total thyroidectomy in MEN-2 carriers is the accepted treatment strategy. Pheochromocytoma in MEN-2 is rarely malignant, and death because of catecholamine crisis is now uncommon with routine monitoring; therefore, prophylactic adrenal surgery is also inappropriate.

RET Proto-Oncogene

The *RET* gene is located on chromosome 10q11.2 near the centromere and includes 21 exons. Takahashi and colleagues[13] first identified *RET* (rearranged during transfection) in 1985 as a proto-oncogene that can undergo activation by cytogenic rearrangement.[13] Three years later, the *RET* gene was cloned by the same investigators.[14] The *RET* gene encodes a plasma membrane-bound tyrosine kinase enzyme, the RET receptor, which is expressed by neuroendocrine and neural cells, including thyroid C-cells, adrenal medullary cells, parasympathetic, sympathetic, and colonic ganglia, cells of the urogenital tract, and parathyroid cells derived from branchial arches.[13–16]

Germline point mutations of *RET* causing activation (gain of function) are responsible for tumor syndromes including MEN-2 and its clinical subtypes.[17–28] Because *RET* is a proto-oncogene, a single activating mutation of one allele is sufficient to cause the disease. The germline mutations in MEN-2 are usually located either in the extracellular cysteine-rich region (exons 10 and 11) of the RET protein, leading to RET receptor homodimerization, or in the intracellular tyrosine kinase domains (exons 13 to 16), which activate the catalytic site of the RET kinase enzyme that alters substrate specificity.[29–31] The first *RET* germline mutations were identified in 1993 in patients with MEN-2A and FMTC.[1,2]

Genotype-Phenotype Correlations

More than 95% of families with MEN-2 have a germline mutation in the *RET* proto-oncogene. The specific *RET* codon mutation (ie, genotype) correlates with the clinical expression (ie, phenotype) of MEN-2 (Figure 1). Moreover, particular mutations correlate with the aggressiveness of MTC, and this association is more predictable within a given family.[32,33] There are examples of mutations in some FMTC families with no known cases of MTC-related death, whereas the same mutations in other families correlate with aggressive MTC, which has led to MTC-related deaths.[34] This observation suggests that other environmental or genetic mechanisms also affect the biologic aggressiveness of MTC.

Mutations at codons 609, 611, 618, and 620 (extracellular cysteine-rich region, exon 10) are responsible for 10 to 15% of cases of MEN-2A and for all cases of MEN-2A/HSCR reported to date. A codon 634 (extracellular cysteine-rich region, exon 11) mutation has been found in approximately 85% of patients with MEN-2A and in all cases of MEN-2A/CLA.[4,35] However, not all patients with codon 634 mutations develop CLA, and not all patients with CLA have been found to carry *RET* mutations. The underlying pathophysiology of CLA may be related to a sensory abnormality in the C6-T6 dermatomes resulting in pruritus and chronic irrita-

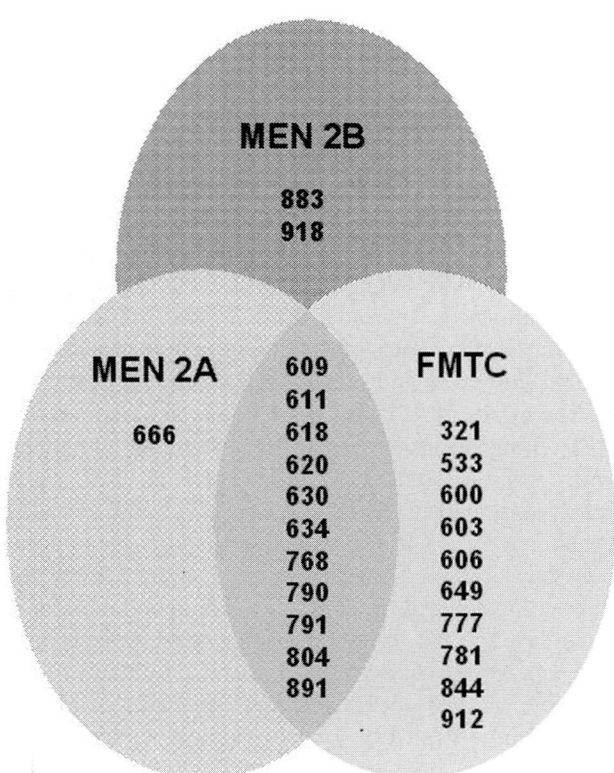

Figure 1 Correlation of specific *RET* codon mutations with the phenotypic expression of hereditary MTC (MEN-2B, MEN-2A, and FMTC). Additional rare *RET* mutations not listed include 532, 534, 635, 636, 638, 639, 778, and 852.

tion.[36,37] HPT, which occurs in up to 20% of MEN-2A patients, is also associated most commonly with codon 634 mutations, specifically the cysteine to arginine mutation (C634R).[35]

Germline mutations reported only in kindreds with FMTC are more equally distributed throughout the *RET* gene and include mutations at codons 321 (exon 5), 533 (exon 8), 600, 603, 606, (exon 10), 649 (exon 11), 777, 781, 844 (exon 14), and 912 (exon 16).[38] Many of these mutations are very rare and have been identified in small numbers of patients.

Some germline mutations in the *RET* gene are commonly associated with both MEN-2A and FMTC. These mutations include 609, 611, 618, 620 (exon 10), 630, 634 (exon 11), 768, 790, 791 (exon 13), 804 (exon 14), and 891 (exon 15). Although mutations at codon 804 were initially believed to be associated only with FMTC, subsequent analysis identified patients with pheochromocytoma harboring this mutation.[39–42] Presently, the V804M mutation has been associated only with FMTC, whereas pheochromocytoma has been reported in a family with the V804L mutation.[40]

A single point mutation at codon 918 (intracellular domain, exon 16) is present in most patients with MEN-2B (95%). Patients with MEN-2B may also rarely have a mutation in codon 883 (intracellular tyrosine kinase domain, exon 15).[4,43–46] Several authors have previously described codon 922 in association with MEN-2B; however, these reports included patients with either somatic codon 922 mutations present only within tumor cells or a compound heterozygous genotype with germline codon 918 and 922 mutations.[47–50] Kitamura and colleagues[50] found that the codon 922 mutation, which was maternally inherited (the codon 918 mutation occurred de novo in the patient), did not cause features of MEN-2B in the patient's mother and, therefore, concluded that the codon 922 mutation is unlikely to seriously affect the function of *RET* and seems not to confer a deleterious effect. Additional *RET* mutations associated with MEN-2B include compound heterozygous mutations of V804M with Y806C and V804M with S904C.[51,52]

Recently it was suggested that the biologic aggressiveness of MTC is associated with the specific *RET* mutation.[33] *RET* mutations have been stratified into 3 groups (levels 1 through 3) based on the biologic aggressiveness of MTC observed in patients with these mutations. Patients with level 1 mutations (codons 609, 768, 790, 791, 804, and 891) have the lowest risk of the development and growth of MTC. Initial clinical observations suggested that mutations at codons 768 and 804 may have low penetrance and, in particular, that patients with codon 804 mutations may develop MTC at an older age. However, subsequently it was found that the age at onset and the aggressiveness of MTC in association with this mutation may vary.[42,53] For example, Frohnauer and Decker reported 1 patient with a V804M mutation who was diagnosed with MTC and distant metastases at age 6 years and ultimately died at age 12 years, whereas another patient from a separate family with a V804M mutation was found to have normal thyroid histology following prophylactic thyroidectomy at age 27 years.[53] Patients with level 2 mutations (codons 611, 618, 620, and 634) have an intermediate risk of the early development and growth of MTC, and invasive MTC may be present as early as 5 years.[32] However, there have been 2 reports of younger patients with a codon 634 mutation in whom focal MTC was found in the thyroid specimen following prophylactic thyroidectomy at ages 15 months and 17 months.[54,55] Finally, patients with level 3 mutations (codons 883 and 918; MEN-2B) have the highest risk of the early development and growth of MTC.[32]

A recent review of the patients with hereditary MTC treated at our institution included 86 patients from 47 kindreds with FMTC or MEN-2; 83% of these patients underwent complete *RET* mutation analysis.[33] This study confirmed that the biologic behavior of MTC can be stratified by the specific *RET* mutations in an MEN-2 population. Because age is an independent predictor of finding advanced disease at the time of thyroidectomy, early thyroidectomy in at-risk patients with level 2 and 3 mutations can potentially reduce the risk of MTC to that for patients with lower-risk mutations. Such data support the practice of early thyroidectomy in higher-risk patients.

Genetic Testing and Genetic Counseling

When MEN-2 has not yet been established in the family and a patient (the "proband") presents with MTC, *RET* testing is indicated to confirm or exclude a hereditary etiology. Approximately 5 to 10% of patients with apparently sporadic MTC (ie, family history is negative) have been found to carry germline *RET* mutations. This is especially likely in patients who are diagnosed with MTC at a young age (< 40 years) or who are found to have bilateral thyroid nodules (multifocal MTC). Importantly, operative management of the neck (extent of lymphadenectomy and the management of the parathyroid glands) is based on the presence or absence of a *RET* mutation and the specific mutation found (Table 2). Correct diagnosis of these patients is also necessary for the early identification of pheochromocy-

toma and to allow the screening of at-risk family members. Therefore, the standard practice of ordering a *RET* test for all patients with a diagnosis of MTC is now supported and recommended by the American Society of Clinical Oncology, the National Comprehensive Cancer Network, and the International MEN99 workshop. *RET* testing is also necessary for carrier screening of relatives from an established MEN-2 family. The rationale for early carrier screening is to allow for the correct timing for prophylactic thyroidectomy, which will hopefully prevent the recurrence of MTC, and thus reduce disease-related morbidity and prevent disease-related death.

The merits of *RET* testing are now well described, and *RET* testing is considered standard of care for all patients with newly diagnosed MTC and for all first-degree relatives of patients with known *RET* mutations. *RET* genetic testing is widely available through many commercially licensed laboratories in the United States and internationally. An updated list of these laboratories including specific mutation testing services, specimen and paperwork requirements, and contact information is available via the GeneTests Web site (genetests.org). The most common practice for *RET* analysis in the United States includes DNA sequencing of exons 10, 11, and 13 to 16 for every patient with MTC, regardless of family history or clinical presentation. This approach will diagnose the overwhelming majority of patients with inherited MTC, missing only those with the rare mutations in exons 5 (codon 321) and 8 (codon 533).

Table 2 Author's Algorithm for the Operative Management of MTC

Patient Classification	Management of Neck*	Management of Parathyroid Glands that are Devascularized/Removed
Prophylactic thyroidectomy in MEN-2A/FMTC	Performance of central (level VI) neck dissection based on *RET* mutation, age, serum calcitonin level, and cervical US findings	• Autograft in neck if *RET* mutation is consistent with FMTC • Cryopreserve/autograft in forearm for *RET* mutations consistent with MEN-2A
Prophylactic thyroidectomy in MEN-2B	• Level VI dissection • Lateral neck (levels IIA, III, IV, V) dissection based on age, serum calcitonin level, and cervical US findings	Autograft in neck as parathyroids are normal in MEN-2B
Therapeutic thyroidectomy in MEN-2A/FMTC; patients with a malignant thyroid nodule(s) and a normal lateral neck by US	• Level 1 *RET* mutation: Level VI dissection • Level 2 *RET* mutation: Level VI dissection; ipsilateral/bilateral levels IIA–V dissection based on age, serum calcitonin level • Level 3 *RET* mutation: Level VI and bilateral levels IIA-V neck dissection	• Autograft in neck if *RET* mutation consistent with FMTC or MEN-2B • Cryopreserve/autograft in forearm for *RET* mutations consistent with MEN-2A
Therapeutic thyroidectomy in sporadic MTC (no *RET* mutation) with a malignant thyroid nodule and a normal lateral neck by US	Level VI dissection and ipsilateral levels IIA–V dissection	Autograft in neck

US = transcutaneous ultrasound.

*It is assumed that if US documents disease in level VI, a level VI dissection would be performed, and if disease is seen by US in the lateral neck, a functional neck dissection would be performed involving levels IIA, III, IV, and V.

If a patient presents with obvious phenotypic evidence of MEN-2B, it is reasonable to request examination of exons 15 and 16 alone, because to date, all patients with MEN-2B have been shown to have mutations only in these exons, and thus targeted exon analysis for MEN-2B patients will yield the same sensitivity with reduced cost and faster turnaround time for laboratory processing. Presymptomatic testing of at-risk relatives from families with a known *RET* mutation can also safely utilize targeted *RET* testing for the sole exon (or more specifically, the exact codon) known to be affected in the family. When a patient with MTC, thought to have a genetic etiology, receives a negative result following standard sequencing of the common 6 *RET* exons, repeat *RET* testing to include sequencing of the entire remaining coding exons should be considered. Analysis of the entire coding sequence of the *RET* gene (21 exons) is only available at selected commercial laboratories and is an expensive test that should be reserved for patients with evidence strongly suggesting a genetic cause.

Prior to ordering a *RET* test, the patient should be counseled regarding the potential risks, benefits, and limitations of genetic testing by a clinician or, preferably, a genetic counselor. A genetic counselor specializes in communicating various aspects of the genetic testing process including legal, ethical, financial, and psychological implications that make ordering a *RET* genetic test far more complicated than that for a standard blood test. When this communication process is completed, the patient can then provide informed consent, which must be documented on a form provided by the laboratory or the ordering institution. Copies of these signed documents should be made available to the patient. In some cases, preauthorization for genetic testing from a patient's health insurance plan may also be required.

Clinical Management of MEN-2-Related Neoplasms Based on Genotype

1. MTC

MTC is a consistent feature of MEN-2, has nearly full penetrance in all clinical subtypes, and is usually the first manifestation of the syndrome.[56,57] Patients with MEN-2A may manifest MTC as early as age 5 years and C-cell hyperplasia at an earlier age. However, when a diagnosis of MEN-2A has not yet been established within a family, newly diagnosed patients typically present with a thyroid nodule or neck mass by the age of 15 to 20 years. In the era before the identification of the *RET* gene as the cause of MEN-2, clinical screening for hereditary MTC consisted of measurements of basal and stimulated plasma calcitonin levels. Unfortunately, calcitonin is not always an accurate marker of MTC because levels of this hormone may also be elevated in patients with C-cell hyperplasia and in patients without MTC who have normal thyroid glands.[58,59] The optimal treatment strategy in patients with an inherited *RET* mutation is to prevent the development of MTC by performing early prophylactic thyroidectomy. The timing of surgical intervention in patients being evaluated for prophylactic thyroidectomy and the extent of surgery in patients with established MTC are based on the specific *RET* mutation (see Table 2). When thyroidectomy is performed for prevention, a total extracapsular thyroidectomy is indicated. Whether prophylactic central neck dissection should be performed depends on the patient's mutation risk group, preoperative plasma CT level, and findings on preoperative ultrasonography.

Patients (probands) with level 1 mutations are often older at presentation and have more indolent tumors than patients with level 2 or 3 mutations. For example, we previously treated a patient with a V804M (level 1) mutation who presented at age 55 years with a palpable thyroid mass. After thyroidectomy and central and bilateral neck dissection, the patient was found to have multifocal, bilateral MTC but no evidence of metastases in the 60 lymph nodes examined. Postoperative calcitonin levels in this patient fell to less than 1 pg/mL. In contrast, we treated a patient with a M918T (level 3) mutation who presented at age 17 years with mucosal neuromas. Pathologic analysis of the thyroidectomy and neck dissection specimen demonstrated multifocal MTC with bilateral metastases in 32 of 71 lymph nodes; this patient developed bone and liver metastases within 5 years. Because patients with level 1 mutations develop MTC with less aggressive metastatic potential and also have an initial delay in the neoplastic transformation of the thyroid C-cells, there is no consensus on the timing of thyroidectomy in these patients; some experts recommend prophylactic thyroidectomy by age 5 years, whereas others suggest that surgery can safely be delayed until age 10 years or beyond.[32] If thyroidectomy is delayed indefinitely, patients with level 1 mutations may develop lymph node and distant metastases. One of our patients with an S891A mutation presented with bone metastases at age 29 years and within 6 years developed metastases in the liver, lung, and breast. Although unusual for a carrier of a level 1 mutation, this case emphasizes the heterogeneity in biologic behavior, which may complicate the management of patients who postpone thyroidectomy.

Patients with level 2 and 3 mutations have a higher risk of the early development and growth of MTC. Thus, early prophylactic thyroidectomy in at-risk individuals represents the standard of care. Current guidelines for the treatment of patients with level 2 mutations include total thyroidectomy by the age of 5 years.[32] Because of our anecdotal experience with a 5-year-old (C634R mutation) who was found to have a 4 mm focus of invasive MTC following thyroidectomy, and the inability of serum calcitonin levels to differentiate between C-cell hyperplasia and invasive MTC, we currently prefer to perform prophylactic thyroidectomy before the age of 5 years in patients with level 2 *RET* mutations.[60] The need for central neck dissection in these patients is obviously based on the estimated risk of invasive MTC; the earlier the thyroidectomy, the lower the risk of invasive MTC.

Patients with level 3 mutations have the highest risk of developing aggressive MTC, and prophylactic total thyroidectomy should be performed by the age of 6 months if possible.[32] In patients who are diagnosed later in childhood, regional lymph node metastases are usually present requiring dissection of the central (level VI) compartment and both lateral neck (levels IIa, III, IV, and V) compartments.

2. PHEOCHROMOCYTOMA

Pheochromocytoma is present in approximately 50% of MEN-2 patients and is usually diagnosed after MTC, although it precedes the MTC diagnosis in up to 10% of patients, particularly those without an established family history of MEN-2. Routine biochemical screening for pheochromocytoma should be performed in all MEN-2 patients. In FMTC kindreds, periodic screening for pheochromocytoma may be warranted as some FMTC families—particularly those that are small, have vague or limited histories, or have a predominance of young individuals—may manifest adrenal disease over time that suggests a phenotype more consistent with MEN-2A. We currently screen all at-risk patients yearly with measurements of plasma-fractionated metanephrines.

Pheochromocytomas in patients with MEN-2 appear to be biologically distinct from pheochromocytomas with a sporadic etiology. MEN-2-related pheochromocytomas may be unilateral but are usually bilateral (up to 78%).[61] They are also frequently multicentric and may be associated with extratumoral medullary hyperplasia.[62] In contrast to sporadic ones, pheochromocytomas in patients with MEN-2 are rarely extra-adrenal or malignant and are diagnosed at a younger age.[63–66] The absence of metastatic pheochromocytoma in patients with hereditary pheochromocytoma, and the risk of morbidity and death from adrenal insufficiency in MEN-2 patients who undergo bilateral total adrenalectomy, support the surgical practice of cortex-sparing adrenalectomy. Prophylactic adrenalectomy is not recommended.

Our experience in the Department of Surgical Oncology, The University of Texas M. D. Anderson Cancer Center suggests that (1) metastatic pheochromocytoma rarely occurs in patients with hereditary pheochromocytoma (0 of 56 patients), (2) cortical-sparing adrenalectomy prevents the need for chronic corticosteroid replacement in the majority (65%) of patients, and (3) the risk of recurrent pheochromocytoma in the remnant adrenal gland after cortical-sparing adrenalectomy is low (20%). We therefore have adopted the following surgical strategy for hereditary pheochromocytoma. In patients with a unilateral pheochromocytoma and a normal contralateral gland, our preferred procedure is a laparoscopic, unilateral total adrenalectomy. In patients who present with bilateral pheochromocytomas, we use a midline incision to perform a unilateral cortical-sparing procedure with removal of the entire contralateral gland. In general, we prefer to preserve the cortex on only one side rather than assume double the risk of recurrent pheochromocytoma by preserving the cortex on both sides. Finally, in patients who present with a metachronous contralateral pheochromocytoma following a previous unilateral total adrenalectomy, we prefer an open cortical-sparing procedure. Short-term follow-up in all patients includes reinforcement of preoperative patient education about adrenal insufficiency and regularly scheduled testing of adrenal reserve. Long-term follow-up includes monitoring of the remaining adrenal gland, or portion of adrenal gland, for recurrent pheochromocytoma with yearly plasma or urinary screening studies.

3. HPT

HPT in MEN-2 is uncommon and has been reported only in patients with MEN-2A. HPT in MEN-2 may be caused by a single adenoma or diffuse hyperplasia of all parathyroid glands. HPT may be associated with symptoms of hypercalcemia or may be subclinical in the setting of mild elevations in serum levels of calcium and parathyroid hormone. Enlarged parathyroid glands encountered during thyroidectomy (prophylactic or therapeutic) for MTC in a eucalcemic patient should be resected.[67] Most endocrine surgeons leave normal-appearing parathyroid glands in situ during thyroid surgery for inherited MTC. Importantly, one should not autograft in the neck if the patient's *RET* mutation is associated with MEN-2A as there remains a risk of the future development of HPT. In this case, resected parathyroid glands should be cryopreserved or autografted into the forearm.

Most MEN-2A patients who develop HPT, develop hypercalcemia many years after they underwent thyroidectomy. The indications for surgical intervention are similar to those for patients with sporadic primary HPT. In patients with asymptomatic HPT and a minimal elevation in serum calcium, we often use bone mineral density changes as an indication for parathyroidectomy. A declining bone mineral density is an indication for operation even in an asymptomatic patient. For those patients with diffuse hyperplasia of all parathyroid glands, either subtotal (3 or 3.5 gland) resection or total parathyroidectomy and autotransplantation is performed.

Conclusion

The management of the MEN-2 patient is complex and requires a combination of an experienced surgeon, endocrinologist, and genetic counselor. Further information regarding the clinical management of patients with MEN and the importance of genetic counseling can be obtained from the Multiple Endocrine Neoplasia Program Web site (www.mdanderson.org/diseases/men).

References

1. Mulligan LM, Kwok JB, Healey CS, et al. Germ-line mutations of the RET proto-oncogene in multiple endocrine neoplasia type 2A. Nature 1993;363:458–60.

2. Donis-Keller H, Dou S, Chi D, et al. Mutations in the RET proto-oncogene are associated with MEN 2A and FMTC. Hum Mol Genet 1993;2:851–6.

3. OMIM (Online Mendelian Inheritance in Man). Johns Hopkins University. Available at: http://www.ncbi.nlm. nih.gov/entrez/query.fcgi?db=OMIM (accessed October 15, 2006.).

4. Eng C, Clayton D, Schuffenecker I, et al. The relationship between specific RET proto-oncogene mutations and disease phenotype in multiple endocrine neoplasia type 2. International RET mutation consortium analysis. JAMA 1996;276:1575–9.

5. Sipple J. The association of pheochromocytoma with carcinomas of the thyroid gland. Am J Med 1961;31:163–6.

6. Steiner AL, Goodman AD, Powers SR. Study of a kindred with pheochromocytoma, medullary thyroid carcinoma, hyperparathyroidism and Cushing's disease: multiple endocrine neoplasia, type 2. Medicine (Baltimore) 1968; 47:371–409.

7. Eng C, Mulligan LM, Smith DP, et al. Low frequency of germline mutations in the RET proto-oncogene in patients with apparently sporadic medullary thyroid carcinoma. Clin Endocrinol (Oxf) 1995;43:123–7.

8. Decker RA, Peacock ML, Watson P. Hirschsprung disease in MEN 2A: increased spectrum of RET exon 10 genotypes and strong genotype-phenotype correlation. Hum Mol Genet 1998;7:129–34.

9. Gagel RF, Levy ML, Donovan DT, et al. Multiple endocrine neoplasia type 2a associated with cutaneous lichen amyloidosis. Ann Intern Med 1989;111:802–6.

10. Gorlin RJ, Sedano HO, Vickers RA, Cervenka J. Multiple mucosal neuromas, pheochromocytoma and medullary carcinoma of the thyroid—a syndrome. Cancer 1968;22: 293–9 passim.

11. Eng C. RET proto-oncogene in the development of human cancer. J Clin Oncol 1999;17:380–93.

12. Farndon JR, Leight GS, Dilley WG, et al. Familial medullary thyroid carcinoma without associated endocrinopathies: a distinct clinical entity. Br J Surg 1986;73:278–81.

13. Takahashi M, Ritz J, Cooper GM. Activation of a novel human transforming gene, ret, by DNA rearrangement. Cell 1985;42:581–8.

14. Takahashi M, Buma Y, Iwamoto T, et al. Cloning and expression of the ret proto-oncogene encoding a tyrosine kinase with two potential transmembrane domains. Oncogene 1988;3:571–8.

15. Pachnis V, Mankoo B, Costantini F. Expression of the c-ret proto-oncogene during mouse embryogenesis. Development 1993;119:1005–17.

16. Tsuzuki T, Takahashi M, Asai N, et al. Spatial and temporal expression of the ret proto-oncogene product in embryonic, infant and adult rat tissues. Oncogene 1995;10:191–8.

17. Takahashi M, Iwashita T, Santoro M, et al. Co-segregation of MEN2 and Hirschsprung's disease: the same mutation of RET with both gain and loss-of-function? Hum Mutat 1999;13:331–6.

18. Donghi R, Sozzi G, Pierotti MA, et al. The oncogene associated with human papillary thyroid carcinoma (PTC) is assigned to chromosome 10 q11-q12 in the same region as multiple endocrine neoplasia type 2A (MEN2A). Oncogene 1989;4:521–3.

19. Grieco M, Santoro M, Berlingieri MT, et al. PTC is a novel rearranged form of the ret proto-oncogene and is frequently detected in vivo in human thyroid papillary carcinomas. Cell 1990;60:557–63.

20. Edery P, Lyonnet S, Mulligan LM, et al. Mutations of the RET proto-oncogene in Hirschsprung's disease. Nature 1994;367:378–80.

21. Romeo G, Ronchetto P, Luo Y, et al. Point mutations affecting the tyrosine kinase domain of the RET proto-oncogene in Hirschsprung's disease. Nature 1994;367:377–8.

22. Angrist M, Bolk S, Thiel B, et al. Mutation analysis of the RET receptor tyrosine kinase in Hirschsprung disease. Hum Mol Genet 1995;4:821–30.

23. Attie T, Pelet A, Edery P, et al. Diversity of RET proto-oncogene mutations in familial and sporadic Hirschsprung disease. Hum Mol Genet 1995;4:1381–6.

24. Eng C. Seminars in medicine of the Beth Israel Hospital, Boston. The RET proto-oncogene in multiple endocrine neoplasia type 2 and Hirschsprung's disease. N Engl J Med 1996;335:943–51.

25. Eng C, Mulligan LM. Mutations of the RET proto-oncogene in the multiple endocrine neoplasia type 2 syndromes, related sporadic tumours, and hirschsprung disease. Hum Mutat 1997;9:97–109.

26. Santoro M, Carlomagno F, Romano A, et al. Activation of RET as a dominant transforming gene by germline mutations of MEN2A and MEN2B. Science 1995;267:381–3.

27. Asai N, Iwashita T, Matsuyama M, Takahashi M. Mechanism of activation of the ret proto-oncogene by multiple endocrine neoplasia 2A mutations. Mol Cell Biol 1995;15:1613–9.

28. Xing S, Smanik PA, Oglesbee MJ, et al. Characterization of ret oncogenic activation in MEN2 inherited cancer syndromes. Endocrinology 1996;137:1512–9.

29. Akhand AA, Ikeyama T, Akazawa S, et al. Evidence of both extra- and intracellular cysteine targets of protein modification for activation of RET kinase. Biochem Biophys Res Commun 2002;292:826–31.

30. Hofstra RM, Landsvater RM, Ceccherini I, et al. A mutation in the RET proto-oncogene associated with multiple endocrine neoplasia type 2B and sporadic medullary thyroid carcinoma. Nature 1994;367:375–6.

31. Eng C, Smith DP, Mulligan LM, et al. A novel point mutation in the tyrosine kinase domain of the RET proto-oncogene in sporadic medullary thyroid carcinoma and in a family with FMTC. Oncogene 1995;10:509–13.

32. Brandi ML, Gagel RF, Angeli A, et al. Guidelines for diagnosis and therapy of MEN type 1 and type 2. J Clin Endocrinol Metab 2001;86:5658–71.

33. Yip L, Cote GJ, Shapiro SE, et al. Multiple endocrine neoplasia type 2: evaluation of the genotype-phenotype relationship. Arch Surg 2003;138:409–16.

34. Gagel RF, Marx S. Multiple endocrine neoplasia. In: Larsen P, Kronenberg S, Melmed S, Polansky K, editors. Williams textbook of endocrinology. 10th ed. Philadelphia: W. B. Saunders; 2003. p. 1717–62.

35. Mulligan LM, Eng C, Healey CS, et al. Specific mutations of the RET proto-oncogene are related to disease phenotype in MEN 2A and FMTC. Nat Genet 1994;6:70–4.

36. Chabre O, Labat F, Pinel N, et al. Cutaneous lesion associated with multiple endocrine neoplasia type 2A: lichen amyloidosis or notalgia paresthetica? Henry Ford Hosp Med J 1992;40:245–8.

37. Wong CK, Lin CS. Friction amyloidosis. Int J Dermatol 1988;27:302–7.

38. Evans DB, Shapiro SE, Cote G. Medullary thyroid cancer: the importance of RET testing. Surgery [In press].

39. Fink M, Weinhusel A, Niederle B, Haas OA. Distinction between sporadic and hereditary medullary thyroid carcinoma (MTC) by mutation analysis of the RET proto-oncogene. Study Group Multiple Endocrine Neoplasia Austria (SMENA). Int J Cancer 1996;69:312–6.

40. Nilsson O, Tisell LE, Jansson S, et al. Adrenal and extra-adrenal pheochromocytomas in a family with germline RET V804L mutation. JAMA 1999;281:1587–8.

41. Fattoruso O, Quadro L, Libroia A, et al. A GTG to ATG novel point mutation at codon 804 in exon 14 of the RET proto-oncogene in two families affected by familial medullary thyroid carcinoma. Hum Mutat 1998;Suppl 1: S167–71.

42. Feldman GL, Edmonds MW, Ainsworth PJ, et al. Variable expressivity of familial medullary thyroid carcinoma (FMTC) due to a RET V804M (GTG—>ATG) mutation. Surgery 2000;128:93–8.

43. Smith DP, Houghton C, Ponder BA. Germline mutation of RET codon 883 in two cases of de novo MEN 2B. Oncogene 1997;15:1213–7.

44. Eng C, Smith DP, Mulligan LM, et al. Point mutation within the tyrosine kinase domain of the RET proto-oncogene in multiple endocrine neoplasia type 2B and related sporadic tumours. Hum Mol Genet 1994;3:237–41.

45. Carlson KM, Dou S, Chi D, et al. Single missense mutation in the tyrosine kinase catalytic domain of the RET protooncogene is associated with multiple endocrine neoplasia type 2B. Proc Natl Acad Sci U S A 1994;91: 1579–83.

46. Rossel M, Schuffenecker I, Schlumberger M, et al. Detection of a germline mutation at codon 918 of the RET proto-oncogene in French MEN 2B families. Hum Genet 1995;95:403–6.

47. Kalinin VN, Amosenko FA, Shabanov MA, et al. Three novel mutations in the RET proto-oncogene. J Mol Med 2001;79:609–12.

48. Jindrichova S, Kodet R, Krskova L, et al. The newly detected mutations in the RET proto-oncogene in exon 16 as a cause of sporadic medullary thyroid carcinoma. J Mol Med 2003;81:819–23.

49. Amosenko FA, Brzhezovskiy VZ, Lyubchendo LN, et al. Analysis of mutations of the RET proto-oncogene in patients with medullary thyroid carcinoma. Russ J Genetics 2003;39:706–11.

50. Kitamura Y, Scavarda N, Wells SA, et al. Two maternally derived missense mutations in the tyrosine kinase domain of the RET protooncogene in a patient with de novo MEN 2B. Hum Mol Genet 1995;4:1987–8.

51. Miyauchi A, Futami H, Hai N, et al. Two germline missense mutations at codons 804 and 806 of the RET proto-oncogene in the same allele in a patient with multiple endocrine neoplasia type 2B without codon 918 mutation. Jpn J Cancer Res 1999;90:1–5.

52. Iwashita T, Murakami H, Kurokawa K, et al. A two-hit model for development of multiple endocrine neoplasia type 2B by RET mutations. Biochem Biophys Res Commun 2000;268:804–8.

53. Frohnauer MK, Decker RA. Update on the MEN 2A c804 RET mutation: is prophylactic thyroidectomy indicated? Surgery 2000;128:1052–8.

54. Sanso GE, Domene HM, Garcia R, et al. Very early detection of RET proto-oncogene mutation is crucial for preventive thyroidectomy in multiple endocrine neoplasia type 2 children: presence of C-cell malignant disease in asymptomatic carriers. Cancer 2002;94:323–30.

55. Machens A, Niccoli-Sire P, Hoegel J, et al. Early malignant progression of hereditary medullary thyroid cancer. N Engl J Med 2003;349:1517–25.

56. Ponder BA, Ponder MA, Coffey R, et al. Risk estimation and screening in families of patients with medullary thyroid carcinoma. Lancet 1988;1:397–401.

57. Easton DF, Ponder MA, Cummings T, et al. The clinical and screening age-at-onset distribution for the MEN-2 syndrome. Am J Hum Genet 1989;44:208–15.

58. Landsvater RM, Rombouts AG, te Meerman GJ, et al. The clinical implications of a positive calcitonin test for C-cell hyperplasia in genetically unaffected members of an MEN2A kindred. Am J Hum Genet 1993;52:335–42.

59. Lips CJ, Landsvater RM, Hoppener JW, et al. Clinical screening as compared with DNA analysis in families with multiple endocrine neoplasia type 2A. N Engl J Med 1994;331:828–35.

60. Yen TW, Shapiro SE, Gagel RF, et al. Medullary thyroid carcinoma: results of a standardized surgical approach in a contemporary series of 80 consecutive patients. Surgery 2003;134:890–901.

61. Koch CA, Pacak K, Chrousos GP. The molecular pathogenesis of hereditary and sporadic adrenocortical and adrenomedullary tumors. J Clin Endocrinol Metab 2002;87:5367–84.

62. Webb TA, Sheps SG, Carney JA. Differences between sporadic pheochromocytoma and pheochromocytoma in multiple endocrine neoplasia, type 2. Am J Surg Pathol 1980;4:121–6.

63. Inabnet WB, Caragliano P, Pertsemlidis D. Pheochromocytoma: inherited associations, bilaterality, and cortex preservation. Surgery 2000;128:1007–12.

64. Neumann HP, Bausch B, McWhinney SR, et al. Germ-line mutations in nonsyndromic pheochromocytoma. N Engl J Med 2002;346:1459–66.

65. Conte-Devolx B, Schuffenecker I, Niccoli P, et al. Multiple endocrine neoplasia type 2: management of patients and subjects at risk. French Study Group on Calcitonin-Secreting Tumors (GETC). Horm Res 1997;47:221–6.

66. Modigliani E, Vasen HM, Raue K, et al. Pheochromocytoma in multiple endocrine neoplasia type 2: European study. The Euromen Study Group. J Intern Med 1995;238:363–7.

67. Simonds WF, James-Newton LA, Agarwal SK, et al. Familial isolated hyperparathyroidism: clinical and genetic characteristics of 36 kindreds. Medicine (Baltimore) 2002;81:1–26.

CHAPTER 51

INDICATION AND TECHNIQUES OF DIAGNOSTIC BREAST BIOPSY

KARI M. ROSENKRANZ, MD

Introduction

A multidisciplinary approach is essential to accurate, expeditious diagnosis of breast cancer. Prior to the routine implementation of mammography and ultrasound for breast cancer screening and diagnosis, breast cancers were detected on physical examination by patients, general practitioners, or gynecologists. Cancers were generally later stage with subsequently worsened prognosis. Multiple surgeries were required for diagnosis and treatment. As imaging and biopsy techniques have improved, general practitioners, gynecologists, radiologists, pathologists, cytopathologists, and surgeons have developed comprehensive algorithms in the diagnosis and management of women with breast abnormalities.

The increasing use of screening mammography for breast cancer diagnosis has resulted in a growing number of detected abnormalities. The American Cancer Society currently recommends annual or biannual screening mammography for all women beginning at the age of 40 and annual screening mammography for all women 50 years and older. Screening mammography results in the identification of earlier-stage breast cancers and a significant reduction in breast cancer mortality. Currently, over 40 million screening mammograms are performed yearly in the United States. Abnormalities are noted on 20% of these studies. Ultimately, 1 to 1.5 million women undergo breast biopsy each year in the United States. Eighty percent of these biopsies are benign.

Historically, abnormalities detected by mammography or physical exam required surgical excision for accurate diagnosis. Over the last 20 years, however, percutaneous biopsy techniques have emerged as safe, precise, and cost-effective methods of tissue acquisition. Biopsy technique, whether fine needle aspiration (FNA), core biopsy, or stereo tactic biopsy, is generally dictated by the location and radiographic qualities of the abnormality as well as by patient factors. Surgery is no longer required for diagnosis; rather, surgery is now implemented for diagnosis only in cases of pathologic-radiological discordance and/or failed percutaneous approaches. Given the high rate of benign biopsy, percutaneous, image-guided biopsy techniques are essential to providing excellent patient care.

Palpable Masses

Palpable masses are the most common presenting symptoms of breast cancer. Approximately 1 in 10 palpable masses represents a cancer. This risk increases significantly with age. Women under the age of 40 with a palpable breast abnormality have a 1% incidence of cancer, whereas those over the age of 55 have a 37% risk.[1] All patients presenting with a palpable breast mass or dominant thickening must undergo standard evaluation including history (focusing on the mass and specific risk factors for breast cancer) and physical examination.

In women under the age of 35 without family history of breast or ovarian cancer, cautious observation of the abnormality over a single menstrual cycle is a reasonable approach. Any persistent mass in a young woman requires imaging. Given the difficulty of mammographic interpretation owing to breast density in young women, ultrasound is a logical first test in this age group. Ultrasound also differentiates solid versus more common cystic lesions. FNA with a 22-gauge needle is used for aspiration of painful cysts for symptomatic relief or for sampling of complex cystic tissue to exclude a cancer diagnosis. Simple cysts are observed unless they are symptomatic. If the simple cyst causes pain or enlarges, FNA is indicated. Bloody fluid cytology should be reviewed by an experienced cytopathologist. Nonbloody aspirate is discarded. Cysts that persist or recur in the same location following aspiration require ultrasound-guided FNA with cytological analysis to exclude a cancer diagnosis.

In women over the age of 35, any dominant, palpable abnormality warrants evaluation with mammography and ultrasound (Figure 1). Between 1 and 3% of women present with synchronous, bilateral breast cancers.[2] Bilateral mammography is therefore recommended despite the presence of a unilaterally palpable process. Routine use of unilateral or bilateral ultrasound significantly increases the 80 to 90% sensitivity of mammography alone. All lesions visualized must undergo biopsy. When feasible, ultrasound offers the most efficient, most comfortable option for patients. The biopsy is performed and documented in real time, capturing images of the biopsy needle within the lesion in longitudinal and transverse planes (Figures 2 and 3). This enhances the accuracy and adequacy of sampling. For solid lesions, we utilize 18-gauge core biopsy rather than FNA. Core biopsy provides information about invasion and tumor grade and enhances surgical planning. Core also obviates the need for experienced cytopathologic interpretation of the sample, which is required for FNA. The skin is prepped and local anesthetic is introduced. Lidocaine is carefully injected under imaging guidance. An 18-gauge core needle is then passed into the lesion as described above. For larger areas of concern, 2 to 6 cores are taken to ensure adequacy of sampling. Metallic

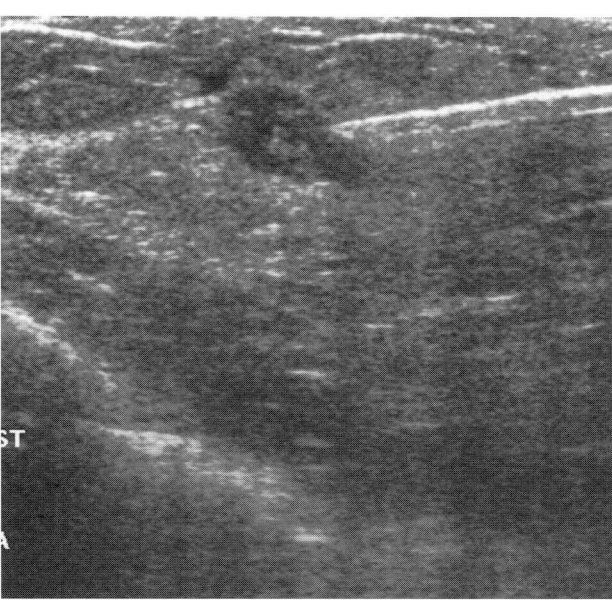

Figure 2 Ultrasound image of a core needle visualized within the targeted lesion in the longitudinal plane.

markers are placed following biopsy. This clip is used to guide surgical excision in patients with complete radiological response to neoadjuvant therapy and in patients in whom complete excision of the lesion is accomplished percutaneously.

The risk of cancer in the setting of a palpable abnormality with a negative ultrasound and Breast

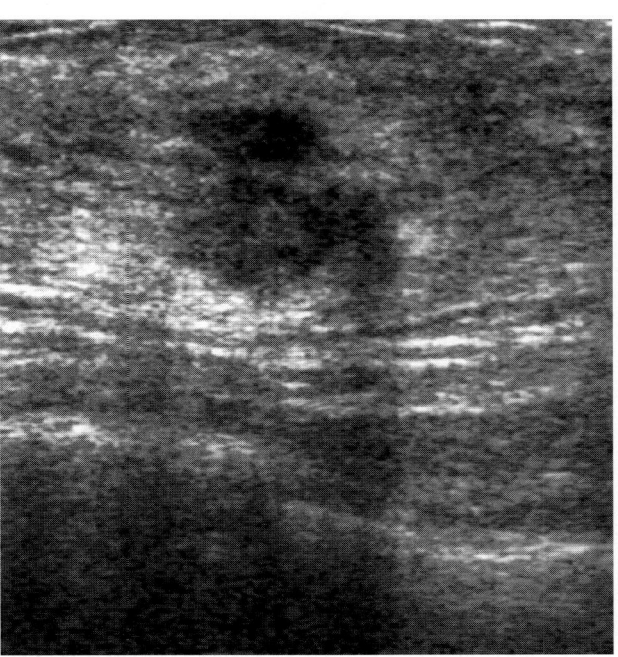

Figure 1 Ultrasound appearance of a 1.5 cm palpable breast mass. Note irregular borders, internal echoes, and posterior acoustic shadowing.

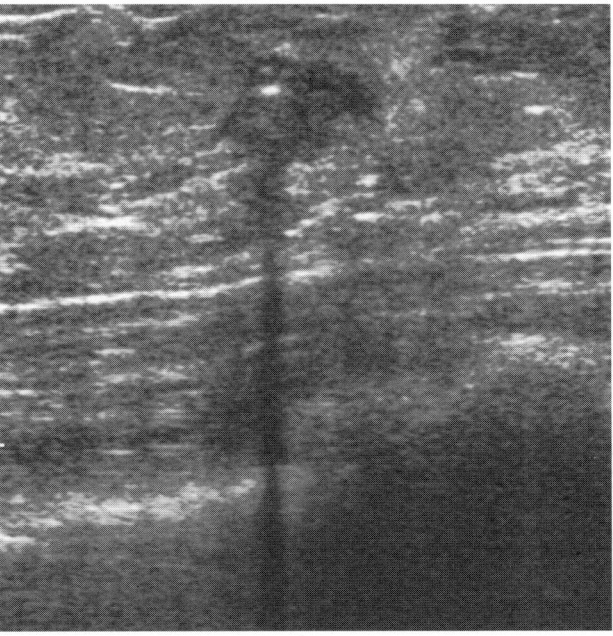

Figure 3 Ultrasound image of a core needle visualized within the targeted lesion in the transverse plane.

Imaging-Reporting and Data System (BI-RADS) category 1 mammogram is 2.7%.[3] Although this risk is low and should provide comfort to patients, all palpable masses must undergo biopsy. If the palpable abnormality is not visualized radiographically, handheld core biopsy with an 18-gauge device must be performed.

If histological or cytological results are insufficient, equivocal, or discordant with clinical or radiographic concern, surgical biopsy offers a definitive option for diagnosis.

Nonpalpable Lesions: Microcalcifications

The increase in mammographic screening has led to a rise in the detection of nonpalpable breast lesions. Patients with BI-RADS 1 and 2 mammograms are recommended for annual follow-up. Women with BI-RADS 3 images should be reevaluated at 6-month intervals with physical exam and repeat imaging. Patients in whom geographic adversity precludes short-interval follow-up or in whom anxiety over a cancer diagnosis is consuming may be offered percutaneous biopsy to exclude cancer on a BI-RADS 3 mammogram. Mammographic lesions of increased concern (BI-RADS 4 and 5) include microcalcifications, discrete masses, and parenchymal densities or distortions. Because most (> 75%) of nonpalpable abnormalities targeted for biopsy are benign, minimally invasive means of biopsy are indicated.

High-risk or suspicious calcifications appear heterogeneous, pleomorphic, linear, or branching. Intermediate (indeterminate) risk calcifications are amorphous, indistinct, clustered, or punctuate (Figure 4). Mammograms demonstrating intermediate-risk calcifications are most often classified as BI-RADS 3. If no suspicious findings are revealed on call-back images (compression and magnified views), these patients are followed with repeat mammogram at 6 months. Suspicious microcalcifications mandate further immediate evaluation with compression and magnification views as well as biopsy. Microcalcifications are generally not well visualized on ultrasound. Stereotactic biopsy is, therefore, the preferred technique of tissue retrieval. Relative contraindications to stereotactic biopsy include very small breasts and lesions close to the skin or chest wall. Stereotactic biopsy requires prone, still positioning of the patient for up to 60 minutes. Patients with anxiety or cardiopulmonary disease may not be able to meet these criteria. Stereotactic equipment also has weight limitations generally under 135 kg. Thus, morbid obesity may represent a contraindication. In these patients, wire

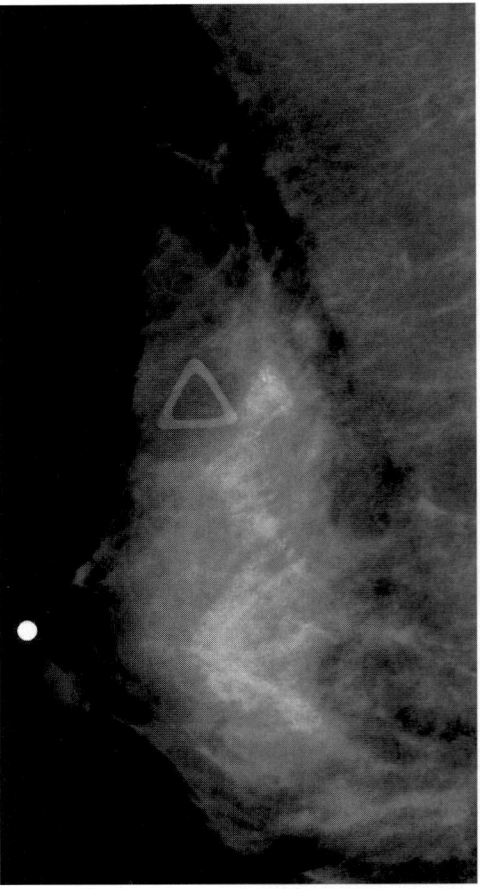

Figure 4 Indeterminate clustered calcifications on magnification view mammogram.

localized excisional biopsy is the only diagnostic technique available.

In patients eligible for and amenable to stereotactic biopsy, a 9-gauge vacuum-assisted device is utilized. After identifying the concerning microcalcifications on scout films, stereotactic digital images are obtained in order to align the core biopsy needle. A minimum of 6 cores are taken. Radiographs of the core samples must reveal the targeted calcification. If the recovery of intended tissue is scant, another 6 core biopsies should be retrieved. A metallic clip is then placed into the targeted area in order to mark the appropriate tissue in the event that surgical excision is necessary (Figure 5).

Pre- or intraoperative needle localization is utilized for patients with microcalcifications who require excisional biopsy for diagnosis and for those who require complete excision of biopsy-proven atypia or malignancy. Metallic clips or visible lesions may be localized preoperatively or intraoperatively using ultrasound guidance. Needle localization is more often performed with mammographic guidance. Two or more bracketing

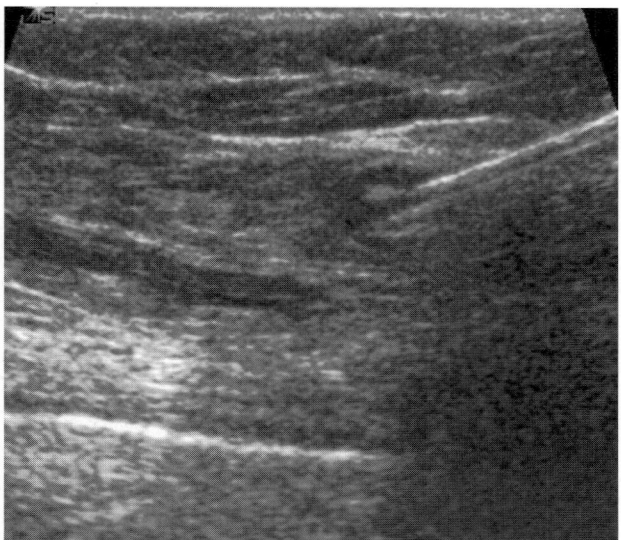

Figure 5 Placement of metallic marker clip under real-time ultrasound guidance.

wires are placed for contiguous areas larger than 2 cm or for multifocal disease (Figure 6). Mammograms with wires in place as well as the radiologist's interpretations are returned to the operating room with the patient to

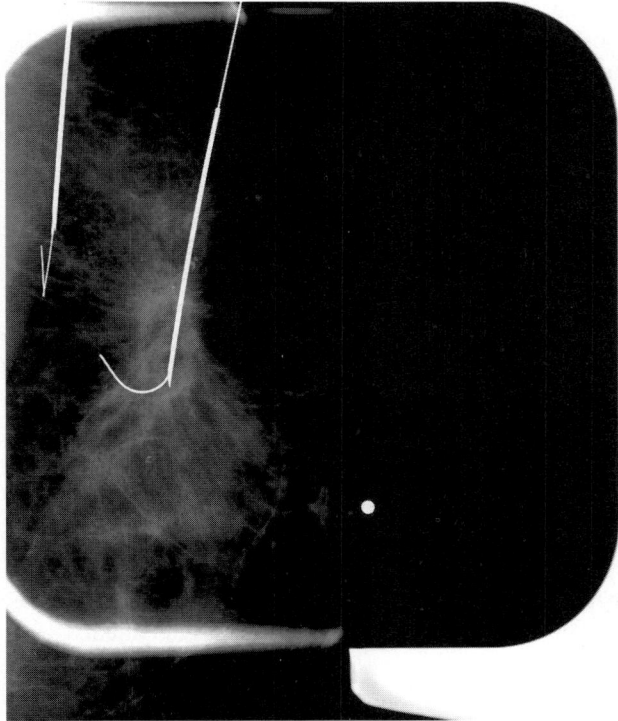

Figure 6 Mammographic wire localization using a bracketed technique for 2.5 cm area of calcifications with associated mass lesion.

facilitate communication between the radiologist and the surgeon. Following surgical excision, the specimen is sent for radiograph to ensure the targeted area of calcifications or the intended marking clips have been removed. Immediate intraoperative pathologic margin assessment in correlation with immediate specimen mammogram decreases the rate of reexcision.

Nonpalpable Lesions: Densities and Masses

Any patient with BI-RAD 4 or 5 mammogram requires a tissue diagnosis to exclude cancer within a mass, or density. Prior to percutaneous intervention, women in this category undergo ultrasound of the ipsilateral breast and nodal basins. If the parenchymal lesion is identified on both mammogram and ultrasound, ultrasound provides the most comfortable and least time-consuming guidance for biopsy. The procedure for ultrasound-guided biopsy for a nonpalpable lesion mirrors that described for a palpable lesion. A linear-array transducer with a frequency of at least 7.5 MHz is used for imaging. After sterilization of the skin, local anesthetic is injected and a small skin incision is made sharply. An 18-gauge core device is then entered into the breast tissue. The ultrasound probe is turned 90 degrees so that the trajectory of the biopsy needle is visualized entering the lesion in both the transverse and longitudinal planes. If nodules visualized on ultrasound are associated with microcalcifications on mammography, core specimens are evaluated by mammography to ensure adequacy of sampling. Multiple cores are taken if the area of concern is large or if calcifications are targeted within the mass. Following the biopsy, the remainder of the breast is then fully evaluated for multicentric disease.

Finally, the axillary, internal mammary, infraclavicular, and supraclavicular nodal basins are inspected for evidence of metastatic disease. Suspicious characteristics in lymph nodes include masses within the node, bulging in the cortical contour (> 2mm), irregulararity of the cortex, round or ovoid shape, hypoechoic core, node enlargement, and compression or displacement of the hyperechoic fatty hilum. Concerning nodes detected by ultrasound (Figures 7 and 8) are evaluated with image-guided FNA using a 21-gauge needle. The needle is entered into the node under guidance and with manual vacuum is passed repeatedly in the node prior to removal from the node. Ultrasound-guided FNA of suspicious lymph nodes carries a sensitivity of 80% and specificity of 100%.[4] Thus, lymph node biopsy is a useful test that may help treatment planning and spare patients the time and expense of unnecessary sentinel lymph node biopsy.

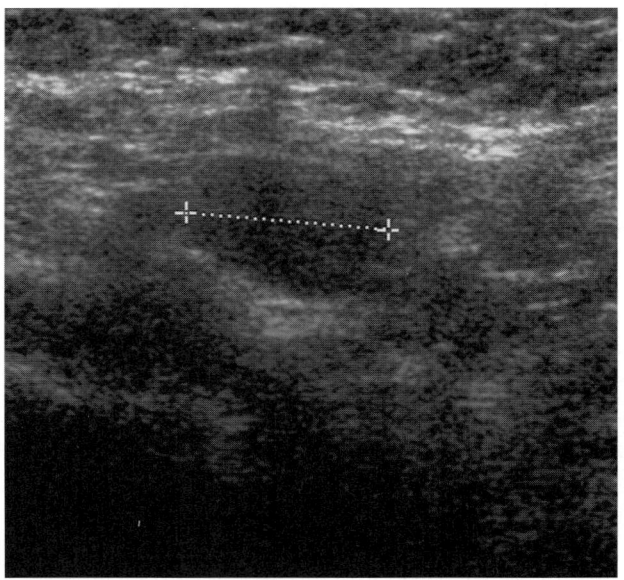

Figure 7 Transverse ultrasound image of suspicious axillary lymph node. Note round shape.

Nonpalpable densities, distortions, and masses visualized by mammography only necessitate stereotactic biopsy. Six indicative biopsy specimens are sufficient if postprocedure mammogram confirms accuracy of the sampling. Again, a metallic marker is placed prior to removal of the biopsy device in order to identify the location for future imaging and treatment. The contra-

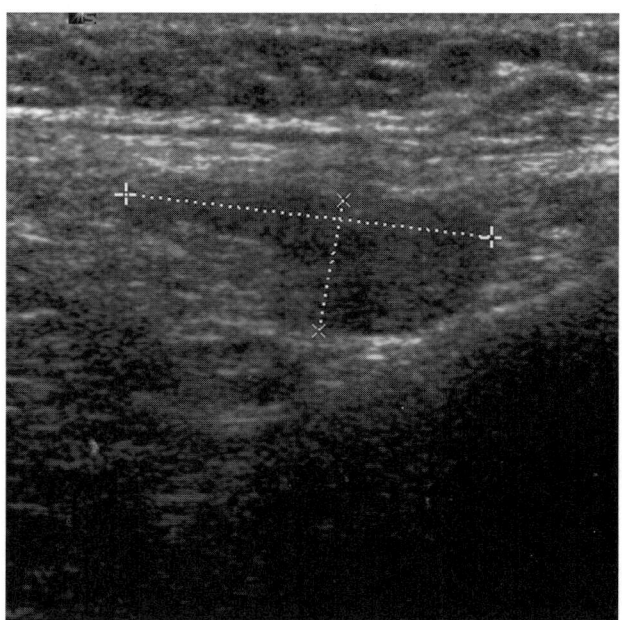

Figure 8 Longitudinal ultrasound image of suspicious axillary lymph node.

indications and technique of stereotactic biopsy in the setting of a nonpalpable mass are as described for microcalcifications. If percutaneous approaches fail, again, surgical biopsy is indicated.

Nonpalpable Lesions: Magnetic Resonance Imaging (MRI) Identification

MRI has been shown to increase cancer detection in women at high risk of developing the disease.[5] Specificity of this test is poor, however. The role of MRI screening in high-risk women remains controversial. Current guidelines from the National Comprehensive Cancer Network support the consideration of screening MRI as an adjunct to clinical breast examination and mammography.[6]

The use of breast MRI mandates capability of MRI-guided localization and biopsy. Currently at our institution we repeat a directed ultrasound examination of suspicious areas identified by MRI. In the majority of cases, ultrasound abnormality is visualized and ultrasound-guided core needle biopsy is performed as described previously. In cases with mammographically and ultrasound occult lesions, MRI-guided biopsy is utilized. MRI-compatible vacuum-guided 9-gauge core biopsy allows accurate sampling of tissue and metallic marker placement. The biopsy is performed in the prone position; patients with cardiopulmonary disease may be unable to tolerate the procedure. Discordant results necessitate surgical excision.

Nipple Discharge

Abnormal or pathologic nipple discharge is spontaneous, arises from a single duct, is persistent, bloody, watery or serous, and unilateral. Physiologic discharge occurs with manipulation only, is white or green, usually bilateral, and is not bloody. The most common etiology of pathologic discharge is a benign intraductal papilloma. Pathologic discharge requires thorough physical examination and radiological evaluation with mammogram, ultrasound, and ductography.

Findings of any mass lesion on imaging studies are assessed with vacuum-assisted core biopsy. Benign papilloma may be associated with amorphorous calcifications or a well-circumscribed mass. Patients with concordant imaging studies and a histologically confirmed benign papilloma are observed. If imaging reveals an irregular mass or suspicious calcifications, benign histology is discordant and excision is required. Atypical features within a papillary lesion mandate excision. Persistent or bloody discharge despite negative imaging studies should be treated with duct excision for accurate tissue diagnosis and symptomatic relief (Figure 9).

Complications of Percutanous Biopsy

Complications of percutaneous biopsy include bleeding, infection, and, rarely, pneumothorax. The overall complication rate of percutaneous biopsy as documented by a multicenter prospective study is negligible and is significantly less than that of surgical biopsy.[7] The use of antiplatelet agents and anticoagulants represents a relative contraindication to percutaneous biopsy and increases bleeding risk. If medical condition permits, antiplatelet agents are held for 5 to 7 days prior to biopsy. Anticoagulants are stopped 3 days prior to biopsy. If the patient's medical team feels that continued use of anticoagulation or antiplatelet agents is mandatory, biopsy can proceed with increased attentiveness to postprocedure compression. Patients with known, uncorrectable bleeding diatheses should be offered open rather than percutaneous biopsy.

Management Issues

ATYPIA

Atypical ductal hyperplasia (ADH) is associated with a 20 to 50% incidence of ductal carcinoma in situ (DCIS) or invasive carcinoma coexistent near the biopsy site.[8,9]

Given the significant likelihood of associated malignancy, we perform needle localized surgical excision in women with biopsy-proven ADH.

The management of lobular neoplasia (atypical lobular hyperplasia [ALH] and lobular carcinoma in situ [LCIS]) identified on core biopsy is controversial and evolving. Lobular atypia is generally asymptomatic and is therefore an incidental finding on screening imaging and subsequent biopsy. Both LCIS and ALH are associated with an increased relative risk of developing breast cancer in both the ipsilateral and contralateral breast. The overall risk of invasive cancer was noted to be 7.1% at 10 years in a study of 4,853 patients from the SEER database.[10] Risk continues to increase over time. A second study determined the relative risk of a breast cancer diagnosis (invasive or in situ) to be increased 8-fold in women in the first 15 years following diagnosis of lobular atypia.[11] The presence of LCIS or ALH in a stereotactic or ultrasound-guided core specimen may reflect an adjacent cancer. The likelihood of upgrading a core biopsy diagnosis after surgical excision of LCIS or ADH ranges from 9 to 38%.[8,12–14] A study from our institution found that the presence of a mammographic mass at the site of core biopsy is predictive of upgraded pathology following surgical excision. Other studies, however, have not identified specific factors that reliably differentiate atypia from cancer on core biopsy.

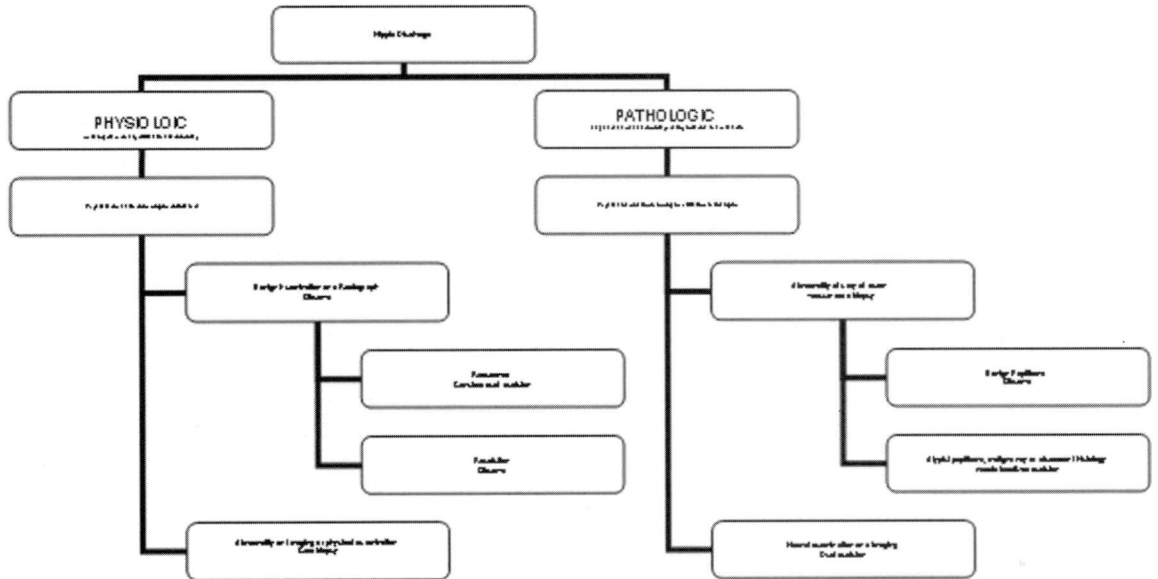

Algorithm for the management of nipple discharge

Figure 9 Management algorithm for nipple discharge.

Decisions regarding management of women with lobular atypia are dictated by the clinical scenario in which the diagnosis is made. Atypia identified on percutaneous core biopsy that is associated with a finding on physical examination, histologic pleomorphism, residual calcifications on mammogram, or a radiographic density mandates surgical excision. If the LCIS or ALH on core biopsy are not associated with any of these risk factors for adjacent cancers, cautious observation is warranted. Physical examination, mammogram, and ultrasound are repeated 6 months following diagnosis (Figure 10).

Radial Scars and Complex Sclerosing Lesions

Radial scars and complex sclerosing lesions are processes that mimic cancer radiographically as areas of architectural distortion. The incidence of coexistent cancer in the setting of a benign percutaneous biopsy is as high as 20 to 35%.[15,16] The historic management of radial scar was, therefore, excision. With improved stereotactic technology, however, controversy has developed in the management of radial scar. All patients diagnosed with radial scar undergo image-guided core biopsy. Often, microcalcifications are associated with these lesions. When calcifications within the lesion are targeted, specimen radiographs confirm appropriate sampling is achieved. Amorphorous calcifications suggest benign papilloma, whereas pleomorphic or fine linear calcifications are associated with atypia and malignancy. A benign result with adequate sampling and concordant radiology/histology merits observation and imaging surveillance in 6 months. Lesions that display atypia on percutaneous biopsy should be excised surgically with needle localization. Discordant findings include suspicious calcifications or irregular masses with benign pathology. These lesions require excision.

Fibroepithelial Lesions

Young women frequently present with palpable, well-circumscribed masses. The most common diagnosis is benign fibroadenoma. Full physical examination and imaging evaluation with biopsy are performed to rule out malignancy. Eighteen-gauge percutaneous core biopsy with ultrasound is generally adequate. Rarely, however, histology reveals fibroepithelial tumor. The differential diagnosis included cystosarcoma phyllodes (benign or malignant) or benign fibroadenoma. When percutaneous biopsy is equivocal, excisional biopsy is performed. Lesions that appear benign on percutaneous biopsy but exhibit rapid growth should also be excised.

Discordant Results

As the number of percutaneous biopsies continues to increase, the importance of interdisciplinary care grows. Pathologists, radiologists, surgeons, gynecologists, and general practitioners may all be involved in the care of

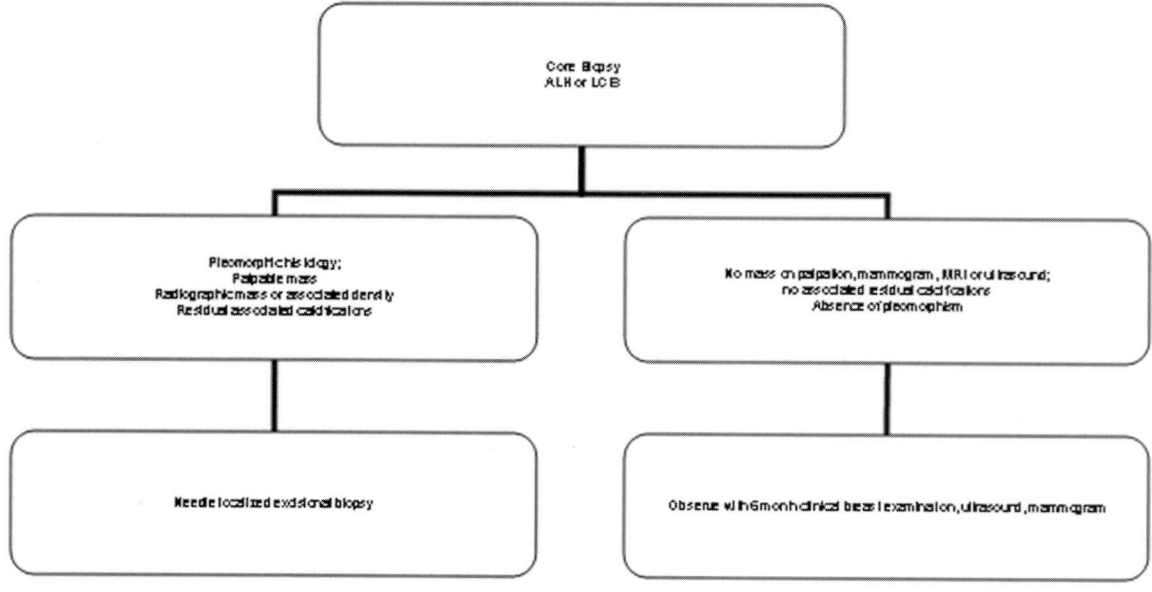

Clinical algorithm for management of lobular atypia

Figure 10 Management algorithm for LCIS identified on core biopsy.

women with breast lesions. An open dialogue is mandatory to ensure concordance between physical examination and histologic and radiographic findings. Any discordance between these parameters requires further evaluation. Occasionally, repeat percutaneous biopsy is sufficient to clarify a diagnosis. Given the large size and number of the biopsies obtained on first attempt, we prefer surgical excision as a definitive diagnostic modality. Surgical biopsy is indicated if any suspicion of occult cancer persists after percutaneous sampling. Open biopsy is also indicated if insufficient material is retrieved during percutaneous biopsy. A regularly scheduled interdisciplinary conference facilitates discussion and planning of challenging or questionable cases.

Percutaneous techniques utilize larger and larger devices for biopsy; complete excision of small lesions is not uncommon. Complete percutaneous excision decreases the incidence of discordant results but does not obviate the need for surgical excision despite resolution of imaging abnormality.[17]

Conclusions

The advent of safe, accurate percutaneous breast biopsy techniques has spared many women the risks, costs, and anxieties of open surgical biopsy. Over the past 20 years, since the incorporation of percutaneous techniques into standard practice, countless surgical procedures and the inherent risks of such procedures have been avoided based on benign percutaneous biopsy capability. Practitioners across the disciplines must remain cognizant of the potential pitfalls of percutaneous techniques. Appropriate imaging modalities and biopsy devices for accurate tissue recovery must be selected based on the radiographic characteristics of lesions. Patient comorbidities may also factor into the decision-making process. Discordant or equivocal results must be verified with surgical biopsy. Insufficient sampling is remedied with repeat percutaneous biopsy or open excision. Placement of marker clips at the time of percutaneous biopsy facilitates future imaging interpretation and surgical planning.

References

1. Kerlikowske K, Smith-Bindman R, Ljung L, Grady D. Evaluation of abnormal mammography results and palpable breast abnormalities. Ann Intern Med 2003;139:274–84.

2. Hungness E, Safa M, Shaughnessy E, et al. Bilateral synchronous breast cancer: mode of detection and comparison of histologic features between the 2 breasts. Surgery 2000;128:702–7.

3. Moy L, Slanetz P, Moore R. Specificity of mammography and US in the evaluation of a palpable abnormality: retrospective review. Radiology 2002;225:176–81.

4. Krishnamurthy S, Sneige Bedi D, et al. Role of ultrasound-guided fine-needle aspiration of indeterminate and suspicious axillary lymph nodes in the initial staging of breast carcinoma. Cancer 2002;95:982–8.

5. Morris E, Liberma L, Ballon DJ, et al. MRI of occult breast carcinoma in a high-risk population. Am J Roentgenol 2003;181:519–25.

6. http://www.nccn.org/professionals/physician_gls/PDF/breast-screening.pdf.

7. Farjardo L, Pisano E, Caudry D, et al. Stereotactic and sonographic large-core biopsy of nonpalpable breast lesions: results of the radiological diagnostic oncology group V study. Acad Radiol 2004;11:293–308.

8. Arpino G, Laucirica R, Elledge RM. Premalignant and in situ breast disease: biology and clinical implications. Ann Intern Med 2005;143:446–57.

9. Harvey JM, Sterrett GF, Frost FA. Atypical ductal hyperplasia and atypia of uncertain significance in core biopsies from mammographically detected lesions: correlation with excision diagnosis. Pathology 2002;34:410–6.

10. Chuba PJ, Hamre MR, Yap J, et al. Bilateral risk for subsequent breast cancer after lobular carcinoma-in-situ: analysis of surveillance, epidemiology, and end results data. J Clin Oncol 2005;23:5534–41.

11. Page DL, Kidd TE, Dupont WD, et al. Lobular neoplasia of the breast:clinical, pathologic and mammographic features. Hum Pathol 1991;22:1232–9.

12. Berg W, Mrose HF, Ioffe OB. Atypical lobular hyperplasia or lobular carcinoma in situ at core-needle breast biopsy. Radiology 2001;218:503–9.

13. Bauer VP, Ditkoff BA, Schnabel F, et al. The management of lobular neoplasia identified on percutaneous core breast biopsy. Breast J 2003;9:4–9.

14. Middleton LP, Grant S, Stephens T, et al. Lobular carcinoma in situ diagnosed by core needle biopsy: when should it be excised? Mod Pathol 2003;16:120–9.

15. Fasih T, Jain M, Shrimanker J, et al. All radial scars/complex sclerosing lesions seen on breast screening mammograms should be excised. Eur J Surg Oncol 2005;31:1125–8.

16. Patterson JA, Scott M, Anderson N, Kirk SJ. Radial scar, complex sclerosing lesion and risk of breast cancer. Analysis of 175 cases in Northern Ireland. Eur J Surg Oncol 2004;30:1065–8.

17. Berg W. Image-guided breast biopsy and management of high-risk lesions. Radiol Clin North Am 2004;42:935–46.

Chapter 52

Treatment of Ductal Carcinoma in Situ

Loren Rourke, MD

Thomas Buchholz, MD

Anthony Lucci, MD

Introduction

Ductal carcinoma in situ (DCIS) is a noninvasive malignant condition in which abnormal cells are found in the lining of the breast duct. Accordingly, DCIS is mainly a local control problem, unlike invasive disease where distant metastases determine outcome. Multiple studies with long-term follow-up show that duct carcinoma in situ (DCIS) metastasizes distantly only 1 to 2% of the time.[1–3] Since by definition DCIS is contained within the structure of origin, some investigators believe that the cases of metastases are examples of undiagnosed occult invasive carcinoma of the breast.

DCIS is highly curable when it is diagnosed prior to the development into an invasive cancer (since invasion carries the concomitant risk of metastases to lymph nodes or distant sites). Prior to the advent of widespread screening mammography programs, DCIS was not usually diagnosed until it was clinically apparent and/or symptomatic. Mammography now plays a key role in the diagnosis of DCIS, since the majority of DCIS lesions are not palpable by exam. Prior to screening mammography, almost all cases of DCIS were treated with mastectomy. Current treatment protocols often involve a combination of segmental resection ("segmental mastectomy") of the breast and whole-breast irradiation therapy (a treatment protocol known as "breast-conserving therapy") when the DCIS is localized. Mastectomy, often performed using a skin-sparing technique combined with immediate reconstruction, is an option for patients with extensive DCIS. Recently, segmental mastectomy alone has been advocated for some patients with DCIS of small volume and low nuclear grade. Surgeons who treat a large number of patients with DCIS will likely utilize each of these surgical techniques at some point. Careful patient selection for each of the appropriate treatment options remains the key to obtaining optimal local control combined with minimal treatment-related morbidity. Interestingly, survival rates for DCIS are similar regardless of the local treatment modality used. In this chapter we will discuss the current evidence-based standards for diagnosis and treatment of DCIS. We will address the possible role of sentinel lymph node dissection (SLND) in the management of DCIS. Finally, the role of breast irradiation in DCIS will be reviewed, as well as possible adjuvant therapies for treatment and prevention of DCIS.

Diagnosis of DCIS

The majority of DCIS diagnosed today is identified mammographically, and usually involves identification of new or progressive microcalcifications. Approximately 90% of cases of DCIS identified mammographically involve calcifications. Malignant type calcifications seen in DCIS typically are pleomorphic, as they vary in size, form, and density. These calcifications are often clustered and may extend in a linear fashion corresponding to their location within the lining of the ductal structures within the breast. In contrast to calcifications associated with DCIS, benign calcifications tend to be more rounded and often are scattered throughout the breast. They may also be more uniform in density than malignant calcifications. All patients with DCIS require mediolateral oblique and craniocaudal mammographic views and magnification views of the suspicious area. This is especially important in those patients desiring breast conservation. Ultrasound is generally not helpful for determining the extent of DCIS but can be useful for further characterization of any mass or density seen in association with suspicious calcifications. Finally, DCIS may present as a palpable mass, but this is relatively rare in clinical practice.

Although mammographic evidence of pleomorphic calcifications often suggests DCIS, obviously the diagnosis can be confirmed only by pathologic evaluation of the tissue in question. The most efficacious course of diagnosis for most cases is stereotactic core needle biopsy with subsequent pathologic evaluation of the tissue, including confirmation of calcifications within the biopsy tissue either by specimen radiograph or by documentation of presence of calcifications in the pathologic specimen. Published studies document a significantly greater likelihood of obtaining negative margins after definitive excision of a lesion diagnosed by a preoperative core needle biopsy, as compared with initial surgical excision for diagnosis. [4,5] Other investigators have documented that patients diagnosed by stereotactic core needle biopsy were 3 times more likely to have only one surgical procedure.[6] Patients whose core needle biopsy demonstrates concordance with benign etiology on pathologic evaluation and confirmed removal of the calcifications by imaging are spared an unnecessary operation and anesthesia. For this reason, we advocate that biopsy of suspicious calcifications be performed by core needle under stereotactic guidance whenever possible to optimize the chances for negative margins of excision at the definitive segmental mastectomy. Only those patients whose calcifications are not amenable to stereotactic biopsy (such as those very close to the skin or the chest wall) are diagnosed with a needle-localized excision at The University of Texas M. D. Anderson Cancer Center. Fine-needle aspiration of lesions should not be considered as an alternative to core biopsy because the resulting cytologic specimens do not allow for the differentiation between DCIS and invasive disease.

Surgical Treatment of DCIS

Once the diagnosis of DCIS is established, treatment options include breast conserving therapy (segmental mastectomy) and radiation, excision alone in select cases, and mastectomy. Regardless of the surgical treatment chosen, it is paramount to obtain negative margins to minimize the chances for local recurrence of DCIS. The National Surgical Adjuvant Breast and Bowel Project (NSABP) B-17 multivariate analyses revealed that tumor margin status was an independent predictor of IBTR (ipsilateral breast tumor recurrence), and that 19 to 43% of patients with < 1 mm were found to have residual disease. Therefore, it is the practice at M. D. Anderson to achieve a 2 mm margin on all segmental mastectomy specimens when possible. The NSABP B-24 trial also noted a significantly higher recurrence rate for patients with positive margins compared with those with negative margins (RR = 1.84).[7,8] Inability to obtain negative margins after attempts at segmental mastectomy may necessitate mastectomy as the next option. Each case of DCIS is different and each patient will require discussion and consideration of all of the options to optimize outcomes and patient satisfaction.

With the institution of screening mammography, DCIS has become a fairly common diagnosis in women. Indeed, data from the American Cancer Society indicate that the incidence of DCIS increased more than 7-fold during 1980 to 2001. This increase was noted across all age groups, although greatest in women older than age 50.[9] Many general surgeons will encounter DCIS as a course of regular practice. In the era prior to screening mammography, DCIS was a far less common diagnosis and usually was treated by mastectomy. Currently, most patients can be treated with breast conservation therapy consisting of segmental mastectomy and breast irradiation. This is especially appropriate in cases of localized DCIS, where negative margins can be obtained with segmental mastectomy. Unfortunately, DCIS may be underestimated by mammography, as microcalcifications are not always present or may be very faint in the area of DCIS. Therefore, preoperative determination of the ability to obtain clear margins by segmental resection is not always accurate. Magnetic resonance imaging (MRI) has been evaluated as a possible means for better delineating the extent of malignant lesions, including DCIS within the breast. The sensitivity of MRI has been reported to be imperfect (87% in one multicenter trial) and often overestimates the size of DCIS in many patients.[10] Because of this, we do not currently routinely utilize MRI to render a decision on the fitness of DCIS patients for breast-conserving therapy.

Since the majority of patients with DCIS have nonpalpable lesions, needle localization is usually required to guide the surgical excision. Occasionally bracketing of the mammographic areas of DCIS is utilized, especially when the area extends over a large distance. After successful needle localization, surgical excision and pathologic evaluation are carried out. Excision specimens are oriented using sutures (ie, short suture marks superior margin, long marks lateral margin) to maintain three-dimensional orientation for the pathologist. This allows the surgeon to return and correctly excise any involved or close (< 2 mm) margins found on permanent pathology. We routinely obtain specimen radiographs to confirm removal of the entire localization wire and to document that calcifications are present within the excision specimen (if applicable). Specimens are inked and sectioned by the pathologist and additional radiographs are taken of the sliced specimen to further evaluate the proximity of suspicious calcifications to the margins. Immediate reexcision of the involved margin is performed when slice radiographs that are obtained during the surgical procedure show calcifications touching or very proximate to specimen margins. Although somewhat time intensive, we feel that this protocol for evaluating DCIS excision specimens reduces the number of repeat operations for reexcision of involved margins.[11]

Although few patients are managed with surgery alone for DCIS, there are some studies that this may be applicable to a specific subset of patients. The National Comprehensive Cancer Network (NCCN) currently lists lumpectomy alone as a treatment option for small (< 0.5 cm), unicentric, low-grade DCIS in its practice guidelines (category 2B recommendation).[12] Unfortunately, there are no data to document which group can be safely excluded from undergoing breast irradiation. Identification of patients who can safely omit irradiation is difficult since irradiation is known to reduce local recurrence in at least two-thirds of all patients with breast cancer.

Proponents of surgery alone for low-grade DCIS argue that using radiation therapy precludes later irradiation use should an invasive cancer develop, and also that a skin-sparing mastectomy for local failure would be technically more challenging in a previously irradiated field. Efforts to define low-grade DCIS, and the lack of consensus on a histopathological classification for DCIS, elicit confusion. The Van Nuys pathologic classification was developed by Silverstein and colleagues, who retrospectively correlated the outcome data from their institutions with a variety of patient, treatment, and disease-related factors. Lesions, if high grade, were placed in the worst prognostic group regardless of comedo status. The nonhigh-grade lesions were then evaluated for the presence or absence of comedonecrosis. This algorithmic division yielded three groups. This pathologic information combined with tumor size, margin, and, lastly, age comprised the Modified USC/Van Nuys Prognostic Index (USC/VNPI). The index provided identified not only those patients likely not to benefit from radiation therapy, but also a subset of DCIS patients who would benefit from mastectomy over breast-conserving therapy. The scoring system ranged from 1 to 3, with 1 being the most favorable and 3 for the least favorable prognosis assigned to the four categories (pathologic classification [nuclear grade + comedo], age, tumor size, margin status). A score of 4 to 12 could be achieved with recommendations of excision alone for the

Table 1 VNPI and proposed treatment

USC/VNPI SCORE	RECOMMENDED TREATMENT	INFLUENCE OF XRT ON LOCAL RECURRENCE
4, 5, or 6	Excision Only	N/A
7, 8, or 9	Excision + XRT	10–12% decrease in local recurrence with XRT
10, 11, or 12	Mastectomy	Statistically significant improvement in recurrence with XRT ($p = 0.0003$)

XRT = external beam radiation therapy (breast irradiation).
Adapted from Silverstein MJ et al.[13]

low-risk group, excision plus radiation therapy for the middle group, and mastectomy for the high-risk group (Table 1).[13]

One reason why VNPI has not gained widespread acceptance is that the tissue-processing protocol within the VNPI is very complex and not easily applicable to all pathology laboratories. In addition, a recent prospective clinical trial from the Dana-Farber/Harvard Cancer Center group was not able to reproduce the results from the Van Nuys group. In this trial, patients with mammographically detected low- or intermediate-grade DCIS that was excised with margins ≥ 1 cm (78% of the participants had reexcisions showing no residual disease) had an ipsilateral local recurrence of 2.4% per patient year for an estimated 5-year rate of recurrence of 12%. This rate crossed the predefined stopping boundary for breast recurrences and led to the data monitoring committee to close the study early. The rate of recurrence was much higher than that reported by the Van Nuys group and more closely approximated the rates of recurrence in the surgery-alone arms of the randomized prospective trials.

If breast conservation is chosen for DCIS, our practice is segmental mastectomy followed by postoperative radiation therapy for DCIS. Table 2 demonstrates results of conservative surgery and radiation for mammographically detected DCIS. In these published series, recurrence rates ranged from 1 to 10%, and in each study, 5-year survival approached 100%.[14] Furthermore, the NSABP B-17 trial showed a reduction of 59% in IBTR with radiation ($p < 0.000005$). Although the incidence was 13.4% for both invasive and noninvasive IBTR in the lumpectomy-alone group, the incidence of invasive IBTR compared with noninvasive was 3.9% and 8.2%, respectively, in the lumpectomy and radiation group. When counseling patients at our institution, we inform them that when radiation is a component of their treatment, recurrence is more likely to be DCIS as opposed to invasive carcinoma. The Eastern Cooperative Oncology Group (ECOG E-5194) trial will evaluate

Table 2 Results of Conservative Surgery and Radiation for Mammographically Detected DCIS

Study	Number of Patients	Actuarial Breast Recurrence %			Cause-Specific Survival %			Median Follow-up Years
		5-year	8-year	10-year	5-year	8-year	10-year	
NSABP B-17	411	10.0	12.1	–	–	96.0	–	7.5 mean
Kuske et al.	44	7.0	–	–	–	–	–	4.0
Fowble et al.	110	1.0	–	15.0	100.0	–	100.0	5.3
Kestin et al.	146	8.0	–	9.2	100.0	–	99.2	7.2
Hiramatsu et al.	54	2.0	–	23.0	–	–	96.0	6.2
Sniege et al.	31	0.0	–	8.0	–	–	–	7.2
Silverstein MJ et al.	133*	7.0	–	19.0	–	–	97.0	7.8
Collaborative Group	110	7.0	–	14.0	100.0	–	96.0	9.3

*Eighty-nine of these patients had mammographically detected cancers.
Adapted from Morrow M et al.[14]

locoregional recurrence in patients with DCIS either ≤ 2.5 cm and low to intermediate grade or ≤ 1 cm and high grade undergoing excision alone.

Although excision alone is certainly attractive and reasonable in the extremely low-risk patient, prospective data must validate the safety of this modality. Table 3 illustrates previously published studies showing results of treatment of DCIS by excision alone. In these studies, recurrence rates ranged from 6 to 21%.[14] Importantly, no published series of DCIS has shown statistically significant differences in breast cancer-specific mortality based on local treatment. Therefore, it is important to identify which subset of patients can be spared the cost and time investment associated with radiation therapy.

Mastectomy remains an option for patients with multicentric disease, or for those with DCIS extending over long distances where complete excision would result in a cosmetically unacceptable outcome. Mastectomy may also be required when the DCIS is central and involves the nipple-areolar complex. However, DCIS in a central location within the breast is not an absolute contraindication for breast conservation, as long as negative margins can be obtained.[15] Mastectomy performed for DCIS is usually skin sparing and amenable to immediate reconstruction in the majority of cases. Patients who underwent excisional biopsy for their diagnosis should have their excisional biopsy scar excised at the time of mastectomy, and this often compromises the cosmetic outcome of the skin-sparing procedure. This is another reason that we do not favor excisional biopsy for the initial diagnosis of DCIS.

The Role of Breast Irradiation in Conjunction with Surgery for Patients with DCIS

Although the benefit of radiation was clearly demonstrated for all subsets of patients analyzed in the NSABP B-17 trial, data suggest that the routine use of radiation for DCIS has not become a standard practice pattern in the United States. The European Organization for

Table 3 Results of Treatment of DCIS by Excision Alone

Study	Number of Patients	Follow-up (months)	% Recurrence	% Invasive
Arnesson and Olsen	169	80†	16/22 (5/10-year actuarial)	
Baird et al.	30	43*	13	25
Carpenter et al.	28	38*	18	20
Cataliotti et al.	99	79*	8/23 (5/10-year actuarial)	38
Eusebi et al.	80	210	20	69
Lagios MD et al.[21]	79	124*	19 (15-year actuarial)	56
Salvadori et al.	74	31*	14	60
Scheer	102	56*	24	42
Schwartz et al.	194	53†	14/25 5/10-year actuarial	18
Sibbering and Blamey	48	58†	6	33
Silverstein et al.	130	45†	21 (8-year actuarial)	33
Kestin et al.	31	71†	7.8/7/8 (5/10-year actuarial)	50

*Mean
†Median
Adapted from Morrow M et al.[14]

Research and Treatment of Cancer subsequently completed an identical trial demonstrating an improvement in 10-year rates of breast recurrence from 26 to 15% ($p < 0.0001$).[16] Additionally, a third randomized trial conducted in the United Kingdom, Australia, and New Zealand evaluated the benefit of radiation therapy and tamoxifen after breast-conservation surgery in patients with DCIS. They reported that radiation therapy reduced the risk of overall breast cancer recurrences (HR = 0.38, $p < 0\ 0.0001$).[17] Data from a survey of the National Cancer Database suggested that, in 1998, 55% of patients with DCIS who received breast-conserving therapy were treated with surgery alone.[18] Furthermore, in a recent survey study of physicians in Australia and New Zealand, only 22% of patients treated with breast-conservation surgery for DCIS were referred for a radiation oncology consultation.[19] Despite the results of randomized phase III trials clearly demonstrating the benefit of radiation therapy for patients with DCIS, there is a profound discrepancy between this level I evidence and practice patterns.

Radiation treatment for women with DCIS is relatively well tolerated, with few side effects and long-term risks. In general, treatment is targeted to the entire ipsilateral breast. Typically, 45 to 50 Gy is delivered in 25 to 28 treatment fractions over a 5-week period. Many centers then add a boost to the site of the original disease within the breast that delivers an additional 10 to 16 Gy in 5 to 8 fractions. Correspondingly, the entire length of therapy lasts 6 to 7 weeks.

Each daily treatment lasts only minutes, and during the treatment period, most patients can continue to work and maintain a near-normal functional status. Patients often experience some generalized fatigue and toward the end of therapy develop some mild irritation of the skin overlying the ipsilateral breast (similar to mild sunburn). These symptoms generally resolve within weeks after treatment is completed. It is not uncommon for the skin to have a residual tan and some degree of edema for months after treatment, but, in general, the long-term expected breast esthetics are good to excellent.

Serious risks from treatment, such as lung injury, heart injury, or second cancer development, are exceedingly rare. Careful treatment planning is critical to minimize these risks. At M. D. Anderson, we use computed tomography treatment planning in every case and carefully design individual fields with the goals of including the target volume, minimizing the volume of the ipsilateral lung irradiated, and completely avoiding the underlying heart. The breast is initially treated with an opposed pair of fields called medial and lateral tangents (because in the axial plane they are tangential to the thorax). Subsequently, we boost the area of the original tumor bed with an appositional field and deliver the radiation with electrons, which have the physical property of rapid dose falloff distal to the tumor bed region.

The Role of Sentinel Lymph Node Dissection for DCIS

With survival greater than 98% at 10 years, systemic treatment for DCIS is not likely to affect survival rates. However, lymph node evaluation remains a point of controversy for surgeons treating DCIS. In a prospective study by Veronesi, only 1.8% (9 of 508) of patients with pure DCIS demonstrated sentinel lymph node metastasis.[20] In our practice, sentinel lymph node dissection is not standard treatment for patients with DCIS and is advocated only in the setting of extensive DCIS requiring mastectomy. Another setting where sentinel node biopsy may be useful is when the diagnosis of DCIS is made with a core biopsy and a significant proportion of the index lesion remains intact. If the lesion is high grade, a significant percentage of patients will be found to have associated invasive disease upon examination of the formal surgical excision specimen. A sentinel node biopsy performed at the time of the definitive resection may avoid a second surgical procedure. Some argue that positive lymph node status in a patient with DCIS suggests a component of invasive carcinoma that has been missed on original pathological evaluation of the primary tumor specimen. Camp and colleagues reported that 80% of patients with extensive DCIS and a positive sentinel node were ultimately determined to have invasive or microinvasive disease in the primary tumor specimen.[21] Others have documented that axillary sentinel lymph nodes can be falsely positive owing to iatrogenic displacement and transport of benign epithelial cells, further confounding the prognostic significance of micrometastases identified in the sentinel nodes of patients with DCIS.[22]

Performing SLND at the time of mastectomy will avoid a second operation to stage the axillary nodes in a significant number of patients with extensive DCIS found to have invasive disease. Lagios and colleagues reported 46% of cases of extensive DCIS requiring mastectomy showed some degree of invasion on final pathology.[23] At our institution we routinely perform SLND for extensive DCIS requiring mastectomy to avoid an additional lymph node staging procedure should invasion be found in the mastectomy specimen. Our practice is to utilize the mastectomy incision to perform the SLND, as even with a skin-sparing circumareolar incision there is almost always adequate exposure to identify and remove the sentinel nodes without a counterincision in the axilla. A small counterincision is an alternative option in patients where exposure and access to the axilla is difficult or limited by a skin-sparing incision. In summary, there are few data to support routine use of SLND for localized DCIS amenable to lumpectomy. Evidence of microinvasion on core biopsy would justify SLND for DCIS. Extensive DCIS requirement mastectomy has a high likelihood of yielding invasive disease, and SLND is warranted in this group of DCIS patients.

Medical Treatments for DCIS

Since survival in DCIS approaches 99%, patients with pure DCIS received little or no benefit from systemic chemotherapy. However, hormonal therapy may offer therapeutic and preventative benefit, since the majority (at least 65–75% in many studies) of DCIS is ER positive. The NSABP B-24 study showed that adjuvant tamoxifen given after breast-conserving surgery and radiation for DCIS significantly decreased the rate of all breast cancer events. The B-35 trial will have similar design but will compare tamoxifen with anastrozole in postmenopausal women.

Summary

In summary, DCIS is a highly curable noninvasive malignancy of the duct system of the breast. Most patients are diagnosed after suspicious microcalcifications are found on screening mammography. We do not routinely advocate use of MRI to evaluate patients for DCIS, as MRI tends to overestimate extent of disease. Diagnosis is obtained by stereotactic core needle biopsy of suspicious calcifications. Needle-localized excisional biopsy remains an option for those patients whose calcifications are not amenable to stereotactic biopsy. Segmental mastectomy with intraoperative margin assessment by slice radiography is the standard at our institution, reducing the number of return operations for margin clearance. Mastectomy is an option for patients with multicentric disease, disease that involves the nipple-areolar complex, or when negative margins cannot be obtained. We prefer negative margins of at least 1 mm on all of our patients with DCIS to optimize local control.

Sentinel lymph node dissection is usually not indicated for localized DCIS amenable to segmental mastectomy, since only a small percentage of these patients will be found to have invasive disease on final pathology. Although positive nodes can be found in patients with pure DCIS, any prognostic significance is doubtful, since the overall 10-year survival rate for the patient with DCIS approximates 99%. SLND is a useful tool when mastectomy is required for extensive DCIS, as a significant number of these patients will be found to have invasion of some degree on the final pathologic assessment of the mastectomy specimen. In this situation, SLND performed at the time of mastectomy for extensive DCIS avoids a second operation to stage the axilla.

Whole-breast irradiation following segmental mastectomy remains the gold standard for DCIS. There is little doubt that radiation decreases local recurrence rates in all breast cancer patients, and at this time it remains unclear which subset of patients can safely omit radiation. Several studies are ongoing to address the question of which patients can be treated with operation alone or possibly with operative resection followed by hormonal therapies. Additionally, clinical trials are now ongoing to evaluate the role of partial-breast irradiation as an alternative to whole-breast irradiation.

Endocrine therapies have been proven to be effective chemopreventive agents in patients at high risk of development of breast cancers, including DCIS. Systemic chemotherapy has essentially no role in the treatment of DCIS owing to the excellent overall survival in the great majority of patients. Future therapies will likely focus on prevention, since medical therapies aimed at treatment are unlikely to change the already excellent outcomes for this disease.

References

1. Julien JP, Bijker N, Fentiman IS, et al. Radiotherapy in breast-conserving treatment for ductal carcinoma in situ: first results of the EORTC randomized phase III trial 10853. EORTC Breast Cancer Cooperative Group and EORTC Radiotherapy Group. Lancet 2000;355:528–33.

2. Silverstein MJ, Barth A, Poller DN, et al. Ten-year results comparing mastectomy to excision and radiation therapy for ductal carcinoma in situ of the breast. Eur J Cancer 1995;31A:1425–7.

3. Solin LJ, Fourquet A, Vicini FA, et al. Long-term outcome after breast-conservation treatment with radiation for mammographically detected ductal carcinoma in situ of the breast. Cancer 2005;103:1137–46.

4. White RR, Halperin TJ, Olson JA Jr, et al. Impact of core-needle breast biopsy on the surgical management of mammographic abnormalities. Ann Surg 2001;233:769–77.

5. Kaufman CS, Delbecq R, Jacobson L. Excising the reexcision: stereotactic core-needle biopsy decreases need for reexcision of breast cancer. World J Surg 1998;22:1023–8.

6. Morrow M, Venta L, Stinson T, et al. Prospective comparison of stereotactic core biopsy and surgical

excision as diagnostic procedures for breast cancer patients. Ann Surg 2001;233:537–41.

7. Fisher ER, Dignam J, Tan-Chiu E, et al. Pathologic findings from the National Surgical Adjuvant Breast Project (NSABP) eight-year update of Protocol B-17: intraductal carcinoma. Cancer 1999;86:429–38.

8. Fisher B, Dignam J, Wolmark N, et al. Lumpectomy and radiation therapy for the treatment of intraductal breast cancer: findings from National Surgical Adjuvant Breast and Bowel Project B-17. J Clin Oncol 1998;16:441–52.

9. American Cancer Society. Breast cancer facts & figures 2005–2006. Atlanta: American Cancer Society; 2005.

10. Bazzocchi M, Zuiani C, Panizza P, et al. Contrast-enhanced breast MRI in patients with suspicious microcalcifications on mammography: results of a multicenter trial. AJR Am J Roentgenol 2006;186:1723–32.

11. Chagpar A, Yen T, Sahin A, et al. Intraoperative margin assessment reduces reexcision rates in patients with ductal carcinoma in situ treated with breast-conserving surgery. Am J Surg 2003;186:371–7.

12. National Comprehensive Cancer Network. Ductal carcinoma in situ. In: NCCN practice guidelines in oncology. NCCN 2006.

13. Silverstein MJ, Woo C. Ductal Carcinoma in situ. In: Bland KI, Copeland EM III, editors. The breast: comprehensive management of benign and malignant disorders, 3rd ed. Philadelphia: W. B.: Saunders: 2004. p. 985–1018.

14. Morrow M, Strom EA, Bassett LW, et al. Standard for the management of ductal carcinoma in situ of the breast (DCIS). CA Cancer J Clin 2002;52:256–76.

15. Simmons RM, Brennan MB, Christos P, et al. Recurrence rates in patients with central or retroareolar breast cancers treated with mastectomy or lumpectomy. Am J Surg 2001; 182:325–9.

16. Bijker N, Meijnen P, Peterse JL, et al. Breast-conserving treatment with or without radiotherapy in ductal carcinoma-in-situ: ten-year results of European Organization for Research and Treatment of Cancer randomized phase III trial 10853—a study by the EORTC Breast Cancer Cooperative Group and EORTC Radiotherapy Group. J Clin Oncol 2006;24:3381–7.

17. Houghton J, George WD, Cuzick J, et al. Radiotherapy and tamoxifen in women with completely excised ductal carcinoma in situ of the breast in the UK, Australia, and New Zealand: randomized controlled trial. Lancet 2003; 362:95–102.

18. Bland KI, Menck HR, Scott-Conner CE, et al. The National Cancer Data Base 10-year survey of breast carcinoma treatment at hospitals in the United States. Cancer 1998;83: 1262–73.

19. Shugg D, White VM, Kitchen PR, et al. Surgical management of ductal carcinoma in situ in Australia in 1995. ANZ J Surg 2002;72:708–15.

20. Veronesi P, Intra M, Vento AR, et al. Sentinel lymph node biopsy for localised ductal carcinoma in situ? Breast 2005; 14(6):520–22.

21. Camp R, Feezor R, Kagraeian A, et al. Sentinel lymph node biopsy for ductal carcinoma in situ: an evolving approach at the University of Florida. Breast J 2005;11(6):394–7.

22. Bleiweiss IJ, Nagi CS, Jaffer S. Axillary sentinel lymph nodes can be falsely positive due to iatrogenic displacement and transport of benign epithelial cells in patients with breast carcinoma. J Clin Oncol 2006;24:2013–8.

23. Lagios MD, Westdahl PR, Margolin FR, et al. Duct carcinoma in situ. Relationship of extent of noninvasive disease to the frequency of occult invasion, multicentricity, lymph node metastases, and short-term treatment failures. Cancer 1982;50:1309–14.

CHAPTER 53

TREATMENT OPTIONS AND SURGICAL TECHNIQUES FOR EARLY-STAGE BREAST CANCER

ROSA F. HWANG, MD

MERRICK I. ROSS, MD

Introduction

As a result of screening mammography and breast cancer awareness programs, early detection has become a reality. Increasing percentages of patients are now being diagnosed with in situ and early-stage invasive disease. Early-stage invasive cancer (stage I and II) is defined by tumor diameter and nodal status. Stage I is defined according to primary tumor size of up to 2 cm, and stage II by any tumor size up to 5 cm with positive nodes or greater than 5 cm with negative nodes. The surgical treatment for patients with early-stage breast cancer has evolved toward a less-invasive approach. For many patients, breast-conservation therapy (BCT)—lumpectomy or segmental mastectomy followed by radiation therapy (RT)—is often the preferred approach. The combination of early diagnosis, the strong desire to avoid the negative impact of mastectomy on women's self-image, and the results of well-designed randomized trials have all contributed to this evolution. For those patients who are not candidates for breast conservation, or would like to avoid radiation therapy, or who just prefer a mastectomy, advances in surgical approaches have emerged that facilitate immediate breast reconstruction and help minimizes and/or overcome the mutilating effects of total mastectomy. Evaluation of the axillary nodal basin can often be accomplished with sentinel lymph node biopsy regardless of how the breast is treated.

This chapter will provide an overview of the role for breast-conserving surgery, including the indications and appropriate selection of patients, technical aspects, and emerging alternative nonsurgical ablative approaches. The indications for and oncologic safety of skin-preserving mastectomy will also be discussed. Sentinel node biopsy in patients with breast cancer is discussed in detail separately in another chapter in this text.

Breast-Conservation Therapy

RATIONALE AND REVIEW OF THE LITERATURE

The earliest reports of treating breast cancer with breast-conserving surgery and RT instead of mastectomy were published in 1924 by Keynes,[1] a surgeon in London, and in 1939 by Peters,[2] a radiation oncologist at the Princess Margaret Hospital in Toronto. The rationale for this combined approach is that surgery removes the bulk of the tumor burden and RT treats any residual disease in the remaining breast tissue.

Evidence to support the use of BCT as an alternative to mastectomy comes from several prospective randomized trials that compared the 2 approaches (Table 1). Two of these pivotal studies are the National Surgical Adjuvant Breast and Bowel Project (NSABP) B-06 study[3] and the Milan-World Health Organization study.[4] After 20 years of follow-up, these 2 randomized trials have failed to show a survival advantage for mastectomy compared with BCT. Four other modern prospective randomized trials comparing mastectomy with BCT for stage I and II breast cancer have also demonstrated that survival is equivalent for the 2 approaches (see Table 1).

Table 1 Prospective Randomized Trials Comparing Breast-Conservation Therapy (BCT) versus Mastectomy (Mx)

Trial	Endpoint	Overall Survival (%)			Disease-Free Survival (%)			Local Recurrence (%)			
		BCT + RT	Mx	p Value	BCT + RT	Mx	p Value	End Point	BCT + RT	Mx	p Value
Milan III[4]	20 years	41.7	41.5	NS	26.1	24.3	NS	Cumulative incidence at 20 years	8.8	2.3	< 0.001
Institut Gustave-Roussy[38]	15 years	73	65	0.19				Cumulative incidence at 15 years	9	14	NS
NSABP B-06[3]	20 years	46	47	NS	35	36	NS	Cumulative incidence	14	10	
NCI[6]	18 years	54	58	NS	63	67	NS	Crude incidence	22.3	0	
EORTC[7]	10 years	65	66	NS				Actuarial at 10 years	20	12	0.01
Danish Breast Cancer Group[39]	6 years	79	82	NS	70	66	NS	Crude incidence at median F/U 3.3 years	3	4	NS

EORTC = European Organization for Research and Treatment of Cancer; F/U = follow-up; NCI = National Cancer Institute; NS = not significant.

A pooled analysis of these 6 major randomized trials by Jatoi and Proschan confirmed that the survival of patients treated with BCT and mastectomy is equivalent.[5]

In addition to survival, the risk of local recurrence is an important end point for patients who may be candidates for BCT. Updated results with long-term follow-up from these 6 randomized trials have shown that the risk of local recurrence is increased for patients undergoing BCT (see Table 1). Data from several trials at earlier follow-up times failed to show a significant difference in local recurrence rates; however, at 20 years of follow-up, the Milan and NSABP B-06 trials demonstrated a higher incidence of local recurrence in the BCT group than in the mastectomy group. In the pooled analysis of these 6 randomized trials, mastectomy was significantly associated with a reduced risk of locoregional and overall recurrence.[5] The current widespread use of adjuvant chemotherapy and endocrine therapy, however, would likely reduce the incidence of local recurrence to even lower rates.

The risk of local recurrence differed greatly among the 6 randomized trials. The highest rates were observed in the National Cancer Institute (NCI) and European Organization for Research and Treatment of Cancer (EORTC) studies, in which local recurrence rates were 20% or higher.[6,7] Variations in patient selection criteria and surgical procedures may have at least partially accounted for these differences. In the NCI study, patients with clinical T1 and T2 tumors were included, and 10% of tumors were larger than 4 cm. Furthermore, negative microscopic surgical margins were not required and often were not reported.[6] Similarly, the EORTC trial did not require negative margins, and 48% of patients in the BCT group had positive microscopic margins.[7] At the other extreme, in the BCT arm of the Milan trial, in which the local recurrence rate was 8.8%, patients underwent quandrantectomy with excision of a 2 to 3 cm margin of normal tissue around the breast tumor.[4] In contrast with surgical procedures, RT delivery was fairly consistent across these 6 randomized trials. In 5 of the trials, whole-breast RT was delivered at doses of 45 to 50 Gy to the ipsilateral breast with a boost to the primary tumor site, whereas in the NSABP B-06 trial, radiation was delivered to the entire breast at a dose of 50 Gy without a boost.

The importance of RT in terms of outcome in patients undergoing breast-conserving surgery has been demonstrated in multiple studies. In a pooled analysis of 15 randomized clinical trials comparing breast-conserving surgery with or without RT, the omission of RT was associated with a 3-fold increase in the rate of ipsilateral breast tumor recurrences (IBTRs).[8] Interestingly, this analysis also found a small mortality increase when RT was omitted. Thus, RT should not be omitted when patients undergo BCT.

Recurrence in the treated breast after BCT can usually be successfully treated with mastectomy. A review of 2,038 breast cancer patients treated with BCT before 1999 and with a median follow-up time of 13.8 years identified 166 patients with IBTR.[9] All patients had been treated with whole-breast irradiation to a median dose of 50 Gy with a 14 Gy boost to the tumor bed following breast-conserving surgery. Most cases of IBTR were detected by mammogram alone, and only 46% were located in the same breast quadrant as the original tumor. Most patients were treated with salvage mastectomy, but 20% were treated with salvage breast-conserving surgery. The survival rate after IBTR was 64.5% at 10 years, and there was no significant difference in survival rates between the salvage mastectomy and salvage breast-conserving surgery groups (65.7% vs 58.0%). Currently, mastectomy is considered the standard treatment for localized recurrence following BCT. However, prospective trials are in development to evaluate the efficacy of salvage breast-conserving surgery with partial-breast irradiation.[9]

SELECTION OF PATIENTS FOR BCT

In its 1990 summary statement, the National Institutes of Health Consensus Development Conference on Treatment of Early-Stage Breast Cancer indicated that BCT is appropriate primary therapy for the majority of women with stage I and stage II breast cancer.[10] To be eligible for BCT, patients should have unicentric disease and an adequate tumor-to-breast-size ratio to allow for an acceptable cosmetic result and negative margins of at least 2 mm.

Absolute contraindications to BCT include multicentric disease, history of prior RT to the breast region, and expected inability to achieve negative surgical margins with breast-conserving surgery. Most radiation oncologists consider collagen vascular disorders such as scleroderma or active lupus erythematous to be absolute contraindications and will not treat patients with such disorders. Historically, diagnosis during the first and second trimester of pregnancy was an absolute contraindication, but with a better appreciation for the appropriate sequence of modalities and evidence concerning the safety of chemotherapy during pregnancy, BCT may be a perfectly safe option, particularly for patients in the second trimester. Allthough it is generally agreed that radiation therapy should not be used at any time during pregnancy, chemotherapy can safely be administered beginning after the completion of fetal organogenesis (the end of the first trimester). Since radiation therapy is not generally administered until surgery and chemotherapy is completed, if chemotherapy is a planned component of the treatment strategy then the time interval necessary to complete these two modalities would include most of the remainder of the pregnancy. Radiation therapy can then be administered in an acceptable time period in the early post partum setting.

In addition, other patient-related factors, such as geographic barriers to receiving RT and psychological concerns about locoregional recurrence should be considered in patient-physician discussions regarding BCT. In a review of 456 patients with breast cancer at a single institution, 21% of patients had contraindications to BCT[11]—10% of patients with stage I disease, 28% of patients with stage II disease, and 33% of patients with DCIS.

Despite the strong evidence supporting the use of BCT and the low proportion of patients with early-stage disease with contraindications to BCT, several population-based studies report that only a minority of patients eligible for BCT actually are treated with breast-conserving surgery. A joint study by the American College of Surgeons and the American College of Radiology reviewed the treatment of breast cancer patients eligible for BCT, most of whom were treated at community hospitals, and found that only 42.6% of eligible patients were treated with BCT.[12] The significant predictors of BCT included northeast location, clinical T1 tumors, and lack of extensive intraductal component in the primary tumor.[12] The practice and perception of surgeons also play a role in adherence to current guidelines on indications for BCT: High-volume surgeons and those who perceived greater quality-of-life benefit from BCT were more likely to favor BCT over mastectomy.[13] In a review of 293 patients eligible for BCT at The University of Texas M. D. Anderson Cancer Center, 69% of patients underwent BCT, and the rest were treated with mastectomy.[14] The only factor that predicted mastectomy over BCT was the patient's being a widow. Other factors that have previously been reported to be significant predictors of BCT,[12] including T1 tumor size and younger patient age, were not significant predictors in this multivariate analysis.

The use of more sensitive imaging modalities could potentially have an impact on the selection of patients to receive BCT. Ultrasound is a critical modality in evaluating the breast for the presence of multicentricity, particularly in young patients with dense breasts in whom the sensitivity of mammography is reduced. Any abnormalities detected can easily be assessed with an ultrasound-guided needle biopsy. Although the role for ultrasound is clear and supported, the use of MRI of the breast in determining the appropriateness of BCT is rather controversial. Although it is clear that MRI is more sensitive than both mammography and ultrasound, some of the additional findings may not only be clinically irrelevant, but also falsely positive. Furthermore, if abnormalities are identified, the technical expertise to perform MRI-guided biopsies is not universally available. Given the excellent local control rates reported with BCT, it is likely that many of the additional findings visualized on MRI that may represent occult extensions of the primary tumor or microscopic foci of multicentric disease would be adequately treated with radiation therapy. Well-designed prospective trials correlating findings on MRI with pathologic specimens or determining long-term recurrence rates after BCT in patients identified to have additional findings on MRI prior to therapy would provide valuable information. Given the cost of MRI and the lack of substantial evidence for its utility in this setting, the routine use of MRI in patients being considered for BCT presently is not justified.

TECHNICAL ASPECTS OF BREAST-CONSERVING SURGERY

Both proper surgical technique and careful examination of the surgical specimen are critical to achieving the goals of complete tumor excision and an optimal cosmetic result. Moreover, it is important to achieve negative margins to decrease the risk of IBTR and potentially improve survival (see "Risk Factors for IBTR" below for a more detailed discussion.)

The skin incision is typically curvilinear and follows Langer's lines, although a radial incision may achieve a better cosmetic result for large lesions in the lower breast and at the 3 o'clock and 9 o'clock positions. The incision should be made as close as possible to the tumor with minimal undermining of tissue. A rim of grossly normal tissue should be excised around the primary lesion. Reapproximation of the breast is occasionally performed in the case of a large defect in an area of the biopsy cavity that can be easily closed without tension. However, it can be difficult to predict what the cosmetic result will be after the patient is awake, upright, and mobile, and thus obliteration of the biopsy cavity is not routinely performed. Placement of drains in the breast after lumpectomy is not recommended. The specimen should be properly oriented by the surgeon prior to sectioning by the pathologist. Titanium clips may be placed in the cavity to aid in identification of the tumor bed during RT planning.

Nonpalpable lesions can be localized preoperatively using mammography, sonography, or, less commonly, magnetic resonance imaging. The lesion should be precisely localized using a guidewire, and films (both craniocaudal and lateral views) should be sent for intraoperative review by the surgeon. Intraoperative ultrasound can also be helpful in localizing nonpalpable breast lesions and allows for direct communication between the ultrasonographer and surgeon.[15] The skin incision for needle localized excision of nonpalpable lesions should be made over the lesion, just as is done for palpable lesions, rather than at the entry site of the guidewire.

Immediate evaluation of the segmental mastectomy specimen by both the surgeon and the pathologist is critical to maximize the chances for complete excision of the tumor. The specimen should be excised en bloc, rather than piecemeal, whenever possible. If any margin appears to be grossly involved with tumor, the surgeon should immediately excise additional tissue at this location. The specimen can be properly oriented with marking sutures, ink, or other marking devices placed by the surgeon to enable the pathologist to identify and comment on specific margins. Gross examination by the pathologist often includes sectioning of the specimen perpendicular to the longest axis through the tumor mass. If, on gross examination, the mass appears to approach a margin, frozen-section analysis can be performed to further examine the margin. For nonpalpable lesions, radiography of the specimen, intact and/or after sectioning, is performed. If the specimen radiograph reveals that the mammographic abnormality has not been completely excised, the radiologist should communicate these findings with the surgeon before wound closure. In addition, in patients who were treated with neoadjuvant chemotherapy and who had a metallic marker placed in the tumor before or during this chemotherapy to mark the tumor location in case of complete or near-complete response, the presence of the marker within the resected tissue should be confirmed with the specimen radiograph.

Risk Factors for IBTR

Although the survival of patients treated with BCT has been shown to be similar to that of patients treated with mastectomy, the risk of local recurrence after BCT is still 0.5 to 1% per year.[3,4] In the NSABP B-06 trial, the majority of IBTRs occurred in the same quadrant as the index lesion and were of the same histologic tumor type and nuclear grade.[16] Local recurrence has been reported to be a predictor of poor survival,[16,17] thus, numerous studies have attempted to identify risk factors for IBTR. Several factors have been cited as significant predictors of IBTR, including patient age, extensive intraductal component, invasive lobular histology, and status of the surgical margins, and these will be discussed in more detail.

PATIENT AGE

Although several studies have found that young patient age is a risk factor for IBTR after BCT, a similar association has been observed between young age and outcome after mastectomy.[4,18] Thus, patient age should not be a factor in clinical decision making regarding local treatment.

INTRADUCTAL TUMOR

Certain tumor characteristics have also been identified as risk factors for IBTR. As mentioned previously, the presence of intraductal tumor was predictive of IBTR in the NSABP B-06 trial; however, IBTR rates were low when negative surgical margins were achieved.[19,20] In a retrospective study of patients with ductal carcinoma in situ (DCIS) who underwent lumpectomy and reexcision, 50% of patients had positive initial excision margins.[21] To reduce the need for reexcision in patients with DCIS,

result of an inherited susceptibility for multiple primary breast cancers rather than radiation induced. Additional findings include similar overall survival and no increased radiation associated toxicity compared with patients with sporadic breast cancer. Although it appears that BCT is safe and effective in *BRCA* cancer patients, these patients need to be made aware of the high rate of second primaries bilaterally before making a decision for BCT

CENTRALLY LOCATED TUMORS

Tumors arising in the subareola location that involve the overlying NAC and Paget's disease represent two clinical scenarios with relative contraindications to BCT because of predicted poor cosmetic outcomes with central segmentectomy and little information concerning its oncologic safety. Two recent studies demonstrated very acceptable rates of local recurrences, less than 10%, when treating these cancers with central segmental mastectomies. In addition, reasonably good cosmetic results and good symmetry can be achieved, particularly in patients without significant breast ptosis. In patients with very large pendulous breasts, after the NAC is resected with the central segmentectomy, bilateral reduction mastopexies can be performed for symmetry, and the NAC can later be tattooed and reconstructed on the cancer side.

LARGE PENDULOUS BREASTS

Patients with very large pendulous breasts were often considered not to be ideal BCT candidates because of the difficulty in designing radiation fields that would effectively treat the entire breast volume and because of the resultant asymmetry. To address both of these concerns these patients may be better treated with bilateral reduction mastopexy-type incisions. Although the best candidates for this approach are those with tumors located in the central regions of the breast (6 and 12 o'clock and deep to the areola, but not involving the NAC), tumors located in other regions of the breast can treated similarly as long as a formal segmental excision can be performed with negative margins through the Wise-pattern incision.

PREVIOUS AUGMENTATION

Although the incidence of breast cancer continues to rise annually, so does the number of breast augmentation procedures performed. Breast augmentation is now the second most commonly performed cosmetic surgical procedure. Therefore, the two events occurring together is becoming increasingly common. Both oncologic and cosmetic issues have been raised. From an oncologic perspective questions are asked about the possibility of delays in diagnosis because of impaired detection and the

effectiveness of BCT. From an aesthetic point of view, concerns relate to long-term cosmesis following radiation therapy.

Unfortunately, most of the available information is from small single-institution experiences reporting stage at diagnosis, percentage of augmented patients receiving BCT, and the aesthetic and oncologic outcomes. These findings were then compared with their own institutional experience with breast cancer patients without a prior augmentation.

Ablative Approaches

Alternatives to surgical excision for patients with early-stage breast cancer include ablative techniques that essentially use either heat or cold to cause cellular damage and destroy the tumor. These techniques include radiofrequency ablation (RFA), cryosurgery, laser ablation, microwave ablation, and focused ultrasound ablation. A common limitation of all of these approaches is that they do not permit assessment of residual tumor burden and margin status. Furthermore, ablation of the lesion precludes analysis of the lesion for histologic features or tumor markers. Since ablative techniques are still considered investigational, only a brief summary of two of the approaches that have received the most attention, RFA and cryosurgery, will be provided here.

RFA destroys tumors using thermal coagulation generated by a high-frequency alternating current flowing from an electrode on an RFA probe. The tumor is usually identified with real-time ultrasound, the probe is inserted percutaneously after induction of local anesthesia, the prongs of the probe are deployed, and the probe is heated to the target temperature. In a pilot study of 10 patients with invasive breast cancer who underwent RFA followed by surgical excision 1 to 3 weeks later, 9 of the 10 patients had no residual viable tumor identified on pathologic evaluation of the surgical specimen.[34] All patients tolerated the procedure well and experienced little discomfort. Another study at M.D. Anderson examined the effectiveness of RFA in the treatment of breast cancers 2 cm or less in size.[35] Ultrasound was performed to exclude patients in whom the tumor was not easily identifiable, directly involved the skin, or was within 1 cm from the chest wall or skin. RFA was performed immediately prior to scheduled surgical excision. In the majority of patients, RFA resulted in effective tumor destruction: No histologic evidence of viable tumor was identified in 20 of 21 patients with T1 invasive breast cancer.[35] The one patient with viable tumor at surgery had received neoadjuvant chemotherapy and was found to have a larger volume of disease than predicted on the basis of ultrasound or mammogram.[35] RFA may be a promising alternative to surgical excision; however, accurate delineation of disease extent may be more difficult following neoadjuvant chemotherapy.

Like RFA, cryotherapy involves use of a probe placed percutaneously under ultrasound guidance. However, whereas RFA uses heat to destroy tumor cells by thermal coagulation, cryotherapy uses cold to disrupt the cell membrane. In a multi-institutional pilot study of cryoablation, 27 patients with T1 invasive breast cancer were treated with cryoablation followed by surgical excision 1 to 4 weeks later.[36] Cryoablation produced complete pathologic destruction of all tumors smaller than 1.0 cm but was unable to destroy tumors larger than 1.0 cm that contained a significant DCIS component. Cryoablation without resection has been approved by the US Food and Drug Administration for treatment of fibroadenomas. With a mean follow-up time of 2.6 years, 97% of patients with fibroadenomas treated with cryoablation were satisfied with the procedure and the long-term results.[37] Cryoablation appears to be useful for treatment of fibroadenomas; however, its oncologic safety in the treatment of invasive breast cancers remains to be determined.

Summary

The evidence from large, randomized trials with 20-year follow-up has demonstrated that survival is equivalent after BCT and mastectomy. Adjuvant RT to reduce the risk of local recurrence is an essential component of BCT. Few patients have true contraindications for BCT. Only a minority of patients who are eligible for BCT receive this treatment, which may reflect surgeons' as well as patients' biases. Technical aspects of breast-conserving surgery, including proper specimen orientation and close communication with colleagues in pathology and radiology, are critical to ensure negative margins and reduce the incidence of IBTR. Finally, although there are relatively few complications related to breast-conserving surgery, alternative approaches for ablation of early-stage breast tumors are under investigation.

Total Mastectomy: A Historical Perspective

Prior to the advent of radiation therapy and systemic chemotherapy, the only effective therapeutic strategy to achieve local and regional control of breast cancer was aggressive surgery, particularly the radical mastectomy. Although the classic descriptions of the radical mastectomy, which included the en bloc removal of the entire breast, its surrounding overlying skin, the pectoralis

major muscle, and the axillary nodes, were attributed to Halsted in the late 1800s, other surgical leaders promoted even more radical practices. Subsequent to Halsted, Meyer modified the approach by including the pectoralis minor muscle in the dissection. This Halsted-Meyer procedure became known as the classic Halsted Radical Mastectomy. In the late 1800s and early 1900s more extensive surgery including removal of the internal mammary nodes (contralateral as well as ipsilateral), and dissection of the supraclavicular nodes was advocated in addition to the Halsted procedure in an attempt to improve the unsatisfactory local-regional control rates. Most of the practicing surgeons in the late nineteenth century and first half of the twentieth century accepted the fact that distant metastases were likely to develop regardless of the surgical procedure because the vast majority of patients presented with advanced (present day stage IIIb) disease. Ultimately, these extended radical procedures were compared directly in a randomized fashion with the Halsted mastectomy without any improvement in survival. The Halsted mastectomy remained the standard practice until the 1970s. Modifications that reduced the extent of surgery were implemented for two reasons: (1) the advent of external beam radiation as a useful tool to reduce the incidence of chest wall recurrence, and (2) more patients being diagnosed with stage I and II disease. These changes to the surgical approach define what is now referred as a "modified" radical mastectomy. The first modification was introduced by Patey, who practiced sparing of the pectoralis major muscle, but still resected the pectoralis minor to facilitate a level III axillary dissection. This approach was further modified by Madden and Auchincloss, who advocated sparing both pectoralis muscles and a level I and II node dissection. In the late 1960s and 1970s two prospective randomized trials were performed comparing radical mastectomy with modified radical mastectomy in stage I and II patients, demonstrating no improvement in overall and disease-free survival or even local control with radical mastectomy. As a result, the modified radical mastectomy is the current standard of care for patients who are not breast-conservation candidates and who have positive axillary nodes. With the advent of sentinel node biopsy as an integral component in the management of clinically node negative patients, the procedure is more accurately referred to as a "total mastectomy," with sentinel lymphadenectomy or axillary dissection depending on the sentinel lymph node status.

Although the classic oncologic indication for mastectomy is multicentric disease, other reasons for mastectomy are predicted poor cosmetic outcome with breast conservation because of large tumor size in a small breast or centrally located tumor, no access to radiation therapy, patient desire to avoid radiation therapy, contraindication for radiation therapy because of underlying collagen vascular disease, inability to obtain negative margins with breast-conserving approaches, and patient fear of in-breast recurrence. In an attempt to optimize the cosmetic outcome and preserve self-image in patients undergoing mastectomy, breast reconstruction techniques have emerged. As the technology for breast reconstruction evolved to using autologous tissue alone or in combination with implants or tissue expander immediately following the mastectomy, the surgical oncology community in parallel developed total mastectomy techniques that preserve the native skin envelope (skin-sparing mastectomy). This approach significantly enhances the ultimate cosmetic success of the reconstruction compared with reconstruction following a conventional nonskin-sparing procedure.

Skin-Sparing Mastectomy

Regardless of how the mastectomy is performed, the objectives of removing all of the breast tissue with adequate margins and minimizing the risk of local recurrence should not be compromised. Compared with a conventional mastectomy, its skin-sparing counterpart facilitates superior cosmesis for the following reasons: preservation of the natural skin envelope, which not only maintains the native shape and contour, but also reduces the need for surgical manipulation of the opposite breast to achieve symmetry; reduced length and number of skin incision scars; avoidance of skin texture and color mismatches; and altered shape that are the inevitable result of patching in a skin paddle from the autologous donor site to replace the skin removed by conventional mastectomy. Although the cosmetic results are clearly superior, many surgeons have been reluctant to adopt the skin-sparing approach because of concerns related to its oncologic safety. Pathologic examinations of clinically normal mastectomy skin flaps have identified an alarming rate of microscopic deposits of carcinoma ranging from 10 to 23% of patients examined. Many of the deposits were located in the skin and subcutaneous tissue close to and overlying the primary tumor. The clinical relevance of these findings is questionable as it relates to stage I and II patients, as many of these specimens were taken from patients with inflammatory cancer, locally advanced breast cancer, and multicentric disease. The most valuable information in regards to safety is derived from actual patient outcomes. Although data derived from comparing local recurrence rates in patients randomly assigned to undergo either conventional or skin-sparing mastectomies in prospective clinical trial settings do not exist, a fairly large experience, with reasonably long-term follow-up from several centers, has been published concerning local control after skin-sparing mastectomy and immediate reconstruction. The incidence of local recurrence compares favorably with that observed in patients who undergo conventional mastectomy and seems to correlate with stage of disease rather than procedure performed. It is very unlikely that a prospective randomized trial will ever be performed to assess the safety of skin-sparing mastectomy, but the large volume of published experience is compelling and supports its continued use.

NIPPLE-AREOLA-SPARING MASTECTOMY

More recently, interest in sparing the nipple-areola complex along with the skin, an approach that has been used primarily in patients undergoing prophylactic mastectomy, has been entertained as an option in patients with early-stage invasive carcinoma. Again, the motivation is to further reduce the impact that mastectomy has on women's self-image by facilitating a reconstruction that more closely resembles a natural breast. In addition to the obvious aesthetic appeal, preserving the nipple and areola offers the potential of preserving normal sensation. Not surprisingly, the safety of this procedure has been strongly challenged. Traditional surgical dogma mandating the removal of the nipple in treating breast cancer is in part based on work by Sappey published in the early 1800s, demonstrating that the breast lymphatics maintain their embryologic connections to the nipple-areola complex. Validating the concern are reports of breast occurrence almost exclusively under the nipple-areola complex in patients undergoing subcutaneous prophylactic mastectomies as well as several studies documenting histologic involvement of the nipple-areola complex with carcinoma in mastectomy specimens from patients with breast cancer. Chapgar identified 14 studies with the incidence of involvement varying greatly from 0 to 50% (median of 17%). The wide range in incidence could be explained by the heterogeneity of the groups studied in terms of the techniques used to evaluate the nipple, the number of patients in the studies, and the distributions of disease stage. Clinical features have been analyzed in an attempt to predict the likelihood of nipple involvement to promote a selective approach to nipple preservation. Decreasing primary tumor distance from the nipple and increasing tumor size appear to be associated with higher rates of nipple involvement, but definitive correlations have not been established. .Some of the more recent literature reports a slightly lower incidence of nipple involvement. From one of the largest published series, Loranga and colleagues demonstrated a 5.6% incidence of nipple involvement in 286 skin-sparing mastectomy specimens from patients with invasive cancer, where the majority of involvement was associated with centrally located and multicentric tumors. A similar incidence was found by Afifi, who reported a 6.3% incidence, which dropped to only 1.2% with occult involvement when the specimens with clinically evident nipple-areola involvement were excluded. Limited patient outcome data exist relative to nipple-areola-sparing procedures. Most studies are very small with relatively short follow-up. Among these studies, similar selection criteria were used: exclusion of patients with clinically evident nipple involvement identified either preoperatively or at the time of surgery and the use of intraoperative frozen-section evaluation of the nipple-areola complex to decide whether or not to resect the overlying nipple and/or areola skin. Probably the most useful insight into the safety of this procedure is derived from a nonrandomized study reported by Gerber, comparing local recurrence rates of patients treated with either total conventional mastectomy ($n = 134$), skin-sparing mastectomy ($n = 51$), or a subcutaneous mastectomy (nipple-areola sparing) ($n = 61$); similar rates were observed, 8%, 6%, and 5%, respectively.

Surgical Techniques

CONVENTIONNAL TOTAL MASTECTOMY

Currently, this surgical approach is more commonly used for patients who have locally advanced disease and generally after preoperative systemic therapy. When it is used for stage I and II disease, it is often reserved for patients who do not desire breast conservation or who are not candidates for BCT because of multicentricity or extensive calcifications and are not interested in immediate reconstruction. The skin incision is made in an elliptical fashion, oriented obliquely or transversely, and extending medially from about 3 to 5 cm lateral to the sternum and laterally to the anterior or midaxillary line. A significant portion of overlying skin is removed en bloc to include the nipple-areola complex, any open or percutaneous biopsy sites, and the skin overlying a superficially located tumor. The sentinel node biopsy or axillary dissection can easily be performed through the lateral extent of the skin incision. If axillary nodal involvement is established preoperatively, then the axillary dissection is performed in an en bloc fashion. Skin flaps are commonly raised with electrocautery to the level of the appropriate anatomic boundaries to ensure

removal of all the breast tissue. The standard anatomic landmarks are superior to the clavicle, inferior to the inframammary fold, medial to the lateral border of the sternum while making sure to spare the main perforating vessels, and lateral to the latissimis dorsi muscle. The skin flaps are raised in the avascular plane at the interface of the breast tissue proper and the subcutaneous tissue. The deep extent of the procedure removes the muscular fascia along with breast tissue as the dissection progresses from medial to lateral. Enough skin is removed to facilitate a smooth skin flap closure over closed suction drains to avoid unsightly and annoying skin redundancies. The vast majority of patients will be discharged from the hospital the next day. The use of paravertebral regional blocks can obviate the need for general anesthesia and improve postoperative pain control, which may in turn facilitate an even earlier discharge.

SKIN-SPARING MASTECTOMIES

These procedures have been popularized over the last 15 to 20 years to optimize the cosmetic appearance of an immediate breast reconstruction. Most of the experience is with techniques that spare as much of the skin envelope as possible, but removes the nipple-areola complex together with the underlying total mastectomy specimen. A circumareolar incision is often preferred in order to minimize the visible evidence of the reconstruction. Sometimes a separate axillary incision is needed to perform the sentinel node biopsy or axillary dissection if this cannot be accomplished through the defect created by the resection of the areola. The axillary incision may sometimes compromise the blood supply to the upper lateral skin flap, resulting in partial flap necrosis. A variety of other incisions may be used, and the approach chosen is often influenced by the location of a previously placed excisional biopsy site, the presence of a superficially located tumor, or the extent of ptosis in the native breast. The incision used for the mastectomy should be planned jointly with the plastic surgeon, taking into account both the oncologic and aesthetic issues. From a technical perspective, these procedures can be challenging. The skin flaps need to be raised in a meticulous fashion to make sure that a safe margin is achieved and that a complete mastectomy can be performed. Careful gross inspection of the specimen is particularly important in patients with relatively superficial tumors, and the use of specimen mammography of the sliced mastectomy specimen is very valuable in patients with nonpalpable tumors and patients with superficial extensions of calcifications. Both maneuvers can direct the pathologist to areas that may require frozen-section margin assessment. Close or positive margins can be addressed by excising additional subcutaneous tissue or more skin before the reconstruction is performed. At the same time, if the flaps are too thin, or if they are uneven and have thinned-out areas with exposed dermis, or if one of the main perforating vessels located superomedially is inadvertently ligated, areas of epidermolysis or full-thickness necrosis may occur. Such events may not only negatively impact the cosmetic result, but may also lead to infections and the eventual removal of the implant or tissue expander if one of these two prosthetic devices were used. The flaps are most commonly raised with electrocautery, but some surgeons prefer sharp dissection to avoid thermal injury. Injections of saline with or without epinephrine or lidocaine performed circumferentially in the subcutaneous tissue may accentuate the subcutaneous/breast tissue interface and facilitate the use of sharp scissor dissection in raising the flaps. Patient selection is important, as certain comorbidities may increase the risk of complications and unfavorable outcomes. Obesity, diabetes, and smoking in particular may increase the risk of flap necrosis. Ideally, cessation of smoking should be implemented at least 1 month prior to the procedure. Whether or not a core biopsy site and needle track needs to be excised is currently an unanswered question. If removal of the biopsy site can be accomplished without significantly compromising the aesthetic result, it is probably prudent to do so. Such a recommendation is influenced by a recent report of 3 patients who developed breast cancer recurrences in the skin and dermis at the entry site of a diagnostic core needle biopsy. These three events were documented on a review of 58 early-stage patients who underwent skin-sparing mastectomy and immediate reconstruction with either a TRAM flap or implant. Interestingly, in this group of 58 patients, only 11 were diagnosed with a core needle biopsy, resulting in almost a 30% incidence of skin biopsy site recurrence in this subgroup. The recurrences developed at a median follow-up of 23 months, and all 3 developed in patients with relatively small primary tumors without any obvious high-risk pathologic features.

The most ambitious skin-sparing approach, in terms of optimizing cosmesis and minimizing external scarring, was recently reported from the group at the University of Arkansas. They performed 50 "total skin-sparing mastectomies" in 31 patients, defined as preserving all of the skin but still removing essentially the entire nipple-areola complex from underneath, but not the overlying nipple and areola skin, followed by an immediate reconstruction with subpectoral tissue expanders. The mastectomy was performed either through an incision made in the inframammary fold or through an incision used to remove an excisional biopsy site. The decision to preserve the nipple and areola skin was made intraoperatively based on frozen-section evaluation of a cored-out nipple excision specimen and areola duct tissue removed with the mastectomy specimen. In 28 patients, the procedure was performed for carcinoma, 79% of which were invasive. In 14% of these patients, the nipple and areola could not be preserved because of a positive frozen section. In 2 additional patients, loss of the nipple and areola occurred owing to necrosis. One patient developed flap necrosis and 5 others superficial epidermolysis. No local recurrences have yet been reported, but the median follow-up time is a very short 7.9 months. As a result, the safety of this approach is still in question.

Another technical variation is to remove just the nipple and its skin en bloc with the mastectomy, but preserve the areola skin. Such an approach requires a linear skin incision extension for a certain distance beyond the areola to achieve adequate exposure for the mastectomy.

Although the goal of optimizing the cosmetic outcome is very important, the goal of not compromising the oncologic outcome is critical and certainly takes precedence. In experienced hands, with the combination of appropriate patient selection, well-planned incisions designed via open communication between the oncologic and plastic surgeons, and the use of meticulous surgical technique, both objectives can routinely be accomplished.

References

1. Keynes G. Conservative treatment of cancer of the breast. BMJ 1937;2:643.

2. Peters M. Cutting the "Gordian knot" in early breast cancer. Ann R Coll Phys Surg Can 1975;8:186.

3. Fisher B, Anderson S, Bryant J, et al. Twenty-year follow-up of a randomized trial comparing total mastectomy, lumpectomy, and lumpectomy plus irradiation for the treatment of invasive breast cancer. N Engl J Med 2002;347:1233–41.

4. Veronesi U, Cascinelli N, Mariani L, et al. Twenty-year follow-up of a randomized study comparing breast-conserving surgery with radical mastectomy for early breast cancer. N Engl J Med 2002;347:1227–32.

5. Jatoi I, Proschan M. Randomized trials of breast-conserving therapy versus mastectomy for primary breast cancer. Am J Clin Oncol 2005;28:289–94.

6. Poggi MM, Danforth DN, Sciuto LC, et al. Eighteen-year results in the treatment of early breast carcinoma with mastectomy versus breast conservation therapy. Cancer 2003;98:697–702.

7. van Dongen JA, Voogd AC, Fentiman IS, et al. Long-term results of a randomized trial comparing breast-conserving therapy with mastectomy: European Organization for

Research and Treatment of Cancer 10801 trial. J Natl Cancer Inst 2000;92:1143–50.

8. Vinh-Hung V, Verschraegen C. Breast-conserving surgery with or without radiotherapy: pooled-analysis for risks of ipsilateral breast tumor recurrence and mortality. J Natl Cancer Inst 2004;96:115–21.

9. Alpert TE, Kuerer HM, Arthur DW, et al. Ipsilateral breast tumor recurrence after breast conservation therapy: outcomes of salvage mastectomy vs. salvage breast-conserving surgery and prognostic factors for salvage breast preservation. Int J Radiat Oncol Biol Phys 2005;63: 845–51.

10. National Institutes of Health Consensus Development Panel. Consensus statement: treatment of early stage breast cancer. J Natl Cancer Inst 1992;11:1–5.

11. Morrow M, Bucci C, Rademaker A. Medical contra-indications are not a major factor in the underutilization of breast conserving therapy. J Am Coll Surg 1998;186:269–74.

12. Morrow M, White J, Moughan J, et al. Factors predicting the use of breast-conserving therapy in stage I and II breast carcinoma. J Clin Oncol 2001;19:2254–62.

13. Katz SJ, Lantz PM, Janz NK, et al. Surgeon perspectives about local therapy for breast carcinoma. Cancer 2005;104: 1854–61.

14. Al-Refaie W, Kuerer HM, Khuwaja A, et al. Determinants of mastectomy in breast conservation therapy candidates. Am J Surg 2005;190:602–5.

15. Fornage B, Ross M, Singletary SE, et al. Localization of impalpable breast masses: value of sonography in the operating room and scanning of excised specimens. AJR Am J Roentgenol 1994;163:569–73.

16. Fisher ER, Anderson S, Tan-Chiu E, et al. Fifteen-year prognostic discriminants for invasive breast carcinoma. Cancer 2001;91:1679–87.

17. Meric F, Mirza NQ, Vlastos G, et al. Positive surgical margins and ipsilateral breast tumor recurrence predict disease-specific survival after breast-conserving therapy. Cancer 2003;97:926–33.

18. Matthews R, McNeese MD, Montague E, et al. Prognostic implications of age in breast cancer patients treated with tumorectomy and irradiation or with mastectomy. Int J Radiat Oncol Biol Phys 1988;14:659–63.

19. Dewar J, Arriagada R, Benhamou S, et al. Local relapse and contralateral tumor rates in patients with breast cancer treated with conservative surgery and radiotherapy (Institut Gustave-Roussy 1970–1982). Cancer 1995;76: 2260–5.

20. Borger J, Kemperman H, Hart A, et al. Risk factors in breast-conservation therapy. J Clin Oncol 1994;12:653–60.

21. Neuschatz AC, DiPetrillo T, Steinhoff M, et al. The value of breast lumpectomy margin assessment as a predictor of residual tumor burden in ductal carcinoma in situ of the breast. Cancer 2002;94:1917–24.

22. Chagpar A, Yen T, Sahin A, et al. Intraoperative margin assessment reduces reexcision rates in patients with ductal carcinoma in situ treated with breast-conserving surgery. Am J Surg 2003;186:371–7.

23. Moore M, Borossa G, Imbrie J, et al. Association of infiltrating lobular carcinoma with positive surgical margins after breast-conservation therapy. Ann Surg 2000;231:877–82.

24. Dillon MF, Hill ADK, Fleming FJ, et al. Identifying patients at risk of compromised margins following breast conservation for lobular carcinoma. Am J Surg 2006;191:201–5.

25. Silverstein M, Lewinsky B, Waisman J, et al. Infiltrating lobular carcinoma. Is it different from infiltrating duct carcinoma? Cancer 1994;73:1673–7.

26. Santiago RJ, Harris EER, Qin L, et al. Similar long-term results of breast-conservation treatment for stage I and II invasive lobular carcinoma compared with invasive ductal carcinoma of the breast. Cancer 2005;103:2447–54.

27. Menes T, Tartter P, Bleiweiss I, et al. The consequence of multiple re-excisions to obtain clear lumpectomy margins in breast cancer patients. Ann Surg Oncol 2005;12:881–5.

28. Park CC, Mitsumori M, Nixon A, et al. Outcome at 8 years after breast-conserving surgery and radiation therapy for invasive breast cancer: influence of margin status and systemic therapy on local recurrence. J Clin Oncol 2000;18: 1668–75.

29. Meric F, Buchholz TA, Mirza NQ, et al. Long-term complications associated with breast-conservation surgery and radiotherapy. Ann Surg Oncol 2002;9:543–9.

30. Harris JR, Levene MB, Svensson G, et al. Analysis of cosmetic results following primary radiation therapy for stages i and ii carcinoma of the breast. Int J Radiat Oncol Biol Phys 1979;5:257–61.

31. de la Rochefordiere A, Abner A, Silver B, et al. Are cosmetic results following conservative surgery and radiation therapy for early breast cancer dependent on technique? Int J Radiat Oncol Biol Phys 1992;23:925–31.

32. Bold R, Kroll S, Baldwin B, et al. Local rotational flaps for breast conservation therapy as an alternative to mastectomy. Ann Surg Oncol 1997;4:540–4.

33. Clough KB, Lewis J, Couturaud B, et al. Oncoplastic techniques allow extensive resections for breast-conserving therapy of breast carcinomas., 2003;237:26–34.

34. Burak WE Jr, Agnese DM, Povoski SP, et al. Radiofrequency ablation of invasive breast carcinoma followed by delayed surgical excision. Cancer 2003;98: 1369–76.

35. Fornage BD, Sneige N, Ross MI, et al. Small (≤ 2-cm) breast cancer treated with US-guided radiofrequency ablation: feasibility study. Radiology 2004;231:215–24.

36. Sabel MS, Kaufman CS, Whitworth P, et al. Cryoablation of early-stage breast cancer: work-in-progress report of a multi-institutional trial. Ann Surg Oncol 2004;11:542–9.

37. Kaufman CS, Littrup PJ, Freeman-Gibb LA, et al. Office-based cryoablation of breast fibroadenomas with long-term follow-up. Breast J 2005;11:344–50.

38. Arriagada R, Le M, Rochard F, et al. Conservative treatment versus mastectomy in early breast cancer: patterns of failure with 15 years of follow-up data. Institut Gustave-Roussy Breast Cancer Group. J Clin Oncol 1996;14:1558–64.

39. Blichert-Toft M, Rose C, Andersen J, et al. Danish randomized trial comparing breast conservation therapy with mastectomy: six years of life-table analysis. Danish Breast Cancer Cooperative Group. J Natl Cancer Inst Monogr 1992;11:19–25.

CHAPTER 54

Accelerated Partial Breast Irradiation after Breast-Conserving Surgery for Breast Cancer

Timothy M. Pawlik, MD, MPH

Henry M. Kuerer, MD, PhD

Introduction

Breast-conserving therapy (BCT) has been established as a standard treatment for women with early-stage breast cancer. BCT, which consists of breast-conserving surgery and radiation therapy (RT), results in survival equivalent to that observed after mastectomy alone.[1–9] A recent 20-year follow-up from the National Surgical Adjuvant Breast and Bowel Project (NSABP) B-06 trial revealed a cumulative rate of recurrence in the ipsilateral breast of 14.3% for women with early-stage breast cancer who underwent lumpectomy and breast irradiation as compared with 39.2% for women who underwent lumpectomy without irradiation—thereby confirming the important role that RT plays in local disease control.[10] Numerous studies have also shown that conservative surgery and irradiation yield satisfactory cosmetic results.[2,7,8,11–15]

Recently, the need for whole-breast RT (WBRT) in BCT has been questioned, and some investigators have advocated accelerated partial breast irradiation (APBI) as an alternative. APBI is delivered over a shorter period than the standard 5 to 6 weeks for WBRT and is delivered to only a portion of the breast. Many health professionals believe that APBI holds promise in terms of a shorter treatment course, greater patient convenience, utilization of fewer resources, and improved cost-effectiveness. Advocates of APBI argue that these advantages may increase the use of RT in general and enhance the likelihood that RT will be used in conjunction with breast- conserving surgery.

The rationale for using WBRT is to eradicate residual tumor foci that are present in the breast after breast-conserving surgery. Some evidence suggests, however, that the overwhelming majority of in-breast recurrences occur in the quadrant of the breast from which the index tumor was excised. Indeed, data from several studies indicate that patients treated with lumpectomy alone have low rates of recurrence at remote sites within the breast and that those rates are similar to the rates seen among patients given WBRT as part of BCT.[16,17] For example, in the NSABP B-06 trial, in which complete excision of the primary tumor was histologically confirmed, virtually all in-breast relapses in the non-irradiated group occurred in the index tumor quadrant.[18] On average, recurrences elsewhere in the breast occur in only approximately 3.3% of patients treated with lumpectomy alone (range, 0.6–5.8%).[1,3,7,8,19–26] Thus, the published data indicate that local relapse occurs overwhelmingly within the index tumor-bearing quadrant and suggest that WBRT may not be necessary for unifocal early-stage breast cancer. APBI, therefore, may provide an equally efficacious, yet more convenient and cost-effective, alternative to WBRT. Several options for delivering APBI are described in the following sections.

Interstitial Brachytherapy

One of the most commonly used and well-investigated methods of APBI is brachytherapy. Brachytherapy permits the delivery of high radiation doses to small volumes that encompass the tumor bed but spare surrounding tissues, including the skin and lung. Brachytherapy traditionally has been delivered via multiple catheters that are implanted at the time of excision or reexcision or as a separate procedure. The radiation source is usually inserted into the catheters surrounding the tumor bed with automated afterloading technology. In the past, many large centers in both the United States and Europe used BCT that comprised breast-conserving surgery, WBRT, and brachytherapy as an alternative to mastectomy. The primary role for brachytherapy was to provide a boost dose of radiation to the tumor-bearing quadrant after breast-conserving surgery and WBRT. Over the past decade, however, the use of brachytherapy as boost therapy has largely been abandoned, and most patients now receive a radiation boost dose with electron beams.[27]

Brachytherapy has more recently been investigated for use as the sole radiation modality after breast-conserving surgery.[28,29] In this setting, brachytherapy is administered with either low-dose-rate (LDR) (Table 1) or high-dose-rate (HDR) radiation sources (Table 2). With LDR brachytherapy, a dosage of 45 to 50 Gy is delivered to the target volume at a rate of about 0.3 to 0.7 Gy/hour over 4 to 5 days on an inpatient basis. HDR brachytherapy, in contrast, can be performed on an outpatient basis and delivers a total dosage of 34 Gy in twice-daily fractions of 3.4 Gy over 5 days. Most studies investigating implant brachytherapy as the sole method of RT are limited by small sample sizes and short follow-up periods.[16,30–34] For example, in the first Guy's Hospital trial,[32] 27 patients who had single operable breast tumors were treated with a rigid iridium-192 implant inserted into the breast at the tumor excision site during surgery. The implant delivered 55 Gy over the ensuing 5 days. In that study, local in-breast relapses occurred in 10 (37%) of the 27 patients. A local relapse rate as high as this for implant brachytherapy would clearly be unacceptable given the 8% relapse rate with WBRT reported in the NSABP-06 trial. However, in the Guy's Hospital trial, no attempt was made to achieve grossly or microscopically clear margins during resection of the primary breast tumor, and in fact 15 of the 27 patients who experienced local relapse had had tumor involvement of the surgical margin.

More recent studies with strict enrollment criteria and well-defined dosimetric parameters have yielded much more promising results. In a prospective trial from the Ochsner Clinic, 52 patients with intraductal or invasive tumors at least 4 cm in diameter with at least 3 positive axillary nodes and negative inked surgical margins were

Table 1 Results of Selected Studies Using Low-Dose-Rate (LDR) Brachytherapy in the Treatment of Early-Stage Breast Cancer

Institution	No. of Cases	Median Follow-Up (months)	XRT Dose (Gy)	Local Recurrence Rate (%)
Guy's Hospital[32,34]	27	72	5.5	37
Oschner Clinic[31]	26	75	4.5	2
William Beaumont[16]	120	82	4.992	1
Ninewells Hospital[58]	11	72	4.6–5.5	0
Massachusetts General Hospital[59]	48	23	5–6	0
RTOG 95-17[44–46]	31	44	4.5	0
Florence[60]	115	50	5–6	6

Table 2 Results of Selected Studies Using High-Dose-Rate (HDR) Brachytherapy in the Treatment of Early-Stage Breast Cancer.

Institution	No. of Cases	Median Follow-Up (months)	XRT Dose (Gy)	Local Recurrence Rate (%)
Oschner Clinic[31]	26	75	3.2	2
London Regional Cancer Ctr (Ontario)[30,61]	39	91	3.72	16
William Beaumont[16]	79	52	3.2	1
RTOG 95-17[44–46]	68	44	3.4	4
National Institutes of Oncology, Hungary[41,62,63]	45	84	4.33–5.2	7
Germany/Austria[64,65]	176	12	5	0.5
Royal Devon and Exeter[33]	45	18	2–3.2	16
(MammoSite RTS)[53]	43	21	3.4	0

treated with brachytherapy by either an LDR (45 Gy over 4 days) or an HDR (32 Gy in 8 fractions over 4 days) technique.[31,35] Only 1 recurrence (2%) in the treated breast and 3 regional nodal failures (6%) were reported. These results compared favorably with those for a comparison group treated with WBRT at the same institution during the same period. At another single-institution study at the William Beaumont Hospital, a total of 199 patients with early-stage breast cancer were treated prospectively with breast-conserving surgery and limited-field interstitial brachytherapy, and 5 experienced ipsilateral breast failure (ie, recurrence).[36] Matched-pair analysis with historical controls who had been treated with WBRT showed no difference in the rates of local recurrence between the 2 groups.[40]

The Radiation Therapy Oncology Group (RTOG) trial 95-17[37-39] was the first multi-institutional trial in which interstitial brachytherapy was used to deliver APBI. The trial sought to examine the brachytherapy given after lumpectomy and axillary lymph node dissection in terms of cosmesis, local control, and disease-free survival.[37-39] Ninety-nine patients were accrued who met all eligibility criteria, and most (87) had T1 tumors. Thirty-one patients were treated with LDR brachytherapy (45 Gy given over 4.5 days) and 68 with HDR brachytherapy (34 Gy in 10 fractions given over 5 days).[37-39] At a median follow-up time of 3.7 years, 3 patients had developed local recurrence, all 3 in patients with T1 disease who had received HDR brachytherapy. The estimated 4-year actuarial in-breast recurrence rate was 3%.

A phase III multicenter brachytherapy APBI protocol was recently developed by the Breast Cancer Working Group of the European Society for Therapeutic Radiology and Oncology.[40] Patients in the control group will be treated with 50 to 50.4 Gy of WBRT plus a 10 Gy boost versus interstitial HDR or pulsed-dose-rate brachytherapy in the experimental group. The planned accrual is 1,170 patients.[40]

Although early reports on the use of brachytherapy as the sole type of RT after breast-conserving surgery show promising results, standard catheter-based interstitial brachytherapy has several disadvantages.[31,41,42] It is technically difficult, and only a limited number of clinicians in the United States are familiar with the technique. In addition, many patients and health care providers find the placement of catheters and the appearance of the multiple puncture sites required for the insertion of traditional brachytherapy catheters disturbing. Collectively, these factors have limited enthusiasm for the use of traditional brachytherapy and have stimulated interest in alternative methods such as balloon-based intracavitary irradiation.

MammoSite Intracavitary Balloon Brachytherapy

The MammoSite device (Proxima Therapeutics, Alpharetta, GA) is a balloon-based applicator that can be used to deliver breast brachytherapy after lumpectomy. The MammoSite device allows an HDR radiation source to be inserted at the center of an inflatable balloon. The device can be placed into the lumpectomy cavity during surgery or after surgery when the definitive margin status is known. The MammoSite Radiation Therapy System (RTS) device looks like a Foley catheter. It is 18.7 cm in length and approximately 0.6 cm in diameter and is available in two versions—one designed to be inflated to a diameter of 4 to 5 cm with a maximum inflation volume of 70 cm³, and the other designed to be inflated to 5 to 6 cm with a maximum inflation volume of 125 cm³. The balloon is usually filled with normal saline combined with a contrast agent to allow radiographic imaging to verify that the device is placed correctly. The MammoSite RTS device has an inflation channel and a central treatment channel that connects to a computerized afterloading device for delivery of the HDR radiation source. The device is pliable and can be worn within a bra (Figure 1), making it potentially more appealing to patients and clinicians than traditional brachytherapy applicators. Because of its simplicity and patient acceptance, balloon-based brachytherapy has been increasingly used for postoperative PBI despite the lack of studies comparing its efficacy

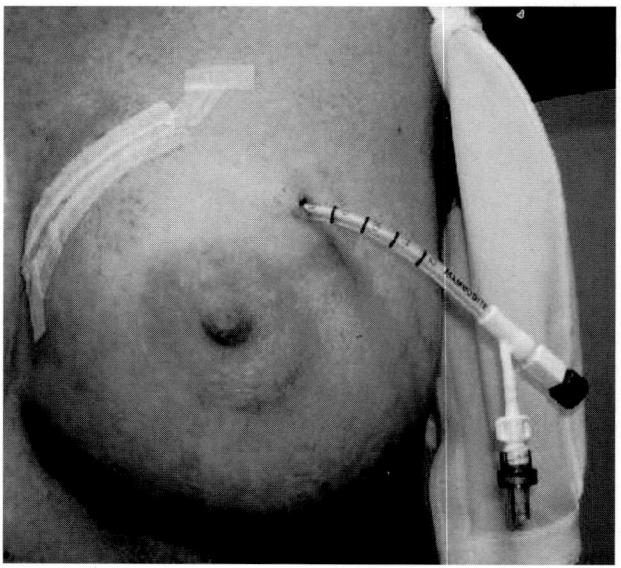

Figure 1 The MammoSite device is pliable and can easily be worn within a bra as shown.

with that of standard postoperative external beam irradiation.

Reproducible placement of the MammoSite RTS device can be easily achieved, and although the mean dose homogeneity index has been shown to be less uniform than that of traditional brachytherapy (0.77 vs 0.93), the coverage of the planned target tissue is better (90% vs 69.8%).[43] The prescribed radiation dose extends to 1 cm beyond the balloon when the balloon conforms to the lumpectomy cavity. The effective radiation penetration, however, may be closer to 2 cm, as the balloon is typically inflated beyond the volume of the lumpectomy cavity, thereby stretching and thinning the surrounding tissue.

In one of the few published studies of the MammoSite RTS device, 70 patients were enrolled in an 8-center prospective trial to evaluate the safety and performance of the device.[44] A dosage of 34 Gy was delivered in 10 fractions over 5 days and was prescribed to be 1 cm from the balloon surface. The device was not implanted in 16 patients because of a cavity that was too large, inadequate skin spacing (eg, less than 7 mm), or final pathology findings. Of the 54 patients who had the MammoSite RTS device placed, 43 (80%) completed brachytherapy, the device was removed in the other 11 patients because of inadequate conformance to the cavity, pathologic findings, patient age, and skin spacing.[44] At this time, no long-term follow-up data are available with respect to cosmesis or local control rates after treatment with the MammoSite RTS device. Although the United States Food and Drug Administration has approved the device for clinical use, a warning was issued stating that "the safety and effectiveness of the MammoSite RTS as a replacement for whole-breast irradiation in the treatment of breast cancer have not been established." The indication for use of the MammoSite RTS device is to provide brachytherapy to deliver intracavitary radiation therapy to the surgical margins after lumpectomy for breast cancer. However, it is critical that the surgical community understand the important ethical and legal considerations that should at a minimum be part of the informed consent process before patients are treated with this new technique in clinical settings. The MammoSite RTS device may actually prove to be equivalent or similar to standard WBRT with respect to local control, but this has yet to be proven in phase III studies. One ongoing study that will help to elucidate the role of the MammoSite device is the MammoSite Patient Registry study sponsored by the American Society of Breast Surgeons. The study will have 7 years of follow-up and enrol approximately 1,300 patients.

Intraoperative Radiation Therapy

Delivery of a single dose of radiation at the time of surgery would be an extremely attractive alternative to postoperative brachytherapy for patients undergoing lumpectomy for breast cancer. Intraoperative radiation therapy (IORT) has been used in patients with breast cancer to give an intraoperative boost dose of 9 Gy to the local tumor bed, followed by additional external beam RT to the whole breast over 6 weeks.[45] Recently some investigators have advocated that IORT be used as the sole method of RT after surgical extirpation of the tumor-bearing tissue. IORT has the advantages of eliminating the possibility of a geographic "miss" and avoiding treatment of the skin, thereby improving cosmesis.

IORT can be delivered by using mobile linear accelerators, which are easily positioned near the operating table and have a movable arm that can be appropriately positioned to deliver the radiation. Mobile linear accelerators usually have a variable spectrum of electron energy (3–10 MeV) and can be used in any operating room without the need for structural modifications. Cylindrical applicators with diameters of 4 to 10 cm and terminal angles between 0° and 45° are used to achieve electron-beam collimation.[46] For radioprotection, mobile shields (2 cm-thick lead) are positioned around and beneath the operating table so that the patient need not be transferred from the operating table. In general, when these devices are used, IORT is easy to perform and only slightly prolongs the surgical procedure. Before IORT can be administered, the breast tissue must be separated from the subcutaneous tissue for 2.5 to 4.0 cm around the wound, with care taken not to compromise the skin vascularity. The breast tissue must also be separated from the pectoralis fascia so that lead shields can be placed between the breast and the pectoralis major muscle. Although this wide mobilization of the breast tissue slightly increases the total time of the operation, some surgeons have argued that it facilitates postresection reconstruction, which improves the cosmetic results.[47]

The European Institute of Oncology in Milan has begun to investigate the feasibility of applying single doses of IORT from 10 Gy up to 22 Gy.[48–50] In the first of these investigations,[48] a portable IORT device with different electron energies was used to treat 65 patients with T1 or T2 (maximum diameter 2.5 cm), N0 or N1 breast cancer. Patients receiving 10 Gy IORT were also given 44 Gy as WBRT, and patients receiving 15 Gy IORT were given 40 Gy as WBRT. Those given IORT doses of 17, 19, or 21 Gy did not undergo WBRT. The authors reported no acute side effects related to IORT and concluded that IORT is feasible and safe.[48] In subsequent studies by the same group, the authors reported that IORT was well tolerated and that most patients did not experience immediate skin erythema or fibrosis. Over the 1-year study period, the mean time needed to perform all the phases of IORT decreased from 40 to 20 minutes. This experience provides preliminary evidence that IORT is simple to use and can be given rapidly, that training staff to perform IORT is easy, and that acute side effects are minimal and not serious.[50]

Another approach, initiated in the United Kingdom, is evaluating definitive IORT with low-energy x-rays as the sole form of RT after segmental mastectomy. In the "TARGIT" (targeted intraoperative radiotherapy) approach, IORT is delivered with a minielectron-beam–driven x-ray source called Intrabeam (currently manufactured by Carl Zeiss). The Intrabeam device was approved by the US Food and Drug Administration for delivery of RT in the United States in 1999. Low-energy x-rays (50 kV maximum) are emitted from the tip of a 10 cm-long, 3.2 mm-diameter probe enclosed in a spherical applicator (available in sizes ranging from 2.5–5.0 cm in diameter) that is inserted into the tumor bed (Figure 2). IORT is delivered over 25 minutes. The prescribed dose at 0.2 cm is 20 Gy and that at 1 cm is 5 Gy. Tungsten-impregnated rubber sheets are placed on the chest wall to protect the heart and lungs and placed over the wound to block stray radiation, and the skin dose is monitored with thermoluminescent detectors. A multinational, multi-institutional randomized trial was begun in March 2000 to compare IORT given with the Intrabeam device plus WBRT with standard WBRT after lumpectomy for women with operable invasive breast cancer (T1 to T3, N0 or N1, M0).[51–54] Several centers in Europe, Australia, and the United States are collaborating to accrue patients on this trial, which will need to enrol approximately 1,000 patients over the next 3 to 4 years to achieve the statistical power to prove equivalence of the 2 treatments.

Use of a low-energy x-ray source has advantages as well as potential disadvantages related to dose attenuation. Because the biologically effective dose of radiation delivered by this source attenuates rapidly, specially designed operating rooms are not needed. However, use of minielectron-beam devices has been criticized because the dose 1 cm from the margin is only 5 Gy, a dose that may be ineffective for eradicating occult carcinoma cells. Concern has also been expressed that tumoricidal doses may be achieved at only about 2 to 3 mm from the x-ray source. Only long-term results of the randomized trial will prove or disprove the validity of these theoretical concerns. The Milan group at the European Institute of Oncology has been using a different device to deliver a

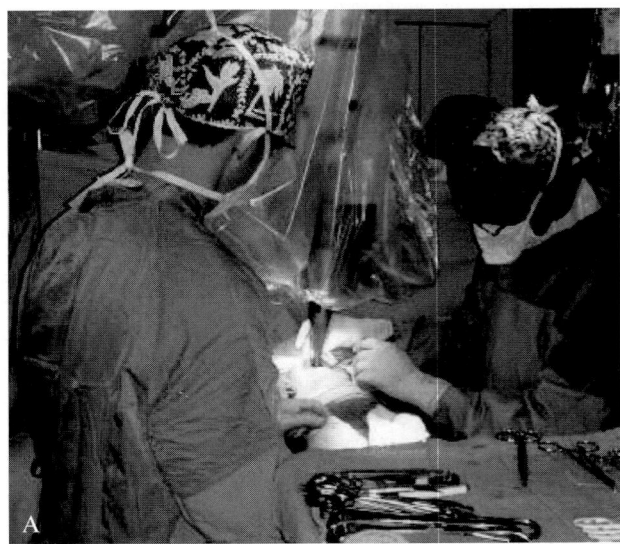

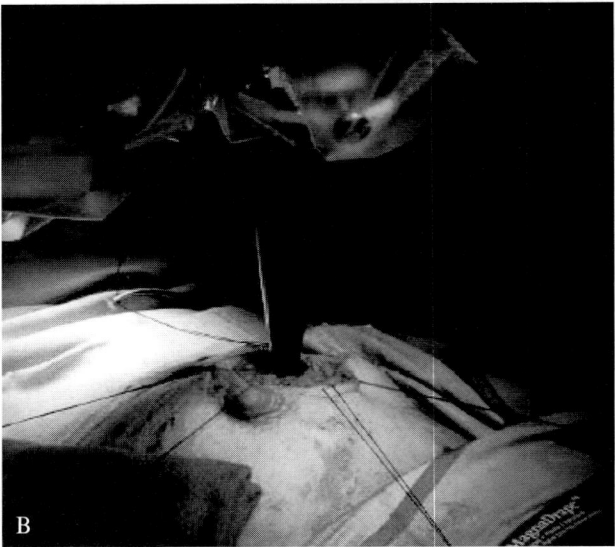

Figure 2 Targeted intraoperative radiation therapy. *A,* Surgical team prepares lumpectomy cavity to deliver IORT. *B,* The applicator is placed in the tumor bed immediately after excision of the tumor and sutured into place to begin radiation delivery. Photos courtesy of Dr. Dennis R. Holmes, Kenneth Norris Comprehensive Cancer Center, Keck School of Medicine, University of Southern California.

larger dose (21 Gy) in a single fraction with electrons. This dose has been criticized as being too high, especially with respect to normal tissues. Adverse effects on normal tissues may also be further exaggerated with the Intrabeam device owing to the very steep dose gradient between the prescription point in the tissue and the surface of the applicator. However, the volume of normal tissues that receives a large single dose from this technique is small, so one might expect a good cosmetic outcome.[51–54]

External Beam Delivery of Highly Conformal Radiation Therapy

Three-dimensional (3-D) conformal RT combines digital diagnostic imaging and postimaging computer analysis to conform the radiation beam to the shape of the tumor. Treatment planning begins with obtaining computed tomography (CT) scans or magnetic resonance (MR) images that show the anatomy of the tumor and the surrounding normal structures. These images are put into a treatment planning computer that produces an accurate 3-D image of the tumor and the surrounding organs so that multiple radiation beams can be aimed at the tumor from different directions, matching the contour of the treatment area. The goal at this approach is to deliver a prescribed dose across all three dimensions (height, width, and depth) of the tumor and to allow the dose to be spread around the surrounding normal tissue, minimizing the dose to any one area and sparing nearby healthy tissue. Three-dimension conformal RT also has the potential advantage of improved dose homogeneity within the target volume, which may improve cosmetic results and reduce the risk of symptomatic fat necrosis. In addition, although implant brachytherapy requires additional training and expertise, most radiation facilities already have the technologic tools required to deliver 3-D conformal RT.

Formenti and colleagues recently reported their early experience with using 3-D conformal external beam PBI in which the patient is imaged and treated with a dedicated CT scanner.[55] In that study, the planned target volume included the tumor bed plus an additional 1 to 2 cm margin defined on a postlumpectomy CT scan. At a minimum follow-up of 36 months (range, 36–53 months), all 10 treated patients were alive and disease-free with good to excellent cosmesis.[55] In the William Beaumont Hospital's experience with 3-D conformal external beam PBI after breast-conserving surgery for 31 patients,[56] cosmetic results were rated as good to excellent in most patients. In addition, the mean coverage of the planned target volume by the 95% isodose line was 100% (range, 97–100%). The authors of that report concluded that 3-D conformal RT is both technically feasible and associated with minimal acute toxicity.

One potential disadvantage of 3-D conformal RT is that the breast moves with respiration, and thus a larger volume of normal breast tissue may need to be irradiated to avoid a geographic "miss" of tumor-containing tissue. The effect of breathing motion on the clinical target volume in 3-D conformal PBI was investigated recently by Baglan and colleagues,[57] who found that 98 to 100% of the clinical target volume was covered by the 95% isodose line at the extremes of inhalation and exhalation

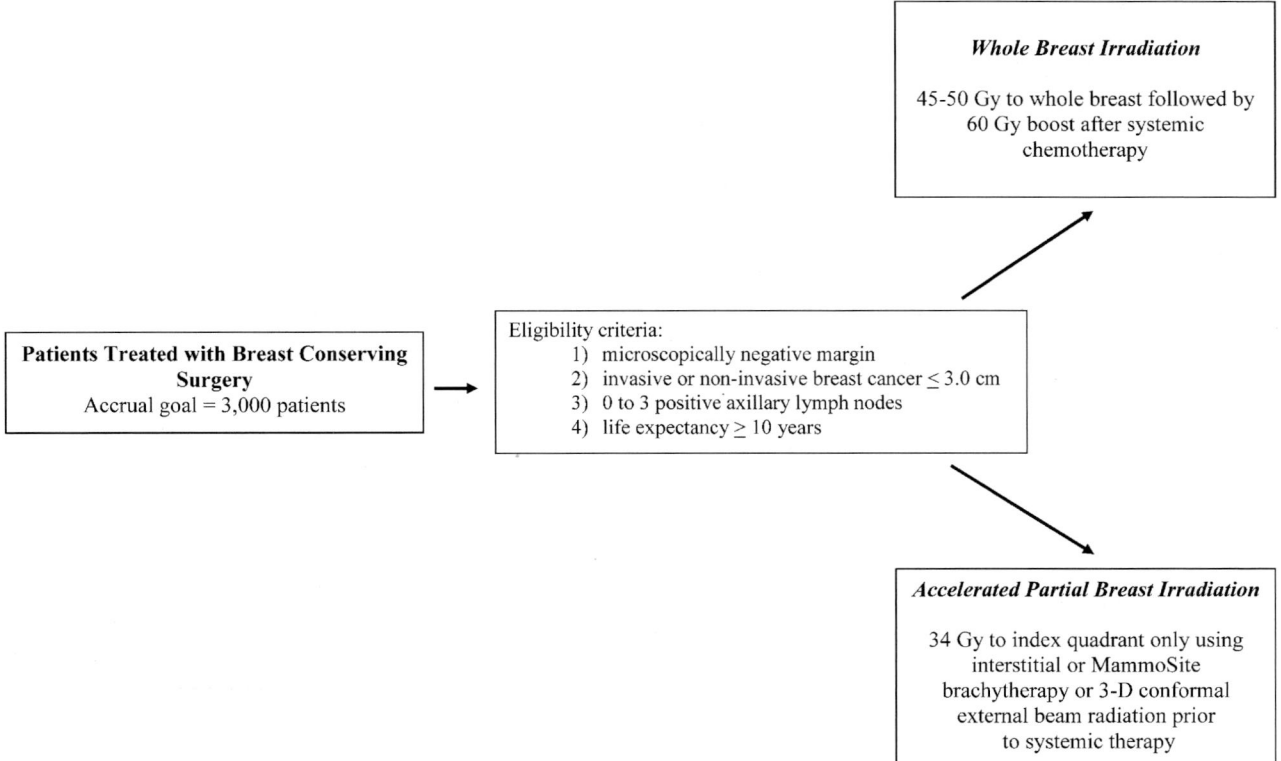

Figure 3 NSABP-RTOG randomized trial evaluating partial breast irradiation after conservative surgery for early-stage breast cancer.

when a 5 mm additional breathing margin was added to the planned target volume. The authors concluded that adding a 10 mm margin to the planned target volume would provide adequate coverage for most patients.

The RTOG recently completed a phase II multicenter trial evaluating 3-D conformal, but the results of that trial had not yet been published when this chapter was written.

Future Perspectives

Regardless of the method of delivery (implant or balloon brachytherapy, IORT or 3-D conformal RT), studies comparing APBI versus standard WBRT with regard to long-term local control and disease-free survival rates are lacking. The American Society of Breast Surgeons has issued a consensus statement on APBI that states that APBI should be performed only as part of an investigational protocol either at an individual institution or as part of a multi-institutional trial and outlines several criteria that may help guide the selection of patients for such NSABP

B-39/RTOG-0413 trials. One such study that recently opened for this purpose is a randomized phase III study of conventional WBRT versus APBI for women with stage 0, I, or II breast cancer (Figure 3). APBI will be delivered as multicatheter brachytherapy, MammoSite RTS brachytherapy, or 3-D conformal external beam RT. Patients requiring chemotherapy will receive it either before undergoing WBRT or after undergoing APBI. The primary end point is in-breast tumor recurrence; secondary end points are overall survival and disease-free survival. Eligibility criteria include microscopically negative surgical margins, invasive or noninvasive breast cancer no larger than 3.0 cm, 0 to 3 positive axillary lymph nodes, and a life expectancy of at least 10 years. The study is cosponsored by the RTOG and has been formally endorsed by the American College of Surgeons Oncology Group and the Southwest Oncology Group. The accrual goal for the study is 3,000 patients. Current efforts should be directed toward enrolling appropriate candidates into large, randomized, prospective trials such as this one so that the efficacy of APBI with regard to local recurrence, survival, cosmesis, and patient satisfaction can be more fully evaluated.

References

1. Gage I, Recht A, Gelman R, et al. Long-term outcome following breast-conserving surgery and radiation therapy. Int J Radiat Oncol Biol Phys 1995;33:245–51.

2. Veronesi U, Salvadori B, Luini A, et al. Conservative treatment of early breast cancer. Long-term results of 1232 cases treated with quadrantectomy, axillary dissection, and radiotherapy. Ann Surg 1990;211:250–9.

3. Kurtz JM, Spitalier JM, Amalric R, et al. The prognostic significance of late local recurrence after breast-conserving therapy. Int J Radiat Oncol Biol Phys 1990;18:87–93.

4. Fisher B, Anderson S, Redmond CK, et al. Reanalysis and results after 12 years of follow-up in a randomized clinical trial comparing total mastectomy with lumpectomy with or without irradiation in the treatment of breast cancer. N Engl J Med 1995;333:1456–61.

5. Sarrazin D, Le MG, Arriagada R, et al. Ten-year results of a randomized trial comparing a conservative treatment to mastectomy in early breast cancer. Radiother Oncol 1989;14:177–84.

6. van Dongen JA, Bartelink H, Fentiman IS, et al. Randomized clinical trial to assess the value of breast-conserving therapy in stage I and II breast cancer, EORTC 10801 trial. J Natl Cancer Inst Monogr 1992;(11):15–8.

7. Fourquet A, Campana F, Zafrani B, et al. Prognostic factors of breast recurrence in the conservative management of early breast cancer: a 25-year follow-up. Int J Radiat Oncol Biol Phys 1989;17:719–25.

8. Fowble B, Solin LJ, Schultz DJ, et al. Breast recurrence following conservative surgery and radiation: patterns of failure, prognosis, and pathologic findings from mastectomy specimens with implications for treatment. Int J Radiat Oncol Biol Phys 1990;19:833–42.

9. Jacobson JA, Danforth DN, Cowan KH, et al. Ten-year results of a comparison of conservation with mastectomy in the treatment of stage I and II breast cancer. N Engl J Med 1995;332:907–11.

10. Fisher B, Anderson S, Bryant J, et al. Twenty-year follow-up of a randomized trial comparing total mastectomy, lumpectomy, and lumpectomy plus irradiation for the treatment of invasive breast cancer. N Engl J Med 2002;347:1233–41.

11. Haffty BG, Goldberg NB, Fischer D, et al. Conservative surgery and radiation therapy in breast carcinoma: local recurrence and prognostic implications. Int J Radiat Oncol Biol Phys 1989;17:727–32.

12. Stotter AT, McNeese MD, Ames FC, et al. Predicting the rate and extent of locoregional failure after breast conservation therapy for early breast cancer. Cancer 1989;64:2217–25.

13. Clarke DH, Edmundson GK, Martinez A, et al. The clinical advantages of I-125 seeds as a substitute for Ir-192 seeds in temporary plastic tube implants. Int J Radiat Oncol Biol Phys 1989;17:859–63.

14. Vicini FA, Recht A, Abner A, et al. Recurrence in the breast following conservative surgery and radiation therapy for early-stage breast cancer. J Natl Cancer Inst Monogr 1992; 11:33–9.

15. Abner AL, Recht A, Eberlein T, et al. Prognosis following salvage mastectomy for recurrence in the breast after conservative surgery and radiation therapy for early-stage breast cancer. J Clin Oncol 1993;11:44–8.

16. Vicini FA, Baglan KL, Kestin LL, et al. Accelerated treatment of breast cancer. J Clin Oncol 2001;19:1993–2001.

17. Vaidya JS, Vyas JJ, Chinoy RF, et al. Multicentricity of breast cancer: whole-organ analysis and clinical implications. Br J Cancer 1996;74:820–4.

18. Fisher B, Redmond C, Poisson R, et al. Eight-year results of a randomized clinical trial comparing total mastectomy and lumpectomy with or without irradiation in the treatment of breast cancer. N Engl J Med 1989;320:822–8.

19. Fortin A, Larochelle M, Laverdiere J, et al. Local failure is responsible for the decrease in survival for patients with breast cancer treated with conservative surgery and post-operative radiotherapy. J Clin Oncol 1999;17:101–9.

20. Boyages J, Recht A, Connolly JL, et al. Early breast cancer: predictors of breast recurrence for patients treated with conservative surgery and radiation therapy. Radiother Oncol 1990;19:29–41.

21. Clark RM, McCulloch PB, Levine MN, et al. Randomized clinical trial to assess the effectiveness of breast irradiation following lumpectomy and axillary dissection for node-negative breast cancer. J Natl Cancer Inst 1992;84:683–9.

22. Liljegren G, Holmberg L, Bergh J, et al. 10-year results after sector resection with or without postoperative radiotherapy for stage I breast cancer: a randomized trial. J Clin Oncol 1999;17:2326–33.

23. Touboul E, Buffat L, Belkacemi Y, et al. Local recurrences and distant metastases after breast-conserving surgery and radiation therapy for early breast cancer. Int J Radiat Oncol Biol Phys 1999;43:25–38.

24. Smith TE, Lee D, Turner BC, et al. True recurrence vs. new primary ipsilateral breast tumor relapse: an analysis of clinical and pathologic differences and their implications in natural history, prognoses, and therapeutic management. Int J Radiat Oncol Biol Phys 2000;48:1281–9.

25. Veronesi U, Marubini E, Mariani L, et al. Radiotherapy after breast-conserving surgery in small breast carcinoma: long-term results of a randomized trial. Ann Oncol 2001; 12:997–1003.

26. Huang E, Buchholz TA, Meric F, et al. Classifying local disease recurrences after breast conservation therapy based on location and histology: new primary tumors have more favorable outcomes than true local disease recurrences. Cancer 2002;95:2059–67.

27. Shank B, Moughan J, Owen J, et al. The 1993-94 patterns of care process survey for breast irradiation after breast-conserving surgery-comparison with the 1992 standard for breast conservation treatment. The Patterns of Care Study, American College of Radiology. Int J Radiat Oncol Biol Phys 2000;48:1291–9.

28. Kuerer HM, Julian TB, Strom EA, et al. Accelerated partial breast irradiation after conservative surgery for breast cancer. Ann Surg 2004;239:338–51.

29. Pawlik TM, Buchholz TA, Kuerer HM. The biologic rationale for and emerging role of accelerated partial breast irradiation for breast cancer. J Am Coll Surg 2004;199:479–92.

30. Perera F, Engel J, Holliday R, et al. Local resection and brachytherapy confined to the lumpectomy site for early breast cancer: a pilot study. J Surg Oncol 1997;65:263–8.

31. King TA, Bolton JS, Kuske RR, et al. Long-term results of wide-field brachytherapy as the sole method of radiation therapy after segmental mastectomy for T(is,1,2) breast cancer. Am J Surg 2000;180:299–304.

32. Fentiman IS, Poole C, Tong D, et al. Iridium implant treatment without external radiotherapy for operable breast cancer: a pilot study. Eur J Cancer 1991;27:447–50.

33. Clarke DH, Vicini F, Jacobs H. High dose rate brachytherapy for breast cancer. In: Nag S, editor. High dose rate brachytherapy. Arnonk, New York: Futura Publishing; 1994. p. 321–9.

34. Fentiman IS, Poole C, Tong D, et al. Inadequacy of iridium implant as sole radiation treatment for operable breast cancer. Eur J Cancer 1996;32A:608–11.

35. Kuske RR, Bolton JS, McKinnon WMP. 5-year results of prospective phase II trial of wide-volume brachytherapy as the sole method of breast irradiation in Tis, T1, T2, N0–1 breast cancer (Abstr.). Int J Radiat Oncol Biol Phys 1998; 42:181.

36. Vicini FA, Kestin L, Chen P, et al. Limited-field radiation therapy in the management of early-stage breast cancer. J Natl Cancer Inst 2003;95:1205–10.

37. Kuske RR, Bolton JS. A phase I/II trial to evaluate brachytherapy as the sole method of radiation therapy for stage I and II breast carcioma. RTOG Publication no. 1055. Philadelphia, PA: Radiation Therapy Oncology Group; 1995.

38. Kuske RR, Winter K, Arthur D. A phase I/II trial of brachytherapy alone following lumpectomy for select breast cancer: toxicity analysis of Radiation Therapy Oncology Group 95-17. Int J Radiat Oncol Biol Phys 2002;54:87.

39. Kuske RR, Winter K, Arthur DW. A phase II trial of brachytherapy alone following lumpectomy for stage I or II breast cancer: initial outcomes of RTOG 95-17. Proc Am Soc Clin Oncol 2004;23:18.

40. Polgar C, Strnad V, Major T. Brachytherapy for parital breast irradiation: the European experience. Semin Radiat Oncol 2005;15:116–22.

41. Wazer DE, Berle L, Graham R, et al. Preliminary results of a phase I/II study of HDR brachytherapy alone for T1/T2 breast cancer. Int J Radiat Oncol Biol Phys 2002;53:889–97.

42. Jewell WR, Krishnan L, Reddy EK, et al. Intraoperative implantation radiation therapy plus lumpectomy for carcinoma of the breast. Arch Surg 1987;122:687–90.

43. Edmundson GK, Vicini FA, Chen PY, et al. Dosimetric characteristics of the MammoSite RTS, a new breast brachytherapy applicator. Int J Radiat Oncol Biol Phys 2002;52:1132–9.

44. Keisch M, Vicini F, Kuske RR, et al. Initial clinical experience with the MammoSite breast brachytherapy applicator in women with early-stage breast cancer treated with breast-conserving therapy. Int J Radiat Oncol Biol Phys 2003;55:289–93.

45. Reitsmaer R, Peintinger F, Sedlmayer F, et al. Intraoperative radiotherapy given as a boost after breast-conserving surgery in breast cancer patients. Eur J Cancer 2002;38:1607–10.

46. Kuerer HM, Chung M, Giovanna G, et al. The case for accelerated partial-breast irradiation for breast cancer. Contemporary Surg 2003;59:508–16.

47. Intra M, Gatti G, Luini A, et al. Surgical technique of intraoperative radiotherapy in conservative treatment of limited-stage breast cancer. Arch Surg 2002;137:737–40.

48. Gatzemeier W, Orecchia R, Gatti G, et al. [Intraoperative radiotherapy (IORT) in treatment of breast carcinoma—a new therapeutic alternative within the scope of breast-saving therapy? Current status and future prospects. Report of experiences from the European Institute of Oncology (EIO), Mailand]. Strahlenther Onkol 2001;177:330–7.

49. Orrechia R, Veronesi U. Intraoperative electrons. Semin Radiat Oncol 2005;15:76–83.

50. Veronesi U, Orecchia R, Luini A, et al. A preliminary report of intraoperative radiotherapy (IORT) in limited-stage breast cancers that are conservatively treated. Eur J Cancer 2001;37:2178–83.

51. Vaidya JS, Baum M, Tobias JS, et al. The novel technique of delivering targeted intraoperative radiotherapy (Targit) for early breast cancer. Eur J Surg Oncol 2002;28:447–54.

52. Vaidya JS, Baum M, Tobias JS, et al. Targeted intra-operative radiotherapy (Targit): an innovative method of treatment for early breast cancer. Ann Oncol 2001;12:1075–80.

53. Vaidya JS, Tobias J, Baum M, et al. Intraoperative radiotherapy for breast cancer. Lancet Oncol 2004;5:163–73.

54. Vaidya JS, Tobias J, Baum M, et al. TARGeted Intraoperative radiotherapy (TARGIT): an innovative approach to partial breast irradiation. Semin Radiat Oncol 2005;15:84–91.

55. Formenti SC, Rosenstein B, Skinner KA, Jozsef G. T1 stage breast cancer: adjuvant hypofractionated conformal radiation therapy to tumor bed in selected postmenopausal breast cancer patients—pilot feasibility study. Radiology 2002;222:171–8.

56. Vicini FA, Remouchamps V, Wallace M, et al. Ongoing clinical experience utilizing 3D conformal external beam radiotherapy to deliver partial-breast irradiation in patients with early-stage breast cancer treated with breast-conserving therapy. Int J Radiat Oncol Biol Phys 2003;57:1247–53.

57. Baglan KL, Sharpe MB, Jaffray D, et al. Accelerated partial breast irradiation using 3D conformal radiation therapy (3D-CRT). Int J Radiat Oncol Biol Phys 2003;55:302–11.

58. Samuel LM, Dewar JA, Preece PE, Wood RAB. A pilot study of radical radiotherapy using a perioperative implant following wide local excision for carcinoma of the breast. Breast 1999;8:95–7.

59. Lawenda BD, Taghian AG, Kachnic LA, et al. Dose-volume analysis of radiotherapy for T1N0 invasive breast cancer treated by local excision and partial breast irradiation by low-dose-rate interstitial implant. Int J Radiat Oncol Biol Phys 2003;56:671–80.

60. Cionini L, Marzano S, Pacini P. Iridium implant of the surgical bed as the sole radiotherapeutic treatment after conservative surgery for breast cancer. Radiother Oncol 1995;35 Suppl:S1.

61. Perera F, Yu E, Engel J, et al. Patterns of breast recurrence in a pilot study of brachytherapy confined to the lumpectomy site for early breast cancer with six years' minimum follow-up. Int J Radiat Oncol Biol Phys 2003;57:1239–46.

62. Polgar C, Fodor J, Major T, et al. Radiotherapy confined to the tumor bed following breast conserving surgery current status, controversies, and future projects. Strahlenther Onkol 2002;178:597–606.

63. Polgar C, Sulyok Z, Fodor J, et al. Sole brachytherapy of the tumor bed after conservative surgery for T1 breast cancer: five-year results of a phase I-II study and initial findings of a randomized phase III trial. J Surg Oncol 2002;80:121–9.

64. Ott OJ, Potter R, Hammer J, et al. Accelerated partial breast irradiation with iridium-192 multicatheter PDR/HDR brachytherapy: preliminary results of the German-Austrian Multicenter Trial. Strahlenther Onkol 2004;180:642–9.

65. Strnad V, Ott OJ, Potter R. Interstitial brachytherapy alone after breast conserving surgery: interim results of 2 German-Austrian multicenter phase II trials. Brachytherapy 2004;3:115–9.

CHAPTER 55

SENTINEL LYMPH NODE DISSECTION: INDICATIONS, TECHNIQUE AND RESULTS

TAMRA MCKENZIE-JOHNSON, MD

AYSEGUL SAHIN, MD

KELLY K. HUNT, MD

Introduction

The goals of axillary lymph node dissection in the treatment of breast cancer are to obtain accurate staging information and to provide regional control in the nodal basin. Although there have been studies that demonstrate improved survival with an increasing number of nodes removed, the general consensus is that there is no benefit to removing healthy (uninvolved) lymph nodes from women with breast cancer. The complications of axillary lymph node dissection may be significant for the individual patient. Potential complications include lymphedema, difficulty with shoulder mobility, paresthesias of the upper extremity and chest wall, chronic pain syndrome, persistent seroma, hematoma formation requiring reoperation and infection. Although the development of these complications after axillary lymph node dissection is relatively infrequent, the incidence of lymphedema has been reported to be as high as 25 to 30%. In addition, lymphedema rates are increased when both surgery and radiation therapy are employed for the individual patient. Shoulder dysfunction is also a significant long-term disability for some patients. The incidence of true shoulder dysfunction has not been well documented in many studies; however, this does seem to occur more frequently in the elderly population and can lead to chronic shoulder dysfunction and arthritic changes within the shoulder joint.

Because of screening mammography and improved public awareness about breast cancer, early detection has become a reality. The incidence of early-stage invasive breast cancer and the percentage of patients diagnosed with ductal carcinoma in situ has increased. As a result, the number of patients presenting with clinically positive axillary lymph nodes or microscopic nodal involvement has dramatically decreased, reducing overall the need for routine axillary dissection for therapeutic or staging purposes. Such trends support the need for a more selective approach to treatment of the axillary lymph nodes.

The use of lymphatic mapping with sentinel lymph node biopsy was popularized by Dr. Donald Morton for the treatment of patients with clinically node-negative melanoma. The definition of the sentinel node is the first node to receive lymphatic drainage from the area of the primary tumor, and, therefore, the status of the sentinel lymph node should be predictive of the remaining lymph nodes in the nodal basin. The concept of lymphatic mapping with sentinel lymph node biopsy for breast cancer was first tested by David Krag and his colleagues and published in 1993.[1] At the same time, Dr. Armando Giuliano developed a significant experience with the use of lymphatic mapping for breast cancer and published his results in 1994.[2] There have now been a number of studies published since these early reports, both single-institution studies and multi-institutional studies, evaluating the identification rates and false-negative rates in the use of sentinel lymph node biopsy for breast cancer. This chapter will review the techniques of sentinel lymph node biopsy for breast cancer and the results of large single institution studies and multi-institutional studies that are now available.

Optimal Technique for Sentinel Lymph Node Biopsy

Successful and accurate completion of lymphatic mapping and sentinel lymph node biopsy procedures involves the integration of several technical components that cross multiple disciplines. These include the injection of sentinel node localizing agents, lymphoscintigraphy, surgical sentinel node harvesting, and finally, careful histologic examination of the sentinel node.

AGENTS FOR LYMPHATIC MAPPING

The initial reports on sentinel lymph node biopsy for breast cancer utilized either isosulfan blue dye as a single agent or technetium-labeled sulfur colloid solution as a single agent. The first published reports on sentinel lymph node biopsy demonstrated identification rates in the 80 to 90% range using a single agent. Investigators soon began to combine the use of these 2 agents, and this proved to be more successful for identification of the sentinel lymph node and also in decreasing the false-negative events. McMasters and colleagues developed a lymphatic mapping registry including 99 surgeons in institutions throughout the United States who performed sentinel lymph node biopsy followed by axillary node dissection as part of their initial experience with the technique.[3] The results from these 99 surgeons demonstrated that in 806 patients who had sentinel lymph node biopsy with axillary dissection, the single-agent technique with blue dye or radioisotope alone was utilized in 244 patients and the dual-agent technique was utilized in 562 patients. Table 1 demonstrates that the identification rate was improved with the use of dual-agent mapping, although this difference was not statistically significant. The number of sentinel lymph nodes recovered at surgery increased with the dual agent and, most importantly, the false-negative events decreased from 11.8% with the single-agent mapping to 5.8% with the dual-agent mapping. This difference was highly statistically significant with a P value less than 0.05.

Interestingly, the radio-pharmaceutical agent used in the United States for localizing the sentinel node and for lymphoscintigraphy, either filtered or unfiltered technetium-labeled sulfur colloid, is not FDA approved for these specific uses. Currently, a new agent with the trade name Lymphoseek is undergoing active investigation as part of an FDA approval process. This agent, (Tc-99) DTPA-mannosyl-dextran is a radiotracer that accumulates in lymphatic tissue by binding to a mannose protein that naturally resides on dendritic cells in lymph nodes. The DTPA component is the chelating site for technetium and the mannose residues are substrates for the receptor on the dendritic cells. It is hypothesized that this is less likely to pass on to secondary echelon nodes because of the specific binding characteristics and in turn reduce the extent of surgery in the nodal basin during the sentinel lymph node dissection.

LEARNING CURVE

The number of procedures necessary for the surgeon learning the technique of sentinel lymph node biopsy for breast cancer has been studied by several investigators. Cox and colleagues of the Moffitt Cancer Center studied the mapping results for 5 different surgeons and noted that 23 cases were required for the surgeon to reach and stay below the 10% failure rate, whereas 53 cases were required for the surgeon to reach the 5% failure rate.[4] Although this defines the failure rate in the surgeon's ability to identify a sentinel lymph node, it does not identify the number of cases necessary to reach the 5% false-negative rate. The Institute for Clinical Systemic Improvement Technology Assessment Committee recently concluded that sentinel lymph node dissection should only be used in clinical settings by an experienced surgeon, and this was defined as a surgeon having an identification rate of greater than or equal to 85%, and a false-negative rate less than or equal to 5%.[5] An international consensus conference of opinion leaders in the field of breast cancer surgery agreed that 20 to 30 cases of sentinel lymph node dissection with axillary dissection would in fact yield a failure and false-negative rate less than 5%.[6] The American Society of Breast Surgeons has issued a consensus statement supporting surgeons performing 20 cases of sentinel lymph node dissection plus axillary dissection prior to abandoning

Table 1 Lymphatic Mapping for Breast Cancer: Single versus Dual-Agent Mapping Technique

Parameter	Single-Agent	Dual-Agent	P Value
SLN ID rate	86%	90%	NS
No. of SLNs	1.5	2.1	0.001
False negative rate	11.8%	5.8%	< 0.05

the standard use of axillary dissection.[7] The Department of Defense (DOD) Multicenter Breast Lymphatic Mapping Trial enrolled participating surgeons from academic and community practices and found that participating surgeons achieved an identification rate of 85% and a false-negative rate of 4% with a validation set of 20 to 25 cases of sentinel lymph node dissection plus axillary lymph node dissection after attending a training course.[8] Cody and colleagues at the Memorial Sloan-Kettering Cancer Center have observed that a surgeon will continue to have false-negative events despite gaining experience with the technique of lymphatic mapping with sentinel lymph node dissection.[9] In fact, tumor and patient factors have recently been described that may impact the false-negative rate, and therefore experienced surgeons may experience false-negative events at any time during their surgical practice of the sentinel lymph node mapping technique. Factors that have been reported to impact the false-negative rate include the presence of multifocality or multicentricity, high S-phase fraction, body mass index, and patient age. Results from the American College of Surgeons Oncology Group (ACOSOG) Z0010 trial recently demonstrated that increasing body mass index and increasing patient age were significant factors that impacted the identification of sentinel lymph nodes in the Z0010 trial.[10] The surgeon-related factors were the number of patients that a surgeon enrolled on the Z0010 trial, with surgeons enrolling more than 50 patients on the trial experiencing a failure rate of less than 1%, whereas those surgeons who enrolled fewer than 50 patients on trial had a failed mapping rate of 2%. Certainly surgeons with higher volume practices are likely to have more experience with the technique, and this will impact not only the identification rate, but presumably the false negative events as well. Cox and colleagues reported that surgeons who perform more than 6 sentinel lymph node dissections per month experience lower failed mapping rates than surgeons who perform fewer sentinel lymph node dissections.[11] One may conclude then that not only the initial credentialing experience is important, but also the ongoing experience in volume of cases within an individual surgeon's practice.

TECHNICAL VARIATIONS IN LYMPHATIC MAPPING

In addition to the agent utilized for breast lymphatic mapping, there can also be variations in the location of the injection of the mapping agent. The initial studies of lymphatic mapping were in large part performed with a peritumoral or parenchymal injection technique. Intratumoral injections have not proved to be useful,

since there is a difficulty in visualizing the mapping agent following intratumoral injection. Both subdermal and intradermal techniques have gained popularity by several groups because of the rapid movement of the mapping agent from this location to the regional lymph nodes. The subareolar injection technique has also been popularized because many tumors are small and non-palpable, and therefore utilizing a subareolar injection does not require the need for any imaging procedures to localize the tumor for preoperative injection. Although subareolar and intradermal injection sites allow for rapid movement of the lymphatic mapping agent to the regional nodes, the type of lymphatic drainage or the nodal basins that receive lymphatic drainage will vary depending on the site of injection. Patients who have intraparenchymal injection of the mapping agent will demonstrate drainage to the internal mammary nodes in 20 to 30% of cases, and in fact will demonstrate drainage to other extra-axillary sites such as infraclavicular and supraclavicular nodes in addition to the axillary nodes. Intradermal/subdermal and periareolar/subareolar injections demonstrate a low rate of internal mammary nodal drainage on the order of 0 to 2%. Subtumoral injections or deep fascial injections that have been utilized by Galimberti and colleagues demonstrate the highest rate of internal mammary nodal drainage, varying anywhere from 20 to 60%.[12] Although the need for biopsy of internal mammary nodes has been questioned by some investigators, it does make sense that surgeons would want to see the true lymphatic drainage pattern of the tumor within the breast and not simply identify an axillary node for removal that may or may not accurately reflect the drainage of the tumor and the metastatic process. In the University of Texas M. D. Anderson Cancer Center experience evaluating over 1,200 patients who have undergone lymphoscintigraphy and sentinel lymph node dissection, we found that 19.8% of the patients had combined drainage to the internal mammary nodes and the axillary nodes, 1.6% had drainage to the internal mammary nodes alone, and 68.1% had drainage to the axillary lymph nodes alone.[13]

PATHOLOGICAL ASSESSMENT OF THE SENTINEL NODES

The sentinel lymph node technique allows pathologists to concentrate their examination on a few select nodes as opposed to examining 15 to 30 lymph nodes that are recovered during a standard axillary lymph node dissection. The standards for pathologic examination of the sentinel lymph nodes have not been well defined. There is no standard in the number of sections for each sentinel lymph node or whether immunohistochemistry for cytokeratin should be performed on the sentinel lymph node as a routine. Giuliano and colleagues compared the rate of metastasis identified within the sentinel nodes in a study where an equal number of patients undergoing sentinel lymph node surgery plus axillary dissection were compared with patients matched for primary tumor factors that were undergoing axillary dissection alone.[14] Approximately 26% of the patients who had sentinel lymph node dissection were upstaged, and a significant percentage of these patients had micrometastasis. Although the clinical significance of micrometastasis has been questioned, the idea of more accurately staging patients with the use of sentinel lymph node dissection has been shown by several investigators. At M. D. Anderson, we performed a study where each sentinel lymph node was examined with a more detailed assessment, including 10 deeper levels through the paraffin block in addition to 2 slides for immunohisto-chemical staining with antibodies to cytokeratin.[15] This study was performed on a population of patients who had undergone sentinel lymph node dissection with axillary lymph node dissection and the sentinel nodes were thought to be negative based on standard pathologic assessment with hematoxylin-eosin (H&E) staining. With the more detailed assessment of serial sectioning and immunohistochemical staining, we identified metastases in 21% of the patients. Many of these metastases were micrometastases; however, this study confirms the fact that a more detailed assessment of the sentinel node by the pathologist will provide a more accurate assessment of the nodal staging. Our pathologists identified that 2 deeper levels through the paraffin block with 1 slide for immunohistochemical staining would be sufficient to identify 98% of the metastases in the study. Our current practice has been modified to include 2 deeper levels through each paraffin block for examination with H&E staining and 1 level reserved for immunohistochemical staining for cytokeratin if the H&E sections are negative for metastasis.

In reporting the findings of the pathological examination of the sentinel node, the pathologist should identify the number of nodes recovered, the type of analysis (H&E staining with or without immunohistochemical staining), the number of nodes with metastasis, and the largest size of the metastasis within the sentinel lymph node. The size of the abnormality is measured and those patients who have only single cells or clusters of cells that measure less than 0.2 mm in size are classified as node negative based on the current AJCC staging system for breast cancer. This type of standardized reporting of the pathologic findings in the sentinel nodes allows clinicians to stage patients accurately and to make treatment decisions based on the number and size of metastases identified.

Intraoperative examination of the sentinel nodes can be performed with touch imprint cytology or frozen-section examination. Our group has preferred the use of touch imprint cytology since this preserves the lymph node tissue for a more detailed assessment with H&E staining or immunohistochemical staining at a later time.[16] Processing of the node for frozen-section examination does eliminate a significant portion of the nodal tissue, since sectioning with the cryostat will cut away portions of the node to produce an appropriate sample for pathologic interpretation. Either technique may provide information to the surgeon allowing for a 1-stage surgical procedure based on the intraoperative findings. One danger of proceeding with completion axillary node dissection based on touch imprint cytology is that small areas of disease within the node may not translate into a pathologic size greater than 0.2 mm on final examination. Both techniques are unlikely to identify micrometastasis at the time of surgery. This shortcoming requires that patients return to the operating room at a second surgery for completion axillary lymph node dissection should the sentinel node prove to be positive. Newer techniques that are being assessed include polymerase chain reaction (PCR) and rapid immunostaining with frozen-section examination. The drawback of PCR technology is that this allows the identification of a signal for the presence of a specific molecular marker (cytokeratin, MUC-1) in the sentinel node, but does not give a histologic assessment of the size of the nodal metastasis. In addition, there are a number of false positives that could result in overstaging the patients. The technique of intraoperative evaluation with rapid immunostaining may be more useful to surgeons, since this provides a sensitive technique in addition to a histologic assessment of the size and number of nodal metastases.

Results of Sentinel Lymph Node Trials

There have now been a number of single-institution reports of sentinel lymph node surgery with patient numbers ranging from 174 to over 500. The sentinel lymph node identification rate ranges from as low as 66% in the initial series reported by Giuliano to as high as 99% in the Italian report from Veronesi and colleagues.[2,17] The false-negative rate ranges from as low as 0.5% to as high as 13%. The Department of Defense (DOD) breast lymphatic mapping study demonstrated that after a learning curve of 20 to 25 cases, surgeons who abandoned the use of completion of axillary lymph node dissection had an identification rate of over 97%, with a nodal failure rate under 5% at last follow-up.[8]

The single-institution reports and registries have by and large reported the identification rates greater than 90% and false-negative rates below 5%. The first multicenter trial published by Krag and colleagues revealed a false-negative rate of 11% with an identification rate of 90%.[18] Although the surgeons participating in this multicenter trial were all experienced breast surgeons, the false-negative rate was higher than that reported to be an acceptable rate for abandoning axillary lymph node dissection. The large randomized trials initiated in the United States, the UK, and Europe were not published until recently, and yet sentinel lymph node surgery was incorporated as standard practice throughout much of the United States despite the high false-negative rate reported in the first multicenter trial.

MULTICENTER TRIALS

The first published trial of a randomized comparison between sentinel node biopsy and standard axillary dissection was published by Veronesi and colleagues in 2003.[17] This group randomized 516 patients with tumors less than 2 cm in size to undergo sentinel biopsy with immediate axillary dissection versus sentinel node biopsy alone. In the sentinel node biopsy alone group, patients who proved to have a positive sentinel node were subjected to axillary lymph node dissection. At a median follow-up time of 46 months, there were no axillary recurrences reported and the sentinel node alone group had less pain and lower morbidity.

The National Surgical Adjuvant Breast and Bowel Project (NSABP) B32 trial was initiated in 1999 and was designed to assess the use of sentinel lymph node biopsy alone compared with sentinel node biopsy with axillary dissection in patients with a clinically negative axilla (Figure 1). Clinical stage I and stage II patients, including those undergoing mastectomy and those undergoing breast-conserving surgery, were eligible for the trial. Patients randomized to the sentinel lymph node biopsy alone group had axillary dissection only if the sentinel node was found to be positive on pathological examination. Pathologically negative sentinel nodes were subjected to immunohistochemical staining, and patients were followed without any specific axillary surgery. Investigators from the NSABP have recently presented their work, demonstrating the ability of surgeons to identify a sentinel lymph node at surgery was 97.2% with an average of 2.9 sentinel nodes recovered.[19] Overall, the sentinel node was positive in 26% of patients and was the only positive node in 61.5% of the patients. The false-negative rate was 9.7% with an equal number of false-negative events in the patients with T1, T2, and T3

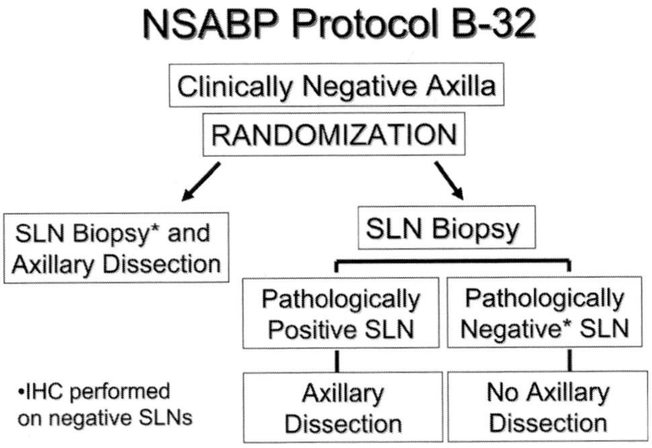

Figure 1

tumors. The identification rate was higher in women under age 50, and the false-negative rate was lower amongst patients less than age 50, although this difference was not statistically significant. There was a higher rate of false-negative events in those patients who had undergone an incisional or excisional biopsy prior to the sentinel node surgery. The false-negative rate was affected by biopsy type, but the false-negative rate did not significantly improve with surgeon experience.

The UK ALMANAC trial was similar in design to the NSABP B32 trial, but patients were randomized to undergo sentinel node biopsy alone versus conventional axillary surgery.[20] In total there were 1,139 patients with T1 to T3 tumors enrolled in this trial, and the investigators reported a failed localization in only 2% of the patients and a nodal positivity rate of 24%. Based on an intention to treat analysis, the sensory changes reported in the group undergoing standard axillary surgery was 47.7% at 1 month and had decreased to 30.3% by 12 months of follow-up. In the sentinel node alone group, the sensory loss was 14.7% at 1 month and dropped to 9.4% at 12 months of follow-up. In addition, the investigators reported that arm swelling was significantly reduced in the group undergoing sentinel node biopsy alone. The investigators concluded that hospital bed stay, drain usage, and infection were significantly less in the sentinel node biopsy alone group.

The American College of Surgeons Oncology Group (ACOSOG) initiated a phase II study of sentinel lymph node surgery in 1999 (Figure 2). This study was designed to evaluate the incidence of micrometastases in both the sentinel lymph nodes and the bone marrow biopsies of women with clinical T1 or T2 breast cancer undergoing breast-conserving surgery with sentinel lymph node biopsy. The trial completed accrual in 2003 with 5,539 patients. The incidence of H&E-positive sentinel nodes in this trial was 24%. The incidence of micrometastasis in the

ACOSOG Z0010

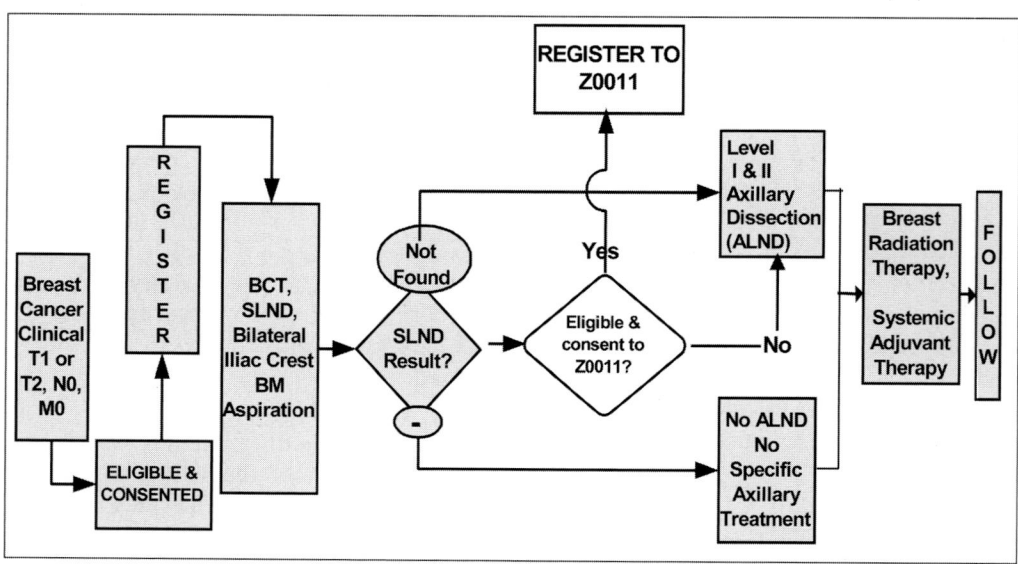

Figure 2

sentinel nodes and bone marrow has not yet been reported. ACOSOG investigators have reported the results of surgical complications related to sentinel lymph node surgery and evaluated both the 30-day morbidity and 6-month morbidity related to this procedure.[21] Overall, the rate of allergic reactions from use of the blue dye was reported at 0.1%. Approximately 3% of the patients suffered hematomas and 0.3% required reoperation. There was a 1.4% incidence of infections, and a small fraction of these patients required hospitalization for treatment of the infection. Approximately 7% of the patients had seroma formation that was reported to be clinically evident by the patient or physician. Overall, about 3% of the patients required placement of a drain or other intervention for the seroma. The morbidities reported at 6 months included range of motion abnormalities, paresthesias in the upper extremity, and the incidence of lymphedema. Lymphedema was defined as a change in arm measurement of 2 cm or greater in the ipsilateral arm, as compared with the pretreatment measurement, and the contralateral upper extremity. Range-of-motion abnormalities were reported to occur in 5% of the patients; however, these had all resolved at 6 months. Paresthesias were evident in 15% of the patients, and these had improved at 6 months of follow-up. Surprisingly, the incidence of lymphedema as documented by arm measurements was 7%. In contrast to the other surgical morbidities that were patient reported, the lymphedema rates were based on arm measurements by the physician or research assistant. This reported

incidence of lymphedema was certainly a surprise to the surgical community; however, it is not clear that this change as documented by arm measurements is clinically significant. It is also unclear how many of the patients required any specific intervention or management for this lymphedema. The risk factors of development of lymphedema in the ACOSOG Z0010 trial were increasing age and increasing body mass index.

The ACOSOG Z0011 trial was initiated in May 1999 as a companion trial to the Z0010 phase II trial. The Z0011 trial was a randomized phase III trial designed to evaluate the need for completion axillary lymph node dissection in women with a positive sentinel node (Figure 3). The Z0011 trial was designed to accrue 1,900 patients to determine whether there was a difference in survival between women who were treated with sentinel lymph node surgery alone versus those who

ACOSOG Z0011

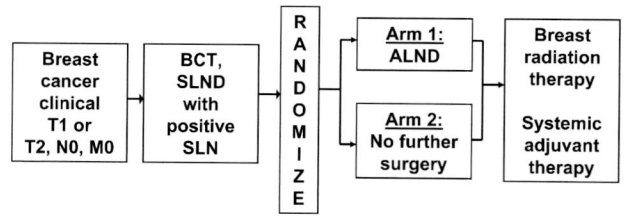

Figure 3

had sentinel lymph node surgery followed by completion axillary lymph node dissection for a positive sentinel node. Unfortunately, the trial was closed early, in December 2004, because of slow patient accrual. The total number of patients accrued was approximately 900. The ACOSOG investigators plan to continue follow-up of these patients, and do intend to assess the differences in locoregional failure rates and survival rates amongst the 2 groups with longer follow-up. Lucci and colleagues reported on the surgical complications between the study groups in Z0011 for short-term surgical complications.[22] There was a difference between the study groups with respect to paresthesias, with more paresthesias reported in the patients undergoing completion axillary lymph node dissection. Interestingly, there was no difference in lymphedema based on the arm measurements between the 2 study groups. Because this initial report was based on 6-month follow-up data, it will be interesting to see if the differences in lymphedema rates between the 2 study groups emerge with longer follow-up.

Although the follow-up times in the cooperative group trials is too short to definitively evaluate locoregional control, the early reports have suggested that the locoregional failure rates are very low in the sentinel node alone study groups. Posther and colleagues reported a 0.3% rate of axillary failures in the Z0010 trial in both the patients with negative sentinel lymph nodes and the patients who had positive sentinel lymph nodes.[10] This low rate of locoregional failures is consistent with single-institution reports that are now being published, demonstrating overall low failure rates following sentinel lymph node surgery for early-stage breast cancer.

The Role of Completion Axillary Dissection in Sentinel Node-Positive Patients

In the cooperative group trials, the incidence of positive sentinel lymph nodes in clinical stage I and stage II breast cancer patients has consistently ranged between 24 and 28%. This nodal positivity rate is based on standard H&E staining. Clearly the incidence of micrometastases may increase as the reports emerge detailing the results of immunohistochemical studies performed on the sentinel lymph nodes. As is true with many of the single-institution reports, the cooperative group trials have demonstrated that the sentinel lymph node is the only positive lymph node in over 60% of these early-stage breast cancer patients. These results, and those of single institutions, have fueled the controversy regarding the need for completion axillary lymph node dissection in all sentinel node-positive patients. Single-institution studies

have identified clinicopathologic factors predicting the presence and/or absence of nonsentinel axillary node metastases for the purpose of promoting a more selective approach to completion dissection. The factors that have been most frequently reported to predict nonsentinel node involvement include primary tumor size, lymphovascular invasion in the primary tumor, the size of the metastasis in the sentinel node, and the method of detection of the sentinel node metastasis.[23–25] Investigators at the Memorial Sloan-Kettering Cancer Center have developed a nomogram that is available on the World Wide Web <www.mskcc.org/nomograms/breastcancer> that estimates the likelihood that a patient with a positive sentinel lymph node will harbor additional disease within the axilla.[26] This nomogram is based on patient, primary tumor and sentinel node-related factors (number of nodes removed and/or involved and extent of tumor burden in the nodes). While the nomogram may help guide patients and physicians regarding the likelihood of additional positive nodes in the axilla, the standard of practice remains that patients with a positive sentinel node should have a completion level I and level II axillary lymph node dissection. The ACOSOG Z0011 trial was designed to answer this question, but, unfortunately, that trial had very slow accrual and therefore will not provide us with the information on survival and recurrence rates for another 5 years. Once again, we resort to the reports of single institutions, where in some cases surgeons have elected to observe patients with a positive sentinel node rather than subject them to the morbidity of a completion axillary lymph node dissection. At M. D. Anderson, we have recently reported our experience with this patient population and demonstrated that the axillary failure rates are less than 1% in women with a positive sentinel lymph node who do not undergo completion axillary lymph node dissection.[27] This is a highly selected group of patients with largely estrogen receptor-positive tumors that were felt to have a low likelihood for harboring additional axillary disease based on the clinician evaluation. At 24 months of follow-up, there have been no axillary recurrences in this group of patients; however, there have been failures in the supraclavicular and infraclavicular nodal basins.

Sentinel Lymph Node Surgery in Special Populations

DUCTAL CARCINOMA IN SITU

The use of sentinel lymph node surgery in patients with ductal carcinoma in situ remains controversial. The history of lymph node surgery in this subgroup of patients suggests that less than 2% of patients with the diagnosis of ductal carcinoma in situ will have node-positive disease. Some groups have suggested that sentinel lymph node surgery is simple and has minimal morbidity, and therefore should be incorporated in the surgical management of all these patients. As we know from the emerging reports from the cooperative group studies, the morbidity rate is low with sentinel lymph node surgery, but it is certainly not zero. This behooves us then to understand which subgroups of patients would potentially benefit from sentinel lymph node surgery at the time of surgical management for ductal carcinoma in situ. The published literature on sentinel lymph surgery in ductal carcinoma in situ has demonstrated a node-positive rate of 0% to as high as 17%. The definition of a positive node within these studies has not always been clearly defined. In some cases, cytokeratin-positive cells within the lymph nodes are considered as positive nodes, and therefore this increases the overall node-positive rate within this patient population. Several studies have demonstrated that it is the patient with large (> 3–4 cm), high-grade tumors who are most likely to harbor microinvasion within the primary tumor, and therefore would most likely benefit from sentinel lymph node surgery. At M. D. Anderson, it has been our practice to perform sentinel lymph node surgery in the setting of total mastectomy for patients with ductal carcinoma in situ.[28] With the increasing use of stereotactic needle core biopsy, we have found that approximately 20 to 25% of patients with a diagnosis of ductal carcinoma in situ will prove to have invasive disease on final pathology of the resected specimen. We have therefore incorporated the use of sentinel lymph node surgery in the setting of total mastectomy, particularly for those patients who have been diagnosed with a stereotactic needle core biopsy. In addition, if an occult focus of carcinoma is found on final pathologic examination after mastectomy, it is not possible for the surgeon to go back and perform a lymphatic mapping procedure. In this instance, only a complete level I and level II axillary lymph node dissection would be possible. Therefore, the patients with a diagnosis of ductal carcinoma in situ who are considered for sentinel lymph node surgery are those undergoing a total mastectomy; those with large tumors (> 3 cm in size), high-grade tumors; and those with findings on pathology that are suspicious for microinvasion.

SENTINEL LYMPH NODE SURGERY AFTER PREOPERATIVE CHEMOTHERAPY

The use of preoperative chemotherapy has evolved from standard practice in patients with locally advanced breast cancer to use in patients with large primary tumors and operable breast cancer. Preoperative chemotherapy has been demonstrated to increase the rates of breast-conserving surgery in women with locally advanced breast cancer, and operable breast cancer, without a significant increase in local failure rates in selected patients. The use of axillary lymph node dissection has been standard practice at the time of breast surgery for patients treated with preoperative chemotherapy. As more patients with operable breast cancer are treated in this fashion, there is a higher percentage of patients who have clinically node-negative disease at presentation and at the time of surgical treatment. The question remains as to whether sentinel lymph node surgery is an appropriate tool in this patient population, and this has been a point of debate amongst clinicians. Some groups have favored performing sentinel lymph node surgery prior to initiating chemotherapy in order to define the lymph node status in these patients. Experience with preoperative chemotherapy at M. D. Anderson has shown that at least 25% of patients who have clinically node-positive disease will be converted to node-negative disease with the chemotherapy treatment. This has led us to incorporate sentinel lymph node surgery into the surgical management of patients following preoperative chemotherapy to define any residual disease after their chemotherapy has been completed.

In our initial experience with sentinel lymph node surgery after preoperative chemotherapy, we reported an identification rate of approximately 88% with a false-negative rate of 12%.[29] This experience paralleled that of the reported experience of Giuliano and colleagues with their initial learning curve in sentinel lymph node surgery.[2] Similar to Dr. Giuliano, we found that, with increasing experience with sentinel lymph node surgery, our identification rate improved, and the false-negative rate decreased. We also noted that there were technical differences in this patient population compared with those patients who present with early-stage disease. Specifically, there is more likely to be fibrosis within the treated breast and within the axilla, and this contributes to poor uptake of the mapping agents and a more challenging search for the sentinel node within the axillary basin. As we have gained experience with sentinel lymph node surgery in this patient population, we now have an identification rate of > 95%, and a false-negative rate of < 8%. We have incorporated sentinel lymph node surgery as a standard in patients who present with clinically node-negative disease, who remain clinically node negative following chemotherapy. In patients who present with clinically node-positive disease that is documented by fine-needle aspiration biopsy, we continue to investigate the use of sentinel lymph node surgery, and are performing axillary lymph node dissection with sentinel lymph node surgery at the time of their primary surgical management.

The largest published experience with sentinel lymph node surgery following chemotherapy was recently reported by the NSABP investigators as a part of the B27 trial.[30] Similar to the M. D. Anderson experience, these investigators reported a lower identification rate in this group of patients than what is typically reported for those with early-stage breast cancer. The false-negative rate in this study was reported to be 11%. Subsequently, there has been a meta-analysis performed of all the published literature on sentinel lymph node surgery after chemotherapy.[31] This meta-analysis demonstrated that the identification rate is 91% and the false-negative rate is < 10%. This experience parallels that of sentinel lymph node surgery for early-stage breast cancer, and therefore it has been suggested that sentinel lymph node surgery is feasible and accurate following chemotherapy. As noted above, the technical aspects of sentinel lymph node surgery following chemotherapy are different from those patients undergoing primary surgery. It is therefore important that each surgeon gains experience in this patient population in the setting of sentinel lymph node surgery with completion axillary lymph node dissection before abandoning axillary lymph node dissection as a standard.

SENTINEL LYMPH NODE BIOPSY IN PATIENTS UNDERGOING BILATERAL PROPHYLACTIC MASTECTOMY OR CONTRALATERAL PROPHYLACTIC MASTECTOMY

Prophylactic mastectomy has been utilized for many years in patients at high risk of developing breast cancer (family history, BRCA1 and BRCA2 mutation carriers, proliferative breast disease) and for those women with a diagnosis of an ipsilateral breast cancer who want to prevent development of cancer in the contralateral breast. In the past, nodal surgery was not routinely performed for these patients since this would have involved an axillary lymph node dissection, which carries a significant risk of development of lymphedema and other complications. With the introduction of sentinel lymph node biopsy, some investigators have incorporated this procedure into the standard surgical management of high-risk patients. Since the incidence of finding an occult cancer in these patients is generally less than 5%, with many of these being in situ carcinomas, we have not routinely advocated the use of sentinel node biopsy in these patients.[32] Boughey and colleagues did identify that older women and those with lobular cancer or LCIS were at higher risk for harboring occult disease, and therefore could be considered for sentinel node surgery at the time of prophylactic mastectomy.[33] Boughey and colleagues also created a decision-analytic model to compare strategies in patients undergoing prophylactic mastectomy. They considered the number of sentinel lymph node biopsies performed per breast cancer detected, the number of sentinel node biopsies attempted to avoid 1 axillary node dissection in a node-negative patient with occult cancer, and the number of axillary complications for each strategy.[34] They concluded that the routine use of sentinel lymph node surgery was not warranted in patients undergoing prophylactic mastectomy, considering the number of procedures required to benefit 1 patient and the potential for complications associated with performing sentinel node surgery in all patients.

SENTINEL LYMPH NODE BIOPSY IN PATIENTS WITH RECURRENCE AFTER PREVIOUS BREAST-CONSERVATION THERAPY

Over the past 2 decades, an increasing number of patients have been diagnosed with early-stage breast cancer allowing for breast preservation to be offered in the majority of patients. Although ipsilateral breast recurrence rates remain relatively low when postoperative breast irradiation is routinely employed, many studies have reported an in-breast failure rate of approximately 10% at 10 years of follow-up. The need for nodal evaluation in patients with recurrence following breast-conserving therapy has not been clearly defined. A number of investigators have begun to explore the use of sentinel node biopsy as a tool for assessing regional lymph node involvement in these patients. The successful identification of a sentinel node in patients with recurrent breast cancer may vary depending on the prior use of radiation therapy and the extent of breast and axillary surgery utilized for treatment of the initial tumor. Port and colleagues at the Memorial Sloan-Kettering Cancer Center reported success in identifying the SLN in 75% of patients who had undergone previous surgery.[35] They reported an 87% success rate in patients with fewer than 10 lymph nodes removed at their initial surgery, and a 44% success rate if greater than 10 lymph nodes had been removed at initial surgery. In our experience with repeat breast and axillary surgery for patients with recurrent breast cancer, we have shown that lymphatic mapping can identify the sentinel node in 65% of patients with ipsilateral breast tumor recurrence following breast-conserving surgery, and 50% of patients with recurrence after mastectomy.[36] In patients who have undergone previous axillary dissection, the sentinel node is more likely to be in an extra-axillary location, and, therefore, preoperative lymphoscintigraphy should be utilized to guide the operative approach. In our series, only 1 patient had a pathologically positive sentinel node and she underwent completion axillary node dissection. The use of sentinel node surgery in patients with recurrent breast cancer appears to be feasible regardless of prior breast or axillary treatment. Lymphoscintigraphy should be considered as an aide to guide the surgical intervention.

SENTINEL LYMPH NODE BIOPSY IN MALE PATIENTS

Male breast cancer accounts for less than 1% of all breast cancer diagnoses in the United States. Because male breast cancer is a rare disease, it is difficult to enrol patients in clinical trials or to develop clinical pathways and guidelines. In general, male patients are treated in a fashion similar to women, although the use of breast-conserving surgery has not been championed in men. Axillary lymph node dissection has long been the standard practice for nodal evaluation in men; however, several studies have been published describing the use of sentinel lymph node surgery in the surgical management of men presenting with clinically node-negative breast cancer.[37–40] These investigators all found that sentinel node surgery was both feasibile and accurate in clinically node-negative male breast cancer patients. We recently compared our experience with sentinel node surgery in male breast cancer patients with our larger experience of sentinel node surgery in women.[41] Over a 6-year time interval we treated 30 men and 2,784 women with sentinel node dissection as part of their surgical management for breast cancer. Males presented at a significantly older age and had larger tumors than their female counterparts. We were able to identify a sentinel node in 100% of males and in 98.3% of females during the study period. The incidence of positive sentinel nodes was higher in men (37.0% vs 22.3%), and in patients with a positive sentinel node, there were additional nonsentinel nodes that were positive in 62.5% of males, compared with 20.7% in females. Male patients had a higher nodal tumor burden reflected in a larger size of nodal metastasis (median size of the largest lymph node metastasis was 10 mm in males and 3 mm in females) and increased risk of harboring additional disease in axillary lymph nodes when the sentinel node was positive. Because of the higher incidence of node-positive disease in men, intraoperative evaluation of the sentinel nodes with frozen-section or touch prep examination is prudent, since they tend to have larger metastases and

these are more likely to be identified with intraoperative assessment. Completion axillary node dissection can then be performed at the same surgery for those patients with a positive sentinel node.

EXTRA-AXILLARY SENTINEL LYMPH NODES

With the increasing use of lymphoscintigraphy in the conduct of sentinel lymph node surgery, the identification of extra-axillary sentinel lymph nodes has become a clinical issue. The most common site of extra-axillary drainage is the internal mammary lymph node basin. Additional sites of drainage are the infraclavicular lymph nodes and the supraclavicular lymph nodes. As noted above in the technical section, the visualization of extra-axillary lymph nodes is most likely to occur when a peritumoral or subtumoral injection technique is utilized. It is rare to see extra-axillary drainage in patients who had an intradermal or subdermal injection technique. Although the need for exploration of these extra-axillary sites of drainage has been questioned, many investigators have begun to routinely biopsy extra-axillary sentinel nodes at the time of the lymphatic mapping procedure. The most recent revision of the AJCC staging system for breast cancer has incorporated internal mammary lymph nodes that are identified on sentinel lymph node biopsy as a component of the lymph node staging. Historically, biopsy of the internal mammary lymph nodes has not been demonstrated to improve the outcome of patients undergoing surgical treatment for breast cancer; however, this was in the setting of radical mastectomy for all patients, regardless of tumor location or lymphatic drainage patterns. Now, with the use of lymphoscintigraphy, and the identification of patients who truly have drainage to the basin, it is more likely to have a clinical impact on those individuals.

There are now several large reported series evaluating internal mammary sentinel lymph node biopsy in the clinical management of patients with early-stage breast cancer (reviewed in Kawase and colleagues[13]). The identification rate of the internal mammary sentinel nodes is typically lower than that reported for axillary sentinel lymph node biopsy, ranging from 60 to 80%. Determining the false-negative rate in this patient population is extremely difficult, since a completion dissection of the entire internal mammary lymph node basin would not typically be performed. The most significant complication reported with this technique has been pneumothorax. Investigators have reported a 10% rate of pneumothoraces; however, this is generally self-limiting as injury to the pleura causes the pneumothorax and there is generally no concomitant injury to the lung to lead to an ongoing air leak. Most importantly, biopsy of the internal mammary sentinel lymph nodes has demonstrated that there is upstaging in approximately 30% of the patients, and a change in the management of patients in approximately 35% of patients. This change in management includes both alteration in radiation fields and use of chemotherapy in patients who would not otherwise have been considered for systemic chemotherapy.

Summary

The introduction of lymphatic mapping and sentinel lymph node biopsy into the surgical management of patients with breast cancer has allowed for more accurate staging of the regional nodes, with a significant reduction in surgical morbidity. This reduced morbidity is realized in both the short-term complications of surgery, such as hematoma formation and infection, in addition to the more significant long-term morbidities of paresthesias and development of lymphedema. Although the question of a survival advantage with the use of axillary dissection remains unanswered, it is important that patients undergo completion axillary lymph node dissection as standard practice in the setting of a positive sentinel node. The use of sentinel lymph node biopsy in the management of patients treated with preoperative chemotherapy appears to be feasible and accurate once the surgeon and multidisciplinary team have gained experience with the technique in this special population. Biopsy of extra-axillary sentinel nodes should be considered in those patients who have dominant drainage to lymph node basins outside the axilla, and in whom a change in management would be expected, should these lymph nodes be positive on pathologic examination.

References

1. Krag DN, Weaver DL, Alex JC, Fairbank JT. Surgical resection and radiolocalization of the sentinel lymph node in breast cancer using a gamma probe. Surg Oncol 1993;2: 335–9.

2. Giuliano AE, Kirgan DM, Guenther JM, et al. Lymphatic mapping and sentinel lymphadenectomy for breast cancer. Ann Surg 1994;220:391–401.

3. McMasters KM, Tuttle TM, Carlson DJ, et al. Sentinel lymph node biopsy for breast cancer: a suitable alternative to routine axillary dissection in multi-institutional practice when optimal technique is used. J Clin Oncol 2000;18: 2560–6.

4. Cox CE, Bass SS, Boulware D, et al. Implementation of new surgical technology: outcome measures for lymphatic mapping of breast carcinoma. Ann Surg Oncol 1999;6: 553–61.

5. Institute for Clinical Systems Improvement Technology. Assessment Update TA#045. Lymphatic mapping with sentinel node biopsy for breast cancer. Institute for Clinical Systems Improvement (ICSI). Breast cancer treatment Bloomington (MN): Institute for Clinical Systems Improvement (ICSI); 2005. p. 57. available at www.guideline.gov.

6. Schwartz GF, Giuliano AE, Veronesi U, et al. Proceedings of the consensus conference on the role of sentinel lymph node biopsy in carcinoma of the breast; 2001 April 19–22; Philadelphia. Cancer 2002;94:2542–51.

7. American Society of Breast Surgeons Consensus Statement on Guidelines for Performance of Sentinel Lymphadenectomy for Breast Cancer. Available at: www.breastsurgeons.org (accessed October 16, 2006).

8. Shivers S, Cox C, Leight G, et al. Final results of the Department of Defense multicenter breast lymphatic mapping trial. Ann Surg Oncol 2002;9:248–55.

9. Cody HS, Hill AD, Tran KN, et al. Credentialing for breast lymphatic mapping: how many cases are enough? Ann Surg 1999;229:723–6.

10. Posther KE, McCall LM, Blumencranz PW, et al. Sentinel node skills verification and surgeon performance: data from a multicenter clinical trial for early-stage breast cancer. Ann Surg 2005;242:593–9.

11. Cox CE, Salud CJ, Cantor A, et al. Learning curves for breast cancer sentinel lymph node mapping based on surgical volume analysis. J Am Coll Surg 2001;193:593–600.

12. Galimberti V, Veronesi P, Arnone P, et al. Stage migration after biopsy of internal mammary chain lymph nodes in breast cancer patients. Ann Surg Oncol 2002;9:924–8.

13. Kawase K, Gayed IW, Hunt KK, et al. Use of lymphoscintigraphy defines lymphatic drainage patterns before sentinel lymph node biopsy for breast cancer. J Am Coll Surg 2006; 203:64–72.

14. Giuliano AE, Dale PS, Turner RR, et al. Improved axillary staging of breast cancer with sentinel lymphadenectomy. Ann Surg 1995;222:394–401.

15. Yared MA, Middleton LP, Smith TL, et al. Recommendations for sentinel lymph node processing in breast cancer. Am J Surg Pathol 2002;26:377–82.

16. Lee A, Krishnamurthy S, Sahin A, et al. Intraoperative touch imprint of sentinel lymph nodes in breast carcinoma patients. Cancer 2002;96:225–31.

17. Veronesi U, Paganelli G, Viale G, et al. A randomized comparison of sentinel-node biopsy with routine axillary dissection in breast cancer. N Engl J Med 2003;349:546–53.

18. Krag D, Weaver D, Ashikaga T, et al. The sentinel node in breast cancer—a multicenter validation study. N Engl J Med 1998;339:941–6.

19. Harlow SP, Krag DN, Julian TB, et al. Prerandomization Surgical Training for the National Surgical Adjuvant Breast and Bowel Project (NSABP) B-32 trial: a randomized phase III clinical trial to compare sentinel node resection to conventional axillary dissection in clinically node-negative breast cancer. Ann Surg 2005;241:48–54.

20. Mansel RE, Fallowfield L, Kissin M, et al. Randomized multicenter trial of sentinel node biopsy versus standard axillary treatment in operable breast cancer: the ALMANAC Trial. J Natl Cancer Inst 2006;98:599–609.

21. Wilke LG, McCall LM, Posther KE, et al. Surgical complications associated with sentinel lymph node biopsy: tesults from a prospective international cooperative group trial. Ann Surg Oncol 2006;13:491–500.

22. Lucci A, Mackie L, Beitsch P, et al. Surgical complications associated with sentinel lymph node dissection (SLND) plus axillary lymph node dissection, versus SLND alone in the American College of Surgeons Oncology Group (ACOSOG) Trial Z0011. Society of Surgical Oncology 59th Annual Meeting, 2006 Mar 23–26; San Diego, CA. Ann Surg Oncol 2006;13:9.

23. Hwang RF, Krishnamurthy S, Hunt KK, et al. Clinicopathologic factors predicting involvement of non-sentinel axillary nodes in women with breast cancer. Ann Surg Oncol 2003;10:248–54.

24. Degnim AC, Griffith KA, Sabel MS, et al. Clinicopathologic features of metastasis in nonsentinel lymph nodes of breast carcinoma patients. Cancer 2003;98:2307–15.

25. Wong SL, Edwards MJ, Chao C, et al. Predicting the status of the nonsentinel axillary nodes: a multicenter study. Arch Surg 2001;136:563–8.

26. Van Zee KJ, Manasseh DM, Bevilacqua JL, et al. A nomogram for predicting the likelihood of additional nodal metastases in breast cancer patients with a positive sentinel node biopsy. Ann Surg Oncol 2003;10:1140–51.

27. Hwang RF, Gonzalez-Angulo AM, Yi M, et al. Low local-regional failure rates in selected breast cancer patients with tumor-positive sentinel nodes who do not undergo completion axillary dissection. 28th San Antonio Breast Cancer Symposium, 2005 Dec 7–11; San Antonio, TX. Breast Cancer Res Treat 2005;94 Suppl 1:402.

28. Yen TW, Hunt KK, Ross MI, et al. Predictors of invasive breast cancer in patients with an initial diagnosis of ductal carcinoma in situ: a guide to the selective use of sentinel lymph node biopsy in the management of ductal carcinoma in situ. J Am Coll Surg 2005;200:516–26.

29. Breslin TM, Cohen L, Sahin A, et al. Sentinel lymph node biopsy is accurate after neoadjuvant chemotherapy for breast cancer. J Clin Oncol 2000;18:3480–6.

30. Mamounas EP, Brown A, Anderson S, et al. Sentinel node biopsy after neoadjuvant chemotherapy in breast cancer: results from National Surgical Adjuvant Breast and Bowel Project Protocol B-27. J Clin Oncol 2005;23:2694–702.

31. Xing Y, Foy M, Cox DD, et al. Meta-analysis of sentinel lymph node biopsy after preoperative chemotherapy in patients with breast cancer. Br J Surg 2006;93:539–46.

32. Goldflam K, Hunt KK, Gershenwald JE, et al. Contralateral prophylactic mastectomy: predictors of significant histologic findings. Cancer 2004;101:1977–86.

33. Boughey JC, Khakpour N, Meric-Bernstam F, et al. Selective use of sentinel lymph node surgery during prophylactic mastectomy. Cancer 2006;107:1440–7.

34. Boughey JC, Cormier JN, Xing Y, et al. Routine sentinel lymphadenectomy in patients undergoing prophylactic mastectomy is not warranted. J Clin Oncol, [Submitted].

35. Port ER, Fey J, Gemignani ML, et al. Reoperative sentinel lymph node biopsy: a new option for patients with primary or locally recurrent breast carcinoma. J Am Coll Surg 2002;195:167–72.

36. Boughey JC, Ross MI, Babiera GV, et al. Sentinel lymph node surgery in locally recurrent breast cancer. Clin Breast Cancer 2006;7:248–53.

37. Albo D, Ames FC, Hunt KK, et al. Evaluation of lymph node status in male breast cancer patients: a role for sentinel lymph node biopsy. Breast Cancer Res Treat 2003;77:9–14.

38. Port ER, Fey JV, Cody HS III, Borgen PI. Sentinel lymph node biopsy in patients with male breast carcinoma. Cancer 2001;91:319–23.

39. Hill AD, Borgen PI, Cody HS III. Sentinel node biopsy in male breast cancer. Eur J Surg Oncol 1999;25:442–3.

40. Cimmino VM, Degnim AC, Sabel MS, et al. Efficacy of sentinel lymph node biopsy in male breast cancer. J Surg Oncol 2004;86:74–7.

41. Boughey JC, Bedrosian I, Meric-Bernstam F, et al. Comparative analysis of sentinel lymph node surgery in male and female breast cancer patients. J Am Coll Surg 2006;203:475–80.

CHAPTER 56

REGIONAL LYMPHADENECTOMY FOR BREAST CANCER: INDICATIONS, EXTENT, AND MORBIDITY

JACKIE JERUSS, MD

MERRICK I. ROSS, MD

Introduction

Recent discoveries in the laboratory have lead to tremendous advances in the understanding of breast cancer biology and prognosis. Nevertheless, lymph node involvement remains the most important clinicopathologic prognostic marker for breast cancer patient outcomes. The significance of nodal involvement stems from the prognostic correlation of regional lymph node involvement with systemic disease, the potential morbidity of untreated nodal disease, and the controversial concept that nodal involvement may facilitate the distant spread of breast cancer.[1] For these reasons, surgeons have been advocating for the removal of regional nodal metastases for more than a century. As our understanding of the natural history of breast cancer has progressed, the radical extent of the nodal resection necessary to benefit patients has been modified. Some ideas that were recently considered arcane are now being revisited, in part as a result of the recent changes in the staging criteria for regional node involvement adopted by the American Joint Commission on Cancer (AJCC). As new information and surgical techniques become available, the indications and the extent of surgical resection for regional nodal disease will continue to evolve.

Over the last several decades there has been a paradigm shift in oncologic surgical therapy from radical resection to increasing levels of tissue preservation. The objective of this approach has been to provide patients with optimal surgical treatment while simultaneously decreasing surgical morbidity. Breast cancer surgery has directly reflected this change in management, as the standard of care for this disease has evolved from the Halstedian radical mastectomy to breast conservation for the majority of patients. This transition has been based on accumulating evidence from large clinical trials, which have established that less radical surgery is safe and effective.[2–4] The introduction of sentinel node biopsy (SNB) into the armamentarium of breast cancer care marks the further progression in our understanding of this disease, and has again permitted a less extensive and less invasive surgical option for many breast cancer patients.[5,6] Although this surgical approach may ultimately prove to be more utilitarian for the management of patients with early-stage breast cancer, the use of SNB as a definitive procedure for the staging and regional control of disease is currently the subject of ongoing studies. In addition, the growing use of neoadjuvant therapy has begun to impact patients with locally advanced disease, who through response to treatment may become eligible for SNB in the place of an axillary dissection. Treatment with neoadjuvant therapy has been associated with a decrease in the incidence of axillary node positivity, as shown by the National Surgical Adjuvant Breast and Bowel Project (NSABP) B-18 trial.[7] The need for completion axillary dissection after SNB, in patients treated with neoadjuvant therapy, is being actively investigated. Nevertheless, subsets of patients presenting with locally advanced disease, particularly those patients who do not respond to neoadjuvant therapy, will benefit from more extensive surgical interventions, such as formal regional lymphadenectomy. Although the survival impact of local disease control may not be significant, the benefits of local control in decreasing the morbidity of bulky nodal disease are definitive.

Typically, regional spread of breast cancer involves the axillary nodal group and the internal mammary nodal chain, and the supraclavicular fossa can also be the sole or additional sites of regional metastases. The pattern of nodal spread is thought to be determined, to some extent, by tumor location. The AJCC staging of nodal disease involving both the internal mammary nodes and the supraclavicular fossa has evolved to reflect a dynamic understanding of the prognostic significance of disease that has spread to these regional locations. Additionally, the use of lymphoscintigraphy, which has become standard in many centers where SNB is performed, has elucidated aberrant lymphatic drainage patterns that would not have been known prior to the era of SNB. This additional preoperative knowledge of tumor drainage patterns has led many surgeons to consider the need for treating the internal mammary chain and supraclavicular regions, based on concerns regarding the patient-specific sentinel lymphatic drainage from the primary tumor. As more surgeons use lymphoscintigraphy to guide the dissection of sentinel nodes in areas of regional nodal spread, the added information gained from this procedure will further contribute to our understanding of the impact of nodal metastases on breast cancer morbidity and prognosis.

The combination of earlier breast cancer diagnosis and, therefore, a higher incidence of node-negative patients, and the global acceptance of SNB as an alternative to axillary dissection has resulted in the quick dilution in the experience with anatomically based formal node dissections. However, patients will still on occasion present with or develop regionally advanced disease in one or more nodal basins, requiring valuable surgical expertise to accomplish durable regional disease control as well as surgery with curative intent. The following discussion will focus on indications for, technical approaches to, and associated morbidity of the major regional lymphadenectomies.

Axillary Node Dissection

RATIONALE AND INDICATIONS

Disease-specific survival has been shown to directly correlate to axillary tumor burden. Crucial treatment decisions have traditionally been predicated on the extent of axillary nodal involvement. For this reason, the

surgical management of axillary nodal disease has been advocated for more than a century. A level I-II axillary dissection has been a standard of surgical care for breast cancer, with the inclusion of a dissection of the level III nodes if they are found to be clinically suspicious or proven to be involved by a prior percutaneous biopsy.[1] Although this surgery has been an important intervention to provide crucial staging information and regional control, it does not appear to confer a major survival benefit.[2] In the NSABP B-04 trial, 18.6% of clinically node-negative patients, who were managed with total mastectomy and axillary observation, developed palpable disease requiring axillary dissection.[2] Yet, axillary recurrence after axillary dissection is an uncommon event, occurring in only 0.5 to 3% of patients.[2,8] Recurrence after axillary dissection has been attributed to anatomic variation in the distribution of axillary nodal tissue, though may also be secondary to an inadequate surgical dissection.[8]

The number of dissected lymph nodes necessary for an axillary dissection to be considered an accurate representation of the patient's disease stage has been examined. In a study of 415 breast cancer patients undergoing a 5-node dissection followed by a concurrent axillary dissection, the 5-node biopsy provided a 97.3% sensitivity to identify lymph node metastases found in the entire axillary dissection.[9] However, Mathiesen and colleagues found that the rate of node positivity increased incrementally up until a total of 10 nodes were removed from the axilla.[10] Although a greater sensitivity for axillary disease detection has been correlated with more extensive surgery, axillary dissection has also been associated with morbid lymphedema, pain, seroma formation, poorer cosmesis, and infection.

The significance of axillary node dissection to guide therapeutic decision making has changed in recent years. Because most patients with tumors greater than 1 cm currently receive some form of systemic therapy, the indication for a complete axillary dissection to define the need for systemic therapy has been called into question. A recent study looking at risk stratification based on patient age, sex, tumor size, hormone receptor status, nuclear grade, and the presence of lymphovascular invasion demonstrated that knowledge of nodal status was not imperative to the decision to administer adjuvant chemotherapy.[11] Thus, as increasing numbers of patients are diagnosed with early-stage disease localized to the breast, and treatment plans are more routinely made based on tumor factors, a complete analysis of the axilla for therapeutic decision making has become less critical.

Simultaneously, the advent of SNB has generated concern based on the potential for undertreatment and understaging of axillary disease, as axillary recurrence occurring within 2 years of axillary dissection has been associated with poor prognosis.[8] The incidence of additional axillary nodal disease, beyond the sentinel nodes, ranges from 34 to 40%.[12,13] The clinical implications of this additional nodal disease in the current era of aggressive systemic therapies have yet to be determined. The extent of nonsentinel nodal involvement has been shown to decrease with smaller primary tumors and decreased axillary SN tumor burden.[14] The role of axillary dissection for patients with microscopic involvement of the sentinel nodes is an area of active debate, though it continues to be the standard of care. The clear indication for axillary dissection remains for patients with palpable disease or disease identified on ultrasound and proven by needle aspiration to be metastatic who stand to benefit from the local control provided by a therapeutic node dissection. The utility of SNB in comparison with axillary dissection in clinically node-negative patients is the focus of the NSABP B-32 trial. Long-term follow-up results from this study and the American College of Surgeons Oncology Group Z0010 study will ultimately be necessary to reveal regional recurrence outcomes in a prospective randomized fashion in node-negative and node-positive patients.[15] Despite

SURGICAL PROCEDURE

The axillary contents are bounded by the axillary vein, the pectoralis musculature, the serrratus anterior muscle, the subscapularis muscle, and the latissimus dorsi muscle. Three levels of axillary nodes have been delineated, based on their anatomic relation to the pectoralis minor muscle. Level I axillary lymph nodes are located inferior or lateral to the pectoralis minor muscle, level II axillary nodes are located posterior to the pectoralis minor muscle, and level III nodes are found medial and superior to the pectoralis minor muscle. Additionally, lymph nodes of clinical significance, known as Rotter's interpectoral nodes, can sometimes be found between the pectoralis minor and major muscles. These lymph nodes may be the passageway for the rare "skip metastasis" found in the level III nodes, despite the level I and II nodes remaining cancer free.

The current surgical practice for axillary dissection has evolved significantly from a surgery that included the removal of several muscle groups bounding the axillary contents as well as the thoracodorsal vessels. Today, the standard axillary dissection involves removal of the level I and level II nodal groups. Positioning for the procedure is important. It is recommended that the intravenous line and anesthesia monitoring equipment be placed on the patient's nonoperative side. This way, the arm involved

in the axillary dissection can be prepped free into the field and easily manipulated should this be necessary. The axillary dissection is performed through an incision that spans from the lateral border of the pectoralis major muscle to the anterior border of the latissimus dorsi muscle. This incision should typically lie just inferior to the hair-bearing area of the axilla. Although some surgeons advocate the use of a curvilinear or lazy-S incision, a transverse incision can also be employed. Alternatively, if the patient is undergoing a total mastectomy, the axillary dissection can be carried out through the lateral-most aspect of the mastectomy incision.

Once the skin incision has been made, the subcutaneous tissue is dissected with the use of electrocautery, and superior and inferior skin flaps are raised. The dissection is taken superiorly to the axillary vein, medially to the juncture of the serratus anterior muscle and pectoralis minor muscle, laterally to the latissimus dorsi muscle, and posteriorly to the subscapularis muscle. The fascia over the latissimus dorsi muscle is incised throughout its length following along superiorly to the tendinous insertion of the muscle. It is at this level that the main intercostobrachial nerve will be identified and just superiorly the axillary vein. As the latissimis dorsi fascia is incised superiorly, an attempt should be made to preserve the intercostobrachial nerve, which spans the width of axilla. This small nerve provides sensation to the medial aspect of the arm and its sacrifice can be particularly bothersome to patients. Nevertheless, if the nerve is involved with bulky disease or precludes a safe and complete dissection, it can be taken. Superiorly, the axillary vein will be identified, avoiding dissection cephalad to the vein, unless obvious bulky disease is found there. The dissection of the vein should be carried medially until the medial pectoral neurovascular bundle is encountered. Branches of this neurovascular bundle that supply the axillary contents must be sacrificed, with care, to preserve the main branches that supply the pectoralis muscle group. Medially, the axillary contents are dissected free from the pectoralis major muscle until the pectoralis minor muscle is identified. At this point, the clavipectoral fascia is incised, and the nodal tissue underneath the pectoralis minor muscle is palpated. If bulky nodal disease is present, the fascia over the medial aspect of the pectoralis minor muscle is incised, permitting the transection of the pectoralis minor muscle from its insertion at the coracoid process.

This maneuver permits a better exposure of the level II and III axillary nodes. Exposure of these nodes can sometimes be enhanced by carefully raising the patient's arm superiorly. The level II axillary nodes are then dissected off the chest wall, from underneath the pectoralis major muscle, progressing from medial to lateral along the anterior boarder of the axillary vein. If palpable level III nodes are found at this point, they too should be included in the dissection. Care should be taken to identify small branches of the axillary vein and to directly ligate these branches. As the dissection continues laterally, the long thoracic nerve will be identified and should be spared and reflected onto the chest wall. The dissection of this nerve should continue inferiorly until the nerve is observed inserting into the seratus anterior muscle. Once the long thoracic nerve has been identified, it is not necessary to insult it by pinching stimulation, as this may only serve to induce injury or temporary neuropraxia. The dissection continues laterally along subscapularis, and if the deep subscapular nodes are found to be clinically suspicious, they too should be included in the dissection at this point. The thoracodorsal neurovascular bundle will then be identified and fascia overlying this structure should be incised. Any branches from this neurovascular bundle extending into the axillary specimen should be ligated and divided, taking care to keep the thoracodorsal nerve out of harm's way. Figure 1 is an intraoperative photograph of a completed axillary dissection illustrating the key anatomic landmarks and preserved structures.

At this point, the axillary nodal contents should be free from any crucial axillary structures and can be passed off the field for pathologic analysis. The wound should be irrigated and meticulous hemostasis achieved. A flexible drain should be placed through a separate incision, inferior but close to the axillary incision, as this drain site will likely be included in tangential radiation

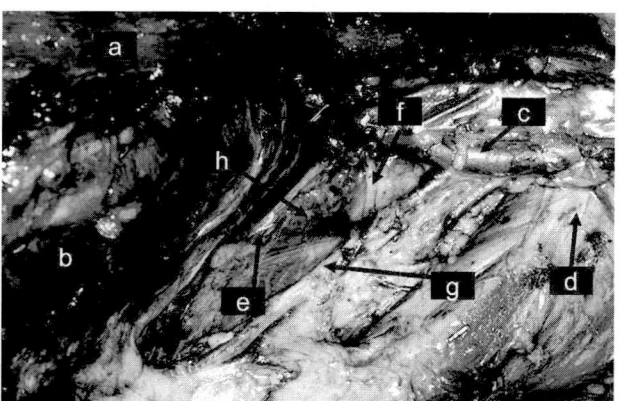

Figure 1 Intraoperative photograph of completed left axillary dissection. The anatomic boundaries and key structures preserved are identified as follows: (a) pectoralis minor muscle, (b) seratus anterior muscle, (c) axillary vein, (d) latissimis dorsi muscle with tendonous insertion exposed, (e) long thoracic nerve, (f) thoracodorsal nerve in a medial position prior to joining the neurovascular bundle proper (g), and (h) subscapularis muscle.

therapy fields, should adjuvant radiation therapy be necessary. The wound should then be closed with interrupted 3-0 Vicryl and running 4-0 PDS sutures.

MORBIDITY

There is a litany of morbidities associated with the axillary dissection procedure, primarily related to the dissection of the axillary nerves and vein. Infections and seroma also occur and tend to develop in the early postoperative period. Other well-known complications include injury to the long thoracic nerve resulting in a "winged scapula," and injury to the thoracodorsal nerve resulting in the compromise of arm adduction. A spectrum of neuropraxias including paresthesias, numbness secondary to sacrifice of the intercostobrachial nerve, and pain are also commonly reported. Some degree of arm and shoulder restriction may also occur, though this tends to be self-limiting. Lymphedematous swelling, which can affect the patient's arm, shoulder, breast, or chest wall can be severe. The pathophysiology of lymphedema is linked to the disruption in axillary lymphatic flow from the affected arm and chest, back toward the axillary vein. Long-standing lymphedema is particularly debilitating for patients, as it significantly limits the functionality of the affected limb and is also disfiguring. Furthermore, the development of lyphangiosarcoma in this setting is often fatal. As expected, patients who undergo SNB experience less associated morbidity.

Internal Mammary Sentinel Lymphadenectomy and Formal Node Dissection

RATIONALE AND INDICATIONS

Perspective on the incidence of internal mammary nodal metastases comes from a review of 7,000 patients who underwent pathologic analysis of both axillary and internal mammary nodes.[1,16] Of these patients, 50% were found to have axillary metastasis, 22% were found to have internal mammary nodal metastases, whereas 5% had isolated internal mammary nodal metastasis without axillary nodal metastasis.[1,16] In the past, dissection of the internal mammary nodes had been performed routinely as the standard therapy for breast cancer, as part of the extended radical mastectomy procedure. This procedure fell out of favor when it was shown through several studies, including prospective randomized trials comparing extended radial mastectomy with radical mastectomy, to confer no patient survival benefit.[17]

A prospective study, performed in the 1960s, did show that patients with central and medially located tumors were more likely to have internal mammary nodal disease, and that parasternal recurrence after resection of internal mammary disease decreased from 3.7 to 0.3%.[1] Overall, the 5-year survival rate for patients with internal mammary node disease is approximately 45%.[18,19] Studies performed from the late 1960s to the early 1980s established that patients with isolated internal mammary disease have outcomes similar to patients with isolated axillary disease.[19] Conversely, patients with simultaneous internal mammary and axillary nodal disease have a worse overall survival rate, when compared with those patients who present with isolated regional lymphatic spread. Consequently, the new AJCC staging system classifies patients with isolated internal mammary disease as N2b, but when internal mammary disease is found in conjunction with axillary disease, it is staged as N3b. When isolated internal mammary disease is detected by sentinel node biopsy, it is categorized as pN1b disease.[19]

With the advent of both sentinel node biopsy and lymphoscintigraphy, surgeons are now in a position to more accurately stage patients who map to alternative regional nodal basins. Using current technology, surgeons can detect smaller-volume internal mammary disease with sentinel node biopsy in those patients who are most likely to benefit from the procedure, sparing those patients who do not drain to the internal mammary chain the unnecessary morbidity of a surgical dissection. Accordingly, we may find that resection of smaller-volume internal mammary disease, guided by sentinel node biopsy, may result in further improved patient outcomes, based on the more precise evaluation of the sentinel nodes and appropriate adjuvant treatment planning. From the data available, an internal mammary node dissection is primarily indicated in patients presenting with isolated sentinel internal mammary disease, particularly if the surgical approach to the breast is a mastectomy. For those patients with isolated sentinel internal mammary disease who also have undergone a breast-conserving approach, breast radiation therapy will be necessary and, therefore, simultaneous internal mammary nodal irradiation can be used as an alternative to surgical resection. Patients who present with gross internal mammary node involvement or who relapse in this nodal group after definitive therapy may be candidates for a formal internal mammary dissection, particularly if no distant disease is identified and if gross disease remains after systemic therapy.

SURGICAL PROCEDURE

The internal mammary sentinel nodes are typically small and located deep in the intercostal space, often intimate to the sternum. Most commonly, lymphatic spread involves one or more of the first through the fourth interspaces for inner quadrant tumors. If the patient is undergoing a modified radical mastectomy at the time of the internal mammary dissection, the mastectomy incision can be used as access for the procedure. Alternatively, if the patient is undergoing breast conservation, a separate incision should be made over the area of maximum detected radioactivity, along the sternal border. This incision should be made in a horizontal fashion for approximately 2 cm in length. The pectoralis major muscle is mobilized and retracted medially; alternatively, the muscle can be divided along the length of its fibers. The intercostal muscles are then divided using electrocautery. Once identified, the internal mammary node is carefully dissected free from the underlying pleura. This can be facilitated with the use of a peanut dissector. After the node has been completely dissected, its vascular supply is controlled through the use of clips or ties. Once the nodal dissection is complete, the lungs are then insufflated to 40 mm Hg to check for evidence of pleural space violation. The dissected intercostal interspace is then irrigated, and meticulous hemostasis should be achieved. This should not be preformed with electrocautery, as the intercostal vessels are at risk of retraction into the chest if they are not directly controlled. The skin incision is then closed with interrupted 3-0 Vicryl and running 4-0 PDS sutures.

When gross disease is detected preoperatively at more than one interspace, a formal internal mammary lymphadenectomy may be performed. This dissection involves removal of the second, third, and fourth costal cartilages from the sternum (Figure 2). Once the costal cartilages are removed, the internal mammary vessels should be visible. The internal mammary vessels must be carefully ligated under the first rib, and then again when they are visualized at the fifth costal cartilage. This is done to ensure that the lymph nodes that span the first through fourth interspaces are safely removed with hemostatic control. Subsequently, the pleura is dissected away from the intercostal vessels and the costal cartilages are divided at the sternal junction, and then again approximately 2 finger breaths laterally. The divided segment of the costal cartilage is then retraced upward to reveal the internal mammary nodes and vasculature. The pluera is then visualized and thoroughly dissected from the overlying structures. This dissection technique is repeated to include the second, third, and fourth costal cartilages. The intercostal vessels and internal mammary nodes are typically located approximately 1 cm lateral to the sternochondral junction. If the pleura is inadvertently disrupted during the dissection, an attempt can be made to repair the defect with a 5.0 or 6.0 suture.

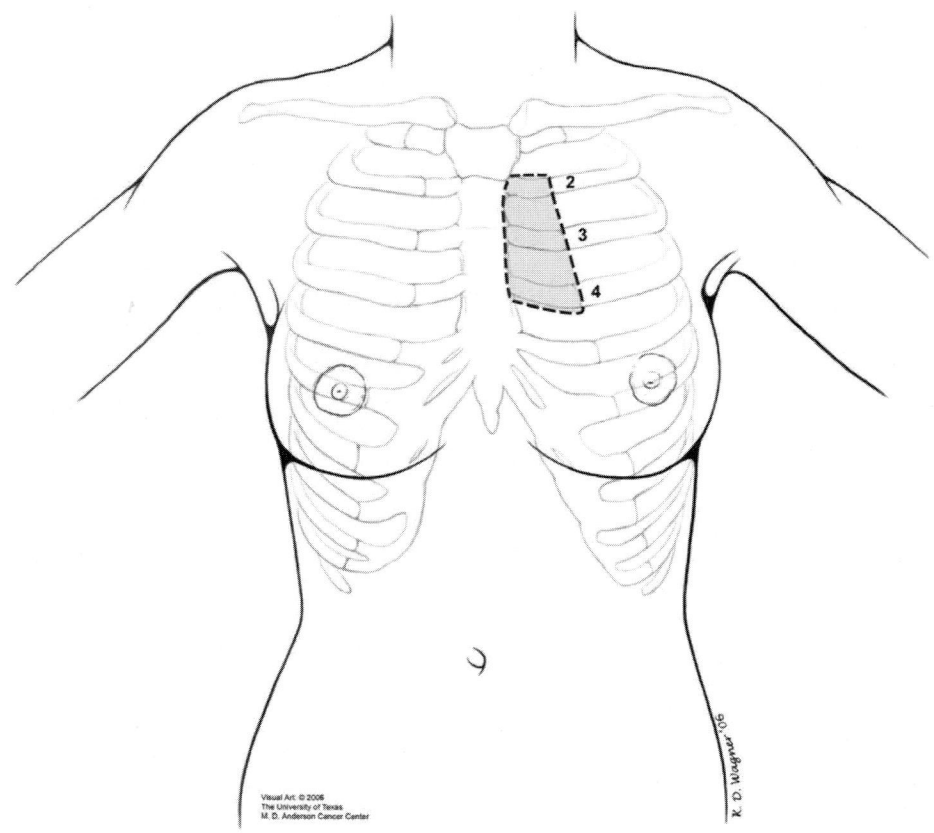

Figure 2 Shaded area depicts the costochondral junctions to be surgically removed as part of a formal internal mammary node dissection. This maneuver provides ample exposure to resect the lymph node bearing tissues in the first through fourth interspaces.

MORBIDITY

The morbidity of an internal mammary node dissection is primarily related to injury to the underlying lung or nearby vasculature. If the pleura, which is intimately associated with the internal mammary nodes, is violated, the patient will typically sustain a pneumothorax. Consequently, a chest x-ray should be obtained postoperatively subsequent to an internal mammary node dissection. The pnemothorax that occurs secondary to an internal mammary dissection is usually small and self-limiting and may not require intervention with a chest tube. Regardless, if a pleural injury occurs, it is recommended that the patient be admitted to an inpatient observation unit, where serial chest x-rays should be taken. Additional morbidity associated with internal mammary dissection is the result of injury to the intercostal arteries and veins. These injuries can be occult at the time of surgery, as the involved vessels tend to retract into the chest cavity. Consequently, the patient may develop a delayed hemothorax requiring either chest tube drainage or thoracotomy. This complication underscores the importance of meticulous surgical technique,

and the need for close postoperative observation. The morbidity of a definitive internal mammary dissection is considerably more debilitating, in regard to postoperative pain and deformity, when compared with a directed sentinel node procedure.

Supraclavicular Node Dissection

RATIONALE AND INDICATIONS

The incidence of isolated supraclavicular disease is rare, occurring in approximately 4% of patients.[20] For nearly a century, the presence of supraclavicular nodal disease has been associated with a poor prognosis, and has been considered a definitive indicator for distant systemic metastases.[21] Several studies have linked the presence of supraclavicular nodal spread with dismal 5-year survival rates, similar to that for patients presenting with stage IV disease.[19,22] These findings had led to the conclusion that patients presenting with supraclavicular involvement would be best managed as stage IV patients with palliative treatments, and to the 1997 AJCC staging classification of supraclavicular nodal involvement as M1 or distant disease.[19]

Recently, a study by Brito and colleagues, examining aggressively treated patients with isolated supraclavicular metastases, has led to a reassessment of the implications of this disease presentation.[23] The idea that the supraclavicular nodal basin is truly distant from the level I, II, and III nodes, based on the anatomic boundary of the clavicle, has been reconsidered. In a small series studied by Harris and colleagues, surgical intervention in patients with supraclavicular disease correlated with a better overall survival.[24] Brito and colleagues have shown that patients with breast cancer and isolated ipsilateral supraclavicular disease treated with chemotherapy, radiotherapy, and surgery had disease-free survival rates at 5 and 10 years of 34% and 32%, respectively, more closely approximating the outcomes for patients with locally advanced breast cancer, rather than patients with stage IV disease.[23] The new findings from the Brito study may reflect the fact that patients treated in earlier studies were considered unsalvageable, and not typically treated with aggressive multimodal local and systemic therapy.[19] The Brito study outcomes prompted a change in the 2002 AJCC staging system to reclassify supraclavicular disease as N3 or regional nodal disease. The intended effect of this new classification is to motivate clinicians to treat patients with supraclavicular disease with a salvageable, curative intent. Therefore, the presence of isolated supraclavicular disease is now an indication for both local therapy, including surgical resection and radiation treatment, as well as systemic chemotherapy. To this end, it will be important to closely follow those patients with supraclavicular nodal involvement, who should now be aggressively managed according to the new AJCC staging guidelines, to ascertain the outcomes for these patients in larger studies with longer follow-up.

SURGICAL PROCEDURE

The supraclavicular node dissection for patients with breast cancer encompasses the cervical levels III through V, as these are the regions where breast cancer metastases have been found most consistently. Although the cervical dissection is selective (limited to specific nodal regions) in its approach, it should be performed in a comprehensive and anatomically based manner to optimize regional control of disease. The extent of the dissection includes the middle jugular nodes (level III), the lower jugular nodes (level IV), and the posterior triangle nodes (level V). Figure 3 illustrates the cervical nodal regions and their relative anatomic locations.

The patient is positioned on the operating table such that the involved side of the neck has maximum exposure, and the operating table is turned to facilitate surgical access. An incision is made along the neck extending from below the mastoid process, along the lateral border of the sternocleidomastoid muscle, and then dropping down inferiorly to approximately 1 cm above the clavicle, in a reversed hockey stick fashion. The incision is made using a knife, through the dermis.

Electrocautery is then used to dissect through the subcutaneous tissue, at which point subplatysmal flaps are raised extending inferiorly to the clavicle and superiorly to the junction of the trapezius muscle and the sternocleidomastoid muscle. Inferiorly, the fascia under the clavicle is then incised exposing the level V lymph nodes. These lymph nodes are then dissected free from the posterior aspect of the posterior triangle, and then carefully dissected from lateral to medial and posterior to anterior to the level of the external jugular vein. At this point, the external jugular vein is dissected, ligated, and divided. Next, the fascia over the sternocleidomastoid muscle is incised to permit the dissection of the level III and IV lymph nodes, medial to the SCM, off the carotid sheath, where they are then passed into the posterior triangle proper. Inferiorly, the internal jugular vein is then skeletonized to the level of the subclavian vein. The carotid sheath is then skeletonized in an inferior to superior direction, extending to the level of the facial vein.

Attention is then turned the area of the brachial plexus, where the dissection continues from inferior to superior, carefully dissecting out the brachial plexus, as well as the medial and superior aspect of the anterior scalene musculature. The dissection then continues medially at the area of the cervical plexus, where care should be taken to avoid the phrenic nerve, and continues proximally to the level of the juncture of the sternocleidomastoid muscle and the trapezius muscle. At this location, the accessory nerve courses from the posterior aspect of the sternocleidomastoid muscle, along the trapezius muscle, and down to the level V lymph nodes. At this point, the greater auricular nerve also courses anterior to the sternocleidomastoid muscle; this nerve should be spared. At the level of the juncture of the sternocleidomastoid muscle and the trapezius muscle, the most superior aspect of the external jugular vein is identified and securely ligated and divided. Any remaining nodes found on the trapezius muscle are removed en bloc. Finally, any remaining vasculature connecting the level III through V lymph nodes to the neck structures is carefully ligated and divided, and the specimen is passed from the field for pathologic analysis. The wound is then carefully inspected for hemostatsis and irrigated with sterile saline (Figure 4). A flexible drain is placed through a separate incision inferior and lateral to the surgical incision. The wound is reapproxi-

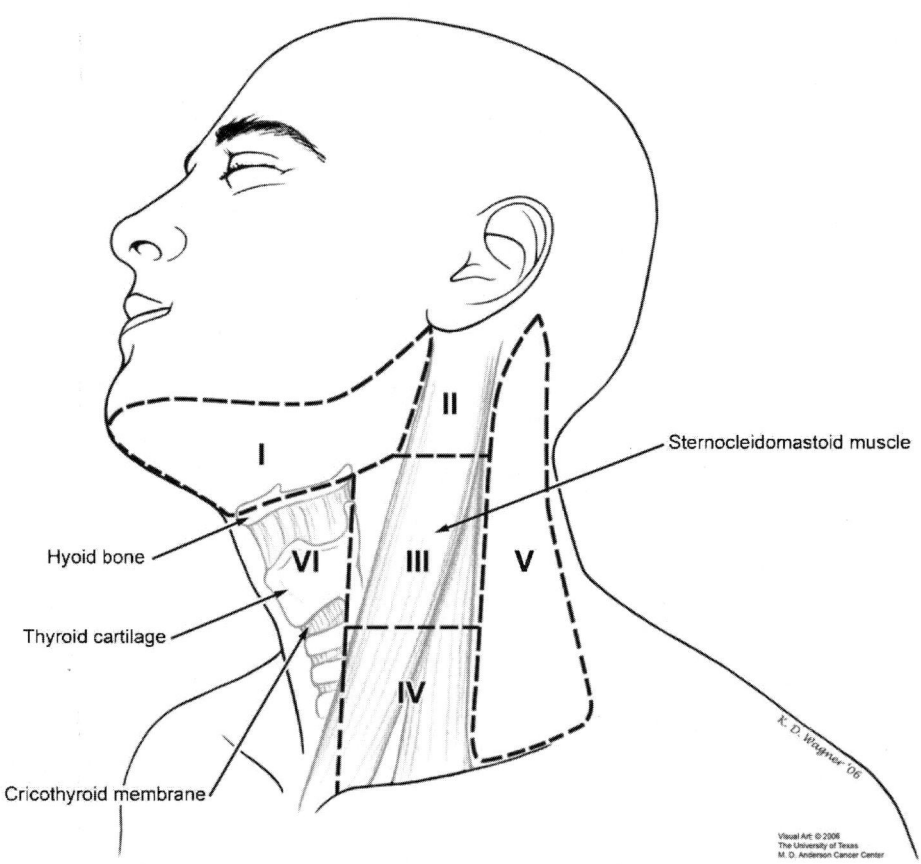

Figure 3 Drawing of the major lymphatic compartments in the neck. Levels III–V are generally dissected en bloc for adequate local control of supraclavicular metastases.

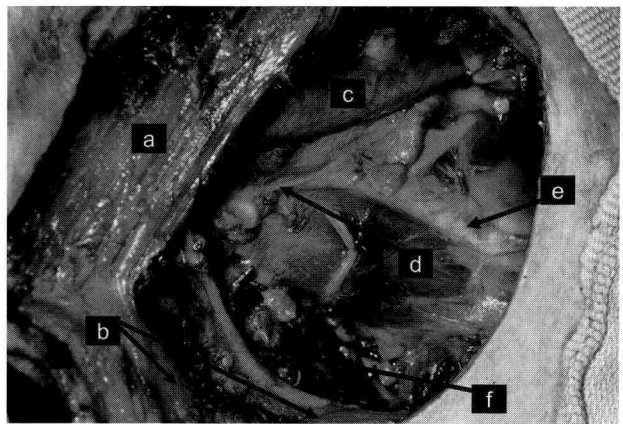

Figure 4 Intraoperative photograph of completed right neck dissection. The head is to the left and the chest to the right. The following anatomic boundaries and preserved structures are designated as follows: (a) sternocleidomastoid muscle, (b) trapezius muscle, (c) internal jugular vein, (d) phrenic nerve, (e) brachial plexus, and (f) spinal accessory nerve.

mated with interrupted 3-0 Vicryl sutures and a running 4-0 PDS suture.

MORBIDITY

The morbidity associated with the supraclavicular next dissection is often minor. A concerning morbidity does include postoperative vascular bleeding, leading to airway compromise. Early postoperative complications also include seroma and infection. Injury to the recurrent laryngeal nerve can result in hoarseness and stridor in conjunction with aspiration and pneumonia. Additionally, damage to the spinal accessory nerve results in both the winged scapula and a shoulder drop. Injury to the phrenic nerve can result in a loss of diaphragmatic control and an elevated hemidiaphram. Furthermore, damage to the thoracic duct in the left neck can result in a chylous fistula that is associated with significant morbidity, including electrolyte imbalances, hypoproteinemia, and immunosuppression. The hypoglossal nerve can also be injured and results in loss of control of the tongue on the affected side. Resection of the sternocleidomastoid muscle may result in some cosmetic deformity.

Conclusions

As the knowledge of breast cancer biology advances both from historical studies and cutting-edge laboratory work, the way in which breast cancer is managed will continue to change and progress. Some practices are abandoned, while others are adopted or modified. Practices that were once thought to be too aggressive may fall back into favor, based on new research findings. The advent of SNB has eliminated the need for the routine use of a formal axillary dissection in clinically node-negative patients, as a sentinel node dissection alone has become the standard therapy for sentinel node-negative patients. Although a formal axillary dissection remains the standard of care for all node-positive patients, a more selective approach to completion dissection in sentinel node-positive patients, who, based on a variety of clinicopathologic factors have a low risk of nonsentinel axillary node involvement, is becoming more commonplace and is the focus of current clinical investigations. Currently, the Memorial Sloan-Kettering nomogram is being used in clinical practice to help predict the likelihood for sentinel node-positive patients to have additional nonsentinel nodal disease, and thus require a completion axillary node dissection.[25] Use of this nomogram has aided in establishing patient surgical expectations and surgical planning. Studies to further determine the significance of positive sentinel nodes, and the need for a completion dissection in patients who are sentinel node positive are ongoing. Nomograms to help predict the likelihood of additional nodal disease in patients who have been treated with neoadjuvant therapy are also in development. Significant controversy exists regarding the appropriate management of patients with micrometastasis and isolated tumor cell identified in the sentinel. Although the standard of care continues to dictate the need to perform a completion axillary dissection in all patients who present with positive sentinel nodes, the goal to manage patients as individuals remains paramount.

The use of lymphoscintigraphy has broadened the scope for understanding the unique sentinel drainage patterns for patients with breast cancer. Consequently, the importance of alternative sentinel drainage patterns to the internal mammary chain and supraclavicular region has been reexamined. Patients found to have isolated internal mammary or isolated supraclavicular lymphatic drainage may stand to benefit from an internal mammary or supraclavicular node dissection.

The recent work demonstrating the more favorable survival outcomes for patients with aggressively managed supraclavicular nodal involvement suggests that this patient population stands to benefit from a formal level III-V neck dissection. The implications of these findings are encouraging, as they indicate that patients who have been deemed terminal in the past may ultimately have more favorable outcomes through aggressive interventions including surgery as an integral part of a multimodality treatment strategy.

References

1. Foster RS Jr. The biologic and clinical significance of lymphatic metastases in breast cancer. Surg Oncol Clin N Am 1996;5:79–104.

2. Fisher B, Montague E, Redmond C, et al. Findings from NSABP Protocol No. B-04-comparison of radical mastectomy with alternative treatments for primary breast cancer. I. Radiation compliance and its relation to treatment outcome. Cancer 1980;46:1–13.

3. Fisher B, Bauer M, Margolese R, et al. Five-year results of a randomized clinical trial comparing total mastectomy and segmental mastectomy with or without radiation in the treatment of breast cancer. N Engl J Med 1985;312:665–73.

4. Veronesi U, Banfi A, Del Vecchio M, et al. Comparison of Halsted mastectomy with quadrantectomy, axillary dissection, and radiotherapy in early breast cancer: long-term results. Eur J Cancer Clin Oncol 1986;22:1085–9.

5. Krag D, Weaver D, Ashikaga T, et al. The sentinel node in breast cancer—a multicenter validation study. N Engl J Med 1998;339:941–6.

6. Giuliano AE, Kirgan DM, Guenther JM, Morton DL. Lymphatic mapping and sentinel lymphadenectomy for breast cancer. Ann Surg 1994;220:391–401.

7. Fisher B, Brown A, Mamounas E, et al. Effect of preoperative chemotherapy on local-regional disease in women with operable breast cancer: findings from National Surgical Adjuvant Breast and Bowel Project B-18. J Clin Oncol 1997;15:2483–93.

8. Wright FC, Walker J, Law CH, McCready DR. Outcomes after localized axillary node recurrence in breast cancer. Ann Surg Oncol 2003;10:1054–8.

9. Ahlgren J, Holmberg L, Bergh J, Liljegren G. Five-node biopsy of the axilla: an alternative to axillary dissection of levels I-II in operable breast cancer. Eur J Surg Oncol 2002; 28:97–102.

10. Mathiesen O, Carl J, Bonderup O, Panduro J. Axillary sampling and the risk of erroneous staging of breast cancer. An analysis of 960 consecutive patients. Acta Oncol 1990; 29:721–5.

11. Marschall J, Nechala P, Colquhoun P, Chibbar R. Reassessing the role of axillary lymph-node dissection in

patients with early-stage breast cancer. Can J Surg 2003;46: 285–9.

12. Voogd AC, Coebergh JW, Repelaer van Driel OJ, et al. The risk of nodal metastases in breast cancer patients with clinically negative lymph nodes: a population-based analysis. Breast Cancer Res Treat 2000;62:63–9.

13. Abdessalam SF, Zervos EE, Prasad M, et al. Predictors of positive axillary lymph nodes after sentinel lymph node biopsy in breast cancer. Am J Surg 2001;182:316–20.

14. Veronesi U, Rilke F, Luini A, et al. Distribution of axillary node metastases by level of invasion. An analysis of 539 cases. Cancer 1987;59:682–7.

15. Wilke LG, Giuliano A. Sentinel lymph node biopsy in patients with early-stage breast cancer: status of the National Clinical Trials. Surg Clin North Am 2003;83: 901–10.

16. Morrow M, Foster RS Jr. Staging of breast cancer: a new rationale for internal mammary node biopsy. Arch Surg 1981;116:748–51.

17. Noguchi M, Tsugawa K, Taniya T, Miwa K. The role of internal mammary lymph node metastases in the management of breast cancer. Breast Cancer 1998;5:117–25.

18. Veronesi U, Marubini E, Mariani L, et al. The dissection of internal mammary nodes does not improve the survival of breast cancer patients. 30-year results of a randomised trial. Eur J Cancer 1999;35:1320–5.

19. AJCC Cancer Staging Handbook. 6th ed. New York: Springer; 2002.

20. Ampil FL, Caldito G, Li BD, Burton GV. Supraclavicular nodal relapse of breast cancer: prevalence, palliation, and prognosis. Eur J Gynaecol Oncol 2003;24:233–5.

21. Halsted W. The results of radical operations for the cure of cancer of the breast. Ann Surg 1907;46:1–5.

22. Debois JM. The significance of a supraclavicular node metastasis in patients with breast cancer. A literature review. Strahlenther Onkol 1997;173:1–12.

23. Brito RA, Valero V, Buzdar AU, et al. Long-term results of combined-modality therapy for locally advanced breast cancer with ipsilateral supraclavicular metastases: The University of Texas M.D. Anderson Cancer Center experience. J Clin Oncol 2001;19:628–33.

24. Harris EE, Hwang WT, Seyednejad F, Solin LJ. Prognosis after regional lymph node recurrence in patients with stage I-II breast carcinoma treated with breast conservation therapy. Cancer 2003;98:2144–51.

25. Van Zee KJ, Manasseh DM, Bevilacqua JL, et al. A nomogram for predicting the likelihood of additional nodal metastases in breast cancer patients with a positive sentinel node biopsy. Ann Surg Oncol 2003;10:1140–51.

CHAPTER 57

Prognostic and Predictive Profiling in Breast Cancer

Funda Meric-Bernstam, MD

W. Fraser Symmans, MD

Introduction

In spite of the advances in breast cancer care, more than 41,000 people die of breast cancer in the United States alone every year.[1] This provides impetus to develop a more personalized approach to medicine in the form of individually tailored therapies that are more effective and less toxic than the current therapies. To accomplish this, new prognostic and predictive markers must be identified, and more efficient methods of doing so must be developed.

Breast cancer treatment is individualized on the basis of markers that provide the clinician with information about the patient's disease. Two kinds of markers are helpful in individualizing breast cancer treatment. Prognostic markers help with identifying patients who are at high risk of disease recurrence and who could, therefore, most benefit from receiving adjuvant therapy. Predictive markers are used to predict individual patients' responses to specific therapeutic regimens, including adverse reactions. The traditional clinical-pathologic markers currently in use, tumor size and pathologic regional node status, provide the basis for the American Joint Committee on Cancer (AJCC) staging criteria. Although these factors provide an estimate of risk of recurrence and death, their usefulness has become increasingly more limited for the following reasons: (1) an increasing percentage of patients are diagnosed with early stage disease (lower incidence of regional node metastases and smaller tumors); (2) a significant percentage of node-negative patients relapse, and a significant number of patients with large tumors are cured and, therefore, these factors are far from ideal in discriminating the relapsing fraction of patients from the cured fraction; (3) a more liberal use of cytotoxic chemotherapy regardless of the estimated risk; and (4) these factors provide no information concerning the likelihood of the effectiveness of specific systemic therapies. As a result, the past few decades have been filled with an intense study of prognostic and predictive markers for breast cancer, and this chapter highlights some of that work and discusses the clinical implications.

How Known Molecular Markers Are Assayed

Breast cancer is driven by an accumulation of genetic alterations that confer a growth or survival advantage to cancer cells. These changes include loss of function of tumor suppressor genes such as *TP53* and gain of function of oncogenes such as human epidermal receptor 2 (*HER2*). Alterations in gene function can result from post-translational modification (eg, phosphorylation) of critical proteins, altered subcellular localization, or other such events, or result from alterations in gene expression leading to changes in protein levels. Gene expression is controlled at several levels, and aberrations can occur at any level, including at the levels of genomic DNA (deletions or amplifications), transcription, messenger RNA stability, translation, and protein stability. Alterations in genes of interest can be assessed individually at the DNA level by approaches such as in situ hybridization (eg, for assessment of *HER2* amplifications), at the RNA level by approaches such as quantitative reverse transcription polymerase chain reaction (RT-PCR), or at the protein level by approaches such as immunohistochemical analysis (eg, for assessment of *HER2/neu* or estrogen receptor [ER]).

Traditional Prognostic and Predictive Markers

Tumor markers routinely used to make decisions for patients with breast cancer include estrogen and progesterone receptor, *HER2*, and proliferation markers such as Ki-67.

ESTROGEN AND PROGESTERONE RECEPTORS

ER and progesterone receptor (PR) intracellularly bind estrogen and progesterone, respectively, and translocate them to the nucleus to induce hormone-dependent gene expression. Estrogen functions through two intracellular receptors, ERα and ERβ. Although ERα is a well-established prognostic and predictive factor, the significance of ERβ is not well established. The use of ER and PR as markers of prognosis and predictors of response to antiestrogen therapy is the standard of care for all patients with primary breast cancer. These markers may also be measured on metastatic lesions if the results would influence treatment planning.

Originally measured with quantitative ligand-binding assays of fresh tumor extracts, hormone receptor levels are now usually measured in tumor tissue by immunohistochemical analysis. ERs are identified in 60 to 70% of breast cancers in premenopausal patients and in 80% of breast cancers in postmenopausal patients. ER levels are often inversely correlated with grade and other measures of proliferation.

Patients with ER-positive tumors have longer disease-free intervals than patients with ER-negative tumors. Progesterone receptor status is a weaker prognostic factor and mainly used as a predictor of response to antiestrogen treatment.

For patients with operable breast cancer, an increased concentration of ER and PR is associated with increased effectiveness of endocrine therapies. A meta-analysis showed that in the adjuvant setting tamoxifen significantly reduced recurrence and death in patients with ER-positive tumors only.[2] Response to tamoxifen is directly related to ER levels, but tumors with as little as 4 to 10 fmol/mg of ER protein or as few as 1 to 10% of cells positive for ER, as determined by immunohistochemical analysis, have responded to tamoxifen.

The role of PR as a predictor of response to endocrine therapy has been more controversial. However, several studies have found that patients with ER-positive/PR-positive tumors benefited much more from adjuvant tamoxifen therapy than patients with ER-positive/PR-negative tumors,[2] and that ER and PR are independent predictors of treatment outcome. In patients with metastatic disease, elevated PR levels are significantly and independently correlated with increased probability of response to tamoxifen, longer time to treatment failure, and longer overall survival.

HER2

HER2 (also called c-erbB-2 or neu) is a receptor tyrosine kinase involved in normal cell growth.[3] The HER2 protein is overexpressed in 15 to 30% of human breast cancers, mostly as a result of gene amplification. HER2 expression is evaluated for every primary breast cancer at the time of diagnosis.

HER2 became clinically relevant when it was demonstrated that HER2-positive breast cancers have a worse prognosis than HER2-negative breast cancers. HER2 overexpression is correlated with shortened disease-free and overall survival and it is an adverse prognostic factor associated with poorly differentiated, high-grade tumors; high rates of cell proliferation; and lymph node involvement. However, tumors overexpressing HER2 have been shown to respond more favorably to doxorubicin-based chemotherapy.

High levels of HER2 expression can be used to identify patients for whom trastuzumab, a monoclonal antibody that targets the extracellular domain of the HER2 protein, may be of clinical benefit. HER2 may be assessed by using immunohistochemical analysis to detect HER2/neu protein overexpression or by using fluorescence in situ hybridization (FISH) to detect *HER2/neu* gene amplification. Both of these methodologies have been validated to have clinical utility. However, demonstration of *HER2* amplification by FISH is thought to be a better predictor of response to trastuzumab-based therapy than HER2 overexpression by immunohistochemical analysis. The predictive values for gene amplification are best for cases that score 3+ on immunohistochemical analysis on a scale of 0 to 3+. Immunohistochemical analysis is often used as a screening tool, and FISH is used to confirm a positive result on immunohistochemical analysis.

KI-67

The nuclear antigen Ki-67, measured by immunohistochemical analysis, is a useful marker of cell proliferation. Its levels correlate well with other markers of proliferation such as S-phase fraction measured by flow cytometry and mitotic index. Ki-67 also correlates with histologic grade. High levels of Ki-67 are associated with poorly differentiated tumors. Overall, Ki-67 appears to be correlated with decreased disease-free survival, but its independent significance is thought to be modest. At this time, the clinical utility of Ki-67 as a prognostic marker is limited to small, node-negative breast cancer where high-grade and high Ki-67 might be used to support a clinical recommendation of adjuvant chemotherapy. Furthermore, there is interest in evaluating Ki-67 as a pharmacodynamic marker of response to endocrine and, potentially, other targeted therapies.

PLOIDY AND S-PHASE FRACTION

DNA content and proliferation as determined by using flow cytometry has also been correlated with outcome. Although neither ploidy nor S phase is accepted as a standard prognostic marker, patients with diploid tumors generally have better disease-free survival rates than those with aneuploid tumors, and a high number of tumor cells in the S phase is associated with a shorter disease-free survival and a higher risk of death.

Investigational Immunohistochemistry-Based Prognostic Markers

Molecular markers shown to have prognostic value but not used routinely include p53, urokinase-type plasminogen activator/plasminogen activator inhibitor type-1, cyclin E, cathepsin D, and microvessel density (MVD). To date, these markers are not widely used in clinical practice, perhaps because they are less likely to influence adjuvant treatment decisions.

Mutations in the *TP53* tumor suppressor gene occur in more than 50% of human cancers. In breast cancer, *TP53* mutations have been found to be associated with worse overall and disease-free survival independently of other risk factors, and they have been implicated in resistance to anticancer therapies.

Urokinase-type plasminogen activator/plasminogen activator inhibitor type-1 overexpression appears to be a very strong prognostic marker for reduced recurrence-free survival and overall survival in breast cancer. Its expression, however, has been determined by enzyme-linked immunosorbent assay, which requires fresh or frozen tissue; this likely limits the widespread use of this marker in the United States, although its use is standard in some countries.

Cyclin E regulates the transition from the G_1 phase to the S phase; high cyclin E levels accelerate the transition through the G_1 phase. Total cyclin E levels and the level of low-molecular-weight forms of cyclin E have been reported to be strongly associated with worse survival among patients with breast cancer.[4]

Cathepsin D is a lysosomal acidic protease. Elevated cathepsin D levels have been proposed to be a predictor of poor prognosis.

MVD is a measure of angiogenesis. MVD can be quantified using immunostaining for factor VIII-related antigen. MVD of the primary tumor may be a predictor of nodal status, disease-free survival, and overall survival.

Micrometastatic Disease

In addition to molecular markers in the tumor, micrometastatic disease in the bone marrow is also being investigated as a potential prognostic marker. Bone marrow micrometastatic disease can be detected by staining bone marrow aspirates with monoclonal antibodies to cytokeratin. Patients with bone marrow micrometastasis have larger tumors, tumors with a higher histologic grade, more lymph node metastases, and more hormone receptor-negative tumors than patients without bone marrow micrometastasis. In 4,700 patients with stage I, II, or III breast cancer, micrometastasis was a significant prognostic factor associated with poor overall survival, breast cancer-specific survival, disease-free survival, and distant disease-free survival during a 10-year observation period.[5] Ongoing work is evaluating the use of routine assessment of bone marrow status in the care of patients with breast cancer.

Currently, researchers are trying to determine whether molecular technologies such as reverse transcriptase-PCR (RT-PCR) can help identify patients with low-volume, subclinical nodal metastases and whether these metastases have prognostic significance.[6] Patients who have a small disease burden (< 0.2 mm) identified by either immunohistochemical analysis of axillary nodes or RT-PCR are considered node negative by the current American Joint Commission on Cancer classification.[7] The accuracy and prognostic value of molecular staging of sentinel nodes for breast cancer is being evaluated in multicenter prospective studies.

There is also a significant amount of data supporting the use of the number of circulating tumor cells (CTCs) as a prognostic factor. In a prospective multicenter trial, the number of CTCs ($\geq$ 5 CTCs vs < 5 CTCs per 7.5 mL of whole blood) before treatment of metastatic breast cancer was an independent predictor of progression-free and overall survival rates.[8] Serial monitoring of CTCs during or after therapy also has been proposed as prognostically useful. This technology, known as CellSearch (Veridex, Warren, NJ), has been approved by the Food and Drug Administration for clinical use. The role of measuring CTCs in guiding therapy for patients with metastatic breast cancer is being evaluated in a prospective trial. The value of identifying CTCs in early-stage breast cancer remains unknown.

Transcriptional Profiling

Recently, high-throughput approaches have been introduced to assay for alterations in gene expression at the level of DNA, RNA, and protein. Hundreds to thousands of genes can be simultaneously assessed with these approaches, of which the most developed is transcriptional profiling. For transcriptional profiling, RNA is extracted from breast tumors and used to generate probes by either reverse transcription of the RNA in the presence of labeled nucleotides or RNA labeling with biotin. The probes are then hybridized to microarrays, which are cDNA or oligonucleotides printed on slides or membranes, and which allow the expression of thousands of genes to be determined simultaneously. From a cancer biology research perspective, transcriptional profiling can help identify individual genes that are important in breast cancer biology, can help identify genes that are coordinately expressed, and can expand our understanding of the networks that drive cancer development and progression. From a clinical perspective, the major goal is to identify transcriptional profiles that predict breast cancer prognosis or response to individual therapeutic regimens. However, biostatistical wisdom holds that identification of profiles from multi-parameter data to predict the future is unreliable, particularly from empirical study designs based on clinical outcomes (eg, relapse vs not). For this reason, findings must be validated in independent studies before they can be trusted.[9,10]

The seminal study using transcriptional profiling technology to evaluate transcriptional profiles of breast cancers was performed by Perou and colleagues.[11] In that study, 65 surgical breast tumor specimens from 42 patients were analyzed using cDNA microarrays representing 8,102 genes. mRNA from the specimens was compared with reference RNA from 11 different cultured cell lines. Genes (1,753) whose abundance varied at least 4-fold from the median in 3 or more samples were used to classify samples further, and the samples were arranged in hierarchical order on the basis of similarity of gene expression. Two tumor samples from the same individual were more similar to each other than were any other samples. Cluster analysis was used to identify an "intrinsic gene set." This gene set represented 496 genes with significantly greater variation between tumors than between paired samples. The molecular classification allowed discrimination of 5 tumor subtypes on the basis of their distinct gene expression profile: luminal epithelial (subtypes A and B), HER2-positive, basal epithelial cell cluster (positive for cytokeratin 5/6 and cytokeratin 17), and normal-like gene expression.

GENE EXPRESSION SIGNATURES FOR PREDICTING PROGNOSIS

With the development of transcriptional profiling, the immediate clinically relevant question was whether molecular classification based on transcriptional profiling can help better predict prognosis. Specifically, the goal would be to identify patients at high risk of disease recurrence so that they could be treated more aggressively, or to identify patients at low risk of disease recurrence so that adjuvant treatment and, thus, the toxicity of adjuvant treatment could be avoided.

One of the early studies of microarray technology was performed by Sorlie and colleagues,[12] who conducted 85 microarray experiments on 78 breast carcinomas. Tumors were classified into 6 subtypes. ER-positive tumors were classified as luminal subtype A, B, or C; ER-negative tumors were classified as normal breast-like, basal-like, or HER2-positive (Figure 1). This classification system remained robust when tumors were classified by two separate gene sets—the intrinsic set previously described and a gene set that classified patients by outcome on supervised analyses. Further, this classification based on tumor subtypes was correlated with overall and relapse-free survival (Figure 2). However, the method of unsupervised clustering that was used to identify these subclasses identifies patterns in a given dataset (analogous to identifying subsets of playing cards after a selection was cast face-up onto the floor) and would be difficult to translate into a clinical diagnostic to evaluate a single sample. Furthermore, the intrinsic gene set continues to change in different studies.

Another landmark study was preformed by van't Veer and colleagues.[13] In that study, node-negative breast tumors smaller than 5 cm from 78 patients less than 55 years of age were used to identify prognostic reporter genes. Thirty-four of the patients had developed distant metastases in less than 5 years, while 44 had developed no distant metastases after more than 5 years. By this classification system, based on distant metastases, a 70-gene expression signature was identified as a predictor of survival. Referred to as the Amsterdam signature, this classification system was cross-validated by the "leave-one-out" strategy. The classifier correctly predicted the actual outcome of disease for 65 of 78 patients (83%). The threshold was adjusted to misclassify no more than 10% of the poor-prognosis tumors.

This 70-gene signature was validated in a separate study by van de Vijver and colleagues[14] of 295 consecutive patients all younger than 53 years old, 61 of whom comprised the lymph node-negative patients from the study by van't Veer and colleagues[13] Patients had stage I or II disease, and 151 were lymph node

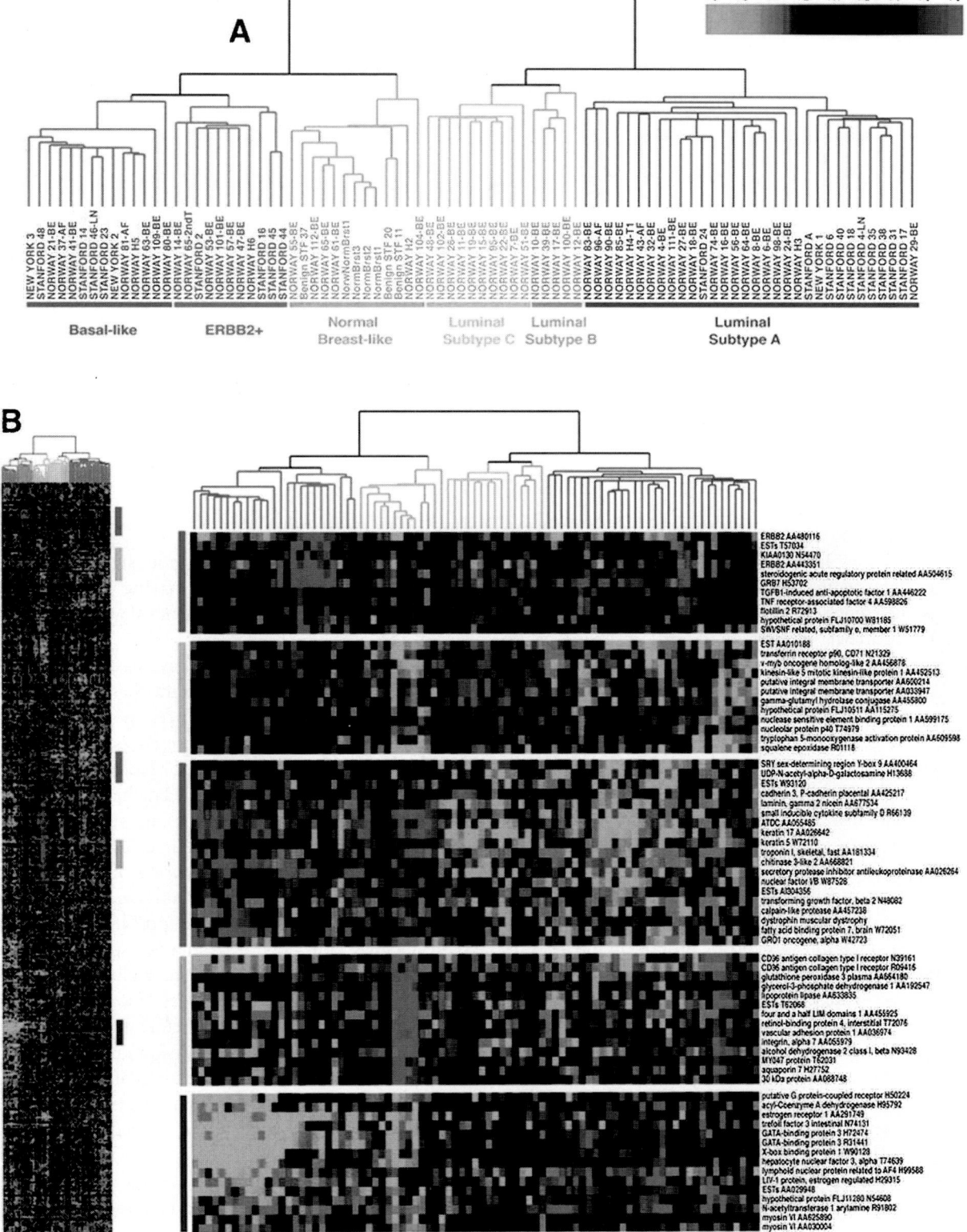

Figure 1 Gene expression patterns of 85 experimental samples analyzed by hierarchical clustering, *A*, identifying different molecular subtypes. *B*, Each column represents a tumor, each row a gene. ERBB2+, *HER2/neu*-positive. Reproduced with permission from Sorlie T et al.[12]

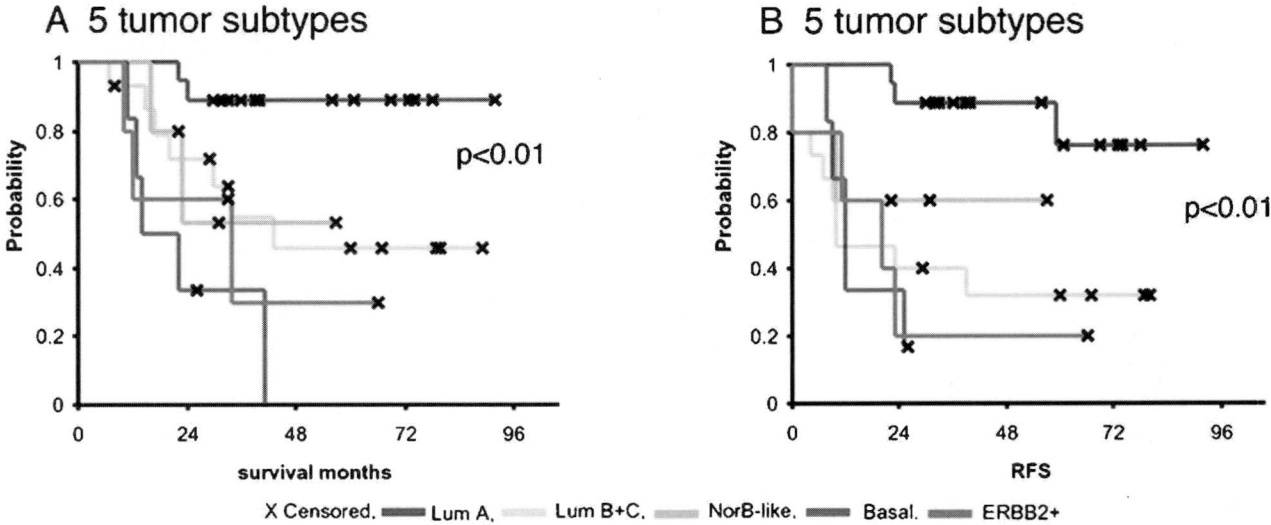

Figure 2 Overall (A) and relapse-free survival (B) analysis of 49 patients with breast cancer uniformly treated in a prospective study grouped by tumor subtypes. ERBB2+, *HER2/neu*-positive; Lum, luminal; NorB-like, normal breast-like; RFS, relapse-free survival. Reproduced with permission from Sorlie T et al.[12]

negative and 144 lymph node positive. One hundred fifteen patients with values of the 70-gene expression were assigned good prognosis based on their 70-gene expression pattern. At 10 years, the probability of remaining free of distant metastasis was 50.5 ± 4.4% in the group with a poor-prognosis signature and was 85.2 ± 4.3% in the group with a good prognosis signature (Figure 3). This gene expression profiling approach more accurately separated low-risk from high-risk patients than either the St. Gallen criteria or the National Institutes of Health (NIH) consensus criteria, which classify patients as low and high risk on the basis of histologic and clinical characteristics.[15,16] Furthermore, patients who were at high risk by the St. Gallen criteria or the NIH consensus criteria could be further subdivided into prognostic groups on the basis of their molecular signature. Using multivariate analysis, van de Vijver and colleagues[14] found that the poor-prognosis signature versus the good-prognosis signature was an independent prognostic variable and had a prognosis with a hazard ratio of 4.6 (95% confidence interval [CI] of 2.3–9.2, $P < 0.001$).

Other groups have obtained similar results using strategies to derive separately prognostic signatures for ER-positive and ER-negative tumors, or to segregate intermediate grade into low-risk and high-risk groups.[17,18,19] Interestingly, many prognostic sets have few genes that overlap; however, some of the prognostic sets have been validated in different datasets. A recent bioinformatic analysis of these different datasets indi-

cated that the different prognostic signatures mostly identify the same patients as having good or poor prognosis, despite the different genes that comprise each signature.[20]

Many transcription profiles have been generated in patients who have received adjuvant therapy, and so for many of these studies, whether the difference in prognosis observed is due to differences in response to therapies or by differences in tumor biology identified by profiling has yet to be elucidated. Furthermore, whether looking at RNA is better than looking at DNA, protein, or all three has not yet been determined. Which prognostic gene set is worth using in the clinic is currently unknown. At the individual institutional laboratory level, some of these profiles indeed seem reproducible,[21] but how to standardize specimen processing and data analysis to ensure reproducibility has not been determined. Whether these more complicated technologies are scalable and whether they can be used nationwide and worldwide remains unknown. The cost-effectiveness of these molecular classification systems has not been determined. Finally, these technologies would be worthwhile only if they can indeed affect clinical management.

To address some of these issues, the European Organization for Research and Treatment of Cancer-TransBreast International Group is conducting a large-scale study, the Microarray In Node negative Disease may Avoid ChemoTherapy trial. Approximately 6,000 patients will be enrolled in this trial. Clinical pathologic

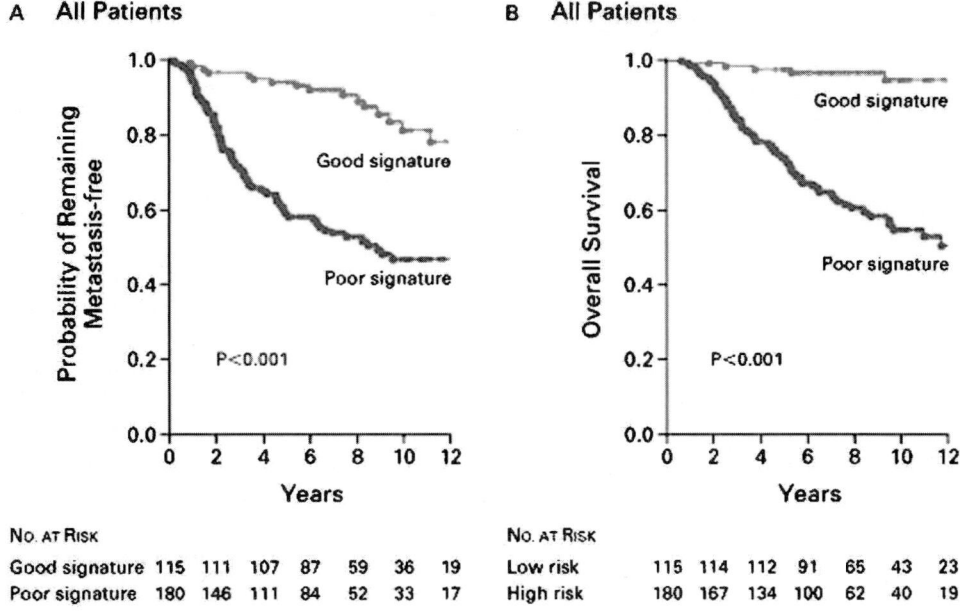

Figure 3 Distant metastasis-free survival (A) and overall survival (B) according to good-prognosis or poor-prognosis signature. Reproduced with permission from van de Vijver MJ et al.[14]

risk assessment will be performed using the Adjuvant! model (www.adjuvantonline.com), and further risk assessment will be performed using the 70-gene transcriptional profile. Patients who are at high risk according to clinical pathologic risk assessment and 70-gene risk assessment will receive chemotherapy. Patients who are at low risk by both risk assessment tools will receive no chemotherapy. Patients who have discordance between their clinical pathologic and 70-gene risk assessments will be randomized to receive or not receive chemotherapy. This study will determine whether the 70-gene prognostic signature should alter our current management and more accurately predict prognosis than our current clinical pathologic evaluation.

GENE EXPRESSION SIGNATURES FOR PREDICTING RESPONSE TO CHEMOTHERAPY

Many studies, including the National Surgical Adjuvant Breast and Bowel Project (NSABP) B-18 trial, have shown that patients who obtain a pathologic complete response to chemotherapy have the best disease-free and overall survival, suggesting that these patients benefit most from a particular chemotherapy regimen. This idea has been the basis for the use of preoperative chemotherapy models for discovery of markers and transcriptional profiles that correlate with complete pathologic response.

Ayers and colleagues[22] have looked at predictors of pathologic complete response to weekly taxanes followed by sequential 5-fluorouracil, doxorubicin, and cyclophosphamide. In their study, 42 patients underwent a fine-needle biopsy procedure prior to starting chemotherapy; 24 of the aspirates were used for predictive marker analyses, and the other 18 were used for validation of the results of the predictive marker analyses. A multigene predictor of 74 genes was identified. The sensitivity of the 74-gene model was 43% (95% CI of 10–82%), the specificity 100% (95% CI of 72–100%), and the overall accuracy 78% (95% CI of 52–94%). This predictive marker set is being validated in an ongoing multicenter trial involving The University of Texas M. D. Anderson Cancer Center and centers in Peru, Spain, and Mexico.

In another study, Chang and colleagues[23] evaluated predictors of docetaxel response. Core biopsies from 24 patients were obtained for pretreatment, and 92 genes were thought to be potentially predictive. Leave-one-out cross-validation analysis demonstrated that the predictive profile had 80% estimated accuracy. This profile was validated in an independent set of 6 patients, and larger-scale validation of this profile is ongoing.

These preliminary studies demonstrate that transcriptional profiles that are predictive of response to treatment can indeed be identified. The long-term clinical implication is that patients who have a nonresponse profile could receive a different agent. Transcriptional profiling may eventually allow for avoidance of chemotherapy in patients who have a no-response signature and a good-prognosis profile. In the future, with advances in anatomic and functional imaging, if a patient has a complete-response profile and complete clinical response in all imaging studies, using local-regional therapy with radiation therapy alone may be contemplated instead of surgery. Alternatively, the molecular signature of the residual breast cancer cells may allow for identification of pathways of chemoresistance, and thus enable the subsequent treatment to be planned accordingly.

GENE EXPRESSION SIGNATURES FOR PREDICTING RESPONSE TO HORMONAL THERAPY

Currently, decisions for endocrine therapy are based on ER and PR status as determined by immunohistochemical analysis. Optimal selection of endocrine therapy for women with ER-positive breast cancer will require biomarkers with better positive predictive value than ER and PR assessment. Therefore, there has been great interest in using genomic technology to identify markers to identify the subset of women with ER-positive breast cancers who would benefit most from hormonal agents. One such proposed predictor is for response to tamoxifen. The predictive marker is the 2-gene expression ratio of homeobox 13 and interleukin-17B receptor, a marker first derived from microarrays of 60 frozen samples of estrogen receptor-positive breast cancer that was associated with distant relapse after adjuvant tamoxifen therapy.[24] However, this result was of borderline significance in a larger analysis of tamoxifen-treated patients.[25] This demonstrated that a number of factors can affect the performance of any prognostic or predictive profile in subsequent validation studies, particularly the initial study design to discover the profile and any subsequent changes to the method of assay performance or interpretation.[26] Several other investigators are pursuing multimarker predictors of tamoxifen sensitivity, while others are pursuing predictors of response to individual aromatase inhibitors.

Other Evolving Molecular Profiling Technologies

Another novel approach to look at multiple genes simultaneously is to perform quantitative RT-PCR using paraffin-fixed tissue. Using a 250-candidate prognostic gene list compiled from the literature, Oncotype DX (Genomic Health, Inc., Redwood City, CA) technology

was used to test the expression of 250 genes from 447 patients who had received tamoxifen with or without chemotherapy. This led to the identification of a 21-gene recurrence score (RS) algorithm. The RS is based on 16 cancer genes and 5 reference genes. The 16 cancer genes comprise proliferation markers (Ki-67, STK15, survivin, cyclin B1, and MYBL2), invasion markers (stromelysin 3 and cathepsin L2), HER2 markers (GRB7 and HER2), estrogen markers (ER, PR, Bcl2, and SCUBE2), GSTM1, BAG1, and CD68. The 5 reference genes are beta-actin, GAPDH, RPLPO, GUS, and TFRC. The RS ranges from 0 to 100 with a score less than 18 classified as low recurrence risk, 18 to less than 31 classified as intermediate risk, and 31 or higher classified as high risk. It should be noted that the calculation of recurrence score is strongly weighted by gene expression related to ER, HER2, and proliferation. Nonetheless, this novel quantitative approach to the evaluation of the best known molecular pathways in breast cancer produced impressive results. Use of this multigene assay to predict recurrence was validated by the NSABP B-14 trial, in which ER-positive, node-negative patients had received tamoxifen. Of the 2,617 patients on the trial who had received tamoxifen, paraffin blocks were available for 675 of them. RT-PCR was successfully completed for 668 of the 675 patients.[27] The RS was indeed able to stratify patients by freedom from distant recurrence (Figure 4). By multivariate Cox proportional analysis, RS was independently associated with recurrence risk, with a hazard ratio of 3.21 (95% CI of 2.23–4.65, $P < 0.001$). In addition, the RS score computed by the Oncotype DX technology predicted benefits from chemotherapy.[28]

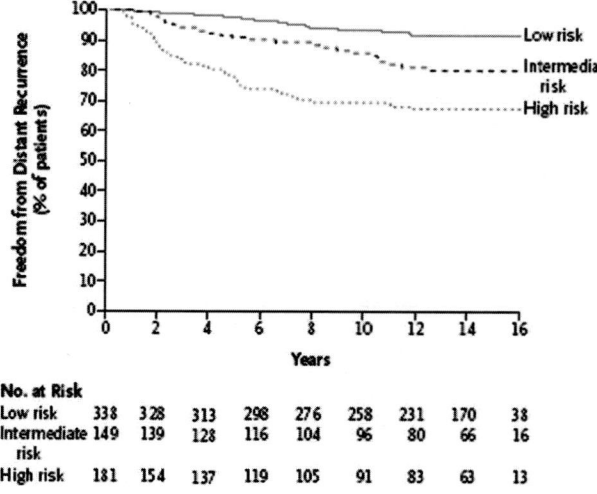

Figure 4 Likelihood of distant recurrence according to recurrence score categories. The difference between the groups was significant ($P < 0.001$). Reproduced with permission from Paik S et al.[27]

Clinical trials will be evaluating the utility of Onco*type* DX for predicting prognosis and response to treatment in patients with ER-positive, node-negative tumors. The hope is that the results of these trials will support a more selective and rational use of systemic therapies.

Other evolving technologies for high-throughput analysis include technologies focused on DNA analyses. These include comparative genomic hybridization arrays, single nucleotide polymorphism arrays, and oligonucleotide arrays for mutational analysis. In addition, there is great interest in developing proteomics approaches, including surface-enhanced laser absorption ionization, mass spectrometry, and reverse phase protein lysate arrays.

Molecular profiling is a potentially powerful approach to predicting prognosis and response to therapy. It is clear that these molecular profiling approaches represent very valuable research tools; however, the gene expression signatures need to be validated in clinical patient care before these approaches are used widely. Molecular markers and molecularly targeted therapies are likely to be the cornerstone of personalized medicine in the near future.

References

1. Jemal A, Siegel R, Ward E, et al. Cancer statistics, 2006. CA Cancer J Clin 2006;56:106–30.

2. Cui X, Schiff R, Arpino G, et al. Biology of progesterone receptor loss in breast cancer and its implications for endocrine therapy. J Clin Oncol 2005;23:7721–35.

3. Meric F, Hung MC, Hortobagyi GN, et al. HER2/neu in the management of invasive breast cancer. J Am Coll Surg 2002;194:488–501.

4. Keyomarsi K, Tucker SL, Buchholz TA, et al. Cyclin E and survival in patients with breast cancer. N Engl J Med 2002;347:1566–75.

5. Braun S, Vogl FD, Naume B, et al. A pooled analysis of bone marrow micrometastasis in breast cancer. N Engl J Med 2005;353:793–802.

6. Backus J, Laughlin T, Wang Y, et al. Identification and characterization of optimal gene expression markers for detection of breast cancer metastasis. J Mol Diagn 2005;7:327–36.

7. Singletary SE, Allred C, Ashley P, et al. Revision of the American Joint Committee on Cancer staging system for breast cancer. J Clin Oncol 2002;20:3628–36.

8. Cristofanilli M, Budd GT, Ellis MJ, et al. Circulating tumor cells, disease progression, and survival in metastatic breast cancer. N Engl J Med 2004;351:781–91.

9. Ransohoff DF. Rules of evidence for cancer molecular-marker discovery and validation. Nat Rev Cancer 2004;4:309–14.

10. Simon R. Development and validation of therapeutically relevant multi-gene biomarker classifiers. J Natl Cancer Inst 2005;97:866–7.

11. Perou CM, Sorlie T, Eisen MB, et al. Molecular portraits of human breast tumours. Nature 2000;406:747–52.

12. Sorlie T, Perou CM, Tibshirani R, et al. Gene expression patterns of breast carcinomas distinguish tumor subclasses with clinical implications. Proc Natl Acad Sci U S A 2001;98:10869–74.

13. van't Veer LJ, Dai H, van de Vijver MJ, et al. Gene expression profiling predicts clinical outcome of breast cancer. Nature 2002;415:530–6.

14. van de Vijver MJ, He YD, van't Veer LJ, et al. A gene-expression signature as a predictor of survival in breast cancer. N Engl J Med 2002;347:1999–2009.

15. Eifel P, Axelson JA, Costa J, et al. National Institutes of Health Consensus Development Conference Statement: adjuvant therapy for breast cancer, November 1–3, 2000. J Natl Cancer Inst 2001;93:979–89.

16. Goldhirsch A, Glick JH, Gelber RD, et al. Meeting highlights: International Consensus Panel on the Treatment of Primary Breast Cancer. Seventh International Conference on Adjuvant Therapy of Primary Breast Cancer. J Clin Oncol 2001;19:3817–27.

17. Foekens JA, Atkins D, Zhang Y, et al. Multicenter validation of a gene expression-based prognostic signature in lymph node-negative primary breast cancer. J Clin Oncol 2006;24:1665–71.

18. Sotiriou C, Wirapati P, Loi S, et al. Gene expression profiling in breast cancer: understanding the molecular basis of histologic grade to improve prognosis. J Natl Cancer Inst 2006;98:262–72.

19. Wang Y, Klijn JG, Zhang Y, et al. Gene-expression profiles to predict distant metastasis of lymph-node-negative primary breast cancer. Lancet 2005;365:671–9.

20. Fan C, Oh DS, Wessels L, et al. Concordance among gene-expression-based predictors for breast cancer. N Engl J Med 2006;355:560–9.

21. Anderson K, Hess KR, Kapoor M, et al. Reproducibility of gene expression signature-based predictions in replicate experiments. Clin Cancer Res 2006;12:1721–7.

22. Ayers M, Symmans WF, Stec J, et al. Gene expression profiles predict complete pathologic response to neoadjuvant paclitaxel and fluorouracil, doxorubicin, and cyclophosphamide chemotherapy in breast cancer. J Clin Oncol 2004;22:2284–93.

23. Chang JC, Wooten EC, Tsimelzon A, et al. Gene expression profiling for the prediction of therapeutic response to

docetaxel in patients with breast cancer. Lancet 2003;362: 362–9.

24. Ma XJ, Wang Z, Ryan PD, et al. A two-gene expression ratio predicts clinical outcome in breast cancer patients treated with tamoxifen. Cancer Cell 2004;5:607–16.

25. Goetz MP, Suman VJ, Ingle JN, et al. A two-gene expression ratio of homeobox 13 and interleukin-17B receptor for prediction of recurrence and survival in women receiving adjuvant tamoxifen. Clin Cancer Res 2006;12:2080–7.

26. Symmans WF. Genomic testing for sensitivity of breast cancer to hormonal therapy. Clin Cancer Res 2006;12: 1954–5.

27. Paik S, Shak S, Tang G, et al. A multigene assay to predict recurrence of tamoxifen-treated, node-negative breast cancer. N Engl J Med 2004;351:2817–26.

28. Gianni L, Zambetti M, Clark K, et al. Gene expression profiles in paraffin-embedded core biopsy tissue predict response to chemotherapy in women with locally advanced breast cancer. J Clin Oncol 2005;23:7265–77.

Chapter 58

Surgical Management of Axillary Metastases from Occult Primary Breast Cancer

Waddah B. Al-Refaie, MD

Eric A. Strom, MD

Lavinia P. Middleton, MD

Gildy V. Babiera, MD

Introduction

Occult breast cancer that presents as disease in the axilla is rare, representing less than 1% of cases of breast cancer in most retrospective series.[1–4] In 1907, Halsted[5] first described this rare entity. In 1909, Cameron[6] advocated the classic surgical treatment of this disease, which consists of an ipsilateral mastectomy and axillary lymph node dissection for palpable axillary masses in the absence of clinical evidence of breast tumors. It wasn't until 1954 that the first retrospective study of 25 patients with axillary metastasis from an unknown primary cancer was reported.[2] Needless to say, because of its rarity, the entity has been described only in small retrospective series that extend over a long period of time, which may help explain the lack of consensus in the management of this uncommon form of breast cancer. And, despite improvements in current diagnostic modalities, patients with this unusual presentation of breast cancer are still encountered. In this chapter, the initial evaluation, diagnostic work-up, and multimodality treatment approach in patients with axillary nodal metastases from occult breast cancer are described.

Clinical Features and Diagnostic Evaluation

It is first important to recognize that clinically or radiographically detected lymphadenopathy is generally due to benign conditions. However, when a malignancy is suspected, one has to be prepared for dealing with a challenging diagnostic dilemma. This is because axillary nodes may become involved with lymphoma and other hematologic malignancies; adenocarcinoma of the breast, lung, colon, uterus, stomach, or thyroid; melanoma; and squamous cell carcinoma of the head and neck, among others. A detailed history and careful physical examination is an important component of the work-up in such patients. For example, patients should be asked about smoking history, prior biopsies or malignancies, family history of cancer, and prior excisions of moles, weight loss, and night sweats. The physical examination should include a detailed examination of both breasts, including the axillary and supraclavicular and infraclavicular compartment and other nodal basins throughout the body, as well as a pelvic and rectal exam (www.nccn.org). However, occult primary breast cancer represents the most common primary histology that can present as axillary lymphadenopathy. A schematic figure (Figure 1) represents the diagnostic work-up and treatment options for patients presumed to have axillary metastases secondary to an occult primary breast cancer.

In general, physical examination of the breasts in patients who present with an occult breast cancer to the axilla yields normal findings, except for those in the axilla. The initial work-up if the breast is felt to be the primary source of the abnormal axillary findings is to typically perform mammography and bilateral breast and axillary ultrasonography in an attempt to identify an area suspicious for breast cancer. In addition, it is imperative that the ultrasound study includes the ipsilateral axillary region as well as the other potentially involved regional lymph node basins, supraclavicular and internal mammary, to assess the extent of regional lymphadenopathy. If these tests fail to identify any suspicious findings in the breast, a percutaneous biopsy of the abnormal axillary lymph nodes (fine-needle aspiration or core-needle biopsy) should be performed. Fine-needle aspiration in such patients requires the skills of an experienced cytopathologist. A core-needle biopsy may also be performed to enable the pathologist to perform multiple histological stains to ascertain the location of the primary

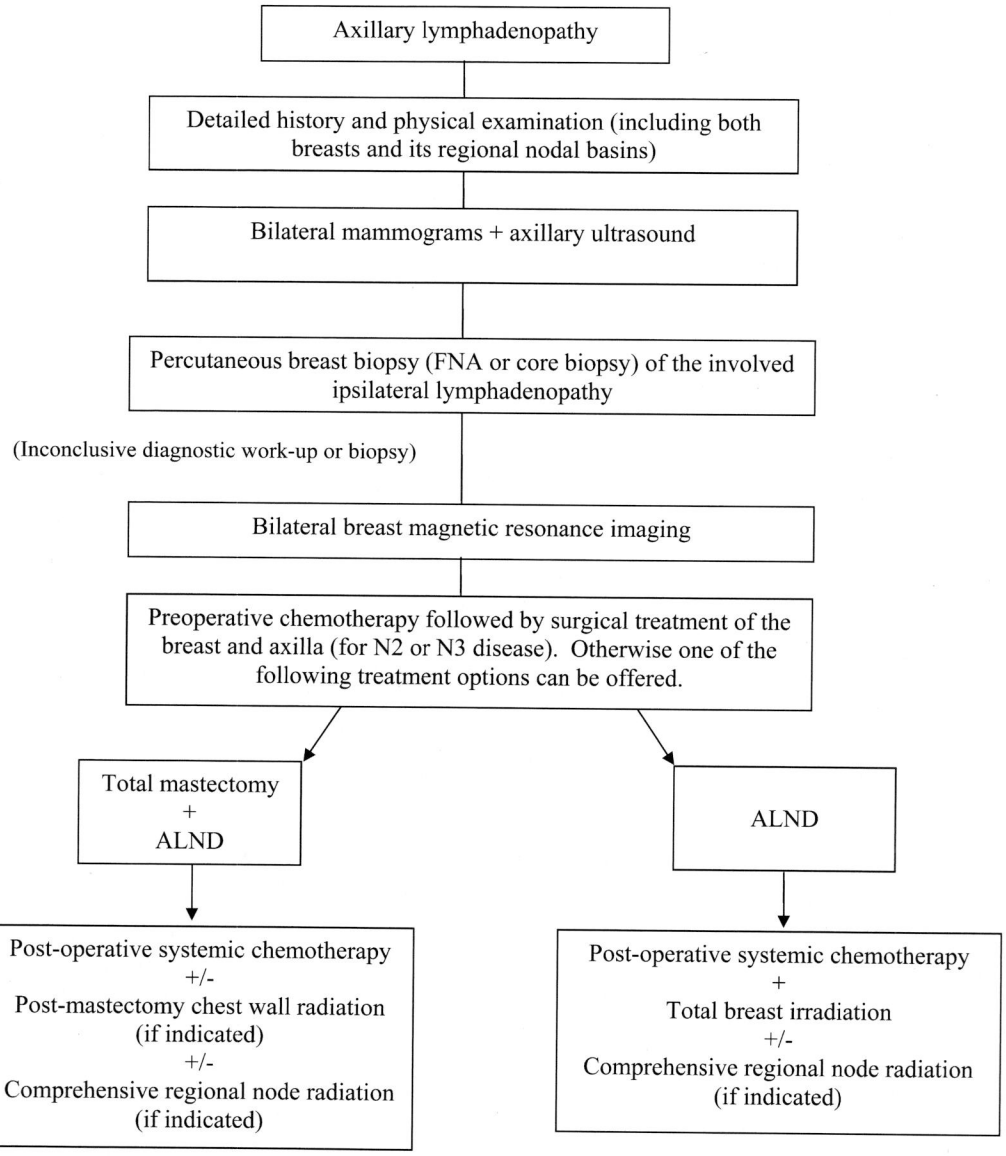

Figure 1

tumor, as will be described later in this chapter. An open excisional biopsy should be performed only when the findings from percutaneous biopsy are not diagnostic.

Once the nodal metastasis is established from a primary breast cancer histologically, patients undergo bilateral breast magnetic resonance imaging in an attempt to further identify the location of the primary breast cancer if routine imaging of the breast is inconclusive.[7,8]

The Importance of Immunohistochemistry Stains Features

The first determination to be made when evaluating an axillary mass pathologically is to ascertain if the mass represents a lymph node or heterotopic breast tissue that resides in the axilla. If normal breast parenchyma cannot be identified surrounding the neoplasm, and, rather, lymphocytes or a nodal capsule is present, an axillary metastasis is favored. The breast and axilla are uncommon sites for nonmammary metastases with almost 90% of axillary metastases originating from a breast primary. The likelihood of finding an occult primary lesion in the breast pathologically is directly related to the extent and thoroughness in which the breast specimen is sampled.[9,10]

By light microscopy a pathologist can determine if the tumor is an adenocarcinoma, squamous cell carcinoma, or lymphoma. If melanin pigment is observed, then the diagnosis of melanoma is suggested. Adenocarcinoma and melanoma make up the majority of metastases to the breast and axilla and may have overlapping morphologic features. Evaluating keratin, S-100, HMB-45, and MART-1, in the tumor can render the appropriate diagnosis. S-100, HMB-45, and MART-1 will be positive in melanoma; HMB-45 and MART-1 are negative in breast cancer. All of these aforementioned tumors can arise primary in the breast. When the histology is that of an adenocarcinoma with no specific discerning features, immunohistochemistry can aid in the evaluation of an unknown primary adenocarcinoma.

GCDFP-15 is a marker of apocrine differentiation, and when present, is highly suggestive of breast origin. Differential cytokeratin expression can also be evaluated; breast tumors are frequently CK7 positive and CK20 negative. The majority of lung carcinomas and many thyroid tumors are TTF-1 positive. To date, no TTF-1 breast cancers have been reported. And although a negative TTF-1 immunohistochemical stain is noncontributory, a positive stain will be more suggestive of a lung primary.

Estrogen and progesterone receptors have been evaluated in axillary nodal metastases harboring occult carcinoma. Two series have shown that in approximately one-third of cases, the tumors are positive for estrogen and progesterone, and 40% of the cases studied were negative for both hormones receptors.

Metastatic thyroid carcinoma has a distinct histomorphology. If a metastasis to the axilla is suspected, then thyroglobulin and TTF-1 immunohistochemistry can be performed. Calcitonin will be immunoreactive in cases of metastatic medullary thyroid carcinoma.

Wilms' Tumor-1 (Wt-1) is a transcription factor that is strongly expressed in ovarian serous and transitional cell carcinomas. Wt-1 immunohistochemical expression in nonmucinous ovarian carcinomas can reliably distinguish this entity from breast carcinoma. Wt-1 analysis is of limited value in discriminating breast carcinoma from ovarian mucinous, clear cell, or endometriod carcinoma, as these latter tumors are negative for Wt-1. For this differential diagnosis, the pathologist must rely on morphology and clinical suspicion.

Gatrointestinal mestastasis to the axilla are extremely uncommon. Metastatic colon carcinoma is histologically distinct, as it forms glands that are filled with eosinophilic debris containing nuclear fragments ("dirty necrosis"). If a metastasis from the colon is suspected by light microscopy, then CEA can be performed in addition to CK7 and CK20. The immunohistochemical profile of colorectal carcinoma is CEA positive, CK7 negative, and CK20 positive.

The Role of Radiation Therapy

Patients with occult breast primaries will often come to medical attention because of bulky lymph node involvement. Since patients with large numbers of involved axillary lymph nodes or those with fixed or matted adenopathy are at high risk for local-regional recurrence with surgery alone, most patients with occult primary tumors will require radiation therapy as a part of their treatment plan. Since local-regional irradiation is likely to be indicated owing to their advanced nodal presentations, few patients will be spared irradiation by performing a mastectomy.

Observation of the breast yields a high probability of subsequent tumor recurrence in the index breast. Thus, breast conservation with radiation is an appropriate option for most patients with axillary metastasis from occult primary breast cancer. Definitive treatment of the breast, at the same time as adjuvant treatment of the regional nodal basins, has proven to be highly successful by multiple investigators.[11–14]

Basic targets for radiation therapy include the skin and soft tissue of the chest wall after mastectomy or the intact breast and the undissected lymph nodes surrounding it. Modern treatment planning utilizes CT-based simulation to determine the specific patient anatomy of these volumes at risk and to identify adjacent critical structures that are to be avoided. After acquisition of the reference CT examination in the treatment position, virtual simulation of the desired fields then is performed. The breast is typically treated by tangential photon fields to a dose of 50 Gy in 25 fractions. In patients who have had an axillary dissection, the axillary apex and supraclavicular nodes are also treated using an anterior "third" field of photons to a dose of 50 Gy in 25 fractions. If the low axilla has not been formally been dissected, supplementation of this area to 50 Gy is indicated. Radiation of the internal mammary lymph nodes is considered elective in this population. However, the use of a separate internal mammary field in the postmastectomy setting may facilitate broad coverage of the anterior chest wall, while minimizing treatment of the interior thoracic contents, especially heart and lung. Additional details on the radiation set-up and technical delivery can be found in the fourth edition of Levitt and Tapley's *Technical Basis of Radiation Therapy*.[15]

Multimodality Treatment Approach for Axillary Metastases from Occult Primary Breast Cancer

The traditional surgical approach for patients with axillary metastases from an occult primary breast tumor has consisted of mastectomy and axillary lymph node dissection (see Figure 1). However, because of the rarity of this entity, it has not been possible to develop a standardized treatment approach guided by treatment outcome in a large population of patients with this entity. Looking to small retrospective studies for guidance has been hampered by a lack of proper standardization in patient selection and treatment approach. Intuitively, total mastectomy is a reasonable surgical treatment. Interestingly, the primary tumor in the mastectomy tumor specimen is identified in only up to 60% of cases. There are several potential explanations for this: (1) the primary breast cancer may have regressed during preoperative systemic therapy; (2) the primary breast cancer may be located somewhere else in the breast; or (3) as alluded to earlier, the primary tumor may have been missed during the histological sectioning and evaluation.

Blanchard and Farley[16] reported on the Mayo Clinic experience in 35 patients who had negative clinical and radiological findings but biopsy-proven axillary metastases from a primary breast cancer. Of these 35 patients, 18 underwent mastectomy, and 16 did not. Of the 16

patients not treated with mastectomy, 8 patients received chemotherapy, radiotherapy, or both, whereas 8 patients received no further treatment. The overall survival in patients who underwent mastectomy (72.7%) was more favorable than that in patients who did not undergo mastectomy (35.7%, $p = 0.047$). Further, the 5-year disease-free survival rate in patients who underwent mastectomy (72.7%) was better than that in patients who did not undergo mastectomy (35.7%, $p = 0.07$). Although the pattern of treatment in the nonsurgical therapy group was not stratified, the local recurrence rates were significantly higher in patients who underwent no surgical treatment (81%) than in those treated with mastectomy (36%). This reinforces the perception that local-regional control should be included in the primary therapy in these patients and that treatment should include chemotherapy, radiation therapy, or both.

Breast-conserving therapy is a feasible treatment option in selected cases, such as in patients with negative initial radiological findings, since they are likely to harbor smaller tumors. The possibility of performing breast-conserving surgery in certain patients is pointed up by the findings of Meterissian and colleagues,[17] who found that postoperative breast tissue specimens contained noninvasive breast cancer and invasive tumors (less than 1 cm) in up to 49% and 75% of cases, respectively. The feasibility of breast-conserving therapy in select patients was demonstrated by the study of Vlastos and colleagues,[13] who analyzed the feasibility of breast-conserving therapy in 45 patients with occult breast cancer. Over 70% of patients underwent breast preservation, with 78% receiving locoregional radiotherapy as well. At a median follow-up of 7 years, there was no significant difference in outcome between patients who underwent breast-conserving surgery and those patients who underwent mastectomy, as shown by the following rates: locoregional recurrence (13% vs 15%), distant recurrence (22% vs 31%), disease-free interval (72% vs 67%), and overall survival (79% vs 75%) ($p > 0.05$ for all previous outcome variables), respectively. These investigators identified that the total number of positive lymph nodes was a main determinant in survival regardless of the type of surgical therapy. That is, the 5-year survival rate was 87% for patients with 1 to 3 positive lymph nodes compared with 42% for patients with 4 or more positive lymph nodes ($p < 0.0001$). Campana and colleagues[11] similarly noted the negative impact of positive lymph nodes on survival in patients with occult breast cancer, as shown by a 5-year survival rate of 91% for those with less than 4 positive lymph nodes versus 65% for those with 4 or more positive lymph nodes ($p = 0.03$).

It is not appropriate to treat only the disease in the axilla (ie, observe the affected breast only), as larger studies have shown that the 5-year risk of recurrence in the nontreated breast approaches 57%.[18] This is underscored by the findings of Foroudi and Tiver,[19] who noted that the median recurrence-free survival in patients who received local treatment to the breast (182 months) was significantly longer than for those patients who were observed only (7 months, $p = 0.003$). Similarly, Shannon and colleagues,[20] from the Royal Marsden Hospital, found that rates of locoregional recurrence were higher in patients who did not receive radiation therapy (69%) than in patients who received radiotherapy (12.5%, $p = 0.02$). Ellerbroek and colleagues[18] likewise found that 57% of patients whose treatment did not include radiation therapy were at 5-year actuarial risk of appearance of primary tumor, whereas this occurred in only 17% of patients who underwent breast irradiation.

Given the current literature, patients with occult primary breast cancer in the axilla should undergo locoregional control of the breast and regional nodes in the form of axillary lymph node dissection with either breast-conserving therapy followed by radiotherapy or modified radical mastectomy, which may include postmastectomy radiation therapy, if indicated. Systemic chemotherapy is usually offered either in the neoadjuvant or adjuvant setting.

Special Considerations

Cross-metastasis to the contralateral axilla is rarely encountered; however, it is certainly an important entity to recognize and treat. Cross-metastases occur when patients have received treatment of their breast cancer and then go on to develop contralateral axillary metastases at a later time. It is postulated that this distinct type of metastases is due to tumor cells crossing the sternum to the contralateral breast via intraparenchymal and dermal lymphatic.[21–25] In a Danish study conducted by Nielsen and colleagues of 84 consecutive autopsies of patients with clinical invasive breast cancer, 16% of patients were found to harbor contralateral metastases to the breast and axilla. Further, 8 out of 84 patients (9.5%) developed contralateral axillary metastases in the absence of breast cancer in the contralateral breast specimens.[26]

The management for cross metastases can be challenging for two reasons. First, there are few published reports describing contralateral axillary cross-metastases, hence our limited understanding of its natural history. Second, physicians are faced with this scenario to decide whether these patients should be approached as stage II or stage IV disease. Prior to embarking on treating these

as stage IV disease, one has to exclude the development of a new contralateral primary breast cancer that has involved its regional lymph node basin or is presenting as second occult breast primary presenting in the axilla. Most investigators agree that patients will be considered to harbor metachronous node-positive contralateral breast cancer (stage II disease) if the histological and molecular markers were not similar between the new primary lesion and original breast cancer.[25] In any case, repeat metastatic work-up is also indicated if the patient presents with a cross-metastasis or new primary with metastasis to the regional nodal basin.

If the patient is felt to have cross-metastases, standardized locoregional treatment of the contralateral regional nodal basin is relatively unknown. Systemic therapy is certainly warranted in addition to a clinical assessment of the patient's long-term prognosis based on the patient's initial stage, time to cross-metastasis, and distant metastases (if present). Whether patients should be treated with surgery and/or radiation and at what time point of systemic treatment is unknown. However, it seems reasonable to suggest locoregional treatment in the setting of palliation or for curative intent if the patient demonstrates adequate control of their systemic disease.

Prognosis

Patients with axillary metastases from occult primary breast cancer are considered to have T0N1/2M0 stage disease, which is designated as AJCC stage II disease. It appears, however, from the several retrospective analyses[10,27] that have been done that the outcome in patients with occult breast cancer involving the axilla is more favorable than that in patients with stage II breast cancer.

Several investigators have evaluated the prognostic factors for patients who present with axillary metastases from an occult primary breast cancer. All have determined that the number of positive lymph nodes, particularly less than 4 positive lymph nodes versus 4 or more positive lymph nodes remains the most reliable predictor of outcome.[11,13]

Conclusions

Axillary metastases from occult primary breast cancer are a rare manifestation of breast cancer. A thorough preoperative diagnostic work-up should be performed in all such patients that include not only standard radiographic imaging with bilateral mammography, but also bilateral breast and regional nodal evaluation with ultrasound and magnetic resonance imaging of the breast in order to establish the location of the primary breast cancer. Although an occult breast cancer may be identified in only up to 60% of patients, treatment of the breast should consist of mastectomy, breast-conserving therapy, or whole-breast irradiation. Patients should also be offered axillary lymph node dissection to provide better local control of disease and complete staging information. Observation of the breast is not recommended, as this is associated with higher rates of locoregional recurrence. Further, patients should be treated with systemic chemotherapy, which may be offered in the preoperative setting. Although patients with occult breast cancer with axillary metastases are considered to have T0 N1/2M0 disease, the overall outcome appears to be more favorable in these patients than in those with stage II disease and an identifiable breast primary.

References

1. Copeland EM, McBride CM. Axillary metastases from unknown primary sites. Ann Surg 1973;178:25–7.

2. Owen HW, Dockerty MB, Gray HK. Occult carcinoma of the breast. Surg Gynecol Obstet 1954;98:302–8.

3. Patel J, Nemoto T, Rosner D, et al. Axillary lymph node metastasis from an occult breast cancer. Cancer 1981;47: 2923–7.

4. Rosen PP. Axillary lymph node metastases in patients with occult noninvasive breast carcinoma. Cancer 1980;46: 1298–306.

5. Halsted W. The results of radical operations for the cure of carcinoma of the breast. Ann Surg Oncol 1907;46:1–19.

6. Cameron H. Some clinical facts regarding mammary cancr. BMJ 1909;1:577–82.

7. Henry-Tillman RS, Harms SE, Westbrook KC, et al. Role of breast magnetic resonance imaging in determining breast as a source of unknown metastatic lymphadenopathy. Am J Surg 1999;178:496–500.

8. Orel SG, Weinstein SP, Schnall MD, et al. Breast MR imaging in patients with axillary node metastases and unknown primary malignancy. Radiology 1999;212:543–9.

9. Baron PL, Moore MP, Kinne DW, et al. Occult breast cancer presenting with axillary metastases. Updated management. Arch Surg 1990;125:210–4.

10. Rosen PP, Kimmel M. Occult breast carcinoma presenting with axillary lymph node metastases: a follow-up study of 48 patients. Hum Pathol 1990;21:518–23.

11. Campana F, Fourquet A, Ashby MA, et al. Presentation of axillary lymphadenopathy without detectable breast primary (T0 N1b breast cancer): experience at Institut Curie. Radiother Oncol 1989;15:321–5.

12. Merson M, Andreola S, Galimberti V, et al. Breast carcinoma presenting as axillary metastases without evidence of a primary tumor. Cancer 1992;70:504–8.

13. Vlastos G, Jean ME, Mirza AN, et al. Feasibility of breast preservation in the treatment of occult primary carcinoma presenting with axillary metastases. Ann Surg Oncol 2001; 8:425–31.

14. Whillis D, Brown PW, Rodger A. Adenocarcinoma from an unknown primary presenting in women with an axillary mass. Clin Oncol (R Coll Radiol) 1990;2:189–92.

15. Levitt SH, Purdy JA, Perez CA, Vijayakumar S, editors. Technical basis of radiation therapy: practical and clinical applications. 4th ed New York: Springer; 2006.

16. Blanchard DK, Farley DR. Retrospective study of women presenting with axillary metastases from occult breast carcinoma. World J Surg 2004;28:535–9.

17. Meterissian S, Fornage BD, Singletary SE. Clinically occult breast carcinoma: diagnostic approaches and role of axillary node dissection. Ann Surg Oncol 1995;2:314–8.

18. Ellerbroek N, Holmes F, Singletary E, et al. Treatment of patients with isolated axillary nodal metastases from an occult primary carcinoma consistent with breast origin. Cancer 1990;66:1461–7.

19. Foroudi F, Tiver KW. Occult breast carcinoma presenting as axillary metastases. Int J Radiat Oncol Biol Phys 2000;47: 143–7.

20. Shannon C, Walsh G, Sapunar F, et al. Occult primary breast carcinoma presenting as axillary lymphadenopathy. Breast 2002;11:414–8.

21. Broet P, de la Rochefordiere A, Scholl SM, et al. [Contralateral breast cancer: metastasis or second primary cancer?]. Bull Cancer 1996;83:870–6.

22. de la Rochefordiere A, Mouret-Fourme E, Asselain B, et al. Metachronous contralateral breast cancer as first event of relapse. Int J Radiat Oncol Biol Phys 1996;36:615–21.

23. Dewar JA, Arriagada R, Benhamou S, et al. Local relapse and contralateral tumor rates in patients with breast cancer treated with conservative surgery and radiotherapy (Institut Gustave-Roussy 1970–1982). IGR Breast Cancer Group. Cancer 1995;76:2260–5.

24. Jaffer S, Goldfarb AB, Gold JE, et al. Contralateral axillary lymph node metastasis as the first evidence of locally recurrent breast carcinoma. Cancer 1995;75:2875–8.

25. Janschek E, Kandioler-Eckersberger D, Ludwig C, et al. Contralateral breast cancer: molecular differentiation between metastasis and second primary cancer. Breast Cancer Res Treat 2001;67:1–8.

26. Nielsen M, Christensen L, Andersen J. Contralateral cancerous breast lesions in women with clinical invasive breast carcinoma. Cancer 1986;57:897–903.

27. van Ooijen B, Bontenbal M, Henzen-Logmans SC, Koper PC. Axillary nodal metastases from an occult primary consistent with breast carcinoma. Br J Surg 1993; 80:1299–300.

LOCALLY ADVANCED AND INFLAMMATORY BREAST CANCER

JUDY C. BOUGHEY, MD

FREDERICK C. AMES, MD

Locally Advanced Breast Cancer

Locally advanced breast cancer (LABC) represents a heterogeneous subgroup of breast cancer that assumes a wide variety of clinical scenarios, often with dismal outcomes. LABC now constitutes a smaller percentage of the breast cancers than was once the case because of the growing use of mammography and the resultant increase in early detection. However, in the underserved populations of the United States and in the populations of developing countries, LABC represents more than half of newly diagnosed breast cancers.

LABC is characterized by tumors that are large. The primary tumor can be > 5 cm (T3) or involve the skin (T4a) or chest wall (T4b). There can also be extensive regional lymph node involvement without metastatic disease. The nodes involved can be infraclavicular (N3a), supraclavicular (N3c), matted or fixed axillary (N2a), or internal mammary (N2b or N3b). LABC includes stages IIB, IIIA, IIIB, and IIIC of the American Joint Committee on Cancer staging system.[1] Despite the advanced stage of the disease at presentation, a significant percentage of these patients can be cured, and they should be treated with curative intent. Inflammatory breast cancer (IBC) is a very aggressive and lethal form of LABC and will be discussed in the second portion of this chapter.

DIAGNOSIS AND DETECTION OF LABC

Because LABC is an advanced form of cancer, most cases are detected by the patients themselves or family members; the remainder are found during routine physical examinations. Presenting signs include a large palpable mass in the breast or axilla, breast enlargement, discoloration, or ulceration. Often these changes have been evident for long before the patient seeks medical attention. Occasionally, patients with LABC may present with a supraclavicular mass or with diffuse induration of the breast in the absence of an easily palpable mass.

The majority of LABC tumors are poorly differentiated and aneuploid, and more than 80% are associated with lymph node involvement. Tumors frequently exhibit necrosis, lymphatic invasion, and vascularity. The majority are hormone receptor positive, and Her-2/*neu* is overexpressed in a proportion of tumors similar to that of other stages of primary breast cancer.

WORK-UP OF LABC

Patients presenting with LABC should undergo full history and physical examination focusing on the breasts and axillary, infraclavicular, supraclavicular, and cervical lymph node basins. The radiographic work-up should include bilateral diagnostic mammograms to assess the extent of disease in the breast, the area involved by calcifications, if any, and the contralateral breast for any abnormalities such as synchronous bilateral breast cancer. Ultrasonography (US) of the breast and regional lymph node basins (axillary, internal mammary, infraclavicular, and supraclavicular) along with fine-needle aspiration (FNA) biopsy of any suspicious lymph nodes provides additional staging information. The primary breast tumor should undergo core needle biopsy either under US or stereotactic guidance to ensure definitive tissue diagnosis of the tumor's histologic type and grade, estrogen receptor (ER) and progesterone receptor (PR) status, and HER2/neu amplification status. All of this information is important in confirming invasive disease and directing treatment.

A full metastatic work-up to stage the disease should include a bone scan, chest X-ray study, and computed tomography scan of the abdomen and pelvis. A complete blood count and renal and hepatic laboratory assessments should also be done. Additional tests should be performed based on the patient's history and any abnormal physical findings.

TREATMENT OF LABC

In the past, LABC was treated initially with a radical mastectomy alone with high rates of regional failure and poor survival. Radiation therapy alone to the breast also failed to achieve local control in the majority of patients, which led to the use of radical surgery and radiation combined, which achieved a high degree of local-regional control, but overall survival (OS) remained poor and the morbidity (especially related to lymphedema) was high. As soon as effective chemotherapy became available with anthracyclines, chemotherapy used in LABC and an improvement in survival was seen. At the same time, we began to explore lesser surgery with preservation of the pectoralis major muscle (modified radical mastectomy) when feasible in an effort to reduce the morbidity. In patients with LABC that was deemed inoperable due to the extent of tumor, clinicians began to use chemotherapy as a first line therapy in the hopes of achieving operable status with response. Initial fears that fungating tumors treated with primary systemic chemotherapy may be associated with septic complications or bleeding were not realized. As experience was gained with chemotherapy in the neoadjuvant setting in inoperable LABC, it became standard of care for most LABCs because neoadjuvant chemotherapy facilitated surgical resection.

NEOADJUVANT CHEMOTHERAPY IN LABC

Neoadjuvant chemotherapy, followed by surgery and radiation therapy and occasionally adjuvant chemotherapy, is the multimodal treatment regimen that has become our standard of care for LABC. One study has shown that there is no difference in local recurrence, distant recurrence, or OS[2] between neoadjuvant and adjuvant chemotherapy; however, patients who achieve a pathologically complete response (pCR) have improved outcomes. In fact, a pCR in the breast and axillary lymph nodes is the best predictor of an improved outcome and prolonged survival. In one study, 75% of patients

achieved a clinical response to neoadjuvant chemotherapy, with a median reduction in tumor size of 50%.[2] Decreasing the size of the tumor can make inoperable cancers operable and also enable up to 45% of the patients who would have required mastectomy to undergo breast conservation therapy (BCT).[3–7]

With neoadjuvant chemotherapy, oncologists can individualize patient treatment based on the tumor's in vivo response to the chemotherapy. If the tumor is not responding it allows us to switch to alternative therapies. Interestingly, it is also possible that leaving the tumor in vivo during chemotherapy initiation inhibits the development or growth of distant metastases.[8] However, if neoadjuvant chemotherapy does not yield a satisfactory response after four cycles, the multidisciplinary team should evaluate the situation and consider switching to an alternative chemotherapy regimen or different treatment modality.

For LABC, chemotherapy used to consist primarily of an anthracycline-based regimen, with 60 to 90% of patients undergoing tumor regression and 8 to 13% experiencing pCRs. Newer agents have improved the response to chemotherapy. For example, treatment with taxanes such as docetaxel and paclitaxel has increased response rates to up to 94%.[9–11] In patients with operable breast cancer receiving neoadjuvant chemotherapy, sequential doxorubicin, cyclophosphamide, and docetaxel were more effective at inducing pCR than concurrent dose-dense doxorubicin and docetaxel.[12] In that study, a negative hormone receptor status and high tumor grade were also predictive factors for pCR.[12] In another study, 10 of 51 patients (20%) experienced a pCR after four cycles of neoadjuvant docetaxel followed by surgery and four cycles of doxorubicin and cyclophosphamide.[13] In that study, single-agent docetaxel was an effective neoadjuvant treatment for patients with LABC, and a clinical response was associated with improved survival. Even more, a review of Phase II and III trials of taxanes as neoadjuvant chemotherapy supported including a taxane in neoadjuvant regimens for patients with LABC.[14] In summary, studies have shown that adding a taxane to therapeutic regimens yields better clinical and pathologic responses than anthracycline-based regimens alone.

SURGICAL MANAGEMENT OF LABC

Patients with inoperable breast tumors, those that are stage IIIB and IIIC, require neoadjuvant chemotherapy prior to surgical resection and radiation. Patients who do not respond to neoadjuvant chemotherapy should then be switched to a different chemotherapeutic regimen if available. If the patient has not responded, but is resectable, mastectomy with flap coverage followed by postoperative radiation is recommended. If the patient remains with disease beyond the surgical field, radiation is often chosen as a last resort, sometimes followed by surgical resection if possible, which may require flap coverage. Once election for radiation is made, the team needs to understand that radiation changes may obscure the skin findings on physical examination due to skin thickening and edema from the radiation therapy.

Although patients with stage IIB and IIIA LABC have potentially operable breast tumors, these patients also benefit from neoadjuvant chemotherapy because it can improve their breast conservation rate and improve their potential for pCR, which improves survival. If a patient's tumor shrinks to less than 2 cm, tumor markers should be placed to avoid a blind surgical excision, which increases the likelihood that residual disease will remain after resection. Even among patients with clinically complete responses (cCRs), 50% are found to have tumor on pathologic examination; therefore, surgical excision is required in all cases.[15] After completing chemotherapy, a patient should undergo mammography, US of the breast and regional nodal basins, and assessment by the surgeon. If the residual tumor is resectable by partial mastectomy, the patient can be offered BCT; if not, a total mastectomy should be performed.

If a patient does not wish to receive neoadjuvant chemotherapy, they can opt to undergo surgical excision—usually a total mastectomy and sentinel lymph node (SLN) surgery or axillary lymph node dissection (ALND) in patients with positive nodal disease. These patients then receive chemotherapy in the adjuvant setting and radiation.

BCT AFTER NEOADJUVANT CHEMOTHERAPY

In 1992, The University of Texas M. D. Anderson Cancer Center performed a study to evaluate the feasibility of BCT in LABC patients after neoadjuvant chemotherapy.[7] In all, 143 patients with stage IIB, IIIA, or IIIB disease or documented supraclavicular nodal disease received vincristine, doxorubicin, cyclophosphamide, and prednisone and underwent total mastectomy and ALNDs. Thirty-three (23%) patients met the BCT criteria of having a complete resolution of skin edema, residual tumors smaller than 5 cm, and an absence of known tumor multicentricity or extensive intramammary lymphatic invasion. In these patients, the initial tumor size decreased from a median of 5 cm to less than 1 cm, with 42% of patients having no residual tumors in their mastectomy specimens and 45% having negative lymph nodes. These 33 patients would have been appropriate

candidates for BCT rather than mastectomy for control of their breast disease.

To be a candidate for BCT, a patient's residual tumor should be smaller than 4 cm, but patients who have larger tumors in larger breasts that appear resectable with a margin of normal tissue can also be offered BCT. Contraindications to BCT include multifocal disease, extensive calcifications on mammography, persistent skin edema, tumors fixated to the skin or chest wall, positive surgical margins, and contraindications to radiation, such as collagen vascular disease.

LABC with initial skin involvement (T4 lesion) is not a contraindication to BCT. In fact, a review of 33 patients with stage IIIB or IIIC breast cancer treated with neoadjuvant chemotherapy, BCT, radiation, and consolidation chemotherapy at M. D. Anderson Cancer Center revealed that a complete resolution of skin changes was seen in 88% of the patients. The 5-year disease-free survival (DFS) rate was 70%, and the breast tumor recurrence rate was 6% at 5 years.[16] Therefore patients with skin involvement (T4 lesion) at presentation can still be candidates for BCT if tumor shrinkage and resolution of skin changes is seen after neoadjuvant chemotherapy.

Generally, patients who are not candidates for BCT or who would prefer a mastectomy should undergo mastectomy. All surgery should be scheduled 2 to 6 weeks after the completion of chemotherapy depending on chemotherapy used. A white cell count (WCC) of greater than 1,000 is preferred, although in the past we have operated on patients with WCCs as low as 800.

MASTECTOMY WITH LOCAL TISSUE FLAP COVERAGE

Patients with inadequate response to neoadjuvant chemotherapy or who have disease progression during chemotherapy should be treated with either surgery or radiation followed by surgical resection. The extent of surgery needs to be guided by intraoperative assessment of the radial and deep margins. On occasion where there is an open contaminated wound preoperatively or a deeper level of involvement is found that requires more extensive surgery than was planned for, such as a chest wall resection, either a temporary skin graft or a wound vac system is used as a bridge until definitive surgery is planned. Full thickness chest wall resection or resection of the pectoral muscles with appropriate flap coverage is feasible in LABC as long as no life threatening distant disease is present.

If significant skin and soft tissue requires resection, local tissue flap coverage, which requires the assistance of a plastic and reconstructive surgery team, is performed.

Skin and soft tissue defects can be covered with autologous tissue transfer such as latissimus dorsi flap or rectus abdominis flap. If only skin coverage is needed, a split-thickness skin graft (STSG) can be placed immediately. Larger coverage areas can benefit from the placement of a vacuum-assisted closure (VAC) device to allow the area to contract and develop a healthy bed of granulation tissue before a STSG is completed. Importantly, a patient who has undergone an STSG may need longer to heal than a patient undergoing primary closure or local tissue flap coverage. This prolonged healing time can delay radiation therapy, and STSGs are not as durable and may break down during radiation therapy. Additionally the cosmetic appearance is better with local tissue flaps; however, the donor site morbidity is greater with autologous tissue transfers than STSG and therefore these options should be assessed with each individual case.

When tumor extends into the chest wall, an en bloc resection for local control of the tumor requires the assistance of a thoracic surgery team. Mesh is used if needed to reconstruct the chest wall. In these situations, pedicled flaps are preferred to avoid the potential loss of the flap and the resultant exposure of the chest wall.

AXILLARY STAGING IN LABC

SLN surgery is feasible and highly accurate for patients with large, intact primary tumors. For example, Bedrosian and colleagues evaluated 87 patients with T2 tumors and 17 patients with T3 tumors who had clinically negative axillac and identified the SLN in 99% of the patients, with a false negative rate of 3%.[17] Another study of 41 patients with tumors 5 cm and larger revealed a 98% accuracy in identifying the SLNs, with a false negative rate of 3%.[18] Overall, the use of SLN surgery can help nearly one-third of LABC patients avoid ALND.[18]

Prior to the widespread use of neoadjuvant chemotherapy, ALND was performed to obtain the staging information required to determine whether chemotherapy, radiation therapy, or both were needed. Since then, it has been established that the use of neoadjuvant chemotherapy results in the downstaging of clinically positive axillary lymph nodes in approximately 32% of cases.[19] Now most patients with LABC receive neoadjuvant chemotherapy and adjuvant radiation regardless of axillary lymph node status. Therefore, the primary reason for ALND in lymph node-positive patients with LABC is to gain local control of the disease. Interestingly, some recent reports have suggested that equivalent local-regional control can be achieved with neoadjuvant chemotherapy followed by ALND or axillary radiation therapy.[20]

SLN Surgery in LABC Treated with Neoadjuvant Chemotherapy

Because the number of metastatic axillary lymph nodes remaining after neoadjuvant chemotherapy is one of the strongest predictors of DFS,[21] and the more positive nodes present after chemotherapy, the worse the prognosis,[22] obtaining accurate staging information is beneficial in patients who have been identified as having axillary disease.

How best to stage the axilla after neoadjuvant chemotherapy remains controversial. In our practice, all patients undergo physical examinations and US to stage their regional nodes (axilla, infraclavicular, supraclavicular, internal mammary) prior to the initiation of therapy.[23] Any nodes that appear suspicious on US undergo an US-guided FNA. The overall sensitivity of US-guided FNA is 86% with a specificity of 100%.[24] And although its sensitivity is somewhat decreased for patients who have had neoadjuvant chemotherapy, US-guided FNA remains a simple, minimally invasive, and reliable technique for the initial determination of axillary lymph node status. Based on the diagnostic results, patients with positive lymph nodes undergo ALND at the time of their surgical resection of their primary tumor. We have confidence in the focused US examination and therefore perform SLN after neoadjuvant chemotherapy in patients without nodal disease documented on US examination at presentation.

Patients without documented axillary disease prior to chemotherapy undergo SLN surgery at the time of their surgical resection. When chemotherapy was first applied as a neoadjuvant treatment, it was not clear whether its effects would impair SLN's reliability; but now that there is more experience with SLN surgery after neoadjuvant chemotherapy at our institution, the SLN identification rate after neoadjuvant chemotherapy has increased from 65% to 94%.[25] Other recent studies have shown SLN surgery to be as reliable in patients who have received chemotherapy as it is in patients who have not.[26,27] Based on that information, we recommend that if the SLN findings are positive, completion ALND be performed, and that if the SLN findings are negative, no further axillary surgery be required.

Nonetheless, some surgeons remain concerned about the reliability of SLN surgery after chemotherapy. For this reason, they may recommend that their patients all undergo SLN surgery at the time of diagnosis, prior to chemotherapy. If the SLN is positive, an ALND is then performed with the surgical resection of the primary tumor after neoadjuvant chemotherapy is completed. If the SLN is negative in these situations, no further axillary staging is required. Studies from Massachusetts General

Hospital reported SLN identification rates of 81% after neoadjuvant chemotherapy compared to 100% identification rates prior to chemotherapy; however, the failure to map correlated with clinically positive nodal disease at presentation and residual disease at the time of ALND.[28]

Recent data from University of Michigan has illustrated that it is possible to perform SLN biopsy after neoadjuvant chemotherapy in patients who were initially lymph node positive prior to chemotherapy. These researchers found residual axillary disease in 35 of 54 patients (65%), with a false-negative SLN rate of 8.6%.[29] The use of SLN surgery in patients undergoing neoadjuvant chemotherapy with known nodal disease remains controversial and is under investigation.

IMMEDIATE RECONSTRUCTION IN PATIENTS WITH LABC

Immediate reconstruction is possible in patients with LABC.[30] An M. D. Anderson study compared 122 patients from 1990 to 1993 with stage IIB, IIIA, and IIIB LABC: 50 underwent immediate breast reconstruction using latissimus dorsi flap, transverse rectus abdominis myocutaneous (TRAM) flap, or implants, and 72 underwent modified radical mastectomy without reconstruction. The study showed that reconstruction was associated with a longer delay before adjuvant chemotherapy could commence, but there was no significant difference in local or distant relapse rates. Autologous tissue is preferred over implants because most LABC patients require postoperative radiation therapy. Of the 15 patients who received implant reconstruction, seven (47%) required subsequent implant removal because of contractures or infections.[30] Another report on 35 patients who underwent mastectomy and immediate TRAM flap reconstruction with postmastectomy radiation showed a 100% flap survival rate and a local recurrence rate of 3% at 4 years. These results further indicated that immediate TRAM breast reconstruction followed by radiation therapy is safe, with minimal morbidity and no significant change in tissue volume.[31]

Currently we prefer to delay breast reconstruction until all therapy for LABC has been completed in order to facilitate delivery of comprehensive chest wall radiation to the chest wall and regional nodal basins. Because this is an advanced stage of breast cancer and metastases and local failure rates are higher with advanced disease, it is preferable to prioritize radiation therapy for local control and chemotherapy for the control of occult metastases and to ensure that the administration of both are timed to maximize the chance of cure. In the past we have considered patients who achieved operable status for immediate reconstruction, as discussed.

At M. D. Anderson, an "immediate delayed" reconstruction[32] has been developed for use in patients with early-stage breast cancer in whom the need for postmastectomy radiation is not known prior to surgery. Currently, an extension of this technique is being investigated at M. D. Anderson: "delayed delayed" reconstruction involves the placement of a subpectoral tissue expander at the time of mastectomy that is expanded while the patient recovers from surgery (and during chemotherapy, if given in the adjuvant setting). During radiation therapy, the expander is deflated so it lies flat on the chest wall. It is then re-inflated after radiation therapy. Finally, the patient's reconstruction is completed with an autologous tissue flap, the skin envelope having been preserved.

RADIATION IN LABC

Radiation is an integral part of therapy for LABC. Although radiation therapy decreases local recurrence rates for all patients undergoing BCT, it is particularly important in patients with LABC because local recurrence risks are greater, and multifocality and multicentricity are more common for this type of breast cancer than any other.[7] Decreasing local recurrences reduces breast cancer mortality.[33]

Patients undergoing mastectomy for LABC are also at increased risk for local failure, and even after neoadjuvant chemotherapy and mastectomy, comprehensive radiation has been shown to enhance both local control and OS in LABC.[34] In fact, even the achievement of a pCR does not preclude the need for postmastectomy radiation,[35] which is recommended for patients who present with T3 or T4 disease and those with four or more involved lymph nodes. It is not yet clear if radiation would benefit women with three or fewer involved lymph nodes. The decision regarding radiation is based on the clinical stage of the disease at presentation, regardless of the response to chemotherapy, and radiation is delivered after any adjuvant chemotherapy regimens are completed.

ENDOCRINE THERAPY IN LABC

Because the majority of LABCs are hormone-receptor positive, endocrine therapy has an important role in the treatment of this disease. Patients with hormone-receptive tumors should receive adjuvant endocrine therapy after the completion of chemotherapy, surgery, and radiation therapy.

Endocrine therapy also has an occasional role as a neoadjuvant agent, especially in patients with substantial comorbidities, which may limit the use of other systemic agents. Neoadjuvant tamoxifen produces tumor regression in 30 to 50% of patients. Neoadjuvant anastrozole is as effective as tamoxifen in ER-positive patients and can make 44% of patients initially eligible for mastectomy only candidates for BCT.[36,37] Neoadjuvant letrozole is associated with response rates of 53 to 60% and a 45 to 47% BCT rate.[38,39] A prospective randomized clinical trial is currently under way that is comparing neoadjuvant exemestane, letrozole, and anastrozole in postmenopausal women with stage II and III ER-positive breast cancer. The best neoadjuvant endocrine agent from that study will then be compared in another trial with neoadjuvant chemotherapy.

Neoadjuvant endocrine therapy takes a longer time, up to 4 to 6 months, to achieve a measurable response and therefore in patients that are not candidates for neoadjuvant chemotherapy, surgery is considered first if the tumor is resectable and endocrine therapy is used in an adjuvant setting.

TRASTUZUMAB IN LABC

Neoadjuvant use of trastuzumab in tumors with Her-2/*neu* overexpression has been shown to increase pCR rates in early-stage breast cancer,[40] but the results of trials with trastuzumab in patients with LABC are still being evaluated. One small study of patients with LABC showed a pCR in the breast in 23% of its patients and a pCR in the breast and axilla in 17% of its patients, with the use of neoadjuvant docetaxel, cisplatin, and trastuzumab. The 4-year progression-free survival (PFS) was 81%, and OS was 86%. Patients who achieved a pCR in the breast and axilla had PFS and OS rates of 100%.[41] Another small neoadjuvant trial involved the administration to 35 patients with LABC once a week as a single agent for 3 weeks, followed by a combination of trastuzumab and docetaxel for 12 weeks before surgery. After the first 3 weeks of trastuzumab, the median tumor volume decreased by 20%.[42]

PROGNOSTIC INDICATORS IN LABC

Many of the established prognostic factors in LABC are similar to those for early-stage breast cancer and include the extent of the disease at presentation (large primary tumors and fixation to the chest wall or skin), involvement of regional nodes, poor differentiation of tumors, and a high proliferative index. Hormone receptor expression confers a slight prognostic advantage, predominantly because it is a predictor of the disease's response to endocrine therapy. Also, baseline serum levels of carcinoembryonic antigen (CEA) and CA 15.3 are independent predictors of outcome in LABC.[43] As detailed in previous sections, the response to neoadjuvant chemotherapy is an independent predictor of survival; specifically, patients with LABC who have a pCR in both the breast and the axilla have significantly improved DFS rates.[44]

PREDICTORS OF LOCAL-REGIONAL RECURRENCE

A review of 542 patients with stage II, IIIA, IIIB, and IV breast cancer treated at M. D. Anderson with neoadjuvant chemotherapy, mastectomy, and postmastectomy radiation therapy demonstrated an overall local-regional recurrence (LRR) rate of 11% at 10 years. Predictors for LRR were skin or nipple involvement, supraclavicular nodal disease, absence of tamoxifen use, extracapsular extension, and ER-negative disease.[40] In the 74% of this population that had two or fewer LRR risk factors, the 10-year LRR rate was less than 8%; in contrast, patients with three or more risk factors had a 10-year LRR rate of 28% despite receiving chemotherapy, surgery, and radiation therapy.

LONG-TERM OUTCOME OF LABC

Patients with LABC have poor prognoses, with 5-year OS rates of 30 to 60% depending on nodal staging and other prognostic indicators as described in a previous section. 15-year OS rates are 50% for stage IIIA cancer and 23% for stage IIIB noninflammatory breast cancer[45]; most of the patients received anthracycline-based chemotherapy. The outcome in patients who receive today's current chemotherapy and endocrine agents is not known.

Inflammatory Breast Cancer

Inflammatory Breast Cancer (IBC), the most aggressive form of primary breast cancer, is a unique clinical entity that is relatively rare, with an incidence rate of 1 to 6% in the United States.[46] It is characterized by rapid disease progression and a poor prognosis. Compared to non-IBC cancers, IBC has lower OS rates.[45,47] Fortunately, the treatment of IBC has improved significantly over the last two decades, as evidenced by increases in local control and survival rates. Standard treatment today is multimodal, with chemotherapy prior to surgery because experience has shown the many limitations of using first-line surgical therapy against IBC.

DEFINITION OF IBC

LABC and IBC are both advanced breast carcinomas with poor prognoses. The two can be difficult to differentiate, especially when LABC presents with secondary IBC features. A diagnosis of IBC requires documentation of the rapid onset of symptoms and signs based on the classic diagnostic criteria for IBC established by

Haagensen.[48] These criteria include diffuse erythema, edema involving more than two-thirds of the breast, peau d'orange, tenderness, induration, warmth, breast enlargement, and diffuseness (or absence) of a tumor on palpation. Often, no mass can be detected on physical examination or mammography owing to the disease's diffuse involvement throughout the lymphatics, although imaging may show a mass or thickening of the breast skin. Although a biopsy of the affected skin may show clusters of tumor cells within the dermal lymphatics, such clusters can be noted in any stage of breast cancer, which makes that pathologic feature neither required nor conclusive of IBC. Classic IBC develops rapidly with signs and symptoms appearing fewer than 3 months before diagnosis.

Primary IBC is the simultaneous development of inflammatory skin changes and carcinoma in a previously healthy breast, whereas secondary IBC is the development of inflammatory changes in a breast that has had a previous malignancy or has a mastectomy scar or changes caused by irradiation. The distinction between classic IBC and noninflammatory LABC with secondary inflammatory features can be extremely difficult to make, even for the most experienced clinician. In addition to documenting the rapid onset of symptoms and signs mentioned above, lymphatic embolization, if present, can be used as a contributory but not pathognomonic criterion. Unfortunately, IBC is often misdiagnosed, and the differentiation between primary and secondary IBC is not often made.

INCIDENCE OF IBC

Data from the Surveillance, Epidemiology and End Results (SEER) program that compared trends and patterns for breast cancer revealed the overall age-adjusted incidence of IBC had doubled (increasing among white women from 0.3 to 0.7 cases per 100,000 person-years between the two periods of 1975 to 1977 and 1990 to1992). This twofold increase in IBC incidence is higher than was observed for non-IBC breast cancers.[47]

AGE, RACE, AND SEX DISTRIBUTION OF IBC

Patients with IBC are significantly younger and more likely to be pre- or perimenopausal than patients with noninflammatory LABC.[47] Among white women, the mean age at diagnosis for IBC is 57 years, compared to 62 years for other breast carcinomas ($p = .0001$).[47] African American women have a higher incidence of IBC than Caucasians and other ethnic groups (10.1%, 6.2%, and 5.1%, respectively)[49] and are affected at a younger age than white women.[47] Within the African American

population, IBC patients' mean age at diagnosis is 52 years, compared to 57 years—the mean age at diagnosis for African American patients with other breast cancers ($p = .0003$).

IBC has been reported in men, but the rarity of breast cancer in men makes the study of IBC in men predominantly anecdotal.

CLINICAL CHARACTERISTICS AND NATURAL COURSE IN IBC

The painless enlargement of the affected breast is generally followed by a sensation of heaviness and slight burning. Within days, redness and thickening of the skin appears, which leads to the classic "peau d'orange" appearance. The rate of growth is rapid, and without treatment the process can soon involve the entire breast. The skin becomes even more reddened, and eventually reddening can spread beyond the borders of the breast. Mild tenderness may or may not be present, and the skin becomes warm to the touch. Nipple retraction is seen when the central portion of the breast is involved with the disease process. Approximately one-half of patients with IBC also experience pain. IBC is often mistaken for an infectious process, such as cellulitis or mastitis, resulting in frequent delays in diagnosis and treatment.

In secondary IBC, a mass has been present, and inflammatory changes occur in the overlying skin. These symptoms usually progress rapidly, and patients frequently have axillary node involvement by the time they seek medical attention. One-third of patients present with diffuse involvement of the entire breast, and axillary lymph nodes are palpable in 50 to 75% of patients. Distant metastases are found in 10 to 36% of cases. Without systemic treatment, the fulminant course of the disease leads to death of more than 90% of patients within 1 year.

CLASSIFICATION, STAGING, AND DIAGNOSIS OF IBC

The evaluation of patients presenting with IBC is multidisciplinary and includes history and physical examination, diagnostic mammography, and US of the breast and regional lymph node basins. A biopsy for diagnosis should include a segment of involved skin because there is usually no dominant mass palpable in a physical examination. Additionally a metastatic work-up should be obtained to rule out distant disease.

PATHOLOGY OF IBC

IBC exhibits all the usual microscopic features of infiltrating ductal carcinoma. Lymphocytic infiltration, although not present in every case, is frequently found in

IBC. There are no special cytologic or architectural characteristics, and no specific dermal lesions are found consistently in the skin biopsies of IBC, although cancer cells penetrating lymphatic channels are frequently seen. Multicentricity is common, especially within the lymphatic spaces. IBCs are poorly differentiated and without evidence of glandular formation. When the nipple is involved, Paget's disease of the nipple can be identified. IBC is an invasive malignancy characterized by high histologic and nuclear grades and by aggressive features such as aneuploidy, high S-phase fractions, negative ER status, and elevated expressions of epidermal growth factor and ErbB-2.

MULTIMODAL TREATMENT OF IBC

In the era of local, single modality treatment, IBC—a systemic process—was nearly always fatal, with early local and distant relapse. The poor outcomes that were seen for these patients led to the development of a combined modality approach as used in LABC. In the United States, M. D. Anderson and National Cancer Institute investigators were among the first to gain experience using multimodal therapy with neoadjuvant chemotherapy to treat IBC. As with LABC, treatment begins with neoadjuvant chemotherapy, followed by surgery, if feasible, and then comprehensive chest wall radiation. This approach has resulted in tumor shrinkage with downsizing making surgical intervention possible. IBC's rapid doubling and hematogenous and local-regional spread necessitate the precise coordination of systemic and local therapeutic modalities. Despite the historically poor prognosis for patients who develop IBC, the disease is now regarded as a moderately curable one, with OS rates at 5 years improved from less than 10% without chemotherapy to between 30 and 55% with multimodal treatment.[49]

Surgical Therapy in IBC

The role of mastectomy in IBC was controversial when recommendations against surgical intervention in IBC were issued[50] because of reports that surgery showed no advantages when combined with chemotherapy and radiation therapy for patients with IBC. However, this stance changed as the result of a review of 178 M. D. Anderson patients by Fleming and colleagues[51] showing that the addition of a mastectomy to combination chemotherapy and radiation therapy improved local control in patients with IBC (local recurrence rate 16.3% with mastectomy versus 35.7% without mastectomy). The same combination improved distant DFS and OS in patients with a cCR or partial response to neoadjuvant chemotherapy.[51] Patients who had no significant

response to neoadjuvant chemotherapy received no survival or local disease-control benefit from the addition of mastectomy to their treatment regimen.[51] "Toilet mastectomy" has no survival benefits, and local control is rarely gained with operative intervention in an inflammatory field. Surgery should be contemplated only when major resolution of the inflammatory change is seen and it is anticipated that negative surgical margins can be achieved.

Most recently, Panades and colleagues reported a retrospective analysis of 485 patients with IBC. Ten-year local-regional RFS rates for patients having mastectomy after chemotherapy, mastectomy before chemotherapy, and without mastectomy were 62.8%, 58.6%, and 34.4% respectively ($p = .0001$). On multivariate analysis, mastectomy was associated with improved local-regional RFS.[52]

Mastectomy after neoadjuvant chemotherapy results in prompt local control and healing. It permits the pathologic assessment of residual tumor burden and axillary lymph node status. Currently, the most effective multimodal approach to achieve local control and control distant disease is neoadjuvant chemotherapy, followed by a mastectomy and then radiation therapy. Radiation therapy is used prior to surgical intervention in patients who are inoperable after neoadjuvant chemotherapy, and more local control is required prior to any surgical resection. It is also used in those patients who are poor operative candidates. Patients with positive margins after resection or extensive axillary lymph node disease receive additional radiation boost for local control.

SLN surgery has no role in IBC. Stearns and colleagues[53] reported on eight patients with IBC treated with chemotherapy followed by SLN and ALND. The SLN was unsuccessful in two cases (25%) and in two other patients the sentinel node was a false negative (25%).[53] Because of cancer infiltrating the dermis and lymphatics, the lymphatic channels in the breast may be occluded. In turn, it may be difficult to identify sentinel nodes, and the false-negative rate is high. The standard of care in IBC remains a modified radical mastectomy despite the increased use of SLN surgery in other stages of breast cancer. BCT still has no role in IBC.

Chemotherapy in IBC

Primary chemotherapy is considered the main component of treatment in IBC. The response to neoadjuvant chemotherapy is an important predictor of outcome. Poor pathologic response (and particularly residual lymph node involvement) following neoadjuvant chemotherapy may be the most powerful predictor of local and systemic recurrence and poor prognosis. A pCR of the breast tumor correlates strongly with both prolonged DFS and OS and occurs in 6 to 31% of patients.

pCR has also been associated with improved prognosis in a large, randomized neoadjuvant chemotherapy trial (National Surgical Adjuvant Breast and Bowel Project Trial B-18),[54] suggesting that quantifying the breast tumor response to preoperative therapy may serve as an intermediate estimate of the effectiveness of neoadjuvant chemotherapy on micrometastatic disease. A study based on M. D. Anderson experience showed that women with IBC who had a pCR to an anthracycline-containing regimen had a 15-year DFS rate of 44% compared to only 7% in patients with less than a partial response.[55]

Anthracyclines and taxanes are the most effective cytotoxic agents available for the management of primary breast cancer and have demonstrated their importance in the management of IBC as well. The addition of taxanes in combination or in sequence with anthracyclines resulted in a significant increase in the rates of overall response, cCR, and pCR. The 3-year OS and PFS rates are higher when patients were treated with paclitaxel than anthracycline-based regimens.[49] The use of a sequence including an anthracyline-containing regimen followed by a taxane (such as docetaxel or paclitaxel) is associated with a higher probability of remission and should be used routinely.

Because the response to neoadjuvant chemotherapy is the most important predictor for local recurrence, DFS, and OS, attempts have been made to improve response rates. These attempts to overcome drug resistance have included high-dose chemotherapy and alternative, non-cross-resistant drugs. High-dose neoadjuvant chemotherapy with autologous bone marrow transplants or peripheral blood stem cell support are a feasible and effective approach to IBC management. This is generally associated with a response rate improvement, but that improvement has not shown a significant impact on DFS or OS compared with standard chemotherapy, probably because of the severity of its adverse effects.

When a patient experiences a poor or minimal response to neoadjuvant anthracyline-containing regimens, taxanes may prove to be an effective alternate way to improve resectability in anthracycline-resistant IBC. In one study of 16 such patients, paclitaxel converted 7 (44%) into candidates for resection, and the patients were able to undergo mastectomy. The use of paclitaxel with high-dose neoadjuvant chemotherapy and peripheral blood stem cell support resulted in a median OS of 36 months (regardless of response to neoadjuvant chemotherapy).[56]

Ueno and colleagues reviewed M. D. Anderson's 20-year experience with 178 patients with IBC who were treated with four different chemotherapy protocols, all of which involved neoadjuvant chemotherapy followed by either radiation therapy or mastectomy, followed by (if mastectomy was performed) chemotherapy and adjuvant radiation therapy.[55] The overall DFS rate was 28% at 15 years with an OS of 29% at 15 years and a median survival of 37 months. There were no significant differences in the DFS or OS among the four different protocols. After neoadjuvant chemotherapy, 74% of the patients achieved major objective tumor response (CR or partial response). After completing combined modality treatments, 92% of the patients were rendered free of disease. The estimated 15-year DFS was 44% for patients who had a CR to chemotherapy, 31% for those who had a partial response, and 6% for those who had any response lesser than a partial one. The estimated 15-year OS rates in these patient groups were 51%, 31%, and 7%, respectively. There was no difference in DFS associated with the type of local therapy, whether that was radiation alone or surgery and radiation. Also in that study, 68% of the patients had breast cancer recurrences (20% had local-regional recurrence, 39% had systemic recurrence, and 9% had central nervous system relapse). The pattern of local failure did not differ by the type of local therapy. However, we recommend mastectomy for local therapy, because it debulks large tumors, resulting in less concern about residual tumors, smaller required doses of radiation, and quicker re-institution of adjuvant chemotherapy.

Radiation Therapy in IBC

A series of prospective trials at M. D. Anderson has demonstrated the usefulness of twice-daily fractionation and radiation dose escalation in IBC. Patients given twice-daily postmastectomy radiation to a total of 66 Gy instead of the more conventional dose of 60 Gy showed improvements over their lower-dose counterparts in local-regional control, DFS, and OS.[57] Local-regional control rates improved with the higher dosage from 58% to 84% at 5 years and from 58% to 77% at 10 years ($p = .028$). The dose given to the entire chest wall and regional nodes was 51 Gy, with a boost dose to the chest wall of 15 Gy (for patients with negative surgical margins), for a total of 66 Gy. Radiation-related complications including arm edema, rib fractures, fibrosis, and symptomatic pneumonitis were comparable between the groups, indicating that the dose escalation did not result in increased morbidity.[57]

The field selection for treatment of the chest wall in IBC requires very broad margins on the chest wall flaps because IBC spreads by dermal lymphatics. The anterior chest skin is treated from just beyond the midline to the posterior axillary line and from below the prior inframammary fold. The regional nodal fields should be tailored according to the volume of disease at presentation.

PROGNOSTIC FACTORS FOR IBC

The majority of patients with IBC will die of their disease, but their specific prognoses can be stratified by several tumor-related factors (such as tumor size, nuclear grade, ER- and Her-2/neu status, and number of involved axillary lymph nodes) and treatment-related factors (such as the use of doxorubicin-containing regimens). The extent of inflammatory changes has been shown to have an effect on prognosis; three indicators of poor prognosis include erythema involving the entire breast at diagnosis, erythema at the end of neoadjuvant chemotherapy, and lymph node involvement.[58] The presence of pathologic residual disease in the breast and lymph nodes after chemotherapy is an important adverse prognostic factor, and a pCR to neoadjuvant chemotherapy is the strongest positive prognostic factor.[22]

Factors found to significantly decrease survival include having tumors larger than 8 cm, ER- and PR-negativity, and lymph node involvement at presentation. OS and RFS are improved in patients who have ER- and PR-positive tumors, fewer than four involved axillary nodes before chemotherapy, and radiation therapy.[59] The finding of dermal lymphatic tumor invasion predicts a high probability of node-positive disease. Researchers at the University of Florida reviewed prognostic factors in 61 women with IBC. They compared the population of IBC patients treated with up-front mastectomy (before multimodal treatment became the standard of care) with patients who received neoadjuvant chemotherapy. They found three factors were significantly associated with improved cause-specific survival: pathologic tumor size < 4 cm, up-front surgery, and local disease control. Factors associated with improved local-regional disease control were pathologic tumor size < 4 cm, age > 55 years and radiation dose > 60 Gy.[60]

There are no statistically significant survival differences between obese and non-obese IBC patients overall or among premenopausal women separately. However, premenopausal women had poorer survival rates than postmenopausal women. Obese postmenopausal women were noted to have poorer survival than leaner postmenopausal patients, whereas obese premenopausal women had better survival (not to a significant degree) than their leaner premenopausal counterparts.[61]

TUMOR MARKERS

P53 is overexpressed in a large percentage of IBC cases. P53-positive tumors exhibit more aggressive biologic behavior and are associated with a shorter median time to progression and shorter median OS.[62] A study conducted at M. D. Anderson reviewed 48 patients with IBC, of whom 58% had p53-positive tumors and 42% p53-negative tumors. The patients with p53-positive tumors were younger ($p = .02$), tended to have tumors of a higher nuclear grade ($p = .09$), lower 5-year PFS rates (35% versus 55%; $p = 0.3$), and lower OS rates (44% versus 54%; $p = 0.4$).[63] In general, the study found patients with p53-positive IBC have a less favorable prognosis than patients with p53-negative IBC.

Human mucin 1 (MUC1) is a mucin glycoprotein expressed in 90% of all breast adenocarcinomas. Seventy-nine percent of the IBCs tested in one study strongly expressed MUC1; those patients had longer times to progression and OS than others.[62]

IBC often exhibits aggressive biomarkers, including high S-phase, aneuploidy, and negative ER and PR status. More recently, reports from the Royal Marsden Hospital (London, UK) cite a 52% incidence of strong Her-2/neu positivity in IBC compared with a 27% incidence in non-IBC breast cancers.[64] The high incidence of Her-2/neu positivity in this study suggests that trastuzumab-based treatment targeted against the Her-2/neu protein is beneficial. The literature already contains isolated reports of the use of trastuzumab in IBC[65–67] and we await future reports.

PROGNOSIS AND LONG-TERM FOLLOW-UP

The National Cancer Institute reported long-term outcomes of 46 patients with IBC who had a median OS of 3.8 years and an event-free survival of 2.3 years (compared with 12.2 and 9.0 years, respectively, for stage IIIA breast cancer patients). One study found the 15-year survival rate for IBC to be 20%,[45] and another study showed 10- and 15-year survival rates of 33% and 29%, respectively.[55] OS is significantly worse for IBC patients than for those with other types of breast carcinoma. This is true among both African American and white women.[47] However, white women experience significantly better survival than their African American counterparts. Between the two periods of 1975 to 1979 and 1988 to 1992, survival among white women with IBC improved significantly—the 3-year survival rates according to SEER data increased from 32% to 42% ($p = .02$).[47]

SUMMARY OF IBC TREATMENT

The management of IBC has changed in the past 20 to 30 years and currently the standard of care requires a team of dedicated and experienced specialists (including a pathologist, surgeon, radiation oncologist, radiologist,

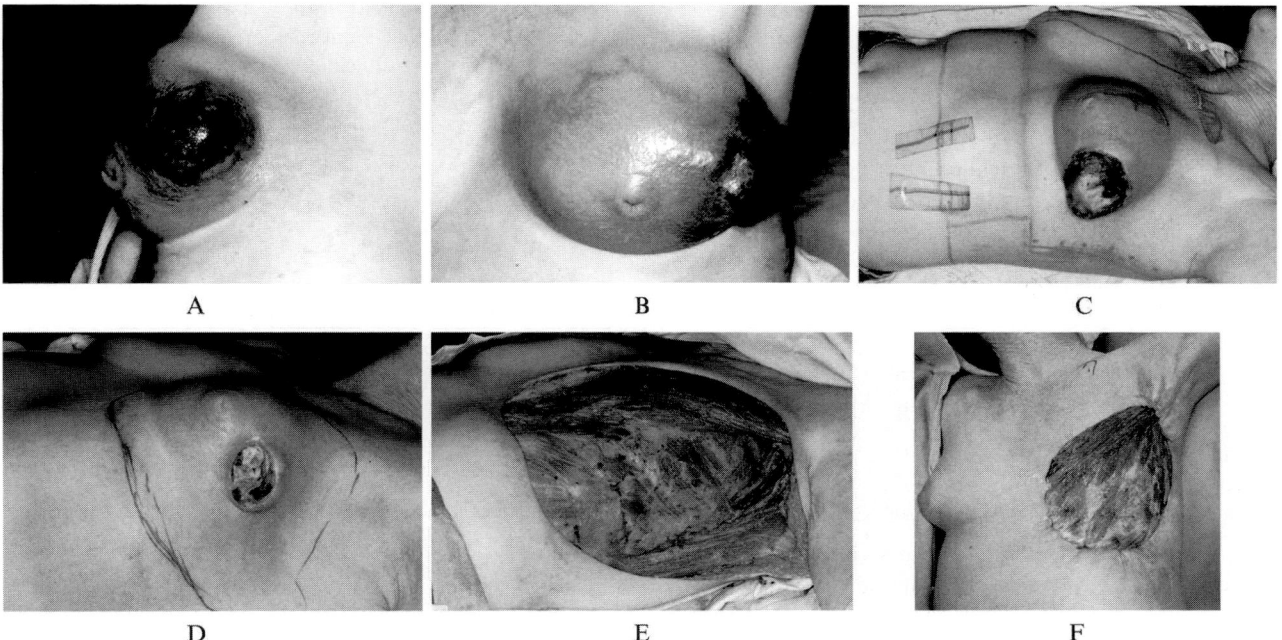

Figure 1 A and B Patient with locally advanced breast cancer, demonstrating diffuse skin thickening and redness involving the majority of the breast with focal ulceration overlying the area of the tumor Figure 1C Radiation fields used to treat this patient. Skin changes remained after chemotherapy; therefore, the patient underwent radiation therapy prior to surgery. Figure 1D Picture showing the preoperative extent of disease. After chemotherapy and radiation, a partial response was seen with decreased area of skin thickening and erythema. Figure 1E Intraoperative photograph showing the chest wall after resection of the breast with overlying skin. The pectoral muscles remained intact. All skin showing any signs of thickening or erythema was resected. Figure 1F Photograph of chest wall after placement of latissimus dorsi flap to cover chest wall.

and medical oncologist) to carry out the complex management of this entity.

In the multidisciplinary treatment of IBC, neoadjuvant chemotherapy is the mainstay of therapy. Local-regional treatment includes surgery followed by comprehensive radiation therapy. The sequence of modalities chosen should depend on the quality of objective response achieved with neoadjuvant chemotherapy. In

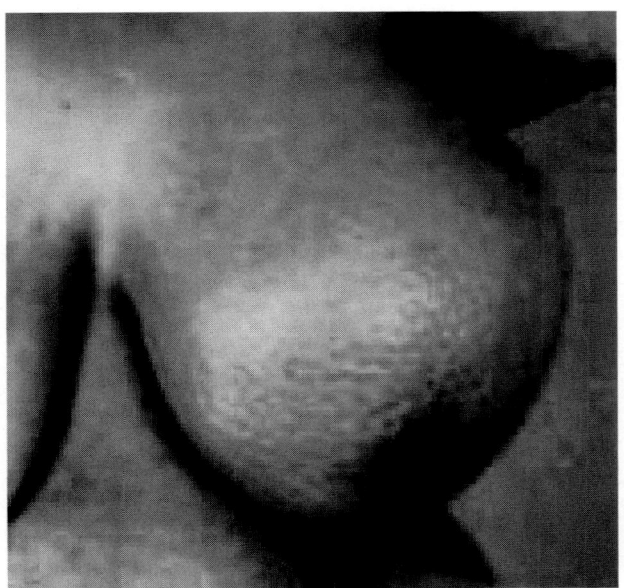

Figure 2 Photograph illustrating skin thickening, peau d'orange, and enlargement of the breast in a patient with inflammatory breast cancer.

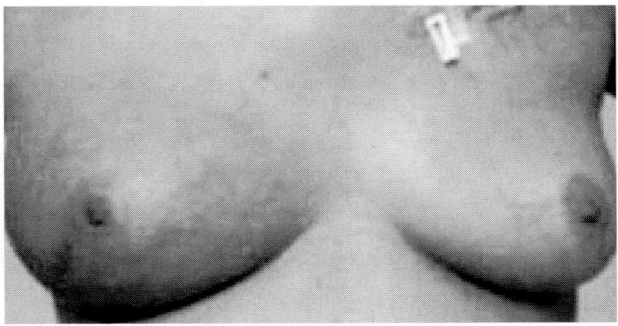

Figure 3 Photograph demonstrating diffuse erythema of the skin of the entire breast in a patient with inflammatory breast cancer.

the majority of cases, after optimal remission—defined as objective clinical disease remission with resolution of the characteristic skin changes—patients are considered surgical candidates and a modified radical mastectomy followed by radiotherapy is recommended. Patients who experience disease progression during chemotherapy should proceed to preoperative radiation therapy. Patients with less than a partial response to chemotherapy but who do not have progressive disease should receive a second chemotherapy regimen and then be reevaluated.

References

1. Singletary SE, Allred C, Ashley P, et al. Revision of the American Joint Committee on Cancer staging system for breast cancer. J Clin Oncol 2002;20:3628–36.

2. Cunningham JD, Weiss SE, Ahmed S, et al. The efficacy of neoadjuvant chemotherapy compared to postoperative therapy in the treatment of locally advanced breast cancer. Cancer Invest 1998;16:80–6.

3. Bonadonna G, Veronesi U, Brambilla C, et al. Primary chemotherapy to avoid mastectomy in tumors with diameters of three centimeters or more. J Natl Cancer Inst 1990;82:1539–45.

4. Mauriac L, MacGrogan G, Avril A, et al. Neoadjuvant chemotherapy for operable breast carcinoma larger than 3 cm: a unicentre randomized trial with a 124-month median follow-up. Institut Bergonie Bordeaux Groupe Sein (IBBGS). Ann Oncol 1999;10:47–52.

5. Touboul E, Lefranc JP, Blondon J, et al. Primary chemotherapy and preoperative irradiation for patients with stage II larger than 3 cm or locally advanced non-inflammatory breast cancer. Radiother Oncol 1997;42:219–29.

6. Merajver SD, Weber BL, Cody R, et al. Breast conservation and prolonged chemotherapy for locally advanced breast cancer: the University of Michigan experience. J Clin Oncol 1997;15:2873–81.

7. Singletary SE, McNeese MD, Hortobagyi GN. Feasibility of breast-conservation surgery after induction chemotherapy for locally advanced breast carcinoma. Cancer 1992;69:2849–52.

8. Fisher B, Saffer E, Rudock C, et al. Effect of local or systemic treatment prior to primary tumor removal on the production and response to a serum growth-stimulating factor in mice. Cancer Res 1989;49:2002–4.

9. Smith IC, Heys SD, Hutcheon AW, et al. Neoadjuvant chemotherapy in breast cancer: significantly enhanced response with docetaxel. J Clin Oncol 2002;20:1456–66.

10. Heys SD, Hutcheon AW, Sarkar TK, et al. Neoadjuvant docetaxel in breast cancer: 3-year survival results from the Aberdeen trial. Clin Breast Cancer 2002;3Suppl 2:S69–74.

11. Bear HD, Anderson S, Brown A, et al. The effect on tumor response of adding sequential preoperative docetaxel to preoperative doxorubicin and cyclophosphamide: preliminary results from National Surgical Adjuvant Breast and Bowel Project Protocol B-27. J Clin Oncol 2003;21:4165–74.

12. von Minckwitz G, Raab G, Caputo A, et al. Doxorubicin with cyclophosphamide followed by docetaxel every 21 days compared with doxorubicin and docetaxel every 14 days as preoperative treatment in operable breast cancer: the GEPARDUO study of the German Breast Group. J Clin Oncol 2005;23:2676–85.

13. Tham YL, Gomez LF, Mohsin S, et al. Clinical response to neoadjuvant docetaxel predicts improved outcome in patients with large locally advanced breast cancers. Breast Cancer Res Treat 2005;94:279–84.

14. Estevez LG, Gradishar WJ. Evidence-based use of neoadjuvant taxane in operable and inoperable breast cancer. Clin Cancer Res 2004;10:3249–61.

15. Kuerer HM, Singletary SE, Buzdar AU, et al. Surgical conservation planning after neoadjuvant chemotherapy for stage II and operable stage III breast carcinoma. Am J Surg 2001;182:601–8.

16. Shen J, Valero V, Buchholz TA, et al. Effective local control and long-term survival in patients with T4 locally advanced breast cancer treated with breast conservation therapy. Ann Surg Oncol 2004;11:854–60.

17. Bedrosian I, Reynolds C, Mick R, et al. Accuracy of sentinel lymph node biopsy in patients with large primary breast tumors. Cancer 2000;88:2540–5.

18. Chung MH, Ye W, Giuliano AE. Role for sentinel lymph node dissection in the management of large (> or = 5 cm) invasive breast cancer. Ann Surg Oncol 2001;8:688–92.

19. Kuerer HM, Newman LA, Fornage BD, et al. Role of axillary lymph node dissection after tumor downstaging with induction chemotherapy for locally advanced breast cancer. Ann Surg Oncol 1998;5:673–80.

20. Perloff M, Lesnick GJ, Korzun A, et al. Combination chemotherapy with mastectomy or radiotherapy for stage III breast carcinoma: a Cancer and Leukemia Group B study. J Clin Oncol 1988;6:261–9.

21. McCready DR, Hortobagyi GN, Kau SW, et al. The prognostic significance of lymph node metastases after preoperative chemotherapy for locally advanced breast cancer. Arch Surg 1989;124:21–5.

22. Kuerer HM, Newman LA, Buzdar AU, et al. Residual metastatic axillary lymph nodes following neoadjuvant chemotherapy predict disease-free survival in patients with locally advanced breast cancer. Am J Surg 1998;176:502–9.

23. Herrada J, Iyer RB, Atkinson EN, et al. Relative value of physical examination, mammography, and breast sonography in evaluating the size of the primary tumor and regional lymph node metastases in women receiving

neoadjuvant chemotherapy for locally advanced breast carcinoma. Clin Cancer Res 1997;3:1565–9.

24. Krishnamurthy S, Sneige N, Bedi DG, et al. Role of ultrasound-guided fine-needle aspiration of indeterminate and suspicious axillary lymph nodes in the initial staging of breast carcinoma. Cancer 2002;95:982–8.

25. Breslin TM, Cohen L, Sahin A, et al. Sentinel lymph node biopsy is accurate after neoadjuvant chemotherapy for breast cancer. J Clin Oncol 2000;18:3480–6.

26. Patel NA, Piper G, Patel JA, et al. Accurate axillary nodal staging can be achieved after neoadjuvant therapy for locally advanced breast cancer. Am Surg 2004;70:696–9; discussion 699–700.

27. Mamounas EP, Brown A, Anderson S, et al. Sentinel node biopsy after neoadjuvant chemotherapy in breast cancer: results from National Surgical Adjuvant Breast and Bowel Project Protocol B-27. J Clin Oncol 2005;23:2694–702.

28. Jones JL, Zabicki K, Christian RL, et al. A comparison of sentinel node biopsy before and after neoadjuvant chemotherapy: timing is important. Am J Surg 2005;190: 517–20.

29. Newman E, Sabel MS, Diehl KM. Sentinel lymph node biopsy performed after neoadjuvant chemotherapy is accurate in patients with documented node-positive disease at presentation. Ann Surg Oncol 2006;13(2 Suppl):10.

30. Newman LA, Kuerer HM, Hunt KK, et al. Feasibility of immediate breast reconstruction for locally advanced breast cancer. Ann Surg Oncol 1999;6:671–5.

31. Foster RD, Hansen SL, Esserman LJ, et al. Safety of immediate transverse rectus abdominis myocutaneous breast reconstruction for patients with locally advanced disease. Arch Surg 2005;140:196–8; discussion 199–200.

32. Kronowitz SJ, Hunt KK, Kuerer HM, et al. Delayed-immediate breast reconstruction. Plast Reconstr Surg 2004; 113:1617–28.

33. Clarke M, Collins R, Darby S, et al. Effects of radiotherapy and of differences in the extent of surgery for early breast cancer on local recurrence and 15-year survival: an overview of the randomised trials. Lancet 2005;366:2087–106.

34. Huang EH, Tucker SL, Strom EA, et al. Postmastectomy radiation improves local-regional control and survival for selected patients with locally advanced breast cancer treated with neoadjuvant chemotherapy and mastectomy. J Clin Oncol 2004;22:4691–9.

35. Buchholz TA, Tucker SL, Masullo L, et al. Predictors of local-regional recurrence after neoadjuvant chemotherapy and mastectomy without radiation. J Clin Oncol 2002;20: 17–23.

36. Smith IE, Dowsett M, Ebbs SR, et al. Neoadjuvant treatment of postmenopausal breast cancer with anastrozole, tamoxifen, or both in combination: the Immediate Preoperative Anastrozole, Tamoxifen, or Combined with Tamoxifen (IMPACT) multicenter double-blind randomized trial. J Clin Oncol 2005;23:5108–16.

37. Cataliotti L, Buzdar AU, Noguchi S, et al. Comparison of anastrozole versus tamoxifen as preoperative therapy in postmenopausal women with hormone receptor-positive breast cancer: the pre-operative "Arimidex" compared to Tamoxifen (PROACT) trial. Cancer 2006;106:2095–103.

38. Ellis MJ, Coop A, Singh B, et al. Letrozole is more effective neoadjuvant endocrine therapy than tamoxifen for ErbB-1- and/or ErbB-2-positive, estrogen receptor-positive primary breast cancer: evidence from a phase III randomized trial. J Clin Oncol 2001;19:3808–16.

39. Eiermann W, Paepke S, Appfelstaedt J, et al. Preoperative treatment of postmenopausal breast cancer patients with letrozole: a randomized double-blind multicenter study. Ann Oncol 2001;12:1527–32.

40. Huang EH, Tucker SL, Strom EA, et al. Predictors of locoregional recurrence in patients with locally advanced breast cancer treated with neoadjuvant chemotherapy, mastectomy, and radiotherapy. Int J Radiat Oncol Biol Phys 2005;62:351–7.

41. Hurley J, Doliny P, Reis I, et al. Docetaxel, cisplatin, and trastuzumab as primary systemic therapy for human epidermal growth factor receptor 2-positive locally advanced breast cancer. J Clin Oncol 2006;24:1831–8.

42. Mohsin SK, Weiss HL, Gutierrez MC, et al. Neoadjuvant trastuzumab induces apoptosis in primary breast cancers. J Clin Oncol 2005;23:2460–8.

43. Martinez-Trufero J, de Lobera AR, Lao J, et al. Serum markers and prognosis in locally advanced breast cancer. Tumori 2005;91:522–30.

44. Kuerer HM, Newman LA, Smith TL, et al. Clinical course of breast cancer patients with complete pathologic primary tumor and axillary lymph node response to doxorubicin-based neoadjuvant chemotherapy. J Clin Oncol 1999;17: 460–9.

45. Low JA, Berman AW, Steinberg SM, et al. Long-term follow-up for locally advanced and inflammatory breast cancer patients treated with multimodality therapy. J Clin Oncol 2004;22:4067–74.

46. Levine PH, Steinhorn SC, Ries LG, Aron JL. Inflammatory breast cancer: the experience of the surveillance, epidemiology, and end results (SEER) program. J Natl Cancer Inst 1985;74:291–7.

47. Chang S, Parker SL, Pham T, et al. Inflammatory breast carcinoma incidence and survival: the surveillance, epidemiology, and end results program of the National Cancer Institute, 1975–1992. Cancer 1998;82:2366–72.

48. Haagensen C. Inflammatory Carcinoma, Diseases of the Breast, 2nd ed. Philadelphia: W.B. Saunders; 1971. p. 576–84.

49. Cristofanilli M, Buzdar AU, Hortobagyi GN. Update on the management of inflammatory breast cancer. Oncologist 2003;8:141–8.

50. De Boer RH, Allum WH, Ebbs SR, et al. Multimodality therapy in inflammatory breast cancer: is there a place for surgery? Ann Oncol 2000;11:1147–53.

51. Fleming RY, Asmar L, Buzdar AU, et al. Effectiveness of mastectomy by response to induction chemotherapy for control in inflammatory breast carcinoma. Ann Surg Oncol 1997;4:452–61.

52. Panades M, Olivotto IA, Speers CH, et al. Evolving treatment strategies for inflammatory breast cancer: a population-based survival analysis. J Clin Oncol 2005;23: 1941–50.

53. Stearns V, Ewing CA, Slack R, et al. Sentinel lymphadenectomy after neoadjuvant chemotherapy for breast cancer may reliably represent the axilla except for inflammatory breast cancer. Ann Surg Oncol 2002;9:235–42.

54. Fisher B, Brown A, Mamounas E, et al. Effect of preoperative chemotherapy on local-regional disease in women with operable breast cancer: findings from National Surgical Adjuvant Breast and Bowel Project B-18. J Clin Oncol 1997;15:2483–93.

55. Ueno NT, Buzdar AU, Singletary SE, et al. Combined-modality treatment of inflammatory breast carcinoma: twenty years of experience at M. D. Anderson Cancer Center. Cancer Chemother Pharmacol 1997;40:321–9.

56. Cristofanilli M, Buzdar AU, Sneige N, et al. Paclitaxel in the multimodality treatment for inflammatory breast carcinoma. Cancer 2001;92:1775–82.

57. Liao Z, Strom EA, Buzdar AU, et al. Locoregional irradiation for inflammatory breast cancer: effectiveness of dose escalation in decreasing recurrence. Int J Radiat Oncol Biol Phys 2000;47:1191–200.

58. Chevallier B, Asselain B, Kunlin A, et al. Inflammatory breast cancer. Determination of prognostic factors by univariate and multivariate analysis. Cancer 1987;60:897–902.

59. Somlo G, Frankel P, Chow W, et al. Prognostic indicators and survival in patients with stage IIIB inflammatory breast carcinoma after dose-intense chemotherapy. J Clin Oncol 2004;22:1839–48.

60. Liauw SL, Benda RK, Morris CG, Mendenhall NP. Inflammatory breast carcinoma: outcomes with trimodality therapy for nonmetastatic disease. Cancer 2004;100:920–8.

61. Chang S, Alderfer JR, Asmar L, Buzdar AU. Inflammatory breast cancer survival: the role of obesity and menopausal status at diagnosis. Breast Cancer Res Treat 2000;64:157–63.

62. Resetkova E, Gonzalez-Angulo AM, Sneige N, et al. Prognostic value of P53, MDM-2, and MUC-1 for patients with inflammatory breast carcinoma. Cancer 2004;101: 913–7.

63. Gonzalez-Angulo AM, Sneige N, Buzdar AU, et al. p53 expression as a prognostic marker in inflammatory breast cancer. Clin Cancer Res 2004;10(18 Pt 1):6215–21.

64. Parton M, Dowsett M, Ashley S, et al. High incidence of HER-2 positivity in inflammatory breast cancer. Breast 2004;13:97–103.

65. Asakura H, Takashima H, Mitani M, et al. Unknown primary carcinoma, diagnosed as inflammatory breast cancer, and successfully treated with trastuzumab and vinorelbine. Int J Clin Oncol 2005;10:285–8.

66. Nomura M, Inoue Y, Fujita S, et al. Pathological complete response to trastuzumab and paclitaxel in a patient with inflammatory local recurrence following breast conserving surgery. Breast Cancer 2005;12:226–30.

67. Okawa Y, Sugiyama K, Aiba K, et al. Successful combination therapy with trastuzumab and Paclitaxel for adriamycin- and docetaxel-resistant inflammatory breast cancer. Breast Cancer 2004;11:309–12.

CHAPTER 60

BREAST RECONSTRUCTION: CURRENT STRATEGIES AND FUTURE OPPORTUNITIES

STEVEN J. KRONOWITZ, MD

Breast reconstruction is a very important component of the multidisciplinary care of patients with breast cancer. Although in some patients, especially those who will require postmastectomy radiation therapy (PMRT), it may be preferable to delay breast reconstruction, immediate breast reconstruction offers aesthetic and technical benefits over delayed reconstruction.[1,2] Immediate breast reconstruction also provides psychological benefits.[3] Patients who undergo immediate breast reconstruction do not have to experience the psychological trauma of not having a breast when they awake from anesthesia. Despite these benefits, many patients continue to present for delayed reconstruction, which is often more complex than immediate breast reconstruction and is associated with an increased risk of complications.

Breast Reconstruction after Partial Mastectomy

Although patients treated with total mastectomy often request breast reconstruction, patients treated with partial mastectomy usually do not inquire about reconstructive options. There are many reasons why patients undergoing partial mastectomy do not routinely ask about reconstruction: for some women, the ability to preserve the breast provides sufficient psychological satisfaction; other women may fear additional operations or may simply not be aware of the reconstructive option.[4]

POTENTIAL BENEFITS OF IMMEDIATE RECONSTRUCTION

In addition to an obvious improvement in aesthetic outcome, immediate repair of partial mastectomy defects offers many other potential advantages. Immediate reconstruction allows the plastic surgeon to participate in the planning of the incisions and the surgical approach to tumor resection and thus simplifies any subsequent breast reconstruction. Even though reconstruction may not ultimately be required (because the defect is smaller than anticipated or the cancer is more extensive than anticipated and precludes partial mastectomy), the involvement of the plastic surgeon in preoperative planning is prudent.

Immediate repair of partial mastectomy defects can also make more large-breasted patients eligible for breast conservation therapy (BCT). Some radiation oncologists are reluctant to treat large-breasted patients because of poor aesthetic outcomes. Radiation delivered to a large breast can lead to increased fibrosis due to difficulties with daily set-up and due to the increased fat content.[5] A reduced breast size allows for a more uniform radiation dose at lower levels, reducing unacceptable late radiation reactions.[6] Immediate repair of a partial mastectomy defect using breast reduction techniques represents an alternative for patients who would not otherwise be considered candidates for BCT.

Immediate reconstruction can also make it easier for the breast surgeon to resect wider margins around the tumor, which in turn has the potential to lower the rates of local recurrence of breast cancer.[7] Immediate reconstruction does not pose a problem with postoperative cancer surveillance.[6] Finally, immediate reconstruction may provide some medical benefits. The contralateral breast reduction for symmetry that is often required in patients who undergo immediate repair of a partial mastectomy defect allows for the sampling of tissue from the contralateral breast. Occult carcinomas have been found in approximately 4.5% of contralateral breast reduction specimens in patients undergoing a symmetry procedure for breast reconstruction.[8]

RECOMMENDATIONS FOR CLINICAL PRACTICE

Immediate repair of partial mastectomy defects before radiation therapy (XRT) is safer than delayed repair after XRT and is the option we prefer at The University of Texas M. D. Anderson Cancer Center. In our recent experience,[9] complication rates were 30% for breast reconstruction overall, 26% for immediate reconstruction, and 42% for delayed reconstruction. The higher risk of complications with delayed reconstruction is mainly related to the fact that irradiated tissues have a decreased capacity for wound healing and respond poorly to surgery.

Reconstruction before Radiation Therapy

In the circumstance of immediate reconstruction, we prefer the use of local breast tissue because of the simplicity of these approaches and because techniques using local tissue maintain the color and texture of the breast. Although the breast reduction technique (Figures 1 and 2) is generally favored over local tissue rearrangement, the breast reduction technique is usually limited to patients with large breasts (D cup or larger). Local tissue rearrangement can be a good alternative for patients with moderate-sized breasts (B or C cup) who have minimal or no nipple ptosis, especially when the partial defect is located in the lower outer quadrant of the breast and involves minimal or no skin resection.

Although we usually prefer immediate reconstruction, if an unexpected deformity results after partial mastectomy or the tumor margin status is unclear, consideration should be given to performing delayed reconstruction prior to XRT. In these circumstances, we also prefer the use of local tissue (Figure 3).

When a large amount of skin needs to be resected, many of the advantages of BCT are lost.[7] When breast skin defects are so extensive that they must be repaired using a flap, further consideration should be given to whether BCT is the best option with respect to breast reconstruction. Although a latissimus dorsi flap can replace a large region of skin, its skin island has a different color and texture than the breast skin,[7] which can lead to a less than ideal aesthetic outcome. Consideration should also be given to whether a latissimus dorsi flap alone can provide an adequate tissue volume for reconstruction. If a breast implant will also be required, it may be preferable to perform a

mastectomy followed by total breast reconstruction because breast implants are not recommended in patients who have had or will have XRT.[10,11] In patients who are not candidates for a transverse rectus abdominis myocutaneous (TRAM) flap breast reconstruction (because of inadequate or excessive abdominal pannus or abdominal scarring), a latissimus dorsi flap may be the only available autologous tissue source should the patient develop a local recurrence of breast cancer or a contour deformity after XRT. Physicians should carefully consider whether a latissimus dorsi flap should be used for primary reconstruction and should warn patients that they might not be able to have further breast reconstruction if local recurrence or contour deformity occurs.

Reconstruction after Radiation Therapy

Unfortunately, in patients who have already undergone XRT, the reconstructive options that can be offered are often limited. In some patients, a contralateral breast reduction is all that is required (Figure 4). However, often there is no choice but to perform a delayed repair of a partial mastectomy defect. Delayed reconstruction after XRT usually requires a latissimus dorsi flap because it provides its own blood supply to assist with healing within the irradiated operative field; however, use of a latissimus dorsi flap may increase the likelihood of lymphedema and leave the patient without autologous tissue options if further reconstruction is required in the future. In addition, in patients with severe cosmetic deformity after partial mastectomy and XRT, the soft tissue requirements are often greater than what a latissimus dorsi flap alone can provide.

Although many of these patients with severe defects after partial mastectomy and XRT have hopes of secondary correction, the aesthetic outcomes are often disappointing.[5]

TRAM Flaps: Better for Total Breast Reconstruction than Defect Repair

The use of TRAM flaps to repair partial breast defects is discouraged. If a patient requires a TRAM flap for reconstruction after partial mastectomy, it is usually better to complete the mastectomy and reconstruct the entire breast with the flap than to discard healthy TRAM flap tissue, especially because the remaining breast tissue is still at risk for development of malignancy.[5] In cases of a severe cosmetic deformity after partial mastectomy and XRT, including a contracted breast skin envelope and malposition of the nipple-areola complex, it also may be preferable to perform a completion mastectomy with total breast reconstruction rather than "waste" a TRAM

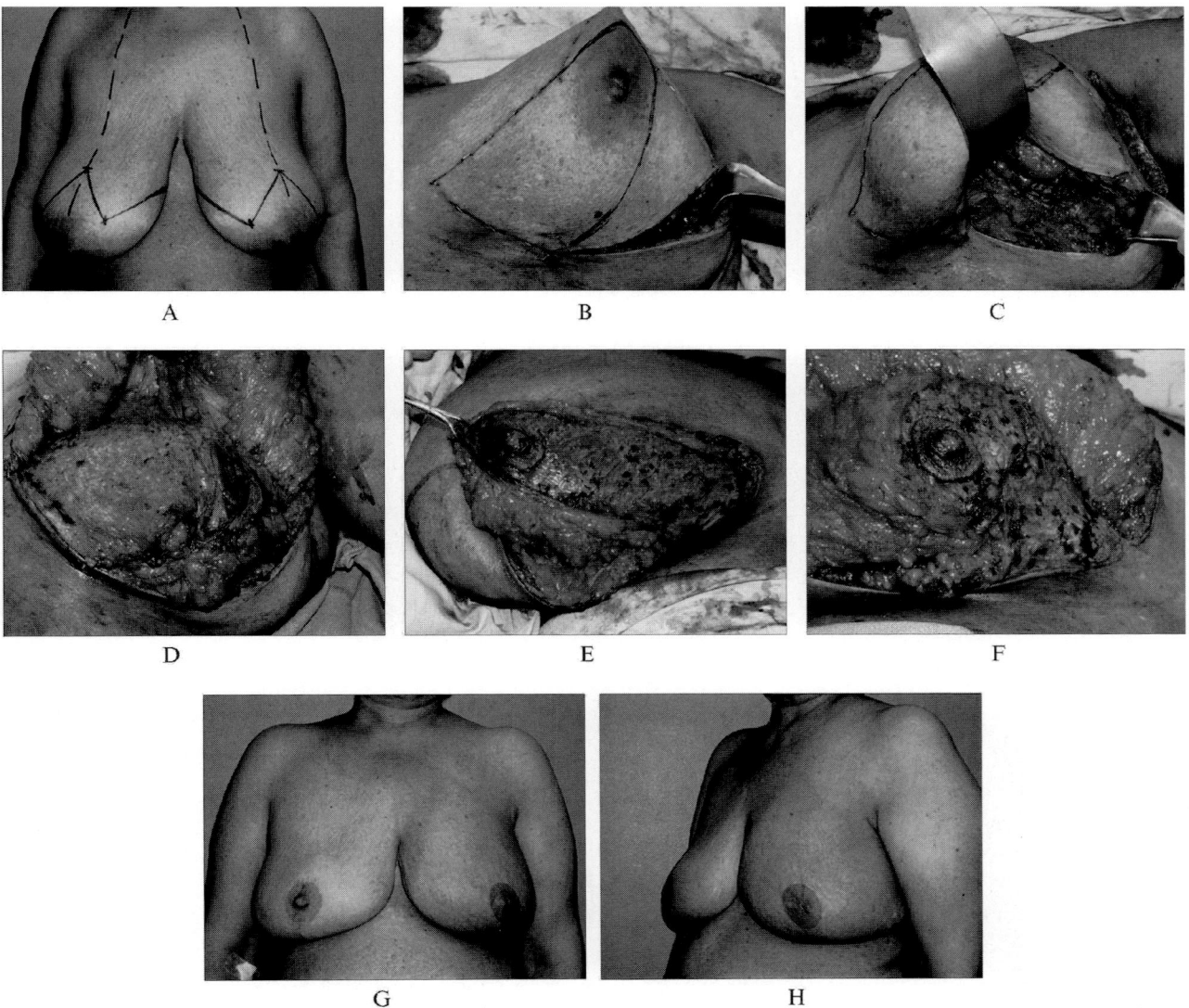

Figure 1 Immediate breast reconstruction after partial mastectomy in a 57-year-old woman with a 38DD bra size who presented with a T3N1 (stage III) invasive ductal carcinoma in the lower outer quadrant of the left breast. The patient had had an excellent response to neoadjuvant chemotherapy and desired breast conservation therapy. *A*, The patient was marked preoperatively with a Wise skin pattern. *B*, The tumor resection was performed through an access incision along the inferior edge of the Wise skin pattern. *C* and *D*, The patient underwent immediate reconstruction with the breast reduction technique (with an inferomedially based parenchymal pedicle) for a defect estimated to be equal to 18% of the breast volume. A right contralateral breast reduction was performed for symmetry. To optimize symmetry, the involved breast was reconstructed first so that the contralateral-breast parenchymal pedicle could be designed to allow the best volume match between the breasts. Also, the parenchymal pedicle design and resection volume for the contralateral breast (*E*) were similar to those for the reconstructed breast. *F*, As shown in the contralateral right breast, with the inferomedial parenchymal pedicle design, the pedicle is rotated to position the nipple-areola complex into its appropriate position in the breast meridian, which maintains the medial fullness of the reconstructed breast. *G* and *H*, Postoperative views 9 months after reconstruction and 6 months after XRT, respectively.

flap on a potentially suboptimal repair of a partial breast defect.

Patient Selection

There are no exact predictors of which patients will or will not benefit from reconstruction after partial mastectomy.

Most patients with medium or large breasts will most likely benefit from immediate reconstruction; however, some patients with small breasts may not. The participation of a plastic surgeon in planning for partial mastectomy is crucial: the plastic surgeon can indicate to patients and referring breast surgeons which patients, from an aesthetic

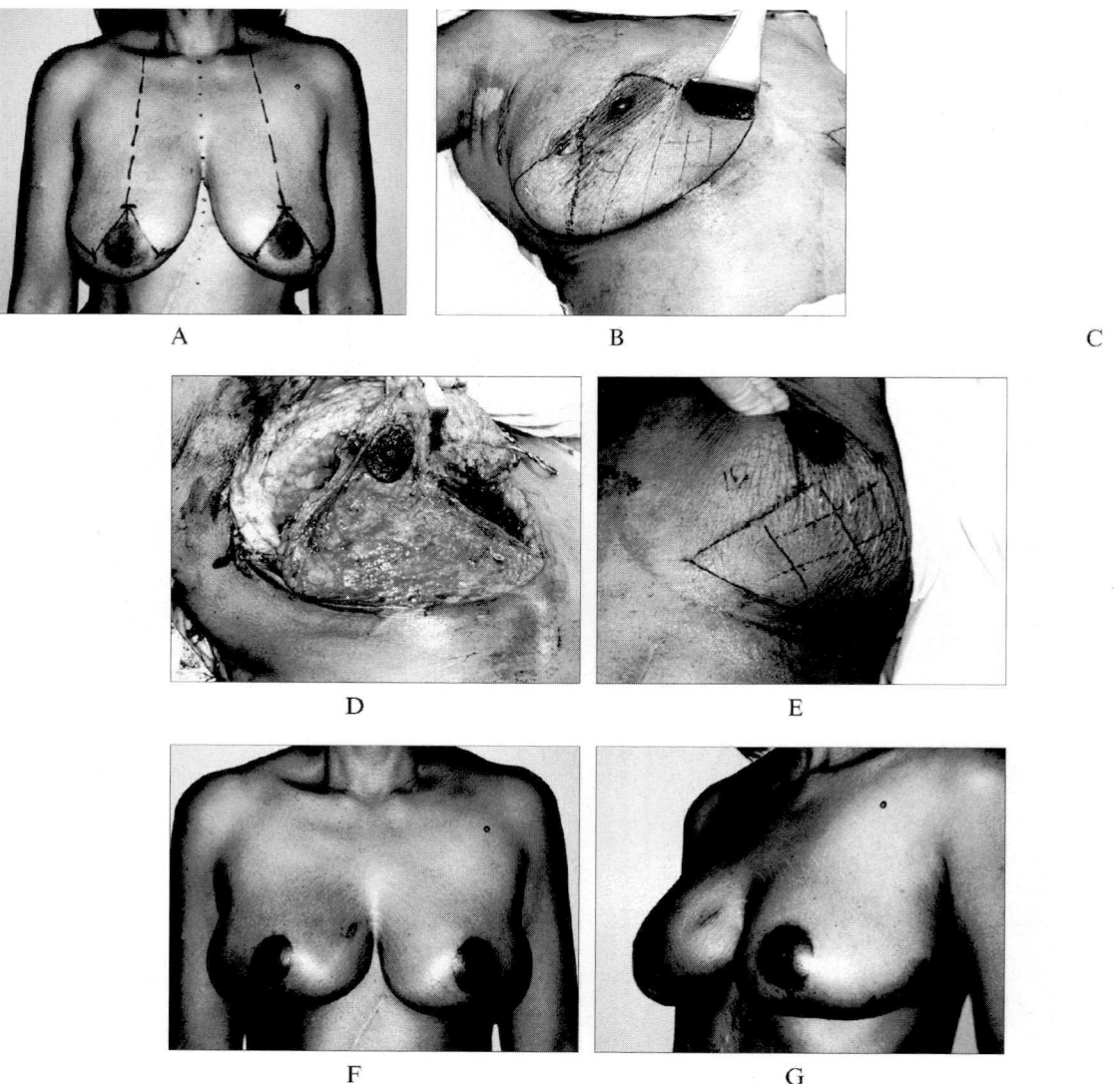

Figure 2 Breast reconstruction after partial mastectomy in a 46-year-old woman with a 38D bra size who presented with a T1N0 (stage I) invasive ductal carcinoma in the upper inner quadrant of the right breast. *A,* The patient was marked preoperatively with a Wise skin pattern in preparation for reconstruction with the breast reduction technique. *B,* Intraoperative view after partial mastectomy (resection volume of 80 grams) shows the defect (7% of the breast volume) in the upper inner quadrant. *C,* Re-excision at the previous biopsy site was performed separately from the tumor resection, which was performed through an access incision along the superior limb of the Wise pattern. *D,* Immediate repair of the defect was performed using an inferomedial parenchymal pedicle design. In this patient, the tumor resection did not encroach on the inferior aspect of the inferomedial pedicle, so it was possible to include both the inferior and medial aspects of the inferomedial pedicle in the reconstruction. *E,* A contralateral breast reduction was performed with the same inferomedial pedicle design to achieve symmetry. *F* and *G,* Postoperative views 6 weeks after reconstruction. The retained medial wedge of breast tissue filled the defect in the upper inner quadrant. In addition, the re-excised biopsy site is barely noticeable and does not detract from the appearance of the reconstructed breast.

point of view, would benefit more from a total mastectomy with breast reconstruction than from a partial mastectomy. Although the recommendations provided should prove useful in the decision-making process, ultimately it is up to the multidisciplinary breast team, along with the patient, to determine which approach is best.

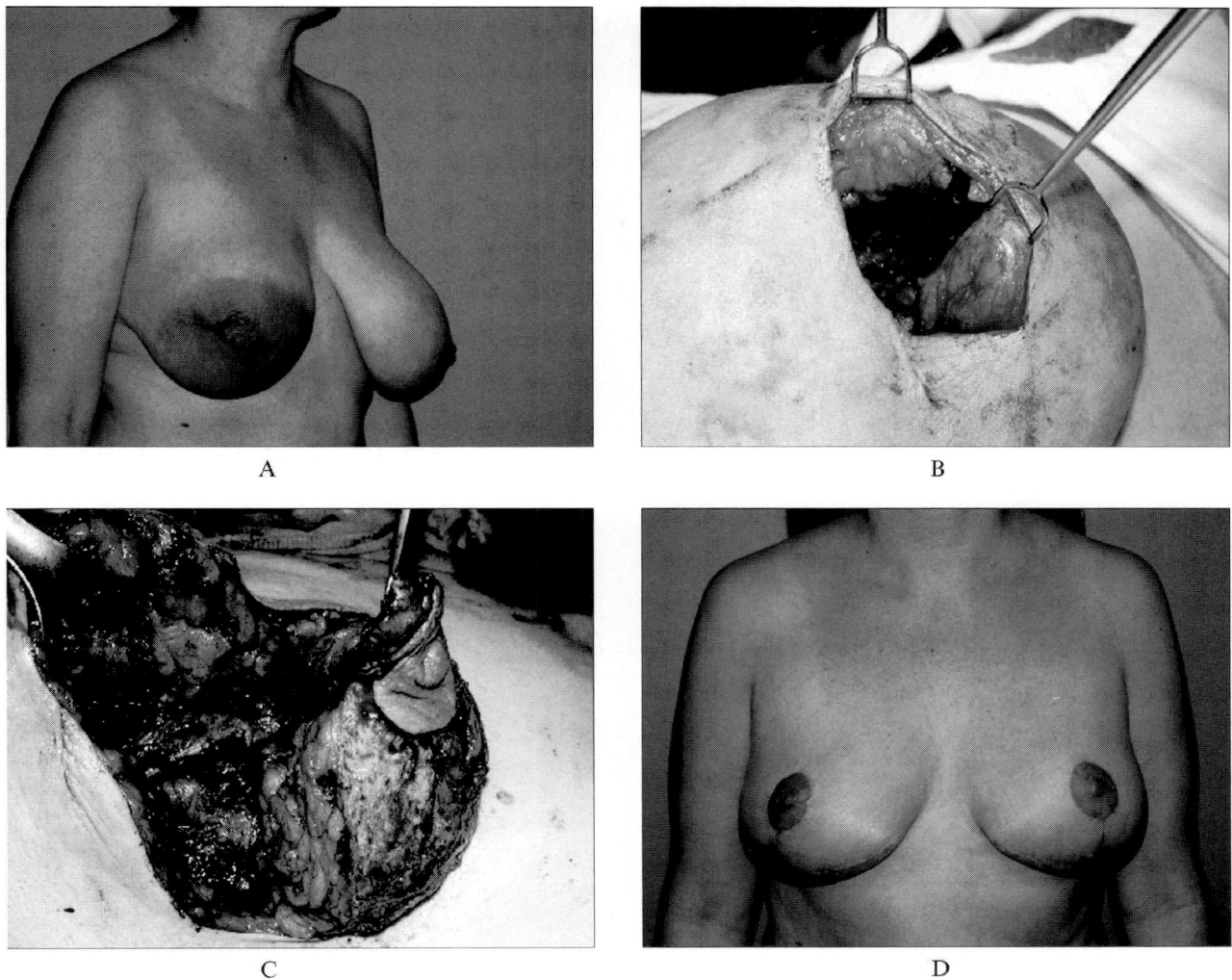

Figure 3 Unexpected deformity after partial mastectomy necessitating delayed reconstruction prior to radiation therapy (XRT). A 41-year-old woman presented 2 weeks after undergoing a partial mastectomy for a central-quadrant tumor. The patient was very dissatisfied with the cosmetic outcome and realized that her outcome would probably be adversely affected by the planned XRT. *A*, Preoperative view. *B*, Intraoperative view. Because the extent and exact location of central resection could not be determined preoperatively, the nipple-areola complex was explored to determine if there was an adequate blood supply for reconstruction with the breast reduction technique. *C*, Intraoperative view demonstrates that the blood supply to the nipple-areola complex was adequate for reconstruction with an inferomedial parenchymal pedicle design. *D*, Postoperative views 3 months after reconstruction. The patient was pleased with the result, and the breast surgeon was relieved that the patient was now satisfied.

Breast Reconstruction after Total Mastectomy

FACTORS AFFECTING SELECTION OF RECONSTRUCTIVE TECHNIQUE

In patients undergoing breast reconstruction after total mastectomy, as in patients undergoing breast reconstruction after partial mastectomy, choosing the best method of reconstruction is essential to optimize the aesthetic outcome and minimize the potential for postoperative complications. Patient desires are extremely important in selecting the reconstructive technique. Unfortunately, sometimes patient's desires cannot be fulfilled because of patient anatomy or other clinical realities.

Breast Cancer Stage

The stage of the breast cancer is critical. Currently, patients with clinical stage I breast cancer are considered to be at low risk for requiring PMRT and are therefore considered candidates for immediate breast reconstruction using any of the available approaches.

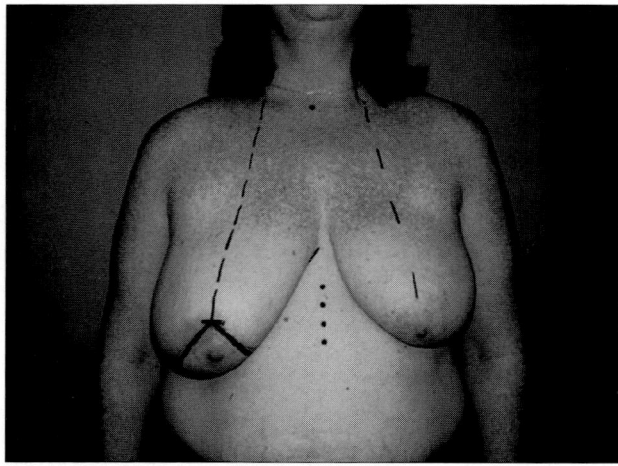

A

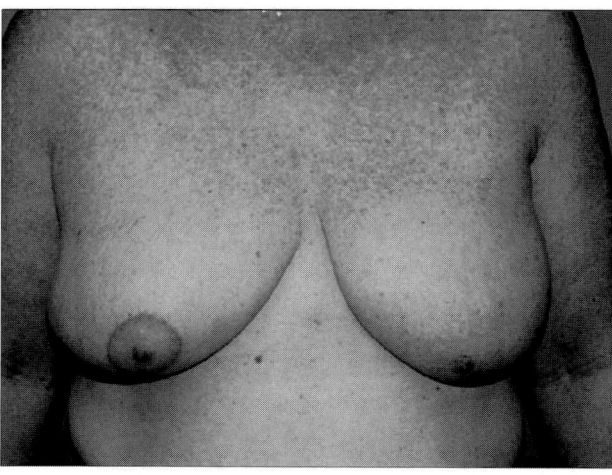

B

Figure 4 A 42-year-old woman presented with breast asymmetry after a left partial mastectomy with subsequent radiation therapy. *A*, Preoperative view. *B*, Postoperative view 3 months after a right breast reduction with a Wise-skin-pattern resection and an inferomedial parenchymal pedicle design.

Patients with clinical stage II breast cancer have a borderline elevated risk of requiring PMRT, and thus are the patients for whom it is most difficult to formulate recommendations regarding breast reconstruction timing.[10,12] It is essential that these patients have a careful preoperative evaluation for risk factors for occult axillary nodal involvement (age younger than 50 years, lymphovascular invasion in the initial biopsy specimen, and T2 tumor)[13] and undetected invasive disease within the breast parenchyma. In patients with any of these risk factors, it may be preferable to avoid the use of breast implants, to perform delayed reconstruction, or to use a delayed-immediate approach (described in detail later in this chapter).

In patients with clinical stage III breast cancer (locally advanced), it may be preferable to delay reconstruction until after mastectomy and PMRT to avoid potential problems with radiation delivery and to avoid the possibility of adverse affects of XRT on an immediately reconstructed breast.[10,14–20] A further consideration in patients with clinical stage III disease is that although breast reconstruction has not been found to delay diagnosis or decrease survival in patients who develop a local recurrence,[21] a nonreconstructed chest wall surface may enhance the ability to examine the chest wall for the purposes of tumor surveillance.

Smoking Status

Smoking is a significant vasoconstrictor and is one of the leading risk factors for complications after breast reconstruction.[22] Smoking can inhibit wound healing, increase the potential for mastectomy skin flap necrosis, and increase the risk of thrombosis of a microvascular flap.

Some studies have shown that in smokers, a microvascular TRAM flap procedure is preferable to a pedicled TRAM flap procedure, in which the flap remains attached to the rectus abdominis muscle and is tunneled to the chest wall.[22] However, consideration should be given to using a more reliable method of reconstruction—use of a latissimus dorsi myocutaneous flap plus a breast implant. A latissimus dorsi myocutaneous flap can provide muscle coverage around a breast implant, which can prevent exposure if skin necrosis occurs post-operatively.[23] This option is preferred to use of a breast implant alone (placement of a tissue expander followed by exchange for a permanent implant).[23] In smokers, consideration should also be given to delaying breast reconstruction until the patient stops smoking. Unfortunately, however, delaying reconstruction denies the patient the opportunity to have the best possible aesthetic outcome—as discussed in detail later in the chapter, less of the breast skin envelope is available when reconstruction is delayed, and thus the shape of the reconstructed breast is not as good as with immediate reconstruction. When delayed breast reconstruction is selected, many reconstructive surgeons advise the patient to stop smoking prior to surgery to decrease the potential for complications.

Anatomy

Anatomy is also a very important factor in selecting the best reconstructive option. In patients who are relatively thin in the lower abdominal region and have large breasts, consideration can be given to performing reconstruction with a TRAM flap combined with an underlying breast implant (Figure 5A).[23] Patients with a diastasis recti with a protuberant abdomen can require more extensive reconstruction of the abdominal wall with synthetic mesh after the harvest of a TRAM flap (Figure 5B). Obese patients have an increased risk of fat necrosis of the TRAM flap as well as wound healing

problems at the abdominal donor site (Figure 5C).[24] Unfortunately, the use of breast implants alone in obese patients usually does not result in a favorable aesthetic outcome. Patients who are extremely thin with small breasts often desire breast augmentation.[23] In this situation, use of a TRAM flap plus an implant is not

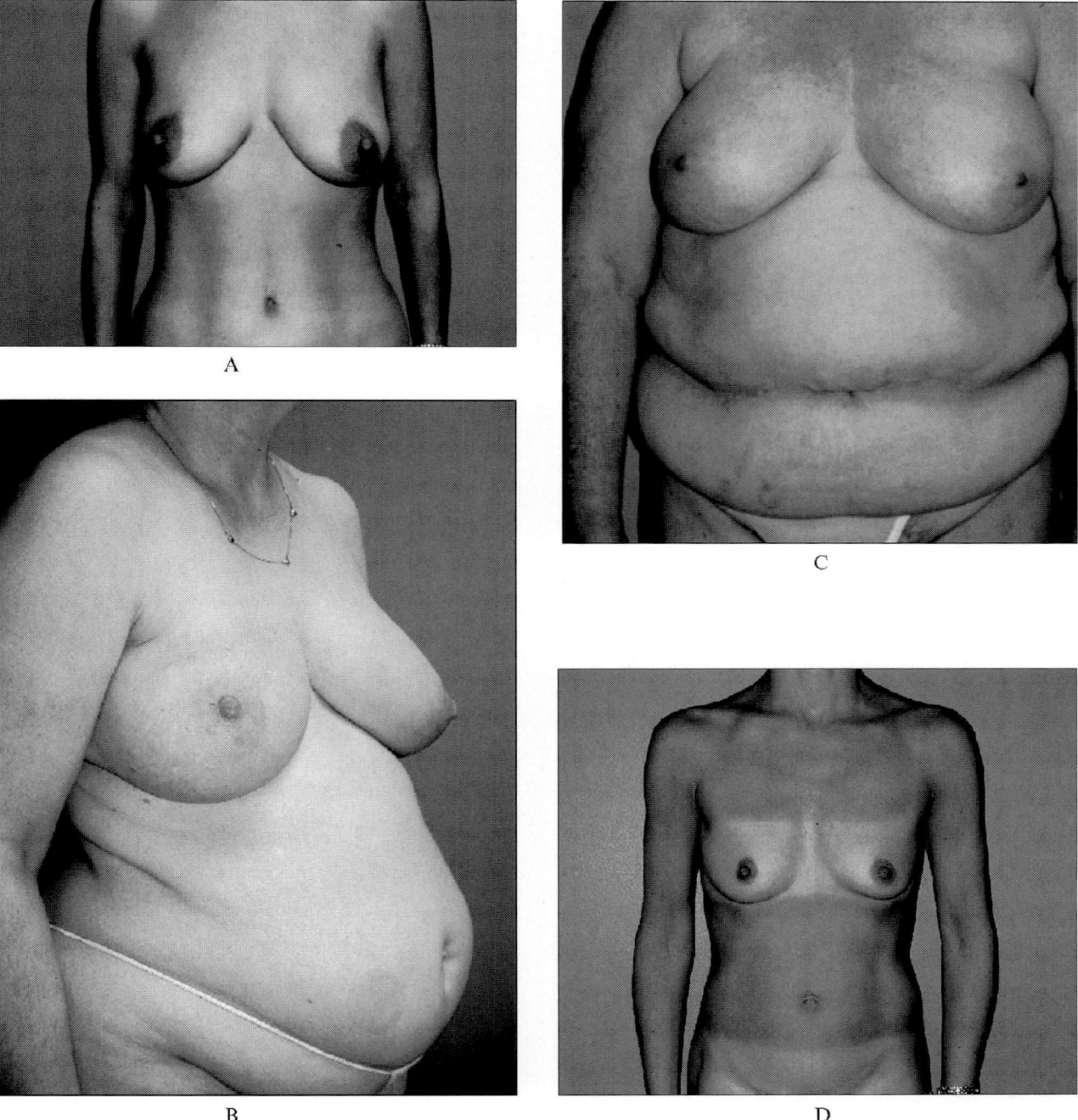

A

B

C

D

Figure 5 Anatomical considerations in determining the appropriate reconstructive method for breast reconstruction after mastectomy. *A*, Relatively thin patient with large breasts. *B*, Patient with a diastasis recti with a protuberant abdomen. *C*, Obese patient. *D*, Extremely thin patient with small breasts.

an option because of the difficulty of closing the abdominal donor site (Figure 5D). In these patients, breast augmentation can be accomplished with tissue expansion followed by insertion of a breast implant, but a better result may be obtained with use of a latissimus dorsi myocutaneous flap combined with a breast implant. A latissimus dorsi myocutaneous flap provides the additional skin needed and provides complete muscle coverage of the breast implant, which may decrease the potential for postoperative rippling (irregularities of the implant wall that can be easily visualized under the skin, especially in thin patients). The use of a silicone implant as opposed to a saline implant can also decrease the potential for rippling.

Preexisting Scars

Preexisting scars from previous surgeries that lie close to potential donor sites must also be taken into account in determining the optimal method of breast reconstruction.[25] This situation occurred with the patient shown in Figure 6. She desired TRAM flap reconstruction, but she unfortunately had previously undergone a nephrectomy (right subcostal incision) as well as several midline laparotomies. Although she could have undergone reconstruction with a hemi-TRAM flap (half of the lower abdominal ellipse of the TRAM flap), performed as either a pedicled or a microvascular procedure on the left side and as a microvascular procedure on the right side, the resultant abdominoplasty (tummy tuck closure) of the abdominal donor site would probably have resulted in the loss of a large triangle of skin on the right side of the abdominal wall, underlying the subcostal scar.

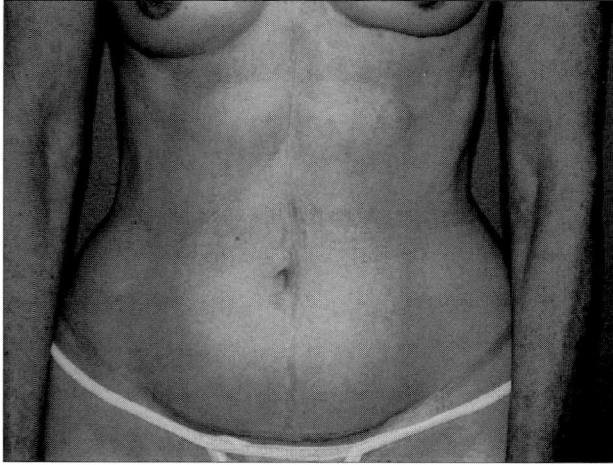

Figure 6 This patient's preexisting abdominal scars, from a nephrectomy (right subcostal incision) and several midline laparotomes, precluded reconstruction with a transverse rectus abdominis myocutaneous flap.

Prior Radiation Therapy

Another important consideration in determining the optimal method of breast reconstruction is that prior XRT to the chest wall increases the amount of tissue—mainly skin—required for delayed breast reconstruction.[12] Delayed reconstruction after XRT usually requires resection of the retained inferior breast skin (between the mastectomy scar and inframammary fold) in order to reconstruct a natural, ptotic-appearing breast. Therefore, delayed reconstruction with a TRAM flap after XRT often requires the use of three-quarters of the lower abdominal ellipse of the TRAM flap, including tissue across the midline of the lower abdominal wall. This situation can be even more complex in a patient who also has a lower abdominal laparotomy scar (Figure 7A). Such patients often require a more complex bipedicled TRAM flap procedure to provide a blood supply on both sides of the lower abdominal vertical scar. The position of a mastectomy scar may also affect the amount of tissue required for delayed breast reconstruction after XRT (Figure 7B). Delayed reconstruction with implants after XRT is not a preferred method because of the potential for capsular contracture,[10] which can result in displacement of the implant and patient discomfort from constriction across the chest wall.

Patient Age

Patient age in and of itself has not been found to independently affect the outcome of breast reconstruction, even in the case of microsurgical reconstruction.[26] Physiologic age is more important than chronologic age. However, significant medical problems must be considered in selecting the appropriate reconstructive technique. For instance, cardiovascular disease may result in intraoperative hypotension, which may increase the potential for microvascular thrombosis of an autologous tissue flap. Medications—like corticosteroids or other agents used for arthritis, such as methotrexate—may inhibit postoperative wound healing. Patients with pulmonary ailments can have difficulties with respiration (atelectasis and pneumonia) after TRAM flap reconstruction, and patients with back ailments can experience worsening back pain.

Planned or Previous Chemotherapy

Immediate breast reconstruction has not been found to delay the start of adjuvant chemotherapy, and administration of neoadjuvant chemotherapy prior to mastectomy and immediate breast reconstruction has not been found to result in an increased incidence of complications.[27]

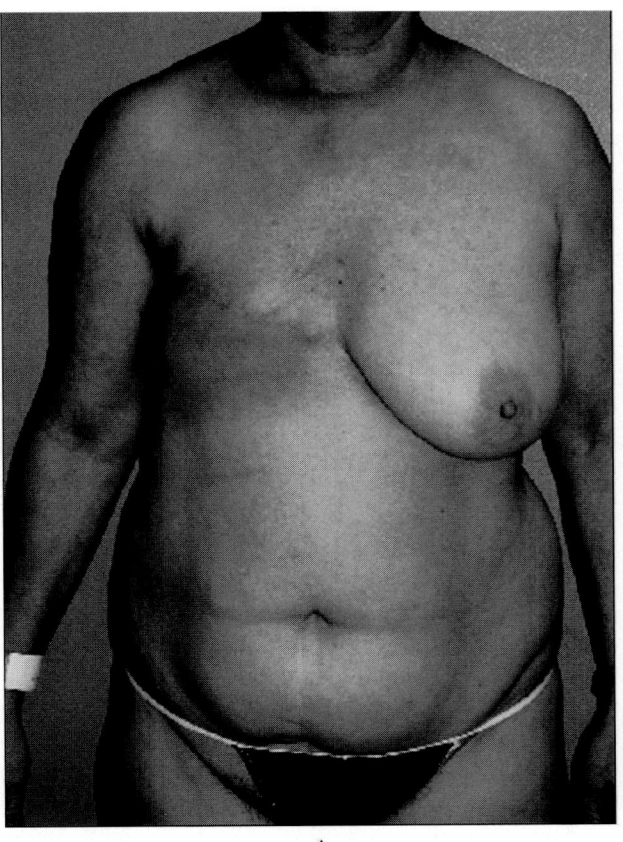
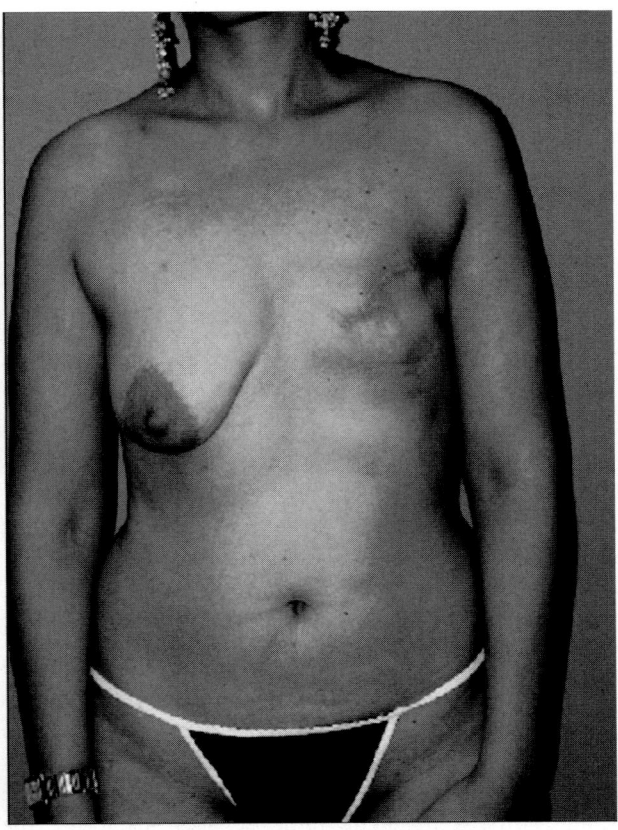

A   B

Figure 7 Challenges in delayed transverse rectus abdominis myocutaneous (TRAM)-flap-based reconstruction after mastectomy and radiation therapy (XRT). *A*, This patient had a lower abdominal midline incision from a previous hysterectomy that limited our ability to use the tissue across the midline. Because reconstruction was performed after XRT, we preferred not to use breast implants, even along with a TRAM flap. Furthermore, we chose not to perform tissue expansion of a breast envelope to decrease the amount of donor-site tissue required because this procedure is associated with a high rate of complications. Because of the need to replace the inferior breast skin, we had to use the lower abdominal tissue across the midline scar (three-quarters of the lower abdominal ellipse). Thus, a more extensive bipedicled TRAM flap was required to provide a blood supply on both sides of the lower abdominal scar. *B*, In this patient, the mastectomy scar was positioned relatively high on the chest wall, necessitating replacement of all the breast skin below the mastectomy incision and the inframammary fold. Given the extensive tissue requirements, a microvascular TRAM flap was used because it provides an enhanced blood supply for large flaps.

IMMEDIATE BREAST RECONSTRUCTION

Immediate breast reconstruction is usually reserved for patients with clinical stage I breast cancer and patients with clinical stage II breast cancer who do not have an increased risk of requiring PMRT. Unfortunately, although the risk of requiring PMRT can be predicted before surgery, the need for PMRT cannot be definitively determined until the final pathologic evaluation is complete.

Immediate breast reconstruction offers many advantages over delayed reconstruction, including a better aesthetic outcome due to preservation of the breast skin envelope[1] and the psychological benefit of awakening from mastectomy with a reconstructed breast.[2] Immediate breast reconstruction also enables patients with active lifestyles to more easily resume their activities of daily living. For example, even while patients are receiving adjuvant chemotherapy, they can still wear their favorite attire to attend social functions. Figure 8 is a timeline of the steps required to complete an immediate breast reconstruction. The figure shows a total time of 1 year; however, there can be much variation depending on the timing of adjuvant therapy, wound healing, technical issues with the breast reconstruction method, and the effects of the patient's personality and lifestyle.

Instead of trying to cover all the available methods of immediate breast reconstruction, this chapter will focus on the methods that are most commonly used.

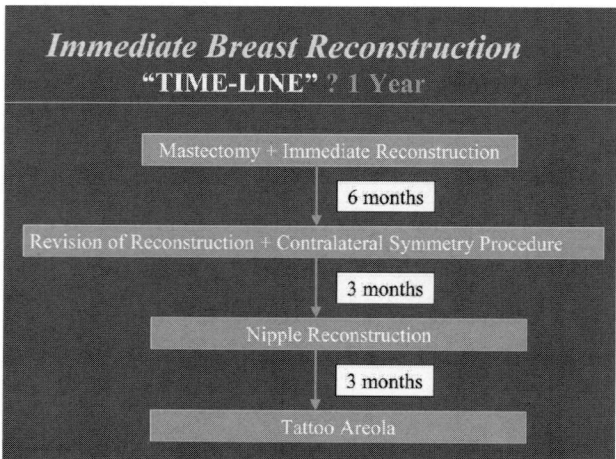

Figure 8 General timeline for immediate breast reconstruction.

Tissue Expansion Followed by Exchange of the Expander for a Permanent Breast Implant

The tissue expansion technique involves the initial submuscular placement of a tissue expander, which is an adjustable breast implant that most commonly has an integrated saline filling port that can easily be accessed by placing a needle through the skin. During postoperative office visits, a magnetic finder is used to locate the integrated port under the skin, and the port is subsequently accessed for saline filling. Tissue expanders are not designed to be used as permanent implants because they preferentially expand the lower pole of the breast and have a more rugged construction than permanent implants to enable them to withstand the forces of expansion.

The tissue expansion technique usually requires multiple postoperative office visits for expansion of the breast skin envelope. The time required to complete the expansion process usually ranges from 3 to 6 months after mastectomy and is mostly dependent on the desired breast size, the thickness of the mastectomy skin flaps, and the patient's ability to tolerate the expansions. Usually the volume of saline that is instilled into the expander at each visit decreases as the breast becomes larger because of increasing discomfort from stretching of the scar capsule and backward pressure on the underlying ribs. Despite discomfort, which can last for several days after each expansion, the process is not usually painful.

A disadvantage of the tissue expansion method as compared with other methods of breast reconstruction is that it is a two-stage approach—a second surgical procedure is required to exchange the tissue expander for a permanent breast implant. Another disadvantage—a disadvantage of implant-based reconstruction in general—is the resultant superior fullness, which makes it difficult to create a ptotic-appearing breast. In addition, with unilateral implant-based reconstruction, obtaining symmetry with the contralateral native breast can be difficult. Patients often require a contralateral mastopexy (breast lift) and a contralateral breast-implant augmentation to obtain adequate symmetry.[28] Bilateral breast reconstruction with the tissue expander technique is an easier way to obtain a symmetric result after breast reconstruction (Figure 9). However, the tissue expansion method can allow for reasonable breast symmetry when the patient wears a bra, which is the goal of reconstruction for some patients who choose this method.

Currently, silicon implants can only be offered to patients as part of an institutional review board–approved protocol. At M. D. Anderson Cancer Center, patients are given the choice of either saline or silicon breast implants. Patients who select silicon implants are given extensive literature to read and are required to give informed consent for the procedure. Although silicon implants offer many advantages, including a softer texture and less implant rippling, patients must be comfortable with the concerns previously raised with the use of silicon breast implants. Another consideration with implant-based reconstruction is that, like a breast implant, a tissue expander is a foreign body and therefore is associated with a risk of infection that could necessitate expander removal.[29]

An advantage of the tissue expansion technique and a reason why many patients prefer this method of breast reconstruction is that the surgical and recovery time tend to be the most rapid. Placement of a tissue expander

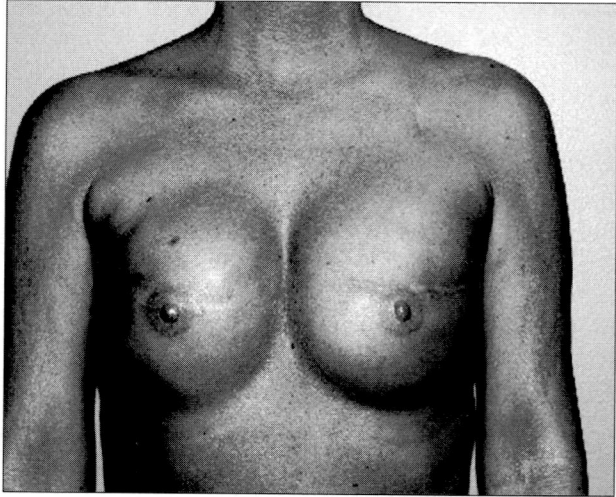

Figure 9 Postoperative views 1 year after bilateral breast reconstruction with tissue expansion followed by placement of permanent silicon breast implants.

usually takes only 1 to 2 hours, and the hospitalization after mastectomy and expander placement is usually just a few days. The out-of-hospital recovery period is approximately 7 to 10 days. However, the subsequent surgical procedure to exchange the expander for the permanent implant is associated with a similar recovery period.

Latissimus Dorsi Myocutaneous Flap Plus a Breast Implant

Reconstruction performed using a latissimus dorsi myocutaneous flap plus a breast implant is more complex than reconstruction performed with an expander and an implant and is associated with a longer recovery period. However, the aesthetic outcome tends to be better—the end result is a more natural-appearing breast.

The latissimus dorsi muscle is located on the back below the tip of the scapula and above the iliac crest. A skin island can be designed overlying the muscle. There can be much variation in skin island design depending on the reconstructive needs and patient anatomy. A small skin island oriented transversely under the scapula can result in a scar that can be camouflaged with a bra and a scar with a fairly good appearance because of the reduced tension on the back closure. The vascular pedicle of the latissimus dorsi flap is the thoracodorsal vessels, which originate from the subscapular vascular system located within the axilla. The combined skin and muscle flap is pivoted under the axilla to the chest wall while remaining attached to the thoracodorsal vessels. The skin island of the flap is used to replace any excised skin, including the nipple-areola complex, and the muscle is draped over a breast implant to soften the texture and appearance of the reconstructed breast.

A latissimus dorsi flap combined with a breast implant is a good option for obese patients, in whom it is not safe to perform a TRAM flap procedure (Figure 10).[23] It is also a good option for thin patients who are not candidates for a TRAM flap procedure because of inadequate tissue for reconstruction or for closure of the abdominal donor site. Unlike the tissue expansion method, breast reconstruction with a latissimus dorsi flap plus an implant can create a ptotic-appearing breast. The skin island that is often included with a latissimus dorsi flap can immediately replace any resected skin, along with the nipple-areola complex, to retain the initial shape of the breast skin envelope. Another benefit of latissimus dorsi flap-based reconstruction as opposed to tissue expansion is that a second surgical procedure is not necessarily required. However, sometimes a revision procedure is required to release the breast implant into the ptotic breast skin envelope. The surgical time with unilateral reconstruction ranges from 3 to 6 hours. Although most patients require only a 2- to 3-day hospitalization, a longer recovery period (4 weeks) is required than with implant-only reconstruction. A disadvantage with latissimus dorsi flap-based reconstruction is that the latissimus muscle tends to atrophy over time, which makes the underlying breast implant more prominent and can reveal even subtle irregularities in the implant caused by capsular contracture.[23]

Autologous Tissue Reconstruction

Breast reconstruction using the patient's own tissues results in the most natural-appearing reconstructed breasts.[30] Although autologous tissue procedures can be lengthy and are associated with the longest recovery period, they often require fewer revision and symmetry procedures (ie, to correct problems resulting from implant malposition secondary to capsular contracture). With autologous tissue reconstruction, it is possible to create a ptotic-appearing breast without the need for a breast implant, and the appearance of the contralateral native breast can be matched without the need for an additional contralateral symmetry procedure.[28] In addition to aesthetic benefits, autologous-tissue-based reconstruction offers extreme versatility in terms of providing extensive tissue replacement and providing a blood supply to assist with healing within an irradiated operative field (Figure 11).[12] Although autologous tissue procedures require a donor site, with the potential for associated morbidity, they avoid implant-related problems, which can worsen over time.[23]

TRAM Flaps

Although breast reconstruction with a TRAM flap can be ideal for motivated patients, it is associated with a long and arduous recovery that requires patients have a good support system. Patients who work must arrange to miss work for 4 to 6 weeks. However, with TRAM flap reconstruction, patients often require fewer follow-up office visits than for tissue expansion and require fewer subsequent surgical procedures.

The fatty tissue of the TRAM flap resembles normal breast tissue and can result in a natural-appearing reconstructed breast. Breasts reconstructed with a TRAM flap also tend to adjust to changes in body weight.[31] If a patient who undergoes an implant-based reconstruction has significant weight loss, an implant exchange may be required to retain symmetry between the reconstructed breast and the normal breast. In a patient who has undergone TRAM flap reconstruction, the reconstructed breast and the contralateral native breast tend to change in tandem in response to changes

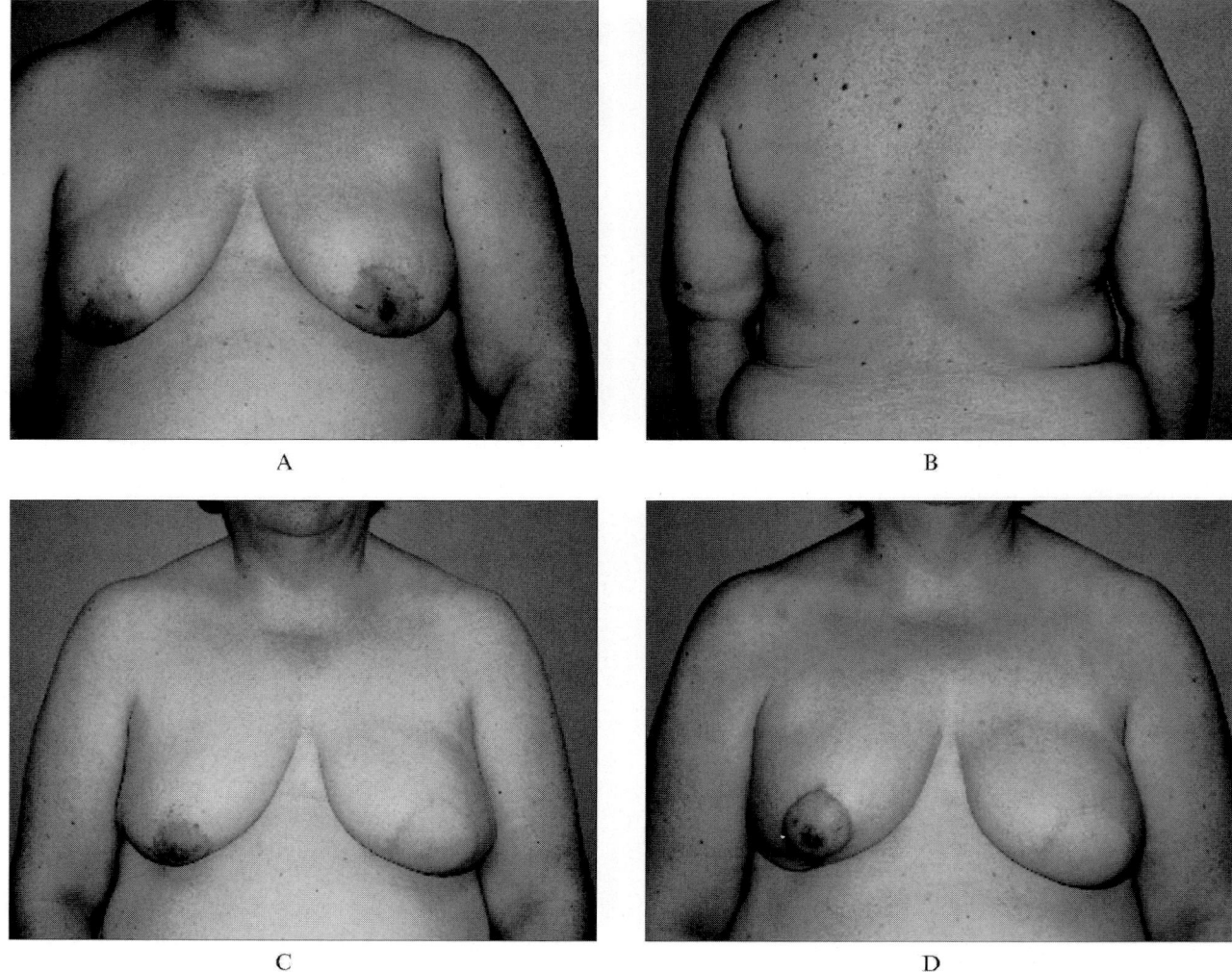

Figure 10 *A* and *B*. A 49-year-old woman with left breast cancer desired breast reconstruction but was obese and therefore not considered a candidate for a transverse rectus abdominis myocutaneous (TRAM) flap procedure. It was also felt that she would not obtain a good aesthetic outcome with breast implants alone. *C*, She underwent a left mastectomy and immediate breast reconstruction with a latissimus dorsi myocutaneous flap and a saline breast implant. *D*, Six months later, she had a right vertical mastopexy with breast implant augmentation for symmetry. She is awaiting the nipple and areola reconstruction.

in body weight. A TRAM flap reconstruction also involves an abdominoplasty (tummy tuck), which patients are always excited about because it allows them to focus on something positive in the midst of otherwise negative changes that are affecting their body image.

Repair of the TRAM flap abdominal donor site is usually technically easier in patients who have borne children because pregnancy results in laxity in their lower abdominal wall and some redundancy of the overlying soft tissues. Obesity and smoking increase the risk of complications after TRAM flap reconstruction.[22,24] A body mass index of less than 30 kg/m^2 is preferred, and patients with a body mass index greater than or equal to 35 kg/m^2 are considered to be at high risk for

complications. These complications are mainly related to a decreased blood supply to the TRAM flap (associated with an increased risk of fat necrosis) and wound healing problems at the lower abdominal donor site. Although with immediate TRAM flap reconstruction it is not always possible to have patients quit smoking prior to surgery, with delayed TRAM flap reconstruction it is prudent to insist that patients quit smoking prior to the procedure.

Pedicled TRAM Flap

The blood supply to a TRAM flap can be provided by any of several methods. One method is to transfer the lower abdominal fatty tissue together with attached underlying

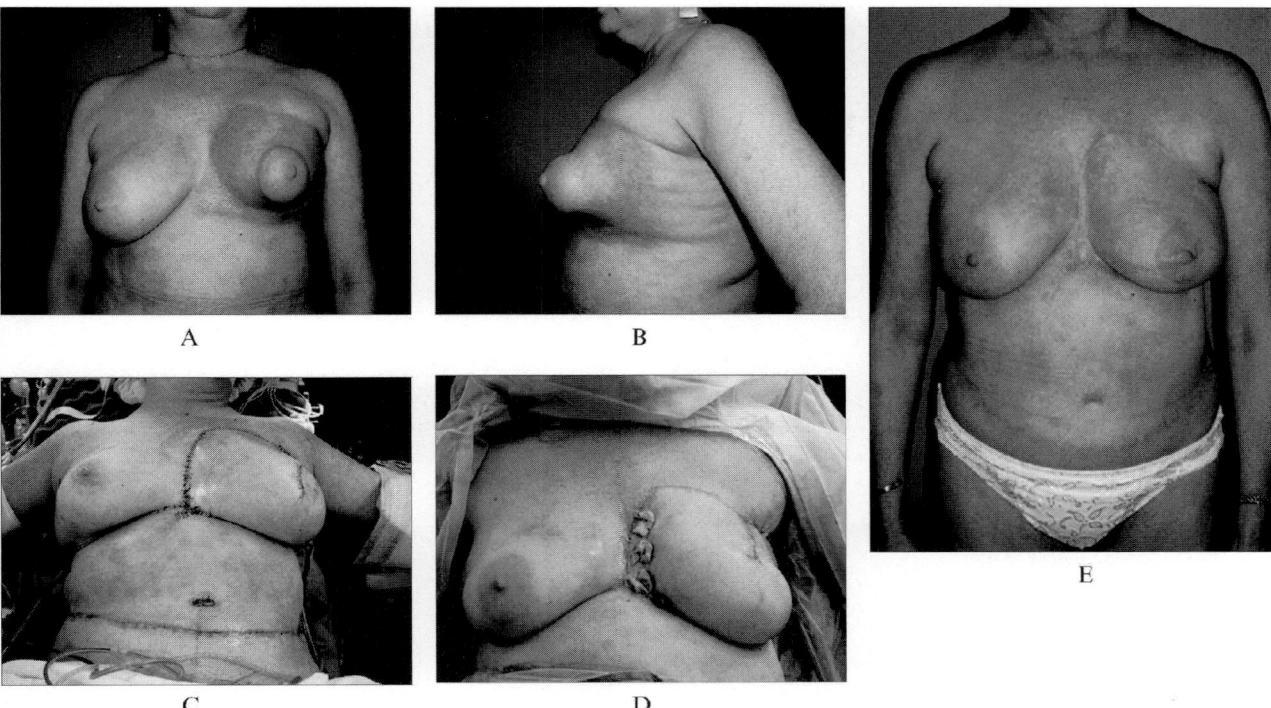

Figure 11 Utility of autologous-tissue breast reconstruction in previously irradiated patients. *A* and *B*, A 50-year-old woman underwent breast conservation therapy for an early-stage left breast cancer. She had an extreme inflammatory and subsequently fibrotic reaction to the radiation therapy that caused not only significant breast deformity but also constant pain. The patient opted for complete mastectomy with immediate breast reconstruction. *C*, The mastectomy was extensive—it entailed removal of all of the breast skin plus a large region of the adjacent chest wall. A complete three-dimensional reconstruction was required. A bipedicled transverse rectus abdominis myocutaneous (TRAM) flap (a combined pedicled right TRAM flap and a microvascular left TRAM flap) was designed, along with an advancement flap of the upper abdomen. The bipedicled nature of the TRAM flap allowed for use of the entire lower abdominal ellipse of the TRAM flap. *D*, Six months after reconstruction, the patient underwent a revision of the reconstructed breast to contour the breast shape and to recreate the cleavage of the breast. *E*, One and a half years after the revision procedure, the patient was without pain and had resumed her active lifestyle.

rectus abdominis muscle. This type of flap is referred to as a pedicled TRAM flap. The blood supply originates from the internal mammary vessels in the thoracic region and travels through the rectus abdominis muscle as the superior epigastric vessels to the umbilical region, where the superior epigastric vessels become the deep inferior epigastric vessels and send perforating vessels into the lower abdominal skin and subcutaneous tissue. With a pedicled TRAM flap, there are limitations on the amount of lower abdominal tissue that can be reliably transferred because of an increased risk of fat necrosis within the TRAM flap. This issue can be especially problematic in obese patients and smokers. Pedicled TRAM flaps require that the entire rectus muscle be elevated and remain attached to the flap. As a result, the inframammary fold must be disrupted to tunnel the flap to the chest wall, which tends to result in a bulge in that region.

Microvascular TRAM Flap

Another method of transferring the lower abdominal fatty tissue, and the method that we prefer at M. D. Anderson, is the microvascular TRAM flap procedure (Figures 12 and 13). A microvascular TRAM flap is completely freed from the underlying rectus abdominis muscle, with its blood supply based inferiorly directly off the deep inferior epigastric vessels, which are branches of the iliac vessels, the predominant blood supply to this anatomic region. This approach avoids the need to use the entire rectus muscle to transfer the flap to the chest wall. At M. D. Anderson, we most commonly use the internal mammary vessels, located on the medial chest wall, as recipient vessels for the microvascular transfer. The internal mammary vessels provide several advantages over the thoracodorsal vessels, which were our previously preferred recipient vessels. In breast cancer patients who

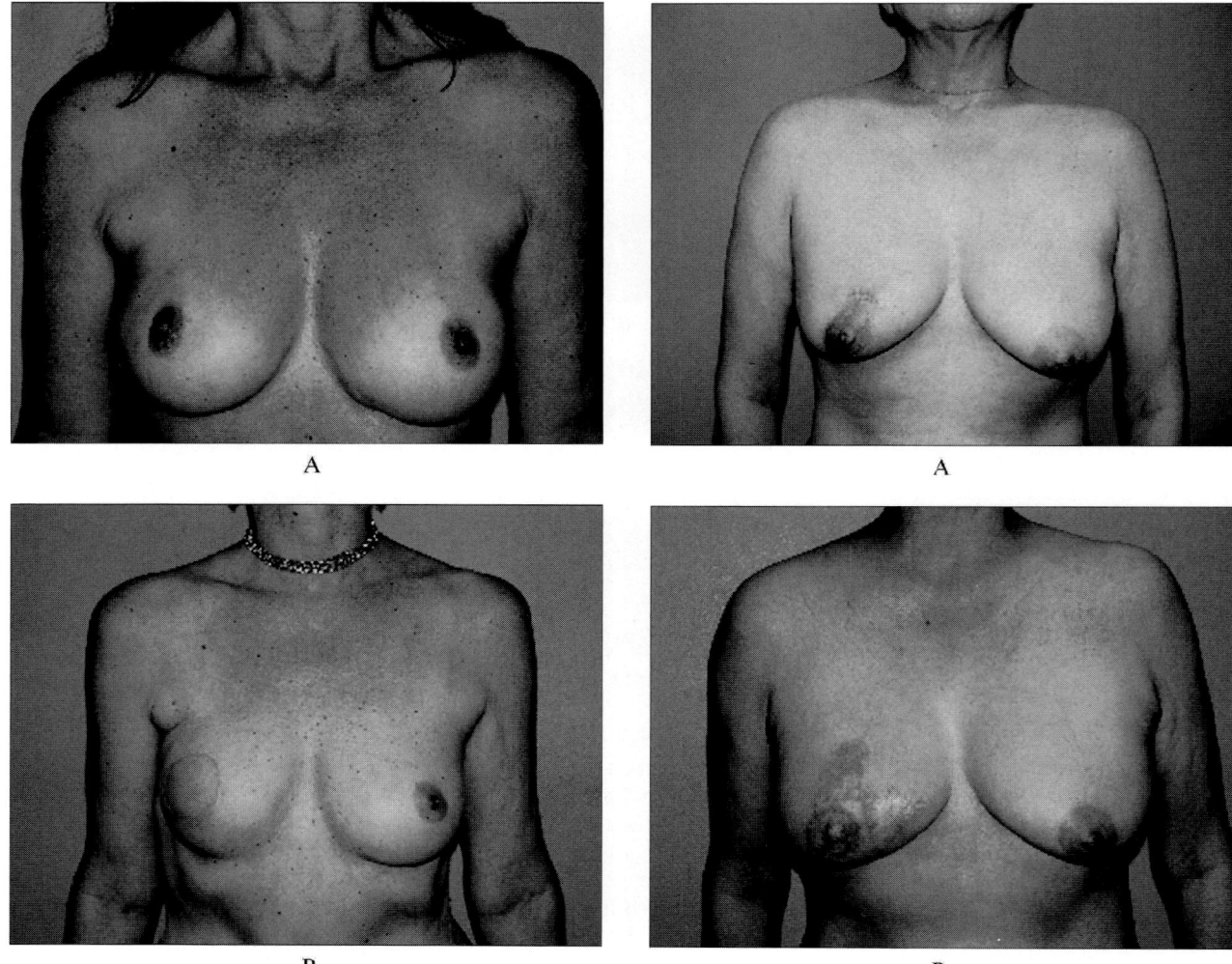

Figure 12 Microvascular transverse rectus abdominis myocutaneous (TRAM) flap reconstruction in a 52-year-old woman with a right-sided breast cancer. *A,* Preoperative view. *B,* Six months after a right skin-sparing modified radical mastectomy with immediate reconstruction using a left microvascular TRAM flap that included the twelfth intercostal nerve. The internal mammary blood vessels were used as recipient vessels, and the medial branch of the third intercostal nerve was used to neurotize the flap. The patient required no revision procedures. Nipple and areola reconstruction were planned.

Figure 13 Microvascular transverse rectus abdominis myocutaneous (TRAM) flap reconstruction in a 56-year-old woman with a right-sided breast cancer. *A* Preoperative view. *B,* One year after a right total mastectomy, right axillary sentinel lymph node biopsy, and immediate breast reconstruction with a left microvascular TRAM flap (the internal mammary artery and vein served as recipient vessels). The patient required no revision procedures. She underwent nipple reconstruction and areola tattooing.

undergo sentinel lymph node biopsy, the thoracodorsal vessels can be damaged, but the internal mammary vessels are not at risk.[13] The use of the internal mammary vessels also allows for more medial positioning of the TRAM flap on the chest wall, which creates a more ideal shape of the reconstructed breast.[32]

After the microvascular TRAM flap is harvested, it is transferred to the chest wall and anastomosed to the internal mammary vessels, which are accessed by removal of the third intercostal cartilage (Figure 14A). Removal of

the cartilage does not usually cause pain or deformity.[32] Occasionally, removal of the cartilage is not required because large perforating vessels from the internal mammary artery and vein perforate between the ribs and are of adequate caliber to serve as recipient vessels (Figure 14B). Although the long-term results are unclear, sensation can be added to a TRAM flap by anastomosis of an intercostal nerve on the chest wall to an intercostal nerve from the abdominal region that is harvested as part of the TRAM flap.[33]

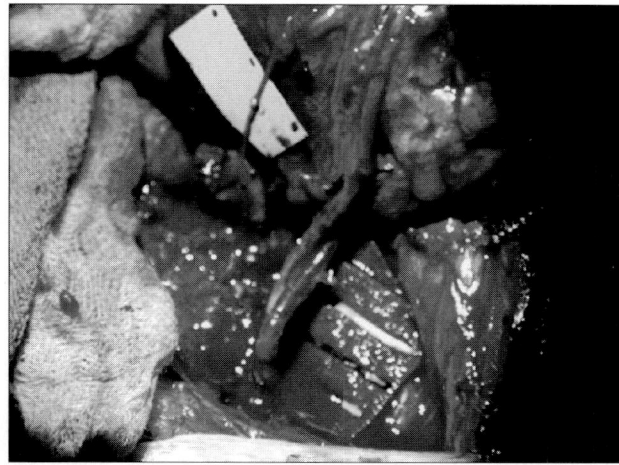

A

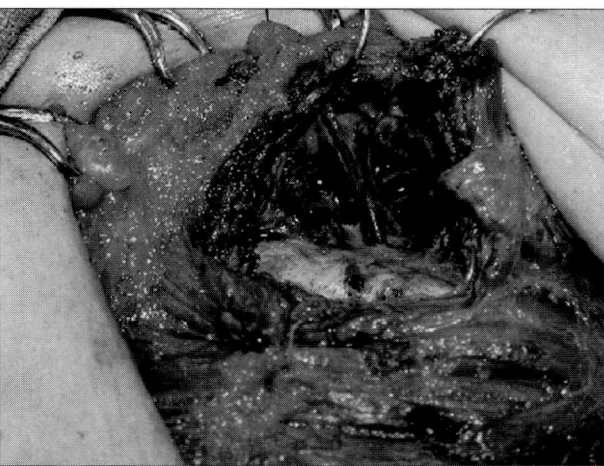

B

Figure 14 Microsurgical aspects of transverse rectus abdominis myocutaneous (TRAM) flap reconstruction. *A* Intraoperative view after microsurgical anastomosis of deep inferior epigastric artery and vein of TRAM flap to internal mammary artery and vein. Also shown is the neurorraphy between the eleventh intercostal nerve, included with the TRAM flap, and the medial branch of third intercostal nerve. *B,* Intraoperative view of large perforating branches from the internal mammary artery and vein dissected away from the pectoralis major muscle in preparation for use as recipient vessels for microsurgical transfer of a TRAM flap.

Unlike the thoracodorsal vessels, which are located within the axilla, the internal mammary vessels can be easily accessed through a small centrally located incision, such as a periareolar mastectomy incision. A periareolar incision can be completely camouflaged by nipple and areola reconstruction, which can decrease the stigma of breast cancer treatment. However, the resultant small skin island can make it difficult to monitor blood flow within the flap with a handheld Doppler probe, the usual

technique. In these cases, an implantable Doppler probe (Cook Vascular Inc., Leechburg, PA) can be placed directly around the vascular pedicle of the flap and monitored through a wire brought out through the skin that is connected to a receiver.

Microvascular TRAM flaps provide some advantages over pedicled TRAM flaps, including less disturbance of the abdominal wall donor site, a more robust blood supply, and the need for less rectus muscle because the flap does not need to be tunneled to the chest wall.[34] Decreased disturbance of the abdominal wall and the need for less muscle may be beneficial for active patients and can avoid the need for synthetic mesh to support the abdominal wall and maintain its contour. Fatty tissue has a very tenuous blood supply, which can become especially evident when we transfer it as a flap. Fat necrosis within a breast reconstructed with a TRAM flap can result in significant atrophy and contour deformities that can cause asymmetry with the normal breast. The microvascular TRAM flap is directly supplied by the deep inferior epigastric system, not a circuitous route depending considerably on the number of choke vessel connections between the superior and inferior epigastric systems located within the umbilical region. The result is less fat necrosis within the microvascular TRAM flap,[34] especially in patients who have a thick abdominal pannus.[24] The enhanced blood supply also allows for the use of a larger portion (three-quarters) of the lower abdominal ellipse of a TRAM flap.

Although the microvascular TRAM flap procedure offers many benefits over the pedicled TRAM flap procedure, the microvascular procedure is more technically demanding and has an all-or-nothing result: if the anastomoses thrombose and the flap cannot be salvaged, the TRAM flap is lost and the patient needs another method of breast reconstruction.

Repair of the TRAM Flap Abdominal Donor Site

There are several approaches to repairing the abdominal wall after harvest of a TRAM flap. The choice of approach depends on the patient's body habitus and the amount of abdominal fascia (anterior rectus sheath) and muscle included with the TRAM flap. Although in many patients we just close the fascial defect primarily, some TRAM harvests require additional fascia to preserve important blood supply to the flap. In these circumstances, synthetic mesh or Alloderm (LifeCell Corp, Branchburg, NJ)—human cadaveric dermis devoid of living cells—is used to replace the fascia that was resected with the TRAM flap (Figure 15). Alloderm avoids a potentially disastrous complication that can occur in patients who have reconstruction of the

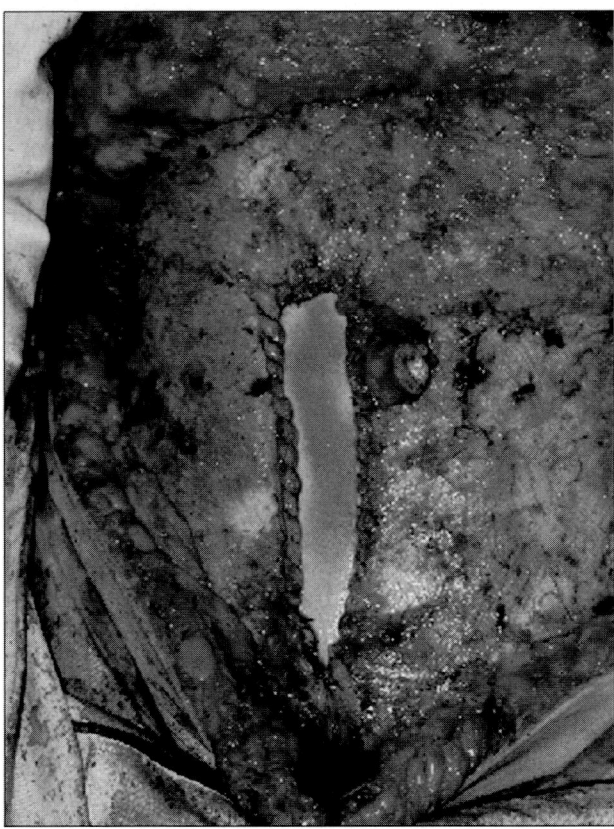

Figure 15 Use of Alloderm (LifeCell Corp, Branchburg, NJ) to replace the fascia resected with a TRAM flap. Intraoperative view after reconstruction of a region of resected anterior rectus sheath fascia with an Alloderm inlay graft.

abdominal wall with synthetic mesh after TRAM flap harvest and subsequently develop an abdominal wall infection: in such patients, poor wound healing at the lower abdominal donor site or umbilical necrosis can require removal of the mesh, which can result in a massive abdominal bulge that can be a source of considerable distress and litigation.

Some patients who have a diastasis recti or a potbelly habitus require a more extensive reconstruction of the abdominal wall to provide support (Figure 16A). In these circumstances, we use both a mesh inlay (to reconstruct the anterior rectus sheath) and a mesh onlay (placed overlying the anterior fascia) (Figure 16B), an approach that we refer to as the "internal girdle." The internal girdle results in long-lasting support with improvement in abdominal contour (Figure 16C) that can allow these patients to maintain an active lifestyle.

Deep Inferior Epigastric Perforator Flaps

Although many patients now present for their breast reconstruction consultation requesting a deep inferior epigastric perforator (DIEP) flap procedure, which comes from the same region as the TRAM flap, DIEP flaps are best used selectively based on the specific needs of the patient (they may be appropriate for athletic patients because the entire rectus abdominis muscle is preserved) and the ability to provide an adequate blood supply to the flap (blood supply is better when a relatively small volume of tissue is needed to reconstruct the breast and when the patient has only a thin or moderately thick lower abdominal pannus). Patients should have relatively large perforating blood vessels from the underlying deep inferior epigastric vessels through the rectus muscle into the lower abdominal skin and subcutaneous tissue. Unfortunately, the caliber of these perforating vessels cannot be reliably predicted preoperatively, so it may be prudent not to assure patients that DIEP flap reconstruction is possible.

The DIEP flap avoids the need to harvest any rectus muscle or abdominal fascia. However, DIEP flaps have been associated with a decreased blood supply compared to TRAM flaps, which can result in an increased incidence of fat necrosis that can significantly affect the shape and contour of the reconstructed breast.[35] Breast reconstruction with a DIEP flap is longer and even more technically demanding than microvascular TRAM flap reconstruction. Although the DIEP flap offers potential functional benefits with regard to the abdominal wall, from an aesthetic point of view the results are essentially the same as those of microvascular TRAM flap reconstruction (Figure 17).

Gluteal Artery Perforator Flaps

Another option for breast reconstruction using autologous tissue is a gluteal artery perforator (GAP) flap. More commonly the superior gluteal tissue is used; however, there has recently been a renewed interest in the use of the inferior gluteal tissue. The superior GAP (SGAP) flap positions the donor scar superiorly on the buttock, away from the region involved with sitting. The design of an SGAP flap resembles that used for an aesthetic buttock lift, with the scar hidden within the bathing suit or underwear line. The flap includes only the skin and subcutaneous tissue harvested based on the superior gluteal artery and vein with no gluteal muscle removed—fibers are just split longitudinally to expose the vessels down to the bony pelvis. However, technical difficulties in performing an SGAP flap procedure, which include problems arising from the relatively short vascular pedicle (superior gluteal artery and vein), have led to an increased use of the inferior GAP (IGAP) flap. Although it is controversial whether the donor scar location with an IGAP flap—within the gluteal crease—is preferable to that with an SGAP flap, IGAP flaps position

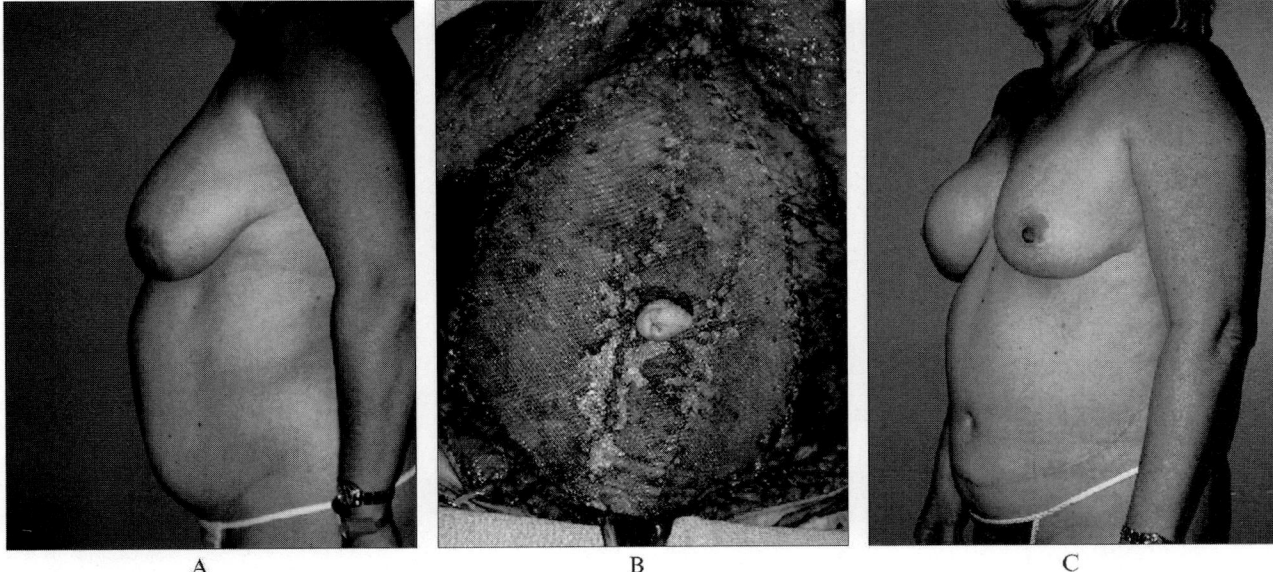

Figure 16 "Internal girdle" reconstruction of the abdominal wall after transverse rectus abdominis myocutaneous (TRAM) flap harvest. *A,* Preoperative view of a 48-year-old mother of three children who presented with right breast cancer and desired breast reconstruction with a TRAM flap. She was especially interested in the associated abdominoplasty; however, she had a diastasis recti with a potbelly habitus. *B,* She underwent reconstruction of her right breast with a neurotized microvascular TRAM flap and reconstruction of the abdominal donor site with both an inlay and an onlay of synthetic mesh ("internal girdle" reconstruction). *C,* Two years after reconstruction, the patient had a good abdominal contour with adequate abdominal support to maintain an active lifestyle with her three children.

the scar in the sitting region of the buttock, which can be especially problematic if the subcutaneous tissue overlying the ischium is included within the flap.

Most reconstructive surgeons consider gluteal flaps to be a second-line option for autologous breast reconstruction, usually in patients who are not candidates for TRAM flap reconstruction.[36] Gluteal flap reconstructions are even more technically complex than DIEP flap reconstructions and are associated with a higher risk of complications. GAP flap reconstruction is usually reserved for patients who have already had a TRAM flap reconstruction for contralateral breast cancer, who underwent a previous aesthetic abdominoplasty, or who have very little abdominal subcutaneous tissue or no laxity in the abdominal musculofascial system (nulliparous women). In these circumstances, gluteal flaps are also useful when the patient has received prior XRT to the chest wall, in which case the use of breast implants is not a preferred option.

Nipple and Areola Reconstruction

Nipple and areola reconstruction is usually performed only after ideal breast symmetry has been achieved because repositioning of a reconstructed nipple can be problematic. Nipple reconstruction is usually an office-based procedure performed under local anesthesia. Many techniques are available for rearranging the local skin and

subcutaneous tissue to create a projecting nipple (Figure 18). Usually the nipples are reconstructed so that they are larger than what will ultimately be required for symmetry because of the significant atrophy that tends to occur over the subsequent 6 to 12 months.[37]

Some surgeons use a skin graft from the groin to reconstruct the areola; the appearance can be very good, but the resultant scar can be painful. At M. D. Anderson, we prefer to only tattoo the areola. We usually wait several months after the nipple reconstruction before tattooing the areola to allow for maturation of the scar so it will absorb the tattoo pigment. It is not uncommon for patients to require some additional pigment to darken the fading tattoo a year or so after the initial application.

DELAYED BREAST RECONSTRUCTION

Delayed breast reconstruction is usually reserved for patients who will require PMRT.

At M. D. Anderson, we prefer not to use breast implants in patients who have received PMRT because of acute problems with wound healing and long-term problems with capsular contracture, which can result in implant displacement and a painful constriction across the chest wall. Thus, we usually perform delayed breast reconstruction using autologous tissue.

Many of the aesthetic outcomes of delayed reconstruction, even when it is performed by experienced

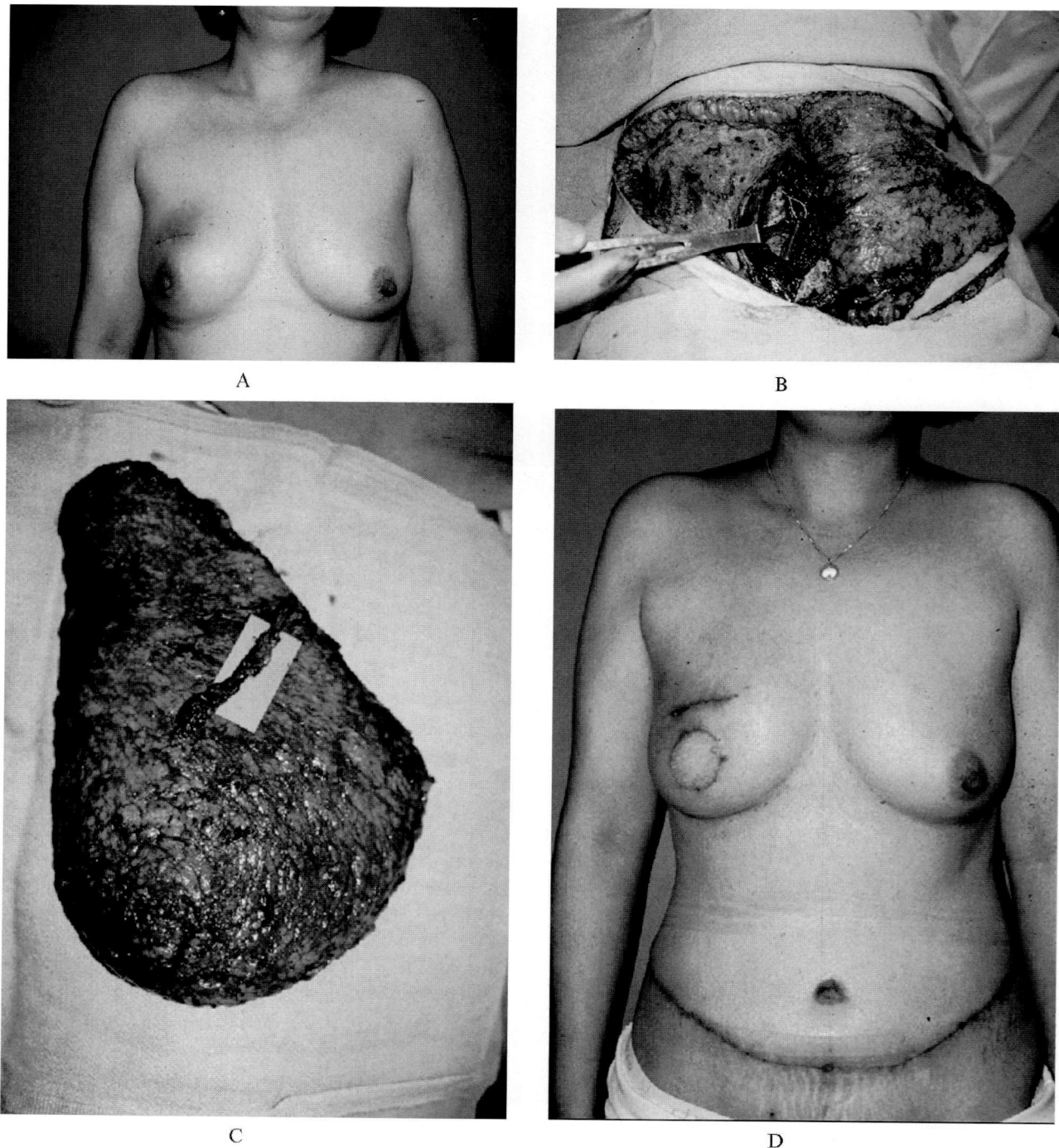

Figure 17 Aesthetic outcomes of DIEP flap breast reconstruction. *A*, A 40-year-old athletic woman with a C bra cup size presented with right-sided breast cancer and desired reconstruction using a deep inferior epigastric perforator (DIEP) flap. *B*, The perforating blood vessels and the deep inferior epigastric vessels were dissected away from the rectus abdominis muscle to their origin in the inguinal region. *C*, The result was a flap with no rectus muscle or abdominal fascia, which allowed for primary repair of the access incision in the anterior rectus sheath. *D*, Six months after DIEP flap reconstruction.

surgeons, are satisfactory at best.[1,2] However, patients who undergo delayed reconstruction after PMRT are the most appreciative because they have had to experience the difficulties of not having a breast. The retained, irradiated, and scarred breast skin located between the mastectomy scar and the inframammary fold is usually

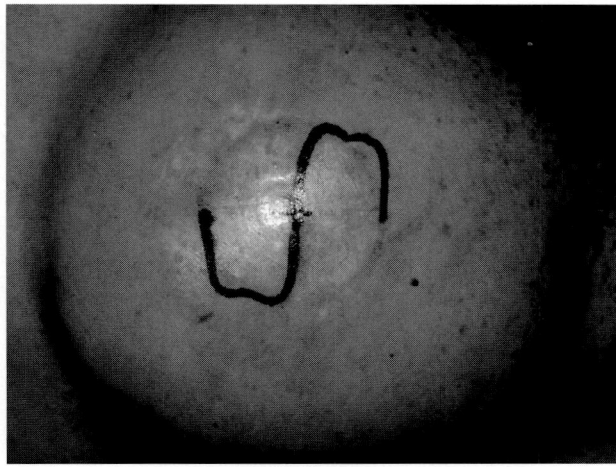

A

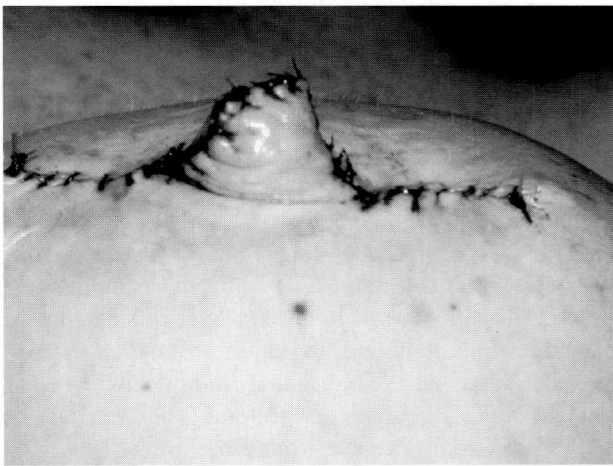

B

Figure 18 Nipple reconstruction after transverse rectus abdominis myocutaneous (TRAM) flap breast reconstruction. *A* Preoperative markings for nipple reconstruction performed using a modified double-opposing tab technique. *B*, Intraoperative view after completion of the nipple reconstruction.

resected at the time of delayed reconstruction because it is inflexible and does not allow for the reconstruction of a curved and ptotic-appearing breast (Figure 19A). This not only requires a much larger volume of flap tissue because of the need for skin replacement but also requires the entire three-dimensional contour of the breast to be recreated (Figure 19B). The need to replace the inferior breast skin means that more flap skin is visible; this appearance is often referred to by patients as the "patch look" (Figure 19C). Because of the increased skin requirements, often three-quarters of the TRAM flap must be used to reconstruct the breast, leaving inadequate tissue for bilateral reconstruction. With delayed breast reconstruction, we also rely more significantly on the ability to perform a contralateral mastopexy (breast lift) to obtain symmetry because it is more difficult to match the ptotic shape of a contralateral native breast.

DELAYED-IMMEDIATE BREAST RECONSTRUCTION

As a consequence of the Danish and Canadian trials,[38,39] there has been an increase in the use of PMRT in patients with early-stage breast cancer. Currently, many centers in the United States routinely recommend PMRT for breast cancer patients with one to three positive lymph nodes. The increasing use of PMRT in patients with early-stage breast cancer has increased the complexity of planning for breast reconstruction. If PMRT is required, delayed reconstruction is usually the best course, but if PMRT is not required, immediate reconstruction is appropriate and permits better aesthetic outcomes. However, because nodal metastases may not be detected until mastectomy[40] and because micrometastases may not be detected until the final pathology review,[40–43] it is often not known until several days after mastectomy whether PMRT will

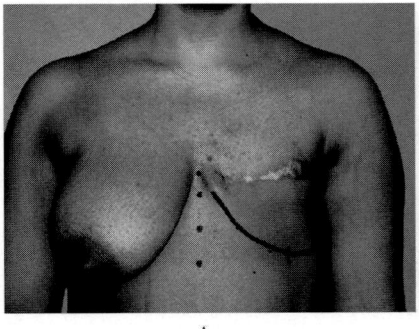

A

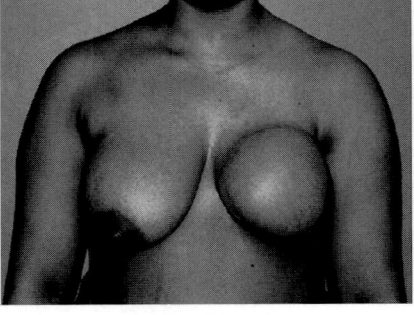

B

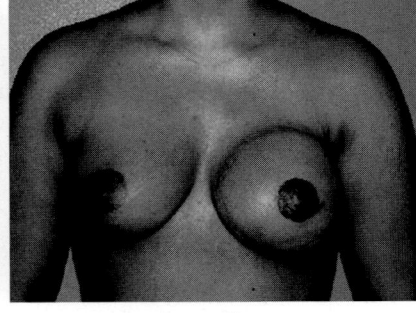

C

Figure 19 Delayed reconstruction after postmastectomy radiation therapy (PMRT). *A*, A 35-year-old woman who had undergone a left modified radical mastectomy presented for delayed reconstruction several years after PMRT. *B*, Six months after delayed reconstruction of the left breast with a right microvascular TRAM flap. *C*, Three months later, after a right vertical mastopexy for symmetry and a left nipple and areola reconstruction.

be required. If breast reconstruction is performed at the time of mastectomy and the patient is found post-operatively to have lymph node involvement, PMRT may adversely affect the aesthetic outcome,[7,14–20] and the reconstructed breast may cause technical difficulties with radiation delivery to the internal mammary nodes, resulting in either increased lung dose or inadequate radiation doses to these nodes.[44,45] On the other hand, if breast reconstruction is delayed because physicians suspect that the patient may require PMRT, but the review of permanent sections reveals that PMRT is not needed, the mastectomy skin and the shape of the breast skin envelope will be lost, along with the chance for the best possible aesthetic outcome.

At M. D. Anderson, we have implemented a two-stage approach, "delayed-immediate breast reconstruction,"[12] to avoid these problems. With delayed-immediate reconstruction, patients who do not require PMRT can achieve aesthetic outcomes similar to those of immediate reconstruction, and patients who require PMRT can avoid the aesthetic and radiation-delivery problems associated with delivery of radiation after an immediate breast reconstruction. Delayed-immediate breast reconstruction also improves patient education by making patients aware preoperatively of the indications for PMRT, which can increase a patient's ability to make treatment and reconstructive decisions.

Indications and Operative Technique

At M. D. Anderson, patients with clinical stage II breast cancer are evaluated by a multidisciplinary breast cancer team (Figure 20) that includes a radiation oncologist. Patients who are deemed to be at increased risk for conditions necessitating PMRT (Figure 21) and who desire breast reconstruction are considered candidates for delayed-immediate breast reconstruction[12] (Figure 22). Stage 1 consists of skin-sparing mastectomy with insertion of a completely filled textured saline tissue expander to preserve the dimensions and shape of the breast skin envelope. After review of permanent sections, patients who do not require PMRT undergo immediate reconstruction (stage 2), and patients who require PMRT undergo this therapy with the expander deflated on the chest wall to result in a flat surface to optimize radiation delivery. After completion of the PMRT, patients undergo re-expansion of the preserved breast skin, an approach to reconstruction that we refer to as "skin-preserving delayed reconstruction."[12]

In patients who are found not to require PMRT, we prefer to perform stage 2 (definitive breast reconstruction) of delayed-immediate reconstruction within 2 weeks after mastectomy. After several weeks, the mastectomy skin flaps may lose their elasticity and retain

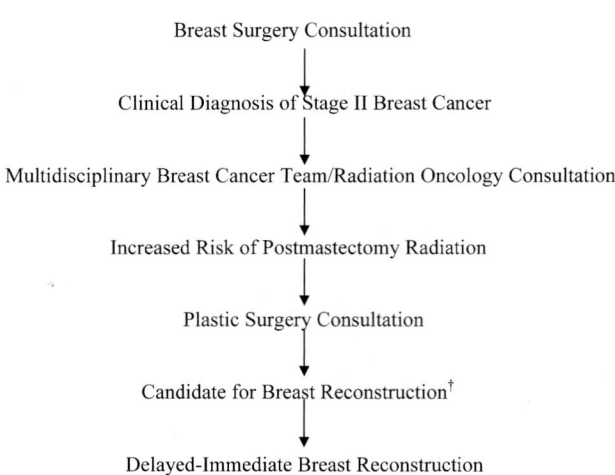

Figure 20 Clinical decision making in patients with clinical stage II breast cancer who desire reconstruction after mastectomy. Reproduced with permission from Kronowitz SJ, Robb GL. Reconstruction and radiation therapy. In: Singletary SE, Robb GL, Hortobagyi GN, editors. Advanced Therapy of Breast Disease. 2nd ed. Hamilton: BC Decker Inc.; 2004.

the shape of the expander. Furthermore, delaying definitive reconstruction longer than 2 weeks may interfere with the initiation of adjuvant chemotherapy, which is usually begun 4 to 6 weeks after mastectomy. In patients who are found to require PMRT and have already undergone neoadjuvant chemotherapy, the 3- to 6-week interval between mastectomy and the start of PMRT allows for adequate wound healing.

Potential Benefits

Delayed-immediate breast reconstruction offers several potential advantages over standard techniques of both

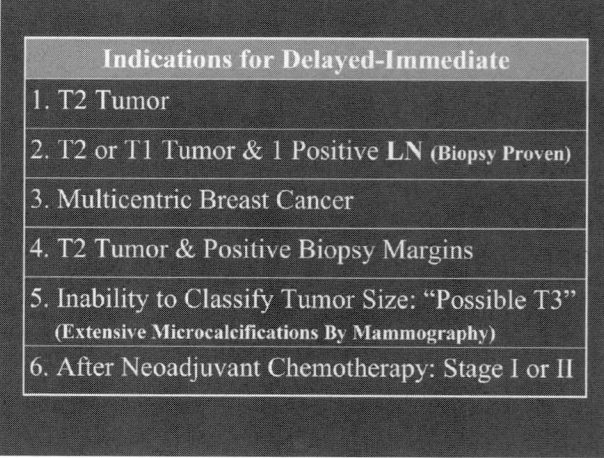

Figure 21 Evolving indications for delayed-immediate breast reconstruction.

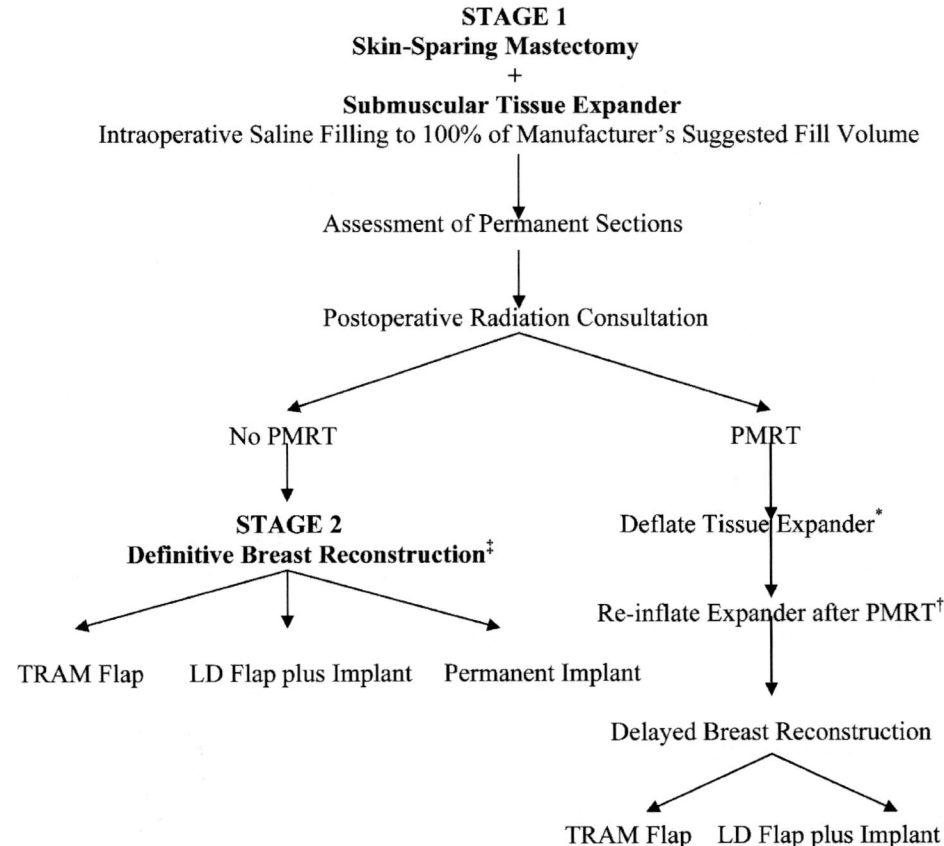

STAGE 1
Skin-Sparing Mastectomy
+
Submuscular Tissue Expander
Intraoperative Saline Filling to 100% of Manufacturer's Suggested Fill Volume

Assessment of Permanent Sections

Postoperative Radiation Consultation

No PMRT | PMRT

STAGE 2
Definitive Breast Reconstruction‡

Deflate Tissue Expander*

Re-inflate Expander after PMRT†

TRAM Flap | LD Flap plus Implant | Permanent Implant

Delayed Breast Reconstruction

TRAM Flap | LD Flap plus Implant

Figure 22 Schema for delayed-immediate breast reconstruction. *After the completion of chemotherapy but prior to the initiation of radiation therapy. If patient had neoadjuvant chemotherapy, leave expander inflated during the 4- to 6-week period before the initiation of radiation therapy. †Allow several weeks for skin desquamation to resolve. The results regarding expander re-inflation are pending. ‡Usually performed 2 weeks after mastectomy and stage 1 of delayed-immediate reconstruction to prevent a delay of chemotherapy. If patient had neoadjuvant chemotherapy, definitive reconstruction may be delayed longer than 2 weeks. Figure shows procedure for patients with unilateral breast cancer not treated with prophylactic contralateral mastectomy and for patients with bilateral breast cancer. In patients with unilateral breast cancer who elect to undergo prophylactic contralateral mastectomy, contralateral mastectomy, and immediate reconstruction are performed at the time of definitive reconstruction of the breast with cancer. PMRT = postmastectomy radiation therapy; LD = latissimus dorsi myocutaneous; TRAM = transverse rectus abdominis myocutaneous. Reproduced with permission from Kronowitz SJ, Robb GL. Reconstruction and radiation therapy. In: Singletary SE, Robb GL, Hortobagyi GN, editors. Advanced Therapy of Breast Disease. 2nd ed. Hamilton: BC Decker Inc.; 2004.

immediate and delayed breast reconstruction. The delayed-immediate technique enables patients to review their final pathology report with a radiation oncologist before committing to a definitive method of breast reconstruction. Placement of the fully inflated expander during stage 1 of delayed-immediate reconstruction prevents retraction of the mastectomy skin and loss of the breast shape. Preservation of the breast skin envelope allows for the reconstruction of a ptotic breast with a shape similar to that of the native breast during stage 2. Delayed-immediate breast reconstruction can be adapted to any clinical practice and modified to comply with various institutional guidelines for PMRT. In addition, delayed-immediate breast reconstruction may afford the opportunity to revise the inframammary fold and

débride any nonviable mastectomy skin prior to insetting of an autologous tissue flap, which may prevent the permanent scarring of breast skin and distortion of breast shape that can occur after an immediate breast reconstruction with secondary healing of mastectomy skin necrosis.

Delayed-immediate reconstruction offers the opportunity for better aesthetic outcomes than are available with standard delayed breast reconstruction. Skin-preserving delayed breast reconstruction is improving the aesthetic outcomes of delayed reconstruction by providing additional usable breast skin for delayed TRAM and GAP flap reconstruction. It is also increasing the eligibility of patients for breast reconstruction: patients who otherwise would not be candidates for delayed breast reconstruction because they are not eligible for a TRAM flap procedure or have insufficient redundant back skin for a standard delayed breast reconstruction can undergo skin-preserving delayed breast reconstruction with a latissimus dorsi flap plus an implant. Delayed-immediate reconstruction also decreases complications that are known to be associated with tissue expansion within an irradiated operative field. Unlike tissue expander insertion after mastectomy and PMRT, which may predispose patients to implant extrusion through an incompletely healed incision,[46] with the delayed-immediate approach, re-expansion of irradiated mastectomy skin occurs after the mastectomy incision is completely healed.

Case Examples: Delayed-Immediate Breast Reconstruction

The following cases illustrate our approach in patients who are found not to require PMRT after skin-sparing mastectomy and subpectoral insertion of a completely filled tissue expander.

Case 1: TRAM Flap Reconstruction

A 55-year-old woman with multicentric left breast cancer underwent neoadjuvant chemotherapy, a left skin-sparing total mastectomy with axillary sentinel lymph node biopsy, and subpectoral placement of a textured saline tissue expander expanded to the manufacturer's suggested intraoperative saline-fill volume of 700 cc (Figure 23A and B). Additional saline filling was performed to a total volume of 900 cc. The review of permanent sections revealed a single positive sentinel lymph node that had been negative on intraoperative imprint cytology. On postoperative day 10, the patient underwent a completion axillary lymph node dissection (Figure 23C). If the patient had undergone immediate breast reconstruction with an axillary-based blood supply, the vascular pedicle of the flap might have been injured during the reoperative axillary surgery.[13] Five weeks after mastectomy the patient underwent delayed-immediate reconstruction of the left breast with a free TRAM flap (Figure 23D and E). The increased interval between mastectomy and TRAM flap reconstruction was due to the additional nodal surgery. Seven months after reconstruction, the patient underwent a left vertical

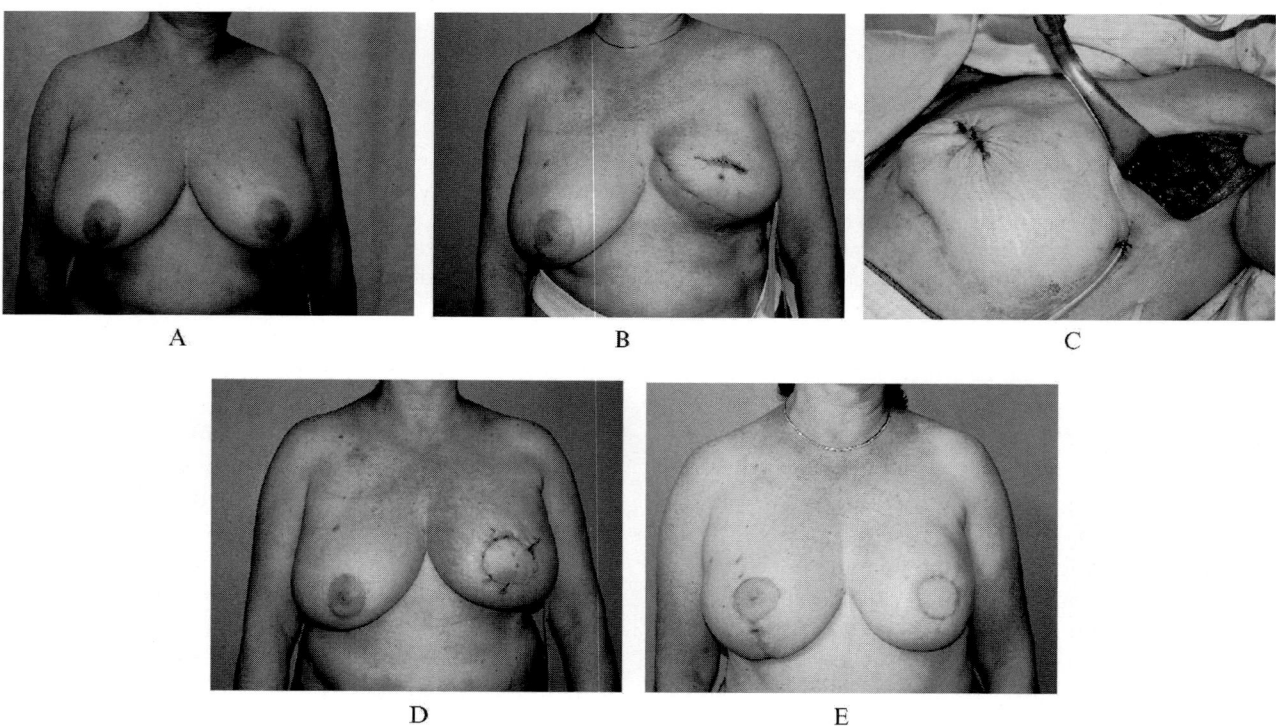

A   B   C

D   E

Figure 23 Delayed-immediate breast reconstruction in a 55-year-old woman with multicentric left breast cancer. *A* Preoperative view. *B*, Four weeks after a left skin-sparing total mastectomy with axillary sentinel lymph node biopsy and subpectoral placement of a textured saline tissue expander expanded to the manufacturer's suggested intraoperative saline-fill volume of 700 cc. *C*, Intraoperative view during complete axillary lymph node dissection performed 10 days after mastectomy. *D*, Ten days after transverse rectus abdominis myocutaneous (TRAM) flap reconstruction. (E) Thirteen months after TRAM flap reconstruction and 6 months after a left vertical breast reduction for symmetry.

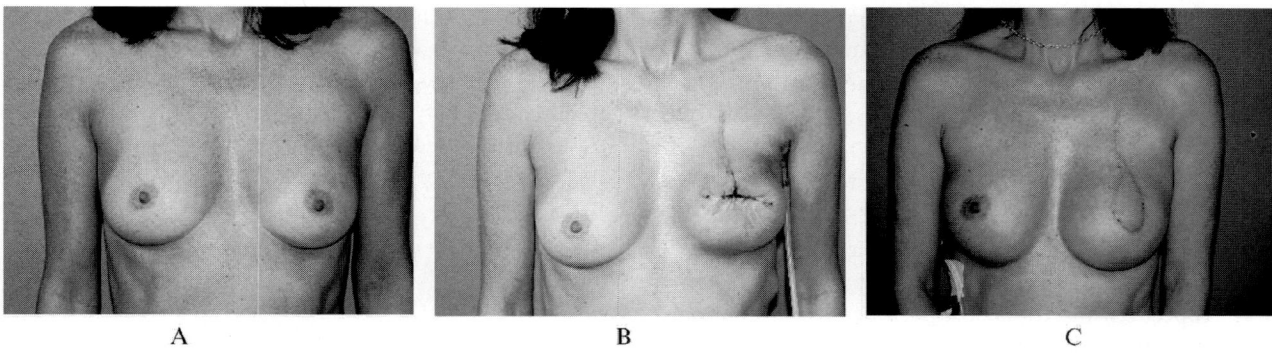

Figure 24 Delayed-immediate breast reconstruction in a 42-year-old woman with extensive microcalcifications in the left breast. *A* Preoperative view. *B*, Three weeks after a left skin-sparing mastectomy with subpectoral insertion of a postoperatively adjustable breast implant with a remote saline-filling port expanded to the manufacturer's suggested intraoperative saline-fill volume of 275 cc. *C*, Seven months after a left delayed-immediate breast reconstruction with a latissimus dorsi myocutaneous flap and a smooth silicon breast implant and a right breast implant augmentation for symmetry.

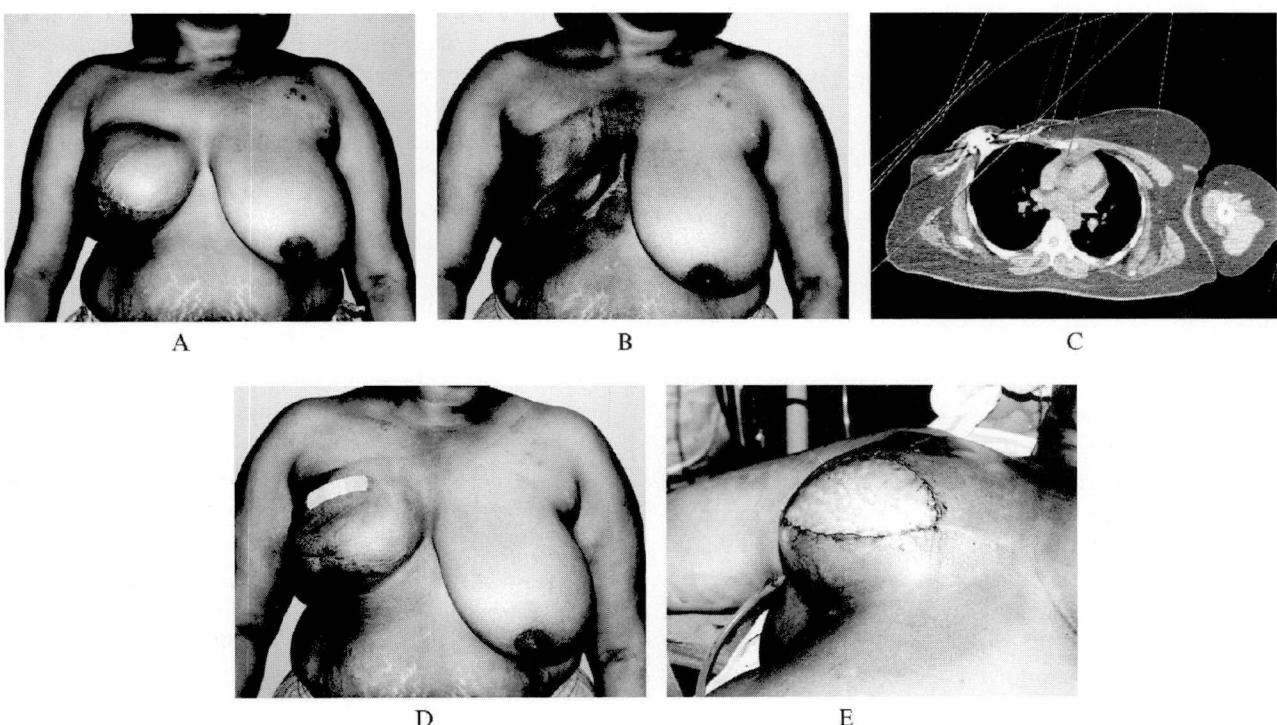

Figure 25 Skin-preserving delayed reconstruction in a 44-year-old woman who presented with an 8 cm region of microcalcifications in the right breast on mammography. *A* Five months after a right modified radical mastectomy with placement of a tissue expander expanded to the manufacturer's suggested intraoperative saline-fill volume of 750 cc and several weeks after completion of adjuvant chemotherapy, during which an additional 200 cc of saline was instilled to bring the total tissue expander volume to 950 cc. *B*, View after complete deflation of the expander before postmastectomy radiation therapy (PMRT). *C*, Computed tomography simulation image of design of radiation delivery fields with the deflated expander on the right chest wall. *D*, Several weeks after completion of PMRT, with the expander re-inflated to 950 cc. *E*, Immediate postoperative view after skin-preserving delayed reconstruction with a free transverse rectus abdominis myocutaneous (TRAM) flap, performed 4 months after completion of PMRT.

breast reduction for symmetry. Although the patient will still require some additional reduction of the right breast, the aesthetic outcome is similar to that of an immediate breast reconstruction.

Case 2: Reconstruction with a Latissimus Dorsi Myocutaneous Flap and a Breast Implant

A 42-year-old woman with extensive microcalcifications in the left breast underwent a left skin-sparing mastectomy and subpectoral insertion of a postoperatively adjustable breast implant with a remote saline-filling port expanded to the manufacturer's suggested intraoperative saline-fill volume of 275 cc (Figure 24A and B). This case illustrates that even with an extensive skin resection with significant scarring, the preservation of breast skin is beneficial. The review of permanent sections revealed that the patient did not require PMRT. The patient then underwent a left delayed-immediate breast reconstruction with a latissimus dorsi myocutaneous flap and a smooth silicon breast implant and, 6 months later, a right breast implant-based augmentation for symmetry (Figure 24C). Again, the aesthetic outcome is similar to that of an immediate breast reconstruction.

Case Example: Skin-Preserving Delayed Breast Reconstruction

The following case illustrates our approach in patients who are found to require PMRT after skin-sparing mastectomy and subpectoral insertion of a completely filled tissue expander.

Case 3

A 44-year-old woman presented with an 8 cm region of microcalcifications in the right breast by mammography. Because the extent of disease within the breast parenchyma was unclear preoperatively, she underwent a right skin-sparing mastectomy and subpectoral placement of an intraoperative expander expanded to the manufacturer's suggested intraoperative saline-fill volume of 750 cc. Review of permanent sections revealed that the entire region of microcalcifications was invasive breast cancer. The patient had additional expansion of the expander during adjuvant chemotherapy, which increased the total fill volume to 950 cc (Figure 25A). The expander was completely deflated immediately before PMRT to allow for treatment of the internal mammary nodes without excessive injury to the heart or lungs (Figure 25B). Even with the relatively large tissue expander (750 cc) used in this patient, complete deflation resulted in a flat chest wall surface (Figure 25C). Several weeks after the completion of PMRT, the tissue expander was progressively re-inflated to the predeflation volume of 950 cc

(Figure 25D). Although this patient required an extensive skin resection at the time of mastectomy and therefore required a larger skin island with the TRAM flap than is usually required, we were still able to perform skin-preserving delayed breast reconstruction 4 months after the completion of PMRT (Figure 25E).

References

1. Kroll SS, Coffey JA, Winn RJ, et al. A comparison of factors affecting aesthetic outcomes of TRAM flap breast reconstructions. Plast Reconstr Surg 1995;96:860.

2. Miller MJ, Rock CS, Robb GL. Aesthetic breast reconstruction using a combination of free transverse rectus abdominis musculocutaneous flaps and breast implants. Ann Plast Surg 1996;37:258.

3. Berger K, Bostwick J. A woman's decision: breast care, treatment and reconstruction. St. Louis: CV Mosby Co.; 1984. p. 45–7.

4. Slavin SA, Love SM, Sadowsky NL. Reconstruction of the radiated partial mastectomy defect with autogenous tissues. Plast Reconstr Surg 1992;90:854.

5. Clough KB, Lewis JS, Couturaud B, et al. Oncoplastic techniques allow extensive resections for breast-conserving therapy of breast carcinomas. Ann Surg 2003;237:26.

6. Losken A, Elwood ET, Styblo TM, et al. The role of reduction mammoplasty in reconstructing partial mastectomy defects. Plas Reconstr Surg 2002;109:968.

7. Clough KB, Kroll SS, Audretsch W. An approach to the repair of partial mastectomy defects. Plast Reconstr Surg 1999;104:409.

8. Rietjends M, Petit JY, Contesso G. The role of reduction mammoplasty in oncology. Eur J Plast Surg 1997;20:246.

9. Kronowitz SJ, Feledy JA, Hunt KK, et al. Determining the optimal approach to breast reconstruction after partial mastectomy. Plast Reconstr Surg 2006;117:1.

10. Kronowitz SJ, Robb GR. Breast reconstruction with postmastectomy radiation therapy: current issues. Plast Reconstr Surg 2004;114:50.

11. Spear SL, Onyewu C. Staged breast reconstruction with saline-filled implants in the irradiated breast: recent trends and therapeutic implications. Plast Reconstr Surg 2000;105:930.

12. Kronowitz SJ, Hunt KK, Kuerer HM, et al. Delayed-immediate breast reconstruction. Plast Reconstr Surg 2004;113:1617.

13. Kronowitz SJ, Chang DW, Robb GL, et al. Implications of axillary sentinel lymph node biopsy in immediate autologous breast reconstruction. Plast Reconstr Surg 2002;109:1888–96.

14. Williams JK, Bostwick J III, Bried JT, et al. TRAM flap breast reconstruction after radiation treatment. Ann Surg 1995;221:756.

15. Kraemer O, Andersen M, Siim E. Breast reconstruction and tissue expansion in irradiated versus not irradiated women after mastectomy. Scand J Plast Reconstr Hand Surg 1996; 30:201.

16. Williams JK, Carlson GW, Bostwick J III, et al. The effects of radiation treatment after TRAM flap breast reconstruction. Plast Reconstr Surg 1997;100:1153.

17. Kroll SS, Schusterman MA, Reece GP, et al. Breast reconstruction with myocutaneous flaps in previously irradiated patients. Plast Reconstr Surg 1994;93:460.

18. Evans GRD, Schusterman MA, Kroll SS, et al. Reconstruction and the radiated breast: is there a role for implants? Plast Reconstr Surg 1995;96:1111.

19. Tran NV, Chang DW, Gupta A, et al. Comparison of immediate and delayed TRAM flap breast reconstruction in patients receiving postmastectomy radiation therapy. Plast Reconstr Surg 2001;108:78–82.

20. Spear SL, Ducic I, Low M, et al. The effect of radiation therapy on pedicled TRAM flap breast reconstruction: outcomes and implications. Plast Reconstr Surg 2005;115:84.

21. Taylor W, Horgan K, Dodwell D. Oncological aspects of breast reconstruction. Breast 2005;14:118.

22. Chang DW, Reece GP, Wang B. Effect of smoking on complications in patients undergoing free TRAM flap breast reconstruction. Plast Reconstr Surg 2000;105:2374.

23. Kronowitz SJ, Robb GL, Youssef A, et al. Optimizing autologous breast reconstruction in thin patients. Plast Reconstr Surg 2003;112:1768.

24. Chang DW, Wang B, Robb GL, et al. Effect of obesity on flap and donor-site complications in free transverse rectus abdominis myocutaneous flap breast reconstruction. Plast Reconstr Surg 2002;109:1199.

25. Takeishi M, Shaw WW, Ahn CY. TRAM flaps in patients with abdominal scars. Plast Reconstr Surg 1997;99:713.

26. Lipa JE, Youssef AA, Kuerer HM. Breast reconstruction in older women: advantages of autogenous tissue. Plast Reconstr Surg 2003;111:1110.

27. Gouy S, Rouzier R, Missana MC, et al. Immediate reconstruction after neoadjuvant chemotherapy: effect on adjuvant treatment starting and survival. Ann Surg Oncol 2005;12:161.

28. Losken A, Carlson G, Bostwick J, et al. Trends in unilateral breast reconstruction and management of the contralateral breast: the Emory experience. Plast Reconstr Surg 2002;110: 89.

29. Nahabedian MY, Tsangaris T, Momen B. Infectious complications following breast reconstruction with expanders and implants. Plast Reconstr Surg 2003;112:467.

30. Kroll SS, Baldwin B. A comparison of outcomes using three different methods of breast reconstruction. Plast Reconstr Surg 1992;90:455.

31. Mandrekas AD, Zambacos GJ, Zervoudis S. TRAM flap breast reconstruction and weight fluctuations: it is alive! Plast Reconstr Surg 2003;112:696.

32. Majumder S, Batchelor GG. Internal mammary vessels as recipient vessels for free TRAM breast reconstruction: aesthetic and functional considerations. Br J Plast Surg 1999;52:286.

33. Isenberg JS. Sense and sensibility: breast reconstruction with innervated TRAM flaps. J Reconstr Microsurg 2002;18:23.

34. Schusterman MA, Kroll SS, Weldon ME. Immediate breast reconstruction: why the free TRAM over the conventional TRAM flap. Plast Reconstr Surg 1992;90:255.

35. Kroll SS. Fat necrosis in free transverse rectus abdominis perforator flaps. Plast Reconstr Surg 2000;106:576.

36. Guerra AB, Metzinger SE, Bidros RS, et al. Breast reconstruction with gluteal artery perforator (GAP) flaps: a critical analysis of 142 cases. Ann Plast Surg 2004;52:118.

37. Shestak KC, Gabriel A, Landecker A, et al. Assessment of long-term nipple projection: a comparison of three techniques. Plast Reconstr Surg 2002;110:780.

38. Overgaard M, Hansen PS, Overgaard J, et al. Postoperative radiotherapy in high-risk premenopausal women with breast cancer who receive adjuvant chemotherapy. N Engl J Med 1997;337:949.

39. Ragaz K, Jackson SM, Le N, et al. Adjuvant radiotherapy and chemotherapy in node-positive premenopausal women with breast cancer. N Engl J Med 1997;337:956.

40. Fisher B, Wolmark W, Bauer M, et al. The accuracy of clinical nodal staging and of limited axillary dissection as a determinant of histologic nodal status in carcinoma of the breast. Surg Gynecol Obstet 1981;152:765–72.

41. Van Diest PJ, Torrenga H, Borgstein PJ, et al. Reliability of intraoperative frozen section and cytological investigation of sentinel lymph nodes in breast cancer. Histopathology 1999;35:14–8.

42. Wiser MR, Montgomery LL, Susnik B, et al. Is routine intraoperative frozen-section examination of sentinel lymph nodes in breast cancer worthwhile? Ann Surg Oncol 2000;7:651–5.

43. Turner RR, Hansen NM, Stern SL, Giuliano AE. Intraoperative examination of the sentinel lymph node for breast carcinoma staging. Am J Clin Pathol 1999;112:627–34.

44. Buchholz TA, Kronowitz SJ, Kuerer HM. Immediate breast reconstruction after skin-sparing mastectomy for treatment of advanced breast cancer: radiation oncology considerations. Ann Surg Oncol 2002;9:820.

45. Strom E. Radiation therapy for early and advanced breast disease. In: Hunt KK, Robb GL, Strom EA, Ueno NT, editors. Breast cancer. The M. D. Anderson Cancer Care Series. Vol 1. New York: Springer-Verlag; 2001. p. 255–81.

46. Mansfield C. Effects of radiation therapy on wound healing after mastectomy. Clin Plast Surg 1979;6:19.

CHAPTER 61

PRIMARY BREAST CANCER PREVENTION: PROPHYLACTIC MASTECTOMY AND CHEMOPREVENTION

ISABELLE BEDROSIAN, MD

THERESE BEVERS, MD

The routine use of screening mammography, promoted as a method of early breast cancer detection in the hope of preventing mortality, is an example of secondary prevention. Although controversy exists concerning its efficacy, because it is applied to all women, and therefore all risk categories, there is little if any associated morbidity. In contrast, primary breast cancer prevention practices attempt to prevent mortality by reducing the incidence of disease. Although the two major approaches, prophylactic mastectomy and chemoprevention target high-risk groups, because of the associated morbidity, particularly with the former, significant controversy exists.

The surgeon, either general or oncologic, will commonly be consulted to offer not only technical expertise, but also intellectual input in helping patients make rational decisions about primary breast cancer prevention. The ensuing discussion will shed some light on the current controversies and the most recent published data to help surgeons negotiate this difficult problem with their patients.

Introduction

Clinicians have long recognized the impact of personal history, family history, and genetics on the risk of developing breast cancer. These risks have been quantified through the use of several different models and, more recently, the identification of specific gene mutations. In the absence of effective medical therapies, efforts at preventing breast cancer in women at high risk have historically favored surgical prophylaxis, but in the past decade, chemoprevention strategies have provided an alternative for women seeking to reduce their likelihood of developing breast cancer. Whether a medical or a surgical prophylactic strategy is optimal for any given patient must be determined on an individual basis. Patients therefore need to be counseled comprehensively, not only on their actual risks of developing breast cancer, but also on the risks and benefits of both chemoprevention and prophylactic mastectomy (PM).

Prophylactic Mastectomy

Removal of the tissue at risk is the most radical intervention for the prevention of breast cancer. Many factors are known to place women at higher-than-baseline risk of developing breast cancer. Chief among these is a personal and/or a family history of breast cancer, which are the most common reasons for pursuing either bilateral or contralateral PM. Although PM has been practiced for over 40 years, definitive recommendations are difficult to make because few studies are available, most are retrospective, and data on the efficacy of PM in preventing death from breast cancer are scarce.

BILATERAL PROPHYLACTIC MASTECTOMY

The efficacy of bilateral PM (BPM) has historically been evaluated in women with a family history of breast cancer. In a large study of 639 patients from the Mayo Clinic, Hartmann and colleagues identified 2 cohorts treated with BPM over a 30-year period: a group of 214 women whose family history suggested a high risk of breast cancer and 425 women considered to be at moderate risk.[1] The outcomes of the patients treated with BPM were compared with the outcomes of sisters of the patients who did not undergo prophylactic surgery, as well as to Gail model predictions. After a median follow-up of 14 years, the authors found that both groups experienced at least a 90% reduction in their risk of developing breast cancer. The absolute risk reduction experienced was 7.9% in the moderate-risk group and 16.1% in the high-risk patients. Furthermore, the number of deaths from breast cancer was reduced in all patients who underwent BPM; no deaths were noted in the moderate-risk group, and only 2 deaths were noted in the high-risk group, compared with 10.4 and 10.5 deaths expected, respectively. Therefore, at least an 80% reduction in the risk of death from breast cancer was seen in the BPM group (absolute risk reduction of 2.4–4%).

In order to understand the impact of the findings from the Mayo Clinic series for an individual patient, Hamm and colleagues analyzed the data regarding the number of patients who need to be treated in order to prevent 1 breast cancer.[2] They estimated that 6 women at high risk and 13 women at moderate risk would need to be treated with BPM to prevent 1 case of breast cancer. In addition, in order to prevent 1 death from breast cancer, 42 women at moderate risk and 25 women at high risk would need to undergo BPM (Table 1). Therefore, a substantial number of women who undergo BPM will receive no benefit from this intervention.

Although studies based on family history have provided important information about the efficacy of BPM for reducing the incidence of breast cancer, they have not taken into account how genetic mutations may affect the patients' risks of breast cancer and, therefore, dilute the impact of BPM. Recent progress in the identification and testing of patients for deleterious BRCA1 and BRCA2 mutations has improved our ability to identify patients genetically disposed to have a very high risk of developing breast cancer. BRCA mutation carriers may have as much as an 85% risk of developing breast carcinoma by age 70.[3,4,5] Therefore, there has been substantial interest in assessing the role of BPM in this genetically defined high-risk population.

Meijers-Heijboer and colleagues prospectively followed a series of 139 women with documented deleterious BRCA1/2 mutations.[6] Seventy-six women in this group had elected to undergo BPM, and 63 women opted for surveillance. A significantly greater number of women who had BPM, compared with those who did not, also opted to undergo prophylactic oophorectomy. After a mean follow-up of only 2.9 years, no cases of breast cancer were observed in the BPM group, although 8 breast cancers had developed in women in the surveillance group. One death from breast cancer was reported in the surveillance group. Using an exponential model and a constant hazard ratio, the authors estimated the 5-year cumulative breast cancer incidence to be 12% in the surveillance group (95% CI, 6–23%) and 0% in the BPM group (Figure 1). BPM was found to significantly decrease the incidence of breast cancer, with a risk reduction of 66 to 100%. The risk reduction remained significant even after adjusting for the effects of prophylactic oophorectomy. The early results of this study show that BPM can prevent breast cancer and increase survival from breast cancer in BRCA1 and BRCA2 mutation carriers. However, given the short duration of follow-up and the small number of events in the study, the accuracy of these estimates of the risk reduction afforded by BPM in BRCA mutation carriers is uncertain, and the results from this study should be interpreted cautiously.

More recent data on the efficacy of BPM in BRCA mutation carriers comes from the prevention and observation of surgical end points (PROSE) study group.[7] This multicenter study enrolled and prospec-

Table 1 Relative Risk Reduction and Number Needed to Treat for the Outcomes of Breast Cancer and Death in High-Risk and Moderate-Risk Women who Underwent Prophylactic Mastectomy

Risk and Outcome	Outcome Rate without Mastectomy	Outcome Rate with Mastectomy	Absolute Risk Reduction	Relative Risk Reduction	Number Needed to Treat
High					
Breast Cancer	0.175	0.014	0.161	0.920	6
Death	0.049	0.009	0.040	0.816	25
Moderate					
Breast Cancer	0.088	0.009	0.079	0.898	13
Death	0.024	0.000	0.024	1.000	42

From Hamm RM et al.[2]

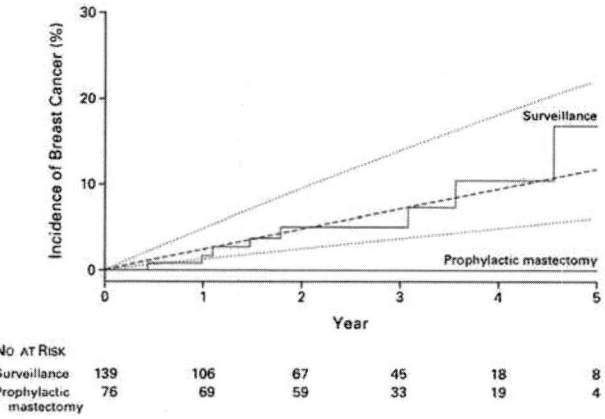

Figure 1 Actuarial incidence of breast cancer among women with a *BRCA1* or *BRCA2* mutation after prophylactic mastectomy or during surveillance. The surveillance group includes data obtained before prophylactic mastectomy in 76 of the 139 women. The dashed line represents the probability of breast cancer during surveillance, and the dotted lines the 95% confidence interval. Values were calculated with the use of an exponential model in which the hazard rate was assumed to be constant. From Meijers-Heijboer H et al.[6]

tively followed 483 women with deleterious germline *BRCA1/2* mutations, 105 of whom underwent BPM. The mean duration of follow-up was 6.4 years. Overall, BPM was found to reduce the relative risk of breast cancer by 95% in women also undergoing bilateral prophylactic oophorectomy and by 90% in women with intact ovaries. Breast cancer was detected in 1.9% of women who had a BPM (2/105) and in 48.7% (184/378) of matched controls, for an absolute reduction in risk of 46.8% during this study period. Therefore, data from the PROSE study group also suggest that BPM reduces the incidence of breast cancer in women who are carriers of deleterious *BRCA1* and *BRCA2* mutations. However, survival end points were not evaluated. Since women who are carriers of *BRCA* mutations often receive close follow-up and surveillance, most are likely to present with early-stage cancer with a high probability for cure. In addition, BPM did not prevent all cases of breast cancer in this population, thus leaving open the possibility of death from breast cancer despite prophylaxis. Therefore, data on survival outcomes for women undergoing BPM compared with those of women in surveillance programs are needed to fully assess the benefits of BPM in preventing death from breast cancer.

CONTRALATERAL PROPHYLACTIC MASTECTOMY

Women with a personal history of breast cancer are at an increased risk of a metachronous malignancy. For most women, this risk is estimated at 0.7 to 1% per year.[8,9,10]

However, additional factors, in particular *BRCA* status and family history, likely influence the magnitude of this risk and, hence, the potential benefit of contralateral prophylactic mastectomy (CPM).

Recent data demonstrate that *BRCA1* and *BRCA2* mutation carriers with stage I or II breast cancer, who do not undergo oophorectomy or receive antiestrogen therapy, have a 43.4% and 34.6% actuarial risk, respectively, of a contralateral breast cancer 10 years after an initial cancer diagnosis.[11] However, with the use of tamoxifen or prophylactic oophorectomy, the risks of contralateral breast cancer at 10 years are reduced to 18.8% in *BRCA1* and 13.1% in *BRCA2* mutation carriers. Although this amounts to a 60% reduction in relative risk, the greatest relative risk reduction was seen in women who underwent CPM, either at the time of initial cancer treatment or at some subsequent interval. With a mean follow-up of 9.2 years, only 1 cancer (0.7%) occurred in this group of 146 women, compared with 97 cancers (28.8%) in 336 women who kept the contralateral breast. Therefore, CPM provided a relative risk reduction of greater than 95%. If CPM is presumed to be equally effective in *BRCA1* and *BRCA2* populations, then, when compared with no surgical ovarian ablation or pharmacologic hormonal manipulation, CPM offered an absolute risk reduction of 42.7% in *BRCA1* mutation carriers and 33.9% in *BRCA2* mutation carriers. The absolute risk reduction in *BRCA1* and *BRCA2* carriers resulting from either oophorectomy or tamoxifen was 24.6% and 21.5%, respectively. Although such data suggest superiority of CPM over tamoxifen, important information about the study population in this series is lacking. First, the estrogen receptor (ER) status could not be verified for many of the patients, and the relative distribution of ER status between the CPM cohorts and those patients who preserved the contralateral breast is unknown. Second, survival end points were not evaluated. This is important because any survival benefit afforded by CPM may be offset by the increased risk of death as a result of the index breast cancer.

The role of CPM in patients with a family history of breast cancer, independent of *BRCA* mutation status, has also been evaluated in a large series of 745 patients from Mayo Clinic.[12] The probability of contralateral breast cancer in this series was estimated by family history, which was stratified as parent/child, sibling, or second-degree relative diagnosed with breast cancer. This probability of contralateral breast cancer was further adjusted to account for the potential effects of adjuvant chemotherapy and tamoxifen. Adjustments were also made for menopausal status at diagnosis of primary breast cancer. Median follow-up was 10 years. Among the entire cohort of 745 patients, 156.5 cases (21%) of breast cancer were expected. However, only 8 (1.1%) were seen. In both pre- and postmenopausal groups, CPM resulted in a 95% reduction in the risk of developing a contralateral breast cancer. The absolute risk reduction, however, was greater in premenopausal women. In this group, 27% of the cohort was predicted to develop breast cancer; however, only a 1.5% incidence of cancer was seen after 10 years of follow-up. In the postmenopausal subgroup, of the 50.3 predicted cancers (14%), only 2 (0.5%) were noted. The survival benefit of CPM was not determined.

A substantial percentage of patients under consideration for CPM are not carriers of deleterious *BRCA* mutations, nor do they have a high-risk family history. As with the higher-risk cohorts, however, CPM reduced the probability of developing a contralateral breast cancer by more than 90% in this population of patients.[13–15] In a retrospective analysis, Peralta and colleagues also reported that such patients undergoing CPM had a 15-year disease-free survival (DFS) rate of 55% compared with 28% in patients who did not undergo CPM.[13] There was no difference, however, in the rates of recurrence and overall survival between the 2 groups. This suggests that the differences in DFS were due largely to differences in the incidence of contralateral breast cancer, and although CPM effectively prevented the development of contralateral disease, this was offset by the risk of death from the index cancer. There was, however, a trend toward improved disease-specific survival in the subgroup of patients with early-stage breast cancer treated with CPM (stage 0-2, $p = 0.06$).[13]

In an attempt to identify patients most likely to benefit from CPM, Goldflam and colleagues retrospectively looked for characteristics in the index tumor that predicted unfavorable histologic findings in the CPM specimen.[14] Significant histologic findings in the contralateral breast were defined as moderate- to high-risk breast lesions, as well as occult malignancies. Among the clinical and histopathologic variables in the index tumor predictive of unfavorable contralateral breast histology were invasive lobular carcinoma (ILC), ER- or progesterone-positive tumor, moderate- to high-risk lesions in the ipsilateral breast, and young patient age (< 40 years old). These results suggest that clinical variables and histologic findings in the index breast may help stratify patients according to their risk of contralateral breast cancer and, thus, help select those most likely to benefit from CPM.

ILC has been reported to have a high propensity for bilaterality, and some have advocated that patients with ILC should undergo CPM. There is, however, very little data regarding the efficacy of CPM in this group of patients. Babiera and colleagues reviewed the survival of 133 patients with ILC; 18 patients underwent CPM and 115 patients were observed only.[15] With a median follow-up of 68 months, 3 contralateral cancers were detected in the observation arm, compared with 0 in the CPM arm; however, no differences were noted in disease-specific survival between the 2 groups. In contrast, data from the Mayo Clinic demonstrated that among 105 patients who were treated with contralateral investigative or prophylactic surgery (either undirected contralateral biopsy or prophylactic mastectomy), there was a small but significant improvement in survival compared with 299 patients who received no surgical intervention to the contralateral breast.[16] These data should be interpreted with much caution, however, given the retrospective nature of the report, the small number of events overall, and the fact that the 2 groups under consideration were not well balanced.

WHO SHOULD UNDERGO PROPHYLACTIC MASTECTOMY?

Data from prospective and retrospective studies indicate that PM is an effective strategy that reduces the relative risk of developing breast cancer by $\geq$ 90% in all cohorts examined. However, this procedure has significant emotional and psychosocial implications for many women. The benefit of prophylactic mastectomy, therefore, needs to be assessed within the context of the individual's overall risk of breast cancer, the absolute reduction in risk offered by the procedure, and the potential impact on survival. Unfortunately, recommendations regarding PM are hampered by a paucity of survival data and lack of direct comparison between medical and surgical risk-reduction regimens.

From the available data, however, it appears that PM is likely to have the most benefit for *BRCA* mutation carriers who have not yet developed breast cancer. Although long-term survival data are lacking, the striking decrease in the absolute odds of developing breast cancer after BPM in this population is likely to result in a substantial reduction in breast cancer mortality as well. Using decision analysis models, survival gains can be shown for young women carriers of *BRCA* mutations who undergo prophylactic surgery.[17] For women who are not *BRCA* mutation carriers but who have a family history of the disease, the survival advantage conferred by BPM appears to be very small, and the majority of these women are not likely to die of breast cancer. Therefore, most such women who undergo BPM are being overtreated, and it is important for these patients to understand their true risks and benefits before committing to surgery.

For patients who have already been diagnosed with breast cancer, the available data point to an even more limited benefit for CPM. In particular, there is little information to compare the survival benefits of CPM with the risk of death from the index carcinoma. Another consideration in these patients is the potential delay in receiving adjuvant therapy secondary to complications associated with the additional surgical intervention of CPM. Subgroups of women, such as those with early-stage disease and/or younger age at diagnosis, may stand to have greater gains from CPM, but in the absence of prospective, long-term data, a general recommendation for CPM cannot be made and such decisions need to be individualized.

Chemoprevention

It is an interesting paradox that prophylactic mastectomy is considered a prevention strategy, whereas the trend for women diagnosed with breast cancer is toward breast conservation therapy. With the advances in breast cancer chemoprevention, most breast cancer prevention experts are shifting the emphasis away from prophylactic surgery toward chemoprevention for women without an inherited predisposition.

Chemoprevention of breast cancer with tamoxifen has been an option for breast cancer risk reduction for women at increased risk of the disease since the publication of the findings of the Breast Cancer Prevention Trial (BCPT) in 1998. On the basis of the 2006 findings of the Study of Tamoxifen and Raloxifene (STAR) for the BCPT, raloxifene is now an additional option for postmenopausal women at increased risk of breast cancer.

TAMOXIFEN

Tamoxifen citrate is a selective estrogen receptor modulator that competes with circulating estrogen for binding to the estrogen receptor. Depending on the tissue and species, tamoxifen acts as an estrogen agonist or an estrogen antagonist. For more than 30 years, tamoxifen has been used in the treatment of breast cancer to reduce the risk of recurrent and contralateral breast cancer.

The BCPT was launched in 1992 by the National Surgical Adjuvant Breast and Bowel Project (NSABP) to investigate the value of tamoxifen in reducing the risk of primary invasive breast cancer in women at increased risk of the disease.[18] A total of 13,388 women age 35 years or older who were at increased risk of breast cancer were entered into the trial and randomly assigned to receive either tamoxifen 20 mg daily or placebo daily for 5 years. Increased risk was defined as a personal history of lobular carcinoma in situ (LCIS), a 5-year risk of developing breast cancer of at least 1.7%, as calculated using the modified Gail model, or age 60 years or older.

Tamoxifen reduced the risk of developing invasive breast cancer by 49%. A 56% risk reduction was seen for women with a history of LCIS, and women with a history of atypical hyperplasia had a dramatic 86% risk reduction. The incidence of ER-positive tumors was reduced 69% in the tamoxifen group, without any impact on the incidence of ER-negative breast cancers (Table 2). Tamoxifen also was suggested to reduce the incidence of osteoporotic fractures.

An increased risk of endometrial cancer, venous thromboembolic events, cataracts, and the need for cataract surgery was seen in patients receiving tamoxifen in the BCPT (Table 3). These risks, although present for all women in the trial, were increased only in women over the age of 50. Common side effects reported included bothersome hot flashes and vaginal discharge. Weight gain and depression were not associated with tamoxifen therapy.

The findings of other tamoxifen prevention trials have been published since the unblinding of the BCPT. The Italian Tamoxifen Prevention Study and Royal Marsden Hospital Tamoxifen Prevention Pilot Trial showed no benefit of tamoxifen over placebo in reducing the incidence of breast cancer.[19,20] Although the results of these two trials differed from those of the BCPT, the differences are most likely due to differences in study population and design. The International Breast Cancer Intervention Study, or IBIS-1, showed a 33% reduction in the incidence of breast cancer, confirming the breast cancer risk reduction benefit of tamoxifen that was seen in the BCPT.[21] A meta-analysis of all the tamoxifen prevention studies demonstrated that tamoxifen reduced the risk of breast cancer by 38% and confirmed the increased risks of endometrial cancer and venous thromboembolic events.[22]

The Food and Drug Administration (FDA) approved tamoxifen for breast cancer risk reduction in 1998. Despite the significant risk reduction conferred by tamoxifen, it has not been widely accepted in the primary care community, and utilization has been limited. Barriers to the use of tamoxifen in the primary care setting include not only the risks of tamoxifen therapy, but also the fact that it is primarily recognized as a treatment for breast cancer. As a result, tamoxifen chemoprevention therapy was never considered for many women who were at increased risk of developing breast cancer.

RALOXIFENE

Raloxifene is a second-generation selective estrogen receptor modulator. The Multiple Outcomes of

Table 2 Outcomes in the Breast Cancer Prevention Trial: Benefits

Outcome	Rate per 1,000 women		
	Tamoxifen	Placebo	Risk Ratio (95% CI)
Invasive breast cancer	3.4	6.8	0.51 (0.39–0.66)
Noninvasive breast cancer	1.4	2.7	0.50 (0.33–0.77)
Invasive breast cancer by patient characteristic			
Age, years			
≤ 49	3.8	6.7	0.56 (0.37–0.85)
50–59	3.1	6.3	0.49 (0.29–0.81)
≥ 60	3.3	7.3	0.45 (0.27–0.74)
History of LCIS			
Yes	5.7	13.0	0.44 (0.16–1.06)
No	3.3	6.4	0.51 (0.39–0.68)
History of atypical hyperplasia			
Yes	1.4	10.1	0.14 (0.03–0.47)
No	3.6	6.4	0.56 (0.42–0.73)
Number of 1st-degree relatives with BrCa			
0	3.0	6.4	0.46 (0.24–0.84)
1	3.0	6.0	0.51 (0.35–0.73)
2	4.8	8.7	0.55 (0.30–0.97)
≥ 3	7.0	13.7	0.51 (0.15–1.55)
Risk of breast cancer by time, years (%)			
≤ 2	2.1	5.5	0.37 (0.18–0.72)
2.01–3.0	3.5	5.2	0.68 (0.41–1.11)
3.01–5.0	3.9	5.9	0.66 (0.39–1.09)
≥ 5.01	4.5	13.3	0.34 (0.19–0.58)
Fractures			
Hip	0.5	0.8	0.55 (0.25–1.15)
Hip, spine, and lower radius combined	4.3	5.3	0.81 (0.63–1.05)

Adapted from Fisher et al.[18]

Raloxifene Evaluation (MORE) trial demonstrated a reduction in the incidence of fractures and an increase in bone density with the use of raloxifene in postmenopausal women with osteoporosis, resulting in FDA approval of the drug for the prevention and treatment of osteoporosis. A subset analysis of the MORE trial demonstrated a 76% reduction in the incidence of breast cancer with raloxifene compared with placebo.[23] Similar to the findings with tamoxifen, an increased incidence in venous thromboembolic events was seen in the raloxifene group. In contrast to the findings with tamoxifen, raloxifene was not associated with an increase in the incidence of endometrial cancer.

These findings from the MORE study served as the basis of the STAR trial. Opened in May 1999, STAR enrolled 19,747 postmenopausal women at increased risk of breast cancer. Women were randomly assigned to receive either tamoxifen 20 mg daily or raloxifene 60 mg daily for 5 years. At the unblinding of the trial in April 2006, raloxifene was found to be equivalent to tamoxifen in reducing the risk of developing invasive breast cancer in postmenopausal women who are at increased risk of the disease.[24] Although tamoxifen has been shown to reduce the incidence of LCIS and ductal carcinoma in

situ (DCIS), raloxifene did not have an effect on these diagnoses (Table 4). This result confirms 2004 data reported in the Continuing Outcomes Relevant to Evista (CORE) trial, a 4-year extension of the MORE trial designed to further assess the effect of raloxifene on breast cancer. Women taking either drug had equivalent numbers of bone fractures.

The incidence of uterine cancer was 38% lower in the raloxifene arm, with the difference approaching, but not reaching, statistical significance. More than half of the women who joined STAR had had a hysterectomy and, therefore, were not at risk of uterine cancer. There was a statistically significant difference between the groups in the incidence of uterine hyperplasia (with and without atypia), with an 84% lower incidence in the raloxifene arm (Table 5). The finding of a lower incidence of uterine hyperplasia in the raloxifene arm suggests that the lower incidence of uterine cancer in this group is a real finding.

Raloxifene resulted in 30% fewer deep vein thromboses and pulmonary embolisms than tamoxifen, a statistically significant finding. The numbers of strokes and transient ischemic attacks occurring in both groups of women were statistically equivalent, as was the

Table 3 Outcomes in the Breast Cancer Prevention Trial: Risks

	Rate per 1,000 women		
Outcome	Tamoxifen	Placebo	Risk Ratio (95% CI)
Invasive endometrial cancer			
Overall	*2.3*	*0.9*	*2.53 (1.35–4.97)*
Age ≤ 49 years	1.3	1.1	1.21 (0.41–3.60)
Age ≥ 50 years	3.0	0.8	4.01 (1.70–10.90)
Thromboembolic events			
Stroke	1.4	0.9	1.59 (0.93–2.77)
Transient ischemic attack	0.7	1.0	0.76 (0.40–1.44)
Pulmonary embolism	0.7	0.2	3.01 (1.15–9.27)
Deep vein thrombosis	1.3	0.8	1.60 (0.91–2.86)

Adapted from Fisher et al..[18]

Table 4 Outcomes in the Study of Tamoxifen and Raloxifene: Benefits

Outcome	Tamoxifen	Raloxifene	Risk Ratio (95% CI)
Invasive breast cancer	163	167	1.02 (0.82–1.27)
Noninvasive breast cancer	57	81	1.41 (1.00–2.02)
Fractures	104	96	0.92 (0.69-1.22)

Adapted from Vogel et al.[24]

Table 5 Outcomes in the Study of Tamoxifen and Raloxifene: Risks

Outcome	Tamoxifen	Raloxifene	Risk Ratio (95% CI)
Invasive uterine cancer	36	23	0.62 (0.35–1.08)
Uterine hyperplasia	84	14	0.16 (0.09–0.29)
Hyperplasia with atypia	12	1	0.08 (0.00–0.55)
Hyperplasia w/o atypia	72	13	0.18 (0.09–0.32)
Hysterectomy	244	111	0.44 (0.35–0.56)
Deep vein thrombosis (DVT)	87	65	0.74 (0.53–1.03)
Pulmonary embolus (PE)	54	35	0.64 (0.41–1.00)
PE and DVT combined	141	100	0.70 (0.54–0.91)
Stroke	53	51	0.96 (0.64–1.43)
Cataracts	394	313	0.79 (0.68–0.92)
Cataract surgery	260	215	0.82 (0.68–0.99)

Adapted from Vogel et al.[24]

number of heart attacks. No difference in the number of deaths from strokes was seen between the 2 groups. The incidence of cataracts and cataract surgery was significantly lower in the raloxifene group (see Table 5).

The side effects of both drugs were mild to moderate in severity, and quality of life was the same for both drugs. The tamoxifen group reported more vasomotor symptoms, vaginal discharge, vaginal bleeding, genital itching or irritation, difficulty with urinary bladder control, and leg cramps. Women on raloxifene reported more vaginal dryness, pain with intercourse, and weight gain.

Although the BCPT was a landmark trial in that it was the first randomized trial to demonstrate that a drug could reduce the incidence of breast cancer, the STAR trial is anticipated to have a greater impact on clinical practice. Postmenopausal women now have 2 options for reducing their risk of developing breast cancer. As previously noted, tamoxifen has not been widely accepted in the primary care community. However, raloxifene is well accepted not only by primary care physicians but also by women. With the new finding of raloxifene's breast cancer prevention benefit, we now have a drug that reduces the risk of 2 diseases of concern to women: breast cancer and osteoporosis.

RISK ASSESSMENT AND COUNSELING

Several mathematical models have been developed to predict the risk of developing breast cancer. The models most commonly used include several hereditary/familial models and the Gail model. The hereditary/familial models assess genetic and familial risk of breast cancer, whereas the Gail model assesses populational risk using nongenetic factors.

Risk factors used in the Gail model include age, age at menarche, age at first live birth (or nulliparity), family history of breast cancer in first-degree relatives, history of breast biopsy, and whether any biopsies identified atypical hyperplasia. Because the incidence of breast cancer differs by race, the current, modified version of the Gail model includes race-specific data. This program is available online at the National Cancer Institute Web site or at <http://www.breastcancerprevention.org> and can be used to facilitate the calculation of a woman's breast cancer risk in the clinical setting. The Gail model is the first multifactorial model that has been made available for clinicians to use for estimating the risk of a specific cancer. Increased risk is defined as a 5-year calculated risk of 1.7% or greater. This is the average risk of a 60-year-old woman, which was the median age of diagnosis of breast cancer at the time the model was developed.

It is important to understand the limitations of the modified Gail model. It is not applicable to women with a personal history of invasive breast cancer, DCIS, or LCIS. In calculating breast cancer risk, the Gail model makes no adjustment for a first-degree relative with premenopausal or bilateral breast cancer. In addition, genetic mutations are not considered in the calculation of breast cancer risk. As a result, risk may be significantly underestimated. For these reasons, the risk calculation cannot be taken out of the context of the patient's overall personal and family history.

Women with a personal history of LCIS or a 5-year risk of 1.7% or greater according to the modified Gail model should be counseled regarding the benefits and risks of risk-reduction therapy. To determine if risk-reduction therapy is appropriate, an attempt must be made to determine the net effect of the therapy, either positive or negative. The greater a woman's breast cancer and osteoporosis risk, the greater the benefit of risk-reduction therapy. The risk of an adverse event associated with risk-reduction therapy is affected by choice of therapy, age, race, and hysterectomy status. For any given race and choice of therapy, the magnitude of the expected effect (be it beneficial or harmful) will increase as a direct function of increasing age. For example, a 60-year-old white woman has a higher risk of a vascular event than a 40-year-old white woman. There also are some substantial differences by race. For example, depending on the age category, the baseline rates of vascular events among black women are between

1.5 and 2.5 times higher than the rates among white women. It also is important to consider other factors that might influence the risks of therapy. For example, although tamoxifen is associated with an increased risk of uterine cancer that is not seen with raloxifene, this is not an issue for women who have had a hysterectomy. Similarly, women who have had cataract surgery with the placement of artificial lenses do not have the risk of cataracts that is associated with tamoxifen therapy.

When all the factors that affect the benefits and risks of tamoxifen are considered, it is possible to identify several groups of women in whom the positive effects of risk reduction will most likely outweigh any negative effects. Premenopausal women at increased risk of developing breast cancer are candidates for tamoxifen therapy, as they will experience the benefits without an increase in the risks of adverse events. The risks and benefits of raloxifene use in premenopausal women have yet to be determined.

Postmenopausal women may consider either tamoxifen or raloxifene for breast cancer risk reduction. In general, postmenopausal women who will significantly benefit from risk-reduction therapy have a greater risk of developing breast cancer and have profiles that put them at a lower risk of adverse events:

1. Women with a very high risk of breast cancer (ie, a personal history of LCIS, atypical hyperplasia, or a significant 5-year predicted breast cancer risk).

2. Women 50 years of age or older with a 5-year predicted risk of 1.7% or more who have had a hysterectomy (if considering tamoxifen) and either are at low risk of vascular events (nonsmoker, not obese, not diabetic, not hypertensive, no prior history of a venous thromboembolic event, and physically active) or are currently taking estrogen replacement therapy. (The risk of vascular events with tamoxifen or raloxifene is comparable with that associated with estrogen replacement therapy; thus, a change from estrogen to either risk-reduction agent would not significantly increase the risk of vascular events.)

Some women may still be considered for risk-reduction therapy, even if the risk/benefit assessment indicates a negative net effect. Consideration should be given to the personal perspectives and desires of the woman. Each individual will have her own perception of how the various beneficial and detrimental effects should be weighed. Many individuals who are at increased risk of breast cancer are willing to incur the potential risks of therapy in exchange for the potential reduction in breast cancer risk. The health care provider should keep in mind that a woman's decision to take a drug for prevention is personal. Except in extreme cases, once a woman fully understands the risks associated with tamoxifen therapy, she should not be denied the opportunity to potentially reduce her risk of breast cancer if she has a strong desire to do so.

References:

1. Hartmann LC, Schaid DJ, Woods JE, et al. Efficacy of bilateral prophylactic mastectomy in women with a family history of breast cancer. N Engl J Med 1999;340:77–84.

2. Hamm RM, Lawler F, Scheid D, et al. Prophylactic mastectomy in women with a high risk of breast cancer. N Engl J Med 1999;340:1837–8.

3. Ford D, Easton DF, Bishop DT, et al. Risks of cancer in BRCA1-mutation carriers. Breast Cancer Linkage Consortium. Lancet 1994;343:692–5.

4. Ford D, Easton DF, Stratton M, et al. Genetic heterogeneity and penetrance analysis of the BRCA1 and BRCA2 genes in breast cancer families. The Breast Cancer Linkage Consortium. Am J Hum Genet 1998;62:676–89.

5. King MC, Marks JH, Mandell JB, et al. Breast and ovarian cancer risks due to inherited mutations in BRCA1 and BRCA2. Science 2003;302:643–6.

6. Meijers-Heijboer HB, van Geel P, van Putten WL, et al. Breast cancer after prophylactic bilateral mastectomy in women with a BRCA1 or BRCA2 mutation. N Engl J Med 2001;345:159–64.

7. Rebbeck TR, Friebel T, Lynch HT, et al. Bilateral prophylactic mastectomy reduces breast cancer risk in BRCA1 and BRCA2 mutation carriers: the PROSE Study Group. J Clin Oncol 2004;22:1055–62.

8. McCredie JA, Inch WR, Alderson M, et al. Consecutive primary carcinomas of the breast. Cancer 1975;35:1472–7.

9. Fisher ER, Land SR, Fisher B, et al. Pathologic findings from the National Surgical Adjuvant Breast Project (Protocol No. 4). XI. Bilateral breast cancer. Cancer 1984; 54:3002–11.

10. Healey EA, Cook EF, Orav EJ, et al. Contralateral breast cancer: clinical characteristics and impact on prognosis. J Clin Oncol 1993;11:1545–52.

11. Metcalfe K, Lynch HT, Ghadirian P, et al. Contralateral breast cancer in BRCA1 and BRCA2 mutation carriers. J Clin Oncol 2004;22:2328–35.

12. McDonnell SK, Schaid DJ, Myers JL, et al. Efficacy of contralateral prophylactic mastectomy in women with a personal and family history of breast cancer. J Clin Oncol 2001;19:3938–43.

13. Peralta EA, Ellenhorn JD, Wagman LD, et al. Contralateral prophylactic mastectomy improves the outcome of selected patients undergoing mastectomy for breast cancer. Am J Surg 2000;180:439–45.

14. Goldflam K, Hunt KK, Gershenwald JE, et al. Contralateral prophylactic mastectomy. Predictors of significant histologic findings. Cancer 2004;101:1977–86.

15. Babiera GV, Lowy AM, Davidson BS, et al. The role of contralateral prophylactic mastectomy in invasive lobular carcinoma." Breast J 1997;3:2–6.

16. Lee JS, Grant CS, Donohue JH, et al. Arguments against routine contralateral mastectomy or undirected biopsy for invasive lobular breast cancer. Surgery 1995;118:640–8.

17. Grann VR, Jacobson JS, Thomason D, et al. Effect of prevention strategies on survival and quality adjusted survival of women with BRCA1/2 mutations: and updated decision analysis. J Clin Oncol 2002;20:2520–9.

18. Fisher B, Costantino JP, Wickerham DL, et al. Tamoxifen for prevention of breast cancer: report of the National Surgical Adjuvant Breast and Bowel Project P-1 Study. J Natl Cancer Inst 1998;90:1371–88.

19. Veronesi U, Maisonneuve P, Costa A, et al. Prevention of breast cancer with tamoxifen: preliminary findings from the Italian randomized trial among hysterectomised women. Italian Tamoxifen Prevention Study. Lancet 1998;352:93–7.

20. Powles T, Eeles R, Ashley S, et al. Interim analysis of the incidence of breast cancer in the Royal Marsden Hospital tamoxifen randomized chemoprevention trial. Lancet 1998; 352:98–101.

21. Cuzick J, Forbes J, Edwards R, et al. First results from the International Breast Cancer Intervention Study (IBIS-1): a randomized prevention trial. Lancet 2002;360:817–24.

22. Cuzick J, Powles T, Veronesi U, et al. Overview of the main outcomes in breast cancer prevention trials. Lancet 2003; 361:296–300.

23. Cummings SR, Eckert S, Krueger KA, et al. The effect of raloxifene on risk of breast cancer in postmenopausal women: results from the MORE randomized trial. Multiple Outcomes of Raloxifene Evaluation. JAMA 1999;281:2189–97.

24. Vogel VG, Costantino JP, Wickerham DL, et al. Effects of tamoxifen vs. raloxifene on the risk of developing invasive breast cancer and other disease outcomes: the NSABP Study of Tamoxifen and Raloxifene (STAR) P-2 Trial. JAMA 2006;295:2727–41.

CHAPTER 62

SURGICAL MANAGEMENT OF RECURRENT BREAST CANCER

ANEES B. CHAGPAR, MD, MSC

MERRICK I. ROSS, MD

One of the primary goals of breast cancer management is local control. Despite surgical, radiation, and systemic efforts to reduce the incidence of recurrence, ipsilateral breast tumor recurrence (IBTR) after partial mastectomy and chest wall recurrence (CWR) after mastectomy continue to pose challenging situations for the multidisciplinary breast team. Surgery remains a mainstay of treatment in these cases.

Management of CWR after Mastectomy

With long-term data demonstrating the survival equivalence of mastectomy and breast-conserving therapy,[1,2] women increasingly have opted for the latter. However, there are circumstances in which mastectomy is preferred either because of multicentric disease, previous radiation therapy, or patient choice.[3,4] Therefore, CWR following mastectomy continues to be a scenario facing clinicians today. Defined as a breast cancer recurrence in the skin, subcutaneous tissue, muscle, or underlying bone, CWR occurs within 10 years of mastectomy in up to 30% of breast cancer patients, even after adjuvant systemic therapy (Table 1). Factors influencing the development of CWR include tumor characteristics such as tumor size, grade, lymphovascular invasion, margin status and nodal

status, and treatment factors such as postmastectomy radiation therapy, which has been found to reduce the incidence of CWR by two-thirds in most series (discussed in greater detail in Chapter 78).[5–10]

The diagnosis of CWR requires a high index of suspicion. Although some recurrences may be obvious (Figure 1), the majority are subtle, often presenting with an asymptomatic nodule in the skin or a slight erythematous rash. More than half of all CWR present as a solitary nodule in the skin; the remainder presenting as multiple nodules or diffuse disease encompassing the chest wall[11] (Figure 2). In 23 to 70% of cases, the recurrence involves the previous mastectomy scar,[7,8,12] and can be mistaken for foreign body granuloma, fat necrosis, or radiation induced injury.[13] The diagnosis is made with a punch biopsy demonstrating malignant cells consistent with breast primary.

Although many CWR occur within 2 to 3 years following mastectomy, local failures after more than 10 years have been reported. Vigilance in surveillance of the chest wall is therefore mandatory following mastectomy, and is accomplished with a thorough chest wall physical examination.

The finding of a CWR was generally considered ominous, as it is accompanied by the presence of distant

TABLE 1 Incidence of CWR after Mastectomy and Adjuvant Chemotherapy

Study	N	Follow-Up	Incidence of CWR
NSABP B-12[27]	1093	5.3 yrs	9%
Ludwig I and II[28]	818	6 yrs	15%
Danish[29]	737	5 yrs	28%
NSABP B-11[27]	697	5.3 yrs	22%
NCCGTC/Mayo[30]	564	8 yrs	20%
ECOG 5177[31]	553	7.7 yrs	28%

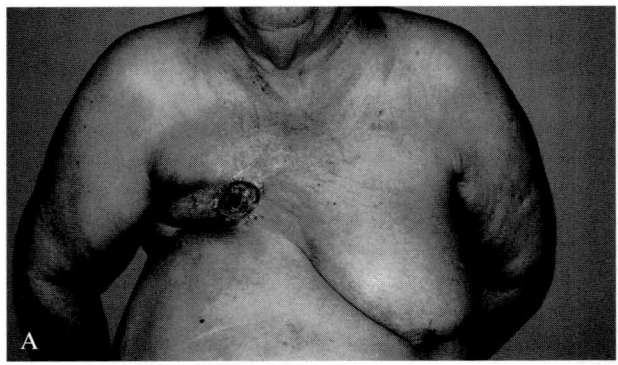

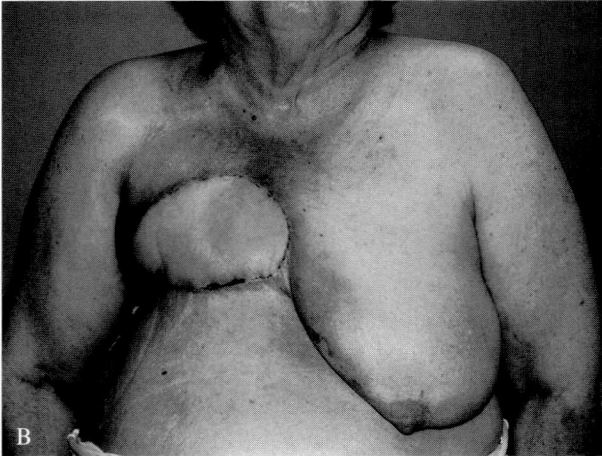

Figure 1 Obvious solitary ulcerated CWR and postoperative resection with latissimus dorsi flap closure. Photos courtesy of The University of Texas M. D. Anderson Cancer Center.

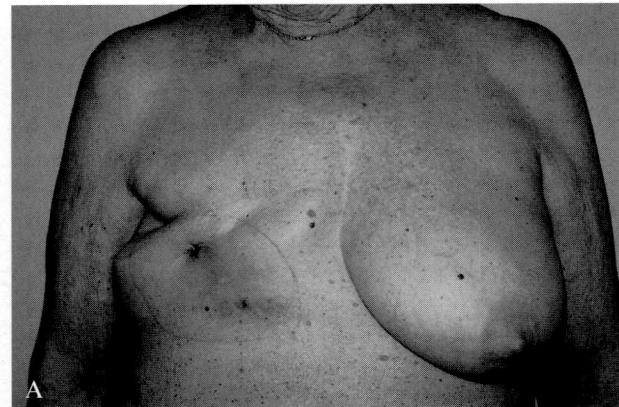

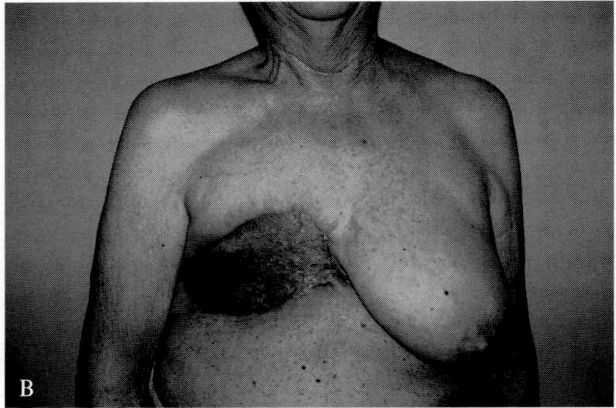

Figure 2 CWR presenting as multiple skin nodules and postoperative resection with skin graft coverage. Photo courtesy of Dr. T. McCurry, University of Louisville.

metastatic disease in up to a third of patients.[13] Therefore, at the time of diagnosis of CWR, evaluation for metastatic disease is warranted, as the presence of distant metastases will dictate the patient's prognosis and treatment. However, the previous notion that all CWR foreshadow a poor prognosis has now been questioned, and there is increasing evidence that this is a heterogeneous population.[5] In patients without distant metastatic disease at presentation of CWR, prognosis varies. It behooves the clinician, therefore, to consider the individual patient's prognosis in planning treatment, as aggressive therapy may be warranted in those with an optimistic prognosis.

PROGNOSTIC STRATIFICATION

Whereas many patients with CWR go on to develop subsequent metastatic disease and succumb to their disease, there is a subgroup of patients with CWR who can be expected to have long-term survival of more than 10 years. Patients with an optimistic prognosis should not therefore be treated with palliative intent. A number of investigators have studied factors that predict prognosis in patients with CWR.[5,7,10]

A recent study from The University of Texas M. D. Anderson Cancer Center analyzed factors that were associated with improved overall and distant disease-free survival in 130 patients presenting with isolated CWR at their institution.[5] On multivariate analysis, initial node-negative status, time to CWR > 24 months, and treatment of the CWR were found to be significant predictors. Using this analysis, the authors categorized patients into a low-risk group (with all 3 favorable features), an intermediate-risk group (with 1 to 2 favorable features), and a high-risk group (with no favorable features). The median overall survival for these 3 groups was 141 months, 54 months, and 16 months, respectively. This corresponded to 10-year actuarial survival rates of 75.4%, 25.1%, and 0% for the low-, intermediate-, and high-risk groups, respectively. Patients in the low-risk group, therefore, have a respectable long-term prognosis, and CWR in these patients must be managed in this context.

A study from the University of Würzberg found that features of the chest wall recurrence were independent predictors of prognosis.[7] In their study, patients with a single chest wall or axillary recurrent nodule with no evidence of tumor necrosis had 5- and 10-year survival rates of 100% and 69%, respectively, in patients older than 50 with disease-free intervals of 1 year or greater. It is therefore clear that some patients can expect a reasonable survival following CWR, and that patients should therefore be treated accordingly.

SURGICAL THERAPY

CWR Following Conventional Mastectomy

Surgery remains a key element in the management of patients with CWR. Although the improvement in survival attributable to surgical resection of CWR is debatable, this modality of therapy provides excellent local control in patients with resectable disease. Surgery is particularly useful in patients who have previously had radiation therapy or those in whom radiation therapy is ill advised.

For patients with isolated recurrences involving only the skin, surgery with resection of the CWR and primary closure is frequently possible, and provides excellent local control. Some patients will have more extensive recurrent disease, however, in which resection with primary closure may not be feasible. In such circumstances, preoperative consultation with a plastic surgeon should be obtained as there are a variety of reconstructive options that exist for coverage. Figure 1 demonstrates a patient who presented with a chest wall recurrence that was resected followed by coverage with a latissimus dorsi flap, whereas Figure 2 demonstrates a patient in whom a skin graft was used. The goal of resection should be the attainment of clear margins, and although there is no consensus on what constitutes a "clear margin" following CWR, we would recommend a minimum of 1 cm.

In patients whose CWR extends to underlying bony structures, including rib and sternum, the value of extensive chest wall resection remains controversial as

TABLE 2 Survival Following Full-Thickness Chest-Wall Resection

Study	N	5-Year Survival
Snyder[32]	24	29%
Shah[33]	52	41%
Miyauchi[34]	23	48%
Faneyte[35]	44	47%
Downey[36]	38	15%
Pameijer[37]	22	71%

this may be associated with significant morbidity. Several authors have reported reasonable long-term results with full-thickness chest wall resection in carefully selected patients, however (Table 2).

CWR Following Mastectomy with Reconstruction

With increased use of skin-sparing mastectomy and immediate reconstruction, there has been some concern regarding the incidence, detection, and management of CWR in this setting. A number of studies have found that there is no significant difference in the local recurrence rate following skin-sparing mastectomy versus conventional mastectomy (Table 3).

The detection of CWR following skin-sparing mastectomy and immediate reconstruction has been controversial. Generally, patients who undergo reconstruction following mastectomy are followed by clinical breast examination. Langstein and colleagues have demonstrated that the majority (72%) of CWR following skin-sparing mastectomy with reconstruction occur under the skin, and are easily palpable on clinical examination.[14] Although some have advocated mammography for surveillance following transverse rectus abdominis muscle (TRAM) flap reconstruction, others have pointed out that fat necrosis may appear as a speculated mass, prompting unnecessary biopsy.

The incidence of CWR does not differ based on type of reconstruction.[14] Although the length of time between mastectomy and finding CWR may be slightly longer in

TABLE 3 Local Recurrence Rates after Skin-Sparing Mastectomy vs Conventional Mastectomy

Study	Follow-Up (months)	N	LR (%) Skin-Sparing Mastectomy	LR (%) Conventional Mastectomy
Murphy[38]	75	1444	1.3	0.7
Newman[39]	50	874	6.2	7.4
Carlson[40]	41	271	4.8	9.5
Simmons[41]	16	231	3.9	3.2
Rivadeneira[42]	49	198	5.6	3.9
Kroll[43]	72	154	7.0	7.5

patients who have had immediate reconstruction, the prognosis between these patients and those who develop a CWR after a conventional mastectomy is not significantly different.[15]

In addition, the management of a CWR in patients with a reconstructed breast does not necessarily mandate takedown of the reconstruction.[15,16] In patients who have had previous TRAM reconstruction, the CWR can be resected with local flap rearrangement to preserve the breast mound. In patients who have had implant-based reconstruction, on the other hand, removal of the implant may be recommended in order to facilitate subsequent radiation therapy.

ADJUVANT THERAPY

It is important to realize that the surgical management of CWR does not occur in a vacuum, but rather a true multidisciplinary approach is critical.

Radiation Therapy

A number of studies have found that the use of radiation therapy in the treatment of CWR is an independent factor that leads to improved prognosis.[5] In such cases, large field radiotherapy encompassing the entire chest wall is preferable to less extensive radiation. In a study of 224 patients with CWR, Halverson and colleagues found that the 5- and 10-year disease-free survival of patients treated with large-field radiation was 75% and 63%, respectively, compared with 36% and 18% when smaller fields were used.[6] Subsequent supraclavicular metastases were also significantly reduced with the use of radiation therapy (16% vs 6% without radiation therapy).[6] For recurrences that were completely excised, good local control could be achieved using doses ranging from 4,500 to 7,000 cGy.[6]

For patients who have previously been treated with radiation therapy to the chest wall, there are few data regarding the efficacy of reirradiation following a CWR. Studies involving limited numbers of patients have demonstrated that reirradiation with electrons to small fields and limited doses may result in significant palliation; however, the utility of such therapy in achieving long-term cure is debatable.[13]

Systemic Therapy

Given that many patients with CWR go on to distant metastases, systemic therapy is often considered part of standard therapy for these patients. Most studies, however, have not found that systemic therapy significantly improves local control when compared with surgery and/or radiation therapy.[13] Some studies have found a nonsignificant trend toward improved survival

using systemic chemotherapy after adequate resection and radiation therapy.[8] Others, however, have found the addition of hormonal therapy after CWR leads to improved survival.[6] In a multicenter trial in which ER-positive patients with isolated CWR were randomized to tamoxifen or placebo after complete local excision and radiation therapy, Borner and colleagues found a significant reduction in second local failures at 5 years.[17] There was, however, no significant overall survival benefit associated with hormonal therapy in this setting.[17] As the hormone receptor status of the CWR is the same as the primary tumor in only 75 to 85% of cases, the biopsy done to confirm the diagnosis of CWR should also be evaluated for estrogen and progesterone receptor status, as well as for *HER2/neu* amplification.

Other Treatment Modalities

Some studies have evaluated hyperthermia in conjunction with radiation therapy. In 4 trials, there was no significant difference in complete response rates between radiation therapy alone and that combined with hyperthermia.[13] Two other trials, however, found a benefit to the addition of hyperthermia.[13] A meta-analysis showed a modest benefit to thermoradiotherapy with complete response rate of 59% versus 49% in patients treated with radiation therapy alone.[18] However, hyperthermia may increase the complication rate following radiation therapy, and therefore the overall value of this modality is questionable.[13]

Photodynamic therapy has resulted in a transient response in some patients, but can lead to superficial skin necrosis.[13] Similarly, intra-arterial regional chemotherapy has been found to result in short-lived responses in some patients.[13] Injection of interferon into the recurrence (either with or without concomitant radiation therapy) has been found to result in good response rates in some studies.[13]

Management of IBTR after Breast Conservation

Tumor recurrence after breast conservation, like CWR, is a challenging clinical scenario. Although clinical trials have demonstrated the utility of radiation therapy in reducing local recurrence following breast conserving therapy, IBTR still occur in up to 20% of patients at 10 years.[1,2,11] At least one-third of all IBTRs are found on surveillance mammography alone; the remaining being detected by physical examination with or without follow-up imaging.[11,13] Most IBTRs have the same mammographic appearance as the original tumor.[19] The majority are of the same histologic subtype and occur in the same quadrant of the breast as the original tumor.[11]

Unlike CWRs, which have a median interval of 2 to 3 years from mastectomy, most IBTRs occur after 3 to 4 years.[11] In addition, CWRs are more often associated with simultaneous distant metastases than IBTRs.[11] As with CWR, initial nodal status and time to IBTR are significant predictors of distant metastasis and outcome.[20–22]

SURGICAL MANAGEMENT OF IBTR

The majority of patients who have breast-conserving therapy as treatment for breast cancer would have had whole-breast radiation therapy. As there is a maximum tolerable dose of radiation to the skin, IBTR in these patients is often treated with mastectomy. For patients who have not been treated with radiation therapy initially, breast conservation with excision of the recurrence and radiation can be considered. A number of studies have compared mastectomy and breast conservation as treatment for IBTR (Table 4). Recent advances in accelerated partial breast irradiation have raised the possibility of using this technique in the management of IBTR.[23]

The possibility of lymph node evaluation with sentinel lymph node biopsy has been found to be feasible in some patients regardless of previous axillary surgery.[24] This may provide additional prognostic information that may be useful in guiding adjuvant management of IBTRs. Clinicians should be cautious, however, to obtain a preoperative lymphoscintigram, as such patients may have altered drainage patterns. The lymphoscintigram shown in Figure 3 is of a patient who presented with an IBTR after breast conservation and axillary dissection, whose sentinel lymph node was found to be in the contralateral axilla.

ADJUVANT THERAPY

As with CWR, there remains controversy regarding the extent to which patients who have previously been treated with radiation ban be reirradiated. However, for

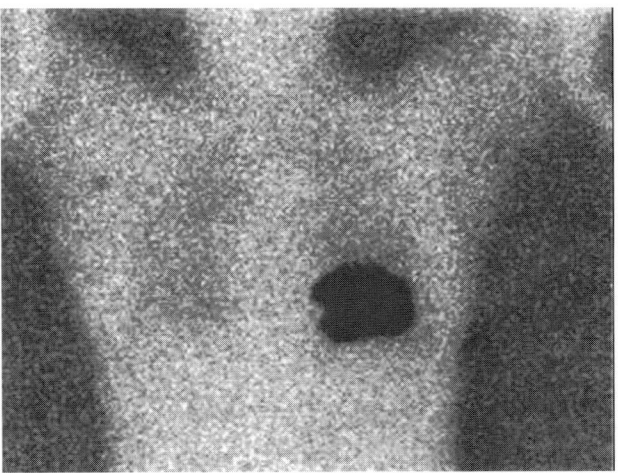

Figure 3 Lymphoscintigraphy of patient with IBTR after breast conservation and axillary dissection, demonstrating altered lymphatic drainage pathways to contralateral axilla. Photo courtesy of Dr. K. Hunt, The University of Texas M. D. Anderson Cancer Center

IBTR, completion mastectomy remains a viable option which avoids further radiation therapy.

Systemic therapy should be used as appropriate. Although Fortin and colleagues have demonstrated that hormonal therapy was more effective than chemotherapy in improving 10-year survival following IBTR (72% vs 47%, respectively),[25] it should be noted that estrogen receptor negative IBTRs have a worse prognosis than those that are estrogen receptor positive.[26] Therefore, in patients who are estrogen receptor negative, use of systemic chemotherapy should be considered.

Conclusion

Local recurrence following breast conservation (IBTR) or mastectomy (CWR) are challenging clinical scenarios. While data are limited as to what constitutes optimal therapy in these patients, it is clear that some of these patients may be expected to have a significant long-term survival. Therapy in such patients should therefore be appropriately aggressive, and should include a multi-

TABLE 4 Surgical Treatment of IBTR after Breast Conservation

		Mastectomy			Breast conservation		
Study	Follow-Up (months)	N	Second Local Recurrence (%)	5-Year Survival (%)	N	Second Local Recurrence (%)	5-Year Survival (%)
Abner[44]	39	106	7	79	16	31	81
Alpert[45]	146	116	7	66	30	7	58
Dalberg[46]	156	65	19	59	14	50	n/s
Kurtz[47]	53	43	12	53	55	32	n/s
Salvadori[48]	73	134	4	70	57	19	85

disciplinary approach. Adjuvant systemic and radiation therapy must be considered as part of the complete management of these patients, and appropriate surveillance implemented.

References

1. Fisher B, Anderson S, Bryant J, et al. Twenty-year follow-up of a randomized trial comparing total mastectomy, lumpectomy, and lumpectomy plus irradiation for the treatment of invasive breast cancer. N Engl J Med 2002;347: 1233–41.

2. Veronesi U, Cascinelli N, Mariani L, et al. Twenty-year follow-up of a randomized study comparing breast-conserving surgery with radical mastectomy for early breast cancer. N Engl J Med 2002;347:1227–32.

3. Chagpar AB, Studts JL, Scoggins CR, et al. Factors associated with surgical options for breast carcinoma. Cancer 2006;106:1462–6.

4. Mastectomy or lumpectomy? The choice of operation for clinical stages I and II breast cancer. The Steering Committee on Clinical Practice Guidelines for the Care and Treatment of Breast Cancer. Canadian Association of Radiation Oncologists. CMAJ 1998;158 Suppl 3:S15–21.

5. Chagpar A, Meric-Bernstam F, Hunt KK, et al. Chest wall recurrence after mastectomy does not always portend a dismal outcome. Ann Surg Oncol 2003;10:628–34.

6. Halverson KJ, Perez CA, Kuske RR, et al. Isolated local-regional recurrence of breast cancer following mastectomy: radiotherapeutic management. Int J Radiat Oncol Biol Phys 1990;19:851–8.

7. Willner J, Kiricuta IC, Kolbl O. Locoregional recurrence of breast cancer following mastectomy: always a fatal event? Results of univariate and multivariate analysis. Int J Radiat Oncol Biol Phys 1997;37:853–63.

8. Schwaibold F, Fowble BL, Solin LJ, et al. The results of radiation therapy for isolated local regional recurrence after mastectomy. Int J Radiat Oncol Biol Phys 1991;21: 299–310.

9. Mora EM, Singletary SE, Buzdar AU, Johnston DA. Aggressive therapy for locoregional recurrence after mastectomy in stage II and III breast cancer patients. Ann Surg Oncol 1996;3:162–8.

10. Kamby C, Sengelov L. Pattern of dissemination and survival following isolated locoregional recurrence of breast cancer. A prospective study with more than 10 years of follow up. Breast Cancer Res Treat 1997;45:181–92.

11. Freedman GM, Fowble BL. Local recurrence after mastectomy or breast-conserving surgery and radiation. Oncology (Williston Park) 2000;14:1561–81.

12. Donegan WL, Perez-Mesa CM, Watson FR. A biostatistical study of locally recurrent breast carcinoma. Surg Gynecol Obstet 1966;122:529–40.

13. Recht A, Come S, Troyan SL, Sadowsky N. Management of recurrent breast cancer. In: Harris JR, Lippman ME, Morrow M, Osborne CK, editors. Diseases of the breast. Philadelphia: Lippincott, Williams and Wilkins; 2000. p. 731–48.

14. Langstein HN, Cheng MH, Singletary SE, et al. Breast cancer recurrence after immediate reconstruction: patterns and significance. Plast Reconstr Surg 2003;111: 712–20.

15. Chagpar A, Langstein HN, Kronowitz SJ, et al. Treatment and outcome of patients with chest wall recurrence after mastectomy and breast reconstruction. Am J Surg 2004; 187:164–9.

16. Howard MA, Polo K, Pusic AL, et al. Breast cancer local recurrence after mastectomy and TRAM flap reconstruction: incidence and treatment options. Plast Reconstr Surg 2006;117:1381–6.

17. Borner M, Bacchi M, Goldhirsch A, et al. First isolated locoregional recurrence following mastectomy for breast cancer: results of a phase III multicenter study comparing systemic treatment with observation after excision and radiation. Swiss Group for Clinical Cancer Research. J Clin Oncol 1994;12:2071–7.

18. Vernon CC, Hand JW, Field SB, et al. Radiotherapy with or without hyperthermia in the treatment of superficial localized breast cancer: results from five randomized controlled trials. International Collaborative Hyperthermia Group. Int J Radiat Oncol Biol Phys 1996;35: 731–44.

19. Philpotts LE, Lee CH, Haffty BG, et al. Mammographic findings of recurrent breast cancer after lumpectomy and radiation therapy: comparison with the primary tumor. Radiology 1996;201:767–71.

20. Komoike Y, Akiyama F, Iino Y, et al. Ipsilateral breast tumor recurrence (IBTR) after breast-conserving treatment for early breast cancer: risk factors and impact on distant metastases. Cancer 2006;106:35–41.

21. Shen J, Hunt KK, Mirza NQ, et al. Predictors of systemic recurrence and disease-specific survival after ipsilateral breast tumor recurrence. Cancer 2005;104:479–90.

22. Brooks JP, Danforth DN, Albert P, et al. Early ipsilateral breast tumor recurrences after breast conservation affect survival: an analysis of the National Cancer Institute randomized trial. Int J Radiat Oncol Biol Phys 2005;62: 785–9.

23. Kuerer HM, Arthur DW, Haffty BG. Repeat breast-conserving surgery for in-breast local breast carcinoma recurrence: the potential role of partial breast irradiation. Cancer 2004;100:2269–80.

24. Port ER, Fey J, Gemignani ML, et al. Reoperative sentinel lymph node biopsy: a new option for patients with primary or locally recurrent breast carcinoma. J Am Coll Surg 2002; 195:167–72.

25. Fortin A, Larochelle M, Laverdiere J, et al. Local failure is responsible for the decrease in survival for patients with breast cancer treated with conservative surgery and postoperative radiotherapy. J Clin Oncol 1999;17:101–9.

26. Haffty BG, Fischer D, Beinfield M, McKhann C. Prognosis following local recurrence in the conservatively treated breast cancer patient. Int J Radiat Oncol Biol Phys 1991;21:293–8.

27. Fisher B, Redmond C, Wickerham DL, et al. Doxorubicin-containing regimens for the treatment of stage II breast cancer: the National Surgical Adjuvant Breast and Bowel Project experience. J Clin Oncol 1989;7:572–82.

28. Goldhirsch A, Gelber RD, Castiglione M. Relapse of breast cancer after adjuvant treatment in premenopausal and perimenopausal women: patterns and prognoses. J Clin Oncol 1988;6:89–97.

29. Overgaard M, Christensen JJ, Johansen H, et al. Evaluation of radiotherapy in high-risk breast cancer patients: report from the Danish Breast Cancer Cooperative Group (DBCG 82) Trial. Int J Radiat Oncol Biol Phys 1990;19:1121–4.

30. Pisansky TM, Ingle JN, Schaid DJ, et al. Patterns of tumor relapse following mastectomy and adjuvant systemic therapy in patients with axillary lymph node-positive breast cancer. Impact of clinical, histopathologic, and flow cytometric factors. Cancer 1993;72:1247–60.

31. Tormey DC, Gray R, Gilchrist K, et al. Adjuvant chemohormonal therapy with cyclophosphamide, methotrexate, 5-fluorouracil, and prednisone (CMFP) or CMFP plus tamoxifen compared with CMF for premenopausal breast cancer patients. An Eastern Cooperative Oncology Group trial. Cancer 1990;65:200–6.

32. Snyder AF, Farrow GM, Masson JK, Payne WS. Chest-wall resection for locally recurrent breast cancer. Arch Surg 1968;97:246–53.

33. Shah JP, Urban JA. Full thickness chest wall resection for recurrent breast carcinoma involving the bony chest wall. Cancer 1975;35:567–73.

34. Miyauchi K, Koyama H, Noguchi S, et al. Surgical treatment for chest wall recurrence of breast cancer. Eur J Cancer 1992;28A:1059–62.

35. Faneyte IF, Rutgers EJ, Zoetmulder FA. Chest wall resection in the treatment of locally recurrent breast carcinoma: indications and outcome for 44 patients. Cancer 1997;80:886–91.

36. Downey RJ, Rusch V, Hsu FI, et al. Chest wall resection for locally recurrent breast cancer: is it worthwhile? J Thorac Cardiovasc Surg 2000;119:420–8.

37. Pameijer CR, Smith D, McCahill LE, et al. Full-thickness chest wall resection for recurrent breast carcinoma: an institutional review and meta-analysis. Am Surg 2005;71:711–5.

38. Murphy RX Jr, Wahhab S, Rovito PF, et al. Impact of immediate reconstruction on the local recurrence of breast cancer after mastectomy. Ann Plast Surg 2003;50:333–8.

39. Newman LA, Kuerer HM, Hunt KK, et al. Presentation, treatment, and outcome of local recurrence afterskin-sparing mastectomy and immediate breast reconstruction. Ann Surg Oncol 1998;5:620–6.

40. Carlson GW, Bostwick J III, Styblo TM, et al. Skin-sparing mastectomy. Oncologic and reconstructive considerations. Ann Surg 1997;225:570–5.

41. Simmons RM, Fish SK, Gayle L, et al. Local and distant recurrence rates in skin-sparing mastectomies compared with non-skin-sparing mastectomies. Ann Surg Oncol 1999;6:676–81.

42. Rivadeneira DE, Simmons RM, Fish SK, et al. Skin-sparing mastectomy with immediate breast reconstruction: a critical analysis of local recurrence. Cancer J 2000;6:331–5.

43. Kroll SS, Khoo A, Singletary SE, et al. Local recurrence risk after skin-sparing and conventional mastectomy: a 6-year follow-up. Plast Reconstr Surg 1999;104:421–5.

44. Abner AL, Recht A, Eberlein T, et al. Prognosis following salvage mastectomy for recurrence in the breast after conservative surgery and radiation therapy for early-stage breast cancer. J Clin Oncol 1993;11:44–8.

45. Alpert TE, Kuerer HM, Arthur DW, et al. Ipsilateral breast tumor recurrence after breast conservation therapy: outcomes of salvage mastectomy vs. salvage breast-conserving surgery and prognostic factors for salvage breast preservation. Int J Radiat Oncol Biol Phys 2005;63:845–51.

46. Dalberg K, Mattsson A, Sandelin K, Rutqvist LE. Outcome of treatment for ipsilateral breast tumor recurrence in early-stage breast cancer. Breast Cancer Res Treat 1998;49:69–78.

47. Kurtz JM, Jacquemier J, Amalric R, et al. Is breast conservation after local recurrence feasible? Eur J Cancer 1991;27:240–4.

48. Salvadori B, Marubini E, Miceli R, et al. Reoperation for locally recurrent breast cancer in patients previously treated with conservative surgery. Br J Surg 1999;86:84–7.

CHAPTER 63

PREGNANCY AND BREAST CANCER

SHAHEENAH DAWOOD, MBBCh, MRCP

RICHARD L. THERIAULT, DO, MBA

Introduction

Pregnancy, normally a joyful time during a woman's life, becomes a challenging situation when complicated by the rare coexistence of cancer. Cancer complicates about 0.02 to 0.1% of all pregnancies, with breast cancer being the most commonly diagnosed (estimated to occur in 1 in 3,000 pregnancies approximately).[1] Most therapeutic recommendations are derived primarily from published retrospective reviews, individual case reports, and small case-control series. Owing to the rarity of the situation and ethical dilemmas involved, prospective trials are sparse with long time intervals required to enrol adequate numbers of patients to derive meaningful information. The purpose of this review is to make clear management recommendations based on the available data, dispel myths surrounding the treatment of pregnant patients with breast cancer, and to address some of the ethical dilemmas that will be faced by both the patient and the treating oncologist.

Diagnosis, Pathology and Staging

A number of physiological changes occur in a woman's body during pregnancy, including engorgement of the breasts, which makes it more difficult to notice small lumps and skin changes that could be indications of an underlying malignant process. As a result, the average delay from first presentation of symptoms to definitive treatment is approximately 5 months, with pregnant patients presenting with more advanced disease than the average nonpregnant patient with breast cancer.[2] The typical presentation is that of a patient complaining of a persistently growing breast mass or breast skin erythema that has not resolved with conventional treatment.

The finding of a suspicious mass should lead to a full history and physical examination, following which a

bilateral diagnostic mammogram with adequate abdominal shielding should be performed. The sensitivity of mammograms may be diminished during pregnancy owing to the increased glandularity and water content of the breasts. However, a retrospective review from The University of Texas M. D. Anderson Cancer Centre showed that mammograms performed in women with stage II and III breast cancer during pregnancy had a 90% pick-up rate despite dense breast parenchymal patterns.[3] Pregnant women and treating physicians are often worried about fetal exposure to potential harmful radiation. However, mammography with modern equipment yields less than 50 mrad (0.5 uGy) exposure to the human embryo/fetus, which is well below the 10 Rad (100 mGy) that is required to increase the risk of fetal malformation by 1%.[4] Sonography of the affected breast and nodal basins, a safe procedure that poses no harm to the developing fetus, may also be used in conjunction with the mammographic imaging and is useful in distinguishing cysts from solid tumors. Breast magnetic resonance imaging (MRI) is not recommended owing to its yet unknown efficacy and concern over safety of gadolinium, which has been shown to cross the placenta.[5] Thus mammography and sonography should be considered standard imaging tools in pregnant women suspected of having breast cancer.

Once a suspicious lesion has been located, obtaining tissue for a diagnosis is imperative before embarking on definitive treatment. Owing to the hyperproliferative state of the mammary tissue during pregnancy, a fine-needle aspiration biopsy of a suspected lesion carries the risk of a false-positive diagnosis of malignancy and the additional risk of missing the malignant lesion.[6] A core or excisional biopsy is recommended as the diagnostic procedure of choice. Although the procedure carries no risk to the mother or fetus, it may be associated with postoperative hematoma, infection, and subsequent development of a milk fistula. To avoid misinterpretation and a false-negative result in doubtful cases, a second opinion slide review at a cancer center is recommended.[7]

Once a definitive diagnosis of breast cancer is made, staging work-up should be based on the clinical tumor-nodes-metastasis (TNM) stage. Staging work-up (Table 1) should include a chest x-ray with abdominal shielding, which is considered safe, as the expected fetal radiation exposure is less than the described threshold for harm.[8] CT (computed tomography) scans should be avoided, whereas sonographic imaging can be used to exclude liver metastasis. When bone metastasis is suspected, bone scans should be avoided. Noncontrast screening MRI of the thoracic and lumbar spine may be used to exclude bone metastases.

The majority of breast tumors diagnosed during pregnancy are high-grade invasive ductal, with lymphovascular invasion being a common phenomenon. The tumors tend to be estrogen receptor negative with 28 to 58% exhibiting overexpression of *HER2/neu*.[9,10]

Management of Early-Stage Breast Cancer

Despite there being scarce data to guide therapeutic management of breast cancer during pregnancy, it is generally agreed that the best outcome will be attained when a multidisciplinary approach is adopted. The managing team should consist of at least an obstetrician gynecologist, radiation oncologist, surgical oncologist, pediatrician, medical oncologist, and psychologist (Table 2).

In order to attain a reasonable chance of cure for patients presenting with early-stage breast cancer, definitive therapy should include surgery, chemotherapy, radiation therapy, and endocrine therapy, if indicated, based on the hormone receptor status of the tumor. The sequence of these therapeutic modalities will depend on the tumor stage, gestational age, and personal decision of the patient (Figure 1). Once a diagnosis of invasive breast

Table 1 Diagnostic and Staging Procedures during Pregnancy

Bilateral mammogram
USS of breasts
Core / Excisional biopsy
Chest X-ray
MRI of Spine
Abdominal ultrasound

Table 2 Members of Multidisciplinary team

Members
Obstetrician/gynecologist
Neonatologist
Medical oncologist
Surgical oncologist
Radiation oncologist
Pathologist
Oncology and obstetrical nurses
Psychologist
Social worker
Genetic counselors
Diagnostic/interventional radiologist

cancer is made, accurate assessment of gestational ultrasound is recommended to assess fetal age and expected date of delivery. When a diagnosis of breast cancer is made during the first trimester of pregnancy (less than 12 weeks gestation), the decision to continue the pregnancy plays an important role. If a decision is made to terminate the pregnancy, management of the breast tumor will be identical to that of a patient who is not pregnant. The following discussion assumes continuation of pregnancy.

SURGERY

Pregnant patients presenting with stage I and II operable breast cancer may be considered for surgery as the first treatment option. The results of large surgical series indicate that breast-directed surgery and axillary lymph node dissection can be performed with minimal risk to the mother, developing fetus, and the continuation of the pregnancy.[11,12] Sentinel lymph node biopsy is a procedure not extensively studied in this setting. The radiation exposure to the fetus through the use of technetium has

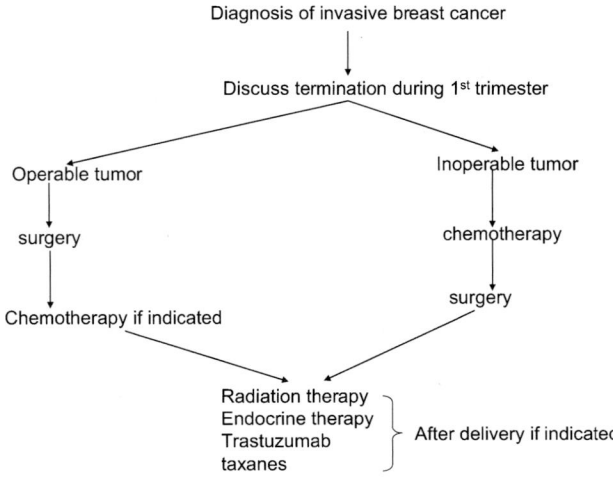

Figure 1 Treatment algorithm.

been estimated to be 4.3 mGy, well below the toxicity threshold.[13] Little if any safety information is available concerning the use of isosulfan blue dye for sentinel lymph node mapping during pregnancy regarding its impact on the developing fetus. This lack of information combined with the rare, but real, associated risk of anaphylactic reactions, the use of isosulfan blue dye is not recommended in pregnant women.[14] Although the sensitivity of sentinel lymph node biopsy may be reduced with the use of only one modality, the use of the radiocolloid is probably the more important of the two available lymphatic mapping agents. Many experienced surgeons have actually moved away from routinely using blue dye for lymphatic mapping; therefore, it is unlikely that pregnant women will be disadvantaged in accurate nodal staging.

The type of breast surgery must take into consideration the gestational age of the fetus and the potential need for systemic therapy and radiation. Modified radical mastectomy with axillary lymph node dissection is the surgery of choice and can safely be performed during all trimesters of pregnancy. Breast-conservative surgery is technically feasible in a pregnant woman, but requires the administration of adjuvant radiation therapy following delivery of the fetus within 8 weeks of the surgery if chemotherapy is not indicated.[15] The option of breast-conservative surgery is thus available for patients presenting in the third trimester of pregnancy or whose stage of presentation warrants the use of either pre- or postoperative chemotherapy[12] such that adjuvant radiation therapy is delivered postpartum.

CHEMOTHERAPY

The indications for systemic therapy in a pregnant patient with breast cancer are the same as those for a nonpregnant woman. However, certain physiological changes during pregnancy may alter the pharmacokinetics and pharmacodynamics of drug metabolism in the mother, resulting in varying efficacy and toxicity profiles. Parameters such as alterations in hepatic metabolism, increased renal clearance, increased blood volume, and altered gastrointestinal function might decrease levels of active drug concentration. Decreased plasma albumin levels associated with pregnancy may increase levels of unbound active drugs. The amniotic fluid may act as a pharmacological third space, delaying elimination of drugs such as methotrexate. Such changes make it difficult to predict appropriate doses and potential toxicities that may be experienced by both mother and fetus. In the absence of appropriate prospective pharmacokinetic studies, pregnant women should receive similar body-surface-area-based doses as women who are not pregnant. Such doses should be adjusted for the continuous weight gain experienced throughout pregnancy.

Administration of chemotherapy during the first trimester of pregnancy is associated with an increased risk of both spontaneous abortion and fetal malformations.[16] The estimated risk of fetal malformations when single-agent chemotherapy is given during the first trimester is up to 17%, with the risk thought to increase with combination regimens. Given the significant risks to the fetus, chemotherapy should generally be avoided during the first trimester.

As organogenesis is completed by the end of the first trimester, fetal malformations are less likely when chemotherapy is administered during the second and third trimester. Small retrospective reviews have been published highlighting the experience of different combination regimens in pregnant patients with breast cancer. The only prospective series comes from M. D. Anderson.[17] This was a single-arm multidisciplinary trial that enrolled 57 women with breast cancer in their second and third trimester of pregnancy. All patients received chemotherapy with FAC (5-Fluorouracil 500 mg/m^2 on days 1 and 4, doxorubicin 50 mg/m^2 as a continuous infusion over 72 hours, cyclophosphamide 500 mg/m^2 on day 1). All women who had delivered had live births, with 1 child born with Down syndrome, and 2 with congenital anomalies, including club foot and congenital bilateral ureteral reflux. Median follow-up was 38.5 months, and thus longer follow-up is needed to evaluate possible long-term side effects on the children, such as impaired cardiac function and fertility. A retrospective review of 28 pregnant patients with breast cancer, who received chemotherapy after the first trimester, 12 of whom received chemotherapy with CMF, reported no deaths or congenital malformations.[18]

Our recommendation is that pregnant patients with breast cancer who require chemotherapy receive it after the first trimester of pregnancy. In the absence of any cardiac dysfunction, FAC should be the chemotherapy of choice. When cardiac dysfunction is a limiting factor for anthracycline, use of CMF may be considered. Individual case reports of taxanes administered after the organogenesis phase of fetal development in pregnant patients have been published that highlight the apparent safety of these agents. However, at the present time there are not enough long-term fetal outcome data to recommend taxanes during pregnancy. Depending on the timing of delivery, taxanes, when indicated, may be administered following delivery in the postpartum period.

RADIATION THERAPY

Adjuvant external beam radiation therapy may be required during the course of treatment. Standard adjuvant doses of 50 to 60 Gy results in the fetus receiving a minimum of 2 cGy during the first trimester, up to 24.6 cGy in the second trimester, and up to 58.6 cGy in the third trimester.[19] These doses are well above the threshold of toxicity. Thus, owing to the risks associated with fetal exposure, adjuvant radiation therapy is contraindicated during pregnancy.

ENDOCRINE THERAPY

Animal studies have shown that tamoxifen potentially may be teratogenic.[20] In addition, there are reports of various birth defects in children born to women exposed to tamoxifen. Abnormalities such as craniofacial defects, Goldenhar's syndrome (oculoauriculovertebral dysplasia), and ambiguous genitalia have been described.[21,22] Therefore, hormone treatment, when indicated, should be started after delivery.

GROWTH FACTOR AND ANTIEMETIC SUPPORT

Granulocyte colony stimulating factor (G-CSF) and erythropoietin may be required during treatment with chemotherapy. Both have been used safely in pregnant patients without immediate complications or associated birth defects.[23] 5HT3 serotonin antagonists have not been associated with fetal malformations[24] and may be used when required. Corticosteroids, commonly used agent for emesis, have been associated with cleft palate in newborns when used in the first trimester.[25] Their use during the second and third trimesters appears safe. Aprepitant, an NK-1 antagonist used to counteract emesis, has not been studied in pregnant women and is not recommended at the present time.

OTHER BIOLOGICAL AGENTS

Recent evidence shows that the use of adjuvant trastuzumab in early-stage breast cancers overexpressing *HER2/neu* improves both disease-free and overall survival.[26] The use of trastuzumab in pregnant women, however, has been limited. Animal studies demonstrate evidence of its placental transfer.[27] Individual case reports, where trastuzumab has been used during pregnancy, have reported an association with the development of oligohydramnios.[28] Pregnant patients with early-stage breast cancer whose tumors overexpress *HER2/neu* should be offered trastuzumab after delivery.

THERAPEUTIC ABORTION

In the past, therapeutic abortion was strongly advocated in pregnant women with breast cancer based on the belief that hormonal changes of pregnancy promoted the growth of breast cancer, and thus would result in worse outcome. Historical case series do not support this belief, revealing no significant reduction in relapse rate or

improvement in survival with termination of pregnancy.[29] It is still, however, reasonable to discuss the option of termination when the fetal teratogenesis is known or suspected, or when the health of the mother is in jeopardy. Regardless of the indication, the decision to continue or terminate the pregnancy should be made by the woman, who should be provided with adequate counseling such that she is able to make an informed, rational decision.

MONITORING THE PREGNANCY

Antenatal care needs the combined effort of both the treating obstetrician and medical oncologist. Evaluation of gestational age before beginning treatment is recommended. Thereafter an assessment of fetal growth should be performed before every cycle of chemotherapy. In case of detection of abnormalities, such as intrauterine growth retardation, oligohydramnios, or severe maternal anemia, Doppler ultrasound of the cord vessels should be performed. When faced with pregnancy-related complications, such as preeclampsia and preterm labor, standard institution-based guidelines should be implemented.

TIMING OF DELIVERY

The treating obstetrician and medical oncologist should work together when deciding the optimal time and method for delivery. Delivery should occur approximately 3 weeks after the last dose of chemotherapy to minimize the risk of maternal and fetal neutropenia and thrombocytopenia, thereby preventing subsequent infectious and bleeding complications, respectively. If chemotherapy and endocrine therapy is continued, postpartum breast-feeding is contraindicated, as most of these agents can be excreted in breast milk.

Prognosis

Breast cancer during pregnancy was once thought to be associated with a poor prognosis, with early reports describing 5-year survival rates of <,20%.[30] With careful multidisciplinary management, prognosis seems to be the same as that of nonpregnant women matched for age and stage of disease.[30]

Metastatic Breast Cancer

The treatment of metastatic breast cancer during pregnancy should follow the same principles as that outlined for early-stage breast cancer. The goal in this setting is palliation. Pregnant patients who have received anthracycline-based regimens in the past are limited to the agents that are available for treatment. There are individual case reports of successful use of vinca alkaloids (eg, vinorelbine),[31] taxanes,[32] and trastuzumab in this setting.[28] The use of bisphosphonates during pregnancy has also been reported as individual case reports where an association with neonatal hypocalcaemia has been documented.[33] The use of these agents will depend on the aggressiveness of the disease and urgency of treatment. Before use, the pregnant patient should be well informed about the lack of long-term fetal outcome data when these therapeutic agents are used in this setting.

The Ethical Triangle

When faced with a pregnant patient with cancer there is always conflict between optimal maternal treatment and fetal well-being. Maternal interests lie in the immediate treatment of a newly diagnosed tumor, which may pose a substantial risk to the fetus. The treating physician and pregnant patient are then faced with the ethical dilemma in choosing the optimal course (Figure 2).

Respect for the pregnant patient's autonomy forms the core of the physician-patient relationship. All possible available therapeutic options, including available outcome data, should be conveyed to the patient in detail. The patient should then be encouraged to make an informed decision based on her values, beliefs, and, in certain instances, cultural restrictions. There is no autonomy-based obligation of the physician toward the unborn fetus. The physician is, however, required to assess all therapeutic options objectively and implement those that will give the mother greatest benefit and offer the fetus least risk. This beneficence-based obligation of the physician to both the mother and fetus and respect for the mother's autonomy may not always be in harmony and can pose an ethical dilemma when in conflict. A multidisciplinary treatment approach and psychological counseling are ways to resolve such conflict.

Pregnancy after Breast Cancer

Pregnancy after treatment of breast cancer is a controversial issue. From the limited, primarily retrospective, data published, it appears that pregnancy does not

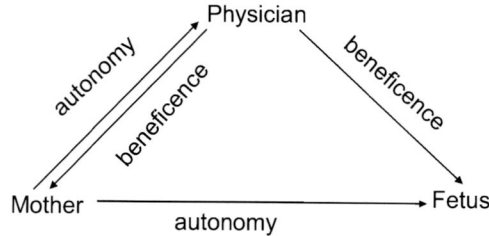

Figure 2 The Ethical triangle.

adversely impact the disease-free or overall survival of patients successfully treated for early-stage breast cancer.[34] Patients with stage IV disease should avoid conception; however, the issue of conception in patients with stage IV breast cancer with no evidence of disease and in long-term remission is a matter of debate.

References

1. White TT. Prognosis of breast cancer for pregnant and nursing women. Surg Gynecol Obstet 1955;100:661–6.

2. Zemlickis D, Lishner M, Degendorfer P, et al. Maternal and fetal outcome after breast cancer in pregnancy. Am J Obstetric Gynecol 1992;166:781–7.

3. Yang WT, Dryden MJ, Gwyn K, et al. Imaging of breast cancer diagnosed and treated with chemotherapy during pregnancy. Radiology 2006;239:52–60.

4. Mazonakis M, Varveris H, Damilakis J, et al. Radiation dose to the conceptus resulting from tangential breast irradiation. Int J Radiat Oncol Biol Phys 2003;55:386–91.

5. Shellock FG, Kanal E. Safety of magnetic resonance imaging contrast agents. J Magn Reson Imagin 1999;10:477–84.

6. Novotny DB, Maygarden SJ, Shermer RW, et al. Fine needle aspiration of benign and malignant breast masses associated with pregnancy. Acta Cytol 1991;35:676–86.

7. Loibl S, Von Minckwitz G, Gwyn K, et al. Breast carcinoma during pregnancy. International recommendations from an expert meeting. Cancer 2006;106:237–46.

8. Osei EK, Faulkner K. Fetal doses from radiological examinations. Br J Radiol 1999;72:773–80.

9. Aziz S, Pervez S, Khan S, et al. Case control study of novel prognostic markers and disease out come in pregnancy/lactation-associated breast carcinoma. Pathol Res Pract 2003;199:15–21.

10. Elledge RM, Ciocca DR, Langone G, et al. Estrogen receptor, progesterone receptor, and HER-2/neu protein in breast cancers from pregnant patients. Cancer 1993;71:2499–506.

11. Mazze RI, Kallen B. Reproductive outcome after anesthesia and operation during pregnancy: a registry study of 5405 cases. Am J Obstet Gynecol 1989;161:1178–85.

12. Kuerer HM, Gwyn K, Ames FC, et al. Conservative surgery and chemotherapy for breast carcinoma during pregnancy. Surgery 2002;131:108–10.

13. Keleher A, Wendt R III, Delpassand E, et al. The safety of lymphatic mapping in pregnant breast cancer patients using Tc-99m sulfur colloid. Breast J 2004;10:492–5.

14. Albo D, Wayne JD, Hunt KK, et al. Anaphylactic reactions to isosulfan blue dye during sentinel lymph node biopsy for breast cancer. Am J Surg 2001;182:393–8.

15. Ruo Redda Mg, Verna R, Guarneri A, et al. Timing of radioatherapy in breast cancer conserving treatment. Cancer Treat Rev 2002;28:5–10.

16. Doll DC, Ringenberg QS, Yarbro JW. Antineoplastic agents and pregnancy. Semin Oncol 1989;16:337–46.

17. Hahn KM, Johnson PH, Gordon N, et al. Treatment of pregnant breast cancer patients and outcomes of children exposed to chemotherapy in utero. Cancer 2006;107:1219–26.

18. Ring AE, Smith IE, Jones A, et al. Chemotherapy for breast cancer during pregnancy: an 18-year experience from five London teaching hospitals. J Clin Oncol 2005;23:4192–7.

19. Mazonakis M, Varveris H, Damilakis J, et al. Radiation dose to conceptus resulting from tangential breast irradiation. Int J Radiation Oncol Biol Phys 2003;55:386–91.

20. Furr BJ, Valcaccia B, Challis JR. The effects of Nolvadex (tamoxifen citrate; ICI 46,474) on pregnancy in rabbits. J Reprod Fertil 1976;48:367–9.

21. Tewari K, Bonebrake RG, Asrat T, et al. Ambiguous genitalia in infant exposed to tamoxifen in utero. Lancet 1997;350:183.

22. Cullins SL, Pridjian G, Sutherland CM. Goldenhar's syndrome associated with tamoxifen given to the mother during gestation. JAMA 1994;271:1905–6.

23. Briggs GC, Greeman RK, Yafee SM. A reference guide to fetal and neonatal risk: drugs in pregnancy and lactation. Philadelphia: Lippincott Williams & Wilkins; 1998.

24. Tincello DG, Johnstone MJ. Treatment of hyperemesis gravidarum with the 5HT3 antagonist ondansetrone (zofran). Postgrad Med J 1996;72:688–9.

25. Rodriguez-Pinilla E, Martinez-Frias ML. Corticosteroids during pregnancy and oral clefts: a case-control study. Teratology 1998;58:2–5.

26. Romond EH, Perez EA, Bryant J, et al. Trastuzumab plus adjuvant chemotherapy for operable HER2-positive breast cancer. N Engl J Med 2005;353:1673–84.

27. Genetech Pharmaceuticals Web site. Full Prescribing Information of Herceptin (Trastuzumab)—Precautions. 2003. Available at: http://www.gene.com/gene/products/information/oncology/herceptin/insert.jsp (accessed October 22, 2004).

28. Watson WJ. Herceptin (trastuzumab) therapy during pregnancy: association with reversible anhydraminos. Obstet Gynecol 2005;10:642–3.

29. White TT. Carcinoma of the breast and pregnancy: analysis of 920 cases collected from the literature and 22 new cases. Ann Surg 1954;139:9–18.

30. Petrek JA, Dukoff R, Rogatko A. Prognosis of pregnancy associated breast cancer. Cancer 1991;67:869–72.

31. Cuvier C, Espie M, Extra JM, et al. Vinorelbine in pregnancy. Eur J Cancer 1997;33:168–9.

32. Desantis M, Lucchese A, De Carolis S, et al. Metastatic breast cancer in pregnancy: first case of chemotherapy with docetaxel. Eur J Cancer care (Engl) 2000;9:235–7.

33. Illidge TM, Hussey M, Godden CW. Malignant hypercalcemia in pregnancy and antenatal administration of intravenous pamidronate. Clin Oncol (R Coll Radiol) 1996;8:257–8.

34. Sankila R, Heinavaara S, Hakulinen T. Survival of breast cancer patients after subsequent term pregnancy: "healthy mother effect." Am J Obstet Gynecol 1994;170:818–23.

CHAPTER **64**

SOFT TISSUE SARCOMAS: TREATMENT ISSUES

PETER W.T. PISTERS, MD

Soft tissue sarcomas (STS) comprise a group of diseases consisting of neoplasms of mesenchymal origin. There are more than thirty different histologic subtypes of soft tissue sarcomas that vary in frequency and anatomic site (Figures 1 and 2). In general, treatment recommendations are based predominantly on anatomic location and secondarily on histologic grade and tumor size. This chapter will review the therapeutic approaches for patients with localized operable soft tissue sarcomas. Other chapters in this monograph will review special considerations in sarcoma treatment.

Standard of Care

The primary local therapy for most patients with extremity and body wall soft tissue sarcomas is surgery with radiation treatment. The evidence base for this comes from two small, single-institution randomized trials that have definitively established that radiation treatment (administered as either brachytherapy or external beam treatment) combined with surgery results in improved local control compared with treatment by surgery alone.[1,2] Neither of these trials demonstrated an

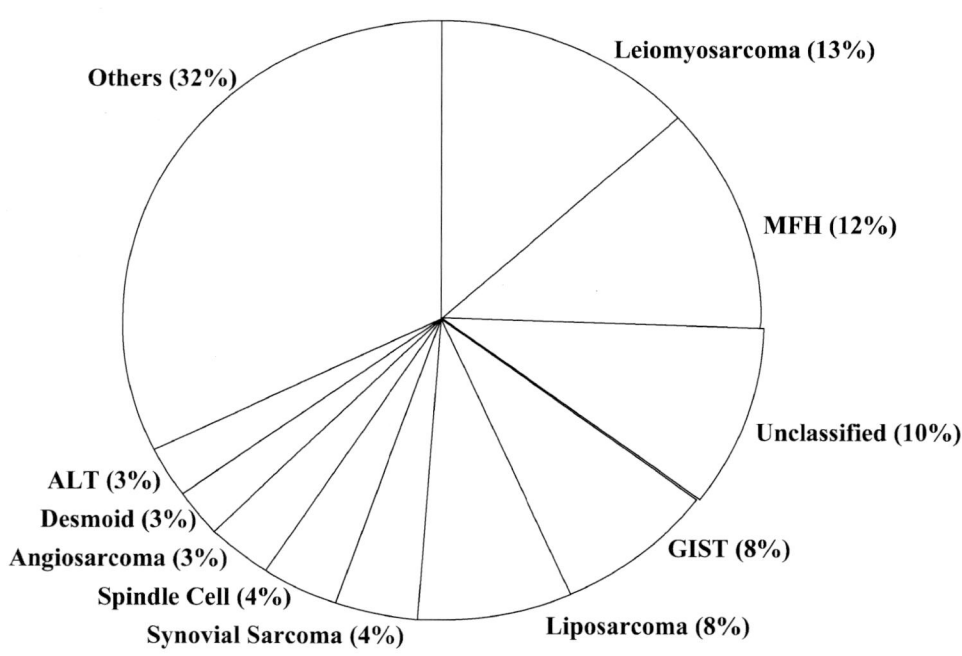

Figure 1 Anatomic site distribution of 6,069 consecutive patients with soft tissue sarcoma referred to The University of Texas M. D. Anderson Cancer Center.

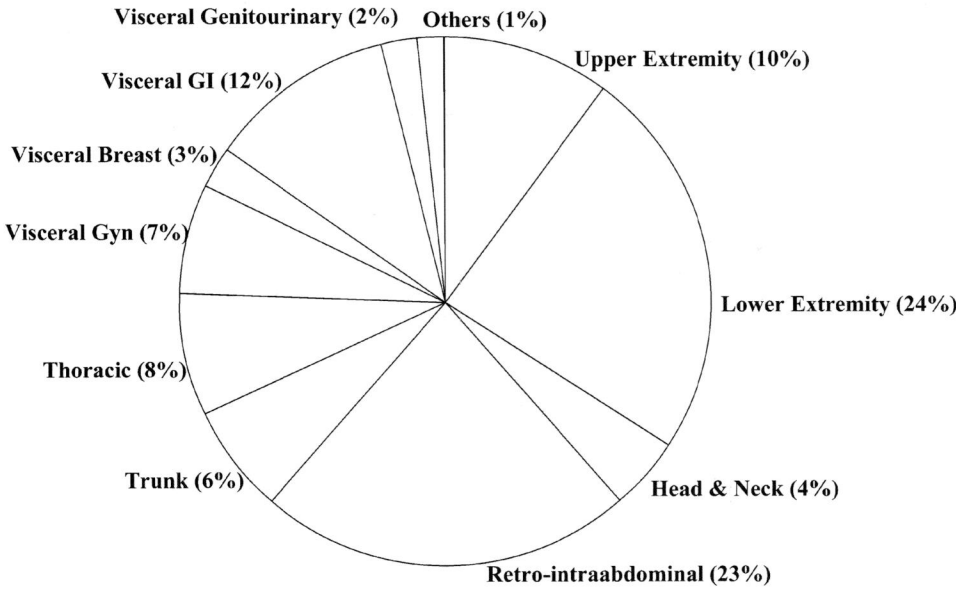

Figure 2 Distribution of histologic subtypes of soft tissue sarcoma in 6,069 consecutive patients with soft tissue sarcoma referred to The University of Texas M. D. Anderson Cancer Center.

impact of radiation treatment on survival, and thus it is believed that the primary clinical benefit of radiation treatment is improved local control. These trials and additional retrospective data demonstrate that local control rates of 85 to 95% can be seen in patients treated with a combination of surgery and radiation treatment.

Over the past decade, one important therapeutic issue that has been addressed is the sequencing of radiation and surgery and the relative merits of preoperative versus postoperative radiation treatment. Historically, postoperative external beam radiation treatment was employed for most patients with extremity and body-wall STS with doses in the range of 60 to 65 Gy. Advantages associated with this approach include the availability of pathologic staging and margin information to assist in treatment planning and the ability to proceed with radiation treatment once the surgical wound is sufficiently healed. This latter issue is important as there are well-established adverse effects of radiation treatment on wound healing, and thus a strategy of upfront surgery allows for satisfactory wound healing before proceeding with adjuvant treatment. In contrast, preoperative radiation treatment can be administered to a lower dose (50 Gy) owing to the ability to treat in a better-oxygenated tumor environment. The resulting treatment volume is smaller, and for radiation treatment planning purposes, the gross tumor volume is easily identified and planned with modern pretreatment cross-sectional imaging. There is also a theoretical possibility that radiation-related response may improve the resectability of preoperatively treated tumors.

The short- and long-term toxicities of radiation treatment administered pre- and postoperatively were carefully investigated in a recently reported randomized clinical trial performed in Canada.[3] This study (often termed "SR2" by the investigators) randomly assigned patients with localized operable extremity soft tissue sarcomas to be treated by preoperative radiation followed by surgery or a program of initial surgery with postoperative external beam treatment. The primary 2end point for the trial was treatment-associated major wound complications. Secondary end points included long-term toxicities (edema and fibrosis), local control, and overall survival. The SR2 trial convincingly demonstrated that treatment-associated major wound complications were significantly more common in patients receiving preoperative radiation treatment. Patients randomized to receive preoperative radiation treatment had a 30% major wound complication rate compared with 17% major wound complication in patients treated with upfront surgery and postoperative radiation treatment. Of interest, radiation-associated wound complications were confined almost exclusively to patients with lower extremity tumors and were exceedingly rare in patients with upper extremity tumors. This site specificity of radiation-associated wound complications has also been noted in a large single-institution report.[4]

The SR2 trial also provided important information on the comparative long-term toxicities of pre- and post-operative radiation treatment. Preoperative radiation was associated with statistically significantly lower rates of treatment-related fibrosis and edema.[3] These late effects of radiation treatment are often clinically significant and are frequently irreversible. This is in contrast to the wound complications associated with preoperative radiation treatment that typically occur over a short time frame and are generally reversible. Local control and survival were similar in both arms of the trial, although it is important to note that the trial was not powered to definitively address these end points.

On the basis of the SR2 trial, there is now fairly convincing evidence to suggest that preoperative radiation treatment is associated with a higher risk of reversible treatment-associated wound complications (approximately 30%), but lower risks of generally irreversible late-treatment effects, including edema and fibrosis. This has resulted in a fairly complicated trade-off for patients and clinicians (Figure 3). The evidence suggests that the optimal treatment approach for patients with localized disease should involve careful assessment of the anatomic site, local anatomy, and the feasibility of preoperative radiation treatment. In clinical settings where preoperative radiation treatment can be administered with low risk of wound complications (eg, upper extremity, preoperative radiation should be considered because late-treatment effects are minimized and wound complications are uncommon. For patients with lower-extremity tumors, treatment sequencing issues are much more complex and require more careful multidisciplinary assessment with careful consideration of the aforementioned short- and long-term toxicities of therapy.

ROLE FOR ADJUVANT CHEMOTHERAPY

There is unequivocal consensus that there is no role for adjuvant chemotherapy treatment for patients with low-risk disease (low grade and/or T1 size). However, the role for adjuvant chemotherapy treatment in the management of patients with localized high-grade sarcoma remains an area of considerable controversy. There remain very divergent opinions regarding the role of adjuvant chemotherapy for higher-risk patients among knowledgeable investigators and opinion leaders in the field.[5] The reasons for this primarily are related to the limitations associated with clinical trials in rare diseases (primarily sample size) and the absence of durable,

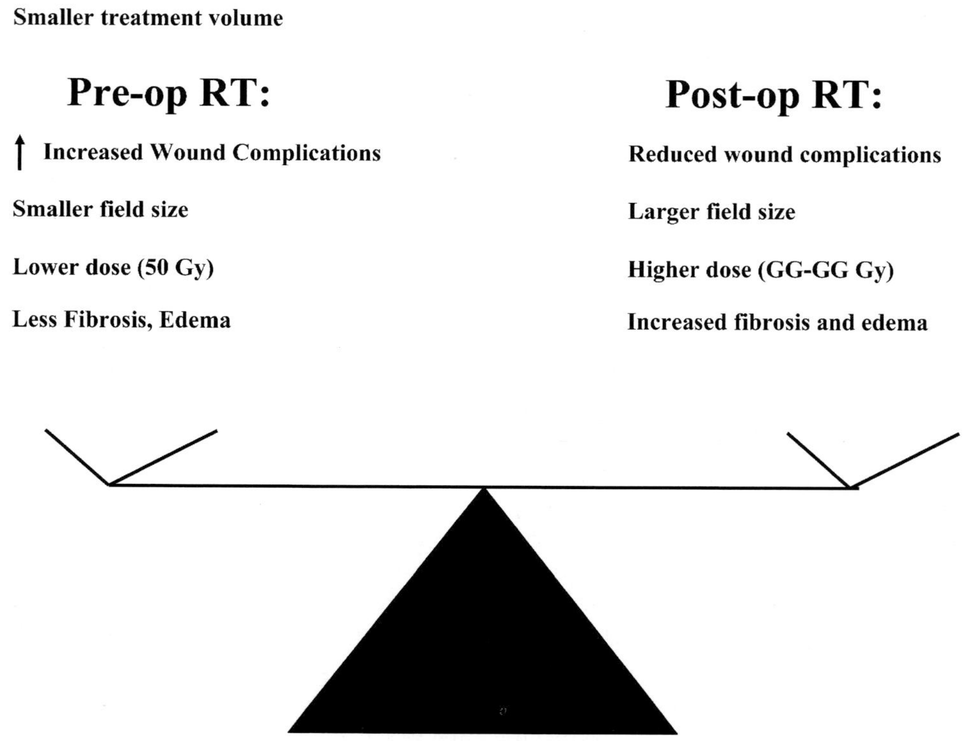

Smaller treatment volume

Pre-op RT:

↑ **Increased Wound Complications**

Smaller field size

Lower dose (50 Gy)

Less Fibrosis, Edema

Post-op RT:

Reduced wound complications

Larger field size

Higher dose (GG-GG Gy)

Increased fibrosis and edema

Figure 3 Trade-off issues to be considered by patients and physicians when considering pre- vs postoperative radiation treatment. Treatment-related wound complications (generally reversible) are less common after postoperative radiation treatment, whereas generally irreversible late effects of radiation treatment (edema and fibrosis) are less common after preoperative radiation. This balance of issues needs to be carefully weighed in individual treatment planning.

clinically significant survival benefit in the published randomized trials.

Over the past decade, the predominant focus has been on the modern generation of randomized trials of adjuvant treatment. These trials have generally included improved eligibility criteria restricting participation to patients with bona fide high-risk disease. Most of these trials have been restricted to patients with high-grade tumors greater than 8 cm in size. This is a patient population that has a risk of disease relapse on the order of 50% or greater. There is unequivocal agreement that this patient population is suitable for studies of adjuvant chemotherapy. In addition, the modern generation of randomized trials has used state-of-the-art chemotherapy agents (primarily the addition of ifosfamide to doxorubicin or epirubicin), dosing, and schedules. As such, the modern generation of adjuvant chemotherapy trials was better designed than the first generation of largely negative trials.

Table 1 summarizes the results of three recent adjuvant studies of anthracycline-based chemotherapy reported since 2000. All of these trials are negative for overall survival, although some trials show a trend in favor of the chemotherapy-treated patients. It could be easily argued that these trials are underpowered and do not definitively address the central question of whether adjuvant chemotherapy improves survival. Nonetheless, none of the presently available randomized studies demonstrate a statistically significantly improved overall survival, and as such the evidence base to substantiate the routine administration of adjuvant chemotherapy is considered weak.

Of the three modern randomized trials, the trial that has generated the most discussion and debate is the report from Frustaci and colleagues. This trial was first reported as positive for overall survival in 2001.[6] At the time of the initial publication, the investigators also published data on the cumulative incidence of distant relapse in chemotherapy-treated patients versus patients treated by local therapy alone (Figure 4). This plot demonstrated convergence of the cumulative incidence of distant relapse at 4 years, suggesting that longer follow-up of the patients in this trial might result in convergence of the survival curves. This possibility was suggested in a prophetic editorial that accompanied

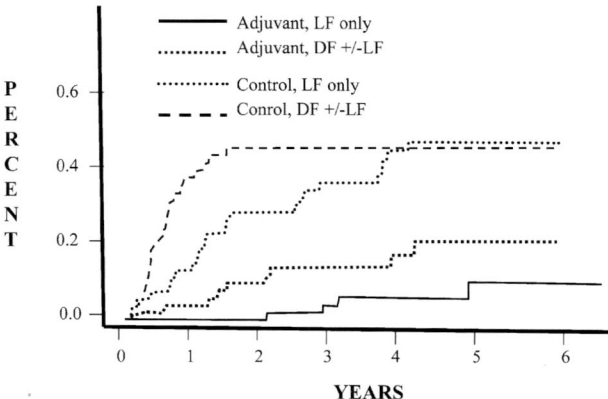

Figure 4 Cumulative incidence function estimates of rates of local and distant failure for patients in the Italian randomized trial of adjuvant epirubicin and ifosfamide-based chemotherapy vs observation in patients with high-risk extremity and limb girdle STS. DF = distant first event; LF = local first event. Note that the rates of distant relapse in the treatment and observation groups converge at 4 years, providing evidence that chemotherapy delays the appearance of, but does not prevent the development of, clinical metastatic disease. Reproduced with permission from Frustaci S et al.[6]

publication of the initial report.[5] Indeed, with longer patient follow-up, the overall survival benefit is no longer seen in the trial that is now considered to be a negative study.[6] This trial suggests that the primary effect of chemotherapy may be to delay the emergence of metastatic disease rather than to eradicate micrometastatic disease.

Additional evidence to support the impression that chemotherapy delays the emergence of metastatic disease rather than eradicating micrometastatic disease is provided by a recent report from The University of Texas M. D. Anderson Cancer Center and the Memorial Sloan-Kettering Cancer Center. These comprehensive cancer centers combined their experience to analyze a consecutive cohort of patients with stage III disease treated at both cancer centers. The patient population was a homogenous group of patients with large high-grade deep extremity soft tissue sarcomas—the group classically considered for adjuvant chemotherapy trials. Interestingly, adjuvant chemotherapy was administered to approximately one-half of the patient population, with

Table 1 Recent Randomized Studies of Adjuvant Chemotherapy

Date	First Author	N	Treatment	Overall Survival
2003	Frustaci[10]	104	E1 vs Obs	NS
2002	Petrioli[11]	88	E or E & I vs Obs	NS
2000	Brodowicz[12]	59	IFACID vs Obs	NS

chemotherapy treatment being more likely at M. D. Anderson and less common at Memorial Sloan-Kettering. The patients treated with chemotherapy and those treated without chemotherapy were balanced for all known prognostic factors except for age. The chemotherapy-treated patients were, on average, a decade younger than the group of patients treated without chemotherapy. Of interest, younger age has been known to be a favorable prognostic factor. Thus, when considering distribution of known prognostic factors, the chemotherapy-treated patients were a more favorable group.

Outcome analysis from the cohort study from MDACC-MSKCC demonstrated varying effects of chemotherapy over time. Over the first year after treatment, chemotherapy was associated with a statistically significant improvement in survival (HR 0.77, 95% C.I., 0.66–0.89, $p < 0.02$). After the first year, however, chemotherapy treatment was associated with a statistically significant inferior survival (HR 1.21, 95% C.I., 1.02–1.69, $p < 0.02$). These data support the observations of the Italian randomized trial, suggesting that the early impact of chemotherapy is to delay the appearance of established metastatic disease. The long-term data from this report do not provide any evidence to suggest that chemotherapy is associated with meaningful clinical benefit beyond 1 year. We do not have clear explanations for the inferior survival seen in chemotherapy-treated patients. However, given the nonrandomized nature of these groups, it is possible that this difference exists as a consequence of an unequal distribution of unknown prognostic factors between the two groups. As noted above, the only known prognostic factors between the two groups are the younger age (a favorable prognostic factor) in the chemotherapy-treated patients. Thus, there should be considerable caution in concluding that chemotherapy treatment is associated with adverse long-term clinical outcome. However, it seems clear that the anthracycline-based chemotherapy treatment is not associated with major clinical benefit definable randomized trials or retrospective cohort analysis of the comprehensive experience in major cancer centers.

Although it seems clear that chemotherapy should be used routinely for patients with high-risk disease, there are specific clinical settings where the administration of chemotherapy should be considered. Examples would include patients with high-risk forms of STS with relative chemosensitive subtype (eg, synovial sarcomas). In this specific situation, the likelihood of chemotherapy-associated response is significantly greater, and there are greater theoretical reasons to believe there may be clinical benefit. Evidence-based treatment recommendations for treatment of patients with localized extremity and body-wall STS are outlined in Figure 5.

Investigational Treatment Approaches

Although the standard treatment for most patients with localized disease consists of surgery and radiation treatment, there continues to be interest in novel treatment approaches, especially for patients who have locally advanced disease not readily treatable with localized surgery. These are often patients with tumors with significant osseous or vascular involvement where treatment-related response may improve resectability. Options that have been utilized in this setting include sequential or concurrent chemoradiation[7] and isolated limb perfusion.[8] The latter has been primarily utilized in Europe where TNFα remains available as a component of the infused chemotherapy that is often part of the isolated limb perfusion. There are no randomized trials evaluating chemoradiation treatment or isolated limb perfusion, and thus these strategies are considered investigational treatments at this time.

Treatment by Surgery Alone

Over the past decade, there has been general recognition that surgery and radiation treatment provides optimal local control for many, if not most, patients with localized disease. However, it is generally recognized that this results in overtreatment of a subset of patients who may be adequately treated by surgery alone. Examples would include small tumors located in favorable anatomic sites where relatively wide, margin-negative resection can be performed without morbidity. This represents a fairly small subset of patients, but certainly a group that could be potentially spared the short- and long-term toxicities associated with radiation treatment.

Several investigators have reported retrospective results of selected patients treated by surgery alone. The selection criteria used by most of these investigators have included tumor size, with this approach often being used for patients with smaller tumors located relatively favorably.

Table 2 summarizes the results of recent series of patients treated by surgery alone. Careful review of the local failure rates in these reports demonstrates relatively low local failure rates, suggesting that with careful patient selection, some patients may be adequately treated by local therapy alone and may not require adjuvant radiation treatment. At this juncture, no firm recommendations can be made about a patient selection for treatment by surgery alone. Reasonable selection criteria certainly must include tumor size, favorable anatomic site, and R0 resection status.

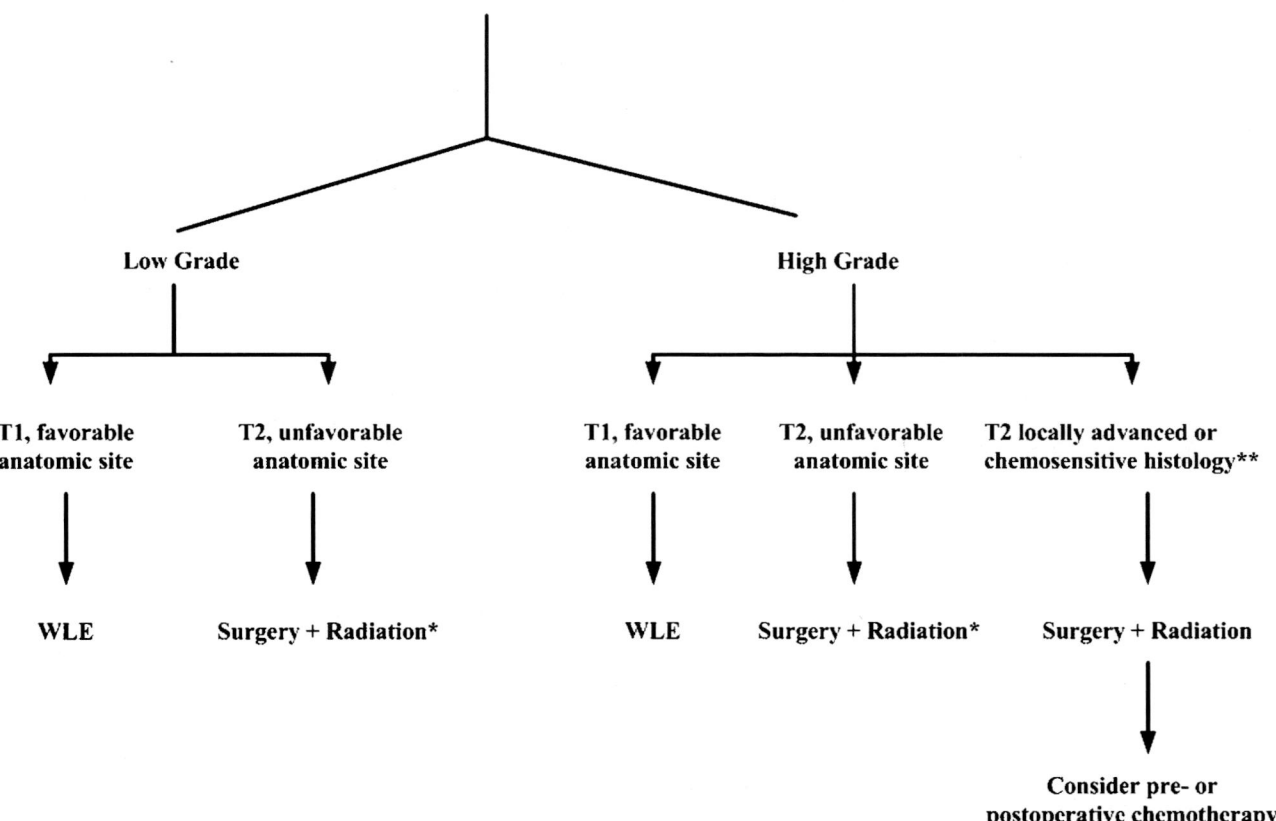

Figure 5 Evidence-based algorithm for management of patients with extremity and body-wall STS. WLE = wide local excision. *Sequencing of radiation and surgery is complex (see text) and requires case-by-case consideration of the complex trade-off issues involved. **Chemosensitive histologies include synovial sarcoma and small cell sarcomas, including those of the Ewing's/PNET family.

Summary

Over the past 2 decades, there has been a general adoption of limb-sparing approaches for most patients with extremity sarcomas. Unfortunately, there is no clear evidence that overall survival has been meaningfully impacted by the changes in sarcoma therapeutics that have occurred in the past 2 decades.[9]

As we move into the new millennium, increased attention must be focused on developing histologies-specific clinical trials for patients with soft tissue sarcomas. Prior trials have not been histology specific and have been open to patients with many different histologic subtypes. This approach is practical but does not take into account the reality that each of these diseases is unique. Histology-specific trials will require novel forms of collaboration, including intrainstitutional collaboration and collaborations through cooperative groups and professional societies such as the Connective Tissue Oncology Society. Increased collaborations and

Table 2 Results of Surgery Alone for Selected Patients with STS

First Author/Institution	No.	Selection Criteria	No. with Adjuvant Radiation	Local Recurrence %	Distant Recurrence %
Geer/MSKCC[13]	174	T1 size, primary tumor	117	10	5
Rydholm/Lund[14]	56	G/M margin negative	0	7	NR
Karakousis/RPCI[15]	116	2 cm G margin	0	10	NR
Respondek/MDACC[16]	57	Size, primary tumor, G/M margin negative	0	2	3
Baldini/Harvard[17]	74	Clinical not specified	0	7	12
Fabrizio/Mayo[18]	34	Clinical not specified	0	15	12

histology-specific trials are two of the most important elements for future progress in soft tissue sarcomas.

References

1. Pisters PW, Harrison LB, Leung DH, et al. Long-term results of a prospective randomized trial of adjuvant brachytherapy in soft tissue sarcoma. J Clin Oncol 1996;14:859–68.

2. Yang JC, Chang AE, Baker AR, et al. A randomized prospective study of the benefit of adjuvant radiation therapy in the treatment of soft tissue sarcomas of the extremity. J Clin Oncol 1998;16:197–203.

3. O'Sullivan B, Davis AM, Turcotte R, et al. Preoperative versus postoperative radiotherapy in soft-tissue sarcoma of the limbs: a randomized trial. Lancet 2002;359:2235–41.

4. Tseng JF, Ballo MT, Langstein H, et al. The effect of preoperative radiotherapy and reconstructive surgery on wound complications after resection of extremity soft-tissue sarcoma. Ann Surg Oncol 2006. [In press].

5. Bramwell VH. Adjuvant chemotherapy for adult soft tissue sarcoma: is there a standard of care? J Clin Oncol 2001;19:1235–7.

6. Frustaci S, Gherlinzoni F, De Paoli A, et al. Adjuvant chemotherapy for adult soft tissue sarcomas of the extremities and girdles: results of the Italian randomized cooperative trial. J Clin Oncol 2001;19:1238–47.

7. Eilber FC, Rosen G, Eckardt J, et al. Treatment-induced pathologic necrosis: a predictor of local recurrence and survival in patients receiving neoadjuvant therapy for high-grade extremity soft tissue sarcomas. J Clin Oncol 2001;19:3203–9.

8. Eggermont AMM, Shraffordt Koops H, Lienard D, et al. Isolated limb perfusion with high-dose tumor necrosis factor-alpha in combination with interferon-gamma and melphalan for nonresectable extremity soft tissue sarcomas: a multicenter trial. J Clin Oncol 1996;14:2653–65.

9. Weitz J, Antonescu CR, Brennan MF. Localized extremity soft tissue sarcoma: improved knowledge with unchanged survival over time. J Clin Oncol 2003;21:2719–25.

10. Frustaci S, De Paoli A, Bidoli E, et al. Ifosfamide in the adjuvant therapy of soft tissue sarcomas. Oncology 2003;65:80–4.

11. Petrioli R, Coratti A, Correale P, et al. Adjuvant epirubicin with or without Ifosfamide for adult soft-tissue sarcoma. Am J Clin Oncol 2002;25:468–73.

12. Brodowicz T, Schwameis E, Widder J, et al. Intensified adjuvant IFADIC chemotherapy for adult soft tissue sarcoma: a prospective randomized feasibility trial. Sarcoma 2000;4:151–60.

13. Geer RJ, Woodruff JM, Casper ES, et al. Management of small soft-tissue sarcoma of the extremity in adults. Arch Surg 1992;127:1285–9.

14. Rydholm A, Gustafson P, Rooser B, et al. Limb-sparing surgery without radiotherapy based on anatomic location of soft tissue sarcoma. J Clin Oncol 1991;9:1757–65.

15. Karakousis CP, Proimakis C, Walsh DL. Primary soft tissue sarcoma of the extremities in adults. Br J Surg 1995;82:1208–12.

16. Respondek P, Pollack A, Feig BW, et al. Prospective trial of conservative surgery and selective use of radiotherapy for AJCC T1 extremity and trunk soft tissue sarcomas. Sarcoma 1997;1:219.

17. Baldini EH, Goldberg J, Jenner C, et al. Long-term outcomes after function-sparing surgery without radiotherapy for soft tissue sarcoma of the extremities and trunk. J Clin Oncol 1999;17:3252–9.

18. Fabrizio PL, Stafford SL, Pritchard DJ. Extremity soft-tissue sarcomas selectively treated with surgery alone. Int J Radiat Oncol Biol Phys 2000;48:227–32.

CHAPTER 65

SARCOMAS OF BONE

PATRICK P. LIN, MD

Introduction

Sarcomas of bone comprise an interesting group of rare tumors. Although they account for less than 0.1% of all malignant neoplasms, they are important in a number of regards. The success of multimodality treatment for these tumors has provided important lessons for surgical oncology, and they offer a paradigm for the treatment of other tumors. Many concepts, such as multiagent chemotherapy and wide en bloc resection, have been validated by the experience with osteosarcoma and Ewing's sarcoma.

Sarcomas of bone differ from soft tissue sarcomas. Many histological subtypes of soft tissue sarcoma, such as liposarcoma, epithelioid sarcoma, and synovial sarcoma, do not occur primarily in bone. Furthermore, sarcomas of bone are not treated like soft tissue sarcomas. In contrast to the latter, sarcomas of bone are not all treated with the same algorithm. Chemotherapy for osteosarcoma is distinct from chemotherapy for Ewing's sarcoma. Some diseases, such as chondrosarcoma, do not benefit from chemotherapy at all. The following chapter is organized into specific diseases, with emphasis on the unique features of each neoplasm.

Staging

The Musculoskeletal Tumor Society (MSTS) staging system for sarcomas of bone is the most widely used system (Table 1).[1] The staging is based on the grade, tumor location, and the presence of metastasis. The grade of the tumor is either low grade (I) or high grade (II). Tumors that are contained completely within the bone compartment are designated intracompartmental (A), whereas tumors that have penetrated the cortical bone are designated extracompartmental (B). Metastatic lesions are stage III.

The staging system of the American Joint Commission on Cancer (AJCC) was similar to the MSTS system in the fifth edition, but significant changes were made in the

sixth edition (Tables 2 and 3).[2] In the fifth edition, tumors were designated as either intracompartmental (T1) or extracompartmental (T2).[3] In contrast, the sixth edition defines tumors based on size (T1 l$\leq$ 8 cm and T2 > 8 cm). A new category T3 denotes skip metastasis in bone and also defines stage III disease (Figure 1).

Staging studies for sarcomas generally include the following. A plain x-ray of the entire bone is necessary to delineate the tumor and to screen for skip metastases. An MRI scan is useful for determining the involvement of surrounding structures. A whole-body bone scan is used to detect distant skeletal metastases. A chest x-ray and chest CT scan are necessary to assess pulmonary metastases, which are the most common type of metastases. PET scans may sometimes be helpful, but their role is still being defined. In addition to screening for skeletal and other metastases, they have the potential to ascertain metabolic activity and monitor response to treatment.

Osteosarcoma

CONVENTIONAL HIGH-GRADE OSTEOSARCOMA

In most cases, the term osteosarcoma (osteogenic sarcoma) refers to "conventional" or "classic" high-grade osteosarcoma arising from intramedullary bone. Historically, osteosarcoma represents one of the great achievements of oncology in the late twentieth century. During the 1960s, the survival rate was about 15% with immediate amputation, but by the turn of the century, approximately two-thirds of patients could be cured with preservation of the limb. The treatment of other rare sarcomas is based in large part on principles that were developed for osteosarcoma.

Clinical Presentation

The incidence of osteosarcoma is 2 to 3 per million per year, and approximately 1,000 cases occur in the United

Table 1 Musculoskeletal Tumor Society (MSTS) Staging System of Sarcomas

Stage	Grade	Site	Metastasis
IA	G1	T1	M0
IB	G1	T2	M0
IIA	G2	T1	M0
IIB	G2	T2	M0
III	G1 or G2	T1 or T2	M1

Grade
  G1 Low grade
  G2 High grade
Site
  T1 Intracompartmental
  T2 Extracompartmental
Metastasis
  M0 No metastasis
  M1 Regional or distant metastasis

States yearly. The peak age is in the latter part of the second decade. Patients under the age of 10 years are uncommon, and patients under 5 years are exceptionally rare. Males are favored by a 3:2 ratio. The most common location is in the metaphyseal region of long bones, particularly the distal femur. The proximal tibia, proximal femur, and proximal humerus are also common locations.

Etiology

Clues to the genetic basis of osteosarcoma came from the study of familial syndromes, including hereditary retinoblastoma and Li-Fraumeni syndrome. The corresponding tumor suppressor genes *RB* and *TP53* are mutated in well over half of all cases. Other genes may exert their effects by their interaction with these genes. For example, amplification of the *MDM2* gene down-regulates *TP53* in about 5% of cases. Unlike Ewing's sarcoma, there is no consistent mutation or chromosomal translocation. The karyotypes of osteosarcoma are quite complex and few recurring patterns have been noted.[4]

Diagnosis and Staging

The plain x-ray suggests the correct diagnosis, and it still remains the most accurate test (apart from biopsy) to make the diagnosis. An osteoblastic lesion is typically present with permeative, poorly demarcated boundaries. When this occurs in the metaphysis of an adolescent, the radiograph is nearly pathognomonic of osteosarcoma (Figure 2).

Needle biopsy is preferable to open surgical biopsy. The accuracy of needle biopsies is high when large core biopsies are obtained, and the risk of recurrence in the needle tract is low when the biopsies are carefully performed.[5] Surgical reexcision of the needle tract is not indicated, and this poses a distinct advantage over open surgical biopsies, which require formal resection of the biopsy scar and bed. Such reexcisions often result in the loss of substantial muscle and skin, which could affect function and wound healing.

In the MSTS staging system, the majority of cases are stage IIB tumors. Relatively few cases have obvious metastases at the time of diagnosis (stage III), and few

Table 2 American Joint Committee on Cancer (AJCC) 5th Edition Staging for Sarcomas of Bone[3]

Stage	Grade	Tumor (primary)	Nodes (regional)	Metastases (distant)
IA	G1-G2	T1	N0	M0
IB	G1-G2	T2	N0	M0
IIA	G3-G4	T1	N0	M0
IIB	G3-G4	T2	N0	M0
III	–	–	–	–
IVA	Any	Any	N1	M0
IVB	Any	Any	Any	M1

Grade (G)
  G1 Well differentiated
  G2 Moderately differentiated
  G3 Poorly differentiated
  G4 Undifferentiated
Primary tumor (T)
  T1 Tumor is confined within cortex
  T2 Tumor extends beyond cortex
Regional lymph nodes (N)
  N0 No regional lymph node metastases
  N1 Regional lymph node metastases
Distant metastases
  M0 None
  M1 Distant metastases

Table 3 American Joint Committee on Cancer (AJCC) 6th Edition Staging for Sarcomas of Bone[2]

Stage	Grade	Tumor (primary)	Nodes (regional)	Metastases (distant)
IA	G1-G2	T1	N0	M0
IB	G1-G2	T2	N0	M0
IIA	G3-G4	T1	N0	M0
IIB	G3-G4	T2	N0	M0
III	Any	T3	N0	M0
IVA	Any	Any	N0	M1a
IVB	Any	Any	N1	Any
			Any	M1b

Grade (G)
   G1 Well differentiated
   G2 Moderately differentiated
   G3 Poorly differentiated
   G4 Undifferentiated
Primary tumor (T)
   T1 Less than or equal to 8 cm in greatest dimension
   T2 Greater than 8 cm
   T3 Skip metastasis (discontinuous tumors in the primary bone site)
Regional lymph nodes (N)
   N0 No regional lymph node metastases
   N1 Regional lymph node metastases
Distant metastases
   M0 None
   M1a Lung only
   M1b Metastasis to other distant sites including lymph nodes

cases are confined within bone (stage IIA). One of the drawbacks of the MSTS system is that it does little to stratify patients and provide prognostic information. The sixth edition of the AJCC has yet to gain widespread acceptance, and it is not clear whether it will prove to be superior.

Pathology

The essential feature of osteosarcoma is the production of osteoid by high-grade, pleomorphic spindle cells (Figure 3). Osteosarcomas are known for their heterogeneity. In any given tumor, there may be regions simulating fibrosarcoma, chondrosarcoma, and angiosarcoma. Sometimes the osteosarcomatous area may comprise only a small fraction of the total. Nevertheless, if osteosarcoma is present, the tumor by definition is an osteosarcoma. Depending on the predominant histology, osteosarcomas are subclassified as osteoblastic, fibroblastic, chondroblastic, telangiectatic, and small cell. With the exception of the rare small cell variant, which fares worse, the different subtypes have similar prognoses.

Treatment

The treatment of osteosarcoma involves high-dose chemotherapy and wide en bloc resection. The disease is resistant to conventional doses of radiation. Although

chemotherapy alone has been tried in a few patients, they usually develop relapse, and chemotherapy without surgery is not considered adequate treatment.

Chemotherapy

Most chemotherapy regimens are based on doxorubicin, which is considered the most effective agent. Other active agents include cisplatin, ifosfamide, and methotrexate. The combination of bleomycin, cyclophosphamide, and dactinomycin (BCD) was used in the 1970s, but these agents are no longer employed routinely since they are relatively weak.

Cisplatin may be given intra-arterially, and this can result in higher concentrations of the drug at the primary site.[6] Although a survival benefit has not been demonstrated, intra-arterial delivery of the drug may facilitate limb-sparing surgery, particularly in cases where the tumor is large and difficult to resect. The preoperative protocol at The University of Texas M. D. Anderson Cancer Center consists of 4 courses of intra-arterial cisplatin (120 mg/m^2 over 2 h) and doxorubicin (90 mg/m^2 over 48 h).

Thus far, studies have not shown much survival difference between preoperative and postoperative chemotherapy. In a randomized study by the Pediatric Oncology Group, the 5-year overall survival was 76% for

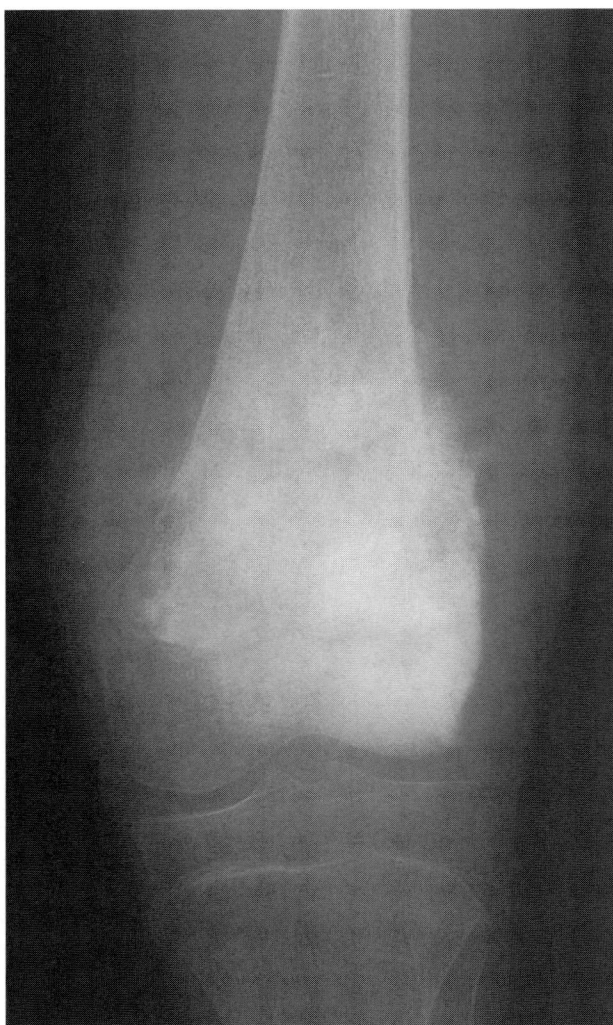

Figure 1 Osteosarcoma of the distal femur in an adolescent female patient. The location of the tumor, the osteoblastic nature of the lesion, and the open growth plates make this x-ray pathognomonic of osteosarcoma.

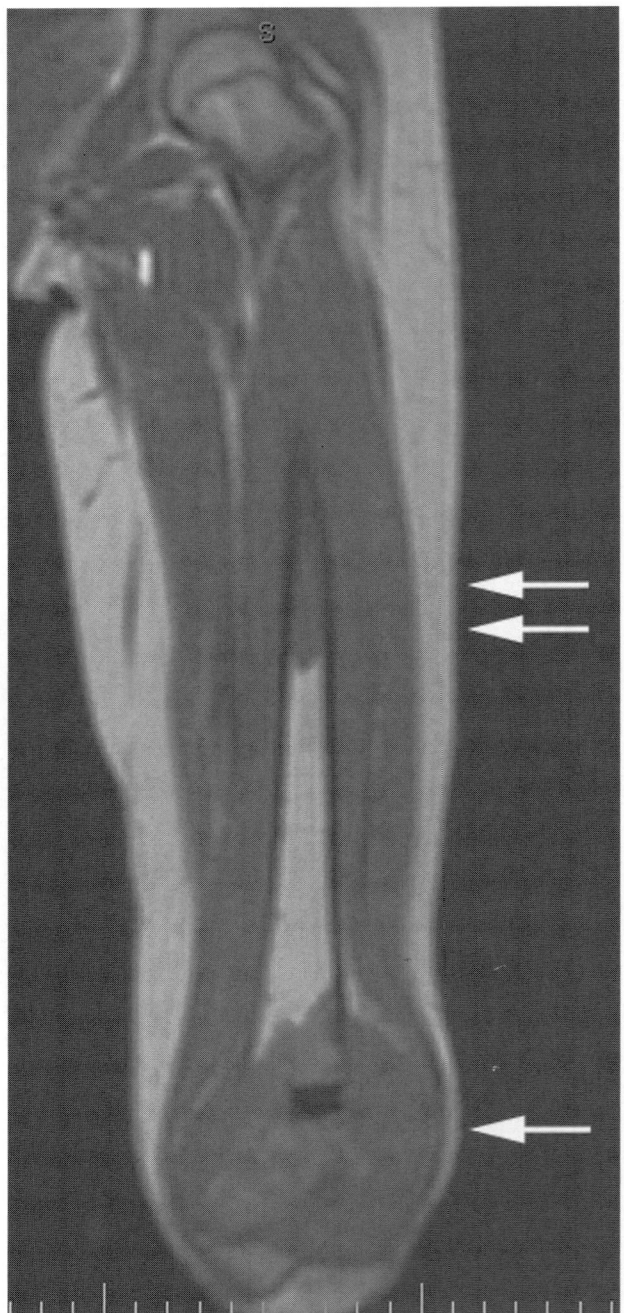

Figure 2 Skip lesion in osteosarcoma is demonstrated well by a coronal view T1-weighted MRI scan. The main tumor is in the distal femur (single arrow). Proximally in the shaft of the femur is a regional metastasis within the same bone (double arrow).

preoperative chemotherapy versus 79% for postoperative chemotherapy.[7] Theoretically, however, there is an advantage to administering preoperative chemotherapy. The response to chemotherapy can be quantified by detailed mapping of the tumor, and the percent necrosis can be calculated.[8] This has been shown in multiple studies to have important prognostic value. Patients who have greater than or equal to 90% necrosis have significantly better survival rates compared with patients with less than 90% necrosis.

The concept of "tailoring" or adjusting postoperative chemotherapy based on the response to the preoperative chemotherapy is attractive. Although initial reports were not positive,[9] more recent data have shown improvement in survival.[10] At M. D. Anderson, patients who did not respond favorably to doxorubicin and cisplatin were switched to high-dose ifosfamide and methotrexate postoperatively. The 5-year continuous disease-free survival increased from 24% to 67% for this unfavorable group ($p = 0.015$).

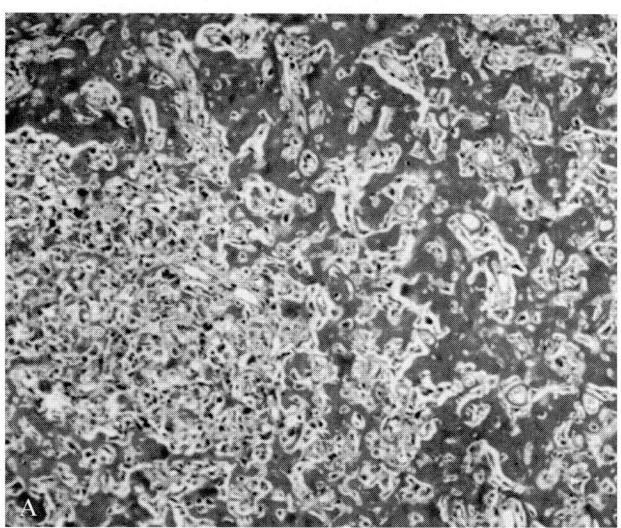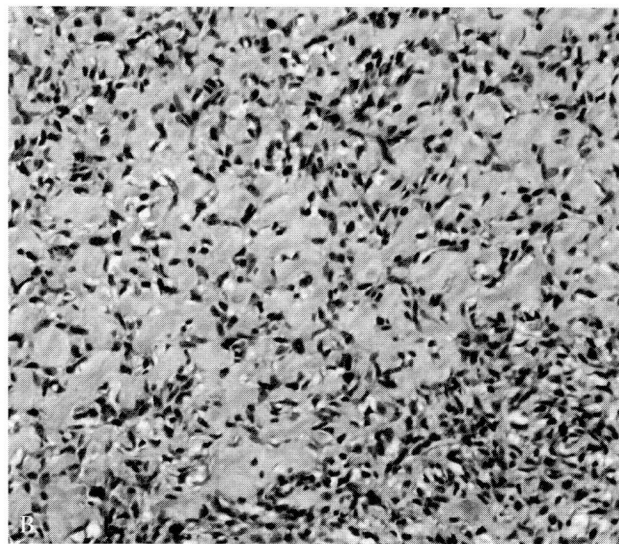

Figure 3 Conventional osteoblastic osteosarcoma. *A*, Low-power view shows abundant, poorly organized, immature bone arising from malignant spindle cells. *B*, Higher magnification shows pink osteoid, which is the extracellular organic matrix that eventually ossifies. The cells are hyperchromatic and pleomorphic.

The results of various large trials have indicated a 5-year disease-free survival of approximately 60 to 75% for nonmetastatic osteosarcoma.[11] Despite attempts at dose intensification of chemotherapy, only modest gains have been made in survival. Interest, therefore, has gained in adding biologically targeted forms of treatment, such as immune modulators.

Surgery

The advent of effective chemotherapy for osteosarcoma heralded the era of limb-salvage surgery. The agents that obliterate the microscopic metastases in the lung also enable limb-preserving surgery to be accomplished safely. In a study comparing limb-salvage and amputation, there was no statistically significant difference in overall survival.[12]

In approximately 10% of cases, limb-preserving surgery is not possible. The primary indication for amputation is the inability to achieve adequate margins. Other indications should be considered relative rather than absolute indications, depending on the clinical situation. These include progression of disease on chemotherapy, very young age, inappropriate previous surgery, and compromise of major nerves. Pathologic fracture is occasionally an indication for amputation, but many patients undergo limb salvage successfully, and the risk of relapse is in large part related to inappropriate treatment of the fracture prior to referral to an oncologist.

With improvements in surgical reconstructive techniques, many problems that previously resulted in amputation can now be addressed. Advances in allografts and modular prostheses have increased the surgical options for restoring skeletal defects (Figure 4). Endoprostheses are now available for young patients that enable noninvasive lengthening of the limb. Microsurgical techniques and free flaps have expanded the potential for restoring major soft tissue defects that result from transverse biopsy incisions and inappropriate prior surgery. Free fibular transfers growing physes can be used in skeletally immature patients (Figure 5).

Surgical excision of pulmonary metastases has the potential to be curative, especially when the metastasis is solitary and presents long after the initial therapy. As the number of metastases increase, the success rate with thoracotomy decreases.[13] An aggressive treatment plan combining chemotherapy and thoracotomy has resulted in 5-year survival rates of 20 to 30% for the patients with metastatic disease.

OSTEOSARCOMA VARIANTS

Parosteal Osteosarcoma

Parosteal osteosarcoma is a form of low-grade osteosarcoma that arises from the surface of the bone. The most common location is on the posterior aspect of the distal femur (Figure 6). Histologically, the tumor is composed of trabeculae of mature and immature bone with an intervening stroma of atypical spindle cells. The cells exhibit much less pleomorphism than high-grade osteosarcoma. The prognosis is generally very good. Patients are usually treated with just wide surgical

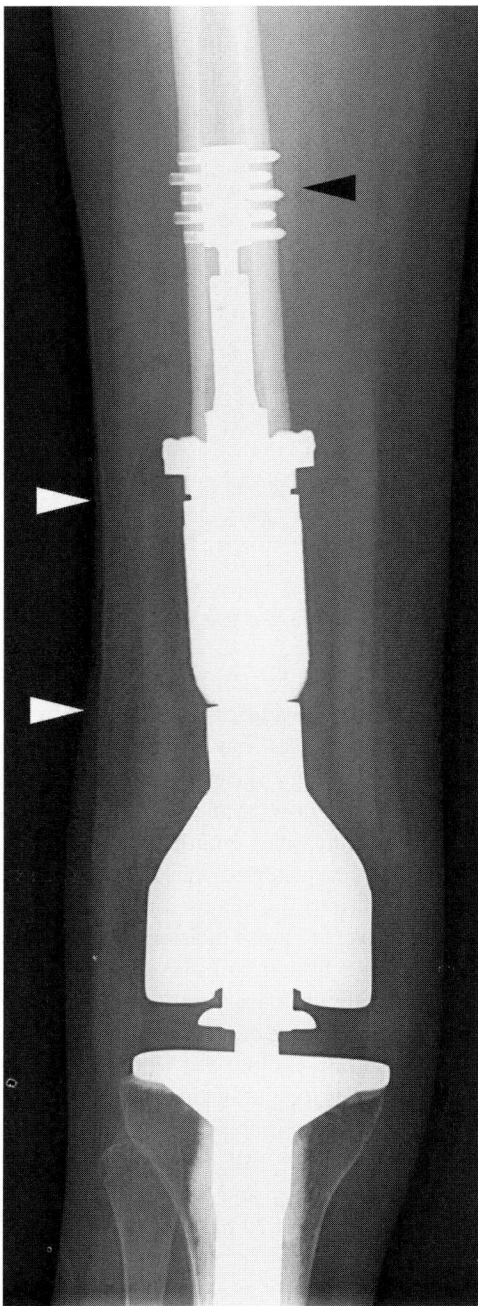

Figure 4 Reconstruction of the distal femur after resection of osteosarcoma was performed by a modular rotating-hinge total knee replacement. Modular stacked components (white arrows) enable the resection length to be restored precisely, and fabrication of a custom implant is no longer routinely necessary. The prosthesis shown (Biomet ComPreSs, Warsaw, IN) utilizes a novel noncemented mechanism for securing the device to the host bone (black arrow).

excision, and long-term survival rates of 90% or better can be expected.[14] A hemicortical allograft is sometimes possible, with preservation of the joint.

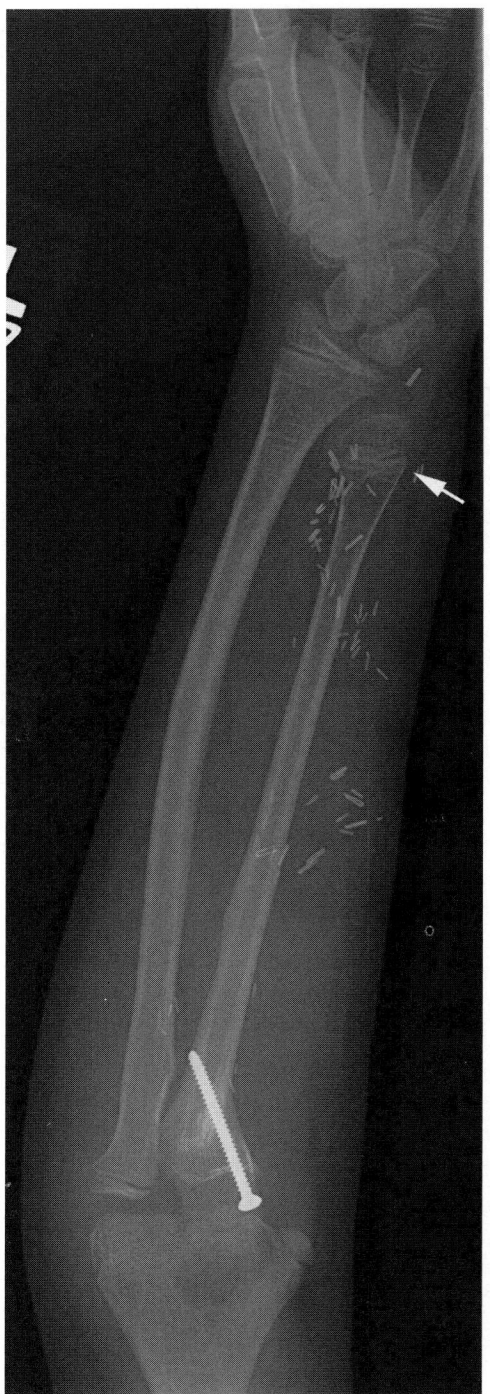

Figure 5 A vascularized fibular graft with live, open physis was used to reconstruct the ulna of a pediatric patient who presented at the age of 8 years with osteosarcoma. The tumor involved nearly the whole ulna. A screw proximally secures the graft to the small remnant of the ulna. The growth plate of the fibula is still open (arrow) at age 12 years.

The diagnostic work-up should include an arterial angiogram. A hypervascular area could signify dediffer-

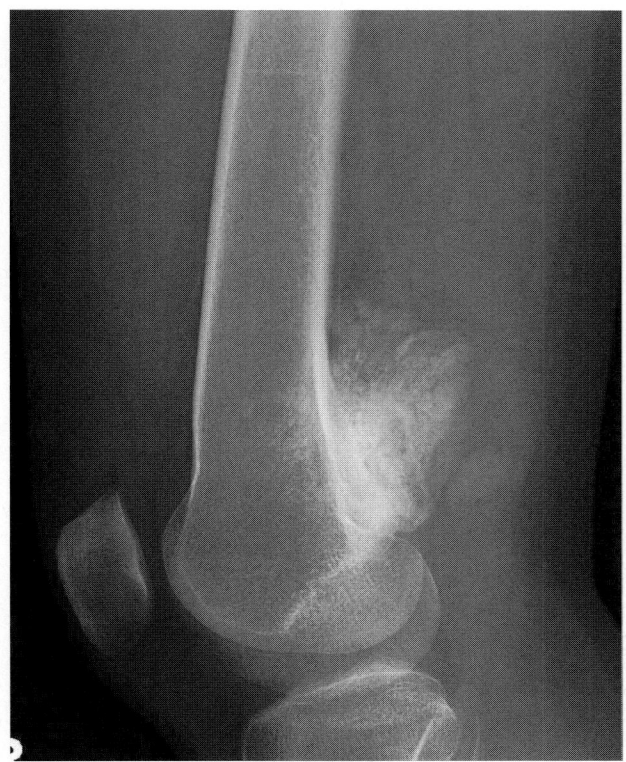

Figure 6 Parosteal osteosarcoma typically affects the posterior cortex of the distal femur. A well-ossified tumor mass is present. The underlying femur appears uninvolved on plain x-ray, but there can be some invasion into the intramedullary canal.

entiation, and the biopsy should be directed to this region.[15] Recognition of "dedifferentiated parosteal osteosarcoma" is vitally important, since the prognosis is significantly worse. It is treated with high-dose chemotherapy similar to conventional osteosarcoma.

Secondary Osteosarcoma

In contrast to conventional osteosarcoma, secondary osteosarcomas usually affects the elderly.[16] The pathogenesis for these tumors involves a pre-existing condition, such as prior radiation treatment, Paget's disease, bone infarcts, and fibrous dysplasia. The prognosis for secondary osteosarcomas is dismal. Most tumors do not respond well to chemotherapy, and the 5-year survival rates are typically 10 to 30%.

Chondrosarcoma

CONVENTIONAL CHONDROSARCOMA

Chondrosarcoma is the second most common sarcoma of bone and is characterized by cartilage-producing chondrocytes. A few notable variants of conventional

chondrosarcoma exist and these are discussed separately below. The exact incidence of chondrosarcoma is subject to debate, since it is not clear what constitutes "low-grade chondrosarcoma." The demarcation between this and a benign enchondroma is altogether clear (Figure 7). There are tumors that may be actively growing and locally aggressive but do not metastasize (Figure 8). Whether these tumors deserve to be called chondrosarcomas is controversial. There has not been much consistency between different centers in the diagnosis and nomenclature of these lesions.

Clinical Presentation

The age range is fairly broad, but most patients present in later adulthood. All bones can be affected, but the femur and pelvis are favored locations. Pain is an important sign, particularly for low-grade chondrosarcoma. Pain implies growth of tumor, and it often correlates with endosteal erosions and expansion of the cortical bone. Such findings are consistent with an active, growing lesion.

Etiology

Primary chondrosarcomas arise from unknown causes. Mutations of *TP53* are uncommon and are associated with a worse prognosis. Mutations of *EXT1* and *EXT2*, which are associated with hereditary multiple exostoses, occur infrequently in conventional chondrosarcomas. Matrix metalloproteinases may be up-regulated in high-grade tumors, but these genes are likely to be more important for the invasiveness of the tumor as opposed to the cause of the tumor.

Diagnosis and Staging

Radiographs are essential to render the diagnosis of chondrosarcomas, particularly low-grade chondrosarcoma. On plain x-rays, worrisome findings include permeative destruction of bone, cortical erosion, and periosteal reaction. Expansion of the bone and endosteal scalloping are not necessarily indicative of malignancy but do suggest active growth (see Figure 8). A purely lytic lesion in bone is more likely to be malignant than one that displays flocculent calcifications in the form of rings and arcs, which are manifestations of more mature cartilage.

MRI scans help identify areas of potential dedifferentiation and erosion through cortical bone. When this invasive behavior is present, the tumor can no longer be considered benign (Figure 9). CT scans are sometimes more helpful than MRI scans for assessing the cortical integrity of bone. Bone scans display increased uptake, but they do not distinguish chondrosarcomas from

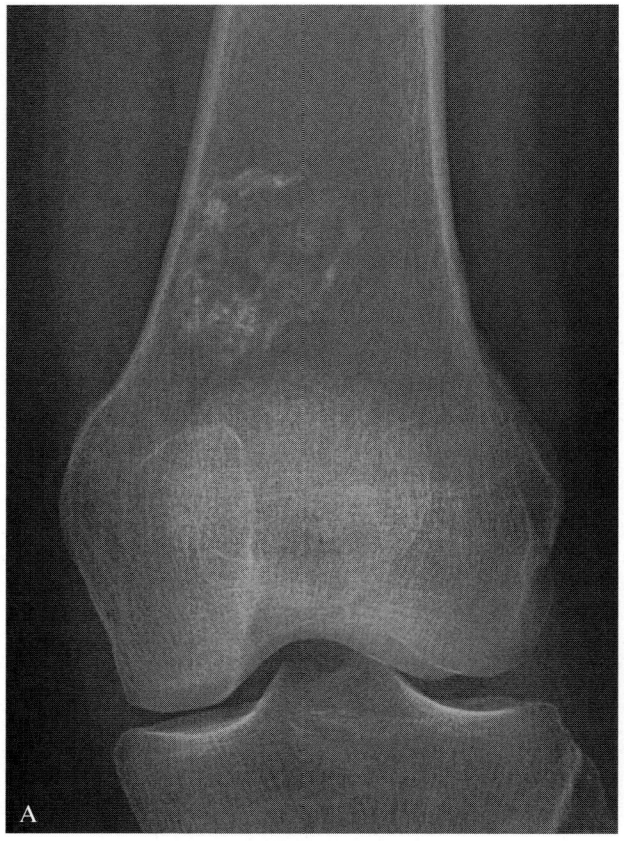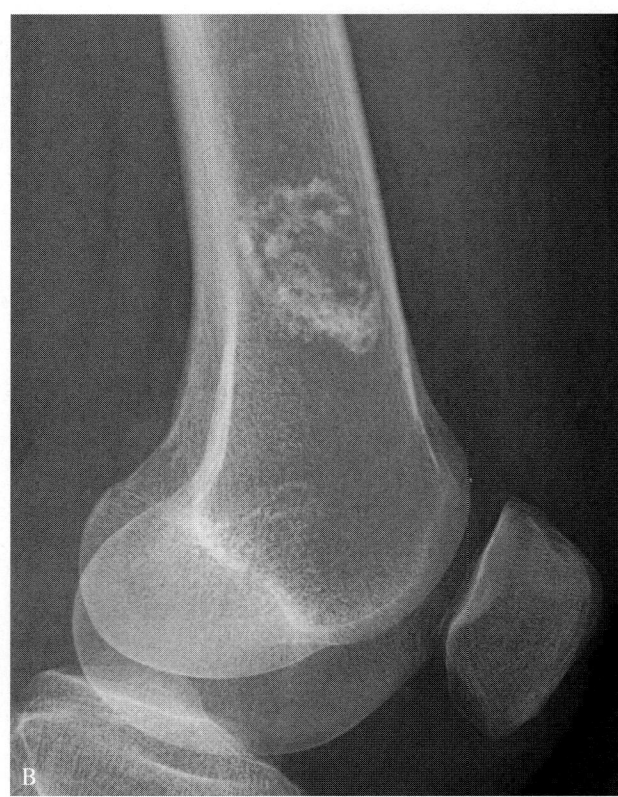

Figure 7 Benign enchondroma of the distal femur. A well-calcified tumor is seen with rings and arcs of flocculent calcification. The tumor is wholly contained within bone. There is no expansion or endosteal scalloping of bone.

enchondromas. In contrast, PET scans may distinguish low-grade cartilaginous lesions from intermediate/high-grade chondrosarcomas, which have significantly higher standardized uptake value (SUV) levels.[17] However, PET scans do not differentiate low-grade chondrosarcomas from enchondromas, which overlap in SUVs.

The staging of chondrosarcoma is problematic since three grades of chondrosarcomas are recognized. In the past, intermediate- and high-grade tumors have been grouped together as high-grade tumors.

Pathology

Chondrosarcomas are composed of aberrant chondrocytes forming chondroid matrix (Figure 10). There are often binucleate cells or multiple cells within a single lacunae, indicating an increased rate of proliferation. Most pathologists designate three grades of chondrosarcoma according to the criteria of Evans and collagues.[18] As the grade of the tumor increases, cellularity increases, and the amount of hyaline cartilage decreases. Myxoid changes often distinguish intermediate-grade tumors from low-grade lesions.

It must be emphasized that the presence of atypia in the chondrocytes is not sufficient to warrant a diagnosis of chondrosarcoma. Cartilage from osteochondromas, enchondromas, chondromas, and other cartilaginous lesions exhibit binucleated cells and other forms of atypia to varying degrees. The diagnosis of low-grade chondrosarcoma can be made only after all radiographic and clinical data are considered.

Treatment

The only curative treatment for intermediate- and high-grade tumors is wide en bloc surgical resection. Surgical margin is of paramount importance, since there is no effective chemotherapy or radiation. Usually, the best chance for cure is with the first operation. Recurrent tumors are much more difficult to eradicate. In unfavorable locations, such as the skull and spine, wide excision may be impossible, and proton beam or ion beam radiation may have a role in therapy.

The prognosis is strongly dependent on the grade. The rate of metastases has been reported to be 0%, 10%, and 71% for low, intermediate, and high-grade tumors,

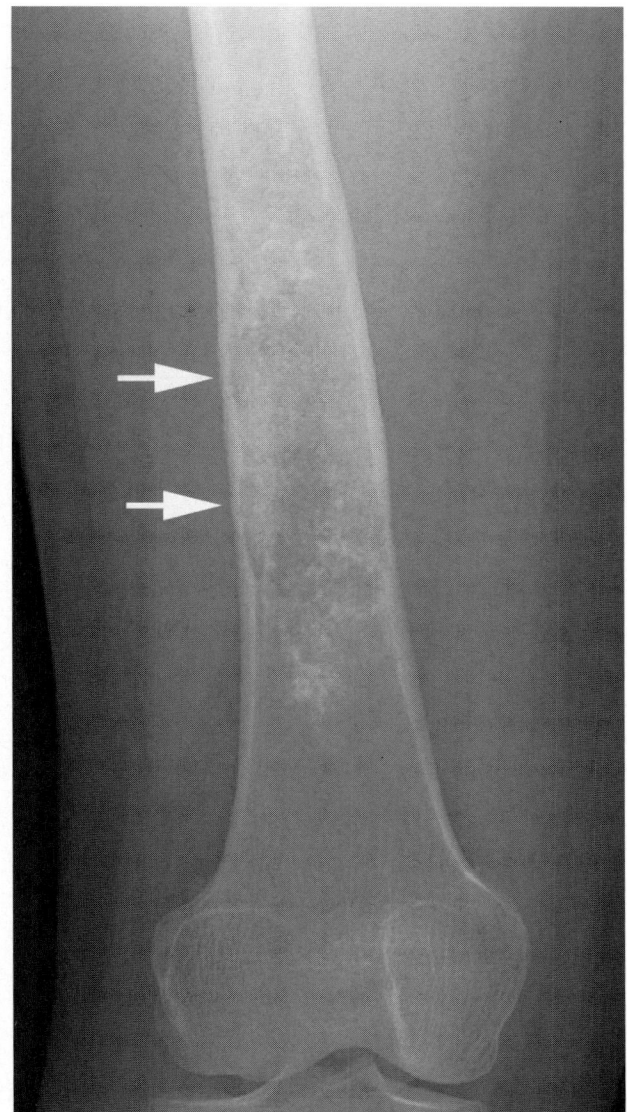

Figure 8 Active low-grade cartilaginous lesion. The x-ray shows endosteal scalloping (arrows) and slight expansion of bone. The typical calcification of cartilage tumors is present. The lesion occupies an extensive portion of the femoral shaft. The PET scan (not shown) demonstrated mild tracer activity with an SUV level of 1.3. The final pathology report indicated the presence of atypical chondrocytes, but a clear diagnosis of grade 1 chondrosarcoma was not made. Some clinicians in the past have called this type of lesion "grade 1/2 chondrosarcoma."

respectively.[18] Patients should be followed for a minimum of 10 years, since local recurrence and metastasis tend to occur late for the more indolent tumors.

The treatment of low-grade chondrosarcomas is problematic. It is not wise to generalize for all sites and patients. En bloc resection entails significant morbidity, and it is not justified for all of these tumors. On the other hand, intralesional treatment (ie, curettage) is not always appropriate. In particular, it is not wise to treat low-grade chondrosarcomas of the pelvis with curettage. These can be very problematic if they recur in the pelvis, and should be treated primarily with wide resection.

In the long bones, small- to intermediate-sized low-grade chondrosarcomas may be suitable for curettage. The surgery should be performed meticulously with minimal contamination of muscle compartments, so that subsequent limb salvage can be performed if the tumor should recur. Preliminary reports suggest that with proper patient selection, the rate of relapse is low. In a study from Scandinavia, the rate of local recurrence was 9% and metastasis 0%.[19]

CHONDROSARCOMA VARIANTS

Clear-cell chondrosarcoma

Clear-cell chondrosarcoma is an exceptionally rare but distinctive tumor that arises in the epiphysis of bones. As the name suggests, the tumor is composed of cells with clear cytoplasm and prominent borders. Some resemblance to chondroblastoma may be present. The tumors are considered low- to intermediate-grade, and the prognosis is favorable. Most patients are cured with wide resection of the tumor.

Dedifferentiated Chondrosarcoma

In rare cases, a low-grade tumor can dedifferentiate into a high-grade sarcoma. For this diagnosis to be made, there must be a low-grade tumor directly adjacent to a high-grade tumor. Most commonly, this is osteosarcoma, but it can also be rhabdomyosarcoma, fibrosarcoma, or malignant fibrous histiocytoma. It is quite possible that the small cell variant known as "mesenchymal chondrosarcoma" represents a form of dedifferentiated chondrosarcoma.

The prognosis for dedifferentiated chondrosarcoma has historically been poor. In 1 study, patients treated by amputation all had metastasis by 12 months, and the median survival was just 6 months.[20] Initially, chemotherapy and radiation were reported to be not effective for the disease. The recent experience with chemotherapy has been more favorable. Patients with localized disease who were treated with preoperative doxorubicin and intra-arterial cisplatin, using osteosarcoma-based protocols, achieved a 5-year continuous relapse-free survival of 51%.[21]

Secondary chondrosarcomas

Secondary chondrosarcomas occur in the setting of a pre-existing lesion such as Ollier's disease (multiple

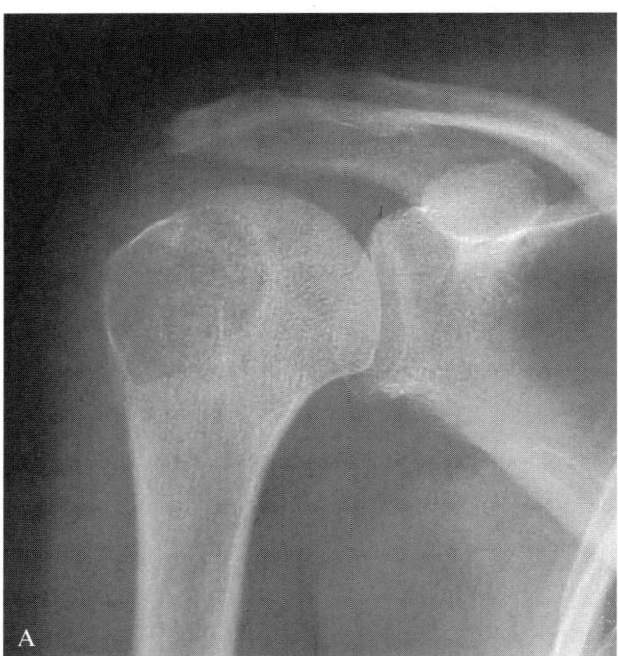
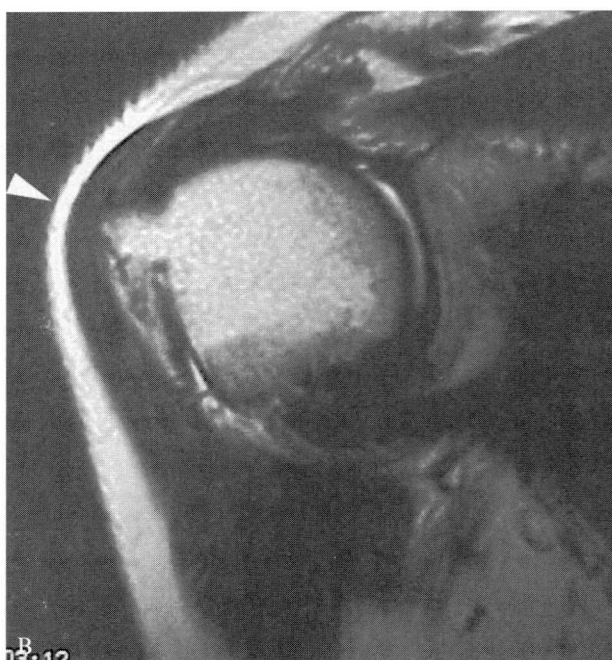

Figure 9 Low grade chondrosarcoma of the proximal humerus. *A,* In contrast to the enchondroma, a lytic, destructive lesion is visible on plain x-ray. Flocculent calcification within the tumor, which is present in enchondromas, is notably absent. (*B*) Coronal MRI scan reveals a small region of cortical perforation and invasion beyond bone (arrow). This is considered evidence for aggressive, malignant potential. The patient was treated with wide resection of the proximal humerus.

enchondromatosis) and hereditary multiple exostoses. Most tumors are low to intermediate grade, with a greater propensity for local recurrence rather than distant metastasis. The prognosis is generally good after wide en bloc resection.

Diagnosis of secondary chondrosarcoma can be difficult histologically. The presence of atypical chondrocytes does not necessarily establish the diagnosis. The best criterion is sudden growth of a lesion. For osteochondromas, this manifests as an increase in the size of the cartilaginous "cap." One cm has arbitrarily been assigned as the limit of normal. Gadolinium-enhanced MRI scans can help distinguish the true cap from the bursa that invariably forms around the lesion.

Ewing's Sarcoma

Ewing's sarcoma is a curious anomaly in the group of bone sarcomas. Ewing's sarcoma is composed of undifferentiated small round blue cells, and there are no clues as to its origin. Other sarcomas, in distinction, recapitulate some type of connective tissue, such as bone or cartilage. It may be relevant to ask whether Ewing's sarcoma is truly a sarcoma, but until its pathogenesis is elucidated, it will continue to be considered a sarcoma of bone.

CLINICAL PRESENTATION

Ewing's sarcoma is not as common as osteosarcoma, but in the pediatric population, the incidence approaches that of osteosarcoma. There is a sharp peak age in the second decade. Cases in the elderly are quite rare but have been documented by molecular tests. The disease has some distinct racial patterns. People of northern European descent are more at risk. In the oriental countries, Ewing's sarcoma is very rare. The disease is more prevalent in African-Americans than native Africans.

Unlike osteosarcoma, which clusters around the knee, Ewing's sarcoma is more widely dispersed, and every bone can be affected. Ewing's sarcoma has a predilection for the shaft of long bones, but it also affects flat bones, such as the pelvis and scapula. Most clinicians do not appreciate the fact that a pediatric patient who presents with a large pelvic tumor very likely has Ewing's sarcoma.

ETIOLOGY

The key genetic aberration is a reciprocal t(11;22) translocation, which results in a fusion gene *EWS-FLI1*. The protein is a modified transcription factor. The C-terminal end of the gene contains the DNA-binding portion of *FLI1* while the N-terminal region is replaced by EWS. *EWS-FLI1* is present in approximately 95% of

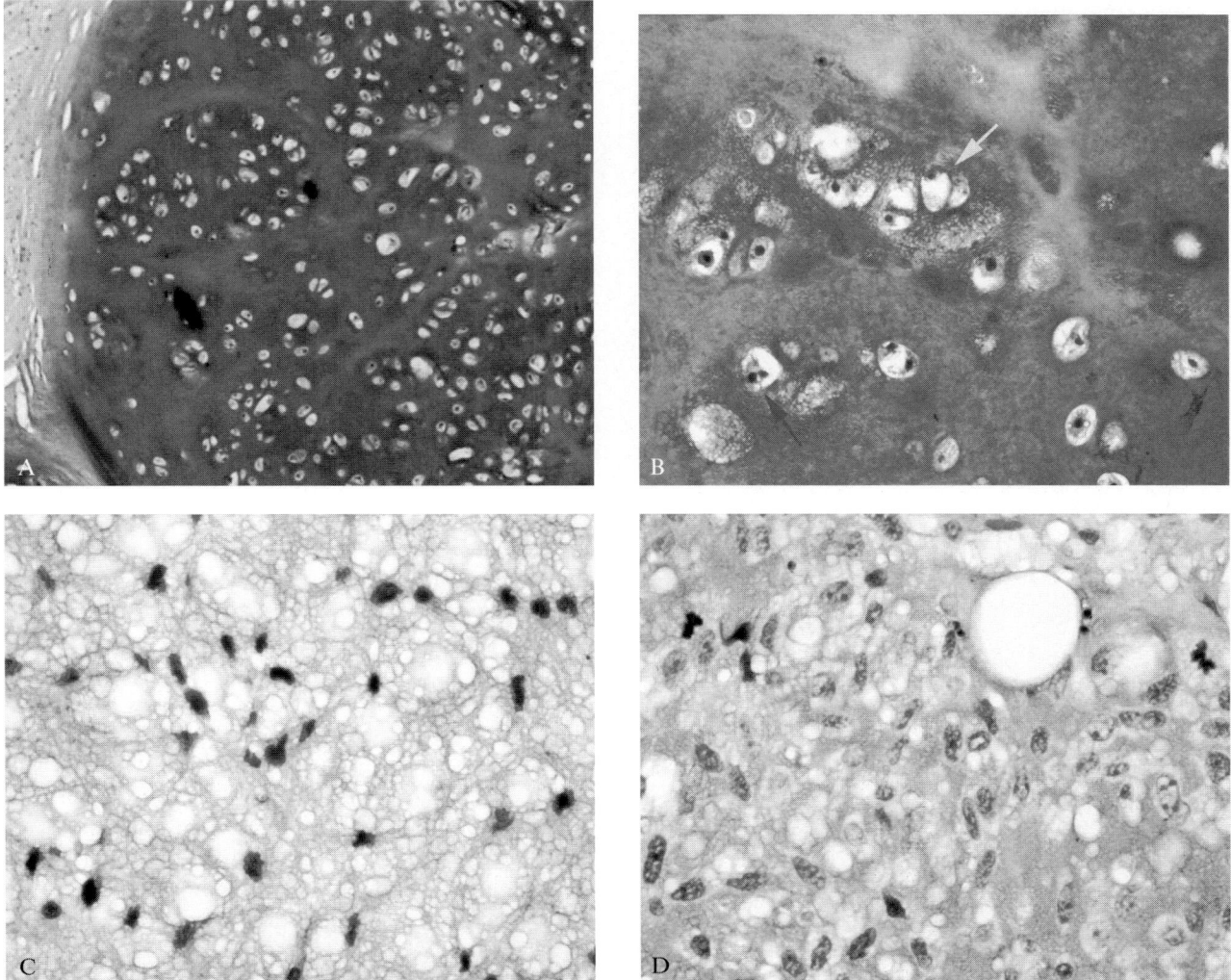

Figure 10 Histopathology of chondrosarcoma. Light microscopy demonstrates increasing cellularity and atypia with grade. *A*, Grade 1 chondrosarcoma under low power shows retention of the lobular nature of the tissue. *B*, Grade 1 chondrosarcoma under high power is notable for abundant hyaline cartilage matrix that stains deeply blue. A few binucleated cells (red arrow) and clusters of multiple nuclei (yellow arrow) are present, but overall there is a paucity of cells. *C*, Grade 2 chondrosarcoma. The extracellular matrix has taken on a looser and more myxoid appearance, with less intense staining. The cells are more abundant and no longer clearly occupying lacunae. *D*, Grade 3 chondrosarcoma. The tumor is clearly more hypercellular. The cells are becoming more spindle shaped and pleomorphic.

cases. In the remaining cases, alternative translocations are present, such as the t(21;22) translocation that produces EWS-ERG. ERG, notably, is identical to *FLI1* in its C-terminal end.

The presence of *EWS-FLI1* has now defined a group of similar small round blue cell tumors, including Askin's tumor of the chest wall, peripheral neuroepithelioma, and primitive neuroectodermal tumor (PNET) of soft tissue. These tumors share many features, including histology and response to therapy.

DIAGNOSIS AND STAGING

Diagnosis of Ewing's sarcoma can be difficult sometimes, and it has the capacity to masquerade as other diseases. The plain radiograph is often the first clue to the disorder. In classic cases, the tumor produces a permeative, lytic lesion in the shaft of a long bone. Some form of periosteal reaction, such as Codman's triangle, is almost invariably present, but onionskin formation is actually not a frequent finding (Figure 11).

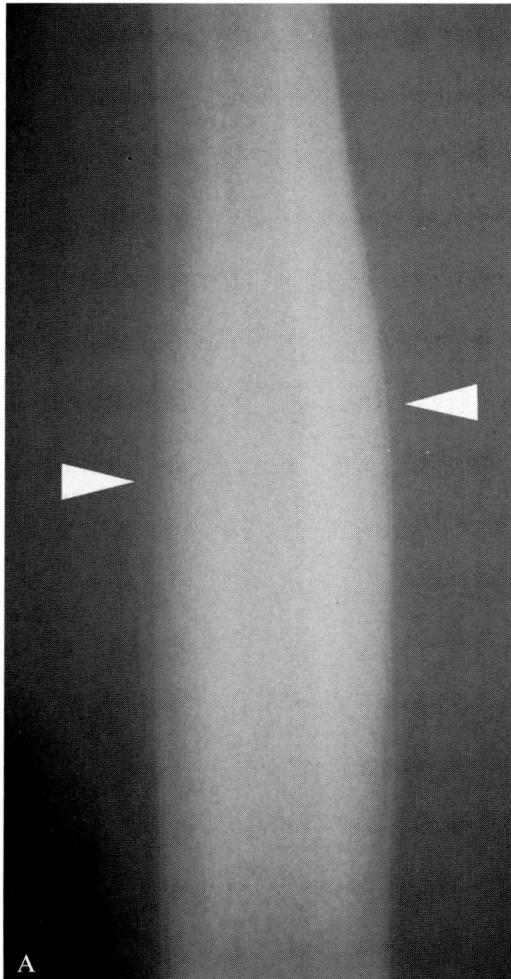

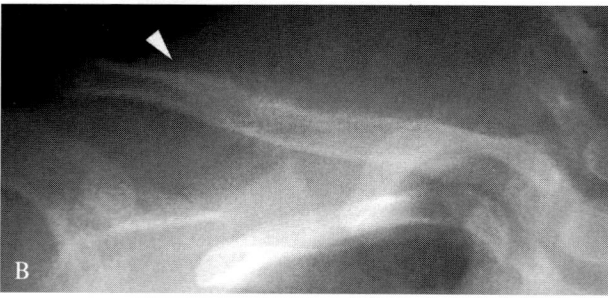

Figure 11 Ewing's sarcoma. Periosteal reaction is the most common radiographic finding on plain x-ray, but contrary to popular belief, it usually does not take the form of onion skin. There are a many ways in which periosteal reaction is manifested, and the clinician must be sensitive to the presence of these findings. *A*, When the extraosseous tumor mass is scant, there may be only a single lamella of periosteal bone formation, which can be quite subtle (arrows). *B*, A sunburst pattern (or "hair on end") is visible, together with a Codman's triangle (arrow) in this case of Ewing's sarcoma involving the clavicle.

Cross-sectional imaging can reveal a large soft tissue mass, which is often invisible on plain x-rays. This tends to be true in flat bones such as the pelvis and scapula, which are favored sites of the disease (Figure 12). A large soft tissue mass is not always present, and an alternative pattern of presentation is permeative growth through the medullary canal of a long bone. This is usually recognized only on MRI scans with coronal or sagittal views of the whole bone.

In a small percentage of cases, Ewing's sarcoma can be present in the bone marrow at multiple sites. Bone scans are relatively insensitive at detecting this mode of spread. PET scans may be somewhat more sensitive at detecting bone disease, but its limit of sensitivity may not yet be sufficient. Iliac crest bone marrow biopsy should be done as part of the staging work-up.

PATHOLOGY

Sheets of uniform small round blue cells characterize the tumor (Figure 13). Mitotic figures are present but not prominent. Genetic tests to detect the presence of *EWS-FLI1* help distinguish the tumor from other malignancies. The tests include RT-PCR, cytogenetics, and FISH. The difficulty with the tests is that variants of the fusion gene exist. The fusion point between *EWS* and *FLI1* usually occurs between exon 7 of *EWS* and exon 6 of *FLI1* (type I fusion), but this is present in only about 60% of cases. Alternative fusion points between *EWS* and *FLI1* or other genes are present in the remaining cases. Therefore, a battery of primers is generally needed to screen for *EWS-FLI1* by RT-PCR.

Immunohistochemistry with monoclonal antibody O13 to detect the CD99 antigen was initially thought to be specific for Ewing's sarcoma, but it has become evident that the antibody can stain lymphomas and other tumors to varying degrees. The antibody is still widely used, but it cannot be relied on exclusively to establish the diagnosis.

TREATMENT

Treatment of Ewing's sarcoma consists of systemic therapy, in the form of high-dose chemotherapy, and local therapy, which could involve surgery and/or radiation. While chemotherapy is of unquestionable necessity, controversy exists over the relative roles of surgery and radiation.

Chemotherapy

Many different protocols have been reported, but most are variants of the VACA regimen (vincristine, doxorubicin [Adriamycin], cyclophosphamide, and dactinomycin). Ifosfamide and etoposide have been recognized

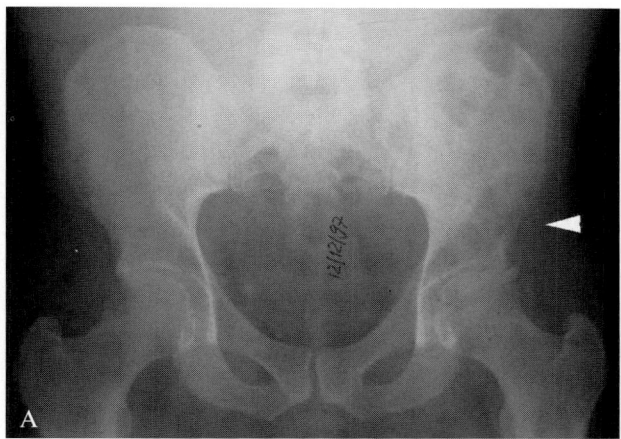
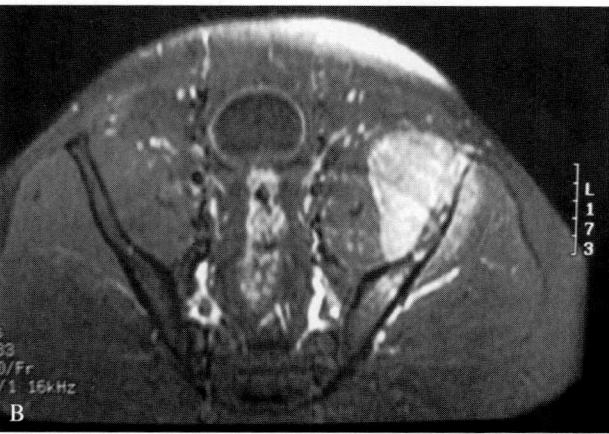

Figure 12 Ewing's sarcoma of the pelvis is a favored location, which is not a widely appreciated fact. *A*, The findings can be easily overlooked on the plain x-ray. An ill-defined, destructive lesion can be seen in the left supra-acetabular region (arrow). *B*, The findings on plain x-ray often belie the large extraosseous mass that is frequently associated with Ewing's sarcoma of flat bones. The MRI scan demonstrates the intrapelvic tumor. This goes unnoticed by the patient and may reach enormous size.

as important therapeutic agents in recent years. In the large CCG/POG trial, patients who received ifosfamide and etoposide in addition to VACA were found to have better 5-year event-free survival (69% vs 54%).[22] In the German CESS-86 trial, chemotherapy for high-risk patients involved substitution of ifosfamide for cyclophosphamide (VAIA vs VACA). This resulted in nearly identical 10-year survival of the high-risk and standard-risk patients.[23]

The trend during recent years has been toward dose intensification, particularly for patients with worse

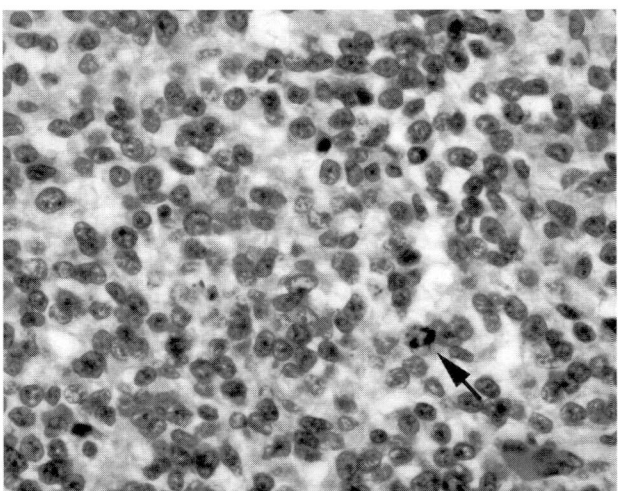

Figure 13 Ewing's sarcoma. Light microscopy reveals sheets of fairly uniform round cells with prominent blue nuclei and scant cytoplasm. There is little if any extracellular matrix. The cytoplasmic borders are indistinct. Mitotic figures (black arrow) are not difficult to find.

prognostic factors. In the IESS-II trial, VACA was administered on either an intermittent high-dose regimen or a moderate continuous dose. Patients with central disease who were placed on the high-dose arm had superior 5-year survival rates compared with conventional dose.[24]

Similar to osteosarcoma, the 5-year survival rates have been in the range of 60 to 70% for most large studies. A significant subset of patients still fares poorly and develops metastases. Myeloablative chemotherapy with stem cell bone marrow rescue transplant has been attempted for patients who relapse, but the experience thus far has been disappointing.[25] Other therapies including whole-lung radiation and surgical resection of metastases have also had only limited success. It is clear that newer agents are needed to treat these patients.

Surgical Treatment

The optimal form of local treatment is a controversial issue. In recent years, there has been a growing preference toward surgery as opposed to radiation.[26] Although no randomized study has been done to date, the available evidence seems to favor surgery, which has lower local relapse rates.

As surgical reconstructive techniques have improved, there are few bones left that cannot be considered expendable. For most sites, such as the femur, tibia, and humerus, a number of different options with endoprostheses and allografts exist (Figure 14). In the long bones, it is important to recognize that the disease can affect a long portion of the shaft of the bone. The preoperative MRI study is important to review carefully to ascertain how far the disease might go. This is

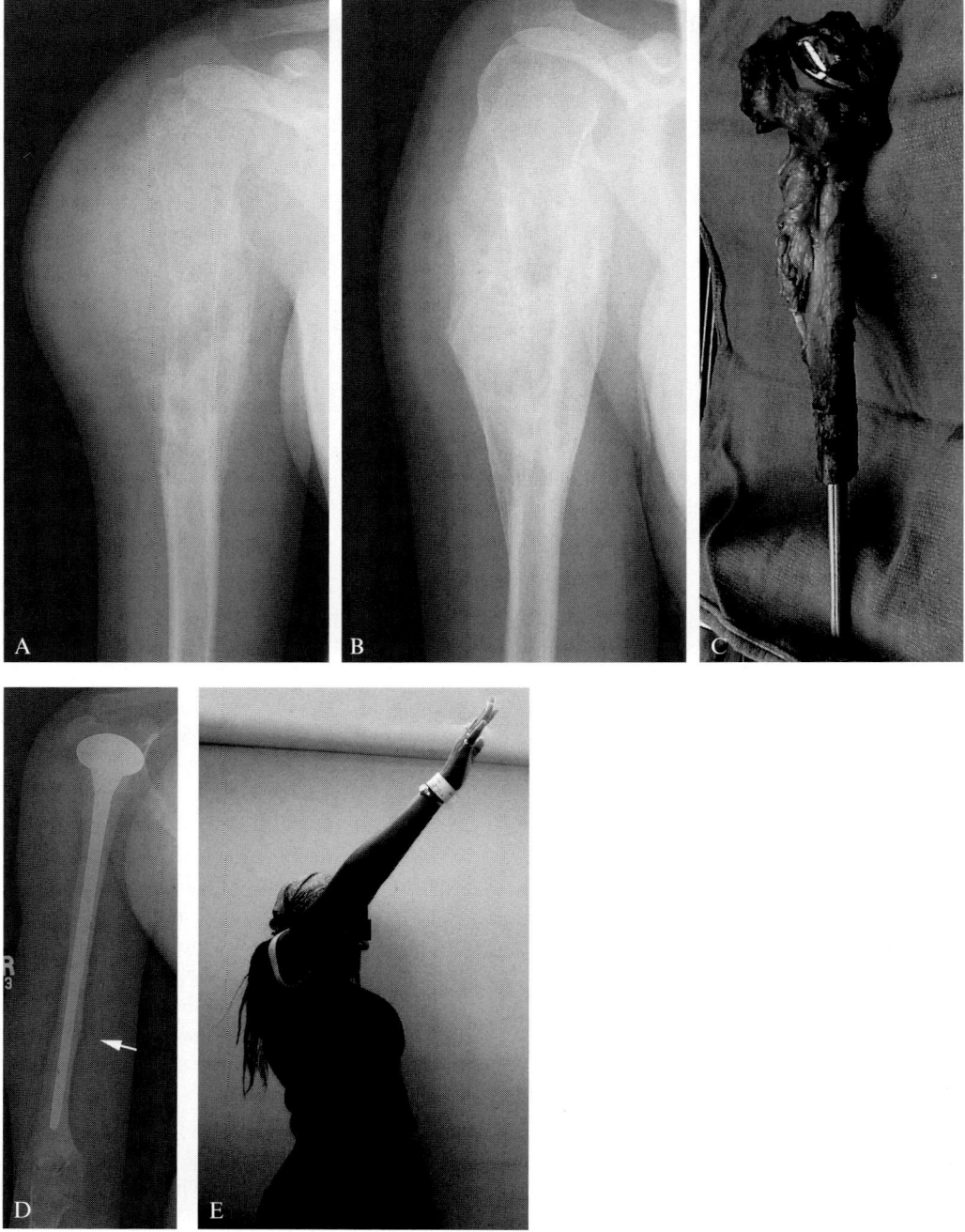

Figure 14 Ewing's sarcoma of the proximal humerus in a 16-year-old girl. *A*, On presentation, the plain x-ray shows typical findings, including involvement of a long portion of the humeral shaft, a large soft tissue mass, and periosteal reaction in the form of onion-skin formation. *B*, After induction chemotherapy, the soft tissue mass has completely ossified, and the periosteal bone formation has matured. This is a favorable sign, suggesting an excellent response to chemotherapy. Notice that the size of the tumor has not appreciably diminished. Unlike the experience with other solid tumors in oncology, reduction of tumor size cannot be used to gauge whether a response to chemotherapy has occurred in sarcomas of bone. Histological mapping subsequently showed 100% tumor necrosis. *C*, Reconstruction for the massive resection was performed with an allograft-prosthesis composite (APC), which is prepared on the back table during surgery. The advantage of the allograft, ironically, is not so much that it replaces bone as that it provides tendons and joint capsules for soft tissue reconstruction. Restoration of shoulder function after proximal humeral resection is extremely difficult to achieve, and the results with artificial metallic prostheses have been poor. *D*, Postoperative x-ray after 2 years shows healing of the osteotomy (arrow). Note the long resection length, which is frequently necessary in Ewing's sarcoma, which tends to percolate down the intramedullary canal. *E*, The patient has regained most, but not all, of forward flexion at the shoulder. This is considered a marked improvement over metallic prostheses for the proximal humerus, which do not enable patients to lift the arm to 90°.

sometimes very difficult to discern because of the frequent use of medications that stimulate bone marrow and cause marrow conversion phenomenon.

For more difficult nonextremity sites, including the pelvis and spine, en bloc resection is possible, but there may be considerable morbidity. For example, en bloc resection of the sacrum may necessitate sacrifice of sacral nerve roots, which would impact on bowel, bladder, and sexual function. Thus, surgery is not always selected for the difficult, central locations.

In the pelvis, allograft resection is associated with a high wound and infection rate. These complications are oncologically detrimental since they may prevent resumption of chemotherapy in a timely fashion. In situations where a patient would benefit from a pelvic reconstruction, it may be prudent to delay surgical treatment until all of the intended chemotherapy has been delivered.

Radiation Treatment

Historically, radiation has occupied an important role in treatment. It was recognized by James Ewing himself that many cases were exquisitely sensitive to radiation. He is credited for pioneering the use of radiation, and this was the first widely accepted treatment for the disease.

The primary advantage of radiation is that it is noninvasive, and no normal anatomic structure has to be removed. This is not an insignificant consideration for the pediatric patient facing ablation of articular cartilage, growth plates, and muscles. Joint replacement in the young patient, whether by endoprosthesis or allograft, does not allow for all of the strenuous activities and athletics that children normally participate in.

There are a number of disadvantages to radiation, including joint contractures, growth retardation, fibrosis, radiation osteitis, and pathologic fractures. Many of these complications are more pronounced with older, less sophisticated methods of delivering radiation, and modern techniques can minimize the side effects.

A serious concern regarding radiation is the potential for secondary malignancies. It is estimated that at 20 years, the risk may be as high as 8 to 9%.[27] Osteosarcomas are the most common secondary malignancies, but other sarcomas and leukemias can also occur. Patients who receive 60 Gy or more appear to be at especially high risk, and current recommendations are for doses of 55 Gy or less.

Local recurrence is another major concern. Early studies such as IESS reported local control rates of 60 to 90%. The reason for the variability in the results was not clear, but may have involved differences in radiation technique. Although it was hoped that advances in radiation oncology would improve results, more recent studies have continued to demonstrate a substantial rate of local relapse in the range of 20 to 25%.[28,29] It should be pointed out that there might be an inherent bias in most studies evaluating radiation. Patients who receive radiation often are the ones who have a worse prognosis, including those with metastatic disease, unresectable tumors, centrally located tumors, and poor response to chemotherapy.

The experience with the combination of surgery and radiation is limited. This is an aggressive form of treatment with a high complication rate, but it is possibly indicated for patients who are at high risk of local relapse, such as those with large, pelvic disease. In an early report from Memorial Sloan-Kettering Cancer Center, the relative risk of relapse was 3.9 for patients who were treated by surgery as opposed to surgery and radiation.[30]

Malignant Fibrous Histiocytoma (MFH)

There has been much confusion over the years regarding MFH and fibrosarcoma. In particular, the distinction between poorly differentiated, high-grade fibrosarcoma and MFH has been hazy at best. Many authorities now consider the terms synonymous. Well-differentiated fibrosarcoma, however, should be distinguished from MFH since these tumors are more indolent and have a good prognosis with surgical treatment alone.

MFH of bone appears to be different from MFH of soft tissue. Although the histological appearance is similar, MFH of bone responds favorably to osteosarcoma-based chemotherapy, whereas MFH of soft tissues tend to be more resistant to chemotherapy. Some clinicians view MFH of bone to be a variant of osteosarcoma. Supporting this notion are documented cases where the primary tumor was designated an MFH, but a subsequent metastasis demonstrated unequivocal osteosarcoma.

MFH of bone differs from osteosarcoma in that patients tend to be older. Indeed, about a third of the cases are secondary to pre-existing conditions, such as bone infarct, fibrous dysplasia, radiation, and Paget's disease. These cases of secondary MFH tend to have a much worse prognosis and do not respond well to chemotherapy, similar to the secondary osteosarcomas. It is important to separate this group of secondary MFH from the group of primary MFH in any analysis of treatment results.

Histologically, MFH is composed of pleomorphic, plump, sometimes foamy spindle cells that are arranged in storiform or cartwheel patterns. There is a conspicuous lack of osteoid formation. Well-differentiated fibrosarcoma, by contrast, tends to have more elongated, fibroblastic-like spindle cells that form a herringbone pattern. Radiographically, the tumor presents as a lytic lesion in bone lacking ossification and calcification (Figure 15).

Primary MFH of bone is treated with preoperative and postoperative chemotherapy, typically with the same protocols used for osteosarcoma. The published literature is sparse but encouraging. The European Osteosarcoma Intergroup reported a 5-year overall survival of 59%.[31]

Chordoma

Chordomas are very challenging tumors to treat, mainly as a result of their site of origin. They occur primarily in the sacrum, but also in the sphenoid and other spinal locations occasionally (Figure 16). The clinical presentation reflects the site of origin. In the sacrum, patients complain of low back pain, sciatica, fecal impaction, and impotence. In the sphenoid, patients often present with headaches, blurred vision, and diabetes insipidus. Most cases affect adults in mid- to later life, and males predominate by a 2:1 ratio.

The tumors bear some resemblance to primitive notochordal tissue. Histologically, they are characterized by the "physaliferous" cell, which has abundant foamy cytoplasm and resembles soap bubbles. Most chordomas are low-grade malignancies. The growth of the tumors is slow, and metastasis uncommon.

The long-term prognosis, in spite of the lack of metastases, is not good. With follow-up of 10 to 20 years, nearly all patients develop local relapse, and this ultimately proves fatal. Morbidity of treatment is high. Surgical resection often requires sacrifice of sacral nerve roots. If S2 and S3 can be preserved on one side, patients have a fair chance of retaining adequate bowel and bladder control.

The surgery is sometimes performed in two stages, particularly when the tumor arises from the S1 segment, which is adjacent to the bifurcation of the aorta and vena cava. In the first stage, anterior mobilization of vascular and other structures is performed. For large tumors, ligation of hypogastric vessels and a diverting colostomy may be necessary. Restoration of spinopelvic stability after a total sacrectomy is a formidable challenge. Instrumentation with spinopelvic rods is augmented by large allografts and vascularized bone transfers. The area is at high risk of wound complications and infection. Muscle flaps are sometimes necessary for adequate coverage.

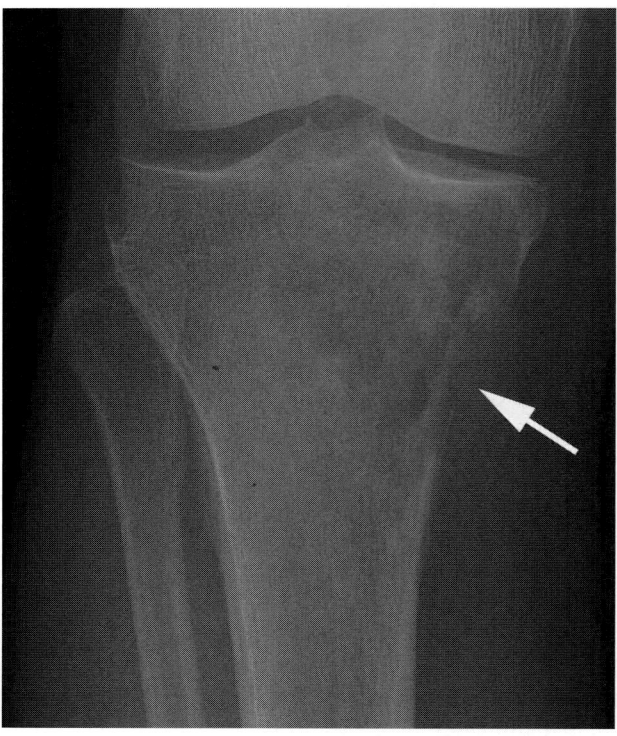

Figure 15 MFH of bone. X-ray of the proximal tibia shows a permeative, poorly delineated tumor (arrow) without the osteoblastic calcifications of osteosarcoma. The patient was 72 years old, which is typical for MFH of bone.

The tumors are not responsive to chemotherapy. Radiation therapy, however, may be helpful.[32] Proton beam or ion beam radiation has been found to be more

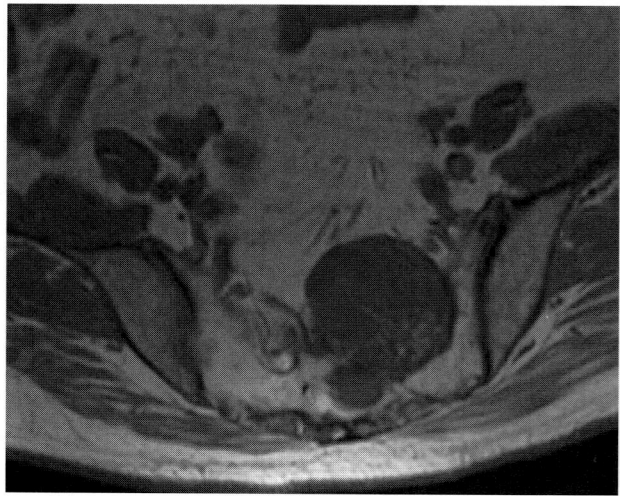

Figure 16 Sacral chordoma. An axial T1-weighted MRI image shows the mass growing out of S2 into the presacral recess.

effective than conventional external beam radiation, with 5-year control rates of 36 to 55%.[33]

Adamantinoma

Adamantinomas are peculiar, low-grade tumors that have a striking biphasic histological pattern. Keratin-positive staining is present in the epithelial-like component, which can take the form of rows of compact cuboidal cells or nests of tubular or alveolar cells. The majority of adamantinomas occur in the tibia. Among other bones affected, there seems to be an odd predilection for the ulna and fibula. The disease usually occurs in adulthood with a mild preference for males. On plain x-ray the tumor appears as a lytic or sometimes bubbly lesion (Figure 17). In up to 10% of cases, there may be a multifocal presentation. The tumors tend to be slow growing, and metastasis is infrequent. Treatment by wide surgical resection is often curative, and the prognosis is favorable, with 10-year survival estimated at 85 to 90%.[34] Metastasis in the lungs is potentially curable by pulmonary resection.

References

1. Enneking WF, Spanier SS, Goodman MA. A system for the surgical staging of musculoskeletal sarcoma. Clin Orthop 1980;153:106–20.

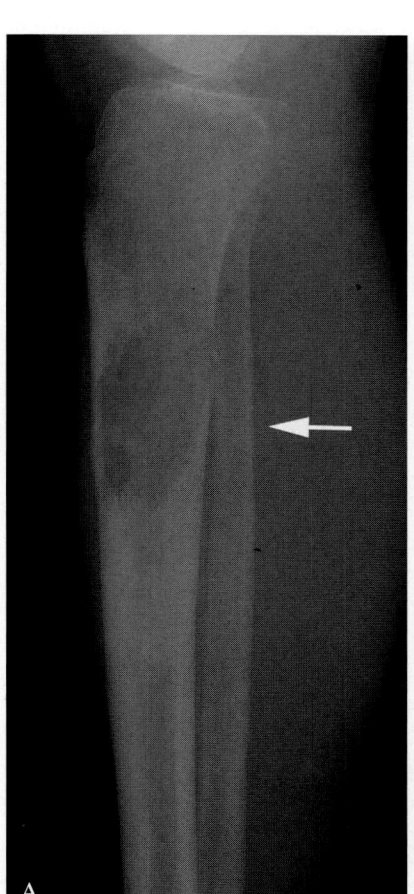
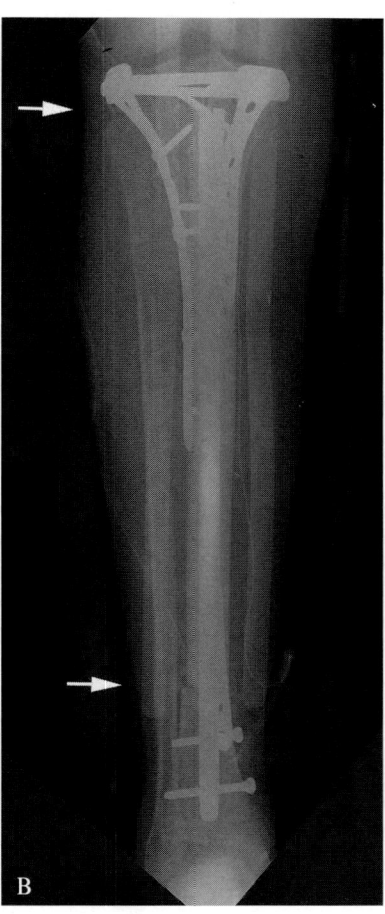
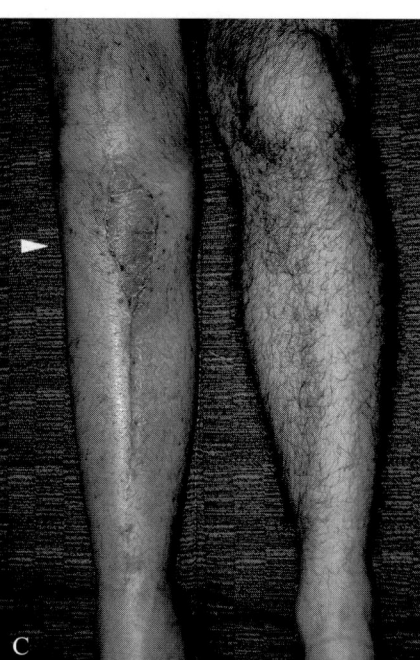

Figure 17 Adamantinoma. *A*, Lateral x-ray reveals a lytic lesion in the tibia of a 49-year-old man. *B*, After wide en bloc resection, the bone was reconstructed with an intercalary allograft. A long resection length was necessary because of intramedullary extension of tumor, and the osteotomies are indicated by arrows. The native knee joint was spared, which is one of the goals of limb-preserving surgery whenever feasible. The allograft was secured with a combination of an intramedullary nail and locking plates. *C*, As a routine part of tibial reconstructions for limb-sparing operations, a medial gastrocnemius flap is frequently needed. A split-thickness or full-thickness skin graft is placed over the exposed portion of the gastrocnemius flap. This provides good muscular coverage of the bone, which decreases the potential for infection. It also enables the wound to be closed without tension. Marked swelling of the calf routinely occurs with limb-sparing oncologic surgery, and this can threaten compartment syndrome or dehiscence of the wound.

2. Greene FL, Page DL, Fleming ID, et al. AJCC cancer staging manual. 6th ed. New York: Springer-Verlag; 2002.

3. Fleming ID, Cooper JS, Henson DE, Hutter RVP. AJCC cancer staging manual. 5th ed. Philadelphia: J.B. Lippincott; 1997.

4. Hoogerwerf WA, Hawkins AL, Perlman EJ, Griffin CA. Chromosome analysis of nine osteosarcomas. Genes Chromosomes Cancer 1994;9:88–92.

5. Ayala AG, Ro JY, Fanning CV, et al. Core needle biopsy and fine-needle aspiration in the diagnosis of bone and soft-tissue lesions. Hematol Oncol Clin North Am 1995;9:633–51.

6. Jaffe N, Knapp J, Chuang VP, et al. Osteosarcoma: intra-arterial treatment of the primary tumor with cis-diammine-dichloroplatinum II (CDP). Angiographic, pathologic, and pharmacologic studies. Cancer 1983;51:402–7.

7. Schwartzentruber DJ, Goorin AM, Gebhart MC, et al. Osteosarcoma: surgical results of POG 8651. Sarcoma 2000.

8. Huvos AG. Bone tumors. Philadelphia: W.B. Saunders; 1991.

9. Meyers PA, Heller G, Healey J, et al. Chemotherapy for nonmetastatic osteogenic sarcoma: the Memorial Sloan-Kettering experience. J Clin Oncol 1992;10:5–15.

10. Benjamin RS, Patel SR, Armen T, et al. The value of ifosfamide in postoperative neoadjuvant chemotherapy of osteosarcoma [Meeting abstract]. Proc Annu Meet Am Soc Clin Oncol 1995;14:A1690.

11. Meyers PA, Gorlick R, Heller G, et al. Intensification of preoperative chemotherapy for osteogenic sarcoma: results of the Memorial Sloan-Kettering (T12) protocol. J Clin Oncol 1998;16:2452–8.

12. Rougraff BT, Simon MA, Kneisl JS, et al. Limb salvage compared with amputation for osteosarcoma of the distal end of the femur. A long-term oncological, functional, and quality-of-life study. J Bone Joint Surg Am 1994;76:649–56.

13. Bacci G, Mercuri M, Briccoli A, et al. Osteogenic sarcoma of the extremity with detectable lung metastases at presentation. Results of treatment of 23 patients with chemotherapy followed by simultaneous resection of primary and metastatic lesions. Cancer 1997;79:245–54.

14. Okada K, Frassica FJ, Sim FH, et al. Parosteal osteosarcoma. A clinicopathological study. J Bone Joint Surg Am 1994;76:366–78.

15. Sheth DS, Yasko AW, Raymond AK, et al. Conventional and dedifferentiated parosteal osteosarcoma. Diagnosis, treatment, and outcome. Cancer 1996;78:2136–45.

16. Huvos AG. Osteogenic sarcoma of bones and soft tissues in older persons. A clinicopathologic analysis of 117 patients older than 60 years. Cancer 1986;57:1442–9.

17. Lee FY, Yu J, Chang SS, et al. Diagnostic value and limitations of fluorine-18 fluorodeoxyglucose positron emission tomography for cartilaginous tumors of bone. J Bone Joint Surg Am 2004;86-A:2677–85.

18. Evans HL, Ayala AG, Romsdahl MM. Prognostic factors in chondrosarcoma of bone: a clinicopathologic analysis with emphasis on histologic grading. Cancer 1977;40:818–31.

19. Bauer HC, Brosjo O, Kreicbergs A, Lindholm J. Low risk of recurrence of enchondroma and low-grade chondrosarcoma in extremities. 80 patients followed for 2–25 years. Acta Orthop Scand 1995;66:283–8.

20. Johnson S, Tetu B, Ayala AG, Chawla SP. Chondrosarcoma with additional mesenchymal component (dedifferentiated chondrosarcoma). I. A clinicopathologic study of 26 cases. Cancer 1986;58:278–86.

21. Benjamin RS, Chu P, Patel SR, et al. Dedifferentiated chondrosarcoma: a treatable disease [Meeting abstract]. Proc Annu Meet Am Assoc Cancer Res 1995;36:A1450.

22. Grier HE, Krailo MD, Tarbell NJ, et al. Addition of ifosfamide and etoposide to standard chemotherapy for Ewing's sarcoma and primitive neuroectodermal tumor of bone. N Engl J Med 2003;348:694–701.

23. Paulussen M, Ahrens S, Dunst J, et al. Localized Ewing tumor of bone: final results of the cooperative Ewing's Sarcoma Study CESS 86. J Clin Oncol 2001;19:1818–29.

24. Evans RG, Nesbit ME, Gehan EA, et al. Multimodal therapy for the management of localized Ewing's sarcoma of pelvic and sacral bones: a report from the second intergroup study. J Clin Oncol 1991;9:1173–80.

25. Pinkerton CR, Bataillard A, Guillo S, et al. Treatment strategies for metastatic Ewing's sarcoma. Eur J Cancer 2001;37:1338–44.

26. Ozaki T, Hillmann A, Hoffmann C, et al. Significance of surgical margin on the prognosis of patients with Ewing's sarcoma. A report from the Cooperative Ewing's Sarcoma Study. Cancer 1996;78:892–900.

27. Kuttesch JF Jr, Wexler LH, Marcus RB, et al. Second malignancies after Ewing's sarcoma: radiation dose-dependency of secondary sarcomas. J Clin Oncol 1996;14:2818–25.

28. Jurgens H, Exner U, Gadner H, et al. Multidisciplinary treatment of primary Ewing's sarcoma of bone. A 6-year experience of a European Cooperative Trial. Cancer 1988;61:23–32.

29. Donaldson S, Shuster J, Andreozzi C. The Pediatric Oncology Group (POG) experience in Ewing's sarcoma of bone. Med Pediatr Oncol 1989;17:283.

30. Wunder JS, Paulian G, Huvos AG, et al. The histological response to chemotherapy as a predictor of the oncological outcome of operative treatment of Ewing sarcoma. J Bone Joint Surg Am 1998;80:1020–33.

31. Bramwell VH, Steward WP, Nooij M, et al. Neoadjuvant chemotherapy with doxorubicin and cisplatin in

malignant fibrous histiocytoma of bone: a European Osteosarcoma Intergroup study. J Clin Oncol 1999;17: 3260–9.

32. Samson IR, Springfield DS, Suit HD, Mankin HJ. Operative treatment of sacrococcygeal chordoma. A review of twenty-one cases. J Bone Joint Surg Am 1993;75:1476–84.

33. Nowakowski VA, Castro JR, Petti PL, et al. Charged particle radiotherapy of paraspinal tumors. Int J Radiat Oncol Biol Phys 1992;22:295–303.

34. Qureshi AA, Shott S, Mallin BA, Gitelis S. Current trends in the management of adamantinoma of long bones. An international study. J Bone Joint Surg Am 2000;82-A:1122–31.

CHAPTER 66

EPIDEMIOLOGY OF SARCOMA

CHANDRAJIT P. RAUT, MD, MSc

Epidemiology

Sarcomas are rare tumors that account for less than 5% of adult malignancies and less than 20% of pediatric neoplasms in the United States.[1] Unlike carcinomas, which are derived from endodermal germ layers, soft tissue and bone sarcomas are derived from mesoderm and ectoderm.[1] They do not generally arise from the degeneration or dedifferentiation of benign soft tissue tumors. Despite different cells of origin and the various histologic subtypes recognized, the clinical behavior of most sarcomas is similar. Staging is dependent on tumor size, histological grade, and anatomic depth rather than specific histology. Lymph node metastases are rare, generally associated with a few histologic subtypes, such as epithelioid sarcoma, synovial sarcoma, rhabdomyosarcoma, clear-cell sarcoma, and angiosarcoma.[2]

The true incidence of soft tissue sarcomas is unknown, in part because sarcomas arising in parenchymal organs are often attributed to those organs rather than to soft tissue. Data from the Surveillance, Epidemiology, and End Results (SEER) program of the National Cancer Institute show average annual age-adjusted incidence rates (per 100,000) for sarcoma of 11.15 for white men, 4.53 for white women, 10.73 for African-American men, and 6.43 for African-American women based on cases identified by histology codes between 1986 and 1990.[2] However, approximately half of the cases in white and African-American men were Kaposi's sarcoma. Data from the Connecticut Tumor Registry and from Canada demonstrate a rising incidence of sarcoma, though much of the increase is due to the dramatic rise in cases of Kaposi's sarcoma in the 1980s.[2,3] Geographic variation may exist, with high rates reported among New Zealand Maoris and low rates among Japanese, though the difficulty in accurately classifying sarcomas may account for some of these differences.[2] A discussion of Kaposi's sarcoma is beyond the scope of this chapter.

Risk Factors

Most sarcomas have no clearly defined etiology, but multiple risk factors and genetic abnormalities have been identified. Genetic abnormalities will be discussed in the following chapter. Recognized risk factors for the development of soft tissue and bone tumors are listed in Table 1.

RADIATION

Exposure to radiation was first described as being associated with the development of soft tissue and bone sarcoma in 1922.[4] In a 1992 review of 160 patients from Memorial Sloan-Kettering Cancer Center, breast cancer (26%), lymphoma (25%), and cervical cancer (14%) treated with radiation were the most common antecedent diseases.[5] In this study, 99% of the patients received external beam radiation therapy, and 14% of them also received additional treatment with temporary or permanent radioisotope implantation. Subsequent sarcomas identified as a second malignancy included osteosarcoma (21%), malignant fibrous histiocytoma (16%), angiosarcoma/lymphangiosarcoma (15%), spindle-cell neoplasm not otherwise classified (10%), fibrosarcoma (7%), liposarcoma (6%), leiomyosarcoma (5%), chondrosarcoma (4%), and desmoids (4%). These patients had an 8-fold to 50-fold increase in the incidence of sarcomas.[2]

The risk of developing sarcoma correlates with the dose of radiation administered. In patients with childhood cancers, the subsequent risk of soft tissue sarcoma is greater than 50-fold excess in those receiving over 50 Gy.[2] Median latency period to the development of sarcoma is 10 years.[6] Radiation-induced sarcomas have a particularly poor prognosis. In the Memorial Sloan-Kettering Cancer Center study, three factors were associated with an unfavorable prognosis on multivariate analysis: presentation with metastatic disease ($p = 0.017$), incomplete resection or no surgery ($p = 0.004$), and tumor size greater than or equal to 5 cm ($p = 0.007$).[5] Site of sarcoma, latency period, and amount

Table 1 Risk Factors for the Development of Soft Tissue and Bone Tumors

Risk Factors	Associated Sarcomas
External beam radiation therapy	Osteogenic sarcoma
	Malignant fibrous histiocytoma
	Angiosarcoma/ lymphangiosarcoma
	Spindle-cell neoplasms, not otherwise specified
	Fibrosarcoma
	Liposarcoma
	Leiomyosarcoma
	Chondrosarcoma
	Desmoid
Lymphedema	
Postmastectomy	Lymphangiosarcoma
Congenital/heritable	Lymphangiosarcoma
Filariasis	Lymphangiosarcoma
Chemicals	
Herbicides containing phenoxyacetic acid	Malignant fibrous histiocytoma
	Leiomyosarcoma
Wood preservatives containing chlorophenols	Various
Vinyl chloride, Thorotrast, arsenic	Hepatic angiosarcoma
Chemotherapy	Pediatric osteogenic sarcoma

of radiation received initially, and the presence or absence of chemotherapy were not significant prognostic factors.

The high prevalence of radiation therapy as a part of breast conservation therapy for the treatment of breast cancer has raised concerns of a potentially increased incidence of sarcomas in these breast cancer patients. A comprehensive review of 122,991 Swedish women with breast cancer treated between 1958 and 1992 identified 116 soft tissue sarcomas.[7] The 40 cases of angiosarcoma correlated with lymphedema and not radiation. The other 76 sarcomas correlated with radiation exposures in a dose-dependent manner.[7,8]

CHEMICAL EXPOSURES

Several studies have reported a relationship between chemical exposure to herbicides containing phenoxyacetic acids and wood preservatives containing chlorophenol and soft tissue sarcomas in agricultural and manufacturing workers. Exposure to these agents was associated with a 6-fold increased risk of soft tissue sarcoma in 2 case-control studies of Swedish agricultural and forestry workers.[9,10] In a study of 251 US cases of sarcoma from 1984 to 1988, exposure to chlorophenol and cutting oil was associated with an increased risk of malignant fibrous histiocytoma and leiomyosarcoma.[11] These data suggest that risk factors may be specific for certain sarcoma subtypes. Similarly, farmers and agricultural

workers in Italy, Britain, and Denmark have a greater risk of soft tissue tumors.[12–14] However, such relationships have not been confirmed in other studies from the United States, New Zealand, and Finland, potentially reflecting differences in specific herbicides used and in accurate assessment of exposure.[15–17] Thus, the overall risk of exposure to these agents remains uncertain.

The potential role of dioxin exposure in the etiology of sarcomas also remains controversial, given the contradictory results in various studies.[18] A US study of over 5,000 manufacturing workers showed a 3-fold increased risk of sarcoma with a 20-year latency period.[19] The risk increased to 9-fold with greater than a 1-year exposure. A multinational study of 19,000 workers demonstrated a 6-fold increased risk 10 to 19 years after exposure.[20] Other studies have failed to demonstrate an increased risk. Nevertheless, the US Environmental Protection Agency's Scientific Advisory Board has classified dioxins as "probably carcinogenic," in part owing to the increased risk of sarcomas in dioxin-exposed workers.[21]

The population around Seveso, Italy reported a 3-fold increased risk of sarcomas after an explosion at a chemical factory in 1976.[22] Although surveys of Vietnam veterans have suggested an excess of soft tissue sarcomas, proportional mortality and case-control studies have not confirmed this.[23] The subset of veterans exposed to the herbicide mixture Agent Orange have also shown no increased risk of sarcoma.

Vinyl chloride exposure (during polyvinyl chloride plastics manufacturing), Thorotrast (colloidal thorium dioxide), and inorganic arsenic are associated with a risk of hepatic angiosarcoma.[24–26] In fact, 22% of the 168 deaths in the United States from hepatic angiosarcoma between 1964 and 1974 were attributable to one of these three agents.[27] The risk of liver tumors (both angiosarcomas and carcinomas) is related to the dose of the alpha-emitting radioisotope Thorotrast delivered to the hepatic parenchyma, with a cumulative risk of 30% at 40 years in those receiving over 20 mL.[28] Sarcomas have also developed along the sites of Thorotrast deposits at injection sites.[28]

Employment in an abattoir was associated with an increased risk of soft tissue sarcoma and hematologic malignancies in two New Zealand case-control studies, potentially through exposure to chemicals used in the treatment of meats and pelts.[29]

Chemotherapy for malignancies has been associated with the development of bone but not soft tissue sarcomas in the pediatric population.[30] The risks from specific chemotherapeutic agents have not been elucidated.

OTHER RISK FACTORS

Lymphedema is a well-described risk factor for the development of sarcomas. Congenital or heritable lymphedema is associated with lymphangiosarcoma, generally of the lower extremities. Lymphedema after mastectomy with axillary dissection and radiation may result in the development of lymphangiosarcoma, an association first described by Stewart and Treves (Stewart-Treves syndrome).[31] Unlike the radiation-induced sarcomas, which are confined to the radiation field, those resulting from lymphedema may develop both within and beyond the field of radiation. Lymphangiosarcoma of the lower extremity is also seen in the setting of filarial infection.

Tissue trauma has also been discussed as a risk factor. World-class hurdlers in a Finnish study had an increased risk of bone and soft tissue sarcomas, leading the authors to consider injuries as a predisposing factor in the development of these tumors.[32] On the other hand, operative trauma after total hip or knee arthroplasty has been investigated as a risk factor. No increased risk of sarcoma was seen, at both the site of surgery nor at other sites.[33,34]

References

1. Mackall CL, Meltzer PS, Helman LJ. Focus on sarcomas. Cancer Cell 2002;2:175–8.

2. Zahm SH, Fraumeni JF Jr. The epidemiology of soft tissue sarcoma. Semin Oncol 1997;24:504–14.

3. Ayiomamitis A. Epidemiology of cancer of the connective tissue in Canada during the period 1950–1985. Cancer Detect Prev 1988;13:149–56.

4. Beck A. Zur frage des Rontgensarkoms, zugleich ein Beitrag zur pathogenese des Sarkoms. Muench Med Wochenschr 1922;69:623.

5. Brady MS, Gaynor JJ, Brennan MF. Radiation-associated sarcoma of bone and soft tissue. Arch Surg 1992;127:1379–85.

6. Cormier JN, Pollock RE. Soft tissue sarcomas. CA Cancer J Clin 2004;54:94–109.

7. Karlsson P, Holmberg E, Samuelsson A, et al. Soft tissue sarcoma after treatment for breast cancer—a Swedish population-based study. Eur J Cancer 1998;34:2068–75.

8. Brennan MF, Alektiar KM, Maki RG. Sarcomas of the soft tissue and bone. In: DeVita VT Jr, Hellman S, Rosenberg SA, editors. Cancer: principles and practice of oncology. Vol 2. Philadelphia: Lippincott Williams & Wilkins; 2001. p. 1841–91.

9. Eriksson M, Hardell L, Berg NO, et al. Soft-tissue sarcomas and exposure to chemical substances: a case-referent study. Br J Ind Med 1981;38:27–33.

10. Hardell L, Sandstrom A. Case-control study: soft-tissue sarcomas and exposure to phenoxyacetic acids or chlorophenols. Br J Cancer 1979;39:711–7.

11. Hoppin JA, Tolbert PE, Flanders WD, et al. Occupational risk factors for sarcoma subtypes. Epidemiology 1999;10:300–6.

12. Balarajan R, Acheson ED. Soft tissue sarcomas in agriculture and forestry workers. J Epidemiol Community Health 1984;38:113–6.

13. Hansen ES, Hasle H, Lander F. A cohort study on cancer incidence among Danish gardeners. Am J Ind Med 1992;21:651–60.

14. Vineis P, Terracini B, Ciccone G, et al. Phenoxy herbicides and soft-tissue sarcomas in female rice weeders. A population-based case-referent study. Scand J Work Environ Health 1987;13:9–17.

15. Hoar SK, Blair A, Holmes FF, et al. Agricultural herbicide use and risk of lymphoma and soft-tissue sarcoma. JAMA 1986;256:1141–7.

16. Riihimaki V, Asp S, Hernberg S. Mortality of 2,4-dichlorophenoxyacetic acid and 2,4,5-trichlorophenoxyacetic acid herbicide applicators in Finland: first report of an ongoing prospective cohort study. Scand J Work Environ Health 1982;8:37–42.

17. Smith AH, Pearce NE, Fisher DO, et al. Soft tissue sarcoma and exposure to phenoxyherbicides and chlorophenols in New Zealand. J Natl Cancer Inst 1984;73:1111–7.

18. Olsson H. An updated review of the epidemiology of soft tissue sarcoma. Acta Orthop Scand Suppl 2004;75:16–20.

19. Fingerhut MA, Halperin WE, Marlow DA, et al. Cancer mortality in workers exposed to 2,3,7,8-tetrachlorodibenzo-p-dioxin. N Engl J Med 1991;324:212–8.

20. Saracci R, Kogevinas M, Bertazzi PA, et al. Cancer mortality in workers exposed to chlorophenoxy herbicides and chlorophenols. Lancet 1991;338:1027–32.

21. U. S. Environmental Protection Agency SAB. Re-evaluating dioxin: Scientific Advisory Board's review of EPA's reassessment of dioxin and dioxin-like compounds. U.S. Government Printing Office 1995.

22. Bertazzi A, Pesatori AC, Consonni D, et al. Cancer incidence in a population accidentally exposed to 2,3,7,8-tetrachlorodibenzo-para-dioxin. Epidemiology 1993;4:398–406.

23. Institute of Medicine. Veterans and Agent Orange: health effects of herbicides used in Vietnam. Washington, DC: National Academy of Sciences, National Academy Press; 1994.

24. Creech JL Jr, Makk L. Liver disease among polyvinyl chloride production workers. Ann N Y Acad Sci 1975;246:88–94.

25. Da Horta JS, Da Motta LC, Abbatt JD, Roriz ML. Malignancy and other late effects following administration of Thorotrast. Lancet 1965;32:201–5.

26. Lander JJ, Stanley RJ, Sumner HW, et al. Angiosarcoma of the liver associated with Fowler's solution (potassium arsenite). Gastroenterology 1975;68:1582–6.

27. Falk H, Thomas LB, Popper H, Ishak KG. Hepatic angiosarcoma associated with androgenic-anabolic steroids. Lancet 1979;2:1120–3.

28. Van Kaick G, Lieberman D, Lorenz D, et al. Recent results of the German Thorotrast study—epidemiological results and dose effect relationships in Thorotrast patients. Health Phys 1983;44 Suppl 1:299–306.

29. Pearce N, Smith AH, Reif JS. Increased risks of soft tissue sarcoma, malignant lymphoma, and acute myeloid leukemia in abattoir workers. Am J Ind Med 1988;14:63–72.

30. Tucker MA, D'Angio GJ, Boice JD Jr, et al. Bone sarcomas linked to radiotherapy and chemotherapy in children. N Engl J Med 1987;317:588–93.

31. Stewart FW, Treves N. Classics in oncology: lymphangiosarcoma in postmastectomy lymphedema: a report of six cases in elephantiasis chirurgica. CA Cancer J Clin 1981;31:284–99.

32. Pukkala E, Kaprio J, Koskenvuo M, et al. Cancer incidence among Finnish world class male athletes. Int J Sports Med 2000;21:216–20.

33. Paavolainen P, Pukkala E, Pulkkinen P, Visuri T. Cancer incidence in Finnish hip replacement patients from 1980 to 1995: a nationwide cohort study involving 31,651 patients. J Arthroplasty 1999;14:272–80.

34. Visuri T, Pukkala E, Pulkkinen P, Paavolainen P. Decreased cancer risk in patients who have been operated on with total hip and knee arthroplasty for primary osteoarthrosis: a meta-analysis of 6 Nordic cohorts with 73,000 patients. Acta Orthop Scand 2003;74:351–60.

CHAPTER 67

GENETICS OF SARCOMA

CHANDRAJIT P. RAUT, MD, MSc

Cytogenetic and molecular genetic abnormalities have been recognized in benign and malignant soft tissue and bone tumors. Although their clinical behavior is similar, most sarcomas arise from different mesodermal and ectodermal cell lines and display distinct histologies. A significant advance in our understanding of sarcomas is in the identification of unique genetic abnormalities corresponding to specific histologic subtypes of sarcoma. Linking oncogene activation, tumor suppressor gene inactivation, expression of growth factors and their receptors, chromosomal analyses, and molecular cytogenetics with specific histologic subtypes of sarcomas enables the clinician to identify the type of tumor involved, and in progressively more situations, provide prognostic information and guide therapy.

Familial Cancer Syndromes

Several known familial cancer syndromes are associated with sarcomas (Table 1). Li-Fraumeni syndrome was first recognized in 4 families with a pattern of soft tissue sarcoma and breast cancer, among other tumors, in both adults and children.[1] Those with germline mutations of *TP53* and Li-Fraumeni syndrome are at greater risk of developing one of a variety of sarcomas, usually before the age of 45.[1] Affected individuals are particularly susceptible to radiation-induced sarcomas.[2]

Individuals with germline mutations of the retinoblastoma (*RB*) gene have a higher incidence of sarcoma, including osteosarcoma, as a second nonocular malignancy diagnosed decades after treatment of their retinoblastoma.[3,4] Furthermore, this risk is enhanced in patients with retinoblastoma treated with radiation therapy.[5]

Neurofibromatosis 1 (NF1) is an autosomal dominant disorder associated with the periodic appearance of benign and malignant growths. Most common tumors in patients with NF1 are in the central nervous system (CNS). In a 42-year follow-up study of individuals with this disorder, 46% developed either a malignant or a benign CNS tumor, and 47% of all malignancies were CNS tumors.[6] Germline loss of the *NF1* gene in neurofibromatosis 1 is associated with a 5% incidence of malignant peripheral nerve sheath tumors (MPNST).[6–8] Affected children are at risk of developing rhabdomyosarcoma, fibrosarcoma, and liposarcoma in addition to CNS tumors.[9] Those with a family history of NF1 have a higher incidence of tumors than those with the sporadic form of the disease, but the risk of developing neoplasms remains high in both groups.

Germline mutations of c-*Kit* are associated with familial gastrointestinal stromal tumor (GIST).[10] Familial adenomatous polyposis and Gardner's syndrome are commonly associated with the development of intraabdominal desmoid and, rarely, fibrosarcoma.[11–13] Carney's triad is a constellation of frequently multicentric gastric leiomyosarcoma, extra-adrenal paraganglioma, and pulmonary chondroma.[14,15] Werner's syndrome, or adult progeria, is an autosomal recessive disorder associated with a shortened life span owing to atherosclerosis and a number of malignancies, including sarcoma.[16] Gorlin's syndrome and tuberous sclerosis are also associated with sarcoma.[2,17–19]

Oncogenes and Tumor Suppressor Genes

Recognized genetic abnormalities include chromosomal deletions, duplications, and translocations and gene rearrangements or mutations resulting in amplification, oncogene activation, or tumor suppressor gene inactivation. Certain translocation break points within genes create novel fusion oncogenes; the functions of the resulting oncoproteins are not fully understood in many circumstances. Other translocation rearrangements adjacent to particular genes result in deregulated expression. Deletions generally result in loss of tumor suppressor genes. Amplifications, classified as either intrachromosomal (homogeneously staining regions) or extrachromosomal (double minute chromosomes), usually signify

Table 1 Genetic Syndromes Associated with Sarcoma*

Syndrome	Gene	Chromosomal Locus	Sarcoma	Reference
Li-Fraumeni	TP53	17q13	Soft tissue, osteogenic	1,50
Retinoblastoma	RB	13q14	Soft tissue, osteogenic	3,51,52
Neurofibromatosis type I	NF1	17q11.2	Malignant peripheral nerve sheath tumor, rhabdomyosarcoma, fibrosarcoma, liposarcoma	7–9
Familial gastrointestinal stromal tumor	KIT	4q11-21	Gastrointestinal stromal tumor	10
Gardner's syndrome	APC	5q21	Fibrosarcoma, desmoid tumor	11,12
Carney's triad	Unknown	Unknown	Gastrointestinal stromal tumor/leiomyosarcoma	14,15
Werner's syndrome (adult progeria)	WRN	8p12	Soft tissue	16
Gorlin's syndrome (nevoid basal cell carcinoma syndrome)	PTC	9q22.3	Fibrosarcoma, rhabdomyosarcoma	2
Tuberous sclerosis (Bourneville disease)	TSC1 TSC2	9q34 16p13.3	Rhabdomyoma, rhabdomyosarcoma	17–19

*Adapted with permission from Brennan MF et al.[53]

increased copies, and thus overexpression, of oncogenes.[20] Identification of the individual abnormalities may help distinguish specific tumor types.[20]

Oncogene overexpression has been documented in soft tissue and bone tumors. Specific oncogenes, the functions of the resultant oncoproteins, and the associated sarcomas are listed in Table 2.[21] Amplification, alteration, or increased expression of genes encoding nuclear transcription factors (c-*myc*, c-*myb*, *gli*), members of the *ras* family (H-, K-, N-*ras*), membrane-bound receptor tyrosine kinases (c-*erb*-B2, *met*, *fms*, c-*Kit*) and nonreceptor tyrosine kinases (*src*, *fes*, *abl*, *FAK*), and growth factors have been reported in benign and malignant soft tissue and bone tumors. The utility in

Table 2 Oncogenes in Soft Tissue and Bone Tumors*

Gene Product	Oncoprotein Function	Sarcoma
Nuclear transcription regulators		
c-Myc	Stimulates cell proliferation	Osteosarcoma, MFH, other
c-Myb	Inhibits cell differentiation	Various
c-Fos	Nuclear transcription factor	Liposarcoma
gli	Nuclear transcription factor	Childhood
ras family		
H-, K-, N-Ras	G-protein pathway regulation	MFH, rhabdomyosarcoma, leiomyosarcoma, vinyl chloride-induced angiosarcoma
Membrane-bound tyrosine kinases		
c-Erb-B2 (HER2)	Homologous to EGFR	Osteosarcoma, other
Met	Receptor for HGF	Various
Fms	Mutant CSF-1 receptor	
c-Kit	Receptor for stem cell factor	Ewing's sarcoma/PNET
Non-receptor tyrosine kinases		
Src	Tyrosine kinase phosphorylation	
Fes	Tyrosine kinase phosphorylation	Low grade
Abl	Tyrosine kinase phosphorylation	Angiomyolipoma, low-grade MFH, low level in leiomyosarcoma
FAK	Tyrosine kinase phosphorylation	Angiomyolipoma, liposarcoma, leiomyosarcoma, neurofibrosarcoma, synovial sarcoma, MFH
Other		
SAS	Regulation of growth-related cellular processes	MFH, liposarcoma
MDM2	Inhibition of wild-type p53	Various

CSF-1 = colony stimulating factor-1; EGFR = epidermal growth factor receptor; HGF = hepatocyte growth factor; MFH = malignant fibrous histiocytoma; PNET = peripheral neuroectodermal tumors.
*Adapted with permission from Slominski A et al.[21]

identifying expression of some of these oncogenes in the management of sarcomas is still under study. Random patterns of oncogene mutations in general limits their use as markers for tumor progression.[21] However, the specificity of individual oncogenes for certain tumors may provide some degree of prognostic data and serve as potential therapeutic targets. For instance, 42% of osteosarcomas express the Erb-B2 oncoprotein, correlating with high metastatic potential and poor prognosis.[22] The significant impact of the KIT receptor tyrosine kinase is discussed in detail below.

Inactivation of tumor suppressor genes has been implicated in the development of sarcomas. Recognized tumor suppressor genes, their chromosomal loci, encoded active protein function, and sarcomas associated with their inactivation are listed in Table 3. The nuclear transcription factor p53 inhibits cell proliferation by inducing arrest at the G_1 stage of the cell cycle by activating the gene encoding p21.[23] Overexpression of the mutant *TP53* gene may be associated with a more aggressive behavior in sarcomas.[24] However, mutant *TP53* gene overexpression in malignant fibrous histiocytoma is common and appears to have no prognostic significance.[25] The nuclear phosphoprotein Rb, encoded by the retinoblastoma gene, binds to transcription regulators to prevent progression of the cell cycle through the G_1 and S stages.[26] However, *RB* gene mutations have a random distribution rather than well-defined mutational "hot spots," thwarting efforts to establish their role in sarcoma formation.[27] Additional tumor suppressor genes encode nuclear cell-cycle regulators, including p16, which inhibits Rb phosphorylation; p18, which inhibits cyclin kinase activities; and p21, which is regulated by p53.[27,28]

Growth Factors

Peptide growth factors help regulate the proliferation and differentiation of mesenchymal cells. Soft tissue tumors may express both growth factors and their receptors; the family of growth factor receptors includes over 50 receptor tyrosine kinases. Implicated growth factors include platelet-derived growth factor (PDGF), epidermal growth factor (EGF), transforming growth factors-alpha and -beta (TGF-α, -β), fibroblast growth factor (FGF), insulin, insulin-like growth factor (IGF), vascular endothelial growth factor (VEGF), and hepatocyte growth factor/scatter factor (HGF/SF).[21] Growth factors and their receptors are inviting therapeutic targets. *In vitro* studies demonstrate that the proliferative effect of PDGF on osteosarcoma cells may be inhibited by antibodies specifically directed against PDGF.[29] Similarly, targeted therapy against the IGF-I pathway may be of benefit in osteosarcoma and Ewing's sarcoma/peripheral neuroectodermal tumors (PNET).[30]

Cytogenetic Abnormalities

A variety of cytogenetic anomalies, which create new fusion proteins, have been described in benign and malignant soft tissue and bone tumors. Cytogenetic anomalies, the resulting fusion protein, and the frequency for each sarcoma are listed in Table 4. The function of many of these fusion genes remains unknown. Specific genetic findings may help distinguish certain tumors or confirm relationships between others. For instance, giant marker and ring chromosomes and abnormalities involving 12q13-15 are seen in atypical lipomatous tumors and dedifferentiated liposarcomas.[31] Unique genetic identities for dermatofibrosarcoma protuberans, giant cell fibroblastoma, and low-grade fibromyxoid sarcoma have been demonstrated.[31] Skeletal and extraskeletal myxoid chondrosarcomas may be distinguished by the specific translocations seen in the latter.[31]

Table 3 Tumor Suppressor Genes in Soft Tissue and Bone Tumors*

Gene	Chromosomal Locus	Protein Function	Sarcomas Associated with Inactivation
TP53	17q13	Nuclear transcription factor inhibiting cell proliferation	MFH, leiomyosarcoma, rhabdomyosarcoma, angiosarcoma, fibrosarcoma, liposarcoma, osteosarcoma, chondrosarcoma, Ewing's sarcoma, synovial sarcoma
RB	13q14	Nuclear phosphoprotein regulating cell proliferation	MFH, leiomyosarcoma, rhabdomyosarcoma, fibrosarcoma, liposarcoma, osteosarcoma, chondrosarcoma, Ewing's sarcoma
p16	9p21	Negative cell-cycle regulators	Osteosarcoma, leiomyosarcoma
p18	1p32	Negative cell-cycle regulators	Leiomyosarcoma
p21	6p21.1	Negative cell-cycle regulators	Leiomyosarcoma

MFH = malignant fibrous histiocytoma.
*Adapted with permission from Slominski A et al.[21]

Table 4 Cytogenetic Abnormalities in Malignant Soft Tissue Tumors

Tumor Type	Cytogenetic Event	Molecular Event	Frequency
Alveolar soft part sarcoma	t(X;17)(p11;q25)	ASPL-TFE3 fusion	> 90%
Angiomatoid fibrous histiocytoma	t(12;16)(q13;p11)	FUS-ATF1 fusion	
Chondrosarcoma, extraskeletal myxoid	t(9;22)(q21-31;q12.2)	CHN-EWS fusion	> 75%
	t(9;17)(q22;q11)	CHN-RBP56 fusion	
Clear-cell sarcoma	t(12;22)(q13;q12)	EWS-ATF1 fusion	> 75%
Desmoplastic small round-cell tumor	t(11;22)(p13;q12)	ESW-WT1 fusion	> 90%
Dermatofibrosarcoma protuberans/giant-cell fibroblastoma	t(17;22)(q22;q13) or ring forms of chromosomes 17,22	COL1A1-PDGFB1 fusion	> 50%; ring > 75%
Endometrial stromal tumor	t(7;17)(p15;q21)	JAZF1-JJAZ1 fusion	30%
Epithelioid sarcoma	Loss of heterozygosity (22q)	unknown	rare
	t(8;22)(q22;q11)	unknown	rare
Ewing's sarcoma/PNET	t(11;22)(q24;q12)	EWS-FLI1 fusion	85%
	t(21;22)(q22;q12)	EWS-ERG fusion	5–10%
	t(7;22)(p22;q12)	EWS-ETV1 fusion	<5%
	t(2;22)(q33;q12)	EWS-FEV fusion	< 5%
	t(17;22)(q12;q12)	EWS-E1AF fusion	< 5%
	t(1;16)(q11-25;q11-24)	unknown	10%
	Trisomy 8	not applicable	50%
	Trisomy 12	not applicable	30%
Fibromyxoid sarcoma, low grade	t(7;16)(q34;p11)	FUS-BBF2H fusion	
Fibrosarcoma, infantile	t(12;15)(p13;q25)	ETV6-NTRK3 fusion	> 75%
Inflammatory myofibroblastic tumor	2p23 rearrangement	ALK fusion genes	50%
Leiomyosarcoma, uterine	t(12;14)(q14-15;q23-24)	unknown	rare
Liposarcoma, well- or dedifferentiated	Ring form, chromosome 12		> 75%
Liposarcoma, myxoid/round cell	t(12;16)(q13;p11)	CHOP-TLS fusion	> 75%
	t(12;22)(q13;q11-q12)	CHOP-EWS fusion	unknown
Rhabdoid tumor, malignant	Deletion 22(q11.2)	INI1 inactivation	50%
Rhabdomyosarcoma, alveolar	t(2;13)(q35;q14)	PAX3-FKHR fusion	> 75%
	t(1;13)(p36;q14), double minutes	PAX7-FKHR fusion	10–20%
Rhabdomyosarcoma, embryonal	Trisomies 2q, 8, 20	unknown	rare
Synovial sarcoma	t(X;18)(p11.2;q11.2)	SYT-SSX1 or SYT-SSX2 fusion	> 90%

PNET = peripheral primitive neuroectodermal tumor.
*Adapted with permission from Brennan MF et al.[53]

Molecular Prognostication of Fusion Genes for Sarcoma

Genetic data are being applied with greater frequency in predicting the behavior of and response to therapy in soft tissue and bone tumors. Cytogenetic analysis has demonstrated a significant correlation between tumor grade and frequency of aneuploidy for high-grade sarcomas.[21] Such aneuploidy is associated with a worse prognosis in patients with malignant fibrous histiocytoma, synovial sarcoma, and clear-cell sarcoma, but with improved prognosis in childhood patients with aneuploid rhabdomyosarcoma.[21]

In tumors with several different mutations, specific mutations may be associated with better prognosis. Molecular prognostication of fusion genes has been addressed in 4 types of sarcoma: synovial sarcoma, Ewing's sarcoma/peripheral primitive neuroectodermal tumor (PNET), alveolar rhabdomyosarcoma, and myxoid liposarcoma. Because of variations in study design,

data modeling, statistical analyses, and evaluated outcomes, it is difficult to reach definitive conclusions.[32] Nevertheless, they demonstrate the potential utility in identifying the molecular biology of sarcoma to enhance prognostication.

The prognostic value of fusion genes in sarcoma was first demonstrated by Kawai and colleagues in synovial sarcoma.[33] In this retrospective study, the authors demonstrated that patients with localized tumors with SYT-SSX1 fusion transcripts had decreased metastasis-free survival. These results have subsequently been confirmed in four other retrospective studies[34–37] and one multi-institutional study,[38] but were not confirmed in the most contemporary study.[39] Thus, the clinical relevance of typing fusion genes in synovial sarcoma remains uncertain.[32]

Two studies in patients with Ewing's sarcoma/PNET have demonstrated that those with the ESWS-FLI1 type I gene fusion involving EWS exon 7 fused with FLI1 exon 6 have a longer relapse-free (local or distant) and overall survival than those with other fusion types.[40,41] However, a third study failed to duplicate this result.[42]

Two retrospective studies demonstrated that patients with alveolar rhabdomyosarcoma with the *PAX7-FKHR* fusion gene have better clinical outcomes.[43,44] Finally, a single study in patients with myxoid liposarcoma failed to demonstrate any association between the structure of the common *TLS-CHOP* fusion gene and disease-specific survival.[45]

Therapeutic Targeting

Mutational analysis is relevant in the clinicopathologic assessment of gastrointestinal stromal tumors (GIST) and deserves special mention. The *KIT* gene, located on chromosome 4q11-21, encodes a type-III receptor tyrosine kinase, CD117.[46] *KIT* mutations have been identified in the majority of patients with GIST, most frequently in the juxtamembrane domain at exon 11, with a smaller number at exons 9 and 13. Germline mutations in exon 11 are seen in familial cases and in patients with multiple GIST.[31] In the majority of patients with GIST, mutations in the *KIT* gene result in a constitutively activate receptor tyrosine kinase. The development of the agents imatinib mesylate and sunitinib malate targeted against the activated KIT protein amongst others has drastically changed the paradigm in the management of this disease. These agents block signaling via KIT (among other tyrosine kinase inhibitors) by lodging in an ATP-binding pocket required for receptor dimerization and activation.[47] In 2001, the first multicenter trial of imatinib mesylate for patients with metastatic GIST documented partial responses in 54%, stable disease in 28%, and disease progression in 14%, with a minimum follow-up of 6 months.[48] Recent reports from phase II studies show that a second agent, sunitinib malate, demonstrates antitumor efficacy in patients resistant to imatinib mesylate.[49]

These promising results with GIST demonstrate how recognized genetic anomalies, resulting in abnormal protein function, may be exploited in treatment strategies. Future studies will uncover additional therapeutic targets.

References

1. Li FP, Fraumeni JF Jr. Soft-tissue sarcomas, breast cancer, and other neoplasms. A familial syndrome? Ann Intern Med 1969;71:747–52.

2. Zahm SH, Fraumeni JF Jr. The epidemiology of soft tissue sarcoma. Semin Oncol 1997;24:504–14.

3. Abramson DH, Ellsworth RM, Kitchin FD, Tung G. Second nonocular tumors in retinoblastoma survivors. Are they radiation-induced? Ophthalmology 1984;91:1351–5.

4. Draper GJ, Sanders BM, Kingston JE. Second primary neoplasms in patients with retinoblastoma. Br J Cancer 1986;53:661–71.

5. Wong FL, Boice JD Jr, Abramson DH, et al. Cancer incidence after retinoblastoma. Radiation dose and sarcoma risk. JAMA 1997;278:1262–7.

6. Sorensen SA, Mulvihill JJ, Nielsen A. Long-term follow-up of von Recklinghausen neurofibromatosis. Survival and malignant neoplasms. N Engl J Med 1986;314:1010–5.

7. Jhanwar SC, Chen Q, Li FP, et al. Cytogenetic analysis of soft tissue sarcomas. Recurrent chromosome abnormalities in malignant peripheral nerve sheath tumors (MPNST). Cancer Genet Cytogenet 1994;78:138–44.

8. King AA, Debaun MR, Riccardi VM, Gutmann DH. Malignant peripheral nerve sheath tumors in neurofibromatosis 1. Am J Med Genet 2000;93:388–92.

9. McKeen EA, Bodurtha J, Meadows AT, et al. Rhabdomyosarcoma complicating multiple neurofibromatosis. J Pediatr 1978;93:992–3.

10. Nishida T, Hirota S, Taniguchi M, et al. Familial gastrointestinal stromal tumours with germline mutation of the KIT gene. Nat Genet 1998;19:323–4.

11. Foulkes WD. A tale of four syndromes: familial adenomatous polyposis, Gardner syndrome, attenuated APC and Turcot syndrome. QJM 1995;88:853–63.

12. Okamoto M, Sato C, Kohno Y, et al. Molecular nature of chromosome 5q loss in colorectal tumors and desmoids from patients with familial adenomatous polyposis. Hum Genet 1990;85:595–9.

13. Posner MC, Shiu MH, Newsome JL, et al. The desmoid tumor. Not a benign disease. Arch Surg 1989;124:191–6.

14. Carney JA. Gastric stromal sarcoma, pulmonary chondroma, and extra-adrenal paraganglioma (Carney Triad): natural history, adrenocortical component, and possible familial occurrence. Mayo Clin Proc 1999;74:543–52.

15. Carney JA, Sheps SG, Go VL, Gordon H. The triad of gastric leiomyosarcoma, functioning extra-adrenal paraganglioma and pulmonary chondroma. N Engl J Med 1977; 296:1517–8.

16. Goto M, Miller RW, Ishikawa Y, Sugano H. Excess of rare cancers in Werner syndrome (adult progeria). Cancer Epidemiol Biomarkers Prev 1996;5:239–46.

17. Povey S, Burley MW, Attwood J, et al. Two loci for tuberous sclerosis: one on 9q34 and one on 16p13. Ann Hum Genet 1994;58(Pt 2):107–27.

18. Sallee D, Spector ML, van Heeckeren DW, Patel CR. Primary pediatric cardiac tumors: a 17 year experience. Cardiol Young 1999;9:155–62.

19. van Slegtenhorst M, de Hoogt R, Hermans C, et al. Identification of the tuberous sclerosis gene TSC1 on chromosome 9q34. Science 1997;277:805–8.

20. Fletcher JA. Molecular biology and cytogenetics of soft tissue sarcomas: relevance for targeted therapies. Cancer Treat Res 2004;120:99–116.

21. Slominski A, Wortsman J, Carlson A, et al. Molecular pathology of soft tissue and bone tumors. A review. Arch Pathol Lab Med 1999;123:1246–59.

22. Onda M, Matsuda S, Higaki S, et al. ErbB-2 expression is correlated with poor prognosis for patients with osteosarcoma. Cancer 1996;77:71–8.

23. Harris CC. The 1995 Walter Hubert Lecture—molecular epidemiology of human cancer: insights from the mutational analysis of the p53 tumour-suppressor gene. Br J Cancer 1996;73:261–9.

24. Drobnjak M, Latres E, Pollack D, et al. Prognostic implications of p53 nuclear overexpression and high proliferation index of Ki-67 in adult soft-tissue sarcomas. J Natl Cancer Inst 1994;86:549–54.

25. Yang P, Hirose T, Hasegawa T, et al. Prognostic implication of the p53 protein and Ki-67 antigen immunohistochemistry in malignant fibrous histiocytoma. Cancer 1995;76:618–25.

26. Mittnacht S, Weinberg RA. G1/S phosphorylation of the retinoblastoma protein is associated with an altered affinity for the nuclear compartment. Cell 1991;65:381–93.

27. Cordon-Cardo C. Mutations of cell cycle regulators. Biological and clinical implications for human neoplasia. Am J Pathol 1995;147:545–60.

28. Dei Tos AP, Maestro R, Doglioni C, et al. Tumor suppressor genes and related molecules in leiomyosarcoma. Am J Pathol 1996;148:1037–45.

29. Benito M, Lorenzo M. Platelet derived growth factor/tyrosine kinase receptor mediated proliferation. Growth Regul 1993;3:172–9.

30. Scotlandi K, Benini S, Sarti M, et al. Insulin-like growth factor I receptor-mediated circuit in Ewing's sarcoma/peripheral neuroectodermal tumor: a possible therapeutic target. Cancer Res 1996;56:4570–4.

31. Hogendoorn PC, Collin F, Daugaard S, et al. Changing concepts in the pathological basis of soft tissue and bone sarcoma treatment. Eur J Cancer 2004;40:1644–54.

32. Oliveira AM, Fletcher CD. Molecular prognostication for soft tissue sarcomas: are we ready yet? J Clin Oncol 2004;22:4031–4.

33. Kawai A, Woodruff J, Healey JH, et al. SYT-SSX gene fusion as a determinant of morphology and prognosis in synovial sarcoma. N Engl J Med 1998;338:153–60.

34. Nilsson G, Skytting B, Xie Y, et al. The SYT-SSX1 variant of synovial sarcoma is associated with a high rate of tumor cell proliferation and poor clinical outcome. Cancer Res 1999;59:3180–4.

35. Inagaki H, Nagasaka T, Otsuka T, et al. Association of SYT-SSX fusion types with proliferative activity and prognosis in synovial sarcoma. Mod Pathol 2000;13:482–8.

36. Mezzelani A, Mariani L, Tamborini E, et al. SYT-SSX fusion genes and prognosis in synovial sarcoma. Br J Cancer 2001;85:1535–9.

37. Panagopoulos I, Mertens F, Isaksson M, et al. Clinical impact of molecular and cytogenetic findings in synovial sarcoma. Genes Chromosomes Cancer 2001;31:362–72.

38. Ladanyi M, Antonescu CR, Leung DH, et al. Impact of SYT-SSX fusion type on the clinical behavior of synovial sarcoma: a multi-institutional retrospective study of 243 patients. Cancer Res 2002;62:135–40.

39. Guillou L, Benhattar J, Bonichon F, et al. Histologic grade, but not SYT-SSX fusion type, is an important prognostic factor in patients with synovial sarcoma: a multicenter, retrospective analysis. J Clin Oncol 2004;22:4040–50.

40. Zoubek A, Dockhorn-Dworniczak B, Delattre O, et al. Does expression of different EWS chimeric transcripts define clinically distinct risk groups of Ewing tumor patients? J Clin Oncol 1996;14:1245–51.

41. de Alava E, Kawai A, Healey JH, et al. EWS-FLI1 fusion transcript structure is an independent determinant of prognosis in Ewing's sarcoma. J Clin Oncol 1998;16:1248–55.

42. Ginsberg JP, de Alava E, Ladanyi M, et al. EWS-FLI1 and EWS-ERG gene fusions are associated with similar clinical phenotypes in Ewing's sarcoma. J Clin Oncol 1999;17:1809–14.

43. Kelly KM, Womer RB, Sorensen PH, et al. Common and variant gene fusions predict distinct clinical phenotypes in rhabdomyosarcoma. J Clin Oncol 1997;15:1831–6.

44. Sorensen PH, Lynch JC, Qualman SJ, et al. PAX3-FKHR and PAX7-FKHR gene fusions are prognostic indicators in alveolar rhabdomyosarcoma: a report from the children's oncology group. J Clin Oncol 2002;20:2672–9.

45. Antonescu CR, Tschernyavsky SJ, Decuseara R, et al. Prognostic impact of P53 status, TLS-CHOP fusion transcript structure, and histological grade in myxoid liposarcoma: a molecular and clinicopathologic study of 82 cases. Clin Cancer Res 2001;7:3977–87.

46. Fletcher CD, Berman JJ, Corless C, et al. Diagnosis of gastrointestinal stromal tumors: a consensus approach. Hum Pathol 2002;33:459–65.

47. Heinrich MC, Griffith DJ, Druker BJ, et al. Inhibition of c-kit receptor tyrosine kinase activity by STI 571, a selective tyrosine kinase inhibitor. Blood 2000;96:925–32.

48. Demetri GD, von Mehren M, Blanke CD, et al. Efficacy and safety of imatinib mesylate in advanced gastrointestinal stromal tumors. N Engl J Med 2002;347:472–80.

49. Demetri GD, Desai J, Fletcher JA, et al. SU11248, a multi-targeted tyrosine kinase inhibitor, can overcome imatinib

resistance caused by diverse genomic mechanisms in patients with metastatic gastrointestinal stromal tumor [abstract 3001]. Proc Am Soc Clin Oncol 2004;23:195.

50. Malkin D, Li FP, Strong LC, et al. Germ line p53 mutations in a familial syndrome of breast cancer, sarcomas, and other neoplasms. Science 1990;250:1233–8.

51. Hovig E, Smith-Sorensen B, Gebhardt MC, et al. No alterations in exon 21 of the RB1 gene in sarcomas and carcinomas of the breast, colon, and lung. Genes Chromosomes Cancer 1992;5:97–103.

52. Scholz RB, Kabisch H, Delling G, Winkler K. Homozygous deletion within the retinoblastoma gene in a native osteosarcoma specimen of a patient cured of a retinoblastoma of both eyes. Pediatr Hematol Oncol 1990;7:265–73.

53. Brennan MF, Alektiar KM, Maki RG. Sarcomas of the Soft Tissue and Bone. In: DeVita VT Jr, Hellman S, Rosenberg SA, editors. Cancer: principles and practice of oncology. Vol 2. Philadelphia: Lippincott Williams & Wilkins; 2001. p. 1841–91.

CHAPTER 68

EVALUATION OF SARCOMA: A PATHOLOGIST'S PERSPECTIVE

BRIAN P. RUBIN, MD, PhD

Introduction

The evaluation of sarcomas is a sophisticated process that involves all members of the multidisciplinary sarcoma treatment team, including surgical oncology, oncology, radiology, nuclear medicine, pathology, and radiation therapy. Analysis of the clinical scenario is absolutely critical in determining the final diagnosis. For example, the differential diagnosis of a large retroperitoneal mass in a 60–year-old woman is very different from the differential diagnosis of a deep-seated soft tissue mass in the thigh of a 25-year-old woman. Another example would be a bluish-red, plaque-like lesion with infiltrative borders on the scalp of a 70-year-old man with substantial sun exposure. This lesion is undoubtedly angiosarcoma until proven otherwise, whereas a lesion with a simlar appearance on the face of a newborn is very likely to be a benign juvenile capillary hemangioma. Similarly, different lesions have different radiologic appearances. For example, a biphasic mass in the retroperitoneum of a 50-year-old woman with a variably fatty and more dense/fleshy appearance on CT scan is likely to be dedifferentiated liposarcoma. It is important to know this, since core biopsies may show only the well-differentiated adipocytic component or, alternatively, the dedifferentiated anaplastic component. These examples are provided to highlight the important point that diagnostic interpretation of sarcomas should not and cannot occur in the vacuum of pathology. There must be integration of all clinical information.

Biopsy of Sarcoma

Biopsy type is another important issue in the diagnosis of sarcomas. Although fine-needle aspiration (FNA) and core needle biopsies may be convenient to obtain for the surgeon and the patient, they may yield insufficient material to make an accurate diagnosis. However, the diagnostic interpretation of sarcoma biopsies is largely dependent on the experience of the pathologist and the surgeon. In Europe, fine-needle aspiration of primary sarcomas is much more common, and, in general, European surgical pathologists have acquired greater experience and are better able to make primary diagnoses using this technique. In contrast, very few pathologists in the United States have sufficient experience to make a primary classification of a sarcoma based on fine-needle aspiration. However, fine-needle aspiration is very useful for triaging a bone or soft tissue mass into the three basic categories of carcinoma/melanoma, hematolymphoid neoplasm, or sarcoma, and these distinctions can be made by all surgical pathologists.

Core needle biopsies are easier to interpret, in general, than fine-needle aspirations, since the pathologist is able to see the architecture of the lesion as well as the cytologic characteristics. These samples are also easy to obtain, and for many lesions, the biopsy can be obtained in the surgical oncologist's office without the need for time in the operating room. Core needle biopsies can also be obtained under CT guidance. However, multiple core needle biopsies are required for the accurate classification of some lesions owing to issues of tumor heterogeneity and sampling. Furthermore, it may be difficult to obtain sufficient tissue for tumor banking and research protocols. Contrary to what is commonly believed, tissue from both fine-needle aspirations and core needle biopsies can be used for cytogenetics and molecular studies.

Open and excisional biopsies have many advantages, owing largely to the greater amount of tissue that is obtained as compared with fine-needle aspiration and core needle biopsy. Furthermore, it is easier to snap freeze or otherwise preserve tissue from open and excisional biopsies for tumor banking or research protocols. Indeed, with the advent of expression array analysis and proteomics, many patients wish to have their tumor tissue banked for use in future studies and genetic analysis. Since many centers perform neoadjuvant chemotherapy for intermediate- and high-grade sarcomas, it is ideal to bank tumor from the biopsy. However, even treated sarcomas should be banked as they may provide additional information regarding molecular aspects of therapy.

Frozen Sections

Frozen sections are useful in the evaluation of sarcoma, but like all techniques, have some limitations. Frozen-section analysis is useful for identifying "lesional" tissue. In other words, it is usually straightforward for the pathologist to determine whether or not the tissue sent for frozen section analysis is neoplastic. Furthermore, once the lesion has been identified, it is useful to triage the tissue into the three basic categories of carcinoma/melanoma, hematolymphoid neoplasm, or sarcoma. In the case of a hematolymphoid neoplasm, tissue can be sent for flow cytometry. In the case of a sarcoma, tissue can be sent for cytogenetics, snap frozen for molecular analysis and tissue banking, and placed in electron microscopy fixative. It is ideal for the pathologist to receive potential sarcomas in an unfixed state, since once the tissue is fixed, it cannot be cultured to yield cytogenetic data or frozen for molecular analysis or tumor banking. It is also reasonable to distinguish benign/low-grade from intermediate- to high-grade sarcomas at the time of frozen section. However, analysis of margins can be a treacherous business at the time of frozen section. The pathologist is unlikely to identify a few atypical cells that are infiltrating normal tissue, whereas it is reasonable to expect the pathologist to identify a flagrantly positive margin. Neoadjuvant radiation therapy makes it especially difficult to determine whether a margin is contaminated by a neoplasm at the time of frozen section. In practical terms, if atypical cells are identified at a margin at the time of frozen section, the margin is usually reported as positive.

Macroscopic Examination

The pathologist and the surgeon should discuss each individual resection specimen immediately after the specimen has been resected. The frozen section laboratory is a good place to have this discussion, since the specimen is fresh and the surgeon is still acutely aware of all the important macroscopic issues. The orientation must be determined and three sutures or other methods of marking can be used to fully orient the specimen. This is important since the specimen often becomes distorted

once it has been fixed. The surgeon should identify any close margins or major structures (major nerves, major blood vessels, etc) that have been resected. It is also important to let the pathologist know of any organs that have been resected along with the sarcoma. This is especially important for abdominal/retroperitoneal resections where large sarcomas frequently engulf kidneys and adrenal glands as well as segments of bowel, and these may be so deeply buried within the specimen that the only way to find them is to "breadloaf" the specimen. This is also a good time to discuss any "special" issues. For instance, if a nodule was noted on preoperative PET scan that remained PET avid after chemotherapy, then this can be noted and an attempt to find the nodule can be performed so that it can be submitted for histologic analysis. After the specimen has been discussed with the surgeon, the pathologist should "breadloaf" the specimen in the manner that permits the most useful analysis of involvement of major structures and analysis of margins. The appearance of the lesion should be described as solid or cystic, hemorrhagic, necrotic, fleshy, myxoid, etc. The pathologist should be able to identify all margins and the macroscopic relationship of the tumor to all margins, since these measurements, performed when the tumor is fresh, may override any measurements that are identified histologically. Furthermore, it is extremely important to note whether the tumor is circumscribed or infiltrative, as this can dictate how many sections of margin are taken and also the orientation of a margin. For instance, with a pushing, circumscribed margin, it is not necessary to take more than one section. However, if the margin is very infiltrative, then more judicious sampling is required. In any case, the microscopic margins should always be correlated with the macroscopic margins. Furthermore, if a margin consists of fascia, bone, or other major anatomic structures, this should be noted and reported in the final diagnosis. The actual distance from the margin should be reported for margins that are less than 2 cm from the neoplasm. Margins should never be reported as "free" of tumor, as this is meaningless and subject to interpretation.

After analysis of the margins, tumor should be snap frozen, placed in electron microscopy fixative, and sent for cytogenetic analysis, if necessary. In addition to tumor, uninvolved "normal" tissue should also be snap frozen, if available. Finally, tissue sections should be submitted for histologic analysis. Generally, one section of tumor is submitted per cm of tumor maximum dimension; however, this is not necessary for very large tumors, especially if they are homogeneous (eg, well-differentiated liposarcoma). Emphasis should always be placed on sampling grossly distinct areas of the neoplasm. Furthermore, a representative section of necrotic tissue should be submitted to verify the macroscopic impression of necrosis. Occasionally, the macroscopic impression of necrosis is incorrect and the neoplasm is found to be myxoid, degenerate, etc after histologic analysis. When this happens, the pathologist needs to return to the gross specimen and submit additional sections of the macroscopically "necrotic" area to fully characterize it under the microscope. The percentage of the neoplasm that is necrotic should be documented, since this has implications on grading and response to therapy. In summary, the gross analysis is used to orient the specimen, document the various components, determine the macroscopic margins, triage tissue for special studies and tumor banking, note the percentage of necrotic tissue, and submit tissue for histologic analysis.

Classification

Classification of sarcomas is accomplished by integrating the clinical information, macroscopic appearance, histologic appearance, immunohistochemical profile, cytogenetic/molecular findings, and in some cases, ultrastructural profile. Histologically, lesions are subdivided into various categories, such as fascicular spindle-cell sarcomas, pleomorphic sarcomas, epithelioid sarcomas, and myxoid sarcomas, each with its own differential diagnosis. For instance, the differential diagnosis of a densely fascicular spindle-cell neoplasm with uniform cells having fine chromatin is fibrosarcomatous dermatofibrosarcoma protuberans, monophasic synovial sarcoma, and malignant peripheral nerve sheath tumor. Immunohistochemistry is useful in further refining the differential diagnosis. For instance, in the above-mentioned differential diagnosis, synovial sarcomas are focally positive for cytokeratins and epithelial membrane antigen, whereas the other two lesions in the differential diagnosis are generally negative for both of these immunohistochemical markers. The modern pathologist has a large arsenal of antibodies available to them that allow determination of line of differentiation into epithelial, muscle, nerve, etc. In general, a panel of antibodies is performed, with pertinent positive and negative immunohistochemical studies. The immunohistochemical profile is interpreted in the context of the histologic appearance and clinical setting to support the final diagnosis. Cytogenetics and molecular studies are also very useful in the classification of sarcomas, since many sarcomas have characteristic cytogenetic findings (Table 1).[1,2] Some sarcomas have overlapping histological and immunohistochemical features, making their precise classification difficult. Furthermore, it is useful to have molecular confirmation of a diagnosis when the lesion is histologically atypical or occurs in an unusual clinical setting. One such example would be Ewing's sarcoma/primitive neuroectodermal tumor in the elderly. Since Ewing's sarcoma/primitive neuroectodermal tumor is rare in the elderly, identification of a t(11;22) translocation by cytogenetics would support this unusual diagnosis very strongly. Alternatively, identification of an *EWS-Fli1* fusion gene by reverse transcriptase-polymerase chain reaction (RT-PCR) would also confirm the diagnosis. RT-PCR has been associated with a lot of false positives when used with paraffin-embedded sections. The tendency for false positives does not seem to be an issue with frozen tissue. However, real-time RT-PCR is being applied to the detection of known translocations from paraffin and appears to be much less error prone, with very few false positives and negatives. Recently, DNA probes for fluorescence in situ hybridization (FISH) have become available commercially that facilitate performing FISH routinely on paraffin-embedded sections for several of the more common translocations. With immunohistochemical and molecular tests, scrupulous attention to quality control is critical and all new tests need to be validated extensively (Cleveland Clinic Paper).

Electron microscopy was used much more extensively in previous times to classify sarcomas. However, with the advent of immunohistochemistry, electron microscopy has largely fallen out of favor. This is due to the high-cost, slow turnover of most electron microscopy laboratories, and the ability to sample only a very limited portion of the specimen.

I recommend classifying sarcomas according to the WHO classification of bone and soft tissue tumors (Tables 2 and 3).[3] According to the recent WHO classification of soft tissue tumors, a recommendation was made to divide tumors into four categories: benign, intermediate (locally aggressive), intermediate (rarely metastasizing), and malignant.

Grading

Unfortunately, there is no generally agreed upon scheme for grading bone and soft tissue tumors.[4] The two most widely used soft tissue grading systems are the French Federation of Cancer Centers Sarcoma Group (FNCLCC) and the National Cancer Institute (NCI) systems.[5,6] Both systems have three grades and are based on mitotic activity, necrosis, and differentiation, and predict clinical behavior very well. However, in addition to these criteria, the NCI system requires the quantification of cellularity and pleomorphism for certain subtypes of sarcomas, which is subjective. In my opinion, the

Table 1 Characteristic Cytogenetic and Molecular Events of Bone and Soft Tissue Tumors

Histologic Type		Cytogenetic Events	Molecular Events
Aneurysmal bone cyst		16q22 and 17p13 rearrangements	
Alveolar soft part sarcoma		t(X;17)(p11;q25)	*ASPL-TFE3* fusion
Aneurysmal bone cyst		t(16;17)q22;p13)	*CDH11-USP6* fusion
Angiomatoid fibrous histiocytoma		t(12;16)(q13;p11)	*FUS-ATF1* fusion
Extraskeletal myxoid chondrosarcoma		t(9;22)(q22;q12)	*EWS-NR4A3* fusion
		t(9;17)(q22;q11)	*TAF2N-NR4A3* fusion
		t(9;15)(q22;q21)	*TCF12-NR4A3* fusion
Chondromyoxid fibroma		Deletion of 6q	
Chondrosarcoma of bone		Complex	
Clear-cell sarcoma		t(12;22)(q13;q12)	*EWS-ATF1* fusion
Desmoplastic small round cell tumor		t(11;22)(p13;q12)	*EWS-WT1* fusion
Dermatofibrosarcoma protuberans		Ring form of chromosomes 17 and 22	*COL1A1-PDGFB* fusion
		t(17;22)(q21;q13)	*COL1A1-PDGFB* fusion
Ewing's sarcoma/PNET		t(11;22)(q24;q12)	*EWS-FLI1* fusion
		t(21;22)(q12;q12)	*EWS-ERG* fusion
		t(2;22)(q33;q12)	*EWS-FEV* fusion
		t(7;22)(p22;q12)	*EWS-ETV1* fusion
		t(17;22)(q12;q12)	*EWS-E1AF* fusion
		inv(22)(q12q12)	*EWS-ZSG*
Fibrosarcoma, infantile		t(12;15)(p13;q26)	*ETV6-NTRK3* fusion
		Trisomies 8, 11, 17, and 20	
Gastrointestinal stromal tumor		Monosomies 14 and 22	
		Deletion of 1p	
			KIT mutation
Inflammatory myofibroblastic tumor		2p23 rearrangement	*ALK* fusion genes
Leiomyoma			
	Uterine	t(12;14)(q15;q24) or Deletion of 7q	*HMGIC* rearrangement
	Extrauterine	Deletion of 1p	
Leiomyosarcoma		Deletion of 1p	
Lipoblastoma		8q12 rearrangement or polysomy 8	PLAG1 oncogenes
Lipoma		12q15 rearrangement	*HMGIC* rearrangement
Liposarcoma			
	Well differentiated	Ring form of chromosome 12	
	Myxoid/Round cell	t(12;16)(q13;p11)	*TLS-CHOP* fusion
		t(12;22)(q13;q12)	*EWS-CHOP* fusion
	Pleomorphic	Complex	
Malignant peripheral nerve sheath tumor		Complex	
Myxofibrosarcoma (myxoid MFH)		Ring form of chromosome 12	
Neuroblastoma			
	Good prognosis	Hyperdiploid, no 1p deletion	
	Poor prognosis	1p deletion	
		Double minute chromosomes	N-*myc* amplification
Osteosarcoma			
	Low grade	Ring chromosomes	
	High grade	Complex	
Rhabdoid tumor		Deletion of 22q	*INI1* inactivation
Rhabdomyosarcoma			
	Alveolar	t(2;13)(q35;q14)	*PAX3-FKHR* fusion
		t(1;13)(p36;q14), double minutes	*PAX7-FKHR* fusion
	Embryonal	Trisomies 2q, 8 and 20	
			Loss of heterozygosity at 11p15
Schwannoma	Benign	Deletion of 22q	*NF2* inactivation
Synovial sarcoma			
	Monophasic	t(X;18)(p11;q11)	*SYT-SSX1* or *SYT-SSX2* fusion
	Biphasic	t(X;18)(p11;q11)	Predominantly *SYT-SSX1* fusion

Table 2 WHO Classification of Soft Tissue Tumors of Intermediate Malignant Potential and Malignant Soft Tissue Tumors

ADIPOCYTIC TUMORS

Intermediate (locally aggressive)
Atypical lipomatous tumor/
Well differentiated liposarcoma

Malignant
Dedifferentiated liposarcoma
Myxoid liposarcoma
Round-cell liposarcoma
Pleomorphic liposarcoma
Mixed-type liposarcoma
Liposarcoma, not otherwise specified

FIBROBLASTIC/MYOFIBROBLASTIC TUMORS

Intermediate (locally aggressive)
Superficial fibromatoses (palmar/plantar)
Desmoid-type fibromatoses
Lipofibromatosis

Intermediate (rarely metastasizing)
Solitary fibrous tumor and hemangiopericytoma (incl. lipomatous
    hemangiopericytoma)
Inflammatory myofibroblastic tumor
Low-grade myofibroblastic sarcoma
Myxoinflammatory fibroblastic sarcoma
Infantile fibrosarcoma

Malignant
Adult fibrosarcoma
Myxofibrosarcoma
Low grade fibromyxoid sarcoma hyalinizing spindle cell tumor
Sclerosing epithelioid fibrosarcoma

SO-CALLED FIBROHISTIOCYTIC TUMORS

Intermediate (rarely metastasizing)
Plexiform fibrohistiocytic tumor
Giant cell tumor of soft tissues

Malignant
Pleomorphic "MFH"/Undifferentiated pleomorphic sarcoma
Giant cell "MFH"/Undifferentiated pleomorphic sarcoma with giant cells
Inflammatory "MFH"/Undifferentiated pleomorphic sarcoma with prominent
    inflammation

SMOOTH-MUSCLE TUMORS

Malignant
Leiomyosarcoma

SKELETAL-MUSCLE TUMORS

Malignant
Embryonal rhabdomyosarcoma (incl. spindle cell, botryoid, anaplastic)
Alveolar rhabdomyosarcoma (incl. solid, anaplastic)
Pleomorphic rhabdomyosarcoma

Table 2 Continued

VASCULAR TUMORS

Intermediate (rarely metastasizing)
Kaposiform hemangioendothelioma
Retiform hemangioendothelioma
Papillary intralymphatic angioendothelioma

Composite hemangioendothelioma
Kaposi's sarcoma

Malignant
Epithelioid hemangioendothelioma
Angiosarcoma of soft tissue

TUMORS OF PERIPHERAL NERVES

Malignant
Malignant peripheral nerve-sheath tumor
Epithelioid malignant peripheral nerve-sheath tumor

CHONDRO-OSSEOUS TUMORS

Malignant
Mesenchymal chondrosarcoma
Extraskeletal osteosarcoma

TUMORS OF UNCERTAIN DIFFERENTIATION

Intermediate (rarely metastasizing)
Angiomatoid fibrous histiocytoma
Ossifying fibromyxoid tumor (incl. atypical/malignant)
Mixed tumour/
Myoepithelioma/
Parachordoma

Malignant
Synovial sarcoma
Epithelioid sarcoma
Alveolar soft part sarcoma
Clear-cell sarcoma of soft tissue
Extraskeletal myxoid chondrosarcoma ("chordoid" type)
PNET/Extraskeletal Ewing's tumor
    pPNET
    extraskeletal Ewing's tumor
Desmoplastic small round-cell tumor
Extrarenal rhabdoid tumor
Malignant mesenchymoma
Neoplasms with perivascular epithelioid
    cell differentiation (PEComa)
    clear-cell myomelanocytic tumor
Intimal sarcoma

Table 3 WHO Classification of Locally Aggressive and Malignant Bone Tumors

CARTILAGE TUMORS
Chondrosarcoma
Central, primary, and secondary
Peripheral
Dedifferentiated
Mesenchymal
Clear cell

OSTEOGENIC TUMORS
Osteosarcoma
Conventional
   chondroblastic
   fibroblastic
   osteoblastic
Telangiectatic
Small cell
Low-grade central
Secondary
Parosteal
Periosteal
High-grade surface

FIBROGENIC TUMORS
Desmoplastic fibroma
Fibrosarcoma

FIBROHISTIOCYTIC TUMORS
Malignant fibrous histiocytoma

EWING's SARCOMA/PRIMITIVE NEUROECTODERMAL TUMOR
Ewing's sarcoma/PNET

HAEMATOPOIETIC TUMORS
Plasma cell myeloma
Malignant lymphoma, NOS

GIANT CELL TUMOR
Giant cell tumor
Malignancy in giant cell tumor

NOTOCHORDAL TUMORS
Chordoma

VASCULAR TUMORS
Angiosarcoma

SMOOTH-MUSCLE TUMORS
Leiomyosarcoma

LIPOGENIC TUMORS
Liposarcoma

MISCELLANEOUS TUMORS
Adamantinoma
Metastatic malignancy

MISCELLANEOUS LESIONS
Langerhans cell histiocytosis

FNCLCC system is easier to use and recent data suggest that it may be slightly better in predicting prognosis than the NCI system.[7] Other systems with two or four grades have also been used. Accurate grading requires an adequate sample of tissue; therefore, it is not always possible for the pathologist to determine the grade accurately on FNA or core needle biopsy or in tumors that have been previously treated with neoadjuvant radiation or chemotherapy.

The FNCLCC grade is based on three parameters: differentiation, mitotic activity, and necrosis. Each parameter receives a score: differentiation (1–3), mitotic activity (1–3), and necrosis (0–2). The scores are totaled and the grade is based on the sum of all scores.

- Grade 1: a total of 3 or less
- Grade 2: a total of 4–5
- Grade 3: a total of 6–8

Tumor differentiation is scored as follows (Table 4):

- Score 1: Sarcomas closely resembling normal, adult mesenchymal tissue
- Score 2: Sarcomas of certain histologic type.
- Score 3: Synovial sarcomas, embryonal sarcomas, undifferentiated sarcomas, and sarcomas of doubtful tumor type

Tumor differentiation is the most problematic aspect of the FNCLCC system. The system is subjective and some diagnostic entities are not included. Nevertheless, it is an important part of the system and an attempt should be made to assign a differentiation score.

Mitosis count: The count is made in the most mitotically active area in 10 successive high-power fields (HPFs) (a high-power field X 400 = 0.1734 mm^2; use the 40X objective):

- Score 1: 0–9 mitoses per 10 HPFs
- Score 2: 10–19 mitoses per 10 HPFs.
- Score 3: ≥ 20 mitoses per 10 HPFs

Tumor Necrosis: Determined on histologic sections:

- Score 0: no tumor necrosis on any examined slides
- Score 1: < 50% tumor necrosis for all the examined slides
- Score 2: > 50% tumor necrosis on the examined slides

The grading of sarcomas of bone is largely driven by the histologic classification, and, traditionally, grading has been based on the system advocated by Broders, which uses cellularity as the major criterion.[8] However, I advocate the following more pragmatic approach to grading aggressive and malignant primary tumors of

Table 4 Tumor Differentiation Score According to Histologic Type in the Updated Version of the FNCLCC System*

Tumor Differentiation

Histologic Type	Score
Well-differentiated liposarcoma	1
Myxoid liposarcoma	2
Round-cell liposarcoma	3
Pleomorphic liposarcoma	3
Dedifferentiated liposarcoma	3
Fibrosarcoma	2
Well-differentiated malignant peripheral nerve-sheath tumor	1
Conventional malignant peripheral nerve-sheath tumor	2
Poorly differentiated malignant peripheral nerve-sheath tumor	3
Myxofibrosarcoma (myxoid MFH)	2
Typical storiform/pleomorphic MFH (pleomorphic sarcoma, NOS)	2
Giant cell and inflammatory MFH (pleomorphic sarcoma, NOS with giant cells or inflammatory cells)	3
Well-differentiated leiomyosarcoma	1
Conventional leiomyosarcoma	2
Poorly differentiated/pleomorphic/epithelioid leiomyosarcoma	3
Biphasic/monophasic synovial sarcoma	3
Poorly differentiated synovial sarcoma	3
Embryonal/alveolar/pleomorphic rhabdomyosarcoma	3
Extraskeletal myxoid chondrosarcoma	2
Mesenchymal chondrosarcoma	3
Extraskeletal osteosarcoma	3
Ewing's sarcoma/PNET	3
Alveolar soft part sarcoma	3
Epithelioid sarcoma	3
Malignant rhabdoid tumor	3
Clear-cell sarcoma	3
Undifferentiated sarcoma	3

MFH = malignant fibrous histiocytoma; NOS = not otherwise specified.
*Adapted from Sobin LH and Wittekind CH.[8]

bone (Table 5). Two benign bone tumors that have a tendency to be locally aggressive but have little to no metastatic potential are giant cell tumor and desmoplastic fibroma. Two bone tumors that are locally aggressive but metastasize infrequently, and thus are definitionally low grade, are low-grade central osteosarcoma and parosteal osteosarcoma. Periosteal osteosarcoma is generally regarded as a grade 2 (intermediate-grade) osteosarcoma. Some primary bone tumors are always high grade and include malignant giant cell tumor, Ewing's sarcoma/PNET, angiosarcoma, dedifferentiated chondrosarcoma, conventional osteosarcoma, telangiectactic osteosarcoma, small cell osteosarcoma, secondary osteosarcoma, and high-grade surface osteosarcoma. Conventional chondrosarcoma is graded based on cellularity, cytologic atypia, and mitotic figures. Grade 1 (low-grade) chondrosarcoma is hypocellular and similar histologically to enchondroma. Grade 2 (intermediate-grade) chondrosarcoma is more cellular than grade 1 chondrosarcoma, has more cytologic atypia, greater hyperchromasia and nuclear size, or has extensive myxoid stroma. Grade 3 (high-grade) chondrosarcoma is

hypercellular, pleomorphic, and contains prominent mitotic activity. Mesenchymal chondrosarcoma, fibrosarcoma, leiomyosarcoma, liposarcoma, and other "soft tissue-type" sarcomas that rarely occur in bone can be graded according to the FNCLCC grading system. Chordomas are ungraded. They are locally aggressive lesions with a propensity for metastasis late in their clinical course. Most adamantinomas tend to have a low-grade clinical course, but this is variable. Fortunately, they are very rare. According to the WHO classification of tumors of bone, adamantinomas are considered low grade.

The AJCC staging system for soft tissue and bone tumors includes a 4-grade system, but essentially collapses into low and high grade.[9,10] Grading in the tumor-nodes-metastasis (TNM) grading system is based on differentiation only, and really does not apply very well to sarcomas. As mentioned above, the FNCLCC system is recommended for grading sarcomas.

GX Grade cannot be assessed

G1 Well differentiated

G2 Moderately differentiated

Table 5 - Bone Tumor Grades

Benign but Aggressive
Desmoplastic fibroma
Giant cell tumor

Always Low Grade (Grade 1)
Low-grade central osteosarcoma
Parosteal osteosardcoma
Adamantinoma

Always Intermediate Grade
Periosteal osteosarcoma

Always High Grade
Malignant giant cell tumor
Ewing's sarcoma/PNET
Angiosarcoma
Dedifferentiated chondrosarcoma
Conventional osteosarcoma
Telangiectactic osteosarcoma
Small cell osteosarcoma
Secondary osteosarcoma
High-grade surface osteosarcoma

Variable Grade
Conventional chondrosarcoma of bone (grades 1–3)
Soft tissue-type sarcomas (eg, leiomyosarcoma)

Ungraded
Chordoma

G3 Poorly differentiated

G4 Poorly differentiated or undifferentiated (4-tiered systems only)

For purposes of using the AJCC staging system, 3-tier systems such as the FNCLCC grading system can be converted to a 4-grade system (TNM grading) as follows: grade 1 = G1, grade 2 = G2, and = grade 3 = G3 and G4. Staging of sarcomas is discussed in detail elsewhere in this book.

Reporting for Sarcomas

The pathology report should summarize all important information necessary to treat and stage sarcomas. Clinical information should include patient identification, birth date, sex, date of procedure, duration of lesion, history of neoadjuvant therapy, relevant radiologic findings (especially important for bone tumors), pre-existing conditions such as Paget's disease of bone, history of tumor predisposition syndrome, and clinical diagnosis. Detailed information regarding the anatomic site should be reported, including whether the lesion is superficial (above fascia) or deep (involving or below fascia) for soft tissue tumors. The location of bone tumors should also be specified regarding epiphysis,

metaphysis, or diaphysis for long bones and surface, cortical, and medullary location for all bone tumors. The type of procedure (core needle biopsy, open biopsy, resection, etc) should also be listed. The size of the tumor in three dimensions, structures and organs that are involved, and the status of all margins should be specified. All ancillary studies, including immunohistochemistry, cytochemistry, electron microscopy, and molecular studies should be reported and interpreted respecting the final diagnosis. I find it helpful to list the percentage of necrosis and the number of mitotic figures, as they are integral parts of the grading and may reflect treatment effect (see below). Lymph node involvement should be reported if present. However, most sarcomas do not metastasize to lymph nodes, so this usually is not an issue.

Assessment of Treatment Response

A universally adopted system for measuring the effect of preoperative (neoadjuvant) chemotherapy/radiation therapy in soft tissue tumors has not been developed. However, owing to the increasing use of neoadjuvant chemotherapy and radiation therapy, it is desirable to quantify these effects, especially in the research setting. In an attempt to satisfy the needs of clinicians regarding whether or not neoadjuvant therapy has had any effect, it is recommended that the proportion of fibrosis and necrosis be quantified and stated in the final diagnosis. Generally, sampling of nonliquified tumor tissue from one cross section through the longest axis of the tumor is recommended. At least 1 section of necrotic tumor should be sampled to verify the gross impression of necrosis. Nonsampled necrotic areas should be included in the estimate of necrosis, and the percentage of tumor necrosis should be reported.

It is essential to estimate the amount of neoadjuvant treatment effect in primary Ewing's sarcoma/PNET and osteosarcoma of bone, as these have been shown to have prognostic significance.[11–13] An entire representative slice of the tumor taken through the long axis should be mapped using a grid pattern diagram, photocopy, or radiologic film to indicate the site for each tumor block. In addition, a section of tumor perpendicular to the long axis should be sampled at the rate of 1 section per centimeter. Areas of soft tissue extension and the interface of tumor with normal tissue should also be sampled. Therapy response is expressed as a percent of total tumor area, which is either necrotic or replaced by fibrous or granulation tissue. Prognostically significant therapy response in osteosarcoma, according to most series, is defined at 90%, with those tumors showing ≥ 90% therapy response associated with a favorable prognosis.[14] Therapy response in Ewing's sarcoma is expressed as grade I (macroscopic viable tumor), grade II (microscopic viable tumor), or grade III (no viable tumor), and is highly correlated with 5-year survival.[13]

Tumor Banking

As mentioned above, tumor banking has become very important for clinical trials and research into rare tumors such as sarcomas. Although there are no agreed upon protocols for banking human tissue, it is recommended that the tumor be cut into 0.1 cm^3 pieces and frozen as quickly as possible. It is also good to freeze as much tissue as feasible, since many researchers are in search of human sarcomas for studies. Normal tissue should also be frozen in the same manner as the tumor. Furthermore, it is good to freeze tumors from biopsies (assuming there is enough tissue) from resection specimens, local recurrences, and distant metastasis. All of these samples provide unique material to answer a litany of biological questions. In the future, it would be very desirable to set up regional tumor banks for the distribution of such tissues for qualified research.

Consultation

Increasingly, academic surgical pathologists are becoming very subspecialized, and thus develop significant diagnostic expertise in their chosen subspecialties. Many of these experts serve as regional, national, and international consultants. These consultants are particularly important in the diagnosis of sarcomas, as they are rare and their classification is extremely complex. It is recommended that general surgical pathologists seek out a consultation pathologist when dealing with unusual lesions with uncharacteristic morphology or clinical scenarios or with lesions that they have not previously seen.

References

1. Ladanyi M, Bridge JA. Contribution of molecular genetic data to the classification of sarcomas. Hum Pathol 2000;31: 532–8.

2. Tomescu O, Barr FG. Chromosomal translocations in sarcomas: prospects for therapy. Trends Mol Med 2001;7: 554–9.

3. Fletcher CDM, Unni KK, Mertens F, editors. WHO classification of tumours. Pathology and genetics: tumours of soft tissue and bone. Lyon: IARC Press; 2002.

4. Oliveira AM, Nascimento AG. Grading in soft tissue tumors: principles and problems. Skeletal Radiol 2001;30: 543–59.

5. Coindre JM, Trojani M, Contesso G, et al. Reproducibility of a histopathologic grading system for adult soft tissue sarcoma. Cancer 1986;58:306–9.

6. Costa J, Wesley RA, Glatstein E, Rosenberg SA. The grading of soft tissue sarcomas. Results of a clinicohistopathologic correlation in a series of 163 cases. Cancer 1984;53: 530–41.

7. Guillou L, Coindre JM, Bonichon F, et al. Comparative study of the National Cancer Institute and French Federation of Cancer Centers Sarcoma Group grading systems in a population of 410 adult patients with soft tissue sarcoma. J Clin Oncol 1997;15:350–62.

8. Sobin LH, Wittekind CH, editors. UICC: TNM classification of malignant tumours. 6th ed. New York: Wiley-Liss; 2002.

9. Inwards CY, Unni KK. Classification and grading of bone sarcomas. Hematol Oncol Clin North Am 1995;9:545–69.

10. Greene FL, Page DL, Fleming ID, et al. AJCC cancer staging manual. 6th ed. New York: Springer; 2002.

11. Bacci G, Ferrari S, Bertoni F, et al. Prognostic factors in nonmetastatic Ewing's sarcoma of bone treated with adjuvant chemotherapy: analysis of 359 patients at the Istituto Ortopedico Rizzoli. J Clin Oncol 2000;18:4–11.

12. Picci P, Sangiorgi L, Rougraff BT, et al. Relationship of chemotherapy-induced necrosis and surgical margins to local recurrence in osteosarcoma. J Clin Oncol 1994;12: 2699–705.

13. Picci P, Bohling T, Bacci G, et al. Chemotherapy-induced tumor necrosis as a prognostic factor in localized Ewing's sarcoma of the extremities. J Clin Oncol 1997;15: 1553–9.

14. Raymond AK, Chawla SP, Carrasco CH, et al. Osteosarcoma chemotherapy effect: a prognostic factor. Semin Diagn Pathol 1987;4:212–36.

CHAPTER 69

EVALUATION: DIAGNOSTIC IMAGING

KEVIN W. MCENERY, MD

Evaluation: Imaging

A multidisciplinary clinical approach and multimodality imaging strategy is necessary for the most effective evaluation and therapy of sarcoma lesions. Surgical and medical oncologists should anticipate the requirement for multiple complementary diagnostic imaging modalities to appropriately stage and assess sarcoma lesions. The radiologist, as a member of the multidisciplinary team, should coordinate imaging findings with pathological findings, especially in the evaluation of bone sarcoma. During pretreatment planning, surgical oncologists should expect consulting radiologists to provide as precise a determination of anticipated surgical margins, and the radiologist can tailor imaging protocols to provide the most optimal preoperative imaging assessment. For sarcoma, the goal of imaging is complete excision of the lesion by enabling precise surgical interventions. In extremity sarcoma there is the additional consideration to preserve the patient's ambulatory function through limb-sparing surgical procedures.

Pretreatment Evaluation

Bone and soft sarcoma are uncommon lesions that require appropriate multimodality management for the best possible patient outcome. Plain radiography has been supplemented in recent years with the availability of imaging modalities of computed tomography (CT), magnetic resonance (MR) imaging, and, most recently, positron emission spectroscopy with concurrent CT (PET/CT) image acquisition and registration. These imaging modalities are complementary, with each providing evaluation of specific clinical aspects of lesion management. Proper sequencing of the imaging evaluation allows the most effective method to identify, stage, and treat sarcomatous lesions.

As most patients are initially imaged in a community setting, it is essential for the initial radiologist to prospectively identify the sarcomatous lesion on initial imaging, or at minimum, include in the differential diagnosis the possibility that the lesion could be a sarcoma. By raising the possibility of a sarcoma rather than a benign process as an explanation for the patient's symptoms, the referring physician or surgeon has the opportunity to consider referral of the patient to a center where a multidisciplinary team is available to provide the opportunity for maximal patient outcome.

Regardless of whether the patient is treated in the local community setting or referred to a tertiary center, all lesion imaging must be completely imaged prior to surgical intervention, especially with regards to MR imaging, as it is impossible to distinguish postoperative soft tissue change from tissue that was preoperatively affected by tumor.

Radiographs

Diagnostic evaluation for an extremity mass is usually initiated when the patient or physician notes a mass on physical examination or the patient notes pain attributable to a bone location without antecedent trauma. Although advanced modalities are available and will likely be employed during the diagnostic work-up, the imaging work-up should begin with a traditional plain radiograph. The limitations of plain radiography to identify soft tissue sarcoma are well documented, but there are certain lesions with a characteristic calcification pattern that can preclude the need for further diagnostic imaging. These include hemangioma with characteristic phleboliths, myositis ossificans with its characteristic peripheral pattern of calcification, and synovial osteochrondromatosis with punctuate cartilaginous calcification. In the case of lipomatous lesions, plain radiographs may be able to detect the presence of a fat-containing mass displacing muscular groups.

It must be emphasized that in the context of a detectable soft tissue mass on physical examination that a negative radiograph is an expected result and must not obviate the need for additional cross-sectional imaging with CT or MR. If calcification is identified in the mass, then CT evaluation may be considered as a more appropriate modality, as MR imaging is relatively insensitive to the detecting calcification. If calcification is absent (the more usual finding) then MR imaging is more appropriate than CT as the next imaging study.

The most common presentation for bone sarcoma is that of pain in an extremity not associated with trauma. Unlike soft tissue sarcoma, plain radiographs are absolutely necessary in bone sarcoma evaluation, and it is essential that initial work-up of bone lesion includes high-quality plain radiographs. Radiographs should be obtained focused on the joint affected as well as additional imaging of the entire bone affected.

As with soft tissue sarcoma, the plain radiograph may reveal a characteristic benign lesion that obviates the need for additional imaging. In general, sarcoma lesions demonstrate cortical destruction, a wide zone of transition between the lesion and normal bone, periosteal reaction at the cortical margin of the lesion, and the presence of an extraosseous soft tissue mass. Radiographic assessment must include lesion location, internal matrix, and margin, periosteal reaction, as well as the patient's age to formulate a precise differential diagnosis.

In most cases, the radiograph is able to identify an aggressive bone sarcoma lesion as well as propose an appropriate differential diagnosis. As will be discussed shortly for bone sarcoma, MR alone does not provide sufficient specificity in the characterization of lesions to reliably provide differential diagnosis. Lesions such as osteomyelitis, giant cell tumor, and osteoid osteoma can have a very aggressive appearance on MR imaging, but are usually readily distinguished from sarcomas based on their radiographic appearance. Therefore, lesion radiographs must be made available for the radiologist who interprets the MR examination. Plain radiographs are also essential for the histologic diagnosis, as most experienced bone pathologists collaborate with the radiologist, and the plain radiograph is an often important discriminator.

With osteosarcoma, the most common location is in the metaphysic adjacent to a large joint, especially around the knee joint (Figure 1A to J). With Ewing's sarcoma, a permeative pattern of bone destruction is expected, usually within the diaphysis of the long bone. Also to be taken into consideration is the age of the patient, as most bone sarcomas have a characteristic age of presentation (Figure 2A to D). For example, osteosarcoma is the most common bone sarcoma in late-

teenaged patients, whereas Ewing's sarcoma is more prevalent in patients of early adolescent age. The characteristic findings for less common bone lesions are well documented and are beyond the scope of this discussion.[1]

Magnetic Resonance Imaging

Magnetic resonance imaging has clearly had the most significant impact on the imaging of sarcoma. MR is uniquely suited for the imaging of sarcoma, with its greater sensitivity for alterations in soft tissue than other available modalities. The advantages of MR over CT include superior soft tissue contrast visualization, direct multiplanar imaging capability, and the lack of radiation exposure for image acquisition.[2,3] For soft tissue sarcoma, MR provides important information regarding the staging of lesions, including extent within the bone marrow as well as involvement of adjacent neurovascular structures.

Although MR has significantly improved the staging and detection of sarcoma lesions, it remains difficult to determine histologic diagnosis.[4,5] The MR appearance of a sarcoma is low-signal intensity on T1-weighted images and increased signal intensity on T2-weighted images with varying amount of surrounding edema[6] (Figure 3A to C). There may be varying heterogeneity of signal from the lesion secondary to the amount of lipomatous tissue on T1-weighted images or the degree of necrosis of the lesion on T2-weighted images. Contrast enhancement is demonstrated to varying amounts in the lesion. Lesions with increased proportion of myxoid tissue can demonstrate intense T2-weighted signal. Fibrosarcomas, with areas of relatively poor cellularity often demonstrate limited areas of contrast enhancement. As it is well accepted that sarcomas can have a heterogeneous tissue components, the reviewer of the MR should focus on the most cellular portion of the lesions (low signal T1 area with contrast enhancement) as representative of the lesion's malignant potential. For this reason, MR imaging protocols should be biased toward precisely defining the lesion's extent and anatomic relationships to neurovascular structures and not at determining the precise sarcoma subtype, as that will be determined in collaboration with the pathologist.

A crucial aspect of MR imaging is that imaging protocols for bone sarcoma must be focused on the evaluation of the sarcoma and not the joint near the sarcoma. The most frequent deficiency noted in MR sarcoma imaging submitted for second opinion is that standard joint imaging protocols were followed with incomplete imaging of the lesion of interest. Standard MR joint protocols are appropriately centered to image

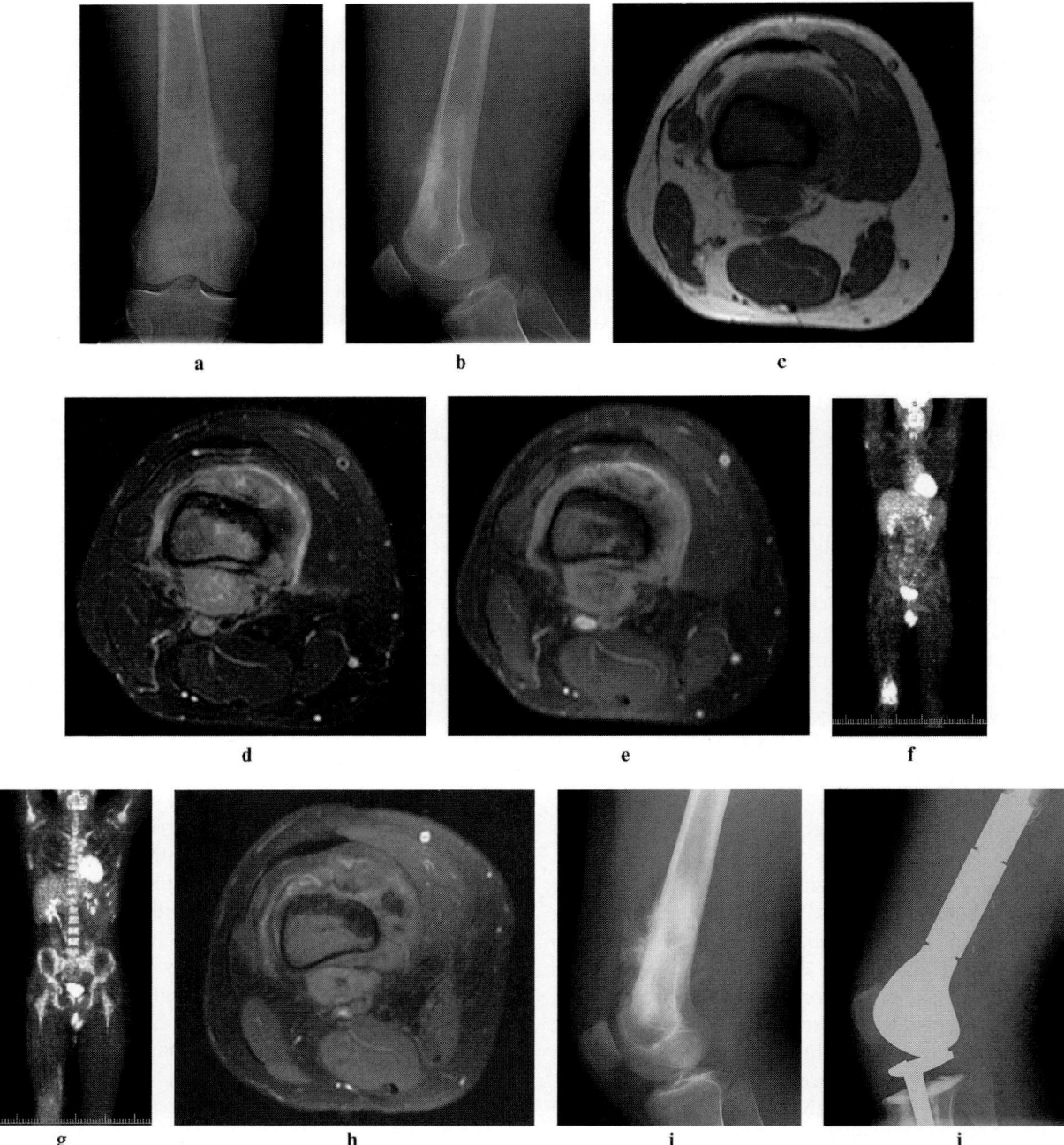

Figure 1 Osteosarcoma of the distal femur: diagnosis, chemotherapy, limb-sparing surgery. Anteroposterior and lateral radiographs of the knee (Figures 1a and 1b) demonstrate an osteoid producing lesion in the distal diaphysis of the femur. There is increased density of the anterior femoral shaft in keeping with direct bone involvement. Subtle soft tissue fullness is demonstrated adjacent to the posterior cortex. Magnetic resonance (MR) axial image through the distal diaphysis reveals circumferential encasement of the distal femur by tumor. Tumor is low signal intensity of T1-weighted images (Figure 1c). Increased signal intensity of T2-weighted (Figure 1d) and also postgadolinium contrast images (Figure 1e). Contrast enhancement indicates vascularized tumor tissue. Normal marrow fat, usually the same signal intensity as subcutaneous fat has been completely replaced by tumor involvement (see Figure 1c). There is a large posterior soft tissue mass that approaches the margin of the popliteal vessels. Coronal PET image pretherapy (Figure 1f) reveals intense metabolic activity in the distal femur. Following 4 courses of chemotherapy (Figure 1g), intensity is markedly diminished on post-therapy imaging. Post-contrast image following therapy reveals a decrease in the contrast enhancement indicating decreased vascularity (Figure 1h) with lateral radiograph (Figure 1i) also demonstrating a maturing of the tumor osteoid, findings indicative of treatment response. Lateral radiograph post-operative imaging (Figure 1j) demonstrates the expected appearance of limb-salvage prothesis.

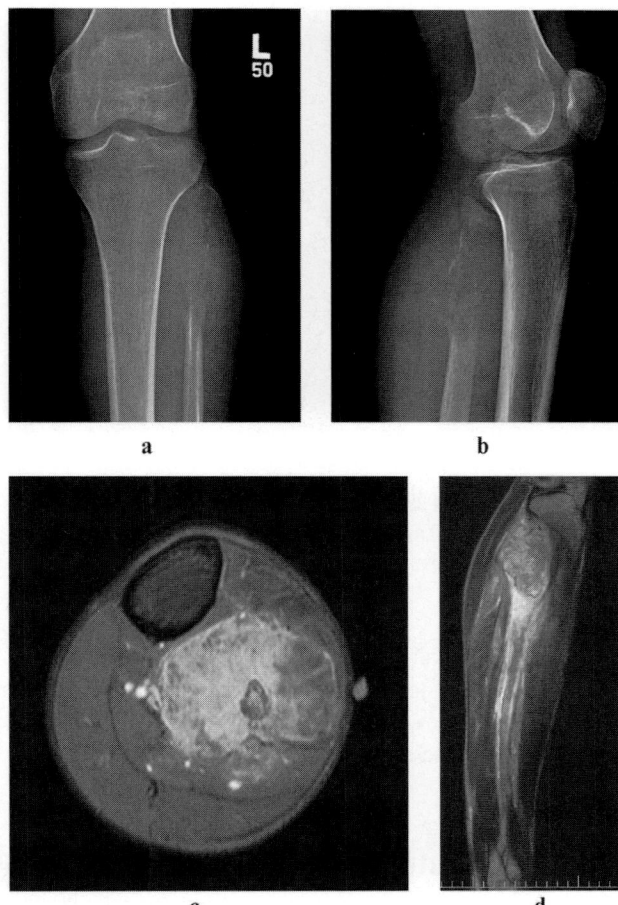

a   b

c   d

Figure 2 Ewing's sarcoma of proximal fibula. AP and lateral radiographs (Figures 2a and 2b) reveal permeative destruction of the proximal fibula with pathologic fracture in keep with Ewing's sarcoma. There is a suggestion of an associated soft tissue mass. Axial, postcontrast MR (Figure 2c) and sagittal T2-weighed sagittal image (Figure 2d) reveal a large soft tissue mass associated with the noted fibula destruction, as well as edema, which is seen extended into the midcalf on the sagittal image.

the joint of interest. For example, standard knee MR protocols are usually optimized to image internal derangements of ligament and assessment of the menisci and cruciate ligaments. In knee MR, sagittal and coronal images are emphasized, and axial imaging plays a subservient role.

Although extremity imaging protocols for sports injuries emphasize coronal and sagittal images, tumor protocols heavily rely on the axial imaging plane as it usually provides the best definition of the lesion's internal matrix, compartmental extent, and relationship to both neurovascular structures and bone. A general rule of thumb for MR tumor imaging is that the field of view should be centered on the location of the suspected lesion. Although axial images focus on the local extent of

the lesion, large field-of-view imaging, usually in the coronal plane, can provide an adequate assessment of sarcoma lesions in the long bones.

High-resolution sarcoma imaging includes the utilization of surface coils, just as with sports injury imaging. However, the coils should be centered on the lesion not on the joint. Bone sarcoma lesions in the metaphysis do require high-resolution imaging of the end of the affected bone for precise determination of lesion extent into the epiphysis. This represents crucial information if epiphysis-sparing limb salvage procedure is being contemplated by the orthopedic oncologist. If disease extends into the epiphysis, then a standard limb salvage procedure is warranted with joint replacement prosthesis.

An often-discussed aspect of MR imaging is whether the diagnostic examination should include the administration of intravenous contrast (gadolinium-DPTA) in the performance of examinations. Authors have correctly argued that in most instances the utilization of MR contrast does not significantly alter their sensitivity or specificity for lesion detection or characterization.[7,8] In general, contrast administration that identifies the expected vascularity increases does not greatly assist formulating the differential diagnosis for identified lesions. However, contrast enhancement patterns are important for two reasons, first to direct the biopsy to the most vascular portion of the lesion, and second to provide baseline assessment of the lesion prior to the administration of chemotherapy.[9] Contrast administration also provides increased accuracy to distinguish the extent of lesion in the soft tissue, as edematous tissue on T2 images should not enhance of postcontrast sequences. When contrast is administered, T1 sequences with fat saturation that minimize fat signal should be acquired to increase the specificity of detecting contrast enhancement. Assessment of the postcontrast sequences should look for satellite lesions in the tissue adjacent to the main lesion, especially in the instance of massive edema or an ill-defined lesion margin.

Authors have often argued the nuances of MR evaluation to delineate the specific histologic lesion make-up. Certain lesions such a liposarcoma do have a characteristic pattern of lipomatous tissue interspersed with vascular elements. However, in my opinion, the primary role of the MR study is to determine with absolute certainly that a lesion can be determined to be benign or, if not, direct the biopsy of the lesion to determine its histologic type.[10,11] Authors have attempted to analyze contrast enhancement patterns to help distinguish between benign and malignant sarcoma lesion with good, but not absolute, success. What must be realized is that biopsy of sarcoma masses in the appropriate hands can be performed with negligible

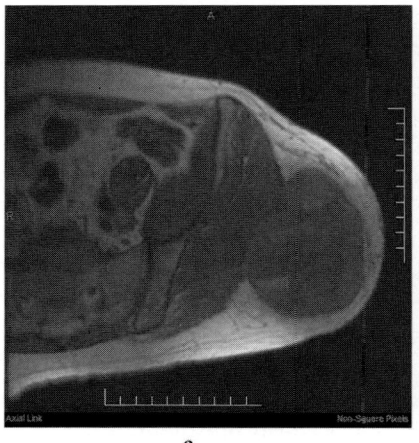 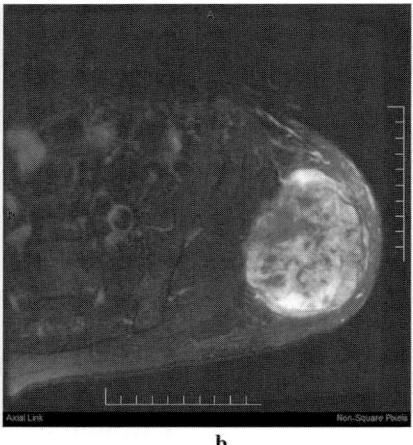 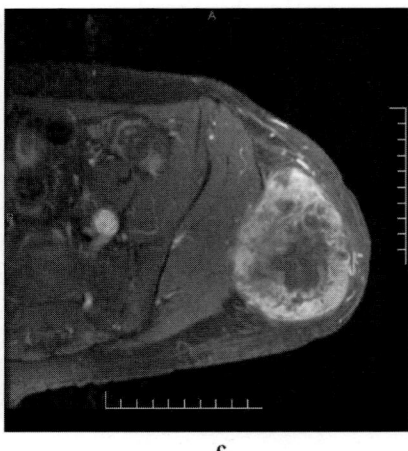

a   b   c

Figure 3 Pleomorphic sarcoma of the buttock. Axial T1- and T2-weighted images Figures 3a and 3b reveal a large mass in the left gluteal region. Heterogeneous contrast enhancement pattern (Figure 3c) suggests areas of both vascularized tissue as well as area of fibrotic and less well-vascularized tissue. Note on both T2 and postcontrast images that the deep margin of the lesion is inseparable from the gluteal muscle, with areas of muscle invasion confirmed during surgical resection.

morbidity and provides a definitive answer as to the histologic grade of the lesion. Unless a soft tissue lesion can be definitely assessed as benign, there is little reason to defer a biopsy in light of the low morbidity of a biopsy.

Authors have attempted to increase the utility of MR imaging with investigation of dynamic contrast enhancement patterns and MR spectroscopy. In dynamic contrast analysis, a specific location in the lesion is serially imaged following the administration of contrast. Postcontrast images are then analyzed for the rate at which the lesion in question demonstrates uptake of contrast material. In theory, contrast uptake occurs in benign lesions at a faster rate than benign lesions. Although studies have demonstrated the potential of the technique, there remains overlap in the patterns of benign versus malignant, and the technique is not specific enough to avoid biopsy in poorly enhancing lesions with otherwise malignant characteristics.[12] As noted previously, unless a lesion can be characterized with certainly that it is benign, then biopsy of the lesion should be performed. MR spectroscopy has also been investigated as an adjunct to increase the specificity of MR lesion characterization, but at present it remains a research application.

The future role of dynamic MR contrast techniques may be in the assessment of treatment response in lesions. In comparing the pretherapy with posttherapy image, it may be possible to obtain a more precise indication of the effectiveness of a chemotherapy specifically selected to address the genetic profile of the lesion under treatment. However, at present there is limited clinical utility to these dynamic

techniques, partially attributable to the limited number of chemotherapy options currently available. Also, the techniques are not able to demonstrate the precision of direct lesion assessment by the pathologist following therapy.

Computed Tomography (CT)

Although MR has clearly supplanted CT in the imaging of soft tissue sarcoma, CT does have important contributions to make in selected cases. As previously noted, if a lesion demonstrates typical calcification of a benign process, then CT examination should be obtained of the extremity in question, as CT is more sensitive than MR in detection and evaluation of calcification. Defining typical benign calcification usually precludes the need to obtain an MR. It is accepted that CT is not as sensitive for detecting exact marrow and soft tissue extent of lesions.[13,14]

When MR is contraindicated, such in a patient with a pacemaker or intracranial aneurysm clipping, CT becomes the modality of choice. Previously, postcontrast CT was demonstrated by the Radiology Diagnostic Oncology Group to be equally effective in defining size of primary lesion and local extent.[15] It is interesting to note that this study dates from the midnineties, when the impact of current generation multidetector CT scanners was just beginning. Current CT scanners are able to acquire 16, 32, and 64 slices in a single, subsecond turn of the gantry. The images obtained are 1 mm or less in thickness compared with the 10 mm standard of last decade. This provides the potential for a reemergence of CT scanning in the imaging of sarcoma.

An especially promising area for CT imaging is in postoperative assessment of patients with limb reconstruction hardware, which limits the imaging capabilities of MR given the metallic artifacts on MR images produced by the metal prosthesis. Therefore, if a patient cannot have an MR examination performed, then a CT scan of the extremity should be obtained. These scans should be performed utilizing thin-section protocols available, with modern multislice CT scanners and multiplanar reconstructions obtained, which provide images in the coronal and sagittal anatomic planes. With multidetector CT, coronal and sagittal reconstructed images approach the anatomic detail available with MR imaging. The contrast enhancement portions of the lesion can also be utilized to direct subsequent biopsy.

Bone Scintigraphy

Bone scintigraphy involves the intravenous administration of technetium 99m pyrophosphate followed by whole-body scanning that demonstrates areas of increased bone metabolism. Bone scanning is useful in scanning the body for osseous metastatic disease both at the time of diagnosis and during preoperative chemotherapy if there is a poor response on MR assessment and clinical concern of developing remote metastatic lesions. It is most appropriate in evaluation of primary bone sarcoma with its higher prevalence of bone-to-bone metastatic disease. In general, bone scanning is of limited value in patients with soft tissue sarcoma.

Bone scanning is not a discriminator of benign versus malignant lesions. Bone sarcomas will invariably demonstrate increased uptake on bone scanning. Benign processes such as osteoid osteoma and bone islands can also demonstrate increased activity. Therefore, any bone with bone scan uptake requires assessment with radiographs to exclude a benign process as the explanation for focal uptake. Technology advances will likely result in an increased prevalence of bone scans with single positron emission computed tomography (SPECT) imaging performed with concurrent CT (SPECT/CT), further increasing the capability to distinguish benign from metastatic lesions.[16]

Positron Emission Tomography/ Computed Tomography (PET/CT)

Imaging with 2-[18F]fluoro-2-deoxyglucose positron emission tomography (FDG-PET), and more recently in combination with concurrent computed tomography scanning (PET/CT), is the latest modality available for the assessment of sarcoma. PET/CT is not appropriate for the diagnosis of sarcoma, but likely will have an ever-growing role, as with other tumors, in monitoring of treatment response.[17] Investigations have demonstrated PET/CT evaluation following initial chemotherapy administration has the potential for short-term assessment of tumor response compared with the weeks necessary to detect a response on contrast-MR evaluation (see Figures 1f and 1g). As noted with dynamic MR techniques, at present this determination may have a limited utility for guiding clinical care given the limited number of chemotherapeutic agents, but as noted with the anticipated increase in more focused chemotherapy interventions, PET/CT imaging may prove invaluable as more targeted chemotherapy regimens are developed and the need for immediate assessment of chemotherapy effect is required.

Ultrasound

At present there is a limited role of ultrasound in the assessment of soft tissue sarcoma. In some hands, Doppler techniques have proved useful for the assessment of tumor vascularity as an indication of a lesion's malignant potential. Ultrasound is utilized in limited cases, with its primary function to assist in instances of image-guided biopsy, where the Doppler ultrasound identifies the most vascular portion of the mass for biopsy.

Evaluation: Sarcoma of Chest, Abdomen, and Pelvis

In the chest, and especially the abdomen and pelvis, CT has an increased role in the management of soft tissue sarcoma, and MR suffers in its imaging capabilities secondarily to motion artifact from breathing and normal peristaltic motion (Figure 4A to C). With the available contrast of abdominal fat and CT's capabilities to negate motion artifact from the visceral organs, CT evaluation with both intravenous and oral contrast is a first-line modality. Thin-section images from modern multidetector scanners provide important information regarding the location of the lesion as well as options for resection, especially with reference to retroperitoneal lesion involvement of kidneys, spleen, pancreas, liver, bladder, and intestinal structures. Lesions affecting the base of the mesentery are particularly problematic from a surgical management perspective, and CT provides information regarding the contiguity of the lesion to critical vascular structures, including the celiac artery, superior and inferior mesenteric arteries, and renal vessels. MRI imaging of the abdomen can provide

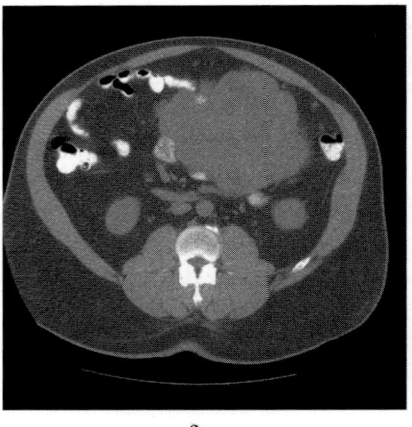 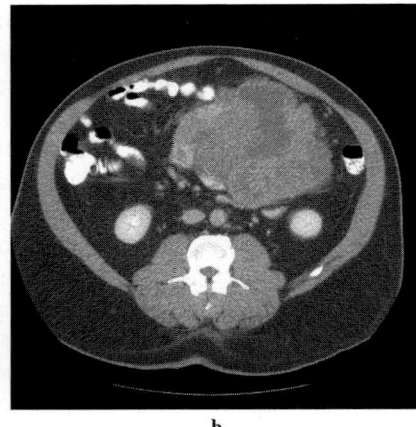 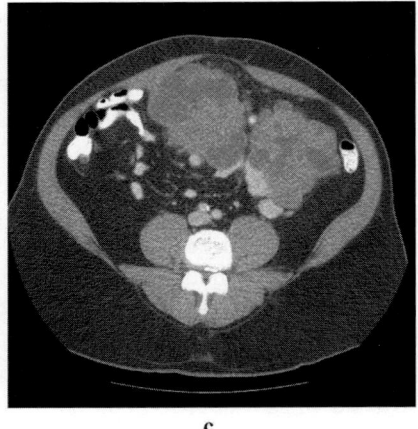

a   b   c

Figure 4 Liposarcoma of abdomen. CT imaging pre- and postcontrast image in the upper abdomen Figures 4a and 4b and postcontrast in the lower abdomen (Figure 4c) reveal a complex mess arising within the small bowel mesentery. The mass demonstrates a heterogeneous enhancement pattern typical of abdominal liposarcoma. Although the mass is greater than 10 cm it does not directly affect central vascular structure (aorta, superior mesenteric artery), and there is a clear area of fat tissue separating the mass from the left kidney.

important information as a supplement to CT study, especially with reference to vascular imaging.

Evaluation: Distant Metastasis

The predilection of bone and soft tissue sarcoma to metastasize to the lungs requires specific assessment. For thoracic metastasis, chest CT remains the most appropriate modality to image the thorax. Intraparenchymal metastases are the most common distant metastatic pattern demonstrated for sarcoma. However, synovial sarcoma is well known for its predilection for pleural-based metastatic spread. A chest radiograph is useful as a screening examination for centimeter or greater lesions. However, it is inadequate for the reliable detection and subsequent assessment of subcentimeter lung metastatic lesions. Current standard of care warrants imaging with multidetector CT imaging capable of producing 2.5 mm or less slice thickness images (compared with the 10 mm standard slice thickness of scanners utilized in the 1990s). In my opinion, every patient should have a chest CT examination at the initiation of therapy to detect metastatic lesions. If no metastases are present, this baseline CT remains available to increase the specificity for metastatic lesion detection of subsequent evaluation.

For bone lesions, there is a predilection for lesion involvement within the affected bone as well as distant osseous metastatic lesions in other bones in the body. As noted previously, at least one MR sequence (usually the coronal plane), should include the entire affected bone to assess for satellite lesions in the affected bone. However, distant metastasis to bone is best demonstrated with

bone scintigraphy. As with chest CT, a baseline bone scan should be acquired to exclude bone metastasis and serve as a baseline for subsequent evaluations. For soft tissue sarcomas, there is little value for bone scan unless there is a known bone metastasis. Bone surveys, obtaining a series of images of the entire skeleton, are insensitive for metastatic lesion detection. If metastasis is suspected on scintigraphy, then formal radiographs of the bone involved in the suspected metastasis should be obtained.

Sarcoma: Lesion Staging

In the assessment of sarcoma, several staging systems have been proposed. However, all staging systems rely on a combination of the physical size of the lesion, location, histologic grade, and the presence of distant metastasis. In the context of the prior discussions, either MR or CT can provide assessment of lesion size.[18] Lesion size of 5 cm or less defines T1 lesions in the American Joint Committee on Cancer's TMN staging system. However, the staging system of the Musculoskeletal Tumor Society, based on the work of Enneking, based the determination of a T1 lesion on the tumor confined to a single anatomic compartment.[19] For this reason, the radiologist should be aware of the staging system employed by referring clinicians and ensure that all aspects of the locally employed staging system are addressed in the diagnostic report.

In both staging systems, assessment of whether the lesion is superficial or invades deep fascial layers is usually readily determined by MR and CT imaging. Regional lymph nodes can also be assessed with CT or MR. A difficulty with MR is that examinations should be optimized for the visualization of the lesion and may not adequately image proximal lymph nodes. This may be more easily accomplished by CT evaluation or obtaining body coil images of either the groin or axillary lymph nodes. PET/CT evaluation can provide imaging of the entire body, including proximal lymph nodes. Distant metastasis is usually to the lungs, and as noted previously, chest CT must be obtained for adequate assessment,

Image-Guided Biopsy

Image-guided biopsy is an important tools in the assessment of soft tissue sarcoma. Biopsy location must be directed into the most vascularized area of the lesion based on MR or CT contrast enhancement, and if PET/CT is available, the most metabolically active region of the lesion. In general, ultrasound is a useful modality to direct image-guided biopsy of the extremity, with CT guidance usually employed for intra-abdominal lesion localization, given the degradation of image quality in areas of the abdomen owing to bowel gas. In my opinion, if the diagnosis of sarcoma is suspected, the biopsy should be performed at the anticipated referral center, as this provides the most optimal coordination between radiologists and pathologist.

Evaluation: Treatment Response

Chemotherapy response is largely determined by MR evaluation with direct comparison with pretreatment evaluation. Ideally, follow-up evaluation should directly emulate the acquisition protocols and procedure obtained on the pretreatment evaluation. Postcontrast imaging is absolutely necessary in the treatment assessment. Ideally, the scan demonstrates a detectable decrease in the bulk of the lesion, especially the proportion of vascularized mass and a subsequent increase in the necrotic areas of the lesion. Lesion size is probably the least important aspect of assessing treatment response. If the lesion remains the same size or smaller, especially in the context of decreased vascularity, this is a reliable indicator of chemotherapy response. If the lesion remains static in both size and vascularity, this is equivocal for response (Figure 5A to C). If the lesion increases in size, but markedly increases the areas of necrosis, the size increase can be attributable to liquefaction of the lesion. However, any increase in size must be confined to the same anatomic compartment, if there is an increase in the lesion's compartmental extent or involvement of neurovascular structure, then the lesion can be characterized as progression during chemotherapy.

The limitation of current imaging is that it cannot accurately distinguish the degrees of necrosis to the 90% certainly needed by most treatment protocols. With current chemotherapeutic agents, most sarcoma lesions do demonstrate response to chemotherapy, and in nonnecrotic lesions, a lesion slowly decreases in size. The surgical intervention of complete excision can provide the pathologist with adequate tissue samples for direct estimation of chemotherapy effect. Current PET/CT imaging provides the most direct assessment of chemotherapy response, but again the precision is not currently to the 90% threshold. However, it is likely that future advances in metabolic and molecular targeted

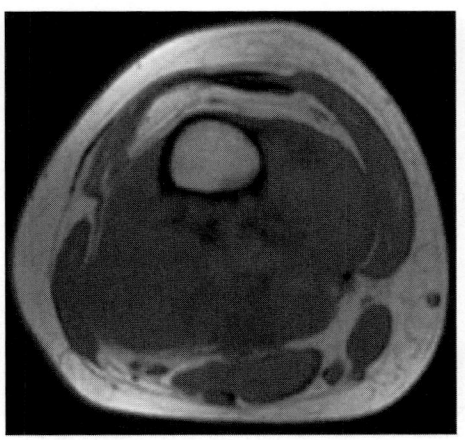 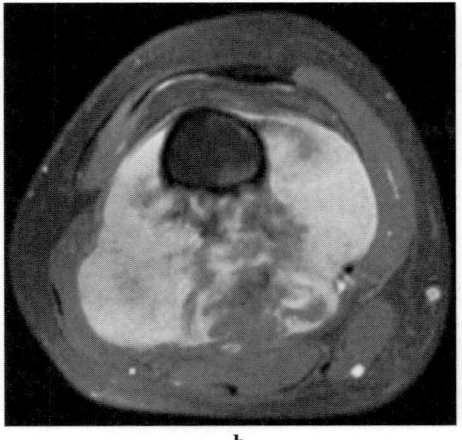 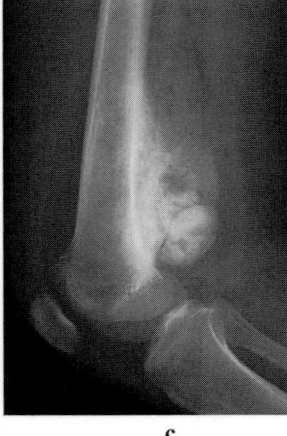

a   b   c

Figure 5 Dedifferentiated periosteal sarcoma: limited treatment response. Pre- and postcontrast axial T1-weighted MR images following 4 courses of chemotherapy demonstrate significant residual contrast enhancement reflecting areas of persistent viable soft tissue (Figures 5a and 5b). Accompanying plain radiograph reveals posterior, nonossified soft tissue mass consistent with limited treatment response (Figure 5c).

imaging will focus even more on the imaging of treatment response to provide a more accurate assessment of initial treatment response and the possibility of quickly altering chemotherapy regimens to provide the most clinical impact.

References

1. Resnick D. Tumors and tumor-like lesions of bone: radiographic principles. In: Resnick D, editor. Diagnosis of bone and joint disorders. Philadelphia: Saunders; 2002. p. 3742–62.

2. Weekes RG, Berquist TH, McLeod RA, Zimmer WD. Magnetic resonance imaging of soft-tissue tumors: comparison with computed tomography. Magn Reson Imaging 1985;3:345–52.

3. Vanel D, Shapeero LG, De Baere T, et al. MR imaging in the follow-up of malignant and aggressive soft-tissue tumors: results of 511 examinations. Radiology 1994;190:263–8.

4. Sundaram M, McLeod RA. MR imaging of tumor and tumorlike lesions of bone and soft tissue. AJR Am J Roentgenol 1990;155:817–24.

5. Dalinka MK, Zlatkin MB, Chao P, et al. The use of magnetic resonance imaging in the evaluation of bone and soft-tissue tumors. Radiol Clin North Am 1990;28:461–70.

6. Boyko OB, Cory DA, Cohen MD, et al. MR imaging of osteogenic and Ewing's sarcoma. AJR Am J Roentgenol 1987;148:317–22.

7. May DA, Good RB, Smith DK, Parsons TW. MR imaging of musculoskeletal tumors and tumor mimickers with intravenous gadolinium: experience with 242 patients. Skeletal Radiol 1997;26:2–15.

8. Verstraete KL, Lang P. Bone and soft tissue tumors: the role of contrast agents for MR imaging. Eur J Radiol 2000;34: 229–46.

9. Sundaram M. The use of gadolinium in the MR imaging of bone tumors. Semin Ultrasound CT MR 1997;18:307–11.

10. Crim JR, Seeger LL, Yao L, et al. Diagnosis of soft-tissue masses with MR imaging: can benign masses be differentiated from malignant ones? Radiology 1992;185:581–6.

11. Moulton JS, Blebea JS, Dunco DM, et al. MR imaging of soft-tissue masses: diagnostic efficacy and value of distinguishing between benign and malignant lesions. AJR Am J Roentgenol 1995;164:1191–9.

12. van Rijswijk CS, Geirnaerdt MJ, Hogendoorn PC, et al. Soft-tissue tumors: value of static and dynamic gadopentetate dimeglumine-enhanced MR imaging in prediction of malignancy. Radiology 2004;233:493–502.

13. Zimmer WD, Berquist TH, McLeod RA, et al. Bone tumors: magnetic resonance imaging versus computed tomography. Radiology 1985;155:709–18.

14. Hogeboom WR, Hoekstra HJ, Mooyaart EL, et al. MRI or CT in the preoperative diagnosis of bone tumours. Eur J Surg Oncol 1992;18:67–72.

15. Panicek DM, Gatsonis C, Rosenthal DI, et al. CT and MR imaging in the local staging of primary malignant musculoskeletal neoplasms: report of the Radiology Diagnostic Oncology Group. Radiology 1997;202:237–46.

16. Utsunomiya D, Shiraishi S, Imuta M, et al. Added value of SPECT/CT fusion in assessing suspected bone metastasis: comparison with scintigraphy alone and nonfused scintigraphy and CT. Radiology 2006;238:264–71.

17. Bastiaannet E, Groen H, Jager PL, et al. The value of FDG-PET in the detection, grading and response to therapy of soft tissue and bone sarcomas: a systematic review and meta-analysis. Cancer Treat Rev 2004;30:83–101.

18. Stacy GS, Mahal RS, Peabody TD. Staging of bone tumors: a review with illustrative examples. AJR Am J Roentgenol 2006;186:967–76.

19. Enneking WF, Spanier SS, Goodman MA. A system for the surgical staging of musculoskeletal sarcoma. Clin Orthop Relat Res 1980;153:106–20.

CHAPTER 70

PROGNOSTIC FACTORS IN SOFT TISSUE SARCOMA

BRIAN O'SULLIVAN, MD

PETER CHUNG, MD

CHARLES CATTON, MD

Introduction

The management of patients with soft tissue sarcoma (STS) has been greatly facilitated by improvements in our recognition of clinicopathologic tumor factors that predict for recurrence and tumor-related death.[1] Notwithstanding this, it is noteworthy that factors not directly related to the tumor also affect the course of disease and the outcomes of interest and will receive some attention in this review. Generally, however, the discussion will concentrate on the most important prognostic factors, especially those that comprise the elements of the tumor (T), regional lymph nodes (N), and distant metastasis (M) of the TNM staging classification,[2,3] and will outline recent knowledge about molecular prognostic factors that may have independent prognostic significance and may be targets for therapeutic interventions. Although the classic oncology outcomes of local control, metastasis, and survival will receive most attention, other outcomes such as limb preservation and function should not be forgotten. This chapter will also commence by acknowledging essential methodologic principles to encourage greater understanding of prognostic factor studies.[1] Of note, although prognostic indexes and nomograms have been implemented in oncology clinical practice, no formal system for classifying prognostic factors exists. For this reason, we will use a framework of tumor-related, patient-related, and treatment/environment-related prognostic factors in the presentation, with further emphasis on their relevance to therapeutic decision making.

Methodologic Issues in Prognostic Factor Evaluation

STATISTICAL ANALYSIS AND VALIDATION OF GENE EXPRESSION STUDIES

There is an important need to encourage an understanding of the statistical methods required to translate new basic discoveries into clinical relevance, and especially the analysis of gene expression in tumor samples. In reality, when a new marker or protein is discovered or investigated, there are often many failings in the initial phase of the development and validation. This area has recently received detailed attention from European and North American groups. Consensus recommendations (Table 1) on how to design and present these studies have been published by several journals simultaneously[4] and are available at <http://www.cancerdiagnosis.nci.nih.gov/assessment/progress/clinical.html>. These timely standards follow a similar approach by some of the same authors for reporting clinical trials (the CONSORT guidelines), where many of the significant statistical formalities are similar.

COMPARISON OF PROGNOSTIC MODELS AND CLASSIFICATIONS

Another underdeveloped area concerns the appreciation of scientific and unbiased methods to compare prog-

Table 1 Clinical Tumor Marker Study Publications Guidelines (REMARK Guidelines)

INTRODUCTION
- State the marker examined and prespecified hypotheses.

MATERIALS AND METHODS

Patients
- Describe the characteristics of the study patients, including their source and inclusion and exclusion criteria.
- Describe treatments received and how chosen (eg, randomized, rule-based).

Specimen Characteristics
- Describe type of biological material used (including controls), and preservation and storage methods.

Assay Methods
- Specify the assay method used and provide (or reference) a detailed protocol, including specific reagents or kits used, quality control procedures, reproducibility assessments, quantitation methods, and scoring and reporting protocols.

Study Design
- State the method of case selection, including whether prospective or retrospective and whether stratified (eg, by stage of disease, age). Specify the time period from which cases were taken, the end of the follow-up period, and the median follow-up time.
- Precisely define all clinical end points examined.
- List all candidate variables initially considered for inclusion in models.
- Give rationale for sample size; if the study was designed to detect a specified effect size, give the target power and effect size.

Statistical Analysis Methods
- Specify all statistical methods, including details of any variable selection procedures and other model-building issues, how model assumptions were verified, and how missing data were handled.
- Clarify how marker values were handled in the analyses; if relevant, describe methods used for cut-point determination.

RESULTS

Data
- Describe the flow of patients through the study, including the number of patients included in each stage of the analysis (a diagram may be helpful) and reasons for dropout. Specifically, both overall and for each subgroup extensively examined report the numbers of patients and the number of events.
- Report distributions of basic demographic characteristics (at least age and sex), standard (disease-specific) prognostic variables, and tumor marker, including numbers of missing values.

Analysis and Presentation
- Show the relation of the marker to standard prognostic variables.
- Present univariate analyses showing the relation between the marker and outcome, with the estimated effect (eg, hazard ratio, survival probability). Preferably provide similar analyses for all other variables being analyzed. For the tumor marker a Kaplan-Meier plot is recommended.
- For key multivariate analyses, report estimated effects (eg, hazard ratio) with confidence intervals for the marker and, at least for the final model, all other variables in the model.
- Among reported results, provide estimated effects with confidence intervals from an analysis in which the marker and standard prognostic variables are included, regardless of their significance.
- If done, report results of further investigations, such as checking assumptions, sensitivity analyses, internal validation, etc.

DISCUSSION
- Interpret the results in the context of the prespecified hypotheses and other relevant studies.
- Discuss implications for future research and clinical value.

REMARK = REporting recommendations for tumor MARKer prognostic studies.
Adapted from <http://www.cancerdiagnosis.nci.nih.gov/assessment/progress/clinical.Html>, and McShane LM et al.[4]

nostic models, and especially stage classifications. Simple "eyeballing" of survival curves or comparison of p-values is not sufficient on a statistical basis.[1] A formal method was used to compare several staging systems in STS, addressing prior and contemporary editions of the International Union Against Cancer (UICC) and the American Joint Committee on Cancer (AJCC) TNM staging system and the surgical staging systems of the Musculoskeletal Tumor Society.[5] This study is mentioned later in this chapter (see "Combining Tumor-Related Factors [The TNM System]") and represents one of the few examples of such an approach.

ADDITIONAL METHODOLOGICAL PROBLEMS IN PROGNOSTIC FACTOR EVALUATION

In STS studies there are many potential end points, each with its own prognostic factors. For example, prognostic factors exist for amputation versus limb preservation, and prognostic factors for local control in extremity STS are not the same as those for distant metastasis and survival.[1] In contrast, failure to control local disease at other anatomic sites (eg, the retroperitoneum, head and neck, or chest) can be equated with tumor-related mortality because of the eventual impact of uncontrolled disease in these locations.

A prognostic factor for a particular end point may be substantially reduced or even eliminated when certain adjuvant treatments are used (eg, radiotherapy in the case of positive resection margins). The continued search for additional therapies will hopefully eliminate some prognostic factors that predict unfavorable outcome in STS.

Another interesting aspect of prognostic factor analysis is the evolution of prognosis over the course of a disease. These include recognition that additional pathologic and clinical factors (such as microscopic surgical margin status, response to chemotherapy, or disease-free interval) become available at variable time sequences over the course of an individual patient's disease. These can be very early after initiation of therapy interventions in the case of surgical margin status, or later in follow-up for other end points; whatever is the case, they can influence subsequent assessment and anticipation of prognosis. It also includes the success or failure of prior treatment, the time between treatment and reemergence of disease (ie, recurrence that may be assessed as time-dependent variables), and the impact of being unable to use certain treatments again because of previous treatments. The temptation also exists to take outcomes that are not contemporaneous with the time of diagnosis or initial treatment planning (eg, clinical or pathological response to therapy) and suggest that these can mimic baseline factors in predicting future outcomes; unappreciated problems of interpretation may be expected from this approach.[1]

INDIVIDUAL VERSUS GROUP PROGNOSIS

The practical management of cancer patients requires predictions and decisions to be made for individuals, and the challenge of prognostication is to link the individual patient to the collective population of patients with the same disease. Traditionally, discussions of cancer prognosis have focused on the outcome of groups of patients for a specific end point, usually survival. Such approaches are appropriate for administrative requirements or researchers, but are not particularly helpful for individual patients. Researchers at Memorial Sloan-Kettering Cancer Center (MSKCC) have constructed and validated a nomogram to predict the probability of 12-year sarcoma-specific death for individual patients based on prospectively acquired data from adult patients with STS. This tool is available at <www.nomograms.org> for downloading to handheld computer devices and is useful for patient counseling, follow-up schedul-

ing, and clinical trial eligibility assessment. It certainly goes a long way toward providing personalized, individual prediction of STS outcome for patients, though must be viewed differently to systems used for predicting outcomes of aggregated groups of patients. Thus the methodologies require an understanding of the statistical uncertainties and differences involved and an appreciation of statistical concepts to estimate prognosis for *individual* patients versus *group* prognosis (eg, the use of prediction intervals rather than confidence intervals in understanding such estimates).

Tumor-Related Prognostic Factors

ANATOMIC FACTORS

Size

A consistent finding in large prospective series of STS patients is the observation that the risk of distant metastasis increases as a function of increasing tumor size.[1] Recent proposals exist for modification of staging systems to acknowledge the additional risk associated with lesions larger than 10 cm instead of the traditional adoption of a 5 cm cut point that is presently used for staging.[2,3] A proposal to subgroup 5 to 10 cm and > 10 cm has been made,[1] and an alternative proposal is to segregate even further with an additional break point beyond 15 cm (Figure 1).[6] Future editions of the stage classifications may include such modifications.

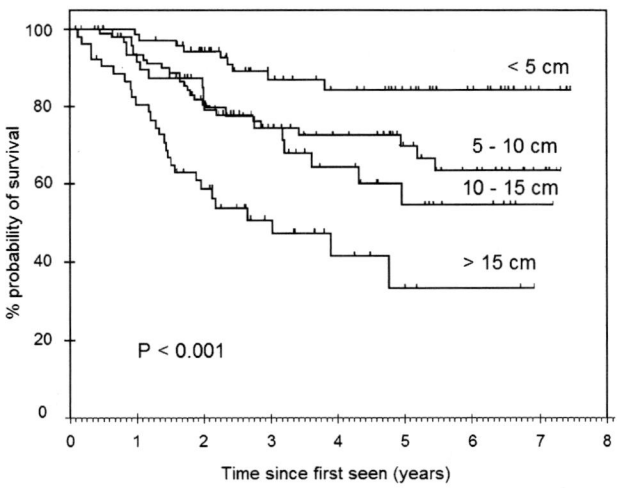

Figure 1 The percentage probability of survival by 4 different size break point in STS. These data are from the Royal Marsden Hospital, United Kingdom, and question whether the tradition size cut point used in the staging systems should be maintained. Reproduced with permission from Ramanathan RC et al.[6]

Depth

Many reports indicate that a tumor's depth of origin superficial or deep to the investing fascia of an anatomic compartment is a valid independent prognostic factor for distant relapse and overall survival in STS.[7] Tumor depth applies to extremity, body wall, and head-neck lesions, but applies equally to lesions of retroperitoneal, mediastinal, or pelvis where they are normally considered to be "deep" lesions.

Anatomic Site

The prognostic impact of anatomic site is complex. Although site is a strong independent factor within many studies,[7] the data are confounded by the vagaries of treatment selection, physician experience in the treatment of uncommon tumors (eg, head and neck or torso lesions compared with extremity lesions), and anatomic constraints limiting optimal surgery or radiotherapy. The latter embrace critical nonexpendable anatomic structures and/or site-specific problems where function and/or cosmetic outcome may predominate decision making (eg, base of the skull). Intra-abdominal lesions such as retroperitoneal sarcomas frequently achieve prodigious size and, despite often exhibiting favorable biologic features in growth and capacity for metastases, may be beyond the capacity for cure. Complete surgical resection is often not possible, and adjuvant radiotherapy is frequently compromised because of dose and volume constraints in the abdomen.

Subsites within Anatomic Regions

Less commonly, variable prognosis has been associated with tumors at different subsites within a major anatomic region. In a recent study of extremity STS, patients with upper extremity tumors had smaller lesions, underwent prereferral "unplanned" excision more often, and received radiotherapy less frequently than patients with lower extremity tumors. Patients with upper extremity tumors had a lower 5-year local recurrence-free rate (82% vs 93%, $p = 0.002$), but a higher 5-year metastasis-free rate (82% vs 69%, $p = 0.013$). The latter finding reflects the larger size of lesions in the lower extremities.[8] It is likely that other examples of variable prognosis according to anatomic subsite exist that are confounded by subtleties in treatment-related factors. In another study, tumors located in the shoulder or groin were defined as "central" location and fared less well on multivariate analysis following brachytherapy, presumably related to the suitability of implant architecture that could be employed at "central" locations. Not surprisingly, this study also showed that upper

extremity lesion and positive margin status were also adverse multivariate characteristics for local control.[9]

Anatomic Invasion

Certain anatomic prognostic factors can directly influence the treatment approach without independently influencing survival. An example is envelopment or invasion of neurovascular structures and/or bone, which would have a direct influence on the surgical approach (eg, amputation), and therefore would be prognostic for an end point such as limb preservation. Differences in definitions and in the ability to precisely determine the presence of neurovascular and osseous invasion in a clinical staging system may account for the discrepancies in the literature.

Microscopic Surgical Margins

The presence of positive resection margins nearly doubles the risk of local recurrence and increases the risk of distant recurrence and disease-related death.[10] However, positive resection margins may have different causes, and also do not constitute a baseline prognostic variable. Patients with microscopically positive margin low-grade liposarcomas have a low risk of local failure, as do patients where a positive margin is anticipated before surgery to preserve critical structures, and radiotherapy is able to sterilize the minimal residual disease. However, two categories of positive surgical margins are associated with a higher risk of local recurrence: (1) patients who present after prereferral unplanned excision and who have a positive margin on subsequent reexcision, and (2) those with unanticipated positive margins occurring during primary sarcoma resection.[11]

Another problem with the unqualified use of "positive resection margins" to determine prognosis is that reports are not always clear about whether radiotherapy or chemotherapy was used as adjuvant therapy, although this could have a significant impact on outcome, especially if radiotherapy was omitted.

Lymph Node Metastasis

Other than for certain histological STS subtypes, lymph node involvement is uncommon. Important exceptions include epithelioid sarcoma, clear-cell sarcoma, angiosarcoma, and rhabdomyosarcoma.[12,13] Selected patients undergoing radical lymphadenectomy for isolated lymph node metastasis had 46% 5-year survival in a series reported from MSKCC.[13] Generally, however, lymph node involvement is considered to have an adverse prognosis rivaling that of distant metastasis and is considered similarly in the TNM classification.[2,3] Despite this prevailing view, recent data suggest that isolated lymph node metastasis may not be as deleterious a factor as was previously thought. Behranwala and colleagues from the Royal Marsden Hospital reported that the 5-year survival of isolated lymph node metastasis was 24% (95% CI, 12.6–37.1%) compared with 0% with lymph node metastasis and distant disease (Figure 2A).[14] At the Princess Margaret Hospital, patients who presented with isolated nodal metastases had a 4-year survival of 71% (see Figure 2B) that equates to stage III disease in the tumor-nodes-netastases (TNM) stage classification described later,[2,3] and which was significantly better than patients with synchronous lymph node metastasis and distant disease.[15] It is possible that such observations may prompt revisions to the TNM, since they may encourage potentially curative approaches in selected patients with lymph node involvement.

BIOLOGIC FACTORS

Tumor Grade

Two of the best known grading systems are the French Federation of Cancer Centers Sarcoma Group and US National Cancer Institute (NCI) systems. Both classify using morphologic criteria-based degrees of necrosis and mitotic rate, but the American system considers histological type or subtype, location, cellularity, and nuclear pleomorphism, whereas the French system relies more on differentiation. Recent impressions are that the French method may be prognostically more useful.[16] Moreover, whether it is characterized by a 2-grade (high vs low), 3-grade, or 4-grade system, it remains one of the most durable and consistent prognostic factor for outcome of STS. The relevance of grade must acknowledge intratumoral variability of this factor (eg, some tumor areas may be relatively low grade, whereas other areas of the same lesion may be high-grade appearance) and grade may change over time. The evolution of dedifferentiated liposarcoma coexisting with well-differentiated liposarcoma is well recognized, as is fibrosarcomatous degeneration associated with multiply recurrent dermatofibrosarcoma protuberans.[1]

Histology

The traditional view of histologic subtypes is that they originate from similar-appearing normal tissue counterparts, and the prevailing view has been that STS histological subtype has little prognostic importance compared with other factors, especially grade.

The concepts of histogenesis and prognosis are now being contested, especially since the determination of a putative cellular origin becomes increasingly difficult with less-differentiated lesions. In fact, the interplay between histologic subtype and grade has already been acknowledged, since some STS subtypes (eg, extraskeletal Ewing's sarcoma and primitive neuroectodermal tumors) are always classified as high-grade lesions in the TNM system; this approach has been extended to other histologies (eg, synovial sarcoma) in some centers.

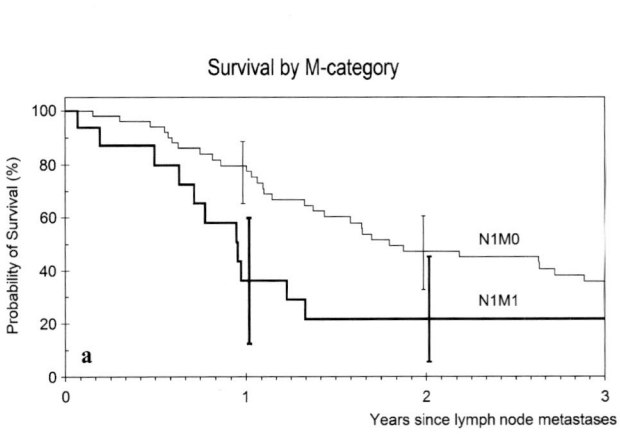

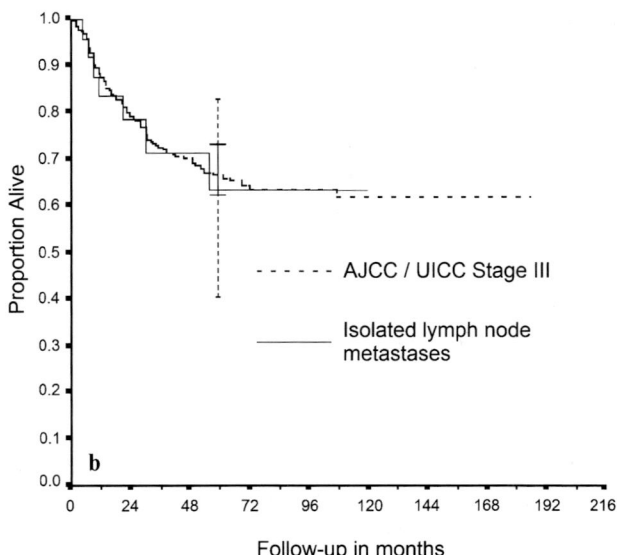

Figure 2 Probability of survival for nodal disease in STS. *A*, Data from the Royal Marsden Hospital, United Kingdom, indicating that patients with isolated regional lymph node metastases fare much better, and some may have long-term survival compared with patients with synchronous distant metastases. Reproduced with permission from Behranwala KA et al.[14] *B*, Data from the Princess Margaret Hospital, Toronto, Canada, indicating that patients with isolated regional lymph node metastases have a similar survival compared with patients presenting with stage III disease. Reproduced with permission from Riad S et al.[15]

Synovial sarcoma also differs from other STS in several respects. For example, it has a reputation for more favourable responses to chemotherapy than most other histologies and has higher risk of lymph node metastasis (< 2–14%).[12,13] It also exhibits unique behavioural features apparently governed by mechanisms linked to molecular characteristics (see below).

Dermatofibrosacoma protruberans (DFSP) is a borderline to low-grade tumor with propensity for local recurrence after simple excision. Its indolence has rendered it exempt from the TNM stage classification system. Malignant mesenchymoma (a diagnostic term no longer in use) is also no longer included in TNM, again illustrating the problem of classical histological typing. For different reasons again, angiosarcoma was also recently excluded from the TNM stage classification largely because its natural history with sinister pattern of growth makes it difficult to control locally (in part owing to difficulty determining the optimal extent of surgical and radiotherapy margins from gross tumor), and because of its propensity to lymph node and distant metastases (at times resembling multifocality) that differ from the general behavior of STS.

Classical rhabdomyosarcoma (RMS) also differs from other STS, being well represented in childhood and less commonly in the adult, where the outcome is significantly less favorable.[17] It commonly involves regional lymph nodes, and rarely but distinctly, there is a tendency for these lesions to develop leptomeningeal disease (in parameningeal lesions), bone marrow involvement, and even synchronous or metachronous metastases in one or both breasts, thereby underlies their unique natural history and different prognosis to other STS. Myxoid liposarcoma has an unusual pattern of recurrence of apparent multifocal presentation or recurrence at two or more anatomically separate soft tissue sites (with predilection for the retroperitoneum and mediastinum) that contrasts with other STS.[18] More favorable survival in a large cohort of liposarcoma patients compared with other histological subtypes was recently reported in a series exceeding 1,000 cases. The observation was independent of other prognostic factors, including grade, depth, and tumor size.[19] Myxoid liposarcoma also appears to manifest an unusually sensitive response to radiotherapy,[18] which may explain the propensity for unexpectedly favorable local control following adjuvant radiotherapy.[20]

Perhaps the best example of unique STS pathology and association with aberrant biological behavior is provided by gastrointestinal stromal tumors (GIST). These lesions have a poor prognosis and rarely respond to conventional systemic chemotherapy. However, they also represent the first solid tumor with a consistent favorable response to molecular targeted therapy in the form of imatinib (Gleevec) that is discussed below (see section, "Specific Molecular Expressions"). The most important prognostic factors for GIST are tumor size, mitotic rate, and the extent of tumor necrosis. In a phase III trial, presence of pulmonary metastases, potential tumor factors such as initial low hemoglobin and low albumin before treatment (related to the influence of disease burden on the host, or alternatively as host factors), nonstomach primary, and a small number of lesions were prognostic for progression within 3 months after treatment initiation.[21]

GISTs also offer additional insights into treatment-related biology in that drug resistance has been studied extensively. Prognostic factors in imatinib-treated GIST patients include overexpression of drug efflux pumps, which confers resistance against imatinib in preclinical models, or activity of imatinib-metabolising enzymes such CYP3A4.[21]

Gene Expression Profiling

With advances in molecular characterization of STS, and the emerging dissatisfaction with traditional methods of classification, researchers have found that a variety of STS subtypes display remarkably distinct and homogenous gene expression profiles.[22] For example, in liposarcoma and malignant fibrous histiocytoma, the two most common histological subtypes, Baird and colleagues found potential clinical differences that could reflect on prognostic outcome.[22] Liposarcomas separate into two divergent groups using unsupervised hierarchical clustering, one being tightly clustered and considered lower-grade lesions, comprising myxoid, round-cell, or well-differentiated tumors. The remainder was dispersed among the malignant fibrous histiocytoma tumors and considered higher-grade tumors, with samples classified as dedifferentiated or pleomorphic liposarcomas. Weighted gene analysis exhibited gene expressions associated with cell adhesion, invasion, cell death, chemotherapy resistance, and metastases among the higher-grade tumor group (Figure 3A).[22]

Similarly, unsupervised hierarchical cluster analysis of malignant fibrous histiocytoma identified two groups where subsequent weighted gene analysis elicited differentially expressed genes carrying a muscle profile in the first group, whereas the second group of tumors revealed an abundance of immune regulatory genes (see Figure 3B). Gene ontology profiling showed that genes expressed in the first group belonged to the ontologic family of motor activity, and the second group of genes belonged to the ontologic family of immune activity and cell adhesion (see Figure 3C). The presence of myogenic differentiation in malignant fibrous histiocytoma and

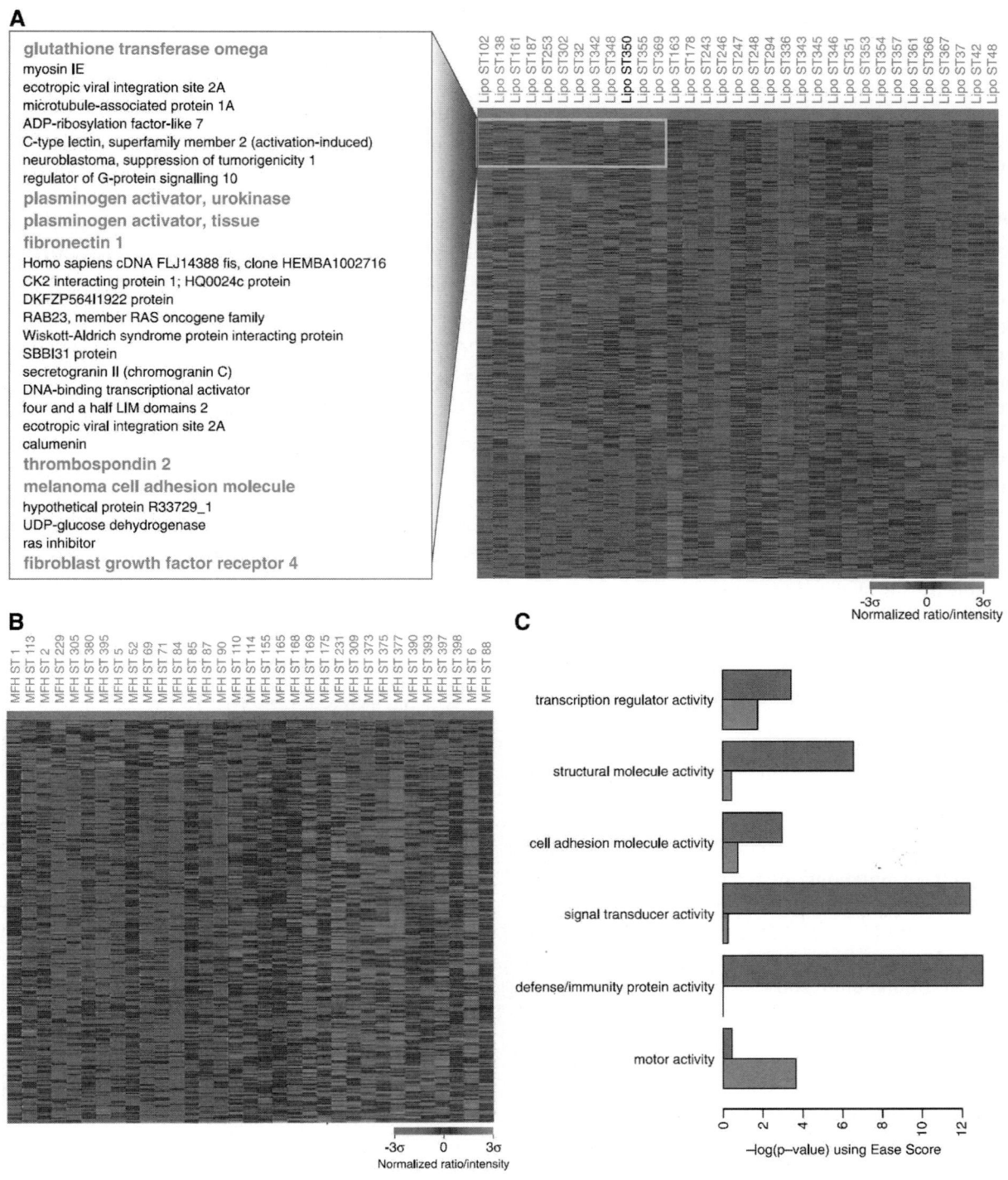

Figure 3 Heat maps and ontologic evaluation of liposarcoma and malignant fibrous histiocytoma. *A*, Weighted gene analysis for the two subgroups of liposarcoma (higher grade indicated by red bar on the left; blue bar indicates lower-grade lesions). The higher-grade liposarcoma indicated by the red bar on the left portion of the heat map reveal that among the most highly weighted genes associated with the higher-grade liposarcomas are several genes known to be associated with cell adhesion, invasion, and metastases. *B*, Weighted gene analysis of the two malignant fibrous histiocytoma groups. The red bar on the left of the diagram indicates tumors with a predominance of muscle-related genes; the blue bar shows the tumors exhibiting an inflammatory profile. *C*, Ontologic evaluation of the two groups of malignant fibrous histiocytoma tumors. The first group (red column) has an abundance of genes associated with muscle and motor activity and presumed to have less favorable prognosis (see text), whereas the second group (blue column) carries an inflammatory profile. Graphs are plotted based on the negative log of the P value of the hypergeometric distribution. Reproduced with permission from Baird K et al.[22]

undifferentiated sarcomas could be clinically relevant, as this feature has been shown to correlate with a more adverse prognosis.[22] It can be anticipated that these methods may enhance or replace "classical" methods of diagnosing or defining subtypes of STS and enhance their prognostic discrimination.

Specific Molecular Expressions

Specific molecular parameters that have been evaluated for prognostic significance include p53, mdm2, and altered expression of the retinoblastoma gene product (pRb).[23] Of these, the most widely studied is Ki-67, a marker of proliferation. but results have also been conflicting, especially when the effect of other factors is taken into account.

In synovial sarcoma, the t(x;18) translocation can almost invariably be detected with the demonstration of a fusion between the SSX and SYT genes, providing a very useful diagnostic tool that is also associated with the two morphological forms of this disease (the SSX1 associated with monophasic histology and the SSX2 gene with biphasic histology). The specific molecular subtypes of the SYT-SSX fusion transcripts have also been associated with prognostic discrimination,[24] although the evidence has recently been overshadowed by observations that morphologically determined tumor grade may override this.[25]

The most dramatic example of molecular prognostic information in STS is represented by GISTs. These lesions harbor so-called gain-of-function mutations in the c-kit or platelet-derived growth factor-α receptor (PDGFRA) genes in 85% and 5% of cases, respectively. Through these mutations, the receptors are constitutively activated, leading to malignant behavior. Patients whose tumors contained exon 11 KIT mutations are more likely to respond to imatinib than those whose tumors have an exon 9 KIT mutation or those with no detectable kinase mutation. Because it appears to govern both the response to specific therapies and represents the initial pathogenetic mechanism, the type of mutation in GIST makes it both a true prognostic marker and a target for intervention. This prognostic observation is notable because of its significance in the influence of histology and biological specificity on decision making in a manner that has not been present previously. Other molecular factors of prognostic importance include several particular DNA copy number alterations, loss of p16 protein, and methylation of the E-cadherin gene.[21]

Another example of molecular-targeted therapy is DFSP, where the presence of t(17;22) translocation in DFSP may predict response to imatinib.[26] Again, this underlines the variable prognosis and rapport between biological processes and histologic subtype through

features that, in part, manifest morphologically by the way lesions are graded.

Tumor Microenvironment

The microenvironment of STSs has been studied. Tissue hypoxia, assessed in various ways, including directly or by CA IX assessment, appears associated with the development of distant metastases independently from depth, size, and grade.[27] At present, useful therapeutic strategies to exploit these findings remain unproven.

COMBINING TUMOR-RELATED FACTORS (THE TNM SYSTEM)

A universally applicable classification based on the tumor-related prognostic factors is desirable. As for many cancers, a classification based predominantly on anatomic factors is the most stable and consistent system for staging STSs and predicting their outcome. The most widely used system for classification is that of the AJCC and the UICC, which partitions the anatomic aspects into those addressing the extent of the primary tumor (T-categories), regional node metastasis (N-categories), and distant metastasis (M-categories) in the TNM classification (Table 2). STS is also almost exceptional in that the TNM classification incorporates a marker of biologic activity (ie, grade), though the incorporation of other factors such as histology, molecular factors, and other indices remains an elusive goal. All soft tissue sarcoma subtypes are included except visceral sarcomas, where an international system is lacking, and certain histologic subtypes noted earlier. Despite this, it is notable that extent of disease remains a major determinant of outcome, even if there is no applicable current staging classification; for example, tumor size and distant metastases are certainly prognostic in GIST.[21]

As for all cancer types, the categories that comprise the TNM system are compiled into prognostic stage groups (see Table 2). The STS TNM system is based on an ascending hierarchy of risk, depending on whether a lesion is deemed to have no adverse features for relapse or 1, 2, or 3 factors present represented by size partitioned at the 5 cm break point, grade (high vs low), and lesion depth as "a" (superficial tumor arising outside the investing fascia) or "b" (a deep tumor that arises beneath the fascia or invades the fascia). Using these criteria, 4 TNM prognostic groups have been compiled that originally showed probabilities of remaining free of distant metastasis at 12 years of 85 ± 8.7%, 69.3 ± 7.3%, 57.1 ± 6.2%, and 24.8 ± 4.0%, respectively.[28] Similar differences were also seen in the survival probabilities and led to the current TNM classification.

Table 2 TNM Staging System of the International Union against Cancer (UICC) and the American Joint Committee on Cancer (AJCC)

T – Primary Tumor

T0	No evidence of primary tumor
T1	Tumor 5 cm or less in greatest dimension
	T1a Superficial tumor*
	T1b Deep tumor*
T2	Tumor more than 5 cm in greatest dimension
	T2a Superficial tumor*
	T2b Deep tumor*

N – Regional Lymph Nodes

N0	No regional lymph node metastasis
N1	Regional lymph node metastasis

M – Distant Metastasis

M0	No distant metastasis
M1	Distant metastasis

G—Histopathologic Grade

Low grade
High grade

Stage Grouping

Stage IA	Low grade	T1a	N0	M0
	Low grade	T1b	N0	M0
Stage IB	Low grade	T2a	N0	M0
	Low grade	T2b	N0	M0
Stage IIA	High grade	T1a	N0	M0
	High grade	T1b	N0	M0
Stage IIB	High grade	T2a	N0	M0
Stage III	High grade	T2b	N0	M0
Stage IV	Any	Any T	N1	M0
	Any	Any T	Any N	M1

*Superficial tumor is located exclusively above the superficial fascia without invasion of the fascia; deep tumor is located either exclusively beneath the superficial fascia, superficial to the fascia with invasion of or through the fascia, or both superficial yet beneath the fascia.
Adapted from Sobin and Wittekind [2] and Greene FL et al.[3]

Formal statistical analysis has shown that the current TNM system was superior to the previous edition of TNM and to the Surgical Staging System of the Musculoskeletal Tumor Society, but was not superior to a staging system in use at MSKCC in predicting systemic relapse in patients with localized extremity STS.[5] Although it is interesting that the two systems that incorporate tumor size, grade, and depth were the most predictive (ie, TNM and MSKCC systems), one must be cautious since the validation of these staging systems was done at the same institution whose research led to their creation. As noted earlier, it may be also useful to add additional size break points in the classification in the future.

A final comment concerns inclusion of resection margins in staging systems and treatment algorithms that address local recurrence.[10] One problem with such a proposal is that staging systems generally address survival alone. Also, although the pathologic TNM classification system could accommodate resection margin as a factor, a correlate in the clinical TNM system (which requires no treatment to have taken place yet) is not available.

Similarly, prognostic variables for prediction of primary curative management are ordinarily determined at baseline, and the resection margin status would not be known at the time a patient presents prior to first treatment.

Treatment/Environment-Related Prognostic Factors

Ironically, the outcome of the patient with STS may be as much related to the setting in which the patient finds him or herself as to specific features of the tumor or the patient. Intercountry differences in survival exist, and regional differences in care may result in adverse outcomes for certain end points.[1] In truth, evidence would appear to support multidisciplinary pretreatment evaluation and management in specialized centers. Patients with extremity STS managed outside of specialty centers had a higher rate of local recurrence than patients treated entirely in specialty centers.[23] A population-based study from the Netherlands reported that initial treatment was based on an erroneous diagnosis in 37% of cases of retroperitoneal sarcoma, with these patients less likely to have complete tumor resection.[23]

In STS, perhaps more than most cancers, the treatment pathway may have been influenced by events that have already taken place. For example, the type of biopsy performed or a prior inappropriate excision may jeopardize the form and outcome of local treatment thereafter.[1]

Another problem concerns how to choose cases for different treatments when more than one option exists, including employing combined modality approaches. Many tumors are readily managed by surgery alone with excellent results, but the variability of sarcoma presentations may provide inconsistent and problematic decisions in this regard in nonspecialty centers. In Scandinavia, long the proponent of surgery alone without radiotherapy for extremity STS, there has been a recent change to an increase in the use of radiotherapy in all tumors, but especially for deep lesions. Not surprisingly, this observation is associated with a reduction in the rate of amputation. Moreover, the change is also associated with alterations in referral patterns and improvement in local control and survival at the Karolinska Hospital in Stockholm, Sweden, where radiotherapy is used more often than at other centers in Scandinavia. This is presently under active scrutiny at the level of the Scandinavian Sarcoma Group Registry.[23]

Patient-Related Prognostic Factors

Intrinsic or acquired patient factors also may affect the outcome of STS. Depending on the end point chosen, patient age may influence outcome,[7] even though patients are usually relatively young, and we already noted that rhabdomyosarcoma in the pediatric population fares better than in the adult.[17] Underlying medical conditions may also affect STS outcome, such as albumin or hemoglobin levels, presumed to be surrogates for *host* debility. In patients with malignant peripheral nerve sheath tumor, staging and follow-up of the peripheral nerve sheath tumor are confounded by the detection of other nodules and masses that often prove to be benign neurofibromas, but may be recurrent disease or a second sarcoma. For example, patients with a peripheral nerve sheath tumor may also have neurofibromatosis 1, which confers an unusually aggressive tumor behavior.[1] Another patient-related prognostic factor (an acquired factor) is radiation-induced STS. Radiation-induced sarcomas are associated with a particularly adverse prognosis, unrelated to the tumor-related characteristics of the new sarcoma and may be associated with a relative paucity of options within tissues previously irradiated, including wide local resection, which is often compromised, in addition to the inability to reirradiate safely.[23]

Table 3 Prognostic Factors in Previously Untreated Localized Soft Tissue Sarcomas

Prognostic Factors	Tumor Related	Host Related	Treatment/Environment Related
Essential	Anatomic site Histologic subtype Tumor size* Histologic grade* Depth of invasion Presence of metastases*		
Additional	Resection margin t(17;22) translocation in DFSP	Neurofibromatosis 1 (NF1) Radiation induced sarcomas Age	Quality of surgery and radiotherapy
New and promising	Ki-67 *TP53* SYT-SSX fusion transcript Tumor hypoxia		

*These variable are incorporated in the TNM staging classification.

Sources: NCCN Clinical Practice Guidelines in Oncology: Sarcoma 2005. <http://www.nccn.org/professionals/physician/sarcoma.pdf>.
ESMO Minimum Clinical Recommendations for diagnosis, treatment, and follow-up of soft tissue sarcoma 2005. >http://annonc.oupjournals.org/cgi/reprint/16/suppl_1/169>.
Note: The factors tabulated generally reflect survival outcome. Other end points may have direct bearing on the treatment to be given for alternative end points, but may not independently influence survival. An example is envelopment or invasion of neurovascular structures ± bone, and which would directly influence the need for amputation, and therefore would be essential factors for an end point such as limb preservation.
Adapted from O'Sullivan B and Catton CN.[23]

Relevance of Prognostic Factors in Clinical Practice

To consider the relevance of prognostic factors in STS clinical practice, prognostic factors have been subdivided into three distinct categories: essential, additional, and new and promising factors.[21,23] Essential factors are those that are fundamental to decisions about the goals and choice of treatment, and include details regarding the selection of treatment modality and specific interventions that should be based on published clinical practice guideline. Additional factors allow finer prognostication, but are not an absolute requirement for the treatment-related decision-making process. Their role is to communicate prognosis, but they do not in themselves influence treatment choice. Finally, new and promising factors are those that shed new light about the biology of disease, or the prognosis for patients, but for which currently there is, at best, incomplete evidence of an independent effect on outcome or prognosis.

Recent tabulations of prognostic factors have recognized the subject categories outlined earlier (tumor, host, and treatment/environment), but also include the clinical relevance strata noted above supported by published STS clinical practice guidelines.[21,23] Using this approach, it is noted that presently not many prognostic factors in STS are indispensable for good practice and reach the "essential" factor criterion. Indeed the only ones to acquiring this level of importance are extent of disease characteristics, grade, and anatomic site (Tables 3, 4, 5,

Table 4 Prognostic Factors in Metastatic Soft Tissue Sarcomas

Prognostic Factors	Tumor Related	Host Related	Treatment/Environment Related
Essential	Interval between diagnosis and metastases Low tumor burden (size and number of metastases)		
Additional			Complete tumor excision
New and promising			

Sources: NCCN Clinical Practice Guidelines in Oncology: Sarcoma 2005. <http://www.nccn.org/professionals/physician/sarcoma.pdf>.
National Cancer Institute: Sarcoma (PDQ): Treatment Guidelines 2005. <http://www.cancer.gov/cancertopics/pdq/treatment/adult-soft-tissue-sarcoma/healthprofessional/>.
Adapted from O'Sullivan B and Catton CN.[23]

Table 5 Prognostic Factors in Previously Untreated Gastrointestinal Stromal Tumors

Prognostic Factors	Tumor Related	Host Related	Treatment/Environment Related
Essential	Tumor size[29] Mitotic rate[29]		
Additional	Resection margin		Quality of surgery
New and promising	DNA copy number changes Loss of p16 protein Extent of tumor necrosis Presence of c-*kit* mutation Mutational site in c-*kit* or *PDGFRA* gene		Application of adjuvant treatment

Adapted from Sleijfer S and Verweij J.[21]

Table 6 Prognostic Factors in Metastatic Gastrointestinal Stromal Tumors

Prognostic Factors	Tumor Related	Host Related	Treatment/Environment Related
Essential	Mutational site in c-*kit* or *PDGFRA* gene Presence of lung metastases Large tumor burden		
Additional			Complete tumor excision
New and promising	Overexpression of drug efflux pumps	Activity of imatinib-metabolizing enzymes	

Adapted from Sleijfer S and Verweij J.[21]

and 6).[21,23] Of course it is important to emphasize that this is only one approach, and it could be misinterpreted as ignoring the important ongoing research that emphasizes the biology of sarcoma, and these may eventually uncover new "essential" categories. Such research should obviously not be discounted on the basis that it does not presently influence therapeutic decision making. We have briefly discussed these concepts in the sections above (see "Gene Expression Profiling" and "Specific Molecular Expressions"), and they serve to emphasize that such work must be supported with the ultimate goal of impacting on clinical management of all STS presentations and that may have potentially different end points.

References

1. O'Sullivan B, Pisters PW. Staging and prognostic factor evaluation in soft tissue sarcoma. Surg Oncol Clin N Am 2003;12:333–53.

2. Sobin L, Wittekind C. TNM classification of malignant tumours. 6th ed. New York: Wiley-Liss; 2002.

3. Greene FL, Page D, Norrow M, et al. AJCC cancer staging manual. 6th ed. New York: Springer; 2002.

4. McShane LM, Altman DG, Sauerbrei W, et al. Reporting recommendations for tumor marker prognostic studies (REMARK). J Natl Cancer Inst 2005;97:1180–4.

5. Wunder JS, Healey JH, Davis AM, Brennan MF. A comparison of staging systems for localized extremity soft tissue sarcoma. Cancer 2000;88:2721–30.

6. Ramanathan RC, A'Hern R, Fisher C, Thomas JM. Modified staging system for extremity soft tissue sarcomas. Ann Surg Oncol 1999;6:57–69.

7. Strander H, Turesson I, Cavallin-Stahl E. A systematic overview of radiation therapy effects in soft tissue sarcomas. Acta Oncol 2003;42:516–31.

8. Gerrand CH, Bell RS, Wunder JS, et al. The influence of anatomic location on outcome in patients with soft tissue sarcoma of the extremity. Cancer 2003;97:485–92.

9. Alektiar KM, Leung D, Zelefsky MJ, et al. Adjuvant brachytherapy for primary high-grade soft tissue sarcoma of the extremity. Ann Surg Oncol 2002;9:48–56.

10. Stojadinovic A, Leung DH, Hoos A, et al. Analysis of the prognostic significance of microscopic margins in 2,084 localized primary adult soft tissue sarcomas. Ann Surg 2002;235:424–34.

11. Gerrand CH, Wunder JS, Kandel RA, et al. Classification of positive margins after resection of soft-tissue sarcoma of the limb predicts the risk of local recurrence. J Bone Joint Surg [Br] 2001;83-B:1149–55.

12. Mazeron JJ, Suit HD. Lymph nodes as sites of metastases from sarcomas of soft tissue. Cancer 1987;60:1800–8.

13. Fong Y, Coit DG, Woodruff JM, Brennan MF. Lymph node metastasis from soft tissue sarcoma in adults. Analysis of data from a prospective database of 1772 sarcoma patients. Ann Surg 1993;217:72–7.

14. Behranwala KA, A'Hern R, Omar AM, Thomas JM. Prognosis of lymph node metastasis in soft tissue sarcoma. Ann Surg Oncol 2004;11:714–9.

15. Riad S, Griffin AM, Liberman B, et al. Lymph node metastasis in soft tissue sarcoma in an extremity. Clin Orthop Relat Res 2004;426:129–34.

16. Borden EC, Baker LH, Bell RS, et al. Soft tissue sarcomas of adults: state of the translational science. Clin Cancer Res 2003;9:1941–56.

17. La Quaglia MP, Heller G, Ghavimi F, et al. The effect of age at diagnosis on outcome in rhabdomyosarcoma. Cancer 1994;73:109–17.

18. Pitson G, Robinson P, Wilke D, et al. Radiation response: an additional unique signature of myxoid liposarcoma. Int J Radiat Oncol Biol Phys 2004;60:522–6.

19. Weitz J, Antonescu CR, Brennan MF. Localized extremity soft tissue sarcoma: improved knowledge with unchanged survival over time. J Clin Oncol 2003;21:2719–25.

20. Hatano H, Ogose A, Hotta T, et al. Treatment of myxoid liposarcoma by marginal or intralesional resection combined with radiotherapy. Anticancer Res 2003;23:3045–9.

21. Sleijfer S, Verweij J. Gastrointestinal stromal tumors. In: Gospodarowiz MK, O'Sullivan B, Sobin L, editors. Prognostic factors in cancer. 3rd ed. New York: Wiley; 2006. p. 187–91.

22. Baird K, Davis S, Antonescu CR, et al. Gene expression profiling of human sarcomas: insights into sarcoma biology. Cancer Res 2005;65:9226–35.

23. O'Sullivan B, Catton CN. Soft tissue sarcomas. In: Gospodarowiz MK, O'Sullivan B, Sobin L, editors. Prognostic factors in cancer. 3rd ed. New York: Wiley; 2006. p. 181–6.

24. Ladanyi M, Antonescu CR, Leung DH, et al. Impact of SYT-SSX fusion type on the clinical behavior of synovial sarcoma: a multi-institutional retrospective study of 243 patients. Cancer Res 2002;62:135–40.

25. Guillou L, Benhattar J, Bonichon F, et al. Histologic grade, but not SYT-SSX fusion type, is an important prognostic factor in patients with synovial sarcoma: a multicenter, retrospective analysis. J Clin Oncol 2004;22:4040–50.

26. McArthur GA, Demetri GD, van Oosterom A, et al. Molecular and clinical analysis of locally advanced dermatofibrosarcoma protuberans treated with imatinib:

Imatinib Target Exploration Consortium Study B2225. J Clin Oncol 2005;23:866–73.

27. Maseide K, Kandel RA, Bell RS, et al. Carbonic anhydrase IX as a marker for poor prognosis in soft tissue sarcoma. Clin Cancer Res 2004;10:4464–71.

28. Gaynor JJ, Tan CC, Casper ES, et al. Refinement of clinicopathologic staging for localized soft tissue sarcoma of the extremity: a study of 423 adults. J Clin Oncol 1992; 10:1317–29.

29. Blay J-Y, Bonvalot S, Casali P, et al. Consensus meeting for management of gastrointestinal stromal tumors. Report of the GIST Consensus Conference of 20–21 March 2004, under the auspices of ESMO. Ann Oncol 2005;16:566–78.

CHAPTER 71

SOFT TISSUE SARCOMA STAGING

BARRY W. FEIG, MD

Introduction

Soft tissue sarcomas are a rare tumor with approximately 8,000 new cases per year in the United States.[1] This group of tumors represents a variety of histologic subtypes. Although there are many similar biologic behaviors shared by the group, there are also a number of clinical patterns that are unique to each specific histologic subtype. It is this rarity and unique nature of soft tissue sarcomas that makes staging a difficult task.

Soft tissue sarcomas are derived embryologically from mesenchymal origin. Because of this derivation, these tumors can involve connective tissue, viscera, and integument and can occur anywhere throughout the body. Approximately two-thirds occur in the extremity, whereas one-third occur in the trunk, retroperitoneum, abdomen, or other locations. As a general rule, the overall survival for patients diagnosed with soft tissue sarcoma is approximately 50% at 5 years.

Surgical excision remains the definitive treatment of soft tissue sarcomas. However, owing to the poor overall survival rate, as mentioned above, chemotherapy and/or radiotherapy are also frequently employed as part of the treatment regimens for this disease. In order to appropriately incorporate these therapeutic modalities into treatment planning, it is necessary to have a staging system that accurately reflects the behavior and outcome of patients with soft tissue sarcoma. Only with accurate staging systems will clinical trials be effective in defining the appropriate use of chemotherapy and radiotherapy in patients with localized, primary disease.

Although local recurrence and distant metastases are a common problem with soft tissue sarcoma, there are patients with these clinical scenarios who can still be successfully salvaged. Local recurrence is not necessarily a forbearance of rapid systemic failure. Many patients with local recurrence of soft tissue sarcoma can still have a significant disease-free interval following effective treatment. In addition, despite the fact that the majority of patients with distant metastases have a poor clinical outcome, there are still approximately 30% of patients who can have a 5-year survival with combined modality therapy. It, therefore, behooves us to find effective staging strategies to define those patients who will benefit from extensive multimodality treatment while avoiding toxic life-altering therapy in patients who have no reasonable chance of responding.

Etiology

No clearly defined etiology has been established for soft tissue sarcomas. There are several clinical scenarios that are known to predispose the development of soft tissue sarcomas, as well as recently identified genetic factors that may play a role in the etiology as well as the behavior of these tumors.

High-dose ionizing radiation has long been known to have a causal relationship with the establishment of soft tissue sarcomas. The most common radiation-induced sarcomas are extraskeletal osteosarcoma (21%), malignant fibrohistiocytoma (16%), and angiosarcoma (15%). The majority of the radiation-induced sarcomas are aggressive, high-grade tumors.[2]

Lymphedema is another known causative factor for the development of lymphangiosarcoma. The syndrome of lymphangiosarcoma developing in a lymphadematous arm status postmastectomy was first described by Stewart and Treves in 1948.[3] Immunocompromised patients, such as those with HIV and organ transplant recipients, have been found to have an increased incidence of sarcomas as well.

Most recently, the majority of the scientific investigation into the etiology of sarcoma has centered on molecular pathologic prognostic factors. These have included both mutations in tumor suppressor genes, as well as oncogenes. The most heavily studied of these include the *TP53* gene and the retinoblastoma gene.[4,5] In addition, cytogenetic malformations have been identified with specific soft tissue sarcomas, such as Ewing's sarcoma, primitive neuroectodermal tumors (PNET), myxoid liposarcoma, alveolar rhabdomyosarcoma, desmoplastic round-cell tumor, and synovial sarcoma.[6-8] These cytogenetic abnormalities are now frequently used to help establish and/or confirm specific histologic diagnoses. Additionally, these specific genetic and molecular alterations are potential future sites for specific targeted therapy.

The involvement of soft tissue sarcomas as a component of inherited cancer syndromes gives further evidence to the importance of the molecular basis for sarcoma pathogenesis. Syndromes that have soft tissue sarcomas as one of the histopathologic features include Li-Fraumeni syndrome, Gardner's syndrome, Wermer's syndrome, Carney's triad, neurofibromatosis type I (von Recklinghausen's disease), and retinoblastoma.

Staging

The identification of accurate and predictable criteria for staging soft tissue sarcomas is imperative to be able to group patients appropriately for clinical trials, report responses to specific treatments, and specifically define prognostic outcome for patients. Unfortunately, the rarity of this tumor type, as well as the variety of histologic subtypes (many with their own unique behaviors and characteristics) has made it extremely difficult to come up with a simplified staging system that encompasses all the tissue types within this broad category of soft tissue sarcoma. Having an established and reproducible staging system is even more important in a rare disease like soft tissue sarcoma, in part, owing to the fact that clinical trials can accrue adequate numbers of patients only with the participation of multiple

centers. Obviously, a reproducible staging system is critical to ensure that all centers in a clinical trial are entering similar patients for evaluation.

These factors have resulted in multiple staging systems being employed for soft tissue sarcomas. The two most commonly used systems are the American Joint Committee on Cancer (AJCC) system[9] and the Musculoskeletal Tumor Society system.[10] The latter is most predominately used by orthopedic oncologists and is shown in Table 1. The most current AJCC system (sixth edition) is shown in Table 2. The presence of multiple staging systems for soft tissue sarcomas further emphasizes the need for a single comprehensive, accurate staging system for this disease.

Despite the fact that the original AJCC staging system was described in 1982, it wasn't until the fourth edition of the staging manual in 1992 that soft tissue sarcoma was included as a specific disease site. Even since that time, there have been several revisions to the soft tissue sarcoma staging within the AJCC staging manual. The initial staging in the fourth edition was based on the grade of the primary soft tissue sarcoma, with stage I being grade 1 tumors, stage 2 being grade 2 tumors, and stage 3 being grade 3 or 4 tumors. Stage 4 represents patients with metastatic disease (Table 3). The fifth edition of the AJCC staging manual took into account the information that there were factors in addition to grade that were important in determining prognosis and outcome. Both the size and location (superficial vs deep) of the primary tumor were now identified as important prognostic factors that were included in the staging criteria. This resulted in a more complex staging system with each stage level being subdivided by both histologic

Table 1 Surgical Staging System by Musculoskeletal Tumor Society

Stage	Grade	Local Extent	Metastasis
I-A	Low	Intracompartmental	None
I-B	Low	Extracompartmental	None
II-A	High	Intracompartmental	None
II-B	High	Extracompartmental	None
III	Any	Any	Present

Table 2 AJCC Staging Manual 4th Edition

IA	G1	T1	N0	M0
IB	G1	T2	N0	M0
IIA	G2	T1	N0	M0
IIB	G2	T2	N0	M0
IIIA	G3-4	T1	N0	M0
IIIB	G3-4	T2	N0	M0
IVA	Any G	Any T	N1	M0
IVB	Any G	Any T	Any N	M1

680 / Advanced Therapy in Surgical Oncology

Table 3 AJCC Staging Manual 5th Edition

IA	G1-2	T1a-b	N0	M0
IB	G1-2	T2a	N0	M0
IIA	G1-2	T2a-b	N0	M0
IIB	G3-4	T1a-b	N0	M0
IIC	G3-4	T2a	N0	M0
III	G3	T2b	N0	M0
IV	Any G	Any T	N1	M0
	Any G	Any T	N0	M1

grade and location. The most recent version of AJCC staging manual (sixth edition) has attempted to simplify the staging categories of soft tissue sarcomas, while still taking into account the complex interrelationship between size, grade, and location of the presenting tumors. These changes have been based on the information obtained from retrospective reviews of large prospective clinical databases, most notably the National Cancer Database of the American College of Surgeons, as well as the Memorial Sloan-Kettering Cancer Center sarcoma database. It is clear from these changes that have occurred over subsequent editions of the AJCC staging manual that we are still learning about the importance of all these prognostic factors, as well as their interrelationships. Only through future careful evaluation of the information from these large databases will we be able to modify and improve our ability to stage and prognosticate the outcome for patients with soft tissue sarcoma.

The specifics of the AJCC staging system are a combination of both clinical and pathologic findings. Pathologic grading is based on the microscopic assessment of presurgical resection biopsy or the surgical specimen itself. Unfortunately, no standardized pathologic criteria are available for the grading of soft tissue sarcomas. A grade is assigned based on a number of pathologic findings, including degree of differentiation, cellularity, mitotic activity, degree of necrosis, and nuclear atypia. This lack of specific defined pathologic criteria has resulted in a high degree of discordance (25–40%) even among expert sarcoma pathologists when assigning histologic grade.[11] It is also common for sarcomas to have significant intratumoral heterogeneity, which can lead to sampling artifacts, particularly when needle biopsies are used to obtain tissue for diagnosis. This is most commonly seen in patients with large retroperitoneal liposarcomas. These tumors will frequently have large areas that appear to be low grade, but can often have small areas of dedifferentiation scattered throughout these low-grade areas. Additionally, histologic subtype needs to be specified for each tumor, and again there is a lack of consistency among sarcoma pathology experts in establishing this

categorization. Multiple additional procedures are often used, including immunohistochemical analysis cytogenetics and electron microscopy, as well as expert peer review to more consistently define histopathologic subtypes in soft tissue sarcomas. Of note, histopathologic subtypes including Kaposi's sarcoma, dermatofibrosarcoma protuberans, desmoid tumors, and sarcomas arising from the dura mater, brain, and viscera are not included in the AJCC staging system. This is due to the fact that these histologic subtypes frequently behave in a unique manner that is dissimilar from the standard behavior of the majority of soft tissue sarcomas. The AJCC staging system uses a grading schema with 4 levels. Grade 1 tumors are defined as well differentiated, grade 2 tumors are moderately differentiated, grade 3 tumors are poorly differentiated, and grade 4 tumors are poorly differentiated or undifferentiated. Three-tiered grading systems also exist, where grade 1 is considered low grade, grade 2 considered intermediate grade, and grade 3 considered high grade. Frequently in the 4-tiered systems, grades 1 and 2 have been considered low grades, whereas grades 3 and 4 are considered high grade. This variability in the grading system only further serves to emphasize the need for standard pathologic evaluation.

Tumor size is also one of the important staging components and a strong predictor of metastases and overall survival. Additionally, data do exist to suggest that primary tumor size greater than 10 cm is a risk factor of subsequent local recurrence. The AJCC staging system defines T1 tumors as those less than or equal to 5 cm and T2 tumors as those greater than 5 cm. Although the AJCC staging system allows tumor size to be determined either by radiologic or physical examination, it is clear that a more accurate evaluation of tumor size is obtained from carefully performed radiologic studies. The tumor size (T) in the AJCC system is further subdivided by the location (depth) of the primary soft tissue sarcoma. Depth of the primary tumor is defined by the location of the tumor relative to the investing fascia at the site of the primary tumor's location. Superficial tumors are designated with an "a" next to the T in the staging system and are defined as a lesion that does not involve the superficial investing muscular fascia. Deep sarcomas are either deep to, or involving the superficial fascia and designated with a "b" next to the T in the staging system. Obviously, all retroperitoneal, intraperitoneal, and intrathoracic tumors are defined as deep lesions.

The presence (N1) or absence (N0) of regional lymph node involvement is an important, albeit rare finding in patients with soft tissue sarcoma. Lymph node involvement with metastatic sarcoma may be suspected on the basis of radiographic evaluation, but must be confirmed by histologic analysis. In the current sixth edition of the AJCC Staging Manual, the presence of regional lymph node involvement is considered stage 4 disease. However, recent studies suggest that lymph node involvement may not result in as poor an outcome as that seen in patients with metastatic disease, with which they are now grouped.[12,13] These studies suggest that patients with lymph node metastases may have outcomes that are similar to patients with AJCC stage 3 disease rather than those with stage 4 disease. This further implies that directed clinical therapy toward the nodal basin may be appropriate in histologic subtypes that are more prone to spread to the lymphatics. Potential clinical interventions would include lymphatic mapping and sentinel lymph node biopsy in patients with histologic subtypes shown to have a predilection for spreading to the lymph nodes, as well as regional lymphadenectomy in patients with documented lymph node involvement.

It is clear that the presence of distant metastases (designated as M1 in the AJCC staging system) is the single strongest predictive factor of survival in patients with soft tissue sarcoma. Although in the current sixth edition of the staging system, both patients with nodal disease and distant metastases are designated as stage 4, further prospective evaluation could potentially result in subsequent changes in the future to the staging system, where patients with isolated nodal involvement would be classified as AJCC stage 3, as suggested by the contemporary analyses mentioned above.

Defining the TNM Components

There is no well-defined clinical scenario associated with the diagnosis of soft tissue sarcomas. The most common finding at presentation is a painless, enlarging mass. Although historically there have been attempts to associate trauma with the development of soft tissue sarcomas, no cause and effect relationship has ever been able to be established. Most likely, a specific episode of trauma serves only to call attention to the presence of the mass in that area. The size of the soft tissue sarcoma at presentation can vary significantly. Tumors of the distal limbs and the head and neck frequently present at small

sizes, as these tumors tend to be identified earlier by patients owing to relatively small, superficial compartments in which they exist. In contrast, tumors of the thigh and retroperitoneum can become extremely large before they are detected. In general, soft tissue sarcomas expand circumferentially, creating a tumor pseudocapsule that consists of a zone of compression of surrounding normal tissue. As a tumor enlarges, localized symptoms such as paresthesia, distal edema, or obstruction may become apparent. The growth rate of sarcomas can be extremely variable, ranging from extremely slow, as seen with a low-grade liposarcoma, to extremely rapid, as seen with high-grade infiltrating tumors such as malignant fibrous hysticytoma and synovial sarcoma.

In general, it is recommended that diagnostic imaging be performed prior to initiating any basic procedure including biopsy. This is to avoid creating imaging artifacts that would decrease the sensitivity of the radiologic studies. The specific radiologic tests that should be performed are based on the findings on clinical examination. Radiologic studies are useful in determining the local and regional extent of the primary tumor. Additionally, radiologic studies can sometimes aid in the determination of histologic diagnosis by suggesting histologic subtypes that have a classic appearance on radiologic imaging studies. For example, plain radiographs may be useful in ruling out primary bone neoplasms or to identify calcifications that can be characteristic of synovial sarcoma. Additionally, computed tomographic (CT) scan of the abdomen often can identify the classic low-grade hypodense fat seen in retroperitoneal liposarcomas. Specific radiologic exams are frequently dictated by the site of the primary tumor. For example, for tumors of the abdomen or retroperitoneum, CT scan is usually performed in order to delineate the exact location of the tumor in relationship to surrounding structures. Magnetic resonance imaging (MRI) may be useful for specific anatomic evaluation, most notably the relationship to major vascular and neurologic structures. For tumors presenting the extremity, MRI is often the radiologic diagnostic test of choice, as the relationship of these tumors to the neurovascular bundles is one of the most critical initial evaluations necessary to determine resectability.[14] Frequently, ultrasound may be helpful in defining the cystic nature of certain pseudotumors such as popliteal cysts, synovial cysts, abscesses, or vascular malformations. Although a chest radiograph is useful as a screening tool to evaluate for the presence of metastatic disease to the lungs, CT scan of the thorax should be employed in patients with high-grade tumors to rule out metastatic disease prior to embarking on definitive treatment regimens. Although recent technological advances in diagnostic imaging techniques have become available, including dynamic enhanced MRI, PET scanning, magnetic resonance spectroscopy, and MR angiography, these specific techniques have not been proven to provide treatment-altering information at this time. Further prospective evaluation is needed to determine whether these imaging modalities can be useful in certain circumstances, such as assessing the viability of tumor following new areas of treatment or better defining the relationship of the tumor to important anatomic structures.

Several notable changes have been included in the most recent sixth edition of the AJCC cancer staging manual. These include the deletion of the histologic subtypes, angiosarcoma and malignant mesenchymoma from the list of histologic subtypes, owing to their distinctly different biologic behavior. In contrast, gastro-intestinal stromal tumor (GIST) and Ewing's sarcoma are now recognized as distinct histologic entities. Fibrosarcoma grade 1 has been replaced by fibromatosis (desmoid tumor) and is not included in the histologic subtypes owing to the fact that desmoids lack metastatic potential. Lastly, tumors designated as G1-2 T2b N0 M0

tumors have been moved from stage 2 to stage 1 based on recently recognized more favorable biologic behavior of these tumors (Table 4).

Future Considerations

There are many clinical factors that occur in patients with soft tissue sarcoma that the AJCC staging system does not incorporate. These include the site of the primary tumor, the margin status at the time of resection, molecular markers, recurrent versus primary tumor, and the definition of tumor size as a continuous variable. Although not included in the AJCC staging system, many of these factors have been shown to influence patient outcome based on retrospective clinical studies, as well as clinical acumen. It is clear that survival rates are affected by many factors, including anatomic location of the primary tumor, anatomic constraints to resection, margin status, and underlying tumor biologic behavior. A recent study from The University of Texas M. D. Anderson Cancer Center has shown that the site of the primary tumor or local recurrence has specific survival implications in an evaluation of 402 patients

Table 4 AJCC Staging Manual 6th Edition

STAGE				
I	G1-2	T1a-b, T2a-b	N0	M0
II	G3-4	T1a-b, T2a	N0	M0
III	G3-4	T2b	N0	M0
IV	Any G	Any T	N1	M0
	Any G	Any T	N1	M0
	Any G	Any T	N0	M1

Primary Tumor (T)		
TX		Primary tumor cannot be assessed
T0		No evidence of primary tumor
T1	T1a superficial tumor	Tumor 5 cm or less in greatest dimension
	T1b deep tumor	
T2	T2a superficial tumor	Tumor more than 5 cm in greatest dimension
	T2b deep tumor	

Regional Lymph Nodes (N)	
NX	Regional lymph nodes cannot be assessed
N0	No regional lymph node metastasis
N1	Regional lymph node metastasis

Distant Metastasis (M)	
MX	Distant metastasis cannot be assessed
M0	No distant metastasis

Histologic Grade (G)	
GX	Grade cannot be assessed
G1	Well differentiated
G2	Moderately differentiated
G3	Poorly differentiated
G4	Poorly differentiated or undifferentiated

with relapsed soft tissue sarcomas.[15] Margin status has been identified as a potential prognostic factor in studies from both Memorial Sloan-Kettering Cancer Center, as well as from M. D. Anderson.[16,17] The importance of local recurrence as a prognostic factor has also been identified in a number of large studies from centers of excellence in sarcoma care.[18] Many investigators have correctly observed that the influence of size on outcome is a continuous variable and that further discrimination of the prognostic significance of tumor size may be obtained by a more specific breakdown of size; specifically, tumors greater than 10 cm and 15 cm may have additional prognostic implications.[19,20]

Conclusions

Sarcomas are a rare group of tumors that present a variety of unique problems to staging. This rare nature places an increased importance on standardized evaluation and reporting. Unfortunately, this is made extremely difficult by the variety of histologic subtypes as well as the unique behavior for many of these different tumors. The AJCC staging system is the most commonly used staging system for soft tissue sarcomas; however, even within this standardized staging system there are several exceptions for sarcomas, such as the addition of grade and depth to the standard TNM classification. These additional prognostic factors have been identified through the use of large prospective sarcoma-specific databases. Current and future emphasis is being placed on the use of molecular-based techniques to help identify additional and more specific prognostic factors.

References

1. Jemal A, Murray T, Ward E, et al. Cancer statistics. Cancer J Clin 2005;55:10–30.

2. Brady MS, Gaynor JJ, Brennan MF. Radiation-associated sarcoma of bone and soft tissue. Arch Surg 1992;127:1379–85.

3. Stewart FW, Treves N. Lymphangiosarcoma in postmastectomy lymphedema: a report of six cases in elephantiasis chirurgica. Cancer 1948;1:64–81.

4. Hieken TJ, Das Gupta TK. Mutant p53 expression: a marker of diminished survival in well-differentiated soft tissue sarcoma. Clin Cancer Res 1996;2:1391–5.

5. Karpeh MS, Brennan MF, Cance WG, et al. Altered patterns of retinoblastoma gene product expression in adult soft-tissue sarcomas. Brit J Cancer 1995;72:986–91.

6. Ladanyi M, Antonescu CR, Leung DH, et al. Impact of SYT-SSX fusion type on the clinical behavior of synovial sarcoma: a multi-institutional retrospective study of 243 patients. Cancer Res 2002;62:135–40.

7. de Alava E, Kawai A, Healey JH, et al. EWS-FLI1 fusion transcript structure is an independent determinant of prognosis in Ewing's sarcoma. J Clin Oncol 1998;16:1248–55.

8. Zoubek A, Dockhorn-Dworniczak B, Delattre O, et al. Does expression of different EWS chimeric transcripts define clinically distinct risk groups of Ewing tumor patients? J Clin Oncol 1996;14:1245–51.

9. Greene FL, Page DL, Fleming ID, et al, editors. AJCC Cancer Staging Manual. 6th ed. New York: Springer-Verlag; 2002.

10. Enneking WF, Spanier SS, Goodman MA. A system for the surgical staging of musculoskeletal sarcoma. Clin Orthop Relat Res 1980;106–20.

11. Coindre JM, Trojani M, Contesso G, et al. Reproducibility of a histopathologic grading system for adult soft tissue sarcoma. Cancer 1986;58:306–9.

12. Riad S, Griffin AM, Liberman B, et al. Lymph node metastasis in soft tissue sarcoma in an extremity. Clin Ortho Related Res 2004;129–34.

13. Behranwala KA, A'Hern R, Omar AM, et al. Prognosis of lymph node metastasis in soft tissue sarcoma. Ann Surg Oncol 2004;11:714–9.

14. Demas BE, Heelan RT, Lane J, et al. Soft-tissue sarcomas of the extremities: comparison of MR and CT in determining the extent of disease. AJR Am J Roentgenol 1988;150:615–20.

15. Zagars GK, Ballo MT, Pisters PW, et al. Prognostic factors for disease-specific survival after first relapse of soft-tissue sarcoma: analysis of 402 patients with disease relapse after initial conservative surgery and radiotherapy. Int J Rad Oncol Biol Phys 2003;57:739–47.

16. Stojadinovic A, Leung DH, Hoos A, et al. Analysis of the prognostic significance of microscopic margins in 2,084 localized primary adult soft tissue sarcomas. Ann Surg 2002;235:424–34.

17. Zagars GK, Ballo MT, Pisters PW, et al. Prognostic factors for patients with localized soft-tissue sarcoma treated with conservation surgery and radiation therapy: an analysis of 225 patients. Cancer 2003;97:2530–43.

18. Eilber FC, Rosen G, Nelson SD, et al. High-grade extremity soft tissue sarcomas: factors predictive of local recurrence and its effect on morbidity and mortality. Ann Surg 2003;237:218–26.

19. Brennan MF. Staging of soft tissue sarcomas. Ann of Surg Oncol 1999;6:8–9.

20. Pisters PW, Leung DH, Woodruff J, et al. Analysis of prognostic factors in 1,041 patients with localized soft tissue sarcomas of the extremities. J Clin Oncol 1996;14:1679–89.

CHAPTER 72

SOFT TISSUE SARCOMA

MATTHEW T. BALLO, MD

GUNAR K. ZAGARS, MD

Introduction

The importance of a multidisciplinary approach to the treatment of patients with soft tissue sarcoma (STS) cannot be overemphasized. Over the years, radical and functionally debilitating surgical procedures have been largely replaced by combinations of conservative surgery and adjuvant radiation therapy. However, surgery performed by an inexperienced surgeon just prior to referral to a tertiary care center may jeopardize optimal treatment. Inappropriately placed biopsy scars or excisional biopsy through the tissue around gross tumor often contaminates large volumes of surrounding tissue, requiring complex surgical reresections. This in turn may complicate the delivery of adjuvant radiation therapy and compromise functional outcome. By routinely referring patients to a tertiary care center, minimally invasive biopsy techniques (eg, core needle biopsy) can be utilized, and patients can be evaluated for preoperative therapies or enrollment on clinical trials. Only through cooperation and mutual respect have surgical and radiation oncologists been able to minimize the functional impact of their treatments, but still obtain acceptable rates of local control for patients with STS.

Natural History and Local Tumor Growth Characteristics

To successfully eradicate STS, the surgical and radiation oncologist must understand its natural history. Radiation therapy, like surgery, is used to address local disease and its potential regional spread. To treat STS without appreciating its unique growth characteristics places patients at risk of local recurrence if treatment is too conservative, and at risk of functional morbidity if treatment is too radical.

Although growth rate depends on histological subtype and grade, the direction of local spread generally occurs along the path of least resistance. Growth begins radially, pushing surrounding tissues into a well-delineated "compression zone," which itself is surrounded by an area of inflammatory reaction, known as a "reactive zone." Combinations of these two zones create what is known as the "pseudocapsule," which invariably contains numerous points of microscopic tumor penetration.[1] Microscopically the reactive zone represents an area of edema, neovascularity, and inflammatory infiltrate that can be visualized on T2-weighted magnetic resonance (MR) imaging as peritumoral edema. Although it is tempting to base surgical resection margins on these MR findings, the extent of microscopic disease is not limited to these edematous areas, and tumor cells may extend up to 4 cm from the dominant contrast-enhancing tumor mass.[2] Any surgical procedure that removes less than this volume of tissue risks leaving viable tumor behind and necessitates adjuvant radiation therapy.

As STSs continue to grow, they typically respect major intermuscular septa and remain confined to the compartment of origin. This growth characteristic results in oblong-shaped tumors, as they grow in the longitudinal direction more than the radial direction. Though extracompartmental extension may occur after surgical manipulation, it is typically a late finding, as local extension occurs through perforating vascular channels.

Several histological subtypes are characterized by unique local growth patterns. Desmoid tumor and epithelioid sarcoma both lack the well-defined pseudocapsule described above, making complete surgical resection difficult. Malignant peripheral nerve sheath tumors may extend in an unpredictable manner along major nerve trunks, and angiosarcoma of the skin has a striking tendency for presentation with widespread dermal involvement that may be clinically occult.

Lymph node metastases are distinctly uncommon, generally occurring in only 5% of patients at diagnosis.[3]

treated postoperatively (48.2% vs 31.5%, $p = 0.07$) because fibrosis, joint stiffness, and edema adversely affect long-term function.[20]

From this data we have concluded that the sequencing of radiation therapy should be based on the site of disease and the likelihood of long-term radiation-related complications rather than the likelihood of local control, which is unrelated to radiation timing. In general, preoperative radiation is preferred because of the lower radiation dose and smaller radiation treatment fields. Although this treatment sequence may result in temporary acute wound problems, it ultimately results in fewer long-term complications.

Radiotherapy Technique

EXTERNAL BEAM

No single radiotherapy guideline can sufficiently address the diverse clinical presentations characteristic of STS. There are, however, general principles based on an understanding of local growth patterns and technical radiotherapy details that are applicable to most clinical situations.

At the time of radiotherapy planning, careful patient positioning and the use of immobilization devices can improve reproducibility and simplify radiation beam orientation. In general, parallel-opposed beams are suitable for extremity lesions, assuming the limb may be positioned appropriately. For retroperitoneal lesions, more complex beam orientations may assist in sparing critical organs while delivering full dose to the primary tumor.

In the preoperative setting, gross tumor is delineated using CT scan, and radiation is delivered to this volume and any additional tissue believed to harbor microscopic spread. It is important to map out the extent of peritumoral edema seen on MR images by either digitally fusing the images to the radiotherapy planning CT scan or manually verifying sufficient coverage by the radiation dose distribution. The required margin of irradiation around the grossly palpable or visible tumor is controversial, but 5 to 7 cm is our recommendation (Figures 1 and 2). In the transverse plane the margin of irradiation is necessarily narrower and is generally 2 to 3 cm. These guidelines may be modified to avoid circumferential irradiation of an entire extremity and spare a generous strip of soft tissue, thereby avoiding unnecessary morbidity. Additionally, care should be taken to not irradiate an entire joint capsule or major tendon. For nonextremity lesions, margins of irradiation have traditionally been much smaller, on the order of 2

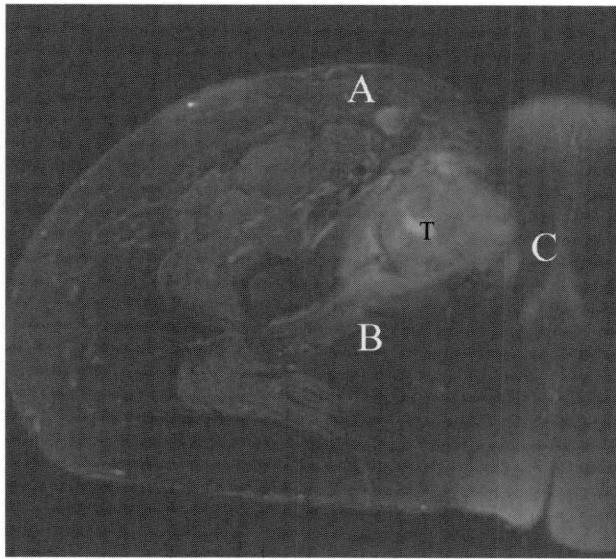

Figure 1 Representative T2-weighted MR image from a patient with an upper thigh soft tissue sarcoma. The dominant tumor mass (T) was associated with a reactive lymph node (A), peritumoral edema that extended toward the femur (B), and a small separate tumor nodule (C).

to 3 cm. The dose of preoperative irradiation is 50 Gy at 2 Gy per fraction.

In the postoperative setting, the appropriate target volume includes the entire surgical cavity, scar, and drain holes, with a 5 to 7 cm margin. After the initial 50 Gy is delivered to this volume, longitudinal margins are reduced ("shrinking-field technique"), and an additional 10 Gy is delivered to the tumor bed and scar. If margins of resection were found to be microscopically positive, the primary tumor bed as outlined by surgical clips placed at the time of resection may be boosted an additional 4 to 6 Gy. The generally agreed on postoperative radiation dose for patients with negative resection margins is 60 Gy. If the resection margins are positive, then the dose is raised to 68 Gy. Patients with recurrent disease after prior surgical resection or head and neck primary sites also benefit from higher doses of radiation, on the order of 64 to 66 Gy.[21]

BRACHYTHERAPY

Although technically demanding and time consuming, brachytherapy has the advantage of delivering a high dose of radiation to a limited volume of tissue while accelerating the time in which the total dose can be delivered. Any successful brachytherapy program requires a dedicated team of physicians, physicists, dosimetrists, and operating room personnel with both experience and interest in performing these procedures.

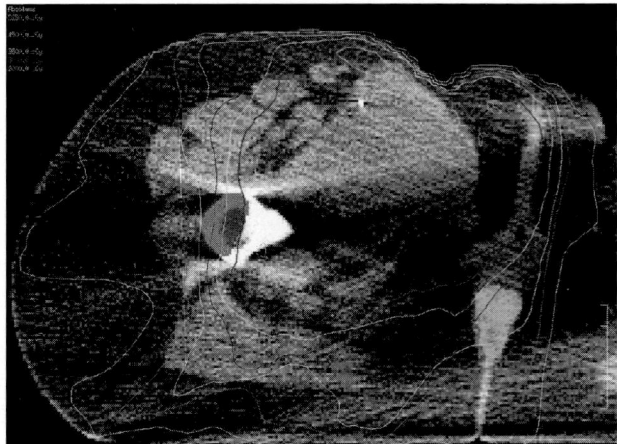

Figure 2 Representative image from the radiotherapy treatment plan Intensity-modulated radiation was used to treat the dominant tumor mass, peritumoral edema, and the tumor nodule with a radial margin of 2–2.5 cm. The total dose was 50 Gy. The femur, rectum, and perineum were contoured as avoidance structures to spare them the full dose of radiation. At the time of surgical resection, the specimen was histologically consistent with malignant fibrous histiocytoma with extensive necrosis (90%) and treatment effect.

After wide local excision and placement of metal clips to outline the areas at risk, a single-plane implant is performed using plastic catheters. This process begins with marking the plane of the implant 1 to 2 cm on either side of the surgical scar using a sterile marking pen. It is then generally recommended to place marks within this plane 1 cm apart to ensure that the correct number of catheters is inserted and that catheters are appropriately spaced. A hollow sharpened metal trochar is then inserted through each entrance site and the plastic catheters, preloaded with the radio-opaque "dummy" source wires, are threaded through. While holding the plastic catheter, the metal trochar is withdrawn and the process is repeated for each exit point.

Once the catheters are placed, they are sutured to the tumor bed using absorbable suture material, and additional metal clips are placed to delineate the clinical target volume and any critical structures such as nerves, vessels, or vascular pedicles in proximity to the implanted volume.

Within 3 to 4 days of implantation, orthogonal localization radiographs are taken of the implant site and the position of the radio-opaque "dummy" sources are digitized into a computerized planning system. Once the clinical target volume is identified, source strengths are chosen based on the geometry of the implant and the "dummy" source wires are replaced by the radioactive wires.

The generally recommended volume around the tumor bed is 2 cm in the superior and inferior dimension and at least 1 cm in the lateral dimension, although anatomic constraints and nearby critical structures may limit the area irradiated.[22] These recommendations appear to be at odds with those for external beam irradiation, where margins are larger to account for the local growth characteristics of STS described earlier, but in practice, these brachytherapy margins have not appeared to be a limitation if patients are selected appropriately (Figure 3).[23]

Brachytherapy has also been used for the management of recurrent STS within a previously irradiated field.[24] In an early review from M. D. Anderson, 26 patients receiving a prior mean external beam dose of 55.6 Gy were managed with wide local excision of the recurrent STS and placement of iridium-192 brachytherapy catheters. The mean brachytherapy dose was 47.2 Gy. The 5-year local recurrence-free survival was 52% for all patients, but for the 17 patients with extremity lesions, the local control was 71%. We have recently reexamined this experience and compared it with a similar cohort of patients managed with surgery alone. In this larger experience with 37 patients receiving reirradiation and 25 patients receiving surgery alone, there were no differences in local control between groups (39% surgery alone vs 58% surgery and radiation at 5 years, $p = 0.4$), but there were clearly more complications associated with the use of radiation (80% vs 17%, $p < 0.001$). This has prompted us to recommend surgery alone as the first salvage therapy for local recurrence within a previously irradiated site. For complex clinical situations where brachytherapy is still recommended, we have explored the use of temporary vacuum-assisted closure over the brachytherapy catheters with delayed plastic surgery reconstruction.

Complications

Although combined modality therapy has resulted in ultimate limb salvage in over 85% of patients, there are complications associated with treatment. Most are temporary and self-limited, but some are lifelong. After the first 3 to 4 weeks of external beam treatment, patients begin to experience a faint erythema with an associated itching sensation within the treatment field. In cases treated postoperatively, this develops into a dry desquamation by week 6. Pain or discomfort requiring medication is unusual. Nausea and fatigue may occur in patients where bowel is irradiated, and moist desquamation may occur in situations where skin folds are treated, but acute reactions requiring medical care are otherwise rare. In most patients, the erythema and dry

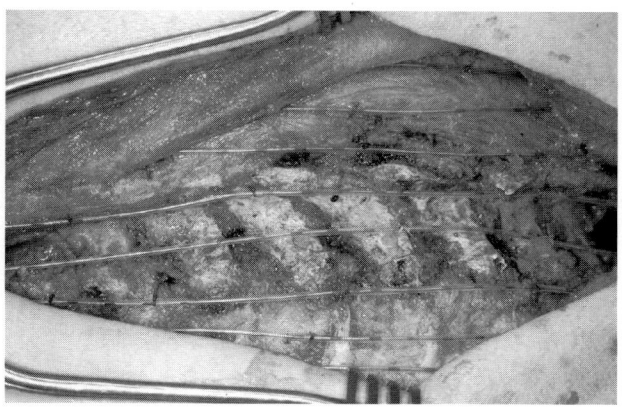

Figure 3 Single-plane brachytherapy implant for recurrent, previously irradiated paraspinal malignant fibrous histiocytoma. For the recurrent disease, a radiation dose of 45 Gy was delivered over 4 days using iridium-192 wire.

desquamation has resolved by 2 to 3 weeks after treatment.

In patients treated postoperatively, wound break-down, infection, or necrosis requiring deep packing or reoperation occurs in less than 10% of patients. An exception would be cases where split-thickness skin grafts have been placed. In these situations, islands of desquamation and loss of portions of the skin grafts are not unusual, and secondary healing over time is required, sometimes over a period of months. Because higher doses of radiation are delivered in the postoperative setting, 50% of these patients go on to develop moderate fibrosis, and approximately 25% will develop some edema within the radiation treatment field.[19] Hyperpigmentation may also be visualized for years.

In patients treated preoperatively, the acute reactions of radiation have generally resolved by the time the patient is taken for surgical resection of the tumor. However, postoperatively, 25 to 30% of these patients will develop some wound breakdown, infection, or necrosis requiring medical management. In our experience, complex plastic surgery reconstructions have not lowered this incidence, a finding also noted in the randomized trial of pre- or postoperative radiation therapy.[17] Because of the lower radiation dose and smaller treatment fields utilized in the preoperative setting, only 30% of patients go on to develop any meaningful long-term fibrosis, and only 15% develop edema.[19]

We have examined the complications of radiation in our lower extremity STS population and found acute wound complications to be associated with the use of preoperative radiation and large tumor size, whereas long-term complications are associated with proximal thigh location and higher radiation doses. We also find

that some patients who develop acute surgical complications go on to develop long-term problems, but in general, the complications of preoperative radiation sequencing are temporary, whereas the complications of postoperative radiation sequencing are long term. This has resulted in our recommending preoperative radiation for most patients with STS.

Results of Treatment

We have maintained a database of all STS patients radiated at M. D. Anderson since 1960 and analyzed their outcome according to patient, tumor, and treatment characteristics.[24] This analysis now includes 1,296 patients with previously untreated, nonmetastatic STS radiated between the years 1960 and 2003. Patients were treated with a conservative surgery and radiation either preoperatively (median radiation dose 50 Gy, 514 patients) or postoperatively (median radiation dose 60 Gy, 728 patients). Two-thirds of the patients were treated for malignant fibrous histiocytoma, liposarcoma, or synovial sarcoma subtypes, and 70% had tumors in an extremity location. There were an additional 241 patients with superficial trunk tumors, 84 with head and neck tumors, and 65 with deep trunk (eg, retroperitoneal) tumors. With a median follow-up of 9.1 years, the local control, distant metastasis-free survival and disease-specific survival was 83%, 68%, and 69%, respectively. Determinants of outcome are shown in Table 2. Although grade and size are the primary determinants of distant spread and disease-specific survival, they have little association with local disease control, which is more closely associated with margin status, primary site, and age. In addition to the characteristics shown in Table 2, patients with recurrent disease have a significantly inferior local control when compared with patients with primary presentation (65% vs 82% at 15 years, $p < 0.001$).

Of interest to the surgical oncologist, we have examined the interval of time between surgery and radiation for patients treated both pre- and postoperatively. Within the range of days studied, there are no clinically significant differences in local control between patients receiving radiation within our standard time frame (4–6 weeks) and those who experience a delay in the initiation of their second phase of treatment. Although there is no clinically significant effect of delayed treatment, it is probably more appropriate to conclude that treatment intensification is unnecessary in patients who have experienced a treatment delay rather than to conclude that there is no effect of treatment delay itself.[26]

Table 2 Primary Determinants of Outcome in 1,296 Patients with Primary, Nonmetastatic Soft Tissue Sarcoma Treated with Conservation Surgery and Radiation

Outcome	Characteristic		Percent at 15 years	p-value
LC	Margin	Positive	60	< 0.001
		Negative	89	
	Location	H&N/Deep trunk	69	< 0.001
		Ext/Superficial trunk	84	
	Age	> 65 years	72	< 0.001
		≤ 65 years	65	
DM	Grade	High	40	< 0.001
		Intermediate	33	
		Low	0	
	Size	≤ 2 cm	11	< 0.001
		> 2 ≤ 5 cm	25	
		> 5 ≤ 10 cm	40	
		> 10 cm	49	

DM = distant metastasis; Ext = extremity; H&N = head and neck; LC = local control.

We have also examined prognostic factors for disease-specific survival after first relapse.[27] Among 402 patients sustaining a first relapse of sarcoma after combined surgery and radiation, the overall disease-specific survival was 25% and 16% at 5 and 15 years, respectively. Disease-specific survival was significantly better in patients with a first local relapse as compared with patients with a first distant relapse. Favorable prognostic factors for survival among the patients with a first local recurrence were extremity site, low or intermediate tumor grade, time to recurrence greater than 12 months, and initial tumor size less than or equal to 5 cm. Among the patients with a first distant relapse, the time to metastasis greater than 12 months was a major determinant of improved survival. Regardless of first local or first distant relapse, long-term survivors tended to be those patients who had disease amenable to surgical resection.

References

1. Enneking WF, Spanier SS, Malawer MM. The effect of the anatomic setting on the results of surgical procedures for soft parts sarcoma of the thigh. Cancer 1981;47:1005–22.

2. White LM, Wunder JS, Bell RS, et al. Histologic assessment of peritumoral edema in soft tissue sarcoma. Int J Radiat Oncol Biol Phys 2005;61:1439–45.

3. Mazeron J, Suit HD. Lymph nodes as sites of metastases from sarcomas of soft tissue. Cancer 1987;60:1800–8.

4. Suit HD, Russell WO, Martin RG. Management of patients with sarcoma of soft tissue in an extremity. Cancer 1973;31:1247–55.

5. Lindberg RD, Martin RG, Romsdahl MM, et al. Conservative surgery and postoperative radiotherapy in 300 adults with soft-tissue sarcomas. Cancer 1981;47:2391–7.

6. Rosenberg SA, Tepper J, Glatstein E, et al. The treatment of soft-tissue sarcomas of the extremities: prospective randomized evaluations of (1) limb-sparing surgery plus radiation therapy compared with amputation and (2) the role of adjuvant chemotherapy. Ann Surg 1982;196:305–15.

7. Pisters PWT, Harrison LB, Leung DHY, et al. Long-term results of a prospective randomized trial of adjuvant brachytherapy in soft tissue sarcoma. J Clin Oncol 1996;14:859–68.

8. Yang JC, Chang AE, Baker AR, et al. Randomized prospective study of the benefit of adjuvant radiation therapy in the treatment of soft tissue sarcomas of the extremity. J Clin Oncol 1998;16:197–203.

9. Zagars GK, Mullen JR, Pollack A. Malignant fibrous histiocytoma: outcome and prognostic factors following conservative surgery and radiotherapy. Int J Radiat Oncol Biol Phys 1996;34:683–94.

10. Zagars GK, Goswitz MS, Pollack A. Liposarcoma: outcome and prognostic factors following conservation surgery and radiation therapy. Int J Radiat Oncol Biol Phys 1996;36:311–9.

11. Mullen JR, Zagars GK. Synovial sarcoma outcome following conservation surgery and radiotherapy. Radiother Oncol 1994;33:23–30.

12. Rydholm A, Gustafson P, Rooser B, et al. Limb-sparing surgery without radiotherapy based on anatomic location of soft tissue sarcoma. J Clin Oncol 1991;9:1757–65.

13. Karakousis CP, Proimakis C, Walsh DL. Primary soft tissue sarcoma of the extremities in adults. Br J Surg 1995;82:1208–12.

14. Baldini EH, Goldberg J, Jenner C, et al. Long-term outcomes after function-sparing surgery without radiotherapy for soft tissue sarcoma of the extremities and trunk. J Clin Oncol 1999;17:3252–9.

15. Fabrizio PL, Stafford SL, Pritchard DJ. Extremity soft-tissue sarcomas selectively treated with surgery alone. In J Radiat Oncol Biol Phys 2000;48:227–32.

16. Robinson MH, Keus RB, Shasha D, et al. Is pre-operative radiotherapy superior to postoperative radiotherapy in the treatment of soft tissue sarcoma? Eur J Cancer 1998;34:1309–16.

17. O'Sullivan B, Davis AM, Turcotte R, et al. Preoperative versus postoperative radiotherapy in soft-tissue sarcoma of the limbs: a randomized trial. Lancet 2002;359:2235–41.

18. Zagars GK, Ballo MT, Pisters PW, et al. Preoperative vs. postoperative radiation therapy for soft tissue sarcoma: a retrospective comparative evaluation of disease outcome. Int J Radiat Oncol Biol Phys 2003;56:482–8.

19. Davis AM, O'Sullivan B, Turcotte R, et al. Late radiation morbidity following randomization to preoperative versus postoperative radiotherapy in extremity soft tissue sarcoma. Radiother Oncol 2005;75:48–53.

20. Davis AM, O'Sullivan B, Turcotte R, et al. Function and health status outcomes in a randomized trial comparing preoperative and postoperative radiotherapy in extremity soft tissue sarcoma. J Clin Oncol 2002;20:4472–7.

21. Zagars GK, Ballo MT. Significance of dose in postoperative radiotherapy for soft tissue sarcoma. Int J Radiat Oncol Biol Phys 2003;56:473–81.

22. Nag S, Shasha D, Janjan N, et al. The American Brachytherapy Society recommendations for brachytherapy of soft tissue sarcomas. Int J Radiat Oncol Biol Phys 2001;49:1033–43.

23. Alektiar KM, Leung D, Zelefsky MJ, et al. Adjuvant brachytherapy for primary high-grade soft tissue sarcoma of the extremity. Ann Surg Oncol 2002;9:48–56.

24. Pearlstone DB, Janjan NA, Feig BW, et al. Re-resection with brachytherapy for locally recurrent soft tissue sarcoma arising in a previously radiated field. Cancer J Sci Am 1999;5:25–33.

25. Zagars GK, Ballo MT, Pisters PW, et al. Prognostic factors for patients with localized soft tissue sarcoma treated with conservation surgery and radiation therapy: an analysis of 1225 patients. Cancer 2003;97:2530–43.

26. Ballo MT, Zagars GK, Cormier JN, et al. Interval between surgery and radiotherapy: effect on local control of soft tissue sarcoma. Int J Radiat Oncol Biol Phys 2004;58:1461–7.

27. Zagars GK, Ballo MT, Pisters PW, et al. Prognostic factors for disease-specific survival after first relapse of soft-tissue sarcoma: analysis of 402 patients with disease relapse after initial conservative surgery and radiotherapy. Int J Radiat Oncol Biol Phys 2003;57:739–47.

CHAPTER 73

MANAGEMENT: CHEMOTHERAPY

ROBERT G. MAKI, MD, PhD

Adjuvant Chemotherapy for Soft Tissue Sarcoma (STS)

The role chemotherapy is much different from that of surgery or radiation. Whereas surgery and radiation play a definite role in the primary treatment of primary sarcomas, the clinical benefit, if any, is modest. Histology becomes important in making this therapeutic decision. For example, for extraskeletal Ewing's sarcoma and rhabdomyosarcoma, without doubt chemotherapy is effective as part of the regimen of treatment to best improve chances for cure, since historical data indicate 80% or more of these patients will die of metastatic disease despite good local control of their tumors. Chemotherapy has improved the cure rate 3-fold or more for these "pediatric" sarcomas, and is mandatory except in patients who could not tolerate the aggressive regimens used in these diseases.[1,2]

As for more the more typical STSs that arise in adults, the role of adjuvant therapy is definitely more limited. The benefit, if there is any, to overall survival, is a small one. In our opinion, the benefits and risks need to be discussed with patients on an individual basis, given conflicting data as to the benefit of what is admittedly toxic therapy.

The utility of chemotherapy in the adjuvant setting has been examined in over 15 randomized studies from the early 1980s to today. Early data were hindered by lack of good markers for the sarcoma pathologist to make diagnoses of sarcomas versus sarcomatoid carcinomas, melanomas, and other tumors. Nearly all of the older studies of adjuvant therapy used a doxorubicin backbone without the other useful drug for STS, namely ifosfamide.

In a meta-analysis of doxorubicin-based chemotherapy adjuvant studies for STS, there was no statistically significant benefit to overall survival with the use of chemotherapy for all sarcomas considered as a whole.[3] However, local and distant disease-free survival and overall disease-free survival were improved with the use of chemotherapy, findings consistent with the bulk of the data from the individual studies. Subset analysis of these data showed a statistically significant benefit for those people who received chemotherapy, but this was done a posteriori, and may not be a legitimate analysis of the data. Furthermore, when pathology was reviewed for one of the largest contributing studies to this meta-analysis, 5% of the tumors were not sarcomas, further complicating the interpretations of this meta-analysis data, in which pathology was not reviewed centrally.[4]

The meta-analysis data show no benefit for the addition of adjuvant chemotherapy for the treatment of intrathoracic, intra-abdominal, or head and neck primary sites. For these anatomical locations, where margins are often an issue, we do not offer adjuvant chemotherapy given the lack of a survival advantage in this subset of patients. We consider breast or trunk locations as more amenable to treatment as extremity sarcomas, since the issues with surgical margins are more typical for those of extremities, and are discussed further below.

To address the question of the addition of ifosfamide to anthracycline-based treatment in the adjuvant setting for patients with extremity sarcomas, three studies have been performed, which show some hints of benefit for adjuvant therapy. The largest is a 2001 study by Frustaci and colleagues that showed a benefit in overall survival for patients with large high-grade extremity sarcomas who received adjuvant ifosfamide and epirubicin. This benefit for survival and disease-free survival is not statistically significant with longer follow-up in an intention-to-treat analysis. However, at 7+ years of follow-up, the 5-year overall survival was still significantly improved in comparison with patients who received no chemotherapy.[5,6] Two other small studies with ifosfamide and doxorubicin-based therapy did not show benefit to overall survival for patients with extremity STS, though there was a trend to improved survival in one of the studies.[7,8]

Other data have come to light based on retrospective analysis of combined prospective sarcoma databases. These data are not randomized, and accordingly it is extremely difficult to make recommendations on such data. In a dataset involving patients treated at UCLA and Memorial Hospital with synovial sarcoma, overall survival benefit was observed for those patients receiving chemotherapy versus those who did not.[9] In a similar compilation of data from Memorial and Dana-Farber Cancer Institute, myxoid/round-cell liposarcoma patients appeared to have superior survival if they received chemotherapy versus those who had local therapy alone.[9]

In contrast, a third compilation of all patients treated at The University of Texas M. D. Anderson Cancer Center and Memorial with all forms of sarcoma appeared to have superior survival intially, but then inferior survival at 2 years or more.[10] The data from this final study are best explained by selection bias. The patients with the sarcomas with worst prognosis were the ones selected to receive chemotherapy. Though patients receiving chemotherapy ultimately had inferior outcome to those receiving local therapy alone, their doing better initially may reflect the response of some of these tumors to chemotherapy, arguing their outcome would have been even worse without chemotherapy. Thus we are again left with difficult decisions as pertains to the use of adjuvant chemotherapy.

We conclude that if there is a benefit to adjuvant chemotherapy for extremity soft tissue sarcomas, it is a small one. Patients who are younger, with relatively chemotherapy-sensitive subtypes of STS such as synovial sarcoma or myxoid/round-cell liposarcoma are the most attractive candidates for such therapy, based on the nonrandomized data above, with the caveat that the ultimate decision has to be individualized.

Chemotherapy for Metastatic STS

For metastatic disease, the situation is diametrically opposed to that in the adjuvant setting—palliation is the goal, except in the small number of patients with resectable metastatic disease, in whom resection of lung or other metastases can be considered. With respect to survival after such resections of metastatic disease, common sense dictates which people fare best with metastatic disease. Those patients with the longest time between initial diagnosis and surgery, fewest nodules (ie, 4 or fewer), and unilateral disease fare the best. Even in this situation the majority of patients will recur elsewhere in the lungs.

For those with metastatic disease without surgical options, doxorubicin and ifosfamide remain the two

workhorses for the medical oncologist. Each has reported response rates in the 20 to 30% range, but more contemporary studies using outside reviews of radiographs and standardized measurement criteria indicate the response rates for these drugs may be as low as the ~10% range.[11] The heterogeneity of patients enrolled on these studies makes interpretation of such studies difficult between regimens. Depending on the blend of patients' sensitive versus resistant sarcoma subtypes treated, the response rate will vary greatly.

Other drugs with activity in STS include dacarbazine and gemcitabine, in particular for leiomyosarcoma in both instances. In rare situations, agents used for epithelial cancers are of benefit in STS; taxanes are active against angiosarcoma and epithelioid hemangioendothelioma, for example. Toxicity also figures into the choice of drugs, in particular in patients with widespread but slowly advancing disease. In this situation, pegylated liposomal doxorubicin (Doxil, Caelyx) is a reasonable option, since in 1 study of 94 patients, it was roughly equivalent to doxorubicin in response rate.[11] The dose of pegylated liposomal doxorubicin that can be administered is lower than that for doxorubicin, but with its very long half-life, the "area under the curve" (the integral of concentration of drug over time) is substantially greater than that for standard doxorubicin.

The subtype of STS predicts the sensitivity to a given treatment. The finding of the combination of two marginally active drugs (gemcitabine and docetaxel) as active in uterine leiomyosarcoma and other sarcomas may highlight the sensitivity of this uterine leiomyosarcoma, the true activity of the combination, or perhaps both.[12,13]

Beyond "pediatric" sarcomas and angiosarcomas mentioned above, one further sarcoma subtype is worth noting. Gastrointestinal stromal tumors (GIST), the tumors rare arising from the interstitial Cajal's cells in myenteric plexus of the stomach and small bowel, recur frequently in the peritoneum or liver, and are resistant to standard chemotherapy. Imatinib, the tyrosine kinase inhibitor shown useful for chronic myelogenous leukemia, is very active in GIST, with 60% response rates or more.[14] This finding points out the importance of the key molecular feature of GIST: a mutated c-kit molecule that can be inactivated by imatinib.[15] It must be noted that other sarcomas (as well as many other cancers) express c-kit, such as Ewing's sarcoma, but do not appear to be sensitive to imatinib. In patients with excellent responses followed by progression in specific sites of tumor, we have occasionally taken people for operations to remove resistant disease, and continued imatinib therapy for the remaining drug-sensitive disease. This pattern of progression appears unique to GIST, and calls for multimodality management of patients even with metastatic disease.

Investigational Therapy

The most advanced of developmental therapeutics for soft tissue sarcomas is arguably ecteinascidin (ET-743, Yondelis), showing a low but consistent 8 to 12% response rate in patients with doxorubicin/ifosfamide refractory disease.[16–18] Patients with liposarcomas or leiomyosarcomas have both responded to this drug, with fewer responses noted in patients with other histologies such as synovial sarcoma and malignant fibrous histiocytoma (MFH). Transaminitis appears 3 to 5 days after drug administration and clears after a further 5 to 10 days. Liver function tests (LFTs) must be monitored serially, as an elevated bilirubin or alkaline phosphatase on treatment predicts for a higher risk of rhabdomyolysis and multisystem organ failure. Elevation in the alkaline phosphatase or bilirubin while on ET-743 is a principal reason for a dose reduction for subsequent cycles of therapy.

Other new agents with hints of activity include brostallicin (soft tissue sarcoma in general)[19] and SU11248 (in phase I/II and phase III studies for GIST).[20] As noted above, tyrosine kinase inhibitors will be increasingly important in the treatment of cancer, and sarcomas are no exception in this regard, especially considering that angiogenic mediatiors such as VEGF are dependent on receptor tyrosine kinases such as VEGFR1 and VEGFR2 for their activity. The recent success of bevacizumab with standard chemotherapy in patients with colon cancer points out the possible utility of such combinations for patients with sarcomas as well.

References

1. Crist WM, Anderson JR, Meza JL, et al. Intergroup rhabdomyosarcoma study-IV: results for patients with nonmetastatic disease. J Clin Oncol 2001;19:3091–102.

2. Grier HE, Krailo MD, Tarbell NJ, et al. Addition of ifosfamide and etoposide to standard chemotherapy for Ewing's sarcoma and primitive neuroectodermal tumor of bone. N Engl J Med 2003;348:694–701.

3. Sarcoma Meta-Analysis Collaboration. Adjuvant chemotherapy for localised resectable soft-tissue sarcoma of adults: meta-analysis of individual data. Lancet 1997;350:1647–54.

4. Verweij J, Seynaeve C. The reason for confining the use of adjuvant chemotherapy in soft tissue sarcoma to the investigational setting. Semin Radiat Oncol 1999;9:352–9.

5. Frustaci S, De Paoli A, Bidoli E, et al. Ifosfamide in the adjuvant therapy of soft tissue sarcomas. Oncology 2003;65Suppl 2:80–4.

6. Frustaci S, Gherlinzoni F, De Paoli A, et al. Adjuvant chemotherapy for adult soft tissue sarcomas of the extremities and girdles: results of the Italian randomized cooperative trial. J Clin Oncol 2001;19:1238–47.

7. Brodowicz T, Schwameis E, Widder J, et al. Intensifed adjuvant IFADIC chemotherapy for adult soft tissue sarcoma: a prospective randomized feasibility trial. Sarcoma 2000;4:151–60.

8. Gortzak E, Azzarelli A, Buesa J, et al. A randomised phase II study on neo-adjuvant chemotherapy for 'high-risk' adult soft-tissue sarcoma. Eur J Cancer 2001;37:1096–103.

9. Eilber FC, Eilber FR, Eckardt J, et al. The impact of chemotherapy on the survival of patients with high-grade primary extremity liposarcoma. Ann Surg 2004;240:686–97.

10. Cormier JN, Huang X, Xing Y, et al. Cohort analysis of patients with localized, high-risk, extremity soft tissue sarcoma treated at two cancer centers: chemotherapy-associated outcomes. J Clin Oncol 2004;22:4567–74.

11. Judson I, Radford JA, Harris M, et al. Randomised phase II trial of pegylated liposomal doxorubicin (DOXIL/CAELYX) versus doxorubicin in the treatment of advanced or metastatic soft tissue sarcoma: a study by the EORTC Soft Tissue and Bone Sarcoma Group. Eur J Cancer 2001;37:870–7.

12. Hensley ML, Maki R, Venkatraman E, et al. Gemcitabine and docetaxel in patients with unresectable leiomyosarcoma: results of a phase II trial. J Clin Oncol 2002;20:2824–31.

13. Leu KM, Ostruszka LJ, Shewach D, et al. Laboratory and clinical evidence of synergistic cytotoxicity of sequential treatment with gemcitabine followed by docetaxel in the treatment of sarcoma. J Clin Oncol 2004;22:1706–12.

14. Demetri GD, von Mehren M, Blanke CD, et al. Efficacy and safety of imatinib mesylate in advanced gastrointestinal stromal tumors. N Engl J Med 2002;347:472–80.

15. Tuveson DA, Willis NA, Jacks T, et al. STI571 inactivation of the gastrointestinal stromal tumor c-KIT oncoprotein: biological and clinical implications. Oncogene 2001;20:5054–8.

16. Yovine A, Riofrio M, Blay JY, et al. Phase II study of ecteinascidin-743 in advanced pretreated soft tissue sarcoma patients. J Clin Oncol 2004;22:890–9.

17. Garcia-Carbonero R, Supko JG, Manola J, et al. Phase II and pharmacokinetic study of ecteinascidin 743 in patients with progressive sarcomas of soft tissues refractory to chemotherapy. J Clin Oncol 2004;22:1480–90.

18. Blay JY, Le Cesne A, Verweij J, et al. A phase II study of ET-743/trabectedin ('Yondelis') for patients with advanced gastrointestinal stromal tumours. Eur J Cancer 2004;40:1327–31.

19. Leahy MG, Blay JY, Verweij J, et al. EORTC 62011: phase II trial of brostallicin for soft tissue sarcoma [abstract 14]. Proc Conn Tiss Oncol Soc 2003. Available at: www.ctos.org (accessed Octobe 22, 2006).

20. Demetri GD, Desai J, Fletcher JA, et al. SU11248, a multi-targeted tyrosine kinase inhibitor, can overcome imatinib (IM) resistance caused by diverse genomic mechanisms in patients (pts) with metastatic gastrointestinal stromal tumor (GIST). J Clin Oncol 2004;22:3001.

CHAPTER 74

SURGICAL TREATMENT OF RETROPERITONEAL SARCOMAS

FARID J. KEHDY, MD

CHARLES R. SCOGGINS, MD

Introduction

Soft tissue sarcomas (STSs) are a heterogeneous group of tumors that may occur anywhere within the body. Unlike carcinomas, which emanate from epithelial tissues, soft tissue sarcomas arise from mesenchymal cells. Sarcomas are rare, and, in fact, the American Cancer Society estimates that approximately 9,000 cases occur in the United States annually.[1] The majority of STSs are located in the extremities, whereas approximately 15% are retroperitoneal.[2] The most common histologies seen in retroperitoneal sarcomas are liposarcoma, leiomyosarcoma, and malignant fibrous histiocytoma[3-5] (Figure 1). Because of the rarity of sarcomas, most surgeons have little experience in the management of these malignancies. As a function of their location, most retroperitoneal sarcomas remain clinically silent for extended periods of time, only to produce symptoms of fullness, pain, obstruction, and a palpable mass when they have achieved a large size. In fact, many retroperitoneal sarcomas are quite large on presentation and may involve multiple organs, making the treatment of these tumors challenging.

Epidemiology

Although soft tissue sarcomas are a rare collection of diseases, some factors have been shown to increase the risk of their development. Patients infected with human immunodeficiency virus (HIV) are prone to developing Kaposi's sarcoma. Radiation, usually given as external beam radiotherapy for a malignancy, is also known to cause soft tissue sarcoma. Patients treated with external beam radiotherapy for cervical, ovarian, testicular, or rectal cancer may have an increased incidence of retroperitoneal and pelvic sarcoma up to 50-fold higher than the rest of the population.[6,7] These radiation-induced STSs, usually leiomyosarcomas and lymphosarcomas, usually occur after a latency period of up to 10 to 20 years. Environmental factors that are linked to the development of sarcomas include polyvinyl chloride, Thorotrast, and arsenic. These agents, however, have been linked to hepatic angiosarcoma, not retroperitoneal sarcomas. In addition, pesticides such as chlorophenol have been shown to increase the risk of STS in a dose-dependent manner.[8]

In addition to these exposure-related risk factors, some patients are prone to the development of sarcomas because of genetic mutations (Table 1). Neuro-fibromatosis type- I (von Recklinghausen's disease), which is a relatively common inherited disease affecting approximately 1 in 3,000 live births, is associated with neurofibroma formation. Patients affected with this disease are at risk of malignant transformation of neurofibromas, especially those with plexiform histology, into malignant peripheral nerve sheath tumors (Figure 2). Additionally, patients with mutations in the tumor suppressor gene *TP53*, whether somatic or as part of the Li-Fraumeni syndrome, are at risk of multiple malignancies, including STS. Patients affected with familial adenomatous polyposis (FAP) and its variant, Gardner's syndrome, are at risk of the development of abdominal and retroperitoneal desmoid tumors. Although desmoids do not harbor metastatic potential, they are often infiltrative and can cause local symptoms with infiltration throughout the retroperitoneum and mesentery. Complete excision is often difficult, and desmoid tumors have a high local failure rate following resection.

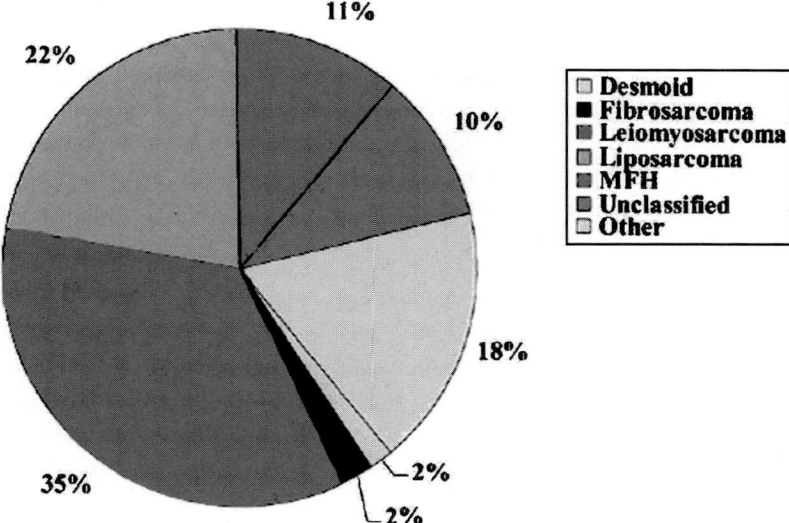

Figure 1 MFH = malignant fibrous histiocytoma. Reproduced with permission from Pisters PW.[4]

Table 1 Inheritable Syndromes Predisposing to Soft Tissue Sarcomas

Syndrome	Gene	Tumor
Neurofibromatosis type −1 (von Recklinghausen's disease)	NF-1	Malignant peripheral nerve sheath tumor
Li-Fraumeni syndrome	TP53	Soft tissue sarcomas, osteogenic sarcoma
Gardner's syndrome	APC	Desmoid tumors*
Hereditary retinoblastoma	Rb	Soft tissue sarcomas

*Although not overtly malignant, many mesenteric and retroperitoneal desmoids behave aggressively with local infiltration and a high rate of local failure following resection.

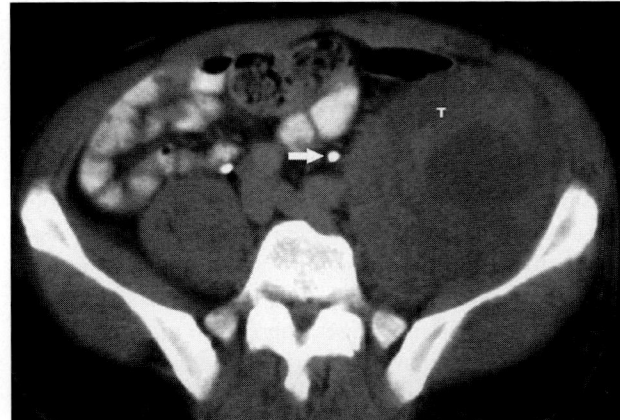

Figure 2 Malignant peripheral nerve sheath tumor arising from the proximal femoral nerve in a patient with neurofibromatosis type-I. Note the left common iliac artery (arrow), which is not involved. T = tumor.

Presentation and Preoperative Evaluation

The majority of retroperitoneal tumors are malignant, and of these, sarcomas represent over 50%, with lymphomas and carcinomas making up the remainder.[9] Most often, retroperitoneal sarcomas are insidious in onset. These tumors remain clinically silent until they either achieve a size large enough to be palpable, or cause symptoms owing to local compression and/or invasion.[10] Additionally, they may cause pain[11] owing to involvement of retroperitoneal or pelvic nerves, or by causing ureteral obstruction. Less common presentations include weight loss, early satiety, nausea and vomiting, lower extremity edema, and varicosities.

Massive retroperitoneal adenopathy seen on imaging studies may be misinterpreted as a retroperitoneal sarcoma. Symptoms suggestive of lymphoma, including fever, night sweats, and weight loss of > 10% body weight (B symptoms) should be elicited. Additionally, patients with lymphoma may have adenopathy in the axilla, cervical, or inguinal basins that may lend clues to the diagnosis and that may be easily biopsied. Enlarged para-aortic lymph nodes in a male patient should prompt a testicular examination, as testicular cancer may metastasize to the retroperitoneal lymph nodes. These patients may be further evaluated with testicular ultrasound and measurement of the alpha-fetoprotein (AFP) and human chorionic gonadotropin (hCG) levels. Another genitourinary malignancy that may present as a retroperitoneal mass is primary renal cell carcinoma (RCC). The classic triad of hematuria, flank mass, and pain occurs in a minority of patients, and, in fact, many patients are asymptomatic and are found to have a renal mass on abdominal imaging for an unrelated cause, or hematuria discovered during urinalysis. Other tumors that may present as retroperitoneal masses include adrenal tumors, angiomyolipomas, and carcinomas, such as a locally advanced colorectal carcinoma with a large extraluminal component or bulky para-aortic adenopathy.

Following a thorough history and physical examination, radiographic assessment is performed. Computed tomography (CT) is the most commonly used modality, as it is readily available in most centers and allows for both tumor characterization as well as assessment of resectability. Magnetic resonance imaging (MRI) may also be used, but probably does not provide additional information over CT for tumors in the abdomen and retroperitoneum. High-quality preoperative imaging is imperative, as many features inherent to the tumor may be determined by careful review of the radiographs. Tumor-organ interfaces can often be determined, allowing for appropriate preoperative planning. In cases where one of the kidneys appears to be involved by a retroperitoneal sarcoma, the clinician must determine if a nephrectomy will be required for complete tumor extirpation.[12] For a patient with a normal serum creatinine and radiographic evidence of contralateral renal perfusion (easily determined on contrast-enhanced abdominal and pelvic CT), removal of the involved kidney seldom results in significant renal impairment. In cases where the preoperative renal function is suboptimal, or when the contralateral kidney is not radiographically normal, further preoperative assessment should be performed.

A careful search for metastatic disease should be performed in all patients suspected of having a retroperitoneal sarcoma. Preoperative CT or MRI may detect peritoneal sarcomatosis or hepatic metastases, and thus minimize the incidence of noncurative explorations. In addition to imaging the abdomen and retroperitoneum, chest radiography should be undertaken, as the lung is the most common site of metastatic disease for patients with soft tissue sarcomas. Plain chest radiographs to rule out pulmonary metastases are generally acceptable, and abnormal results may be followed up with chest CT. In cases of very large or high-grade retroperitoneal sarcomas, chest CT should be the primary imaging modality.

The role of preoperative biopsy for retroperitoneal tumors is controversial. In general, most retroperitoneal tumors are malignant, and thus require resection when appropriate. Preoperative attempts at biopsy, usually performed under radiologic guidance, rarely alter the overall therapeutic plan. In fact, the heterogeneous nature of these tumors often makes pathologic diagnosis difficult on needle biopsy specimens, thus misleading clinicians into a trial period of observation.[4] However, patients in whom the diagnosis is in question should be considered for an image-guided percutaneous biopsy, provided an expert cytopathologist is available for interpretation of the specimen. In addition, patients being considered for either neoadjuvant radiation or chemotherapy as part of a clinical trial need preoperative biopsy. Also, patients that are inoperable or whose tumors are unresectable should undergo percutaneous biopsy. Biopsies can be obtained using fine-needle aspiration (FNA) under CT guidance. Core needle biopsy may be more accurate, and yields enough tissue for multiple diagnostic tests. Incisional biopsy may be performed when percutaneous biopsy is nondiagnostic. Meticulous hemostasis is essential to prevent dissemination of the tumor cells through tissue planes from an expanding hematoma.

Staging of Retroperitoneal Sarcomas

The American Joint Committee for Cancer (AJCC) stages sarcomas based on tumor size, histological grade, and the presence of regional lymph node and distant metastases[13] (Table 2). Most retroperitoneal sarcomas are larger than 5 cm when diagnosed, and are by definition deep to the investing fascia, making T2b the most common T classification in this disease. Regional lymph node metastasis in soft tissue sarcoma is rare ($< 10\%$)[14] and carries the same poor prognosis as distant metastases, thus placing the patient in stage IV disease. Because of the rarity of nodal metastases, there is no role for routine lymphadenectomy in retroperitoneal sarcoma surgery. Nodal metastases may occur slightly more frequency with specific sarcoma histologies, including synovial sarcoma, clear-cell sarcoma, angiosarcoma, rhabdomyosarcoma, and epitheliod sarcoma;[14] however, these sarcomas are most commonly found in the extremity. Since patient outcome is heavily influenced by the adequacy of surgery,

Table 2 Soft Tissue Sarcoma Staging System*

Primary Tumor (T)

TX	Primary tumor cannot be assessed	
T0	No evidence of primary tumor	
T1	Tumor 5 cm or less in greatest dimension	
	T1a	superficial to the investing fascia
	T1b	deep to the investing fascia†
T2	Tumor more than 5 cm in greatest dimension	
	T2a	superficial to the investing fascia
	T2b	deep to the investing fascia†

Regional Lymph Nodes (N)

NX	Regional lymph nodes cannot be assessed
N0	No regional lymph nodes metastasis
N1	Regional lymph nodes metastasis

Distant Metastasis (M)

MX	Distant metastasis cannot be assessed
M0	No distant metastasis
M1	Distant metastasis

Histologic Grade (G)

GX	Grade cannot be assessed
G1	Well differentiated
G2	Moderately differentiated
G3	Poorly differentiated (4-tiered systems include undifferentiated as G4)

Stage Grouping

Stage I	Any T	N0	M0	G1-2 (Low grade)
Stage II	T1a, T1b, T2a	N0	M0	G3-4 (High grade)
Stage III	T2b	N0	M0	G3-4 (High grade)
Stage IV	Any T	N0	M1	Any grade
	Any T	N1‡	M0	Any grade

†All retroperitoneal sarcomas are by definition deep to their investing fascia, and thus "b" tumors.
‡The presence of nodal metastasis is considered M1 disease.
*Reprinted with permission from Greene FL et al.[13]

and the AJCC does not factor resection into the staging system, an alternative classification system has been proposed by van Dalen and colleagues.[15] This post-surgical system is a clinicopathologic classification based on completeness of resection, tumor grade, and the presence or absence of distant metastasis.[15] Although this system accurately stratifies patients based on tumor biology and the quality of surgical resection, it is dependent on surgical resection, and may be more useful as an adjunct to the current AJCC staging system rather than a surrogate.

Surgical Therapy for Primary Retroperitoneal Sarcomas

Surgical therapy remains the treatment of choice for primary retroperitoneal sarcoma and offers the best outcome for patients.[5,16,17] Indeed, the dictum that the first operation is the best chance for a cure is based more

on fact than on surgical dogma. In general, the resectability rate of primary retroperitoneal sarcomas treated at experienced referral centers ranges from 79 to 96%.[5,18–21] Resectability appears to not be governed by biologic factors, such as tumor size, grade, or histologic subtype,[5] but more by anatomic factors, such as invasion into vital structures, and the presence or absence of distant metastases. It is difficult to compare resectability rates from different institutions because the data are a function of whether the series included primary or recurrent tumors, the referral pattern of the reporting institution, institutional criteria of resectability, and the skill and experience of the surgical team. Some authors have noted improved patient outcomes when treatment of retroperitoneal sarcomas occurs at tertiary referral centers, citing a higher rate of complete resection as the major factor.[15]

Most surgeons approach retroperitoneal sarcomas via a midline incision. Bulky sarcomas of the upper abdominal quadrants may be approached through a thoracoabdominal incision with a midline extension.[22] Similarly, pelvic tumors are usually approached via a midline incision, and additional exposure may be gained by either separating the rectus sheath from the pubis or with a transplant-type flank incision. Complete tumor extirpation may require visceral resection. The organ most frequently resected is the kidney (32–46%), followed by the colon (25%), adrenal (18%), pancreas (10–15%), and spleen (10%)[12,22] (Figure 3). In general, an organ should be resected en bloc with the tumor if it will allow for a margin-negative resection. It is not advisable to "separate" tumors from organs that are involved or invaded by a sarcoma. Often, the tumor resection is facilitated by commencing dissection away from vascular structures and vital organs, leaving these more complicated portions of the case for last. In addition to organ involvement that may necessitate visceral resection, many retroperitoneal sarcomas involve large vascular structures. Indeed, leiomyosarcomas of the great vessels of the retroperitoneum or pelvis may be safely resected and reconstructed. Preoperative assessment should include determination of patency of the inferior vena cava and iliac veins in cases where the tumor involves these structures. When the vena cava and/or iliac vein is thrombosed preoperatively, simple resection without attempts at reconstruction should be performed. Often this is facilitated with the aid of a linear vascular stapler. In cases of aortic and/or iliac arterial involvement, reconstruction should be performed using standard vascular surgical techniques (Figure 4).

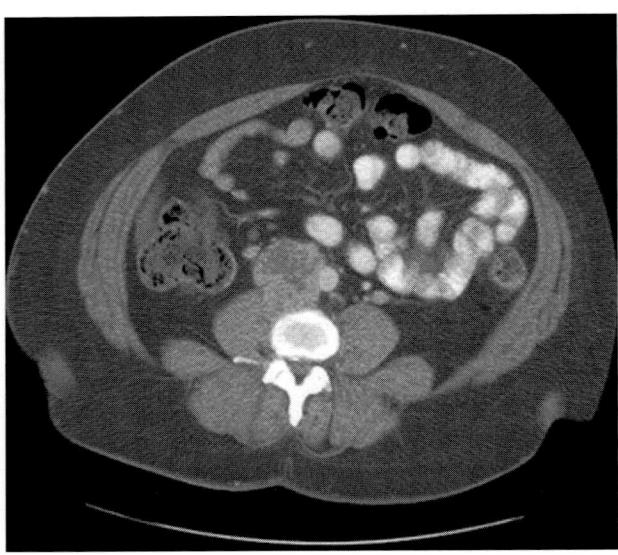

Figure 4 *A,* Staging CT demonstrating an IVC leiomyosarcoma involving the lateral wall of the distal aorta just before the bifurcation. The IVC is thrombosed. *B,* Leiomyosarcoma from (A) involving the aorta. *C,* Vena cava resection done with vascular staplers with en bloc aortic resection. The aorta was reconstructed with an interposition graft.

A balance of surgeon-controlled factors and tumor biology dictates patient outcome in oncologic surgery (Figure 5). This is especially true for patients affected with retroperitoneal sarcomas, where the tumor often reaches a large size, involves multiple structures, and the confines of the retroperitoneum and pelvis may hinder exposure. Of all the factors that impact outcome for patients with retroperitoneal sarcomas, the three most important are margin status, tumor grade, and tumor histology.

THE EFFECT OF MARGIN STATUS ON OUTCOME

Complete surgical resection is the mainstay of therapy for retroperitoneal sarcomas. The most important surgeon-controlled factor that determines outcome is completeness of resection (Figure 6). Patients with positive margins following resection have shorter survival times[5,19–21] and develop metastatic disease more frequently[5] than patients with negative margins. As with all malignancies, the goal of surgical treatment of retroperitoneal sarcomas is a margin-negative (R0) resection. Realistically, however, the true status of the entire margin from a large retroperitoneal sarcoma is difficult, if not impossible, to document pathologically. Therefore, in the majority of cases the goal of surgery should be a "gross total excision." This includes wide excision of the tumor

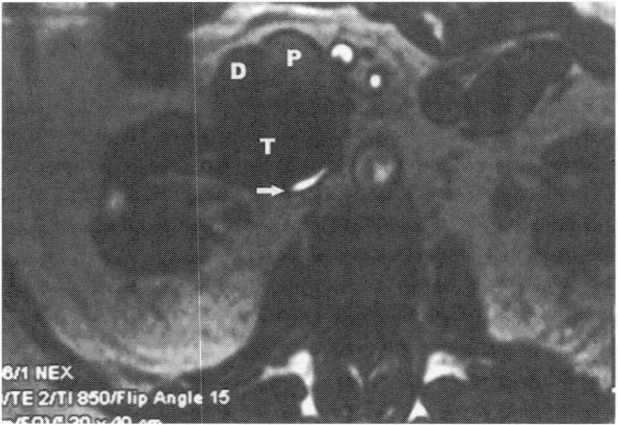

Figure 3 MRI demonstrating a leiomyosarcoma (T) of the inferior vena cava that invades the right renal hilum, duodenum (D), and pancreas (P). Note that the IVC remains patent (arrow). This sarcoma required a pancreaticoduodenectomy with en bloc right nephrectomy and vena cava resection with reconstruction.

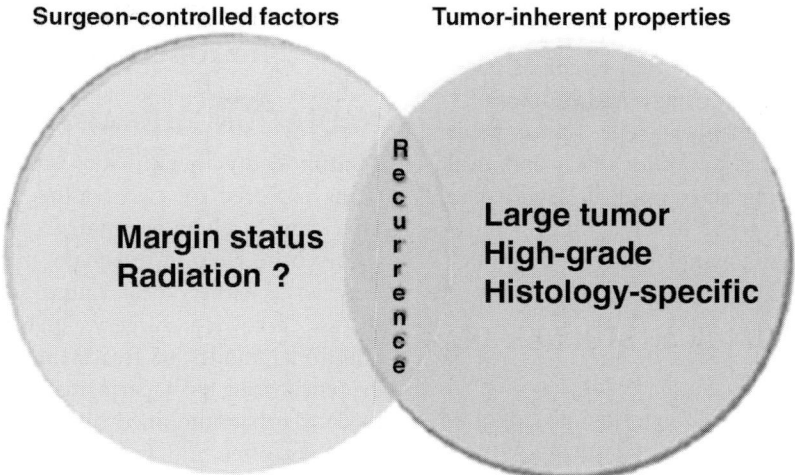

Figure 5 Local failure following resection of retroperitoneal sarcomas is determined by the interplay of the factors that are surgeon controlled and those inherent to the tumor.

with en bloc resection of adherent or invaded structures, when possible. Enucleation or "shelling out" of retroperitoneal sarcomas should be discouraged owing to the poor results. In fact, partial resection of a retroperitoneal sarcoma offers a similar median survival as an incisional biopsy.[21] One possible exception to this rule, however, is in cases of retroperitoneal liposarcoma where complete resection of the entire tumor is not feasible. Incomplete resection may provide prolongation of survival and successful symptom palliation for this specific tumor type.[23] This represents a function of tumor biology, in that the main case of symptoms and death from low-grade retroperitoneal liposarcoma is local disease, not

distant metastasis. Partial resection should be reserved for patients with low-grade liposarcomas who have significant symptoms that can be palliated by debulking, such as bowel or ureteral obstruction.

THE EFFECT OF TUMOR GRADE ON OUTCOME

Numerous studies on retroperitoneal sarcomas demonstrate the importance of tumor grade on prognosis.[5,11,18–20,24,25] In fact, grade is one of the components of the American Joint Committee on Cancer (AJCC) staging system.[13] As a reflection of tumor

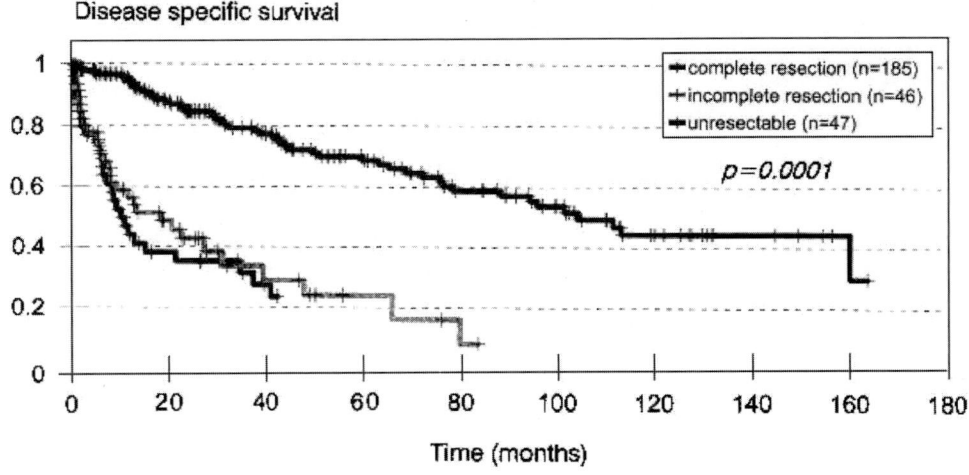

Figure 6 Disease-specific survival for retroperitoneal sarcomas based on margin status. The median survival of patients with grossly negative surgical margins was 103 months versus 18 months for patients who underwent an incomplete resection. There was no difference between patients who underwent incomplete resection and those deemed unresectable. Reproduced with permission from Lewis JJ et al.[5]

biology, grade has a huge impact on survival following resection. This is illustrated by the fact that resected patients with low-grade retroperitoneal sarcomas survive twice as long as patients with high-grade tumors[5,19,21] (Figure 7). Additionally, it appears that tumor grade's influence on survival applies to both primary and locally recurrent disease following resection.[19] It is not clear, however, whether tumor grade has a significant impact on the local failure rate following curative resection.[19]

THE EFFECT OF TUMOR HISTOLOGY ON OUTCOME

In addition to tumor grade, histology plays an important role in patient outcome following treatment of retroperitoneal sarcomas. Clinical behavior between the various types of sarcomas is as variable as the sarcomas themselves. Some sarcomas have a more insidious behavior, such as retroperitoneal liposarcomas.[21,23] These tumors often grow at a modest rate and have relatively long periods where they do not metastasize, despite achieving enormous tumor sizes. In fact, local recurrence without evidence for distant metastasis is relatively common following potentially curative resection for retroperitoneal liposarcomas,[5] as precise distinction between normal retroperitoneal fat and tumor often becomes impossible. Other histologies behave more aggressively with high rates of local failure following resection and a tendency for early metastasis. One of the most aggressive histologies is leiomyosarcoma.[20,21] These tumors have a high local recurrence rate and are often metastatic early in the disease course.

Multimodality Therapy for Retroperitoneal Sarcomas

RADIATION THERAPY

Multimodality therapy for retroperitoneal sarcomas is being explored for two reasons. First, disease outcome after surgery alone is unsatisfactory, with high rates of recurrence. Despite adequate margins, many patients experience either local failure or develop metastatic disease following surgery, highlighting the need for additional modes of treatment. Second, there is good evidence from trials performed on extremity and trunk sarcomas that combined modality therapy may improve recurrence-free and possibly overall survival compared with surgery alone.[26–29] These data, plus retrospective reports[3,30,31] suggest that there may be a role for radiation therapy in the treatment of retroperitoneal sarcomas. One of the major problems with delivering adequate doses of radiation to the retroperitoneum, however, is the dose-limiting toxicity of the gastrointestinal tract and spinal cord.

Radiation therapy may be delivered preoperatively, as part of a neoadjuvant regimen; intraoperatively; or postoperatively, as a component of adjuvant treatment. There are several potential advantages that neoadjuvant therapy may have over adjuvant therapy. First, when delivered preoperatively, radiation treatments may be more accurately delivered to the correct tissues, as the tumor accurately defines the treatment planes. In addition, the tumor may act as a tissue expander, thus preventing radiosensitive viscera from entering the

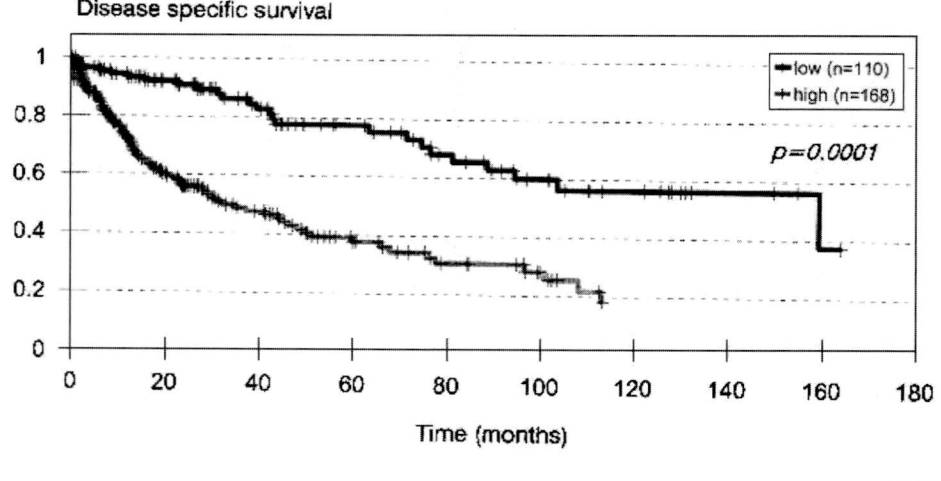

Figure 7 Disease-specific survival for retroperitoneal sarcomas based on tumor grade. The median survival of patients with low-grade tumors was 149 months vs 33 months for those with high-grade tumors. Reproduced with permission from Lewis JJ et al.[5]

radiation field. The effectiveness of the treatment may be determined, as radiographic assessment of the tumor's response can also be made. Additionally, postoperative scarring may alter the effectiveness of adjuvant radiation, as effective tissue oxygen delivery is important for radiation therapy. More patients may finish the entire course of treatment when delivered preoperatively, as some patients will inevitably have serious postoperative complications that limit their tolerance to adjuvant treatment. Finally, the dose of radiation therapy necessary to treat the tumor field may actually be lower when delivered preoperatively.[32]

Several groups have reported on the use of neoadjuvant radiotherapy for retroperitoneal sarcomas.[33,34] These data help to establish the feasibility of neoadjuvant radiotherapy for this disease. Based in part on these data, the American College of Surgeons Oncology Group (ACOSOG) has begun enrolling patients on a randomized, phase III protocol to formally evaluate preoperative radiation for retroperitoneal sarcomas. These data will hopefully clarify the role of preoperative radiation in this disease.

Another delivery strategy that has been studied is intraoperative radiation therapy (EB-IORT). Theoretically, EB-IORT may limit the dose-related toxicities to the surrounding tissues that would result from standard external beam radiotherapy. In a specially equipped operating room, the tumor bed is treated with focused radiation following tumor extirpation. Several small studies have been conducted on EB-IORT for retroperitoneal sarcomas. The results for local control following resection are conflicting,[35–37] in part owing to the small sample sizes. Further evaluation must be done before definitive conclusions can be made regarding EB-IORT.

There are no definitive data regarding adjuvant radiotherapy for retroperitoneal sarcomas. As previously discussed, the small bowel often becomes adherent to tumor resection beds, thus increasing the volume of normal tissue at risk of toxicity. It remains unknown what the role of postoperative radiation is for patients with positive margins following resection. Additionally, the use of adjuvant radiation based on tumor grade has not been elucidated. Selected histologic subtypes of retroperitoneal sarcomas may benefit from adjuvant external beam radiotherapy. Patients with completely resected inferior vena cava leiomyosarcomas appear to benefit from radiation with an improvement in local control.[38]

NEOADJUVANT CHEMORADIATION

Several groups have investigated the role of neoadjuvant chemoradiation in retroperitoneal sarcoma. The cyto-toxic agents most commonly studied are doxorubicin, ifosfamide, and idoxuridine. In highly selected cases, the majority of patients treated with this strategy are able to complete the chemoradiation and undergo the surgery as planned.[34,39] Interestingly, tumor downstaging sufficient enough to impact surgical therapy may occur in a minority of patients.[40] In addition, radiographic response to neoadjuvant chemoradiation may predict improved local control and overall survival following margin-negative resection.[40] Currently, however, neoadjuvant chemoradiation for retroperitoneal sarcomas remains investigational.

CHEMOTHERAPY

The use of chemotherapy for patients with resectable sarcomas is controversial. To date, no chemotherapy regimen has been proven to significantly improve survival for patients with retroperitoneal sarcoma. Additionally, the agents commonly used for STS have significant toxicities with limited response rates. As with radiation therapy, much of the literature evaluating chemotherapy is focused on extremity sarcomas. Most studies have not demonstrated a significant survival advantage. Several retrospective studies on postoperative chemotherapy for retroperitoneal sarcoma have demonstrated no survival benefit[20,41] and, in fact, has been associated with worse survival in small numbers of patients.[18,21] This was likely a result of the chemotherapeutic agents being reserved for patients with poorer prognostic factors, but nonetheless is quite intriguing.

Management of Recurrent Retroperitoneal Sarcomas

Despite adequate primary surgery, local recurrence remains a significant problem, and with accurate long-term follow-up, the true rate of local recurrence may exceed 70%.[3] Recurrence of a retroperitoneal sarcoma following resection is often a harbinger of disseminated disease and a marker for shortened survival.[5,20,21] Patients presenting with primary disease fare much better than those presenting with local recurrence.[19,21] Additionally, patients initially treated with adequate surgery who subsequently develop locally recurrent disease have a shortened survival.[18] Overall and disease-free survivals are worse for patients resected for recurrent disease, even when a curative resection is performed[5,19,20] (Figure 8). Additionally, the curative resection rate is lower for patients with recurrent disease when compared with primary tumors.[5,19,20]

A patient with locally recurrent disease should undergo thorough restaging, including CT of the abdo-

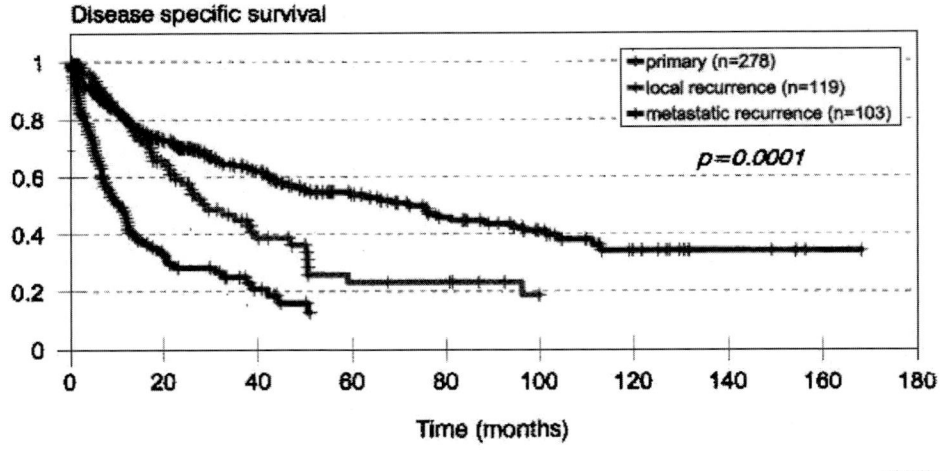

Figure 8 Disease-specific survival for retroperitoneal sarcomas based on presentation status. Medial survival was 72 months for those patients with primary disease, 28 months for those with recurrence, and 10 months for patients with metastatic disease. Reproduced with permission from Lewis JJ et al.[5]

men and pelvis. CT of the chest should be performed if there are abnormalities on plain chest radiographs or in cases of intermediate- or high-grade histology. Additional symptoms, such as bone pain or neurological symptoms should be evaluated individually with appropriate imaging modalities. In the absence of distant metastases, resection of the recurrence should be entertained. Similar to patients with primary disease, patients in whom complete resection of local recurrence can be performed survive longer than those who are not resectable.[5,18,20] Despite seemingly adequate surgery, some patients experience multiple recurrences. Repeat resection may have a role in patients with true local recurrences, as demonstrated by improved survival in highly selected cases.[42]

Conclusions

Retroperitoneal sarcomas are a rare, heterogeneous group of malignancies that pose significant management challenges to even the most experienced surgeons. Patients suspected of having a retroperitoneal sarcoma should undergo a thorough staging work-up and an evaluation by a surgeon experienced in the management of these tumors. Curative surgery is the best chance for cure, and often necessitates resection of multiple organs to achieve gross total excision. Biological factors inherent to the tumor, including tumor grade and histologic subtype significantly impact patient outcome. Despite seemingly adequate surgery, however, recurrence remains common, and patients found to have a true local recurrence should be evaluated for reresection. At this

time, there is no definitive evidence to support the routine use of chemotherapy or radiation therapy for resectable disease. Ongoing clinical trials will hopefully better define the roles of multimodality therapy for retroperitoneal sarcomas.

References

1. American Cancer Society. Cancer facts & figures 2004. Atlanta, GA: American Cancer Society: 2004.

2. DeVita VT Jr, Hellman S, Rosenberg SA. Cancer: principles and practice of oncology. Philadelphia, PA: Lippincott Williams & Wilkins; 2001.

3. Catton CN, O'Sullivan B, Kotwall C, et al. Outcome and prognosis in retroperitoneal soft tissue sarcoma. Int J Radiat Oncol Biol Phys 1994;29:1005–10.

4. Pisters PW. Staging and prognosis. In: Pollock RE, editor. American Cancer Society atlas of clinical oncology: soft tissue sarcomas. Hamilton, ON: BC Decker; 2002. p. 80–8.

5. Lewis JJ, Leung D, Woodruff JM, Brennan MF. Retroperitoneal soft-tissue sarcoma: analysis of 500 patients treated and followed at a single institution. Ann Surg 1998;228:355–65.

6. Brady MS, Gaynor JJ, Brennan MF. Radiation-associated sarcoma of bone and soft tissue. Arch Surg 1992;127:1379–85.

7. Zahm SH, Fraumeni JF Jr. The epidemiology of soft tissue sarcoma. Semin Oncol 1997;24:504–14.

8. Hoppin JA, Tolbert PE, Herrick RF, et al. Occupational chlorophenol exposure and soft tissue sarcoma risk

among men aged 30–60 years. Am J Epidemiol 1998;148: 693–703.

9. Arlen M, Marcove RC. Retroperitoneal sarcomas. In: Arlen M, Maarcove RC, editors. Surgical management of soft tissue tumors. Philadelphia: WB Saunders; 1987. p. 220.

10. Cormier JN, Pollock RE. Soft tissue sarcomas. CA Cancer J Clin 2004;54:94–109.

11. Alvarenga JC, Ball AB, Fisher C, et al. Limitations of surgery in the treatment of retroperitoneal sarcoma. Br J Surg 1991;78:912–6.

12. Russo P, Kim Y, Ravindran S, et al. Nephrectomy during operative management of retroperitoneal sarcoma. Ann Surg Oncol 1997;4:421–4.

13. Green FL, Page DL, Fleming ID, et al, editors. AJCC cancer staging manual. 6th ed. New York: Springer; 2002.

14. Skinner KA, Eilber FR. Soft tissue sarcoma nodal metastases: biologic significance and therapeutic considerations. Surg Oncol Clin N Am 1996;5:121–7.

15. van Dalen T, Hennipman A, Van Coevorden F, et al. Evaluation of a clinically applicable post-surgical classification system for primary retroperitoneal soft-tissue sarcoma. Ann Surg Oncol 2004;11:483–90.

16. Bevilacqua RG, Rogatko A, Hajdu SI, Brennan MF. Prognostic factors in primary retroperitoneal soft-tissue sarcomas. Arch Surg 1991;126:328–34.

17. Cody HS III, Turnbull AD, Fortner JG, Hajdu SI. The continuing challenge of retroperitoneal sarcomas. Cancer 1981;47:2147–52.

18. Karakousis CP, Gerstenbluth R, Kontzoglou K, Driscoll DL. Retroperitoneal sarcomas and their management. Arch Surg 1995;130:1104–9.

19. Ferrario T, Karakousis CP. Retroperitoneal sarcomas: grade and survival. Arch Surg 2003;138:248–51.

20. Chiappa A, Zbar AP, Biffi R, et al. Primary and recurrent retroperitoneal sarcoma: factors affecting survival and long-term outcome. Hepatogastroenterology 2004;51: 1304–9.

21. Hassan I, Park SZ, Donohue JH, et al. Operative management of primary retroperitoneal sarcomas: a reappraisal of an institutional experience. Ann Surg 2004;239:244–50.

22. Karakousis CP, Pourshahmir M. Thoracoabdominal incisions and resection of upper retroperitoneal sarcomas. J Surg Oncol 1999;72:150–5.

23. Shibata D, Lewis JJ, Leung DH, Brennan MF. Is there a role for incomplete resection in the management of retroperitoneal liposarcomas? J Am Coll Surg 2001;193: 373–9.

24. Dalton RR, Donohue JH, Mucha P Jr, et al. Management of retroperitoneal sarcomas. Surgery 1989;106:725–32.

25. Kilkenny JW III, Bland KI, Copeland EM III. Retroperitoneal sarcoma: the University of Florida experience. J Am Coll Surg 1996;182:329–39.

26. Andrews SF, Anderson PR, Eisenberg BL, et al. Soft tissue sarcomas treated with postoperative external beam radiotherapy with and without low-dose-rate brachytherapy. Int J Radiat Oncol Biol Phys 2004;59:475–80.

27. Pearlstone DB, Janjan NA, Feig BW, et al. Re-resection with brachytherapy for locally recurrent soft tissue sarcoma arising in a previously radiated field. Cancer J Sci Am 1999; 5:26–33.

28. Pisters PW, Harrison LB, Leung DH, et al. Long-term results of a prospective randomized trial of adjuvant brachytherapy in soft tissue sarcoma. J Clin Oncol 1996;14: 859–68.

29. Yang JC, Chang AE, Baker AR, et al. Randomized prospective study of the benefit of adjuvant radiation therapy in the treatment of soft tissue sarcomas of the extremity. J Clin Oncol 1998;16:197–203.

30. Harrison LB, Gutierrez E, Fischer JJ. Retroperitoneal sarcomas: the Yale experience and a review of the literature. J Surg Oncol 1986;32:159–64.

31. Tepper JE, Suit HD, Wood WC, et al. Radiation therapy of retroperitoneal soft tissue sarcomas. Int J Radiat Oncol Biol Phys 1984;10:825–30.

32. Zagars GK, Ballo MT. Sequencing radiotherapy for soft tissue sarcoma when re-resection is planned. Int J Radiat Oncol Biol Phys 2003;56:21–7.

33. Pisters PW, Ballo MT, Fenstermacher MJ, et al. Phase I trial of preoperative concurrent doxorubicin and radiation therapy, surgical resection, and intraoperative electron-beam radiation therapy for patients with localized retroperitoneal sarcoma. J Clin Oncol 2003;21:3092–7.

34. Robertson JM, Sondak VK, Weiss SA, et al. Preoperative radiation therapy and iododeoxyuridine for large retroperitoneal sarcomas. Int J Radiat Oncol Biol Phys 1995;31: 87–92.

35. Alektiar KM, Hu K, Anderson L, et al. High-dose-rate intraoperative radiation therapy (HDR-IORT) for retroperitoneal sarcomas. Int J Radiat Oncol Biol Phys 2000;47: 157–63.

36. Sindelar WF, Kinsella TJ, Chen PW, et al. Intraoperative radiotherapy in retroperitoneal sarcomas. Final results of a prospective, randomized, clinical trial. Arch Surg 1993;128: 402–10.

37. Willett CG, Suit HD, Tepper JE, et al. Intraoperative electron beam radiation therapy for retroperitoneal soft tissue sarcoma. Cancer 1991;68:278–83.

38. Hines OJ, Nelson S, Quinones-Baldrich WJ, Eilber FR. Leiomyosarcoma of the inferior vena cava: prognosis and comparison with leiomyosarcoma of other anatomic sites. Cancer 1999;85:1077–83.

39. Sondak VK, Robertson JM, Sussman JJ, et al. Preoperative idoxuridine and radiation for large soft tissue sarcomas: clinical results with five-year follow-up. Ann Surg Oncol 1998;5:106–12.

40. Meric F, Hess KR, Varma DG, et al. Radiographic response to neoadjuvant chemotherapy is a predictor of local control and survival in soft tissue sarcomas. Cancer 2002;95:1120–6.

41. Glenn J, Sindelar WF, Kinsella T, et al. Results of multimodality therapy of resectable soft-tissue sarcomas of the retroperitoneum. Surgery 1985;97:316–25.

42. Bautista N, Su W, O'Connell TX. Retroperitoneal soft-tissue sarcomas: prognosis and treatment of primary and recurrent disease. Am Surg 2000;66:832–6.

CHAPTER 75

SARCOMA SPECIAL SITUATIONS: HEAD AND NECK

THOMAS D. SHELLENBERGER, DMD, MD

ERICH M. STURGIS, MD, MPH

Sarcomas of the head and neck are a heterogeneous group of malignancies that display a spectrum of clinical behavior from slow growing to locally aggressive and regionally destructive lesions with the potential for systemic metastases. Like sarcomas of other sites of origin, those arising in the head and neck comprise a diverse array of histologic types with variable biologic behavior. Sarcoma affects a multiplicity of subsites within the head and neck, each with unique anatomical implications on form and function. While sarcomas are uncommon malignancies overall, these tumors occur even less commonly in the head and neck region; only about 10% of primary tumors arise from this region. Therefore, treatment recommendations are drawn from the results of multi-institutional trials representing small subgroups of patients with head and neck sarcoma and from the few retrospective series from single institutions. Together these factors contribute to the formidable challenge posed by these malignancies for the surgeon, the radiation oncologist, and the medical oncologist managing sarcomas in the head and neck region.

Epidemiology

Approximately 9% of soft tissue sarcomas in adults originate in the head and neck, while most arise in an extremity (59%), the trunk (19%), or the retroperitoneum (15%).[1] Like sarcoma in general, head and neck sarcoma occurs in a wide range of age groups, though most often in children, adolescents, and young adults. Indeed, in children, as many as 35% of rhabdomyosarcomas arise in the head and neck.[2] Sarcomas are very rare among head and neck neoplasms, representing only 1% of all primary tumors located within the head and neck region.[3] The vast majority of head and neck sarcomas

arise sporadically in patients without identifiable predisposing genetic risk factors, and exposure to a known environmental carcinogen can be identified in less than 10% of patients with head and neck sarcomas.[4]

Evaluation

Considering the preponderance of benign soft tissue masses and the relative frequency of cervical metastases from squamous cell carcinoma of the upper aerodigestive tract, a diagnosis of sarcoma is rare in the head and neck. Moreover, the nonspecific nature of presenting symptoms, sometimes brought to attention by antecedent trauma, typically fails to raise the suspicion of sarcoma, resulting in delay in diagnosis. Together these factors contribute to the difficulty in diagnosis of sarcoma at most head and neck sites. A minority of patients develop tumors at subsites that produce symptoms early and allow earlier detection. The subsite of origin determines the clinical presentation and subsequent diagnostic evaluation of patients with sarcoma of the head and neck.

Among 1,161 patients evaluated with sarcoma of the head and neck at The University of Texas M. D. Anderson Cancer Center between 1970 and 2004 (Table 1), the most frequent subsites of origin included the scalp or face (30%) and the sinonasal tract or anteromedial skull base (31%). The parotid gland or neck accounted for 19% of these tumors and the upper aerodigestive tract (oral cavity, oro/hypopharynx, and larynx) for 18%; sarcomas arising from the ear or posterolateral skull base were exceedingly rare (only 1%).

Like soft tissue sarcomas of the extremity and trunk, those arising in the neck commonly present as a painless mass. While a solitary neck mass is a frequent presentation of head and neck sarcoma, it is only rarely diagnosed

Table 1 Head and Neck Sarcomas at The University of Texas M. D. Anderson Cancer Center (1970–2004)

Histologic Type	No.	%	Scalp & Face	Sinonasal Tract Anteromedial Skull Base	Ear Posterolateral Skull Base	Upper Aerodigestive Tract	Parotid & Neck
Bony							
Osteosarcoma	173	14.9	0	95	1	76	1
Cartilagenous							
Chondrosarcoma	75	6.5	1	50	0	22	2
Fibrous							
Malignant fibrous histiocytoma	111	9.6	37	24	3	13	34
Fibrosarcoma	42	3.6	13	15	0	7	7
Dermatofibrosarcoma protruberans	60	5.2	48	0	1	0	11
Muscular							
Rhabdomyosarcoma	150	12.9	21	82	4	29	14
Leiomyosarcoma	33	2.8	7	8	0	8	10
Vascular							
Angiosarcoma	135	11.6	115	5	3	3	9
Hemangiopericytoma	23	2.0	6	8	0	2	7
Neural							
Neurogenic sarcoma	59	5.1	20	6	0	1	32
Fatty							
Liposarcoma	28	2.4	7	3	0	4	14
Histogenesis Unclear							
Synovial sarcoma	46	4.0	11	3	0	11	21
Ewing's sarcoma	13	1.1	4	5	0	0	4
Alveolar soft part sarcoma	6	0.5	1	3	0	1	1
Unclassified	207	17.8	58	56	2	32	59
Head & Neck Sarcoma (Totals)	1,161	100	349	363	14	209	226

as a primary soft tissue sarcoma. Although the presentation of a patient with a painless neck mass raises a broad range of diagnostic possibilities, the clinical setting alone can often narrow the differential diagnosis. Tumors of the neck can impinge on vital structures, causing dysphagia, hoarseness, and even dyspnea. Physical examination typically reveals a subcutaneous mass with possible distortion or destruction of adjacent structures. Associated signs and symptoms of pain and fixation to deep structures are ominous. Like painless masses arising in the neck, those in the parotid region do not frequently raise suspicion of sarcoma on differential diagnosis. Sarcoma of the scalp and face may present with skin and soft tissue manifestations that suggest the pathologic type. For instance, erythematous or violaceous macular lesions, which are often described as a spreading bruise, suggest angiosarcoma, while a raised, sclerotic, reddish-blue plaque-like nodule is associated with dermatofibrosarcoma protruberans.

Imaging studies augment the physical examination with more accurate assessment of the size and location of tumors in the head and neck.[5] Imaging studies also delineate bony involvement, intracranial extension, and regional nodal disease. High-resolution computed tomo-graphy (CT) and magnetic resonance imaging (MRI) scans are the studies of choice in nearly all cases. CT scanning is rapid and presents fewer problems with motion artifact than MRI. CT also offers greater sensitivity for bony abnormalities, another advantage of this modality. Furthermore, CT imaging is less expensive than MRI. MRI does, however, offer much better soft tissue resolution and is therefore better able to evaluate the primary lesion, perineural extension, dural involvement, bone marrow replacement, and orbital invasion. Multiplanar imaging also provides more accurate views of the tumor and adjacent structures. Other advantages of MRI are the lack of exposure to radiation and iodinated contrast material. Because of the unique qualities of CT and MRI, they can often be used in a complementary fashion, especially for surgical planning for skull base tumors. Imaging characteristics can differentiate between various histologic entities to predict specific pathologic features that assist in diagnosis. For example, osteosarcoma classically causes radial periosteal and extracortical bone deposition that produce a sunburst appearance on plain radiographs or CT scan.

Upon completion of imaging studies, a biopsy should be performed to establish a definitive tissue diagnosis and histologic classification for optimal planning of therapy, regardless of how strongly the history, physical findings, and radiographic studies suggest sarcoma. While an initial biopsy can be done with simple fine-needle aspiration (FNA), core needle biopsies provide adequate tissue to accurately subtype the tumor. Nevertheless, some institutions and pathologists prefer an open biopsy. When an open approach is required, the technique should be carefully considered to avoid contamination of uninvolved adjacent fascial compartments. Complete surgical excision is preferred over incisional biopsy for small masses in the neck or parotid. Incisional biopsy should be reserved for cases in children and for large masses when dysfunction or disfigurement might result from complete surgical resection. The incision for any biopsy should be oriented to easily incorporate future definitive surgical approaches. Moreover, the extent of tissue dissection and tumor resection should be limited to achieve only the goals of obtaining representative tissue. All specimens from current and previous biopsies, along with clinical and radiographic features, must be reviewed by a pathologist with experience in sarcoma subtyping. Special immunohistochemical stains and cytogenetic studies can greatly assist in identifying the tissue of origin. Because few centers have extensive experience in sarcoma evaluation, a second opinion from an outside facility can aid in resolving any diagnostic dilemmas.

Sarcomas are classified pathologically by tissue of origin to aid in determining prognosis and optimal treatment strategies. Head and neck sarcomas arise from bony or soft tissue elements depending on the mesenchymal cells from which they are derived. Among our series of patients with head and neck sarcomas at the University of Texas M. D. Anderson Cancer Center, most tumors, approximately 80%, were of the soft tissue type, and only 20% were of bony or cartilaginous origin (see Table 1). The tumor subtypes arising in the head and neck are no less heterogeneous than those arising from more frequent extremity, trunk, and retroperitoneal sites. In addition to their diverse origins from muscle, vessels, nerve, fat, and fibrous tissue, approximately 1 in 5 sarcomas is of unclear histogenesis or of unclassified subtype. The most common subtypes of sarcoma found within the head and neck region are osteosarcoma, pleomorphic sarcoma (malignant fibrous histiocytoma), angiosarcoma, and rhabdomyosarcoma.

Osteosarcoma is a primary malignancy of osteoblastic tissue that is defined by the direct formation of bone or osteoid by tumor cells. About 10% of osteosarcomas occur in the head and neck region.[5] These malignancies accounted for 15% of head and neck sarcomas in our series (see Table 1). Patients typically present in the third or fourth decade of life, some 10 to 15 years older on average than those presenting with osteosarcoma of the long bones. The mandible and maxilla are the sites most frequently affected in the head and neck region, followed by bones of the skull. At least one-third of osteosarcomas of the head and neck are of low histologic grade, perhaps explaining their lower potential for distant metastasis compared with primary tumors of other sites.[6] However, the ability of obtaining wide surgical margins is often limited for osteosarcoma of the head and neck region, making local recurrence more common.

Malignant fibrous histiocytoma, also known as pleomorphic sarcoma, the most common histologic subtype of soft tissue sarcoma overall,[7] represents a significant proportion of head and neck sarcomas—14% of head and neck soft tissue sarcomas in our series (see Table 1). With the increased accuracy of ultrastructural and immunohistochemical subtyping, the diagnosis of malignant fibrous histiocytoma currently includes tumors of a broadened range of cellular origins. In the head and neck region, these lesions present as subcutaneous or submucosal lesions in the parotid, sinonasal tract, or upper aerodigestive tract, and rarely in bone.

Angiosarcoma is a malignancy of vascular endothelial cell origin that, while rare, occurs in the head and neck region in about 50% of cases.[8] These lesions classically present as bruise-like macules and plaques on the forehead and scalp of elderly white men.[9] The correct diagnosis is often delayed by the similarity to more common, benign dermatologic conditions. Immunohistochemical markers such as CD31, CD34, factor VIII, and von Willebrand factor aid in the histologic classification.[10–12] The growth pattern of angiosarcoma is characterized by extensive radial invasion within the dermis.

Rhabdomyosarcoma, while rarely affecting adults, represents the most common form of sarcoma in children and arises in the head and neck region in about 40% of cases.[13] Unlike other types of soft tissue sarcoma, these tumors carry significant potential for metastasis to regional lymph nodes in the neck. A thorough investigation is warranted because as many as 23% of patients harbor disease at distant sites.[14–17]

Staging

The current American Joint Committee on Cancer staging system for soft tissue sarcoma is based on histologic grade, tumor size and depth, and the presence of regional nodal or distant metastasis.[18] While the staging system is optimally designed for staging extremity tumors, a major limitation is its lack of consideration for anatomic and histologic heterogeneity among soft tissue sarcomas. These concerns apply especially to head and neck sites where primary tumors are relatively smaller at presentation but commonly lie deep to the deep fascia. Therefore, the system lacks stage discrimination and thus may provide less accurate prognostic information for head and neck sarcomas than for sarcomas of other sites.

Prognostic Factors

For adult soft tissue sarcomas of all sites, size (> 5 cm), high grade, local extension (to skin, major neurovascular structures, or bone), and positive surgical margins have been linked in multivariate analysis to increased rates of local recurrence and distant failure, and decreased disease-specific survival (DSS).[19,20] Soft tissue sarcomas arising in the head and neck region are associated with the highest local recurrence rates and lowest DSS rates of all soft tissue sarcomas. Several studies of head and neck soft tissue sarcomas of various histologic types have attempted to quantify outcomes associated with tumor factors. The majority of series have reported a correlation between tumor size (> 5 cm) and high histologic grade and decreased DSS.[3,21–23] A few studies have evaluated the impact of local tumor extent on outcome. Farhood and colleagues found a univariate association of bony involvement with decreased overall survival (OS),[24] while LeVay and colleagues demonstrated by multivariate analysis that local extent predicts rates of local recurrence, distant metastases, and disease-free survival (DFS).[25] In five studies, surgical margin status was linked to both local control and survival, and two of these confirmed the association in multivariate analyses.[19,21] While outcome may vary among subsites of origin within the head and neck, this factor appears less predictive than other prognostic indicators. The strongest prognostic factors for sarcoma of the head and neck appear to include tumor size, local extent, grade, and margin status, and these factors provide a basis for comparing results of treatment strategies and for determining the role of adjuvant therapies.

Management

The treatment approach toward sarcoma of the head and neck is determined by the tumor type, location, and grade, along with consideration of patient age and performance status. The treatment goals are determined by resectability. Surgery alone or combined with adjuvant radiotherapy is the mainstay of treatment for sarcomas of the head and neck. A multimodal approach offers improved local control in the management of head and neck sarcoma, especially for those lesions with high histologic grade or anatomic limitations to en bloc resection. An optimal approach is best planned in a multidisciplinary setting with consideration for the timing and sequence of modes of therapy, reconstructive strategies, and plans for rehabilitation. In parallel with limb-sparing surgical approaches permitted by multimodal therapy for extremity sarcomas, functional organ preservation has emerged in the treatment strategies for head and neck sarcoma.

SURGERY

Surgical resection with wide margins, alone or combined with adjuvant radiotherapy, provides the best chance for cure of head and neck sarcoma in the absence of metastatic disease. The unique anatomical considerations of the head and neck allow smaller tumors to involve critical neurovascular structures, limiting complete en bloc resection, with implications for both local control and survival. Therefore, the operation should be planned by an experienced surgical team with the expertise of specialized radiologists and pathologists. Moreover, consultation with neurological, ophthalmologic, and plastic surgeons is often warranted.

Surgery for sarcoma of the head and neck should follow the same sound oncologic principles applied to sarcoma operations at other sites. The conduct of surgery for sarcoma of any site of origin is dictated by a growth pattern in which centrifugal expansion occurs with infiltration along tissue planes formed by fascia, muscle, and bone. Compressed tissue surrounding the enlarging mass forms a pseudocapsule that is penetrated by malignant cells extending a considerable distance from gross tumor.[26] Therefore, excision along involved planes leaves extracapsular microscopic disease in situ at the circumference of the resection margin, leading to the possibility of multicentric recurrence, and such extracapsular enucleation of sarcoma carries a local recurrence rate of up to 90%.[27] Conversely, complete excision may be accomplished by limiting dissection to uninvolved tissue planes and resecting the tumor en bloc with wide (2 to 3 cm) margins including, when possible, at least one uninvolved tissue plane circumferentially. The resection may include skin, subcutaneous tissue, and soft tissue or bone adjacent to the tumor. Any incisions and tracts of a previous biopsy should be excised en bloc with the specimen. Major neurovascular structures should be widely exposed proximally and distally to allow meticulous assessment of the perineural or adventitial planes in determining resectability. The resected specimen margins are carefully inked for pathologic assessment of microscopic clearance. Residual disease is a powerful predictor of local recurrence and disease-related mortality.

Surgery for sarcoma of the head and neck combines these oncologic principles with basic tenets that apply to surgical procedures at each subsite. Though guided by similar sound oncologic principles, surgery in the head and neck poses additional challenges because of the unique anatomic considerations of the site. Operations for sarcoma of the head and neck vary with the subsite of tumor. The primary surgical goal, however, remains the same as that for sarcomas at other sites—complete en bloc excision.

Sarcomas presenting as a mass in the neck often arise from tissue within the fascial compartment of the neck. Tumors may be contained within the fascial compartment or expand to involve superficial or deep structures. Complete resection is attained more easily for soft tissue sarcomas of the neck than for those arising at other head and neck sites. The primary goal of en bloc resection can usually be achieved by neck dissections defined by the boundaries of uninvolved structures. When the mass is contained within a fascial compartment, the mass can be removed by excision of the involved compartment and its structures by modifications of standard oncologic neck dissection. Such an approach adheres to the oncologic principles of compartment dissection of the neck defined by tissue planes rather than the goal of complete lymphadenectomy. Neck wounds can typically be closed primarily. When primary closure places undue tension on wound edges, however, larger skin defects can occasionally be closed with local rotation flaps or split thickness skin grafts. Larger defects and those requiring bulk are best handled by pedicled myocutaneous flaps from pectoralis major and trapezius muscle donor sites. These more complex reconstructive options should also be considered to abrogate the potential risk for complications related to preoperative radiotherapy or subsequent postoperative radiotherapy.

Sarcomas may arise as a mass in the parotid gland. For tumors arising in the superficial lobe of the parotid gland, superficial parotidectomy can be performed with preservation of the facial nerve. Those tumors arising from the deep lobe often present as a parapharyngeal space mass and may be excised by a transcervical approach. Tumors involving both the superficial and deep lobes of the parotid often present with facial paralysis and require radical parotidectomy, sacrificing the facial nerve to obtain complete resection. Moreover, mastoidectomy may be required to obtain negative surgical margins.

Wide local excision is the initial step in treatment for the majority of soft tissue sarcomas of the scalp and face. The ability to achieve clear surgical margins is, however, hampered by the propensity for radial spread (particularly for angiosarcoma), and the desire to preserve form

and function. For most lesions of the scalp and some of the face, the procedure of choice is wide local excision down to bone, including the periosteum, with meticulous frozen sections to ensure negative margins. For scalp tumors with bony involvement of the calvarium, craniectomy is required. For lesions overlying the parotid gland, the excision is extended to include superficial parotidectomy with facial nerve dissection to preserve the main trunk and uninvolved branches. With eyelid involvement, total lid resection may be required, whereas extension beyond the periorbita or orbital septum may require orbital exenteration for complete resection. While conservative surgery followed by adjuvant therapy may preserve a globe, the implications of incomplete resection on survival must be considered. Extension of tumor to the bony and cartilaginous structures of the midface may require maxillectomy and rhinectomy for adequate resection. Perineural spread of tumor along major cranial nerve branches is an ominous sign, often limiting complete resection owing to skull base involvement and the unreliability of frozen section assessment of involved nerves. While such perineural extension is common for other head and neck histologic types (squamous cell carcinoma and adenoid cystic carcinoma), it is rare for sarcomas of the head and neck.

The approach to reconstruction of defects resulting from surgical resection of soft tissue sarcoma of the scalp and face is determined by the size and complexity of the defect. Options vary from simple primary closure to more advanced techniques, such as microvascular free-tissue transfer. The primary reconstructive goals are to restore form by providing coverage of exposed bone and preventing radiotherapy-associated complications. Additional goals include restoration of eyelid function, oral competence, and a patent nasal airway. Well-executed reconstruction is critical to maximizing form, function, and quality of life. Primary closure with local rotation or advancement flaps is often adequate for facial soft tissue defects. Scalp defects more commonly require split-thickness skin graft coverage. For defects widely exposing cortical bone, removal of the outer table can provide a well-vascularized medullary bone surface capable of supporting a skin graft. Larger defects resulting from resection of facial bones and overlying soft tissue often require microvascular free flap reconstruction. Moreover, prostheses may be invaluable in restoring facial form and oronasal separation after orbital exenteration, total rhinectomy, or maxillectomy without major loss of skin and soft tissue. For sarcomas of the upper aerodigestive tract, more classic procedures such as laryngectomy or mandibulectomy may be required.

RADIOTHERAPY

The rationale for adjuvant radiation in the management of head and neck soft tissue sarcoma in adults has stemmed from the results of limb-sparing surgery combined with postoperative radiotherapy for extremity sarcoma. Indeed, that approach offers improved functional results and local control rates similar to those of radical amputation without compromising OS.[28] While adjuvant radiation therapy for management of the extremity sarcoma is supported by randomized trials and large institutional series, patients with head and neck sarcoma were either excluded or insufficient in number to allow meaningful subgroup analysis. Moreover, no similar studies focusing on the treatment of head and neck sarcoma are available to define the optimal role of radiation therapy. Therefore, support for the use of adjuvant radiation therapy for the head and neck soft tissue sarcoma is largely empirical, extrapolated from the experience at other sites of origin or based on retrospective reviews of head and neck series.

Despite such limitations, adjuvant radiotherapy has evolved over the last several decades as an important means of improving local disease control after surgery for adult soft tissue sarcoma of the head and neck. The need for adjuvant local therapy is strongly supported by the high rate of local recurrence linked to the difficulty in obtaining microscopically negative margins after resection of tumors in close proximity to vital structures within the head and neck region. Bentz and colleagues reported a series of adult soft tissue sarcomas of the head and neck from Memorial Sloan Kettering Cancer Center in which final pathologic findings demonstrated positive margins in 42% of patients overall and 63% of patients presenting after prior treatment.[29] A high rate of local recurrence was attributed to the predominance of patients treated with surgery alone (77%) and, more importantly, demonstrated a close relationship between local recurrence and survival. Thus, adjuvant radiotherapy appears to improve local control rates with the potential of increasing DFS.

Our standard approach administers adjuvant radiotherapy after surgery for head and neck soft tissue sarcoma in patients with high-grade and some intermediate-grade tumors of any size. Only patients with small (< 5 cm), previously untreated, low-grade tumors resected with negative microscopic margins may be considered adequately treated by wide local excision alone. As for soft tissue sarcomas of other sites, the optimal mode and sequence of radiation therapy have not yet been determined.

External beam therapy is delivered postoperatively to total doses similar to hose employed in sarcoma of the extremity, 60 to 70 Gy in standard fractions over 4 to 6 weeks. High-grade tumors and positive margins require an additional 5 to 10 Gy, up to 75 Gy. While the optimal margins of radiotherapy remain undetermined, wider coverage beyond 5 to 7 cm from the surgical bed is warranted for increasing tumor size and grade. Metallic clips placed in the tumor bed during surgery have been used to define the resection limits and identify the location of positive margins for optimal planning of radiotherapy.

Brachytherapy is an alternative approach to adjuvant radiotherapy in patients with head and neck soft tissue sarcoma, involving placement of multiple catheters within the tumor resection bed to deliver iridium[192]. Brachytherapy offers the theoretical advantage of delivering an adequate dose of ionizing radiation to the surgical bed while sparing adjacent vital structures of the head and neck region based on the radiobiology of the inverse square law. Additional benefits include a shorter overall treatment time (4 to 6 days) and lower overall costs than external beam therapy. The utility of brachytherapy in head and neck sites can be inferred from the report of Harrison and colleagues of a prospective trial in which surgery plus adjuvant brachytherapy improved local control rate to 90% from 65% with surgery alone for completely resected high-grade sarcomas of the extremities and trunk.[30] Furthermore, brachytherapy is particularly useful in treating recurrent disease after prior external beam therapy and planned positive margins at vital structures such as the carotid artery.

Like the mode of radiotherapy, the optimal timing of radiotherapy has not been determined. Preoperative radiotherapy offers several theoretical advantages over postoperative radiotherapy.[31] First, radiation therapy delivered early in the course of a multidisciplinary approach can improve planning and ensure that treatment is delivered without the delays imposed by perioperative complications. Second, a lower total dose of radiation can be delivered to a smaller field of tumor that may have greater tissue oxygenation. Finally, preoperative radiation can result in a tumor response that facilitates surgical resectability. A randomized trial of soft tissue sarcoma of the extremities found a higher rate of wound complications in patients treated with preoperative radiation (35%) than patients treated with postoperative radiation (17%), with similarly high rates of local control and progression-free survival.[32] Nonetheless, wound healing complications in the head and neck may be offset by a generally better regional blood supply and more frequent use of primary reconstruction with vascularized tissue.[33] Moreover, intensity-modulated radiotherapy techniques have improved the ability to deliver highly localized radiotherapy in the head and neck region and may offer further advantages for preoperative targeting and delivery.

Preoperative radiation may also be justified in selected patients whose soft tissue sarcoma of the head and neck has been deemed unresectable or inoperable, if conservative resection can offer palliation. De Paoli and colleagues reported the use of preoperative radiation therapy prior to resection of skull base sarcomas that had been considered unresectable. In each of seven patients, an initially inoperable tumor was conservatively resected in order to preserve function or maximize palliation.[34]

CHEMOTHERAPY

Despite adequate local tumor control with surgery and radiotherapy, mortality from head and neck sarcoma occurs from distant metastasis, most commonly to lungs. Thus, the goals of chemotherapy for sarcoma have been directed toward systemic control in an attempt to prolong DFS. Such efforts have been approached with therapeutic, adjuvant, and palliative intentions. The use of traditional generic approaches to chemotherapy belies the heterogeneity of soft tissue sarcomas in that chemosensitivity varies according to the tumor subtype.[35] Head and neck sarcomas range according to histologic subtype from highly responsive to universally resistant to cytotoxic chemotherapy. The likelihood of a response is further influenced by tumor grade, the patient's age and performance status, and the timing of metastatic disease.[35] Therefore, major obstacles to the use of adjuvant chemotherapy have been the risks of toxicity in patients who are unlikely to respond to therapy and the difficulty in identifying patients who are most likely to benefit from therapy.

The use of postoperative chemotherapy for head and neck soft tissue sarcoma bears a burden of proof similar to that for localized, resectable soft tissue sarcoma of other sites. A lack of benefit from adjuvant chemotherapy for head and neck sarcoma may be implied from the Sarcoma Meta-analysis Collaboration, which evaluated 14 trials of doxorubicin-based adjuvant chemotherapy, several of which included head and neck sites.[36] The analysis revealed significant increases in time to local and distant recurrence and rates of recurrence-free survival for patients who received chemotherapy; however, there was no significant difference in OS. While subset analysis revealed a greater benefit for patients with extremity sarcoma, no clear benefit was evident at other sites owing to wide confidence intervals reflecting small numbers of patients. Thus, there is still no conclusive evidence for the use of adjuvant chemotherapy following resection for patients with head and neck soft tissue sarcoma.

Findings of the European Organisation for Research and Treatment of Cancer (EORTC) trial in 468 soft tissue sarcoma patients comparing an adjuvant regimen of CYVADIC (cyclophosphamide, vincristine, doxorubicin, and dacarbazine) with no chemotherapy carry implications in the treatment of head and neck soft tissue sarcoma.[37] Relapse-free survival rate was significantly increased (56% versus 43% for controls) and local recurrence rate significantly reduced (17% versus 31%) by adjuvant chemotherapy despite similar rates of distant metastasis and OS. The reduction in local recurrence rate was apparent only in head and neck and trunk tumors but not in extremity tumors. Thus, these findings suggest a potential for adjuvant chemotherapy to improve local control in high-risk disease sites such as the head and neck where radical surgery and radiation are less feasible.

Based upon the currently available data from these trials, evidence is insufficient to support the standard use of adjuvant chemotherapy in the management of head and neck sarcoma. However, in selected patients for whom the completeness of resection or the intensification of radiation therapy is limited, adjuvant chemotherapy appears to improve local control. Thus, further evaluation in trials of adjuvant chemotherapy is warranted in these settings and in patients whose tumor is of high histologic grade.

Preoperative chemotherapy for head and neck sarcoma offers several of the same theoretical advantages proposed for chemotherapy at other disease sites and for preoperative radiotherapy.[38] First, delivering systemic therapy earlier in the disease course may be more effective against smaller tumor burdens of micrometastatic disease. Second, induction therapy may result in a response that improves the likelihood of complete resection with negative margins that might not be possible otherwise. Another advantage is the ability to assess a tumor response in situ by radiologic imaging and pathologically after resection and thus tailor subsequent treatment approaches while providing additional prognostic information. The feasibility of surgery after neoadjuvant chemotherapy has been demonstrated by Meric and colleagues in a retrospective review of 309 patients who underwent surgery for extremity or retroperitoneal/visceral soft tissue sarcoma.[38] Patients who received neoadjuvant chemotherapy had no increase in early or delayed surgical complications compared to those who underwent surgery without neoadjuvant therapy. Our experience with surgery in the head and neck after neoadjuvant chemotherapy has been similar and may be attributed to a more reliable regional blood supply in the head and neck than in the extremities and retroperitoneum.

While preoperative chemoradiation strategies has been investigated in the treatment of extremity and retroperitoneal soft tissue sarcomas over the last two decades, similar approaches for head and neck tumors have been less studied. Such strategies are based primarily upon maximizing local control while preserving function and secondarily upon early treatment of potential micrometastatic disease. The rationale is directed toward prolonging recurrence-free or even OS in selected patients. Pisters and colleagues cite the promise of future investigation supported by (1) the favorable response rates and acceptable toxicity profiles in preliminary reports of extended-duration chemotherapy with concurrent radiation, (2) local control rates in excess of 95% with concurrent (intravenous or intra-arterial) doxorubicin-based chemoradiation for locally advanced soft tissue sarcoma, and (3) favorable preliminary survival data from RTOG 95-14.[39] This multi-institutional phase II trial has shown a 2-year actuarial OS rate of 95% among 66 patients with high-risk extremity sarcoma treated by preoperative sequential chemotherapy and split-course radiation.[40] Furthermore, novel approaches to radiosensitization, including doxorubicin-, gemcitabine-, idoxuridine-, razoxane-, and ifosfamide-based regimens, have shown promise in selected patients with soft tissue sarcomas of various sites. Though limited by the local complications of intra-arterial delivery to tumors of the head and neck, chemotherapy with doxorubicin-based regimens delivered by intravenous routes and combined with concurrent or sequential radiation may offer similar promise. Furthermore, the comparability of response rates between head and neck and extremity sites of soft tissue sarcoma warrants the inclusion of patients with head and neck tumors in future multi-institutional trials.

FOLLOW-UP

The major objectives for surveillance after curative therapy for head and neck sarcoma parallel those outlined by Patel and colleagues for soft tissue sarcoma: (1) early identification of curable recurrences and reversible/treatable complications of therapy, (2) identification of second primary tumors, and (3) increasingly, reassurance of the patient. These objectives are met by careful consideration of prognostic factors and patterns of recurrence.[41]

After curative therapy for head and neck sarcoma, the major determinant of survival is the control of local and distant recurrence. In contrast to patients with a primary tumor of the extremity or trunk, patients with head and neck sarcoma have a greater tendency toward local recurrence rather than distant metastases. In series reported by Weber and colleagues[3] and by Tran and colleagues[42], the lung was the most common site of distant metastasis, and the majority of local recurrences occur within 2 years of treatment. While patients with isolated local recurrence have had 5- and 10-year DSS rates of 51% and 48%, respectively, the rates for patients with distant relapse are dismal at 16% and 10%.[41] Nonetheless, the overall 5-, 10-, and 15-year DSS rates of 27%, 22%, and 19%, respectively, for patients after first relapse attest that a small group of patients can be long-term survivors.[41] Surveillance strategies should thus attempt to identify favorable subsets of these patients with resectable recurrences.

We monitor patients who have undergone curative therapy for head and neck soft tissue sarcoma with history, physical exam, chest X-ray, and cross-sectional imaging every 3 to 4 months for the first 2 years, every 4 to 6 months for the next 2 years, and every 6 to 12 months for the fifth year. Laboratory tests may include a complete blood count, electrolytes, liver function tests, and creatinine at each follow-up visit. Cross-sectional imaging, especially for surgical sites difficult to examine clinically, may be performed by CT alone or by MRI. Ultrasonography provides an additional means of surveillance and offers the advantage of FNA biopsy to aid in the evaluation of suspect findings. While its role in surveillance after therapy for sarcoma remains to be defined, positron emission tomography scanning offers promise in differentiating recurrent disease from postoperative scar tissue in selected cases.

References

1. DeVita VT Jr, Hellman S, Rosenberg SA. Sarcomas of the soft tissues and bone. In: DeVita VT Jr, Hellman S, Rosenberg SA, editors. Cancer: principles and practice of oncology, 6th ed. Philadelphia: Lippincott Williams and Wilkins; 2005. p. 1841–91.

2. Lawrence W Jr, Anderson JR, Gehan EA, Maurer H. Pretreatment TNM staging of childhood rhabdomyosarcoma: a report of the Intergroup Rhabdomyosarcoma Study Group. Children's Cancer Study Group. Pediatric Oncology Group. Cancer 1997;80:1165–70.

3. Weber RS, Benjamin RS, Peters LJ, et al. Soft tissue sarcomas of the head and neck in adolescents and adults. Am J Surg 1986;152:386–92.

4. McClay EF. Epidemiology of bone and soft tissue sarcomas. Semin Oncol 1989;16:264–72.

5. Potter BO, Sturgis EM. Sarcomas of the head and neck. Surg Oncol Clin N Am 2003;12:379–417.

6. O'Sullivan B, Audet N, Catton C, Gullane P. Soft tissue and bone sarcomas of the head and neck. In: Harrison LB, Sessions RB, Hong WK, editors. Head and neck cancer: a

multidisciplinary approach, 2nd ed. Philadelphia: Lippincott Williams and Wilkins; 2003. p. 786–824.

7. Enzinger FM. Malignant fibrous histiocytoma 20 years after Staout. Am J Surg Pathol 1986;10(Suppl 1):43–53.

8. Lydiatt WM, Shaha AR, Shah JP. Angiosarcoma of the head and neck. Am J Surg 1994;168:451–4.

9. Morrison WH, Byers RM, Garden AS, et al. Cutaneous angiosarcoma of the head and neck. A therapeutic dilemma. Cancer 1995;76:319–27.

10. Mark RJ, Tran LM, Sercarz J, et al. Angiosarcoma of the head and neck. The UCLA experience 1955 through 1990. Arch Otolaryngol Head Neck Surg 1993;119:973–8.

11. Loos BM, Wieneke JA, Thompson LD. Laryngeal angiosarcoma: a clinicopathologic study of five cases with a review of the literature. Laryngoscope 2001;111:1197–202.

12. Aust MR, Olsen KD, Lewis JE, et al. Angiosarcomas of the head and neck: clinical and pathologic characteristics. Ann Otol Rhinol Laryngol 1997;106:943–51.

13. Callender TA, Weber RS, Janjan N, et al. Rhabdomyosarcoma of the nose and paranasal sinuses in adults and children. Otolaryngol Head Neck Surg 1995;112: 252–7.

14. Nayar RC, Prudhomme F, Parise O, et al. Rhabdomyosarcoma of the head and neck in adults: a study of 26 patients. Laryngoscope 1993;103:1362–6.

15. Kraus DH, Saenz NC, Gollamudi S, et al. Pediatric rhabdomyosarcoma of the head and neck. Am J Surg 1197;174:556–60.

16. Anderson GJ, Toth GK, Gibbons WA. Protein engineering of the IgE receptor and its subunits by solid-phase synthesis and spectroscopy. Biochem Soc Trans 1990;10: 1306–7.

17. Feldman BA. Rhabdomyosarcoma of the head and neck. Laryngoscope 1982;92:424–40.

18. Green FL, Page DL, Flemming FD, et al. Soft tissue sarcoma. In: Page DL, editor. American Joint Committee on Cancer: Cancer Staging Manual, 6th ed. New York: Springer; 2002. p. 221–6.

19. LeVay J, O'Sullivan B, Catton C, et al. Outcome and prognostic factors in soft tissue sarcoma in the adult. Int J Radiat Oncol Biol Phys 1993;27:1091–9.

20. Cakir S, Dincbas FO, Uzel O. Multivariate analysis of prognostic factors in 75 patients with soft tissue sarcoma. Radiother Oncol 1995;37:10–6.

21. Kraus DH, Dubner S, Harrison LB, et al. Prognostic factors for recurrence and survival in head and neck soft tissue sarcomas. Cancer 1994;74:697–702.

22. Wanebo HJ, Koness RJ, MacFarlane JK, et al. Head and neck sarcoma: report of the head and neck sarcoma Registry. Society of Head and Neck Surgeons Committee on Research. Head Neck 1992;14:1–7.

23. Greager JA, Patel MK, Briele HA, et al. Soft tissue sarcomas of the adult head and neck. Cancer 1985;56:820–4.

24. Farhood AI, Hajdu SI, Shiu MH, Strong EW. Soft tissue sarcomas of the head and neck in adults. Am J Surg 1990; 160:365–9.

25. LeVay J, O'Sullivan B, Catton C, et al. An assessment of prognostic factors in soft-tissue sarcoma of the head and neck. Arch Otolaryngol Head Neck Surg 1994;120:981–6.

26. Bowden L, Booher RJ. The principles and technique of resection of soft parts form sarcoma. Surgery 1958;44:963–76.

27. Enneking WK. In: Enneking WK, editor. Musculoskeletal tumor surgery. New York: Churchill Livingstone; 1983. p. 1–23.

28. Yang JC, Chang AE, Baker AR, et al. Randomized prospective study of the benefit of adjuvant radiation therapy in the treatment of soft tissue sarcomas of the extremity. J Clin Oncol 1998;16:197–203.

29. Bentz BG, Singh B, Woodruff J, et al. Head and neck soft tissue sarcomas: a multivariate analysis of outcomes. Ann Surg Oncol 2004;11:619–28.

30. Harrison LB, Franzese F, Gaynor JJ, Brennan MF. Long-term results of a prospective randomized trial of adjuvant brachytherapy in the management of completely resected soft tissue sarcomas of the extremity and superficial trunk. Int J Radiat Oncol Biol Phys 1993;27:259–65.

31. Cormier JN, Pollock RE. Soft tissue sarcomas. CA Cancer J Clin 2004;54:94–109.

32. O'Sullivan B, Davis AM, Turcotte R, et al. Preoperative versus postoperative radiotherapy in soft-tissue sarcoma of the limbs: a randomized trial. Lancet 2002;359:2235–41.

33. O'Sullivan B, Gullane P, Irish J, et al. Preoperative radiotherapy for adult head and neck soft tissue sarcoma: assessment of wound complication rates and cancer outcome in a prospective series. World J Surg 2003;27: 875–83.

34. De Paoli A, Bertola G, Boz G, et al. Radiation therapy and conservative surgery for soft tissue sarcomas of the extremities, torso and head and neck. Ann Oncol 1992;(3 Suppl 2):S97–101.

35. Clark MA, Fisher C, Judson I, Thomas JM. Soft-tissue sarcomas in adults. N Engl J Med 2005;353:701–11.

36. Adjuvant chemotherapy for localised resectable soft-tissue sarcoma of adults:meta-analysis of individual data. Sarcoma Meta-analysis Collaboration. Lancet 1997;350: 1647–54.

37. Bramwell V, Rouesse J, Steward W, et al. Adjuvant CYVADIC chemotherapy for adult soft tissue sarcoma—reduced local recurrence but no improvement in survival: a study of the European Organization for Research and Treatment of Cancer Soft Tissue and Bone Sarcoma Group. J Clin Oncol 1994;12:1137–49.

38. Meric F, Milas M, Hunt KK, et al. Impact of neoadjuvant chemotherapy on postoperative morbidity in soft tissue sarcomas. J Clin Oncol 2000;18:3378–83.

39. Pisters PW, Ballo MT, Patel SR. Preoperative chemoradiation treatment strategies for localized sarcoma. Ann Surg Oncol 2002;9:535–42.

40. Kraybill WG, Spiro IJ, Harris JA, et al. Radiation Therapy Oncology (RTOG) 95-14: a phase II study of neoadjuvant chemotherapy and radiation therapy in high risk, high grade, soft tissue sarcoma of the extremities and body wall: a preliminary report. Proc Am Soc Clin Oncol 2001;20:348a.

41. Patel SR, Zagars GK, Pisters PW. The follow-up of adult soft-tissue sarcomas. Semin Oncol 2003;30:413–6.

42. Tran LM, Mark R, Meier R, et al. Sarcomas of the head and neck. Prognostic factors and treatment strategies. Cancer 1992;70:169–77.

CHAPTER 76

RETROPERITONEAL SARCOMAS: TREATMENT ISSUES

PETER W.T. PISTERS, MD

Patients with retroperitoneal sarcomas comprise approximately 15% of patients with soft tissue sarcoma referred to a tertiary care center.[1] These patients represent a significant challenge to treating physicians owing to the large size of these tumors and their complex anatomy (Figure 1). The primary pattern of failure for patients with retroperitoneal sarcomas is local recurrence. Distant recurrence occurs considerably less commonly than for patients with extremity soft tissue sarcomas where the risk for local recurrence for patients with primary disease is on the order of 10% and risks for distant relapse approach 50% for patients with high-grade disease.[2]

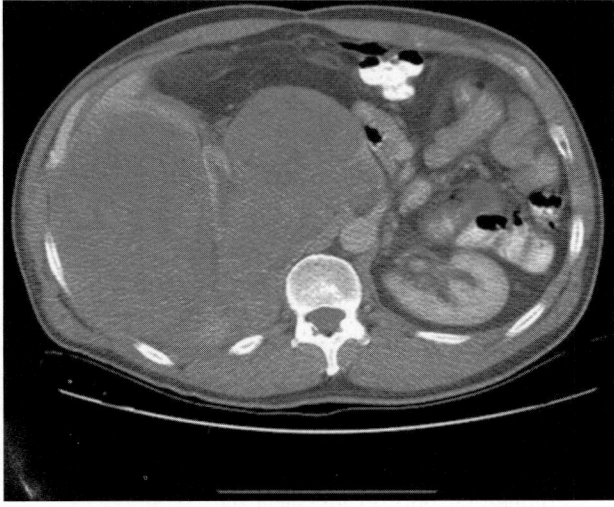

Figure 1 Abdominal computed tomography scan of a 53-year-old male who presented with a right retroperitoneal sarcoma. Resection required en-bloc right hepatectomy, right nephrectomy, and resection of the lateral chest wall. Note the right kidney sandwiched in between lobes of the tumor.

Surgical resection remains the mainstay of therapy for patients with localized retroperitoneal sarcoma. The therapeutic goal is macroscopically complete resection. This often requires multivisceral resection either because of contiguous extension of disease to involve adjacent organs (or their blood supply) or because (often in the case of the colon) the organ lies anterior to the tumor and often requires resection in order to afford exposure of the tumor. The organs most commonly included as part of the surgical resection include the kidney and colon and less commonly the pancreas, spleen, adrenal gland, and muscle including the diaphragm.

The technical aspects of surgical resection are beyond the scope of this chapter but are well addressed in other monographs devoted exclusively to technical issues.[3] Often, multispecialty teams provide for optimal treatment with members that may include vascular surgery, thoracic surgery, hepatic surgery, urology, and plastic and reconstructive surgery. The need for one or more specialties is predicated on pretreatment imaging and the likely need for expertise provided by one or more specialties.

Radiation Treatment for Localized Disease

Given the fact that many patients with retroperitoneal sarcoma are at risk for local recurrence, there remains considerable interest in treatment involving surgery plus radiation. For patients with retroperitoneal sarcomas, preoperative radiation has many potential advantages. These include:

1. The ability to target the gross tumor volume with precision avoiding radiation treatment to radiosensitive viscera including the small bowel.

2. Radiation treatment can be administered to a lower total dose (often 45 to 50 Gy) with less toxicity.
3. Radiation treatment may cause some degree of treatment-related fibrosis of the tumor capsule and may eradicate viable tumor cells at the periphery of the tumor.

Several single-institution reports have evaluated the feasibility and safety of preoperative radiation treatment and have demonstrated that preoperative radiation can be administered safely to doses on the order of 45 to 50 Gy.[4–6]

In contrast, postoperative radiation treatment usually involves administration of radiation to a large treatment volume that frequently includes bowel that has migrated into the radiation treatment field following resection of the tumor. This results in significant radiation to the small intestine that is fixed in the radiation treatment field by surgical adhesions.[7,8] Consequently, postoperative radiation treatment is associated with significant risks for treatment-related toxicities. In the absence of defined clinical benefit associated with radiation treatment we do not recommend postoperative radiation treatment for patients referred to our center for consideration of adjuvant treatment after complete resection of retroperitoneal sarcomas.

At this juncture, there are no studies that directly establish a role for radiation treatment. A recent randomized trial comparing surgery alone to preoperative radiation plus surgery (American College of Surgeons Oncology Group Z9031) was closed by the NCI Cancer Therapy Evaluation Program as a result of insufficient accrual. Thus, it appears unlikely that there will be future phase III trials conducted in North America to investigate the potential role of radiation treatment. This will result in the unfortunate situation where clinicians will be left to extrapolate from the small randomized trials evaluating radiation treatment in patients with extremity sarcomas.[9,10] These trials demonstrate improvement in local control with radiation treatment. It therefore may be reasonable to hypothesize that this local control benefit may also exist in other anatomic sites for patients with tumors of the same histologic subtypes as those included in the randomized trials for patients with extremity and body wall sarcomas. This remains unproven speculation but reasonable conjecture given the absence of controlled trials.

Adjuvant Chemotherapy Treatment

Adjuvant chemotherapy should not be considered for the majority of patients with retroperitoneal sarcomas. This recommendation is largely based on the absence of any randomized data establishing a role for chemotherapy treatment and the fact that the primary pattern of failure for patients with this disease is local rather than systemic. Exceptions to this recommendation certainly include specific histologic subtypes that are known to be more sensitive to chemotherapy, such as synovial sarcoma and desmoplastic small round cell tumor. The latter are uncommon histologies in the retroperitoneum accounting for less than 5% of patients. Thus, for the majority of patients with retroperitoneal sarcoma who have liposarcoma, leiomyosarcoma, or the less commonly applied diagnosis of malignant fibrocystic sarcoma, there is no role for routine administration of pre- or postoperative chemotherapy.

Summary

Patients with retroperitoneal sarcoma remain a significant management challenge. Optimal care is provided in the context of the multidisciplinary environment where patients may undergo a thorough pretreatment staging evaluation and pretreatment multidisciplinary case review. This allows for careful treatment planning and consideration of a preoperative radiation treatment where appropriate. Moreover, this approach allows for multispecialty surgical resection in clinical settings where this is appropriate.

References

1. Pisters PWT, O'Sullivan B. Soft-tissue sarcomas. In: Kufe D, Bast R Jr, Hait W, et al, editors. Cancer medicine. Hamilton: B.C. Decker, Inc.; 2006. p. 1694–720.

2. Brennan MF, Casper ES, Harrison LB. Soft tissue sarcoma. In: Vita V, Helman S, Rosenberg S, editors. Cancer: Principles and practice of oncology. Philadelphia: Lippincott-Raven; 1997. p. 1738–88.

3. Karakousis CP. Surgery for soft tissue sarcomas. In: Bland KI, Karakousis CP, Copeland EM, editors. Atlas of surgical oncology. Philadelphia: WB Saunders; 1995. p. 283–400.

4. Jones JJ, Catton CN, O'Sullivan B, et al. Initial results of a trial of preoperative external-beam radiation therapy and postoperative brachytherapy for retroperitoneal sarcoma. Ann Surg Oncol 2002;9:346–54.

5. Pisters PW, Ballo MT, Fenstermacher MJ, et al. Phase I trial of preoperative concurrent doxorubicin and radiation therapy, surgical resection, and intraoperative electron-beam radiation therapy for patients with localized retroperitoneal sarcoma. J Clin Oncol 2003;21:3092–7.

6. Pawlik TM, Pisters PW, Mikula L, et al. Long-term results of two prospective trials of preoperative external beam radiotherapy for localized intermediate- or high-grade retroperitoneal soft tissue sarcoma. Ann Surg Oncol 2006; 13:508–17.

7. Stoeckle E, Coindre JM, Bonvalot S, et al. Prognostic factors in retroperitoneal sarcoma: A multivariate analysis of a series of 165 patients of the French Cancer Center Federation Sarcoma Group. Cancer 2001;92:359–68.

8. Gilbeau L, Kantor G, Stoeckle E, et al. Surgical resection and radiotherapy for primary retroperitoneal soft tissue sarcoma. Radiother Oncol 2002;65:137–43.

9. Pisters PW, Harrison LB, Leung DH, et al. Long-term results of a prospective randomized trial of adjuvant brachytherapy in soft tissue sarcoma. J Clin Oncol 1996;14: 859–68.

10. Yang JC, Chang AE, Baker AR, et al. A randomized prospective study of the benefit of adjuvant radiation therapy in the treatment of soft tissue sarcomas of the extremity. J Clin Oncol 1998;16:197–203.

CHAPTER 77

SPECIAL SITUATIONS: METASTASIS (LUNG METS)

SHANDA H. BLACKMON, MD, MPH

ARA A. VAPORCIYAN, MD

There are an estimated 8,000 to 9,000 new cases of sarcoma diagnosed in the United States each year.[1,2] In spite of the progress that has been made with multi-modality treatment, approximately half are expected to die, mostly of metastatic disease.[1-3] Eighty percent of metastatic lesions will involve the lung.[4] Of patients with extremity sarcoma, approximately 20% will have isolated pulmonary metastatic disease at some point in the course of their disease.[5,6] Therefore, control of the intrathoracic disease is an important component for patient survival. After complete pulmonary resection, reported 3-year survival rates range from 20 to 54%,[5,7-9] making resection the treatment of choice when possible.[7,8,10] Multiple or repeated resections of pulmonary lesions are also possible. Five-year survival approaches 0% when patients cannot be rendered disease-free at operation.[6] Although chemotherapy may shrink sarcomas in 30 to 50% of patients, local relapse in spite of systemic pre- and post-op chemotherapy is routine, making nonsurgical management of good candidates inappropriate (Figure 1).[11-16]

In this chapter, we will discuss the indication, advantages, and disadvantages of metastectomy. The outcomes after mega-metastectomy and extended resections will also be discussed. In patients with unresectable pulmonary metastases from sarcoma, systemic chemotherapy is usually offered. Because of dose-limiting toxicities, other novel techniques will also be discussed, such as isolated lung perfusion and inhalation techniques.

Pathology

The relation between histology and frequency of pulmonary metastasis is not well defined. There is evidence that patients with extremity spindle cell sarcoma and extra-skeletal osteosarcoma are more likely to develop pulmonary metastases.[8] All sarcomas can metastasize to the lung, and it is the tumor most likely to spread to lung. In a series of 242 patients with sarcoma, those with tenosynovial sarcoma had the highest incidence of pulmonary metastases.[17]

The most common types of sarcoma are malignant fibrous histiocytoma, liposarcoma, and leiomyosarcoma. The frequency of these differs depending on the site. For example, leiomyosarcomas are the most common abdominal sarcoma, while liposarcomas and malignant fibrous histiocytomas are most common in the legs.

Complete resection of isolated pulmonary metastases is generally associated with improved patient survival regardless of the primary histology. This metastatic process may take place via hematogenous, lymphatic, direct invasion, or aerogenous routes, and thus complete resection with negative margins should be paramount. For further details about pathologic subclassification, please refer to Chapters 70 and 71.

Symptoms

Pulmonary metastases rarely cause symptoms. Most of these lesions are discovered during routine screening after the primary tumor has been resected. When present, the most common symptoms are dyspnea, pain, cough, or hemoptysis. Although parietal pleural invasion and thus pain is rare, palliation may become necessary for the occasional tumor invading the chest wall.

Diagnosis

Although a wide spectrum of pulmonary findings may be present in patients with lung metastases, the more typical

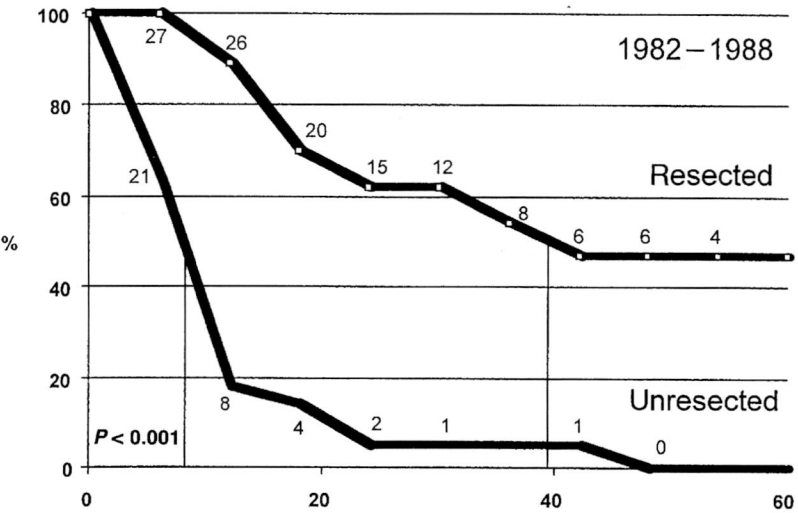

Figure 1 Lung metastasectomy in a consecutive series of childhood osteosarcomas: overall survival from the time of detection lung metastases according to salvage surgery, in the years 1982–1988.

characteristics include small, well-circumscribed, peripheral nodules in the patient with a known primary malignancy. The typical screening includes chest X-ray or helical computed tomography (CT) scanning every 3 to 6 months during treatment, followed by further evaluation for suspicious lesions (Table 1).

Magnetic resonance imaging may be as sensitive as CT scanning, but adds little information and is not recommended unless extended resections are planned. When evaluating new pulmonary nodules, it is also important to consider other pathology, such as tuberculosis, benign granulomatous disease, or primary lung cancer. In this case, positron emission tomography (PET) scanning is particularly advantageous. PET scanning is also helpful when trying to quantify interval

response to therapy or new growth of a tumor, or to rule out extra-thoracic nonprimary lesions.

Treatment

SURGERY

It is important to note the primary goal of surgery for metastatic sarcoma to the lung is to enhance long-term survival. Not all patients will be considered optimal candidates, but surgical resection can still be offered if the postoperative mortality and morbidity remain low. The best candidates for resection are described below. There are other patients who have a much worse prognosis, but may still benefit from surgical resection as a palliative measure because no other treatment options exist.

In a recent report from the international pulmonary metastases registry,[19] soft tissue sarcomas were the most common type of pulmonary metastases resected; they accounted for 42% of all patients undergoing metastectomy. Forty percent of patients were rendered disease-free 3 years after resection.[19] Despite the near uniform acceptance of surgical resection of pulmonary metastasis, there is no definitive evidence that it confers a survival advantage. No randomized trial has been conducted to prove the advantage of early resection of occult disease. However, considerable retrospective evidence appears to support its use, especially when the indications below are used.

Indications for Resection

The therapy for pulmonary metastases remains complete resection of all disease in patients who meet all of the

Table 1 Indications for Imaging Studies for Sarcoma Patients with Lung Metastases

Imaging Study	Indication	Sensitivity/Specificity
CXR	Limited surveillance occasionally	low/low
Helical CT Scan	Routine surveillance*	100/96
	Identification of known nodules	
MRI	Evaluate chest wall invasion	88/96
	Evaluate mediastinal invasion	
PET Scan	Discriminate benign lesions	87/100
	Identify extra-thoracic metastases	
	Evaluate response to therapy	

(18-Lucas, 1998)
*Every 3 months during systemic therapy to evaluate for treatment response, then every 6 months thereafter.
CT = computed tomography; MRI = magnetic resonance imaging; PET = positron emission tomography.

Table 2 Indications for Pulmonary Resection

Absolute	Control of the primary tumor has been achieved
	All nodules are potentially resectable
	Adequate postoperative pulmonary reserve established
	No evidence of extrathoracic disease
	Pulmonary nodules are consistent with the diagnosis
Relative	Diagnosis is needed
	Tissue markers are needed for further therapy
	Immunohistochemical studies are needed for further therapy
	Relief of "tumor tamponade"
	Removal of residual nodules after chemotherapy
	Decrease tumor burden

[9] Putnam

following criteria: the primary site of disease is controlled, imaging studies consistent with metastatic disease, ability to have all intrathoracic disease resected,[20–22] ability to tolerate the operation or operations physiologically, and no extra-thoracic evidence of disease[23–26] (Table 2). Other indications for partial or incomplete resection include diagnosis, removal of residual nodules after chemotherapy, relief of tumor tamponade, to obtain tissue markers or immunohistochemical studies, or to decrease tumor burden.[9] Clinical features such as the histological type and grading, disease-free interval, doubling time or number of lesions represent potential prognostic factors but cannot be used to select patients for surgery.

Surgical Approaches

The approach for surgical resection depends on the location of tumor(s) burden, bilaterality, and patient pulmonary reserve. The goal of resection is complete removal of detectable disease. The lesser invasive techniques such as thoracoscopy are not adequate for complete resection but may be beneficial when diagnosis

is needed. For a comparison of available approaches, see Table 3.

THORACOTOMY

Thoracotomy is the standard approach to metastectomy (Figure 2). In patients presenting with basilar tumors or centrally located tumors involving both lungs, sequential thoracotomy approach would be required. Sequential thoracotomies for bilateral disease begin with the least diseased side followed by the more diseased side.[27] The time between sequential thoracotomies is usually 2 to 4 weeks, depending on patient reserve. Our institution now incorporates a muscle-sparing thoracotomy and a more limited skin incision (Table 4).

The thoracotomy is performed with single-lung ventilation to allow complete palpation of the lung. After positioning of the double-lumen endotracheal tube has been confirmed with fiberoptic bronchoscopy, the patient is placed into the lateral decubitus position. Prior to making an incision, an intercostal and subcutaneous nerve block is performed with local anesthesia. Our choice for resection is a posterior muscle-sparring thoracotomy. This incision affords adequate exposure with limited functional deficit that accompanies division of the latissimus muscle performed during a posterolateral thoracotomy. The incision is made from the tip of the scapula extending to the posterior edge of the latissimus. Mobilization of the latissimus muscle is performed, retracting the muscle anteriorly. Limiting the dissection on the superficial surface of the latissimus prevents excess dead space reducing the incidence of postoperative seroma formation. The serratus anterior muscle may also need to be mobilized anteriorly in a similar fashion. Once the fifth intercostal space has been identified, the lung is deflated and the intercostal muscle is separated from the superior edge of the rib as the chest

Table 3 Comparison of Different Surgical Approaches for Metastectomy

Description	Staged Thoracotomy	Median Sternotomy	Bilateral (Clamshell)	Video-Assisted Thoracoscopy
Exposure	****	**	***	***
Palpation	****	**	***	*
Pain	***	**	****	*
LOS	****	**	***	*
Qualifier				
Single metastasis	****	**	*	****
Bilateral mets	****	**	***	***
Upper lobe mets	****	****	***	**
Lower lobe mets	****	*	**	**
Numerous mets	****	**	***	*
Central mets	****	***	**	*
Poor pulmonary reserve	**	****	**	****

*Indicates degree of variable.

LOS = length of stay.

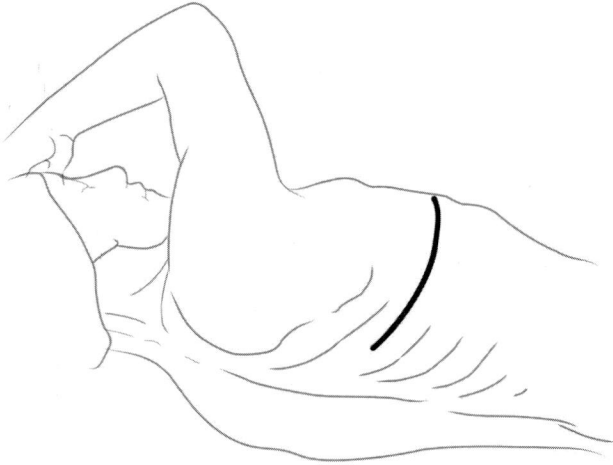

Figure 2 Thoracotomy incision.

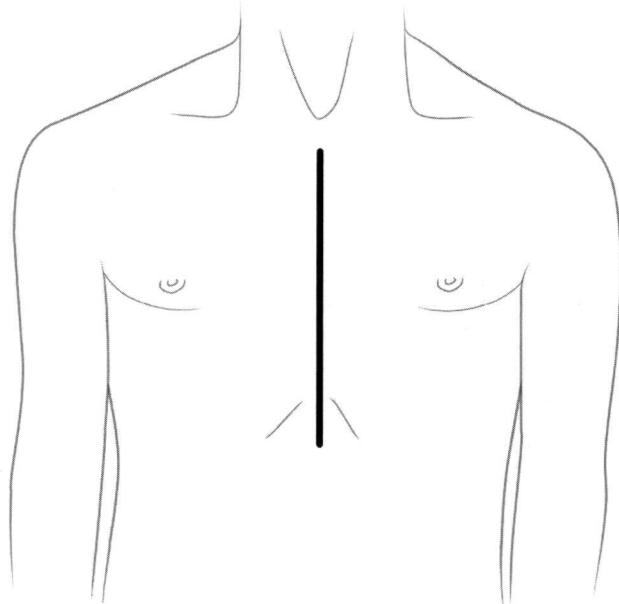

Figure 3 Median sternotomy incision.

is entered. A 1 cm segment of the posterior aspect of the sixth rib may be excised to facilitate rib spreading. This approach provides excellent exposure of all lobes of the lung and hilar structures as well.

MEDIAN STERNOTOMY

In those patients with disease limited to bilateral upper lobes, simultaneous resection with a median sternotomy can be used (Figure 3). The technique of median sternotomy has several advantages, including the ability to inspect both pleural spaces in one surgery, the ability to avoid division of the intercostals muscle and post-operative splinting, and the lack of pleural adhesions, which may complicate re-resection in the event of recurrence.[27]

For this technique, the patient is positioned supine. The skin prep should include the entire anterior thorax with abdomen and both groins prepped but covered. The pulmonary ligament is mobilized bilaterally to enhance mobility of the lung. The lungs are sequentially deflated and palpated. After the metastatic lesions are resected,

the lung is re-inflated and after a few minutes attention is turned to the other lung. When both sides are complete chest tubes are placed and the sternum is closed. Internal mammary retractors are useful to improve access to each thorax (Table 5).

CLAMSHELL OR BILATERAL ANTERIOR THORACOTOMY OR TRANSVERSE STERNOTOMY

Like the median sternotomy, a clamshell or bilateral anterior thoracotomy will also provide bilateral pleural access (Figure 4). Unlike the former technique, this approach also provides better access to both lower lobes of the lung and more posterior structures. Bilateral anterior thoracotomy with and without a transverse sternal incision may therefore be preferred in selected cases where bilateral pleural access is desired and access to all lobes of the lung is also needed (Table 6).[28]

Table 4 The Advantages and Disadvantages of Staged or One-Sided Thoracotomy

Advantages	Standard approach
	Access to all lobes of the lung and hilar structures
	Open approach provides good exposure for palpation
	Muscle-sparing technique can be used (including vertical anterior thoracotomy)
	Excellent for unilateral lesions: should not change survival if contralateral thoracotomy is delayed until lesions are visualized
Disadvantages	2 surgeries for bilateral disease, prolonging hospitalization
	May cause increased splinting or discomfort

Table 5 The Advantages and Disadvantages of Median Sternotomy

Advantages	Bilateral approach with one incision
	Less splinting due to patient discomfort
	Fewer pleural adhesions in the event of re-resection
Disadvantages	Hilar access is limited, especially posterior lesions
	Lower lobar lesion may be difficult to expose, in selected cases
	(CHF, obese patients, COPD)

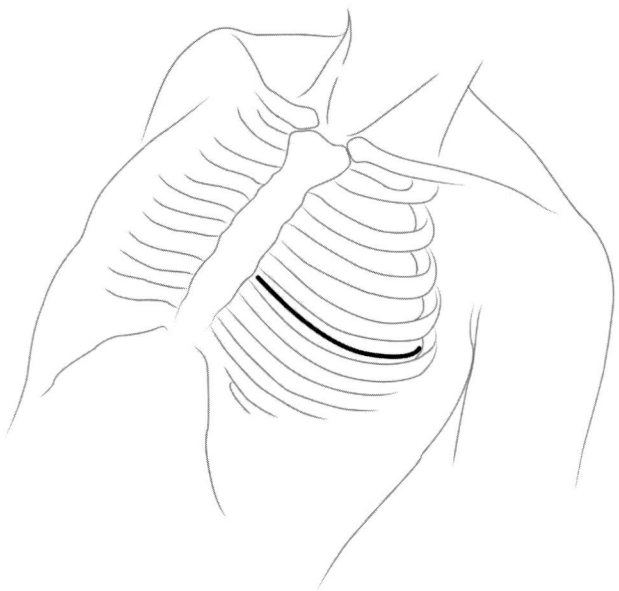

Figure 4 Bilateral anterior thoracotomy incision.

These patients are also kept in the supine position and the skin prep should include the entire anterior thorax and the abdomen and groins as well. A curvilinear incision is made underneath both inframammary creases, connecting these two incisions in the middle with a slight upward curve. The pectoral muscles are reflected superiorly to provide access to the fourth intercostals space. The sternum is divided with a saw in a transverse fashion. Traditional thoracic retractors may be used to provide access to the pleural spaces.

VIDEO-ASSISTED THORACOSTOMY

Video-assisted thoracoscopy (VATS) is a newer technique that has specific uses (Figure 5). The best uses of this approach for metastatic sarcoma to the lung remain diagnosis or preliminary evaluation for resectability. We recommend that this technique should not be used for attempted complete resection of sarcoma metastasis,

Table 6 The Advantages and Disadvantages of Clamshell or Bilateral Anterior Thoracotomy/Transverse Sternotomy

Advantages	Bilateral access to pleural spaces
	Only one incision; may be a more cosmetic incision for females
	Better access to all lobes of the lung (especially LLL) than median sternotomy
Disadvantages	Painful incision
	Larger incision
	Approximation of the sternum and intercostal spaces is difficult
	Requires division of the internal mammary arteries

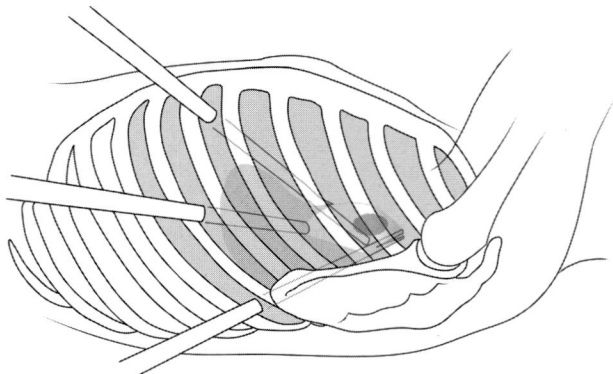

Figure 5 Video-assisted thoracoscopy.

which may have an up to 40 to 60% rate of occult metastasis. Adequate palpation is difficult, and lesions deep within the parenchyma and close to hilar structures may be missed completely with VATS. There are reports of a substernal handport being used to assist in bilateral palpation of lung nodules during VATS metastectomy, but this technique has yet to be standardized (Table 7).

Techniques of Resection

Once the chest has been entered, there are several ways to resect the actual tumors. The surgeon may use electrocautery, a stapled technique, or laser-assisted resection. Determining the degree of resection necessary has not been shown to influence recurrence as long as the surgical margins are negative. When lesions involve other vital structures, extended resections may become necessary. The number of nodules being resected should not deter a surgeon from operating as long as the patient is believed to have adequate pulmonary reserve after resection. It is for this reason that a staged thoracotomy

Table 7 The Advantages and Disadvantages of VATS

Advantages	Small incision
	Probably less pain
	Potentially less immunosuppressive
	Excellent visualization
	Can identify pleural dissemination without a large incision
	Better for diagnostic procedures
Disadvantages	Many lesions may remain undetected
	Poor choice for sarcomas, which have 40–60% rate of occult metastasis[29]
	Adequate palpation is difficult[30]
	Small nodules deep within the lung parenchyma are not reachable
	Late chest wall port site recurrences have been reported[31]

VATS = video-assisted thoracoscopy.

Table 8 The Advantages and Disadvantages of Electrocautery Resection

Advantages	Simple and easy to use
	May enhance preservation of lung parenchyma
	Better adapted for hypermetastectomy
Disadvantages	Prolonged air leaks
	Increased bleeding

may be preferred when a higher number of lesions are to be resected (hyper-metastectomy); the patient may have a chance to declare how they will recover from the first part of the planned resection without undergoing the more extensive entry into the contralateral pleura.

BOVIE ELECTROCAUTERY RESECTION

Dr. Urschel was the first thoracic surgeon to describe resection of pulmonary lesions with Bovie electrocautery. The advantages of this technique remain the ease-of-use and the ability to stay close to the tumor as it is resected, thus preserving lung parenchyma. The use of Bovie may lead to increased blood loss as deeper lesions are excised and division of larger terminal bronchioles may translate into prolonged postoperative air leak (Table 8).

STAPLED WEDGE RESECTION

With the advent of the surgical stapler, most surgeons have adopted this technique for the majority of their resections. Control of bleeding and bronchioles are obtained in a simple and consistent fashion. In emphysematous lungs the use of reinforcing strips may further reduce the postoperative leakage of air. Unfortunately, for deeper lesions a significant portion of uninvolved tissue may also be resected with the stapled wedge (Table 9).

LASER-ASSISTED RESECTION

Laser-assisted techniques are sometimes advocated above stapling or bovie electrocautery because they may spare more of the parenchyma and at the same time lessen the duration of air leak. Although this technique frequently takes longer to perform, it also provides a more precise excision (Table 10).

Table 9 The Advantages and Disadvantages of Stapled Wedge Resection

Advantages	Less bleeding
	Better for deeper parenchymal lesions
Disadvantages	Additional uninvolved lung tissue resected

Table 10 The Advantages and Disadvantages of Laser-Assisted Resection

Advantages	May enhance preservation of lung parenchyma
	More precise incisions
Disadvantages	Prolonged operating time
	Prolonged air leaks

EXTENDED RESECTION

Extended resections can safely be performed[35]. Less than 3% of metastectomy patients will require this type of resection. Due to the extended resection being performed, this approach is recommended only for patients who have had a long disease-free interval, young patients, and single or dominant metastatic lesions. Pneumonectomy is the most morbid of the extended resections involving the lung (Table 11).

Five-year survival after pneumonectomy for completely resected metastatic lesions is reported to be from 16 to 25%.[19,35,36] Our institution has performed several right atrial resections with bovine pericardium reconstruction and the use of cardiopulmonary bypass in highly selected cases with good results and acceptable mortality.

HYPER-METASTECTOMY (TABLE 12)

Results of Surgical Resection

Pulmonary metastectomy has become a standard treatment for selected patients with isolated pulmonary metastases from extrathoracic primary sarcoma. Although all the data is retrospective, the consensus is that roughly 30% of patients will achieve long-term survival with complete resection. Surgical resection is believed to have improved survival when compared to patients who do not have their pulmonary metastases resected,[7,20,37–39] although randomized data addressing this are not available.

Table 11 The Advantages and Disadvantages of Extended Resections

Advantages	Structures that can be resected include:
	Chest wall
	Diaphragm
	Pericardium
	Superior vena cava
	Entire lung
	Can be safely performed[35]
Disadvantages	Higher mortality and pulmonary insufficiency
	Cardio-pulmonary reserve
	Life expectancy gain may not favor an extended resection
	Quality of life effect

Table 12 The Advantages and Disadvantages of Hyper-Metastectomy

Advantages	Can be safely performed
	Cytoreduction and prolongation of survival
Disadvantages	Patient may not have adequate postoperative pulmonary reserve

Furthermore, the morbidity of pulmonary metastectomy should be quite low with reported rates of 0 to 2%.[21,22,43] Although permanent cure is usually achieved in less than one-third of these patients, 5-year survival averages about 36%.[19] Complete lung resection is optimal, but even in these cases there is a 53% relapse with a median time to recurrences noted at 10 months.[19] If complete resection cannot be achieved, the 5-year survival decreases to 15%.[19] Several prognostic variables have been identified that are associated with favorable survival after pulmonary metastectomy. Favorable factors include an extended disease-free interval,[6,7,9] three or fewer pulmonary nodules,[6,9] and a longer tumor doubling time.[8,44] In a more recent study by Brennan and colleagues, the number of pulmonary nodules did not appear to be a significant prognostic indicator if all disease was resected.[5,45] The most consistent favorable prognostic factor is metastatic disease that is amenable to resection.[7,44,46] Prognostic factors specific to sarcomas include the grade of tumor and presence of local recurrence.[19]

In spite of newer imaging technology improving detection, an open technique remains the gold standard for resection of metastatic lesions. Although high-resolution CT scanners can reduce the number of undetected lesions from 40% to 22%, this rate is still unacceptable[47]. Based on this, VATS resection should be reserved for patients in whom a single lesion is being resected for diagnosis, where pleural dissemination remains a question, or in patients who would not tolerate an otherwise open technique.

Adjuvant Treatment

CHEMOTHERAPY

Chemotherapy is primarily used to eliminate potential micrometastatic disease, which can enhance the local control achieved by cytoreduction. The effectiveness of cytotoxic drugs for metastatic parenchymal pulmonary sarcoma may be limited by the toxicities that occur before the therapeutic dose is reached. Newer techniques such as isolated lung perfusion remain experimental and are discussed in a following section within this chapter.

Please refer to Chapter 79 for further details.

RADIATION THERAPY

The effectiveness of radiation therapy for metastatic parenchymal pulmonary sarcoma is limited by the concomitant lung toxicity. When complete resection is not possible, radiotherapy may be recommended. The primary utility of radiotherapy here is palliation of symptoms of advanced metastases. Prophylactic radiotherapy is also not recommended.

Please refer to Chapter 78 for further details

Cost-Effectiveness of Treatment

For surgical candidates with pulmonary metastases from soft tissue sarcoma, pulmonary resection was the most cost-effective treatment strategy. The incremental cost-effectiveness ratio was $14 versus $104,000 per life-year gained for pulmonary resection versus systemic chemotherapy patients, respectively. The cost-effectiveness ratio for combined therapy (surgery and chemotherapy) was $51,000 per life-year gained. Even with favorable assumptions regarding its clinical benefit, systemic chemotherapy alone, compared with no treatment, was not a cost-effective treatment strategy for sarcoma patients with lung metastases.[48]

Experimental Treatment Strategies

Pulmonary artery (antero- or retrograde) infusion of chemotherapeutics, using isolated lung perfusion tech-

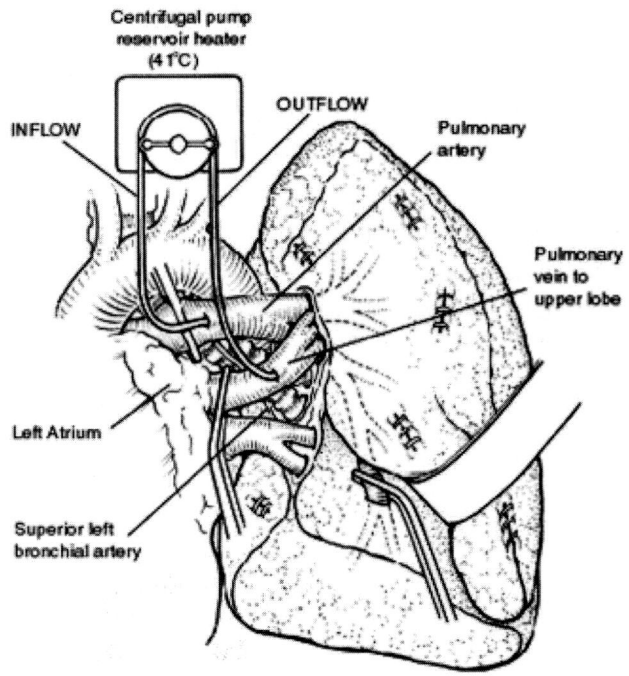

Figure 6 Selective lung perfusion.

niques (ILP)[49–51] have been used to intensify therapy while limiting systemic toxicity following surgery (Figure 6). Because of their technical complexity, attendant potential morbidity, and lack of documented efficacy, it has not gained widespread application. It is well known that the therapeutic index of cisplatin, one of the most effective single drugs in the treatment of sarcoma, is limited by its systemic toxicity.[49] Based on this rationale, Schröder recently developed a surgical technique for the isolated lobar or lung perfusion with high doses of cisplatin under hyperthermic (41°C) conditions in patients with recurrent or unresectable lung sarcoma metastases. In patients with resectable metastasis, surgery should be performed before resorting to ILP. Hyperthermic ILP deserves further investigation for patients with advanced, drug resistant, and/or surgically refractory lung sarcoma metastasis. Inhalational techniques and RFA are other forms of treatment also being investigated,[50,51] but these remain experimental as well.

References

1. Jemal A, Siegel R, Ward E, et al. Cancer statistics 2002. CA Cancer J Clin 2002;52:23–47.

2. American Cancer Society. Cancer facts and figures, 2006. Atlanta: American Cancer Society; 2006.

3. Landis SH, Murray T, Bolden S, Wingo PA. Cancer statistics, 1998. CA Cancer J Clin 1998;48:6–29.

4. Potter DA, Glenn J, Kinsella T, et al. Patterns of recurrence in patients with high-grade soft-tissue sarcomas. J Clin Oncol 1985;3:353–66.

5. Gadd MA, Casper ES, Woodruff JM, et al. Development and treatment of pulmonary metastases in adult patients with extremity soft tissue sarcoma. Ann Surg 1993;218:705–12.

6. Casson AG, Putnam JB, Natarajan G, et al. Five-year survival after pulmonary metastasectomy for adult soft tissue sarcoma. Cancer 1992;62:662–8.

7. Jablons D, Steinberg SM, Roth J, et al. Metastasectomy for soft tissue sarcoma. Further evidence for efficacy and prognostic indicators. J Thorac Cardiovasc Surg 1989;97:695–705.

8. Verazin GT, Warneke JA, Driscoll DL, et al. Resection of lung metastases from soft-tissue sarcomas. A multivariate analysis. Arch Surg 1992;127:1407–11.

9. Putnam JB, Roth JA, Wesley MN, et al. Analysis of prognostic factors in patients undergoing resection of pulmonary metastases from soft tissue sarcomas. J Thorac Cardiovasc Surg 1984;87:260–8.

10. Glenn J, Kinsella T, Glatstein E, et al. A randomized, prospective trial of adjuvant chemotherapy in adults with soft tissue sarcomas of the head and neck, breast, and trunk. Cancer 1985;55:1206–14.

11. Chang AE, Kinsella T, Glatstein E, et al. Adjuvant chemotherapy for patients with high-grade soft tissue sarcomas of the extremity. J Clin Oncol 1988;6:1491–500.

12. Omura GA, Major FJ, Blessing JA, et al. A randomized study of Adriamycin with and without dimethyl triazenoimidazole carboxamide in advanced uterine sarcomas. Cancer 1983;52:626–32.

13. Lerner HJ, Amato DA, Savlov ED, et al. A comparison of adjuvant doxorubicin and observation for patients with localized soft tissue sarcoma. J Clin Oncol 1987;5:613–7.

14. Rosenberg SA. Prospective randomized trials demonstrating the efficacy of adjuvant chemotherapy in adult patients with soft tissue sarcomas. Cancer Treat Rep 1984;68:1067–78.

15. Lanza LA, Putnam JB Jr, Benjamin RS, Roth JA. Response to chemotherapy does not predict survival after resection of sarcomatous pulmonary metastases. Ann Thorac Surg 1991;51:219–24.

16. Casper ES, Gaynor JJ, Harrison LB, et al. Preoperative and postoperative adjuvant combination chemotherapy for adults with high-grade soft-tissue sarcoma. Cancer 1994;73:1644–51.

17. Temple LK, Brennan MF. The role of pulmonary metastasectomy in soft tissue sarcoma. Semin Thorac Cardiovasc Surg 2002;114:35–44.

18. Lucas JD, O'Doherty MJ, Wong JCH, et al. Evaluation of fluorodeoxyglucose positron emission tomography in the management of soft-tissue sarcomas. J Bone Joint Surg Br 1998;80:441–7.

19. Pastorino U, Buyse M, Friedel G, et al. Long-term results of lung metastasectomy: prognostic analyses based on 5206 cases. The International Registry of Lung Metastases. J Thorac Cardiovasc Surg 1997;113:37–49.

20. Sadoff JD, Detterbeck FC. Pulmonary metastases from extrapulmonary cancer. In: Detterbeck FC, Rivera MP, Socinski MA, Rosenman JG, editors. Diagnosis and treatment of lung cancer: an evidence-based guide for the practicing clinician. Philadelphia: W.B. Saunders; 2001. p. 450–64.

21. Koong HN, Pastorino U, Ginsberg RJ. Is there a role for pneumonectomy in pulmonary metastases? International Registry of Lung Metastases. Ann Thor Surg 1999;68:2039.

22. Mountain CF, McMurtrey MJ, Hermes KE. Surgery for pulmonary metastasis: a 20-year experience. Ann Thorac Surg 1984;38:323–30.

23. Todd TR. The surgical treatment of pulmonary metastases. Chest 1997;112:287S–290S.

24. Rusch VW. Pulmonary metastasectomy. Current indications. Chest 1995;107:322S–331S.

25. Vogt-Moykopf I, Krysa S, Bulzebruck H, Schirren J. Surgery for pulmonary metastases. The Heidelberg experience. Chest Surg Clin N Am 1994;4:85–112.

26. Harvey JC, Lee K, Beattie EJ. Surgical management of pulmonary metastases. Chest Surg Clin N Am 1994;4:55–66.

27. Roth JA, Pass HI, Wesley MN, et al. Comparison of median sternotomy and thoracotomy for resection of pulmonary metastases in patients with adult soft tissue sarcomas. Ann Thorac Surg 1986;42:134–8.

28. Bains MS, Ginsberg RJ, Jones WG 2nd, et al. The clamshell incision: an improved approach to bilateral pulmonary and mediastinal tumor. Ann Thorac Surg 1994;58:30–3.

29. McCormack PM. Role of video-assisted thoracic surgery in the treatment of pulmonary metastases: results of a prospective trial. Ann Thorac Surg 1996;62:213–6; discussion 216–7.

30. Mack M. 1992 Thoracoscopy for the diagnosis of the indeterminate solitary pulmonary nodule. Ann Thorac Surg 1993;56:825–30; discussion 830–2.

31. Walsh GL, Nesbitt JC. Tumor implants after thoracoscopic resection of a metastatic sarcoma. Ann Thorac Surg 1995;59:215–6.

32. Chang AE, Schaner EG, Conkle DM, et al. Evaluation of computed tomography in the detection of pulmonary metastases: a prospective study. Cancer 1979;43:913–6.

33. Schaner EG, Chang AE, Doppman JL, et al. Comparison of computed and conventional whole lung tomography in detecting pulmonary nodules: a prospective radiologic-pathologic study. AJR Am J Roentgenol 1978;131:51–4.

34. Urschel HC. Discussion of Cooper et al. Precision cautery excision of pulmonary lesions. Ann Thorac Surg 1986;41:53.

35. Putnam JB. 1993 Extended resection of pulmonary metastases: is the risk justified?.

36. Spaggiari L, Grunewald DH, Girard P, et al. 1998 Pneumonectomy for lung metastases: indications, risks, and outcome. Ann Thorac Surg 1998;66:1930–3.

37. Tafra L, Dale PS, Wanek LA, et al. Resection and adjuvant immunotherapy for melanoma metastatic to the lung and thorax. J Thorac Cardiovasc Surg 1995;110:119–29.

38. Carter SR, Grimer RJ, Sneath RS, Matthews HR. Results of thoracotomy in osteogenic sarcoma with pulmonary metastases. Thorax 1991;46:727–31.

39. Martini N, Huvos AG, Mike V, et al. Multiple pulmonary resections in the treatment of osteogenic sarcoma. Ann Thorac Surg 1971;12:271–80.

40. Thrasher JB, Clark JR, Cleland BP. Surgery for pulmonary metastases from renal cell carcinoma. Army experience from 1977–1987. Urology 1990;35:487–91.

41. Staren ED, Salerno C, Rongione, et al. Pulmonary resection for metastatic breast cancer. Arch Surg 1992;127:1282–4.

42. Friedel G, Hurtgen M, Penzenstadler M, et al. Resection of pulmonary metastases from renal cell carcinoma. Anticancer Res 1999;19:1593–6.

43. Stewart JR, Carey JA, Merrill WH, et al. Twenty years' experience with pulmonary metastasectomy. Am Surg 1992;58:100–3.

44. Van Geel. 1994 Repeated resection of recurrent pulmonary metastatic soft tissue sarcoma. Eur J Surg Oncol 1994;20:436–40.

45. Billingsley KG, Burt ME, Jara E, et al. Pulmonary metastases from soft-tissue sarcoma: analysis of patterns of disease and postmetastasis survival. Ann Surg 1999;229:602–12.

46. Creagan ET. 1979 Pulmonary resection for metastatic nonosteogenic sarcoma. Cancer 1979;44:1908–12.

47. Parsons AM, Detterbeck FC, Parker LA. Accuracy of helical CT in the detection of pulmonary metastases: is intraoperative palpation still necessary? Ann Thorac Surg 2004;78:1910–8.

48. Porter GA, Cantor SB, Walsh GL, et al. Cost-effectiveness of pulmonary resection and systemic chemotherapy in the management of metastatic soft tissue sarcoma: a combined analysis from the University of Texas M. D. Anderson and Memorial Sloan-Kettering Cancer Centers. J Thorac Cardiovasc Surg 2004;127:1366–72.

49. Wechsler, Ng B, Lenert JT, Burt ME. Isolated single-lung perfusion with doxorubicin is pharmacokinetically superior to intravenous injection. Ann Thorac Surg 1993;56:209–14.

50. Akeboshi M, Yamakado K, Nakatsuka A, et al. Percutaneous radiofrequency ablation of lung neoplasms: initial therapeutic response. J Vasc Interv Radiol 2004;15:463–70.

51. Hershey AE, Kurzman ID, Forrest LJ, et al. Inhalation chemotherapy for macroscopic primary or metastatic lung tumors: proof of principle using dogs with spontaneously occurring tumors as a model. Clinical Cancer Research 1999;5:2653–9.

CHAPTER 78

SURGICAL TREATMENT OF SARCOMA LIVER METASTASES

STEVEN A. CURLEY, MD

FRANCESCO IZZO, MD

Unlike colorectal or neuroendocrine cancer liver metastases, the role for surgical treatment of sarcoma liver metastases is not well established. Most published reports of liver resection for sarcoma metastases are limited by a small number of patients, inclusion of patients who underwent concomitant resection of nonhepatic metastatic disease, short periods of follow-up inadequate to establish a survival benefit, inclusion of a variety of histologic subtypes of sarcoma, or inclusion of patients with nonsarcoma liver metastases.[1–11] However, there is mounting interest in establishing a role for metastectomy in patients with sarcoma liver metastases based on improved safety of liver resection and on established data for a survival benefit in some patients undergoing metastectomy for sarcoma lung metastases.[12,13]

Extremity and trunk soft tissue sarcomas have a propensity to metastasize to the lungs. In contrast, gastrointestinal (GI) and retroperitoneal sarcomas frequently metastasize to the liver. Between 20 to 60% of patients with GI or retroperitoneal sarcomas will develop liver metastases as a component of their disease process.[14–17] As with colorectal cancer (CRC), a subset of these patients will have metastatic disease isolated to the liver that may be amenable to surgical treatment. In fact, surgical treatment provides the only potentially curative option in these patients because standard cytotoxic systemic chemotherapy drugs or hepatic arterial chemoembolization is associated with low response rates, is palliative at best, and yields median survival times of 11 to 14 months.[14,18–20]

Histologic Subtypes of Sarcoma Liver Metastases

Prior to 1998, the most common soft tissue sarcomas associated with liver metastases were classified as leiomyosarcomas.[3,4,9,11,15,17] The site of origin of these leiomyosarcomas was usually the GI tract, genitourinary organs, or the retroperitoneum. In 1998 Hirota and colleagues described gain-of-function mutations in exon 11 of the *c-kit* proto-oncogene.[21] The *c-kit* proto-oncogene encodes a cell-surface trans-membrane receptor with tyrosine kinase activity. The recognition that constitutive activation of the *c-kit* receptor tyrosine kinase stimulates proliferation and enhances survival of gastrointestinal stromal tumor (GIST) cells led to two important changes in the management of some sarcoma patients. First, many patients who were initially categorized as having leiomyosarcomas were reclassified as GIST patients based on presence of mutation in the *c-kit* proto-oncogene.[22] Secondly, clinical trials of an oral tyrosine kinase inhibitor, imatinib mesylate, were performed with the results indicating a significant improvement in antitumor response rates.[23–25] Prior to the discovery of the *c-kit* proto-oncogene, chemotherapeutic agents used to treat metastatic sarcomas (regardless of histologic subtype) included dacarbazine, mitomycin C, doxorubicin, ifosfamide, and cisplatin.[22,23] The measurable antitumor response rates to these chemotherapeutic agents were generally less than 15%, with little or no improvement in survival rates but with significant toxicities and resultant negative impact on the quality of life in these patients. It is now recognized that treatment of primary or metastatic GIST with imatinib mesylate yields dramatic objective response rates of 70% or more with minimal associated toxicity. However, despite prolonged durable response in a subset of patients with GIST treated with imatinib mesylate, it is now clear with longer follow-up that tumor recurrence or development of new metastatic disease develops in the majority of GIST patients.[25–27]

An analysis of our prospective hepatobiliary tumor surgery database for a 10-year period from 1996 to 2005 yielded 66 patients with sarcoma liver metastases treated surgically.[28] Of these patients, 36 (54.5%) had metastatic GIST, 18 (27.3%) had metastatic leiomyosarcoma, and 12 (18.2%) had a sarcoma that was not otherwise classified. The preponderance of metastatic GIST in our patients is consistent with other series reported since the identification of the *c-kit* proto-oncogene, and metastatic GIST is likely to be the most frequently encountered histologic sarcoma subtype to be considered for surgical treatment of liver metastases.[23,26]

Surgical Treatment of Sarcoma Liver Metastases

As is true for carcinomas metastatic to the liver from a number of organ sites, there are no randomized trials comparing surgical treatment with medical treatment of sarcoma liver metastases. Thus, the few reports describing the long-term outcome after surgical treatment of sarcoma liver metastases represent a highly selected subset of patients with a relatively rare histologic type of primary malignancy, ie, visceral or retroperitoneal sarcoma. One study reported that the long-term survival after resection of leiomyosarcoma liver metastases in 26 patients was superior to patients with liver metastases treated with conventional cytotoxic chemotherapy or hepatic arterial chemoembolization.[8] The 5-year survival rate in these 26 patients who underwent liver resection was 13% overall, and was 20% in the patients who underwent margin-negative, complete tumor resection (RO) resection. The authors stated these results compared favorably to historical and published reports with essentially no chance for 5-year survival in patients treated with systemic or regional chemotherapy. However, the authors did not compare the 26 surgical patients to a matched cohort of sarcoma liver metastasis patients treated medically at their institution. The 26

patients who underwent a total of 34 surgical treatments were accrued over a 15-year period, indicative of the small number of patients with sarcoma liver metastases who are candidates for aggressive surgical treatment.

Review of 200 GIST patients from a prospective sarcoma database revealed that 61 patients (30.5%) presented with or developed liver metastases.[16] This study indicated that there were not any patient or tumor-specific prognostic factors that were predictive of long-term survival. Patient age, gender, tumor number, and whether resection was performed for recurrent or initial metastatic disease did not influence survival. Patients who underwent a complete gross surgical resection of all primary and metastatic GIST had a better median survival than patients who underwent incomplete resection.

The evaluation of our experience with surgical treatment of sarcoma liver metastases at the University of Texas M. D. Anderson Cancer Center showed that the site of the primary sarcoma was the abdomen or retroperitoneum in 22 patients (33.3%), stomach in 18 (27.3%), small or large bowel in 17 (25.8%), pelvic structures in 4 (6.1%), the uterus in 3 (4.5%), or some other site in 2 (3.0%).[28] In contrast to other reports that considered only patients who could be treated with resection, we expanded the population of patients that could be treated with surgical intent by using radiofrequency ablation (RFA) in some of our patients. Complete surgical treatment with resection alone was possible in 35 of our 66 patients (53.0%), RFA alone was used for lesions in unresectable locations in 13 patients (19.7%), and resection of large or dominant lesions combined with RFA of additional smaller tumors was performed in 18 patients (27.3%). The two latter groups of patients are individuals who otherwise would have not been considered candidates for surgical treatment because of the location, number, or involvement of multiple hepatic segments by tumor prior to the addition of RFA to our surgical treatment armamentarium. Patients who underwent less than a hemihepatectomy more frequently had RFA as a component of their surgical treatment (54.2%), while patients who had a hemihepatectomy or extended hepatectomy also underwent RFA in a minority of the cases (22.7%, $p = .03$). Of the 53 patients who underwent resection as a component of their surgical treatment, no patient had a positive margin. The perioperative complication rate in these 66 patients was 15.2%, however, three patients died within 90 days of surgical treatment for a perioperative mortality rate of 4.5%.

Most of the patients in our study (n = 52, 78.8%) received some form of systemic chemotherapy, generally both preoperative and postoperative treatment.[28] Patients with GIST diagnosed in the last 5 years of our study received imatinib mesylate, but the patients diagnosed with leiomyosarcoma or unclassified sarcomas received eight different systemic chemotherapy regimens. Of the 36 patients with GIST, 26 received imatinib mesylate while 10 patients underwent surgical treatment before this drug was available. At a median follow-up of 36 months, 44 of the 66 patients (66.7%) had developed recurrent disease. The sites of recurrent disease in these patients is listed in Table 1. The median time to development of recurrent disease was 13.5 months (range 2 to 59 months). Univariate and multivariate analysis of factors that might predict risk of recurrence demonstrated that the type of surgical resection, the primary tumor histology, primary tumor site, primary tumor size, surgical treatment of initial versus recurrent liver metastases, number of liver metastases treated, number of lesions treated with RFA, number of liver metastases and size of liver metastases were not predictive of an increased risk to develop recurrent disease. The only factor we found that was a statistically significant predictor of disease recurrence was the use of RFA. Patients who underwent RFA alone or resection plus RFA were more likely to develop recurrent disease (84.6% and 88.9%, respectively) compared to patients who underwent resection alone (57.1%, $p < .05$).

The 1-, 3-, and 5-year disease-free survival (DFS) rates in our patients were 52.1%, 20.6%, and 16.4%, respectively. The median overall survival (OS) in our 66 patients was 47.2 months and the 1-, 3-, and 5-year OS rates were 91.2%, 65.4%, and 27.1%, respectively (Figure 1). Only two factors were found to have an impact on DFS and OS. First, patients who underwent RFA as a component of their surgical treatment had a shorter disease-free interval (7.4 months) and overall median survival (33.2 months) compared with patients who were treated with only surgical resection (18.6 months and 54.0 months, respectively, $p < .01$). Secondly, patients treated with preoperative, postoperative, or both pre- and postoperative chemotherapy had an improved DFS (36.3 months with chemotherapy versus 22.7 months with no chemotherapy, $p = .01$) and had a longer median OS time (51.8 months) compared to patients treated with only surgical therapy (18.4 months,

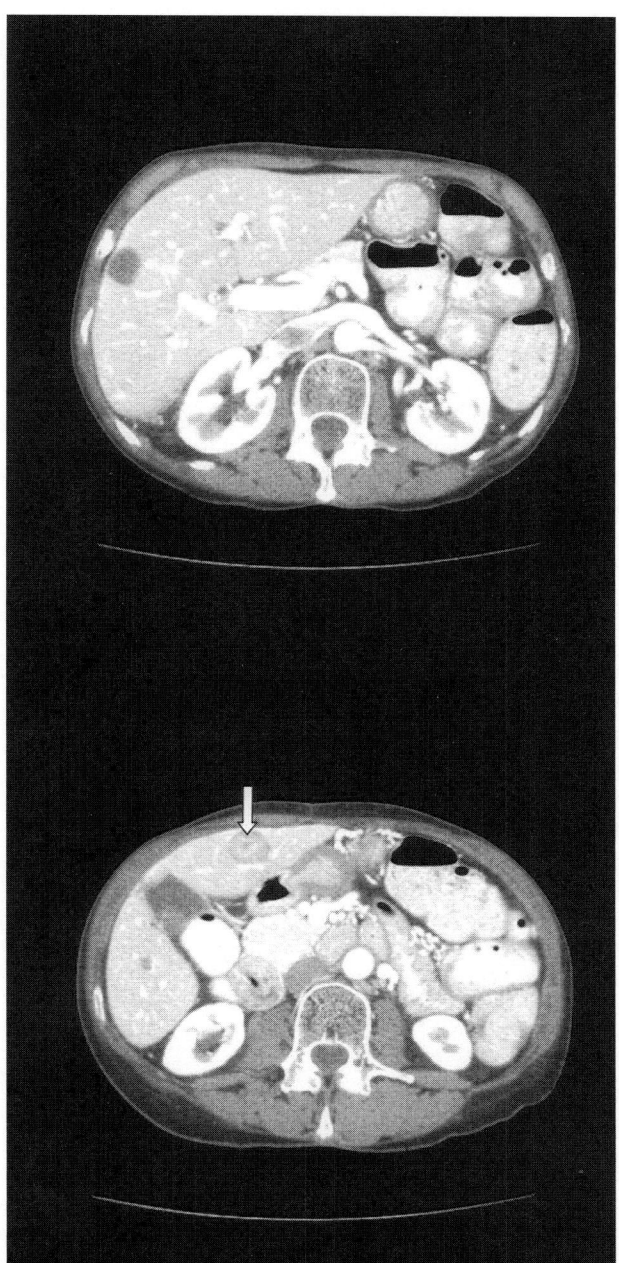

Figure 1 Overall survival in 66 patients with sarcoma liver metastases treated surgically (resection, radiofrequency ablation (RFA) only, resection plus RFA). Median overall survival was 47.2 months.

$p = .02$).[28] Interestingly, patients with GIST who were treated with imatinib mesylate have not yet reached their median survival, and this group of patients appears to have the best survival of the sarcoma liver metastases patients in our study.

It is important to emphasize that a direct comparison of patients in our study who underwent resection alone,

Table 1 Site of Recurrence in 44 of 66 Patients Who Underwent Surgical Treatment of Sarcoma Liver Metastases

Location	Number of Patients (%)
Liver	33 (50.0)
Lung	15 (34.1)
Local recurrence at primary tumor site	9 (20.5)
Peritoneum	3 (6.8)
Bone	2 (4.5)

RFA alone, or resection combined with RFA is problematic at best. We had only 66 patients who underwent surgical treatment of sarcoma liver metastases over a 10-year period. The type of surgical treatment chosen was based on the number, extent, and location of metastatic lesions and it would be impossible to perform a randomized, prospective study of this unusual group of patients to determine differences in outcome comparing resection with RFA. Our finding that patients treated with RFA of sarcoma liver metastases had a higher risk of recurrence and subsequently, reduced disease-free and overall median survival times is consistent with our larger series of 348 patients with CRC liver metastases.[29] In the patients with CRC liver metastases, treatment with RFA alone or combined with resection was associated with a significantly shorter disease-free interval and a reduced probability of long-term survival.

Surgical treatment should certainly be considered as a component of the treatment of patients with GIST liver metastases. The availability of imatinib mesylate and other targeted therapies for patients with GIST have improved the response and survival rates. However, most patients with an initial response will tend to develop disease that is resistant to tyrosine kinase inhibitors and when appropriate, these patients should be considered for surgical treatment of residual or recurrent disease (Figure 2). The role for surgical treatment of GIST liver metastases will be further elucidated by trials such as the Radiation Therapy Oncology Group S-0132 trial, which is evaluating the role of imatinib mesylate as adjuvant therapy in patients with potentially resectable metastatic GIST.

Conclusions

Liver metastases from GIST and non-GIST sarcomas may be amenable to surgical treatment in a subset of patients. However, patients with non-GIST sarcoma liver metastases have a lower probability of long-term survival benefit from surgical therapy in part because of a lack of active systemic chemotherapy drugs. The data available from the few studies that have evaluated surgical treatment of sarcoma liver metastases indicate that surgical treatment is associated with an improved DFS and OS rate. It must again be emphasized that these are highly selected and rare patients, and confirmation of these impressions in randomized, prospective trials will likely not be possible. We are proponents of aggressive surgical treatment of properly selected patients with sarcoma liver metastases when they can be rendered surgically free of disease. Surgical treatment should be performed as one component of a multidisciplinary approach using systemic chemotherapy drugs, particularly in patients with GIST who appear to derive a very significant long-term survival benefit from combined modality approaches.

References

1. Hemming AW, Sielaff TD, Gallinger S, et al. Hepatic resection of noncolorectal nonneuroendocrine metastases. Liver Transpl 2000;6:97–101.

2. Foster JH. Survival after liver resection for secondary tumors. Am J Surg 1978;135:389–94.

3. Chen H, Pruitt A, Nicol TL, et al. Complete hepatic resection of metastases from leiomyosarcoma prolongs survival. J Gastrointest Surg 1998;2:151–5.

4. Karakousis CP, Blumenson LE, Canavese G, Rao U. Surgery for disseminated abdominal sarcoma. Am J Surg 1992;163:560–4.

5. Tepetes K, Tsamandas AC, Ravazoula P, et al. Survival for 5 years after repeat liver resections and multimodality treatment for metastatic intestinal leiomyosarcoma: report of a case. Surg Today 2002;32:925–8.

6. Kamoshita N, Yokomori T, Iesato H, et al. Malignant gastrointestinal stromal tumor of the jejunum with liver metastasis. Hepatogastroenterology 2002;49:1311–4.

7. Shima Y, Horimi T, Ishikawa T, et al. Aggressive surgery for liver metastases from gastrointestinal stromal tumors. J Hepatobiliary Pancreat Surg 2003;10:77–80.

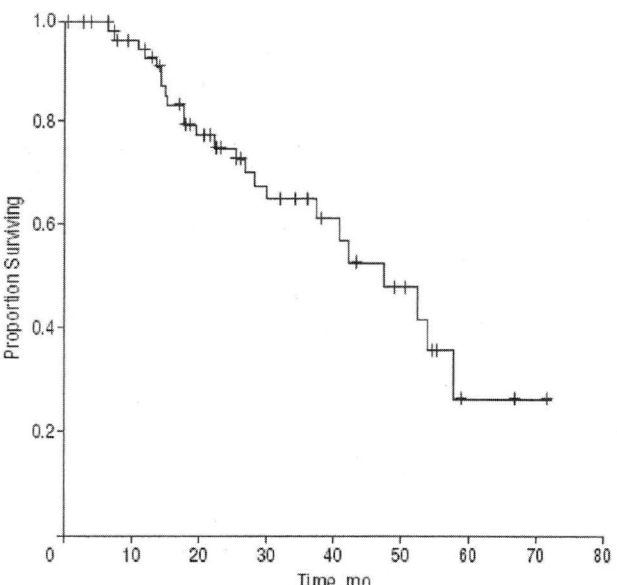

Figure 2 A computed tomography scan of a patient with multiple gastrointestinal stromal tumor liver metastases. Cystic degeneration of the lesions related to treatment with imatinib mesylate is seen, however, after 18 months of treatment progressive disease in one area (arrow) developed. This recurrent tumor was resected.

8. Lang H, Nussbaum KT, Kaudel P, et al. Hepatic metastases from leiomyosarcoma: a single-center experience with 34 liver resections during a 15-year period. Ann Surg 2000; 231:500–5.

9. Schwartz SI. Hepatic resection for noncolorectal nonneuroendocrine metastases. World J Surg 1995;19:72–5.

10. Weitz J, Blumgart LH, Fong Y, et al. Partial hepatectomy for metastases from noncolorectal, nonneuroendocrine carcinoma. Ann Surg 2005;241:269–76.

11. Elias D, Cavalcanti de Albuquerque A, Eggenspieler P, et al. Resection of liver metastases from a noncolorectal primary: indications and results based on 147 monocentric patients. J Am Coll Surg 1998;187:487–93.

12. Billingsley KG, Burt ME, Jara E, et al. Pulmonary metastases from soft tissue sarcoma: analysis of patterns of diseases and postmetastasis survival. Ann Surg 1999;229: 602–10; discussion 610–2.

13. Weiser MR, Downey RJ, Leung DH, et al. Repeat resection of pulmonary metastases in patients with soft-tissue sarcoma. J Am Coll Surg 2000;191:184–90; discussion 190–1.

14. Mudan SS, Conlon KC, Woodruff JM, et al. Salvage surgery for patients with recurrent gastrointestinal sarcoma: prognostic factors to guide patient selection. Cancer 2000;88:66–74.

15. Ng EH, Pollock RE, Romsdahl MM. Prognostic implications of patterns of failure for gastrointestinal leiomyosarcomas. Cancer 1992;69:1334–41.

16. DeMatteo RP, Lewis JJ, Leung D, et al. Two hundred gastrointestinal stromal tumors: recurrence patterns and prognostic factors for survival. Ann Surg 2000;231:51–8.

17. Jaques DP, Coit DG, Casper ES, Brennan MF. Hepatic metastases from soft-tissue sarcoma. Ann Surg 1995;221: 392–7.

18. Van Glabbeke M, van Oosterom AT, Oosterhuis JW, et al. Prognostic factors for the outcome of chemotherapy in advanced soft tissue sarcoma: an analysis of 2,185 patients treated with anthracycline-containing first-line regimens—a European Organization for Research and Treatment of Cancer Soft Tissue and Bone Sarcoma Group Study. J Clin Oncol 1999;17:150–7.

19. Le Cesne A, Judson I, Crowther D, et al. Randomized phase III study comparing conventional-dose doxorubicin plus ifosfamide versus high-dose doxorubicin plus ifosfamide plus recombinant human granulocyte-macrophage colony-stimulating factor in advanced soft tissue sarcomas: a trial of the European Organization for Research and Treatment of Cancer/Soft Tissue and Bone Sarcoma Group. J Clin Oncol 2000;18:2676–84.

20. Mavligit GM, Zukwiski AA, Ellis LM, et al. Gastrointestinal leiomyosarcoma metastatic to the liver. Durable tumor regression by hepatic chemoembolization infusion with cisplatin and vinblastine. Cancer 1995;75:2083–8.

21. Hirota S, Isozaki K, Moriyama Y, et al. Gain-of-function mutations of c-kit in human gastrointestinal stromal tumors. Science 1998;279:577–80.

22. Goss GA, Merriam P, Manola J, et al. Clinical and pathological characteristics of gastrointestinal stroma tumors (GIST). Prog Proc Am Soc Clin Oncol 2000;X: 599a.

23. Dematteo RP, Heinrich MC, El-Rifai WM, Demetri G. Clinical management of gastrointestinal stromal tumors: before and after STI-571. Hum Pathol 2002;33:466–77.

24. Demetri GD, von Mehren M, Blanke CD, et al. Efficacy and safety of imatinib mesylate in advanced gastrointestinal stromal tumors. N Engl J Med 2002;347:472–80.

25. Gorre ME, Mohammed M, Ellwood K, et al. Clinical resistance to STI-571 cancer therapy caused by BCR-ABL gene mutation or amplification. Science 2001;293:876–80.

26. Wu PC, Langerman A, Ryan CW, et al. Surgical treatment of gastrointestinal stromal tumors in the imatinib (STI-571) era. Surgery 2003;134:656–65; discussion 665–6.

27. Mauro MJ, O'Dwyer M, Heinrich MC, Druker BJ. STI571: a paradigm of new agents for cancer therapeutics. J Clin Oncol 2002;20:325–34.

28. Pawlik TM, Vauthey JN, Abdalla EK, et al. Results of a single-center experience with resection and ablation for sarcoma metastatic to the liver. Arch Surg 2006;141:537–44.

29. Abdalla EK, Vauthey JN, Ellis LM, et al. Recurrence and outcomes following hepatic resection, radiofrequency ablation, and combined resection/ablation for colorectal liver metastases. Ann Surg 2004;239:818–25; discussion 825–7.

CHAPTER 79

SPECIAL SITUATIONS: LOCAL RECURRENCE

FRITZ C. EILBER, MD

WILLIAM D. TAP, MD

FREDERICK R. EILBER, MD

Despite improvements in multimodality therapy, local recurrence remains a significant problem for patients with soft tissue sarcomas. In most series, the local recurrence rate after the treatment of primary extremity soft tissue sarcomas is about 10 to 15% and about 40 to 50% after the treatment of primary retroperitoneal sarcomas.[1–8] In addition, 30 to 40% of the patients who present to university hospitals or cancer centers do so with locally recurrent disease.[1–8] It is thus critical for a surgical oncologist treating soft tissue sarcomas to understand how to handle the challenging situation of a local recurrence.

As is true in all areas of surgical oncology, effective treatment is predicated on understanding the biology of the malignancy being treated and where surgery fits in the context of other treatments available to the patient. This is particularly true in the setting of locally recurrent soft tissue sarcomas. Locally recurrent disease is very different from primary disease, and understanding how is important. This chapter will primarily focus on locally recurrent extremity soft tissue sarcomas because this is the most common site of disease. However, many if not all of the principles that are touched upon can be translated to sarcomas of other sites.

Proper Treatment of Primary Disease

The optimal management of locally recurrent disease is preventing it. This is best done in the setting of the primary disease with an aggressive multimodality treatment paradigm devised by an experienced team of physicians at a specialty sarcoma center.[1–8]

A common pitfall in the setting of the primary disease is centered on the patient referred to the university hospital or cancer center after having an unplanned (no cross-sectional imaging or tissue diagnosis) excision of a presumably benign tumor only to find out that it is a sarcoma. In addition to reviewing the outside pathology, we will re-image the surgical site to see if there is any residual gross disease. Finally, the surgical site should be re-resected. This is done for two reasons. First, about half of the time there is residual macroscopic disease is in the reoperative specimen. In a study looking at planned reoperation after unplanned total excision of soft tissue sarcoma, 44 of the 91 patients (49%) in this study had macroscopic residual disease in the reoperative specimen[9] Second, re-resection is associated with an improved survival. In a study looking at the effect of re-resection in extremity soft tissue sarcomas, re-resection was a highly significant ($p = .005$, RR = 0.6) independent predictor of improved disease-specific survival.[10]

An additional pitfall is centered on the patient who undergoes suboptimal treatment (surgery, radiation, and/or chemotherapy) for their primary disease with the belief that they can be referred to specialty center if or when the patient recurs. This is a morbid and often lethal misconception that unfortunately occurs not infrequently. The morbidity of a local recurrence is readily apparent and is shown in Figure 1. In patients who presented with primary extremity soft tissue sarcomas to University of California, Los Angeles (UCLA), the amputation rate was 5%. The amputation rate increased to 38% with the development of a local recurrence.[4] The amputation rate for patients who presented to UCLA with locally recurrent disease was 13%, almost three

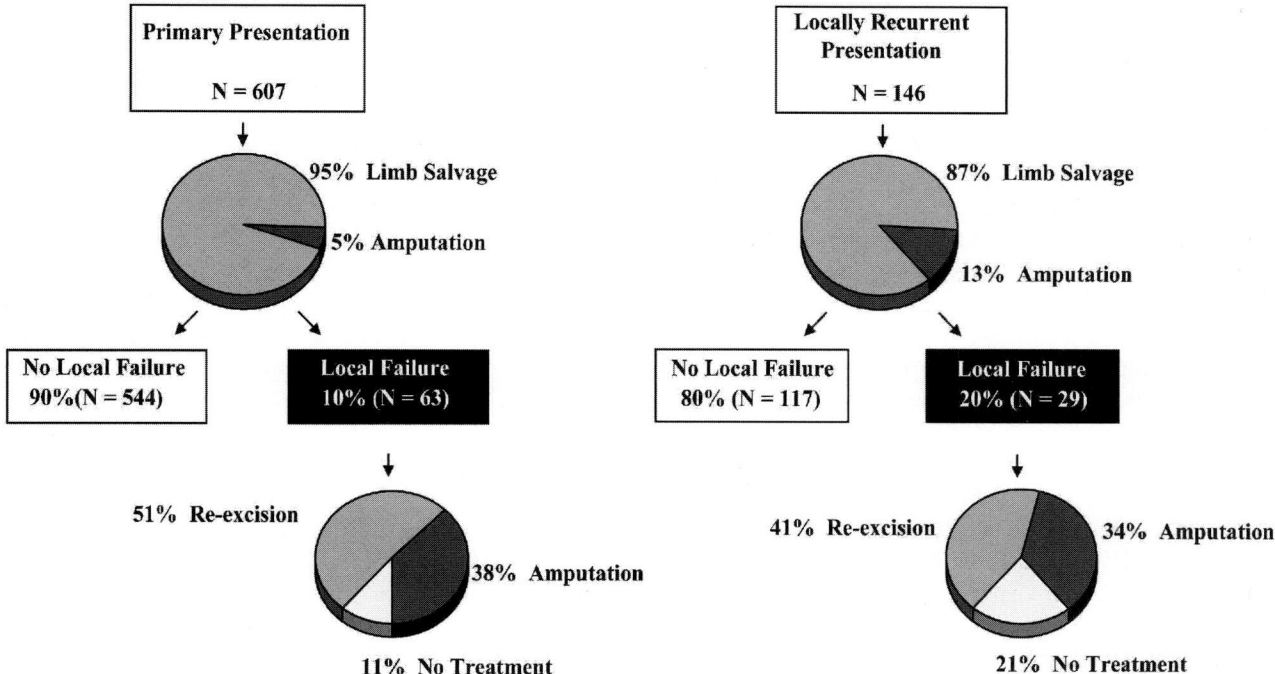

Figure 1

times that for patients presenting with primary disease. In addition, these patients were twice as likely to develop an additional local recurrence and twice as likely to develop subsequently metastatic disease.[4]

Local recurrence, similar to grade and size, is in and of itself a significant independent adverse prognostic variable associated with a decreased disease survival. This has been clearly shown by several large database analyses. A patient that develops a local recurrence is two to three times more likely to die of disease compared to patients who do not. [4,11] While these studies show that local recurrence is associated with decreased survival, it is difficult to draw any conclusions regarding the causal relationship between local recurrence and survival. This association most likely exists because local recurrence is a reflection of a biologically aggressive tumor and is not causal. Regardless, the best opportunity to cure a patient with soft tissue sarcoma is in the setting of their primary disease and underestimating the significance of local control is a morbid and often lethal misconception.

Biology and Management

It is quite evident that local recurrence is morbid and is associated with a significant decreased disease-specific survival compared to patients with primary disease. The next questions are: When do they occur? How bad are they? What are the differences between the primary and local recurrence tumor characteristics, if any? and Are there any characteristics of these patients with locally recurrent disease that predict better or worse outcomes? In other word, what is the biologic behavior of locally recurrent disease?

A number of studies that have looked at local recurrence in extremity soft tissue sarcomas, the majority of which have focused on whether or not local recurrence, in and of itself, is a prognostic variable associated with decreased survival.[1,2,6,7,11–14] Few studies have looked at the factors predictive of survival in patients with locally recurrent extremity soft tissue sarcomas, and these studies are limited by small numbers, short follow-up and a mixture of initial presentation status.[4–8,12,13–16] Accurate analysis of locally recurrent extremity soft tissue sarcomas is dependent upon the population of patients studied. It is important to make a distinction between patients who present with locally recurrent disease after having undergone treatment for the primary at another institution and patients who develop a local recurrence after having undergone treatment for the primary at the same institution. Patients who present with locally recurrent disease can have a long interval between initial treatment and presentation with locally recurrent disease. A recent publication found the mean interval between treatment of the primary at another institution and presentation to UCLA with locally recurrent disease to be 30 months.[4]

Additionally 40% of the patients with primary disease that subsequently locally recurred, died within 2 years of their local recurrence. This suggests that patients who present initially with locally recurrent disease are a highly selected population, particularly if their interval to local recurrence is long.[4] Further difficulty in drawing conclusions from such a population include limited information about the primary tumor pathologic characteristics and an unknown extent of initial surgery.

The ideal population of patients to study is one that has developed a local recurrence while being followed at the same institution that performed the primary operation. Unfortunately, the studies on locally recurrent extremity soft tissue sarcomas have either analyzed a selected population of patients who presented initially with locally recurrent disease, or patients with a mixture of initial presentation status.[5–8,12,13,15] Finally, none of these studies have identified and compared both the primary and the local recurrent tumor characteristics.[4–8,11–16] As such, the factors predictive of survival in patients with locally recurrent extremity soft tissue sarcoma had not been well defined.

A recent analysis addresses these questions using a study population of patients who developed a local recurrence while being followed at the same institution, which performed the primary operation. 179 patients with extremity soft tissue sarcomas who underwent complete surgical resection of both the primary and subsequent local recurrence at Memorial Sloan-Kettering Cancer Center (MSKCC) during 1982 to 2002 were analyzed.[17] Clinicopathologic characteristics of these 179 patients were similar to large series of patients with primary extremity soft tissue sarcomas. No histology was disproportionately represented.[1–5] Interestingly, there was not a significant difference between the grade of the primary and the grade of the local recurrence. Only four patients who presented with a low-grade primary tumor progressed to a high-grade local recurrence, and this occurred in four different histologies.[17] Additionally, there was not a significant difference between the number of patients with a microscopically positive margin following resection of the primary tumor and resection of the local recurrence. There was a significant difference between the depth and size of the primary tumor and the depth and size of the local recurrence. There were 161 (90%) deep tumors at local recurrence compared to 142 (72%) deep primary tumors ($p <$ .0001). The median tumor size at local recurrence was 5 cm compared to a median primary tumor size of 7 cm ($p <$ .0001).[17]

The median interval to local recurrence was 16 months, with 65% developing a local recurrence by 2 years and 90% by 4 years (Figure 2).[17] Vigilant follow-up of patients for at least the first 4 years following resection

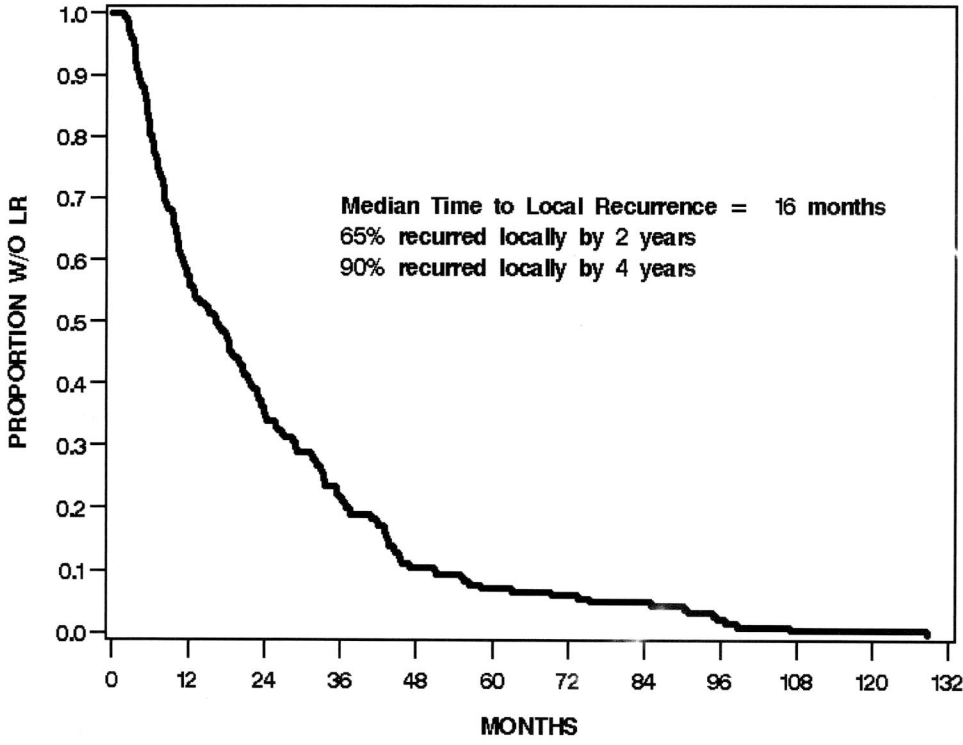

Median Time to Local Recurrence = 16 months
65% recurred locally by 2 years
90% recurred locally by 4 years

Figure 2

of their primary extremity sarcoma is clearly warranted because 90% of the local recurrences developed within this time period. At UCLA, we perform a physical exam, chest X-ray, and cross-sectional imaging (computed tomography [CT] or magnetic resonance imaging) of the surgical site every 6 months for the first 5 years following surgery. Whether discovering a local recurrence at a smaller size in a shorter interval impacts the limb salvage rate or the survival of these patients is not entirely clear; however, we do feel that it is easier to surgically address a smaller local recurrence rather that a larger one.[18,19]

The disease-specific survival for all 179 patients was 68% at 2 years and 55% at 4 years.[17] The fact that 45% of all patients died of disease within 4 years of developing a local recurrence demonstrates the high-risk biology of these patients. As expected, patients with high-grade tumors had a significantly worse disease-specific mortality compared to patients with low-grade tumors (Figure 3).[17] Interestingly, six (15%) patients with low-grade primary tumors died of disease, three (7.5%) of which had myxoid liposarcomas, suggesting that low-grade tumors of this histologic subtype warrant particular attention.[17]

Analysis of the clinicopathologic characteristics associated with disease-specific survival revealed that high histologic grade (primary and local recurrence), large local recurrence tumor size, and short local recurrence free interval were all independently associated with decreased disease-specific survival. Unexpectedly, primary tumor size was not significant on multivariate analysis.[17] This, in conjunction with the fact that tumor grade remained essentially unchanged, allows for prompt treatment planning to occur at presentation with locally recurrent disease. Specifically the surgeon needs date of primary surgery, original pathology slides to confirm histology and grade, and cross-sectional imaging of the extremity to assess local recurrence size.

Local recurrence does offer a unique glimpse of the biology of the specific patient's disease. Because the time it took for the tumor to grow to a pathologically defined size is known, an assessment of growth rate can be made. These growth rate characteristics are predictive of disease-specific survival and represent an expression of tumor aggressiveness independent of histologic grade. The profound significance of these characteristics is illustrated in Figure 4.[17] Patients who developed a local recurrence > 5cm in ≤ 16 months had a 4-year disease-specific survival rate of 18%. By comparison, patients who developed a local recurrence < 5 cm in > 16 months had a 4-year disease specific survival rate of 81%.[17]

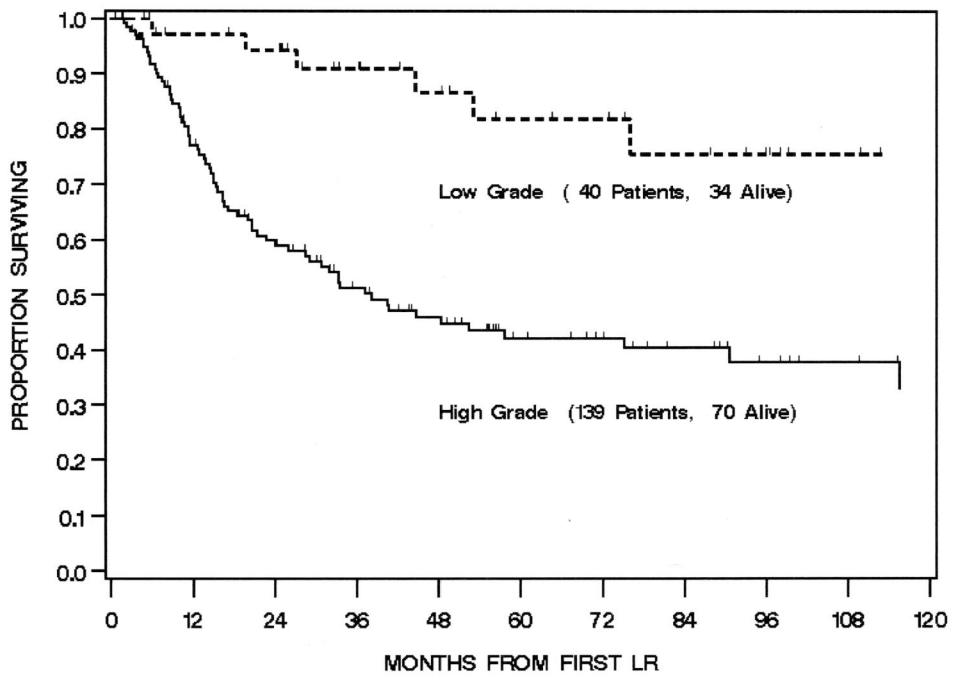

Tick mark(I) indicates last follow-up

Figure 3

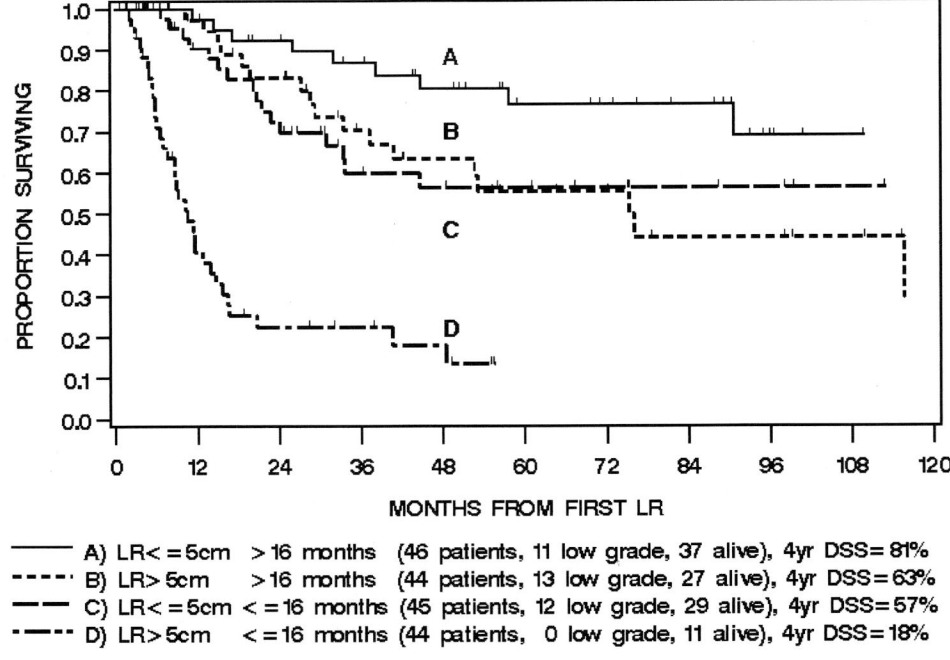

A) LR< =5cm   >16 months   (46 patients, 11 low grade, 37 alive), 4yr DSS= 81%
B) LR>5cm   >16 months   (44 patients, 13 low grade, 27 alive), 4yr DSS= 63%
C) LR< =5cm < =16 months   (45 patients, 12 low grade, 29 alive), 4yr DSS= 57%
D) LR>5cm   < =16 months   (44 patients, 0 low grade, 11 alive), 4yr DSS= 18%

Tick mark(I) indicates last follow—up

Figure 4

Treatment

Locally recurrent extremity diseases usually presents as either a nodular mass in the surgical bed detected by physical exam or as a deeper mass detected by cross-sectional imaging. Locally recurrent retroperitoneal disease is almost exclusively detected by cross-sectional imaging. CT guided core biopsy is occasionally warranted to confirm the presence of a local recurrence, particularly if the recurrence is small. Once a local recurrence is confirmed, treatment planning can begin.

SURGERY

Just as with primary disease, surgery is the cornerstone of treating locally recurrent disease. Complete surgical resection is the goal. Although the amputation rate increases in the setting of locally recurrent disease, the vast majority (> 80%) are able to undergo limb-sparing surgery, and amputation is still considered a last resort.[4,20,21] Amputation is basically never used in the setting of a recurrent low-grade lesion. It may be necessary in the setting of a recurrent high-grade lesion with neurovascular involvement. In this setting, we will treat the patient with neoadjuvant therapy (chemotherapy and or chemo-radiation therapy) for two reasons. The neoadjuvant treatment can shrink the lesion allowing for limb salvage. More importantly, the treatment-induced pathologic necrosis in the resected specimen indicates the effectiveness of that particular therapy for the patient.[22]

RADIATION THERAPY

Although radiation therapy is rarely if ever used for low-grade primary soft tissue sarcomas, we will often use it for recurrent low-grade lesions both in the extremity and retroperitoneum.[23] This treatment is predominantly postoperative external beam radiation therapy (5,000 Gy) to the effected area. Occasionally in the setting of a large low-grade local recurrence we will use neoadjuvant radiation therapy. All locally recurrent high-grade soft tissue sarcomas are treated with radiation therapy if they did not receive it in the setting of their primary disease. We do not use brachytherapy.

CHEMOTHERAPY

We believe that high-grade locally recurrent soft tissue sarcomas should be treated with neoadjuvant systemic chemotherapy. These are very high-risk lesions that reflect a biologically aggressive malignancy that likely have subclinical micrometastatic disease.[4,17] As was shown in the setting of locally recurrent extremity soft tissue sarcomas, these high-grade local recurrences can be stratified by the size and interval of the local recurrence.

Patients who developed a local recurrence > 5cm in ≤ 16 months had a two-year disease specific mortality of about 80% (see Figure 4).[17] Although not as well studied in the setting of retroperitoneal sarcomas, we believe the same principles apply.

Our first line chemotherapy is high-dose ifosfamide base chemotherapy at a dose of 2 $gm/m^2/day$ as a continuous venous infusion over seven days for a total dose of 14 gm/m^2.[22,24,25] Two cycles of this are given prior to surgery. If the patient has previously been treated with this regimen for his or her primary tumor, or if the patient is not able to undergo such intensive treatment, we will use gemcitabine/docetaxel as our second-line treatment. These treatments are always given neoadjuvantly for the reasons touched on above. If there has been a good response to treatment, assessed by pathologic necrosis in the resected specimen, then the patients are treated with two additional cycles postoperatively.[22] If there has been a poor response to treatment, then no additional chemotherapy is given. Because patients with locally recurrent high-grade extremity soft tissue sarcomas die of systemic disease, we do not perform isolated limb perfusion.

Conclusion

Optimal management of locally recurrent disease is preventing it. This is best done with proper and aggressive treatment in the setting of the primary tumor by an experienced, multidisciplinary group of physicians at specialty sarcoma centers. Underestimating the significance of local control is a morbid and often lethal misconception. Sixty-five percent of patients develop a local recurrence within 2 years of the primary surgery. Histologic grade, local recurrence size, and local recurrence-free interval are independent predictors of survival in patients with locally recurrent extremity soft tissue sarcomas. A large local recurrence that develops in a short interval indicates a biologically aggressive tumor with a tumor specific mortality of close to 80%. Patients who develop such recurrences should be treated with neoadjuvant systemic therapy.

References

1. Brennan MF. The enigma of local recurrence. Ann Surg Oncol 1997;4:1–12.

2. Pisters PWT, Leung DHY, Woodruff J, et al. Analysis of prognostic factors in 1,041 patients with localized soft tissue sarcomas of the extremities. J Clin Oncol 1996;14: 1679–89.

3. Lewis JJ, Leung D, Woodruff JM, et al. Retroperitoneal soft tissue sarcoma: analysis of 500 patients treated and followed at a single institution. Ann Surg 1998;228:355–65.

4. Eilber FC, Rosen G, Nelson SD, et al. High grade extremity soft tissue sarcomas. Factors predictive of local recurrence and its effect on morbidity and mortality. Ann Surg 2003; 237:218–26.

5. Stotter AT, Ahern RP, Fisher C, et al. The influence of local recurrence of extremity soft tissue sarcoma on metastases and survival. Cancer 1990;65:1119–29.

6. Gustafson P, Rooser B, Rydholm A. Is local recurrence of minor importance for metastases in soft tissue sarcoma? Cancer 1991;67:2083–6.

7. Trovik CS. Local recurrence of soft tissue sarcoma. A Scandinavian Sarcoma Group project. Acta Orthop Scand 2001;72:1–31.

8. Ramanathan RC, A'Hern R, Fisher C, et al. Prognostic index for extremity soft tissue sarcomas with isolated local recurrence. Ann Surg Oncol 2001;8:278–89.

9. Giuliano AE, Eilber FR. The rationale for planned reoperation after unplanned total excision of soft tissue sarcomas. J Clin Oncol 1985;3:1344–8.

10. Lewis JJ, Leung D, Espat J, et al. Effect of reresection in extremity soft tissue sarcoma. Ann Surg 2000;231:655–63.

11. Giuliano AE, Eilber FR, Morton DL. The management of locally recurrent soft-tissue sarcoma. Ann Surg 1982;196: 87–91.

12. Karakousis CP, Proimakis C, Rao U, et al. Local recurrence and survival in soft-tissue sarcomas. Ann Surg Oncol 1996; 3:255–60.

13. Potter DA, Kinsella T, Glatstein E, et al. High-grade soft tissue sarcomas of the extremities. Cancer 1986;58:190–205.

14. Lewis JJ, Leung D, Heslin M, et al. Association of local recurrence with subsequent survival in extremity soft tissue sarcoma. J Clin Oncol 1997;15:646–52.

15. Midis GP, Pollock RE, Chen NP, et al. Locally recurrent soft tissue sarcoma of the extremity. Surgery 1998;123:666–71.

16. Stojadinovic A, Yeh A, Brennan MF. Completely resected recurrent soft tissue sarcoma: primary anatomic site governs outcome. J Am Coll Surg 2002;194:436–47.

17. Eilber FC, Brennan MF, Riedel E, et al. Prognostic factors for survival in patients with locally recurrent extremity soft tissue sarcomas. Ann Surg Oncol 2005;12:228–36.

18. Whooley BP, Gibbs JF, Mooney MM, et al. Primary extremity sarcoma. What is the appropriate follow-up? Ann Surg Oncol 2000;7:9–14.

19. Brennan MF. Follow-up is valuable and effective: true, true, and unrelated? Ann Surg Oncol 2000;7:2–3.

20. Eilber FR, Mirra JJ, Grant TT, et al. Is amputation necessary for sarcomas? A seven-year experience with limb salvage. Ann Surg 1980;192:431–8.

21. Rosenberg SA, Tepper J, Glatstein E, et al. The treatment of soft-tissue sarcoma of the extremities: prospective randomized evaluation of (1) limb-sparing surgery plus radiation therapy compared with amputation and (2) the role of adjuvant chemotherapy. Ann Surg 1982;196: 305–15.

22. Eilber FC, Rosen G, Eckardt J, et al. Treatment induced pathologic necrosis: a predictor of local recurrence and survival in patients receiving neoadjuvant therapy for high grade extremity soft tissue sarcomas. J Clin Oncol 2001;19: 3203–9.

23. Pisters PW, Harrison LB, Leung DH, et al. Long-term results of a prospective randomized trial of adjuvant brachytherapy in soft tissue sarcoma. J Clin Oncol 1996;14: 859–68.

24. Eilber FC, Eilber FR, Eckardt JJ, et al. The impact of chemotherapy on the survival of patients with high-grade primary extremity liposarcoma. Ann Surg 2004;240:686–95.

25. Eilber FC, Tap WD, Nelson SD, et al. Advances in chemotherapy for patients with extremity soft tissue sarcoma. Orthop Clin North Am 2006;37:15–22.

26. Hensley ML, Maki R, Venkatraman E, et al. Gemcitabine and docetaxel in patients with unresectable leiomyosarcoma: results of a phase II trial. J Clin Oncol 2002;20:2824–31.

CHAPTER 80

GASTROINTESTINAL STROMAL TUMOR

ERIC KLEINBAUM, MD

JONATHAN C. TRENT, MD, PhD

Over the past 60 years, basic science, pathology, and clinical investigators have studied gastrointestinal stromal tumors (GISTs) with minor advances in patient care. Recent discoveries made by basic scientists, pathologists, and clinical investigators have led to an understanding of the biological role of Kit in GISTs and the development of one of the most exciting examples of targeted therapy to date. The success of the Kit tyrosine kinase inhibitor imatinib mesylate (Gleevec, formerly STI-571) has caught the attention of the medical community. With the use of targeted therapy in a targetable disease, new developments in our understanding of the medical and surgical management of GIST have become apparent. Intense study of GIST may lead to new paradigms in the management of cancer.

Using modern histopathologic methods including immunohistochemical analysis of KIT expression, Swedish investigators reevaluated a series of intra-abdominal sarcomas and estimated the incidence of GIST to be 14.5 cases per million people, equating to about 5,000 new cases per year in the US.[1,2]

The peak incidence of GIST occurs in the late sixth and early seventh decades of life, and there is a slight male predominance. This tumor rarely occurs before the age of 20. In a large retrospective study there was a suggestion of an increased risk among African-Americans and Asian/Pacific Islanders, but this has not been validated in other studies.[3] Approximately 60% of GISTs occur in the stomach, 25% in the small intestine, 10% in the large bowel, rectum, appendix, and esophagus, and rarely in extra-intestinal sites such as the gallbladder, omentum, and mesentery. GISTs make up 2.2% of all gastric malignancies, 13.9% of all small intestine malignancies, and 0.1% of all colonic malignancies.[4] Gastric GIST has a better prognosis than extragastric GIST.[5] The common metastatic sites for GIST include the liver and omentum, less frequently to the lung, and rarely to the regional lymph nodes and bone.[6]

Histopathology

The neoplastic cells in GISTs are thought to arise from the interstitial cells of Cajal (ICC) or its progenitor cell. Sarlomo-Rikali and colleagues noted in 1998 that GISTs stained nearly universally positive for *CD117* (KIT) as compared to other mesenchymal tumors such as leiomyoma, leiomyosarcomas, and schwannomas.[7] It is now estimated that nearly 95% of GISTs stain for KIT.[2] Other positive immunohistochemical markers include *CD34* (70%), *smooth muscle actin* (35%), *S-100* (10%) and rarely *desmin* (5%).[2] Although these antigens are useful to distinguish GIST from smooth muscle tumors, desmoid fibromatosis, and schwannoma, they should not be relied upon to the exclusion of tumor cell morphology and clinical findings.

Three major histological subtypes are characteristic of GIST. These include spindle cell (70%), epithelioid (20%), and a mixed subtype (10%).[8] Epithelioid variants are more often seen in the stomach and in some studies have been linked to expression of *Bcl-2*[9] and adverse outcomes.[10]

Many factors have been looked at in estimating the malignant potential of primary GIST. While many studies have looked at the site of the tumor and mucosal invasion, the two most predictive factors appear to be tumor size (greatest diameter) and number of mitoses per high-powered field. Consensus histological criteria have been formulated (Table 1). Despite these criteria, the true malignant or benign activity of primary GIST is

Table 1 European Society for Medical Oncology (ESMO) Risk of Malignancy Classification of Primary Gastrointestinal Stromal Tumors

Risk	Size	Mitotic Count
Very low	< 2 cm	< 5/50 hpf
Low risk	2–5 cm	< 5/50 hpf
Intermediate risk	< 5 cm	6–10/50 hpf
	5–10 cm	< 5/50 hpf
High risk	> 5 cm	> 5/50 hpf
	> 10 cm	Any mitotic rate
	Any size	> 10/50 hpf

hpf = high powered field.

unpredictable because even small (< 1 cm) tumors may recur 10 years or more after diagnosis.

Pathophysiology of the Kit Receptor Tyrosine Kinase

The Kit tyrosine kinase receptor, when stimulated by its native ligand, steel ligand, or stem cell factor (SCF), functions in a host of cellular processes including cellular proliferation, differentiation, maturation, survival, chemotaxis, and adhesion (Figure 1). Transmission of these various processes is mediated through the dimerization of Kit tyrosine kinase. Dimerization of the Kit receptor leads to phosphorylation and activation of several transduction pathways including the Phosphoinositide 3' kinase (PI3K), Jak-Stat, Ras-Erk, and Phospholipase C pathways.[11]

Genetic mutations in specific exons of the *kit* genome lead to a gain of function of this tyrosine kinase receptor in GIST. Kit is constitutively active in the absence of stimulation by SCF or via homodimerization resulting ultimately in oncogenesis.[11] Most mutations occur in the juxtamembrane region encoded by exon 11 (71%) or extracellular region encoded by exon 9 (14%), and less frequently in exon 13 (4%) or 17 (4%), which encode the tyrosine kinase domain.[12] The remainder of the mutations occur predominantly in another tyrosine kinase receptor, namely PDGFRα.[13,14]

Radiology

COMPUTED TOMOGRAPHY

GISTs have characteristic features on computed tomography (CT) imaging. These tumors tend to grow extraluminally, and as a result generally do not usually present as obstructing lesions with the exception of large tumors or those that arise in the esophagus or rectum. GISTs arise in the myenteric plexus between the circular

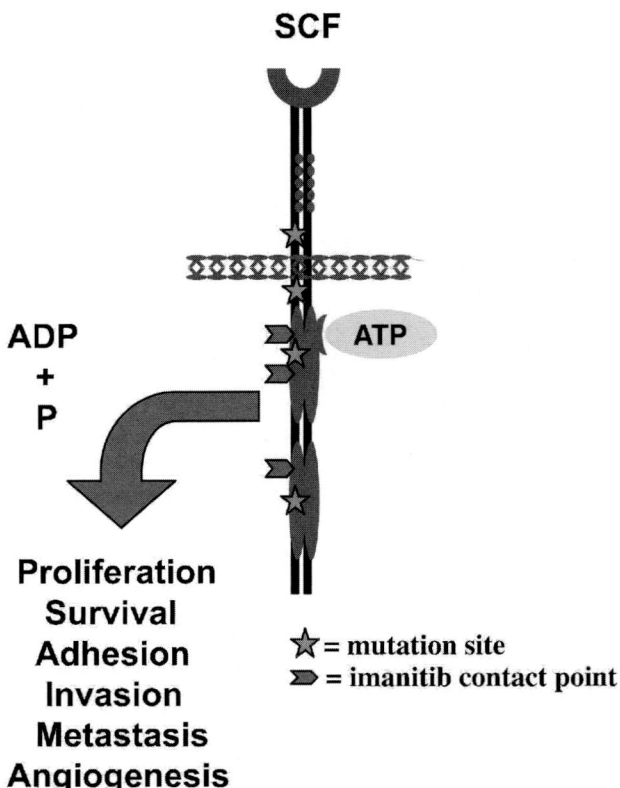

Figure 1 Graphic representation of KIT tyrosine kinase receptor homodimer. Stem cell factor (SCF) is the native ligand of the KIT receptor, but when mutant KIT is expressed in gastrointestinal stromal tumors, adenosin triphosphate (ATP)-dependent signal transduction occurs in the absence of SCF.

and longitudinal muscularis layers, which may give rise to the appearance of aneurysmal dilatation of the bowel wall.[15] Mucosal ulceration is a finding identified by free air or oral contrast within the tumor (Figure 2B). Other findings on CT imaging include intratumoral hemorrhage, which is more commonly seen in larger tumors. Tumor calcification and invasion into surrounding viscera and vessels are rare.[15] CT is the most valuable imaging tool, not only in the initial diagnosis of GIST, but also in assessing the efficacy of therapy. On initial appearance, GISTs are often large, heterogenous, masses (see Figure 2B). The small, nonenhancing portions of the untreated GIST contain necrotic tissue. When patients initiate therapy with imatinib, lesions that respond to therapy change in character on CT imaging (Figure 2C). Radiographically, gastrointestinal (GI), mesenteric, and hepatic lesions become hypovascular and appear cystic in radiodensity. These lesions may initially increase or not change in size and when analyzed pathologically they contain myxoid material with no viable cellular material.[16,17] Even after several month of therapy, the tumor

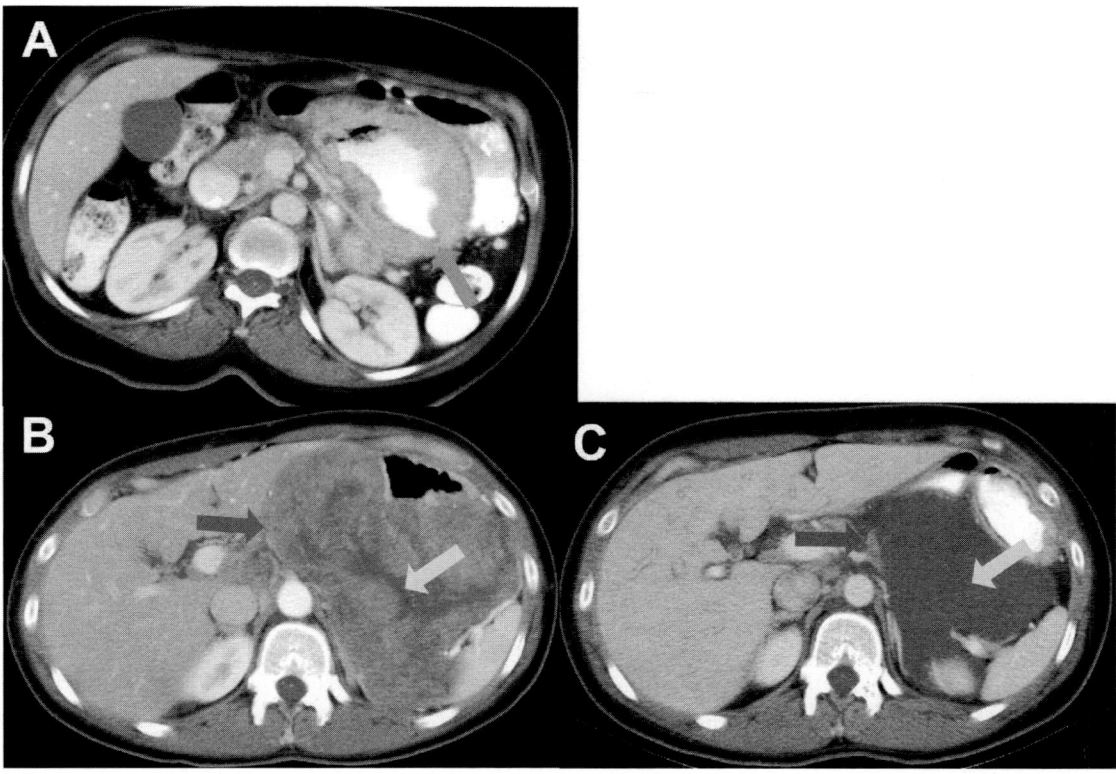

Figure 2 *A*, The large gastrointestinal stromal tumor (GIST) arising from the stomach wall has ulcerated and contains air and oral contrast. *B*, The GIST arising from the small bowel (yellow arrow) is large and heterogeneous with central necrosis (pink arrow). *C*, After initiation of imatinib therapy, the viable portion of the tumor (yellow arrow) is markedly decreased in size while the necrotic portion of the tumor has enlarged to compose the majority of the mass (pink arrow).

size may not change appreciably, although there has been marked reduction in the CT radiodensity.

Metastatic disease within the peritoneum is a frequent manifestation of GIST but may be underestimated by imaging. Peritoneal implants are often small and may be difficult to differentiate from unopacified bowel, lymph nodes, or small blood vessels.[15] Although three-phase CT scan is the best imaging modality in GIST, additional metastatic lesions in the liver or peritoneal cavity may be found at laparotomy.

Metastatic disease of the liver is a common phenomenon in GIST. The lesions, unlike their mesenteric and omental counterparts, are frequently hypervascular and enhance with contrast. The most sensitive means of detecting hepatic metastases remains the three-phase CT scan. Single-phase venous contrast may miss lesions and underestimate the extent of disease in the liver. Ascites in GIST occurs late in the disease and may be difficult to distinguish from the ascites seen as a complication of imatinib therapy.

Metastases outside the abdomen seldom occur and are associated with advanced disease. Lymphatic spread is also rare and in the presence of lymphadenopathy clinicians should entertain other diagnoses.

PET IMAGING

Positron emission tomography (PET) imaging is a functional imaging modality with limited utility in GIST.[17] PET imaging evaluates the metabolic rate of tumors by the uptake of a radiolabelled glucose molecule fluourodeoxy glucose (FDG). PET imaging has been used to detect metabolic changes very early in therapy. For instance, Figure 3 depicts a pre-imatinib PET scan showing uptake of FDG by the tumor ,which is completely abrogated after only 3 days of therapy. Additionally, PET imaging may be useful in interpreting the results of an ambiguous CT or MRI study. As patients with GIST are treated with imatinib, enlarging or stable lesions would be misclassified as stable or as an indication of progressive disease if relying solely on tumor size. However, with the noted metabolic changes on PET scanning and the correlative pathological findings of myxoid degeneration, the standard response criteria of tumor size in this malignancy is invalid.[17]

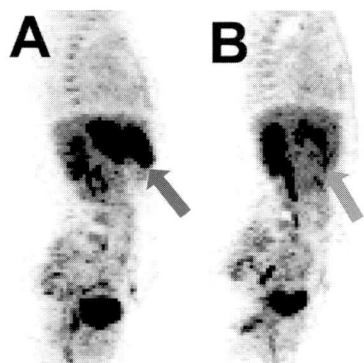

Pre-imatinib Post-imatinib

Figure 3 *A*, Prior to imatinib the patient was found to have an fluourodeoxy glucose -avid gastrointestinal stromal tumor on positron emission tomography imaging that underwent complete metabolic response after initation of imatinib (B).

The utility of PET scanning also has a role in surgical planning of initial unresectable or metastatic disease. In patients who are initiated on imatinib therapy, the clinical response can have a bearing on whether patients should undergo surgical resection. In patients with unresectable disease, decreased FDG-PET signaling may make resection at the primary GI site an option. In metastatic disease, PET scanning can be used to detect which lesions are active tumor and if they are few in number and technically feasible surgical intervention can be pursued.

Despite the benefit of PET scanning in the management of GI stromal tumors, drawbacks and limitations exist. First, low-grade lesions may be negative on PET imaging. Second, smaller tumors may not be detected by PET imaging.[17] In addition, Scaife and colleagues at MD Anderson Cancer Center have questioned the validity of PET scans as a measure of tumor response.[18] In a study conducted by Scaife and colleagues, 17 patients who received neoadjuvant imatinib had surgery performed on previously nonresectable GIST.[18] The pathological findings were then correlated with the radiological response to imatinib. Eleven of these patients had a PET scan and six demonstrated no evidence of metabolic activity on FDG-PET scan after imatinib therapy and prior to surgery. The review of the pathologic specimens revealed viable tumor in 5 of the 6 specimens. These scans were obtained within 3 months of surgical intervention and the therapeutic response may have changed during this time to explain this discrepancy.[18] However, the findings in this study do raise the question of the validity of this imaging modality in assessing tumor response. The utility of this imaging modality, while promising, requires further investigation.

EMERGING CONCEPTS IN RADIOGRAPHIC INTERPRETATION

Limited Progression

An emerging concept that has arisen in the treatment of GIST with imatinib is that of limited progression. Imatinib therapy, when administered to GIST patients, often elicits a complete metabolic response by PET imaging with gross residual water-density abnormality on CT imaging. At the time of progression, some lesions will continue to demonstrate quiescent stable disease, while a single lesion may demonstrate radiographic evidence of tumor growth. The following patient illustrates such a concept. A patient with metastatic disease to the liver is started on imatinib. This patient has an initial response in all lesions and is clinically stable. However, on reevaluation after 6 months of treatment, one of the patient's liver lesion starts to grow (Figure 4A-D). The dose of imatinib is increased, but this one solitary lesion still continues to grow. This scenario illustrates the limited progression of disease. The lesion in this scenario is best treated with local therapy such as surgical resection, radiofrequency ablation, or selective hepatic arterial embolization or chemoembolization. The patient should continue to take imatinib to treat the stable lesions.

Patients who fail to respond to imatinib therapy or who have a significant number of GIST lesions that progress on imatinib and are not amenable to local therapy. These patients have widespread progression. Therapeutic options for these patients include increasing the dose of imatinib or clinical trials with some of the alternative tyrosine kinase inhibitors under current investigation.

Therapy of Metastatic GIST

The discovery of the KIT tyrosine kinase receptor and the development of imatinib to block the activity of this receptor have changed the treatment and the outlook of this malignancy. Prior to this discovery, surgery was the only viable treatment option. Chemotherapy was largely ineffective with poor response rates and radiation therapy often impractical because of extent and location of the disease.

Primary Systemic Therapy: Imatinib Mesylate

The use of imatinib in the therapy of metastatic GIST has changed the course of this disease. From the initiation of its compassionate use in a 50-year-old patient with

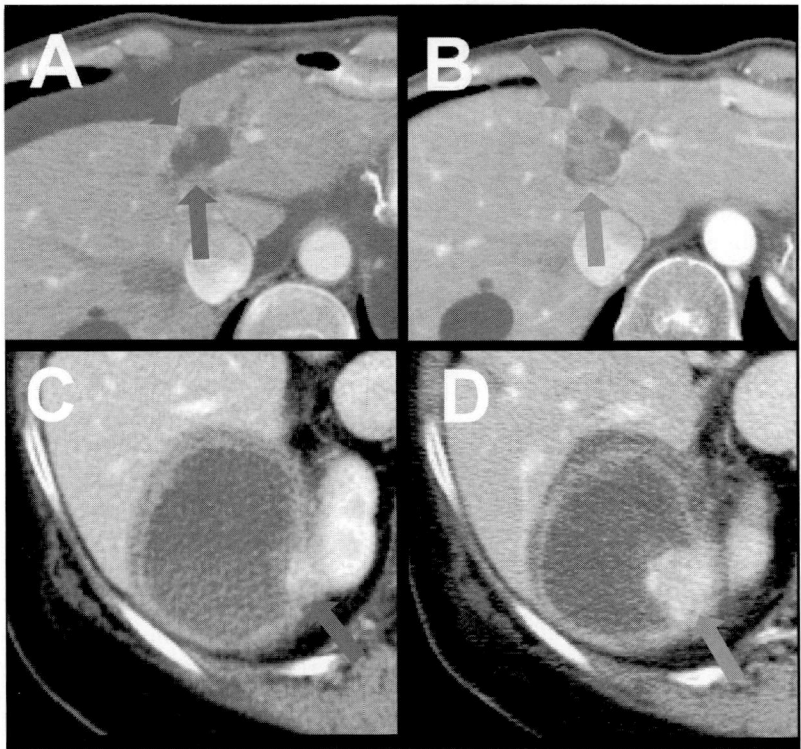

Figure 4 *A*, The patient has multiple, bilobar hepatic metastases that appear cystic due to imatinib therapy. *B*, While on imatinib therapy, the liver lesion has drastically increased in size while the remainder of the liver lesions are controlled by continuation of imatinib therapy. *C*, The gastrointestinal stromal tumor patient has a large, necrotic appearing hepatic metastasis except for one peripheral radiodense nodule. *D*, After increasing the patient's imatinib dose to 800 mg, the enhancing nodule continued to increase in size with no measurable decrease in radiodensity.

metastatic GIST in March 2000 to its position as the standard of care in patients with metastatic or unresectable disease, patients can now experience prolonged disease-free and overall survival (OS).[6,16,19] The standard dose of imatinib was established in a European Organisation for Research and Treatment of Cancer (EORTC) trial by Van Oosterom and colleagues,[20] which looked at 36 patients with GIST who were randomized to a dose of 400 mg/d, 300 mg bid, 400 mg bid, or 500 mg bid. Toxicity and efficacy were monitored and the findings showed that the best tolerated dose was 400 mg/d. The side effects were manageable and most commonly included edema, nausea, diarrhea, malaise, and fatigue. Rare side effects included myelosuppression, hemorrhage, and elevated transaminases, which required interruption or discontinuation in treatment.[20] Several phase II and III clinical trials have been designed to assess the efficacy of imatinib in the metastatic setting. Based on the data from these studies, the observed response to imatinib ranges from 48 to 71% and disease stabilization in 70 to 85% of patients. The median progression-free survival (PFS) ranges from 20 to 24 months.[6,19,21,22]

Two large international studies randomized patients with metastatic GIST to standard dose or high dose imatinib (400 mg/d versus 800 mg/d, respectively).[6,19] The North American Sarcoma Intergroup study S0033 consisted of the US cooperative oncology groups (Southwest Oncology Group, Cancer and Leukemia Group B, and the Eastern Cooperative Group) and the National Cancer Institute of Canada Sarcoma Group. Seven-hundred and forty-six patients were randomized to receive the 400-mg daily dose and were allowed to cross over to the 800 mg daily dose if they had progression of disease. Early results of this trial were presented at the American Society of Clinical Oncology (ASCO) annual meeting in 2004.[23] Median OS had not been reached in either arm after a median follow-up of 25.6 months. Although *p* value was greater than .05, there was a superior PFS rate for patients with metastatic GIST treated at an initial dose of 800 mg/d. PFS rate estimates at 2 years were 50% for the 400 mg arm and 53% for the 800 mg arm. Survival estimates at 2 years were equivalent between the two arms (78% for the 400 mg arm and versus 73% for the 800 mg arm). Interestingly, of the 106 patients who crossed over to the higher dose after having progression of disease on the 400 mg daily dose, 7% had a partial response and 32% had stable disease, indicating that patients benefit from dose escalation at the time of progression. The EORTC Soft Tissue and Bone Sarcoma Group, Italian Sarcoma Group, and Australasian Gastro-Intestinal Trials Group conducted a similarly designed phase III trial of imatinib mesylate in patients with unresectable or metastatic GIST. Nine-hundred and fifty-two patients with GIST were randomized to receive imatinib mesylate at a dose of either 400 or 800 mg daily. The objective response rates were 50% and 54% for the 400 mg and 800 mg arms, respectively. The 2-year OS estimate was 69% for patients treated at an initial daily dose of 400 mg and 74% for those patients started at 800 mg daily. PFS rates were significantly superior (52%) ($p = .026$) for patients allocated to 800 mg daily of imatinib compared to those who received the lower dose (44%). It is possible that different results in the two studies are due to the greater number of patients enrolled in the EORTC study, thus allowing more power to detect statistical differences. The combined observations of superior PFS with high dose imatinib and benefit from dose escalation at the time of progression suggest that there is a dose-response relationship for imatinib in GIST. Determining which patients will benefit from higher doses of imatinib is important in view of the greater toxicity at higher doses.

Imatinib-Resistant GIST

Resistance to imatinib while on therapy appears to occur as the result of acquired mutations that develop during the course of therapy. In patients with imatinib-naïve GIST, most mutations occur in the juxtamembrane (exon 11) or extracellular domain (exon 9). In patients with acquired resistance, the mutations are predominantly located in the intracellular kinase domain. Six rapidly progressive imatinib-resistant implants from five patients were found to encode an identical novel *kit* missense mutation, 1982T to C, that resulted in Val654Ala in the KIT tyrosine kinase domain 1. This novel mutation was not present in pre-imatinib or post-imatinib residual quiescent GISTs and strongly correlated with clinical imatinib resistance. Allelic-specific sequencing data show that this new mutation occurred in the allele that harbored the original activating mutation of KIT.[24] The end result is thought to be the formation of a stable activated form of the Kit homodimer most commonly due to mutations in exon 17 and less commonly a mutation at the binding site of imatinib in exon 14 changing the three-dimensional conformation of the homodimer and preventing binding and activity of imatinib.[25] In patients for which no secondary mutations in kit or PDGFRα are found, it is thought that other events such as mutations in other tyrosine kinase genes or activation of survival pathways may play a role in resistance.[25]

Systemic Therapy of Imatinib-resistant Metastatic GIST

Widespread progression of disease generally requires systemic therapy. The initial approach should be to maximize the dose of imatinib to 800 mg daily. As discussed previously, patients who undergo dose increase to 800 mg daily from 400 mg daily were found to experience a 7% partial response rate and a 32% stable disease rate.[19] After progression on the maximum tolerated dose of imatinib, patients should be evaluated for a clinical trial or may be treated with a recently Food and Drug Administration-approved tyrosine kinase inhibitor called sunitinib. Sunitinib (SU11248) possesses potentially both anti-angiogenic and anti-oncogenic properties because it inhibits the vascular endothelial growth factor receptor and the KIT receptor, respectively. Sunitinib was investigated in 97 patients with imatinib-resistant GIST. Each patient has received 50 mg daily of the drug and after 1 year 22 patients obtained either a partial response or stable disease.[26] In a phase III study in metastatic, imatinib-resistant GIST sunitinib was found to have a 7% partial response rate and a 58% stable disease rate after imatinib discontinuation. This phase III study randomized patients to receive either sunitinib or placebo so that the benefit of sunitinib over continued imatinib remains unknown.[27] AMG 706 is another multitargeted tyrosine kinase inhibitor with high affinity for the VEGFR and KIT. The safety and efficacy of this agent has not been published to date. The use of newer KIT inhibitors and agents that inhibit imatinib-resistance pathways may soon add to the therapeutic armamentarium for the treatment of resistant GIST.

Combined Modality Studies of Imatinib with Surgery in Patients with Primary GIST

Neoadjuvant Imatinib

Although its use is compelling, the use of imatinib in patients with resectable primary GIST is investigational. Neoadjuvant imatinib allows assessment of imatinib sensitivity and potential down-staging of surgical procedure as well as an opportunity to avoid a potentially morbid surgical procedure in patients with aggressive, imatinib-resistant GIST. Additionally, preoperative administration of imatinib allows reliable administration of therapy prior to the difficulty a patient may have with oral intake postoperatively. Moreover, the pharmacokinetics of imatinib in patients with dumping syndrome or who have had portions of their stomach and small intestine removed is not known. Other possible benefits of preoperative imatinib include decreases in tumor rupture and hemorrhage during the surgical procedure. The largest retrospective study published to date was performed at the M. D. Anderson Cancer Center (MDACC), which evaluated 126 patients with pathologically confirmed and unresectable GIST. All patients received neoadjuvant imatinib and 17 patients subsequently had surgical resection of their GIST. These patients received imatinib for a median of 10 months and response to imatinib was assessed preoperatively by CT imaging. Prior to surgery, the radiographic overall response was 76% (1 CR, 12 PR) per CT scan. Two patients were found to have no viable tumor cells at the time of surgical resection.[18] This study demonstrated that preoperative imatinib may be of utility in a certain subset of patients with initially surgically unresectable GIST and patients with a partial response to imatinib may be found to have a complete histopathologic response. However, no long term follow-up data have yet been accrued to see if there is a survival benefit in patients who underwent surgical consolidation.

Adjuvant Imatinib

Imatinib therapy may be potentially beneficial in the elimination of micrometastatic disease after surgical resection. Experience in the administration of adjuvant imatinib is limited and published data are scarce Two trials by the American College of Surgeons Oncology Group (ACOSOG Z9000 and Z9001) are evaluating the role of adjuvant imatinib therapy in patients with primary GIST. Two other trials being conducted by the EORTC Soft Tissue and Bone Sarcoma Group and the Scandinavian Sarcoma Group are evaluating duration of imatinib therapy in the adjuvant setting with survival as the primary endpoint. At this current time, accrual of data is still underway and analysis of the data not yet complete. Adjuvant imatinib is currently investigational and should be given on a clinical trial.

Combined Neo-adjuvant and Adjuvant Imatinib

The combined use of neoadjuvant and adjuvant imatinib and its role in the therapy of GIST is appealing and is under evaluation in two clinical trials. Studies currently in progress at The University of Texas, MDACC,[28] and the Radiation Therapy and Oncology Group (RTOG)[29] take the approach of treating patients with preoperative imatinib, surgical resection, and postoperative imatinib for 2 years (Table 2). These trials provide innovative approaches with important biologic correlates that may provide insight into the mechanism of action of imatinib in GIST. In MDACC ID03-0023, patients with resectable GIST undergo preoperative imatinib for 3, 5, or 7 days, surgical resection, and subsequent adjuvant imatinib mesylate for 2 years. In order to understand the early molecular and pathologic changes in GIST tumors treated with imatinib mesylate with respect to PET response, patients undergo baseline studies including a

Table 2 Preoperative and Postoperative Trials of Imatinib in GIST

Trial	Phase	Design	Objective
ACOSOG-Z9000 (closed to accrual)	II	Adjuvant imatinib for 1 year in patients with high-risk, completely resected GIST	Determine OS, 2- and 5-year RFS, safety of adjuvant imatinib
ACOSOG-Z9001	III	Adjuvant imatinib for 1 year in patients with completely resected GIST versus placebo	Comparison of RFS, OS, and safety of adjuvant imatinib
EORTC 62024	III	Adjuvant imatinib for 2 years in completely resected intermediate or high risk GIST versus placebo	Comparison of PFS and OS
Scandinavian Sarcoma Group Trial SSGXVIII	III	Adjuvant imatinib for 1 or 3 years in completely resected, high/very high-risk GIST	Comparison of RFS, GIST-specific survival, OS, and toxicities of treatment
RTOG-S0132	II	Neoadjuvant and adjuvant imatinib in KIT positive patients with operable GIST	Analysis of the safety of adjuvant imatinib, PET tumor response, molecular biological correlate of response, PFS, and OS
MDACC ID03-0023	II	Neoadjuvant and 2 years of adjuvant imatinib in patients with CD117 positive primary, recurrent, or resectable metastatic GIST	Determination of mechanism of tumor response, optimal radiological modality to monitor tumor response, DFS, and safety and tolerability of pre- and postoperative imatinib

ACOSOG = American College of Surgeons Oncology Group; DFS = disease-free survival; EORTC = European Organization for Research and Treatment of Cancer; GIST = gastrointestinal stromal tumor; MDACC = The University of Texas, M. D. Anderson Cancer Center; OS = overall survival; PET = positron emission tomography;
PFS = progression-free survival; RFS = recurrence-free survival; RTOG = radiation therapy oncology group.

tumor biopsy followed by therapy with imatinib mesylate and surgical resection. Genomic changes, KIT signaling, tumor vascularity, and apoptosis are evaluated before and after imatinib. RTOG S0132 has a similar design, although patients are treated to maximum clinical benefit prior to surgical resection.

Surgical Therapy of Metastatic Disease

GIST frequently metastasizes to both the liver and peritoneum. Metastatic disease in the setting of disease recurrence is the most common scenario for surgical resection. In nearly one-third of patients with loco-regional recurrence, metastasis to either the liver or peritoneum appears concomitantly.[30] The most sensitive means of detecting metastatic disease is CT scan, which frequently underestimates the extent of peritoneal disease. Such a shortcoming can result in identification of extensive viable tumor implants when the patient undergoes laparotomy.[25] The role of surgical intervention in metastatic disease is limited and isolated to solitary metastatic lesions. In a study performed by Mudan and colleagues, where 60 patients with metastatic GIST underwent surgery of these isolated metastases, the median survival was only 20 months and were not influenced by tumor-free margins.[30] These statistics reflect metastectomy in the pre-imatinib era and may change with the institution of imatinib therapy and conversion of nonresectable metastatic or locally advanced disease to resectable disease.

Hepatic Artery Chemoembolization and Radiofrequency Ablation of Metastatic Disease

With the emergence of imatinib and its efficacy in the treatment of metastatic disease, the role of hepatic artery embolization has decreased. Hepatic artery embolization should be considered in patients who either are refractory to treatment with imatinib or patients with liver lesions not amenable to surgical intervention. Optimal candidates for such intervention include patients without portal vein thrombosis, ascites, or hyperbilirubinemia.

Hepatic artery embolization capitalizes on several characteristics of tumor pathophysiology. First, tumors are angiogenic entities that require an ample blood supply to survive and grow. Gastrointestinal stromal tumors are known to be highly vascular tumors. By embolizing the segment of the hepatic artery supplying the tumor, it causes ischemia leading to cell death. Second, the introduction of chemotherapy along with a

device (poppy seed oil or polyvinyl alcohol sponge particles) can increase the intratumoral concentrations and minimize systemic exposure and toxicities of the chemotherapeutic agents. In the setting of intratumoral ischemia, much of the resistance to systemic chemotherapy is thought to be overcome. Decreased production of such proteins like p-glycoprotein known to be implicated in chemotherapy resistance in GIST is thought to improve the efficacy of such agents like adriamycin. Third, with the introduction of agents such as alcohol, direct cytotoxicity to the tumor cells occurs.[31]

Median survival in patients who undergo this procedure ranges from 18 to 20 months and a mean duration of response of 10 months.[32] The risks associated with this procedure include postembolization syndrome (fever, abdominal pain, nausea and ileus), sepsis, hepatic necrosis, abscess, cholecystitis, pancreatitis, or death. In summary, hepatic artery embolization offers moderate benefit to GIST patients with end-stage disease.

Radiofrequency ablation (RFA) is another surgical alternative in patients with unresectable hepatic metastases. This technique has been successful in the treatment of hepatic metastases from other solid malignancies, most notably colorectal cancer. RFA utilizes hyperthermia administered via a catheter to cause local tissue destruction and cell death. The procedure may be performed percutaneously, laparoscopically, or via laparotomy. The percutaneous approach is the preferred approach in patients with easily accessible peripheral hepatic metastases. Laparoscopy affords the surgeon a better perspective on the size and the location near any major blood vessel to better direct the catheter. It also provides information on metastatic disease within the peritoneal cavity that may preclude intervention. An open surgical approach is taken in patients with large lesions (> 5 cm), adhesions from prior surgery or lesions abutting major blood vessels.[33] The benefit of RFA in gist has not been specifically studied but several large studies have evaluated the efficacy of this technique in an array of metastatic lesions. One study conducted by Curley and colleagues at MD Anderson Cancer Center evaluated 123 patients that received RFA. Seventy-five of these patients had hepatic lesions secondary to metastases from a variety of tumors. At a median follow-up of 15 months, the local recurrence rate was noted to be 1.8% and the metastatic disease developed in 27.6%.[34] Other studies have noted that the risk of local tumor recurrence occurs in larger lesions (> 4 cm) and that local recurrence occurs at the edge of previously treated lesions.[33] Complications from this procedure include fever, hepatitis, and hepatic abscess. While the experience of treating unresectable GIST is predominantly limited to major academic centers, and the number of cases is few in number, the procedure appears to offer disease control with minimal morbidity.

Conclusion

The understanding of the molecular pathogenesis and the therapeutic interventions for gist have changed dramatically over the past decade. The tumor has evolved from a poorly understood, under-diagnosed, and treatment-refractory tumor to an accurately diagnosed, well understood, and treatment-responsive tumor. The understanding of the role of KIT tyrosine kinase in the pathogenesis and the ability of imatinib to block the signaling of the KIT tyrosine kinase oncogenic activity has led to an improvement in the survival and quality of life of patients with metastatic or unresectable gist. Imatinib's greatest effect has been seen in the metastatic setting but may prove to be beneficial in patients with locally unresectable disease. Optimal candidates to receive neoadjuvant or adjuvant therapy are still being defined. The development of alternative tyrosine kinase inhibitors and other drugs may benefit patients who are either refractory to imatinib, or it can be used in combination with imatinib to improve response rates. The flurry of clinical advances in gist makes the outlook for these patients very bright now and in the future.

References

1. Nilsson B, Bèumming P, Meis-Kindblom JM, et al. Gastrointestinal stromal tumors: the incidence, prevalence, clinical course, and prognostication in the preimatinib mesylate era—a population-based study in western Sweden. Cancer 2005;103:821–9.

2. Corless CL, Fletcher JA, Heinrich MC. Biology of gastrointestinal stromal tumors. J Clin Oncol 2004;22: 3813–25.

3. Emory T, Sobin LH, Lukes L, et al. Prognosis of gastrointestinal smooth muscle (stromal) tumors: dependence on anatomic site. Am J Surg Pathol 1999;23:82–7.

4. Fletcher CD, Berman JJ, Corless C, et al. Diagnosis of gastrointestinal stromal tumors: a consensus approach. Int J Surg Pathol 2002;10:81–9.

5. Miettinen M, Sobin LH, Lasota J. Gastrointestinal stromal tumors of the stomach: a clinicopathologic, immunohistochemical, and molecular genetic study of 1,765 cases with long-term follow-up. Am J Surg Pathol 2005;29:52–68.

6. Verweij J, Casali PG, Zalcberg J, et al. Progression-free survival in gastrointestinal stromal tumours with high-dose imatinib: randomised trial. Lancet 2004;364:1127–34.

7. Sarlomo-Rikala M, Kovatich AJ, Barusevicius A, Miettinen M. CD117: a sensitive marker for gastrointestinal stromal tumors that is more specific than CD34. Mod Pathol 1998;11:728–34.

8. Blay JY, Bonvalot S, Casali P, et al. Consensus meeting for the management of gastrointestinal stromal tumors: report of the GIST consensus conference 20–21 March 2004, under the auspices of ESMO. Ann Oncol 2005;16: 566–78.

9. Steinert DM, Oyarzo M, Wang X, et al. Expression of Bcl-2 in gastrointestinal stromal tumors: correlation with progression-free survival in 81 patients treated with imatinib mesylate. Cancer 2006;106(7):1617–23.

10. Trupiano JK, Stewart RE, Misick C, et al. Gastric stromal tumors: a clinicopathologic study of 77 cases with correlation of features with nonaggressive and aggressive clinical behaviors. Am J Surg Pathol 2002;26:705–14.

11. Lennartsson J, Jelacic T, Linnekin D, Shivakrupa R. Normal and oncogenic forms of the receptor tyrosine kinase kit. Stem cells 2005;23(1):16–43.

12. Heinrich MC, Corless CL, Demetri GD, et al. Kinase mutations and imatinib response in patients with metastatic gastrointestinal stromal tumor. J Clin Oncol 2003;21: 4342–9.

13. Duensing A, Medeiros F, McConarty B, et al. Mechanisms of oncogenic KIT signal transduction in primary gastrointestinal stromal tumors (GISTs). Oncogene 2004;23: 3999–4006.

14. Heinrich MC, Corless CL, Duensing A, et al. PDGFRA activating mutations in gastrointestinal stromal tumors. Science 2003;299:708–10.

15. Sandrasegaran K, Rajesh A, Rushing DA, et al. Gastrointestinal stromal tumors: CT and MRI findings. Eur Radiol 2005;15:1407–14.

16. Joensuu H, Roberts P, Sarlomo-Rikala M, et al. Effect of the tyrosine kinase inhibitor STI571 in a patient with a metastatic gastrointestinal stromal tumor. N Engl J Med 2001;344(14):1052–6.

17. Choi H, Charnsangavej C, de Castro Faria S, et al. CT evaluation of the response of gastrointestinal stromal tumors after imatinib mesylate treatment: a quantitative analysis correlated with FDG PET findings. Am J Roentgenol 2004;183:1619–28.

18. Scaife CL, Hunt KK, Patel SR, et al. Is there a role for surgery in patients with "unresectable" cKIT+ gastrointestinal stromal tumors treated with imatinib mesylate? Am J Surg 2003;186:665–9.

19. Rankin C, von Mehren M, Blanke CD, et al. Dose effect of imatinib (IM) in patients (pts) with metastatic GIST—Phase III Sarcoma Group Study S0033. Am Soc Clin Oncol 2004;23:815 (abstract 9005).

20. van Oosterom AT, Judson I, Verweij J, et al. Safety and efficacy of imatinib (STI571) in metastatic gastrointestinal stromal tumours: a phase I study. Lancet 2001;358:1421–3.

21. von Mehren M, Blanke C, Joensuu H, et al. High incidence of durable responses induced by imatinib mesylate (Gleevec) in patients with unresectable and metastatic gastrointestinal stromal tumors (GISTs) (abstract # 1608) Proceedings of the American Society of Clinical Oncology 2002.

22. Demetri GD, von Mehren M, Blanke CD, et al. Efficacy and safety of imatinib mesylate in advanced gastrointestinal stromal tumors. N Engl J Med 2002;347:472–80.

23. Rankin C, von Mehren M, Blanke C, et al. Dose effect of imatinib in patients with metastatic GIST—a phase III sarcoma group study S0033 Am Soc Clin Oncol, 2004;23: 815.

24. Chen LL, Trent JC, Wu EF, et al. A missense mutation in KIT kinase domain 1 correlates with imatinib resistance in gastrointestinal stromal tumors. Cancer Res 2004;64:5913–9.

25. Trent J, Dhupart J, Zhang W. Imatinib mesylate: targeted therapy of gastrointestinal stromal tumors. Curr Canc Ther Rev 2005;1:93–108.

26. Maki RG, Fletcher JA, Heinrich MC, et al. Results from a continuation trial of SU11248 in patients (pts) with imatinib (IM)-resistant gastrointestinal stromal tumor (GIST) (abstract 9011) Am Soc Clin Oncol 2005;24:24.

27. Demetri GD, Oosterom ATv, Blackstein M, et al. Phase 3, multicenter, randomized, double-blind, placebo-controlled trial of SU11248 in patients (pts) following failure of imatinib for metastatic GIST (Abstract 4000) Am Soc Clin Oncol 2005;24:24.

28. Trent J. A prospective, randomized, phase II study of preoperative plus postoperative imatinib mesylate (Gleevec, Formerly STI-571) in patients with primary, recurrent, or metastatic resectable, kit-expressing, gastrointestinal stromal tumor (GIST), 2004.

29. Trent J. A phase II trial of neoadjuvant/adjuvant STI-571 (Gleevec NSC #716051) for primary and recurrent operable malignant GIST expressing the KIT receptor tyrosine kinase (CD117) (ACRIN 6665), 2004.

30. DeMatteo RP, Lewis JJ, Leung D, et al. Two hundred gastrointestinal stromal tumors: recurrence patterns and prognostic factors for survival. Ann Surg 2000;231:51–8.

31. Sullivan KL. Hepatic artery chemoembolization. Semin Oncol 2002;29:145–51.

32. Rajan DK, Soulen MC, Clark TW, et al. Sarcomas metastatic to the liver: response and survival after cisplatin, doxorubicin, mitomycin-C, Ethiodol, and polyvinyl alcohol chemoembolization. J Vasc Interv Radiol 2001;12:187–93.

33. Curley SA. Radiofrequency ablation of malignant liver tumors. Ann Surg Oncol 2003;10:338–47.

34. Curley SA, Izzo F, Delrio P, et al. Radiofrequency ablation of unresectable primary and metastatic hepatic malignancies: results in 123 patients. Ann Surg 1999;230:1–8.

CHAPTER 81

PEDIATRIC SURGICAL ONCOLOGY

ANDREA A. HAYES-JORDAN, MD

CHARLES S. COX JR, MD

KEVIN P. LALLY, MD

Cancer is the second-leading cause of death in children in most developed countries. Significant advances have been made in the treatment of many of these malignancies, with dramatic improvements in survival over the past 50 years. These improvements have caused a shift in focus to some of the treatments from highly intensive protocols with hope for cure to evaluating less toxic therapies and protocols in attempts to limit morbidity and maintain high survival rates.

A discussion of all of the tumors in children is beyond the scope of this text; thus, we will focus on three of the most common solid tumors in children: neuroblastoma, Wilms' tumor, and rhabdomyosarcoma (RMS).

CHAPTER 81a

Neuroblastoma

GENERAL INFORMATION/BACKGROUND

Neuroblastoma is a tumor of early childhood. The majority of cases are in children younger than 5 years. It is the most common extracranial solid childhood cancer.[1,2] The origin and migratory fate of fetal neuroblasts accounts for the anatomic locations of neuroblastoma. Tumors may appear in the abdomen (adrenal or paraspinal ganglia) or extra-abdominal sites in the thorax, pelvis, or neck. Infants more frequently have thoracic and cervical tumors. The reported incidence of neuroblastoma is 8.6 cases/million. There are approximately 500 new cases of neuroblastoma annually in the United States.

NEUROBLASTOMA BIOLOGY

Numerous biologic variables have been noted to be predictive of outcome in patients with neuroblastoma. Age has been a component of most systems that predict clinical outcome. Children younger than 12 to 18 months tend to have improved prognoses.[3–5] The principally important variables are Shimada histologic classification (Table 1), deoxyribonucleic acid (DNA) ploidy, and N-MYC oncogene amplification. The Shimada classification evaluates tumor specimens for the amount of stroma, degree of differentiation, and the mitosis-karyorrhexis index (MKI). The histologic classification combines these variables to determine favorable or unfavorable histology.[6–8] The DNA index is a more important prognostic factor in older children. Hyperdiploid DNA is associated with a favorable prognosis in infants. N-MYC gene amplification (> 10 copies) is associated with a poor prognosis; fewer than three copies is considered non-amplified. In contrast, N-MYC gene expression (protein) does not predict prognosis. There are a host of other biologic variables, such as TRK-A (a gene coding for a neurotrophin receptor), serum LDH, and serum ferritin; chromosomal abnormalities may have some biologic predictive value, but they are not routinely used to influence risk group assignment that determines initial treatment.

CLINICAL PRESENTATION

The clinical signs and symptoms of neuroblastoma vary according to the site of the disease. General symptoms may include weight loss, malaise, anorexia, fatigue, and diarrhea. The most common symptoms are due to the

Table 1 Shimada Pathologic Classification

	Favorable Histology	Unfavorable Histology
Stroma-rich	Well differentiated Intermixed	Nodular
Stroma-poor		
Age < 18 mo	MKI < 200/5,000	MKI < 100/5,000
Age 18–60 mo	MKI > 100/5,000 Differentiated	MKI < 100/5,000 Undifferentiated
Age > 5 yr	None	All

MKI = mitosis-karyorrhexis index.

tumor mass or bone pain/limp due to metastases. Other symptoms depend on the relationship of the tumor mass to vital structures. Abdominal tumors may be noted as an asymptomatic abdominal mass. Tumors arising in the thorax may compress the stellate ganglion, producing Horner's Syndrome. Posterior mediastinal tumors may cause mild airway obstructive symptoms or cough. Dumbell tumors that extend into the spinal cord may produce signs/symptoms of cord compression, including paralysis, incontinence, etc. Proptosis and periorbital ecchymosis are due to retrobulbar metastases. Approximately 2% of patients demonstrate the para-neoplastic syndrome of opsoclonus/myoclonus.[9,10] This immunologic phenomenon is clinically characterized by myoclonic jerking and random eye movements. These findings may persist after resection of the primary tumor. This syndrome is mediated by an incompletely defined immunologic mechanism and is associated with more pervasive neurologic/neuropsychiatric symptoms.

DIAGNOSTIC STUDIES

Neuroblastoma is usually detected on imaging studies obtained to evaluate a specific symptom or sign. Further imaging is obtained to more accurately define the character or anatomic relationships of the mass. Once neuroblastoma is suspected, a tissue sample is required to both confirm the diagnosis and assist in staging/risk stratification. The diagnosis is confirmed by pathologic evaluation on light microscopy or a bone marrow aspirate/biopsy containing tumor cells and elevated urinary catecholamines. The tissue sample may be obtained at the time of complete resection, or if determined unresectable, a biopsy may be taken.

METASTATIC EVALUATION

Prior to initiating treatment, a complete metastatic evaluation should be undertaken. A computed tomo-graphy scan of the chest, abdomen, and pelvis (neck if this is the primary site) should be obtained. Bone should be evaluated with MIBG scanning; bone marrow aspirate/biopsy will define the presence of bone marrow

involvement. Lumbar puncture should not be performed routinely.

STAGING AND RISK GROUPING

The treatment of neuroblastoma is based on the clinico-pathogenic staging using the International Neuroblastoma Staging System (INSS) that combines elements of pre-viously used Pediatric Oncology Group (POG) and Children Cancer Group (CCG) Staging Systems.

INSS

INSS combines certain features of the previously used POG and CCG systems and has identified distinct prognostic groups.

- Stage 1: Localized tumor with complete gross excision, with or without microscopic residual disease; representative ipsilateral lymph nodes negative for tumor microscopically (ie, nodes attached to and removed with the primary tumor may be positive)
- Stage 2A: Localized tumor with incomplete gross excision; representative ipsilateral nonadherent lymph nodes negative for tumor microscopically
- Stage 2B: Localized tumor with or without complete gross excision, with ipsilateral nonad-herent lymph nodes positive for tumor; enlarged contralateral lymph nodes must be negative microscopically
- Stage 3: Unresectable unilateral tumor infiltrating across the midline, with or without regional lymph node involvement; or localized unilateral tumor with contralateral regional lymph node involvement; or midline tumor with bilateral extension by infiltration (unresectable) or by lymph node involvement; the midline is defined as the vertebral column; tumors originating on one side and crossing the midline must infiltrate to or beyond the opposite side of the vertebral column
- Stage 4: Any primary tumor with dissemination to distant lymph nodes, bone, bone marrow, liver, skin, and/or other organs, except as defined for stage 4S
- Stage 4S: Localized primary tumor, as defined for stage 1, 2A, or 2B, with dissemination limited to skin, liver, and/or bone marrow (ie, limited to infants younger than 1 year); marrow involve-ment should be minimal (ie, < 10% of total nucleated cells identified as malignant by bone biopsy or by bone marrow aspirate); more extensive bone marrow involvement would be considered to be stage 4 disease; the results of the

MIBG scan, if performed, should be negative for disease in the bone marrow

The other staging systems (POG, CCG, and St. Jude's) are rarely used today.

TREATMENT OUTLINE (TABLE 2)

- Low Risk: Low-risk patients are treated primarily with surgery alone. Platinum-based chemotherapy is used in 4% of patients with respiratory failure due to hepatic infiltration or patients with spinal cord compression.
- Intermediate Risk: These patients are treated with surgery within 12 to 24 weeks of chemotherapy.
- High Risk: As opposed to the lower-risk groups, high-risk patients are treated with ifosfamide and cis-platinum. After neoadjuvant chemotherapy, the primary tumor should be resected if at all possible. Myeloablative chemotherapy, TBI, and autologous stem cell rescue/transplantation follows. After recovery, patients are treated with 13-cis-retinoic acid. The role of surgical intervention in managing high-risk neuroblastoma is contro-

versial. Some reports suggest improved survival with gross total resection of residual disease, while others dispute this claim.[11–14] The Children's Oncology Group high-risk protocol recommends attempted gross total resection if possible. The surgeon must weigh the benefits of this against potential renal or other organ loss that may delay or preclude further chemotherapy

PROGNOSIS

Patients in the low-risk group, the intermediate-risk group, and the high-risk group have an overall 3-year survival of $> 90\%$, 70 to 90% and $\sim 30\%$.

SURGICAL RESECTION OF NEUROBLASTOMA

Abdominal: As noted above, abdominal neuroblastoma arises principally from the adrenal gland. Typically, both of the abdominal tumor types (adrenal and midline) are approached through a supra-umbilical transverse incision. Localized tumors are removed as if doing a standard adrenalectomy from an anterior approach. The tumor is

Table 2 Children's Oncology Group Neuroblastoma Risk Group Assignment Schema

INSS Stage	Age	MYCN Status	Shimada Histology	DNA Ploidy	Risk Group
1	0-21y	Any	Any	Any	Low
2A/2B*	<365d	Any	Any	Any	Low
	≥365d-21y	NonAmp	Any	-	Low
	≥365d-21y	Amp	Fav	-	Low
	≥365d-21y	Amp	Unfav	-	High
3***	<365d	NonAmp	Any	Any	Intermediate
	<365d	Amp	Any	Any	High
	±365d-21y	NonAmp	Fav	-	Intermediate
	≥365d-21y	NonAmp	Unfav	-	High
	≥365d-21y	Amp	Any	-	High
4***	<365d	NonAmp	Any	Any	Intermediate
	<365d	Amp	Any	Any	High
	≥365d-21y	Any	Any	-	High
4S**	<365d	NonAmp	Fav	>1	Low
	<365d	NonAmp	Any	=1	Intermediate
	<365d	NonAmp	Unfav	Any	Intermediate
	<365d	Amp	Any	Any	High
Biology Defined By:	MYCN Status: Amplified (Amp versus NonAmplified [NonAmp])				
	Shimada Histopathology: Favorable (Fav) versus Unfavorable (Unfav)				
	DNA Ploidy: DNA Index (DI) ≥ 1; hypodiploid tumors (with DI < 1) will be treated as a tumor with a DI >1 (DNA index < 1 (hypodiploid) to be considered favorable ploidy).				

* **INSS 2A/2B symptomatic patients with spinal cord compression, neurologic deficits, or other symptoms are treated on the LOW RISK NB Study with immediate chemotherapy for 4 cycles (Course 1).**

** **INSS 4S infants with favorable biology and clinical symptoms are treated on the LOW RISK NB Study with immediate chemotherapy until asymptomatic (2 to 4 cycles). Clinical symptoms defined as: respiratory distress with or without hepatomegaly or cord compression and neurologic deficit or inferior vena cava compression and renal ischemia; or genitourinary obstruction; or gastrointestinal obstruction and vomiting; or coagulopathy with significant clinical hemorrhage unresponsive to replacement therapy.**

*** **INSS 3 or 4 patients with clinical symptoms as above (or if in the investigator's opinion it is in the best interest of the patient) will receive immediate chemotherapy.**

often quite adherent to the lateral IVC at the confluence with the renal vein on the right. Laparoscopic resection of adrenal neuroblastoma has been advocated. Caution in interpreting these claims is warranted because in one report, 4 of 6 patients had differentiated ganglioneuroblastoma.[15] Ganglioneuroblastoma is more differentiated and a much less infiltrative tumor, thus, it is a technically simpler operation. It is critical to employ an incision that allows for extension to achieve resection. An example is a thoracoabdominal approach for high, central tumors at the hiatus.

MIDLINE ABDOMINAL TUMORS

A primary principle is to avoid permanent damage to surrounding structures (nephrectomy), if at all possible. Neuroblastoma that is centrally located can encase the aorta, SMA, celiac, and renal vessels. While there is an infiltrative character of this tumor, it rarely invades the media of the vessel. Thus, sharp dissection on the vessels and bi-valving the tumor to allow subsequent dissection is a viable strategy to achieve gross total resection. Obviously, en-bloc resection is not feasible, but the tumor is still resectable. The cavitron ultrasonic surgical aspirator (CUSA) is of little value, and the harmonic scalpel is not precise enough for this dissection. Care must be taken to avoid tangentially going ever deeper into the vessel, leading to the need for a patch vascular repair. Also, precise identification of the main aortic branches may require medial visceral rotation as used for trauma and retroperitoneal spine exposures. This may require detaching the diaphragm for the superior exposure. Care should be taken to preserve the lumbar vessels or intercostal vessels in cases where a component of the tumor is posterior. After resecting the tumor, titanium clips can be left in the tumor bed/margin as a guide for future radiotherapy.

MEDIASTINAL

Most mediastinal tumors arise along the sympathetic chain. Therefore, a posterior lateral thoracotomy is the typical incision to approach these lesions. A special circumstance involves patients with neurologic symptoms consistent with cord compression and a dumbbell-type tumor. In these cases, a combined or staged approach may be undertaken with a laminectomy and excision of the extradual tumor occurring first. The thoracic portion of the tumor may then be approached. In asymptomatic patients, preoperative chemotherapy may reduce the need or extent of the spinal portion of the procedure. Apical tumors often involve the stellate ganglion, thus they may either present with Horner's Syndrome or develop Horner's Syndrome as a consequence of a complete gross excision. Apical tumors that extend into the neck may require more innovative exposures. Pranikoff and colleagues have advocated the trapdoor incision as used occasionally for subclavian vascular injuries.[16] Recently, Sauvat and colleagues illustrated a transmanubrial technique that dissects the hemimanubrium at its origin, rotating it en-bloc with the clavicle (after detaching the SCM), to allow exposure and control of the subclavian vessels and the root of the neck.[17]

References

1. Grosfeld JL, Baehner RL. Neuroblastoma: an analysis of 100 cases. World J Surg 1980;4:29–38.

2. Young JL, Ries LG, Silverberg E, et al. Cancer incidence, survival, and mortality for children younger than 15 years of age. Cancer 1986;58:598–602.

3. Morris JA, Shochat S, Smith EI, et al. Biological variables in thoracic neuroblastoma: a Pediatric Oncology Group Study. J Pediatr Surg 1995;30:296–303.

4. Franks LM, Bollen A, Seeger RC, et al. Neuroblastoma in adults and adolescents: an indolent course with poor survival. Cancer 1997;79:2028–35.

5. Schmidt ML, Lal A, Seeger RC, et al. Favorable prognosis for patients 12–18 months of age with stage 4 nonamplified MYCN neuroblastoma: a Children's Cancer Group Study. J Clin Oncol 2005;23:6474–80.

6. Cotterill SJ, Pearson AD, Pritchard J, et al. Clinical prognostic factors in 1277 patients with neuroblastoma: results of the European Neuroblastoma Study Group Survey 1982–1992. Eur J Cancer 2000;36:901–8.

7. Look AT, Hayes, Shuster JJ, et al. Clinical relevance of tumor cell ploidy and N-myc gene amplification in childhood neuroblastoma: a Pediatric Oncology Group study. J Clin Oncol 2000;18:1260–8.

8. Schmidt ML, Lukens JN, Seeger RC, et al. Biologic factors determine prognosis in infants with stage IV neuroblastoma. A prospective Children's Cancer Group study. J Clin Oncol 2000;9:581–91.

9. Connolly AM, Pestronk A, Mehta S, et al. Serum autoantibodies in childhood opsoclonus-myoclonus syndrome: an analysis of antigenic targets in neural tissues. J Pediatr 1997;130:878–84.

10. Rudnick E, Khakoo Y, Antunes NL, et al. Opsoclounus-myoclonus-ataxia syndrome in neuroblastoma: histopathologic features—a report from the Children's Cancer Group. Med Pediatr Oncol 2001;36:623–9.

11. Hasse GM, O'Leary MC, Ramsay NK, et al. Aggressive surgery combined with intensive chemotherapy improves survival in poor-risk neuroblastoma. J Pediatr Surg 1991;26:1119–23.

12. Kiely EM. The surgical challenge of neuroblastoma. J Pediatr Surg 1994;29:128–33.

13. Castel V, Tovar JA, Costa E, et al. The role of surgery in stage IV neuroblastoma. J Pediatr Surg 2002;37:1574–8.

14. Von Schweinitz D, Hero B, Berthold F. The impact of surgical radicality on outcome in childhood neuroblastoma. Eur J Pediatr Surg 2002;12:402–9.

15. Saad DF, Gow KW, Milas Z, Wulkan ML. Laparoscopic adrenalectomy for neuroblastoma in children: a report of 6 cases. J Pediatr Surg 2005;40:1948–50.

16. Pranikoff T, Hirschl RB, Schnaufer L. Approach to cervico-thoracic neuroblastoma via trap-door incision. J Pediatr Surg 1995;30:546–8.

17. Sauvat F, Brisse H, Magdeleinat P, et al. The transmanubrial approach: a new operative approach to cervicothoracic neuroblastoma in children. Surgery 2006;139:109–14.

CHAPTER 81b

Wilms' Tumor

GENERAL INFORMATION/BACKGROUND

Named for the pathologist, Wilms' tumor is the second most common solid tumor in children. The tumor occurs in 1 in every 10,000 children in North America.[1] Wilms' tumor is one of the solid tumors where multimodal therapy has made a dramatic improvement in survival for most patients. Two large study groups—the National Wilms' Tumor Study Group (NWTSG) (now the Renal Tumors Committee of the Children's Oncology Group) and the International Society of Pediatric Oncology (SIOP)—have published a number of studies that have led to this improved survival, and both now focus on identifying low-risk patients who can receive less therapy as well as identifying the high-risk patients who may need more intensive therapy. Both study groups differ in several respects, but the role of preoperative chemotherapy is an area of significant difference.

Diagnosis

Wilms' tumor is most commonly seen in children under the age of 5 years, although it can present in older children. Often the patients present with an asymptomatic abdominal mass. Other presenting symptoms can include pain, anorexia, and vomiting, and less than one-third will have hematuria. Physical examination will demonstrate the abdominal mass, and up to 25% of the children will have hypertension. While some congenital syndromes such as Beckwith-Wiedemann, WAGR, and Denys-Drash are associated with Wilms' tumor, most of the patients have isolated disease and have been otherwise healthy. Approximately 10% may have bilateral tumors. There is no specific diagnostic serum test.

The diagnosis is usually made with an abdominal ultrasound and computed tomography (CT) scan. The CT scan will show a unilateral or bilateral tumor arising from the kidney (Figure 1). Occasionally, Wilms' tumor can be confused with a neuroblastoma, but the diagnosis

is usually evident. CT of the chest should be performed as well to evaluate the patient for pulmonary metastases. There is no clear role for a routine chest radiograph, nor is there an established standard for routine magnetic resonance imaging (MRI) or positron emission tomography scanning at this time.

Staging

The prognosis for patients with Wilms' tumor is determined by the stage of the tumor (Table 1) as well as the histology of the tumor. As noted in the table, regional lymph node disease is important and regional lymph node sampling (ie, hilar and perihilar) should be performed in all patients at the time of nephrectomy.

Histologic evaluation of the tumor is also important in determining treatment. Most patients with Wilms' tumor will have a favorable histology. Anaplasia, which is defined as tumors with large, polypoid nuclei, carries a much worse prognosis except in patients with Stage I disease. Anaplastic tumors are more common in African-Americans and older patients.[2]

Treatment

Most patients with Wilms' tumor in the United States are treated using protocols established by the NWTSG. More recent protocols are being developed by the Children's Oncology national cooperative group (COG). As mentioned above, the approach in the United States is to attempt resection of unilateral disease if little risk of

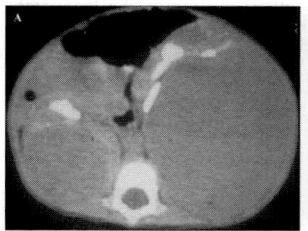 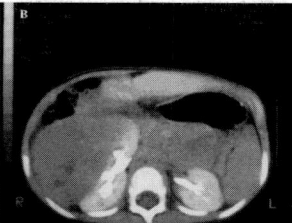

Figure 1a Bilateral Wilms' tumor. Figure 1b Right-sided Wilms' tumor.

Table 1 Wilms' Tumor Staging

Stage I (43% of patients)
The tumor is confined to the kidney and is completely resected. The renal capsule is intact, the tumor is not ruptured or biopsied, and there in no involvement of the renal sinus vessels.
Stage II (23% of patients)
The tumor is completely resected with no evidence of tumor beyond the margins of resection including the regional lymph nodes. One of the following criteria is also met: There is penetration of the renal capsule.   There is invasion of the renal sinus vessels.   There was local spillage of the tumor or a biopsy was performed.   The tumor was biopsied or there was local spillage during nephrectomy.
Stage III (23% of patients)
There is gross or microscopic residual disease following nephrectomy. This includes positive surgical margins, tumor spillage, penetration of the peritoneal surface, regional lymph node metastases, or transected tumor thrombus. There was local tumor spillage or a biopsy was performed.
Stage IV (10% of patients)
There is hematogenous metastases (lung, liver, bone, brain, etc.) or lymph node metastases outside the abdominopelvic region.
Stage V (5% of patients)
Bilateral involvement. (An attempt should be made to stage each side according to the above criteria.)

tumor spillage exists. The arguments for this approach are to allow for accurate staging, including nodal disease, and to avoid treating patients purely on the basis of radiographic findings because some patients in the SIOP trial were found to not have malignant disease. The trade-off for this approach, however, is a higher incidence of tumor rupture at the original operation. Tumor rupture of any kind necessitates postoperative abdominal radiation, and it is estimated that 8% of Wilms' tumor patients will recur with unresectable abdominal disease.

The current guidelines for therapy are summarized in Table 2. The National Cancer Institute maintains an excellent Web site with current information on treatment regimens. This can be found at <http://www.cancer.gov/cancertopics/pdq/treatment/wilms/HealthProfessional>.

The current recommendations are based on a compilation of information from the NWTS studies I–V as well as the SIOP studies. These studies have resulted in a gradual decrease in toxicity and more targeted therapies depending on stage and histology. Future studies will include trials designed to target patients whose tumors have a specific genetic phenotype, reserving highly toxic therapy for the highest-risk patient.

Special Situations

BILATERAL TUMORS

As noted in Table 2, the approach to bilateral tumors is initial surgical exploration. Both kidneys are carefully evaluated, and biopsies as well as lymph node sampling

are performed. Treatment after initial operation is tailored to the histology of the more aggressive side. After 6 weeks of therapy, the tumors are reevaluated with imaging studies. A laparotomy may be done at this point, or further biopsy and treatment may be done depending on the response of the tumor. Partial nephrectomy should be attempted for each side if at all feasible. In the upcoming trials, a new approach is being investigated. Because the initial treatment for stage V Wilms' tumor is the same, a patient may begin treatment without an initial biopsy. Then, after two cycles of chemotherapy, a laparotomy is performed for restaging. At this time, resectable disease is removed using a nephron-sparing approach. If disease is unresectable, bilateral biopsies are performed at this time and treatment is modified based on biopsy histologic results. Up to 10% of patients with bilateral tumors may have anaplastic tumors, and these warrant an aggressive approach.

INTRAVASCULAR EXTENSION

All patients with Wilms' tumor should be evaluated preoperatively for evidence of intracaval or intra-atrial extension. This is best achieved with ultrasound, but may be seen on MRI. Between 4 and 10% of patients will have some level of intracaval tumor thrombus.[3] The extent of intracaval involvement will affect management. Tumors that are low in the vena cava can be removed at initial operation with vascular control and cavotomy. More extensive disease is best treated with preoperative chemotherapy followed by resection. Patients with suprahepatic and intra-atrial disease may require cardi-

Table 2 Current Therapy of Wilms' Tumor by Stage and Histology

Stage I

Favorable histology and focal or diffuse anaplasia
Nephrectomy with lymph node sampling and 18 weeks of chemotherapy with vincristine and pulse-intensive dactinomycin

Stage II

Favorable histology
Nephrectomy with lymph node sampling and 18 weeks of chemotherapy with vincristine and pulse-intensive dactinomycin
Focal anaplasia
Nephrectomy with lymph node sampling, abdominal radiation, and 24 weeks of chemotherapy with vincristine, doxorubicin, and pulse-intensive dactinomycin
Diffuse anaplasia
Nephrectomy with lymph node sampling, abdominal radiation, and 24 weeks of chemotherapy with vincristine, doxorubicin, etoposide, cyclophosphamide, and mesna

Stage III

Favorable histology or focal anaplasia
Nephrectomy with lymph node sampling, abdominal radiation, and 24 weeks of chemotherapy with vincristine, doxorubicin, and pulse-intensive dactinomycin
Diffuse anaplasia
Nephrectomy with lymph node sampling, abdominal radiation, and 24 weeks of chemotherapy with vincristine, doxorubicin, etoposide, cyclophosphamide, and mesna

Stage IV

Favorable histology or focal anaplasia
Nephrectomy with lymph node sampling, abdominal radiation according to local stage of renal tumor, bilateral pulmonary radiation for patients with chest X-ray evidence of pulmonary metastases, and 24 weeks of chemotherapy with vincristine, doxorubicin, and pulse-intensive dactinomycin

Stage V

Patients should be staged at initial laparotomy for each kidney. Treatment is individualized depending on histology, location of tumor and response. Partial nephrectomy should be attempted if feasible in both kidneys.

---

opulmonary bypass with an atriotomy for excision. Mortality after this approach is low, but has been reported to be up to 5% in one series.

PULMONARY METASTASES

Patients who present with pulmonary metastases and favorable histology still have a significant salvage rate. Initially, patients were treated with whole lung irradiation as well as chemotherapy. Some data suggested prolonged survival for patients with more intensive chemotherapy, prompting the question of whether chemotherapy alone may be curative in a subset of children with pulmonary metastases detectable only on CT scan. This will be addressed in the next national Wilms' tumor study. Patients who do not respond to the initial chemotherapy in 6 weeks will have a more intensified regimen. Resection of unchanged or residual pulmonary disease is warranted in this setting because some may have nonviable tumor. A recent report has demonstrated the value of biopsy in some patients because not all CT-imaged lesions are metastases.[4] Because of the morbidity noted in NWTSG-5, pulmonary radiation of children less than 6 months of age will be omitted in the next prospective study. Questionable pulmonary lesions seen on CT scan should be biopsied; however, biopsy is not required to initiate therapy for pulmonary metastasis in Wilms' tumor.

RECURRENT DISEASE

Most patients who relapse after treatment for Wilms' tumor do so within the first 2 years after therapy.[5] The most common site for relapse is the lungs, with the abdominal bed a distant second. Other sites include the liver, bones, and lymph nodes. Initial reports from the NWTS did not show benefit from surgical excision of pulmonary metastases compared to chemotherapy alone. We have taken a generally aggressive approach to management. If there is isolated or persistent disease after therapy, we will perform a thoracotomy to remove residual disease. Abdominal relapse carries a worse prognosis than lung recurrence. Surgery is used as an adjunct to chemotherapy and radiation in this setting. Experimental cytoreductive surgery followed by continuous hyperthermic peritoneal perfusion is being evaluated in this setting. The role of high-dose chemotherapy followed by autologous bone marrow transplant can be considered, but there is a lack of sufficient data to warrant firm conclusions in this setting.

OUTCOME

Survival for Wilms' tumor is generally good except in patients with unfavorable histology. Overall survival is 85%, and patients with localized disease and favorable histology have a 4-year survival of over 90%. Even patients with pulmonary metastases and favorable histology have approximately a 70% chance of survival. Patients with anaplastic, advanced disease however, have survival rates below 50% with current therapies.

In terms of long-term outcomes, most children do well. There is a dose-dependent risk of cardiac toxicity in patients who have received anthracyclines. The cardiac risk increases with combined whole lung radiation. Pulmonary function in patients who receive whole lung radiation can be affected with total lung and vital capacities at 50 to 70% predicted.[6] Second malignancies are uncommon, but the risks are higher with radiation and the use of alkylating agents or doxorubicin. Both chemotherapy- and radiation-induced long-term effects have been markedly diminished with newer protocols aimed at decreasing toxicity.

Renal failure is uncommon is most patients with Wilms' tumor.[7] The reported incidence is 0.6% for 5,347 patients who had a unilateral nephrectomy and no other underlying disease. The incidence increases markedly for patients with underlying urinary disorders and syndromes. End-stage renal disease can occur in 12% of patients with bilateral disease who have undergone nephron sparing surgery.

References

1. Rivera MN, Haber DA. Wilms' tumour: connecting tumorigenesis and organ development in the kidney. Nat Rev Cancer 2005;5:699–712.

2. Bonadio JF, Storer B, Norkool P, et al. Anaplastic Wilms' tumor: clinical and pathologic studies. J Clin Oncol 1987;3:513–20.

3. Lall A, Pritchard-Jones K, Walker J, et al. Wilms' tumor with intracaval thrombus in the UK Children's Cancer Study Group UKW3 Trial. J Pediatr Surg 2006;41:382–7.

4. Ehrlich PF, Hamilton TE, Grundy P, et al. The value of surgery in directing therapy for patients with Wilms' tumor with pulmonary disease. A report from the National Wilms' Tumor Study Group. J Pediatr Surg 2006;41:162–7.

5. Firoozi F, Kogan BA. Follow-up and Management of Recurrent Wilms' tumor. Urol Clin N Am 2003;30:869–79.

6. Kalapurakal JA, Dome JS, Perlman EJ, et al. Management of Wilms' tumour: current practice and future goals. Lancet Oncol 2004;5:37–46.

7. Breslow NE, Collins AJ, Ritchey ML, et al. End stage renal disease in patients with Wilms tumor: results from the National Wilms Tumor Study Group and the United States Renal Data System. J Urol 2005;174:1972–5.

CHAPTER 81c

Rhabdomyosarcoma

GENERAL INFORMATION/BACKGROUND

Childhood rhabdomyosarcoma (RMS) is a soft tissue malignant tumor of skeletal muscle origin that can arise in any skeletal muscle group in the body. RMS is the most common soft tissue sarcoma in children and adolescents, accounting for nearly 250 cases of childhood cancer in the United States each year. This accounts for approximately 3.5% of the cases of cancer among children 0 to 14 years and only 2% of cases among adolescents and young adults 15 to 19 years of age.[1] Since the original description of RMS by Weber in 1854, uniform diagnostic criteria and specific risk-based therapies have been developed by the Intergroup Rhabdomyosarcoma Study Group (IRSG).[2] The first IRSG was a national cooperative group began in 1972. During the course of four consecutive IRSG clinical trials, the outcome for children and adolescents with RMS has improved significantly.[3–7]

In the 1960s, less than one-third of the children with RMS survived regardless of surgery, radiation, or the single agent chemotherapy that was given at the time. In the present day, collectively, survival from RMS, using multimodality therapy and multiagent chemotherapy, is greater than 70%.[8–12] This improvement in outcome is multifactorial and can be attributed to improvement in multiagent chemotherapy, supportive care, and risk-adapted therapy based on prognostic factors such as age, extent of disease at diagnosis, histology, and tumor site. Because of the rarity of RMS and the histologic, clinical, and genetic heterogeneity, national cooperative groups from which data could be aggregated were needed. The IRSG began when three pediatric cancer study groups pooled their patients and resources to form the Intergroup Rhabdomyosarcoma Study (IRS) committee. The protocols from IRS now form the backbone of treatment for all children with RMS throughout the United States and Canada. The IRS is now part of the Children's Oncology Group (COG) and continues to develop new risk-based protocols to advance the treatment of childhood RMS.

ETIOLOGY

Most cases of RMS occur sporadically with no clear recognized risk factors. However, a small percentage is clearly associated with genetic conditions. These include Li Fraumeni cancer susceptibility syndrome, Neurofibromatosis type 1, and Beckwith Weidemann syndrome.[13–19] Chemical or environmental exposure during pregnancy has not been clearly associated with RMS.

HISTOLOGY

The histologic classification is based on the tumors resemblance to fetal skeletal muscle. The first histologic classification was described by Horn and Eternline.[20] This classification has been adapted by the World Health Organization and the IRS committee and includes embryonal, botryoid a subset of embryonal) and alveolar and pleomorphic. Approximately 60% of RMS tumors are embryonal and 20% alveolar. The remainders are pleomorphic or undifferentiated.

Microscopically embryonal RMS is characterized by primitive round cells that may by tightly packed or loosely dispersed. The rhabdomyoblast is the mature component of this cell that has a bright eosinophilic cytoplasm. After treatment with chemotherapy, remaining lesions may have rhabdomyoblasts that should not be confused with active tumor.

In contrast, alveolar RMS is characterized by fibrovascular septa that form spaces that look similar to lung alveoli. The free spaces contain monomorphous round malignant cells with abundant eosinophilic cytoplasm. Tumors can have components of both alveolar and embryonal histology. In the past, pathologists required at least 50% of the tumor to have alveolar pathology to be categorized as alveolar RMS. However, the IRS committee pathologists have concluded that if any portion of the tumor contains alveolar pathology, it will be categorized as alveolar RMS.

Pleomorphic RMS were identified in only 5 of 1,600 tumors studied from the first IRS study group.[21,22] This has since led to the elimination of this histologic classification. The COG sarcoma committee now recognizes a new histologic variant that can occur in either alveolar or embryonal RMS—anaplastic. This anaplastic variant is newly described and may have critical implications for prognosis and treatment of patients with RMS. On preliminary review, histologically the patients with embryonal tumors that have an anaplastic component have a poorer survival rate than patients whose tumors demonstrate embryonal histology only.

GENETIC AND MOLECULAR FEATURES

Heterogeneic chromosomal abnormalities have been seen in RMS. Hyperdiploid DNA is usually found in embryonal cases and tumors with tetraploid DNA are almost exclusively alveolar. Cases with hyperdiploid DNA may be more sensitive to chemotherapy and radiation therapy.[23] Ploidy has not been incorporated into the clinical management of RMS. In alveolar RMS, characteristic translocations have been found involving chromosome 2 and 13 t(2; 13)(q35; q14). This affects the PAX3 gene in band 2q35 and the FKHR gene in band 13q14. (14,15). PAX 3 is a transcription factor that is expressed during embryonic development of mesenchymal precursors that will become myoblasts. The reciprocal translocation of t(2; 13) fuses PAX 3 to FKHR gene, which is also a transcription factor. This chimeric structure of PAX 3 or PAX 7 and FKHR (FOX01a gene) functions as an oncoprotein by inappropriately activating PAX 3 and PAX 7 transcriptional targets, which affects cell growth.[3] These translocations and fusion proteins uniquely identify alveolar RMS, although less than 25% of ARMS are fusion protein negative.[24,25]

STAGING AND CLASSIFICATION

The staging system for RMS includes clinical group (Table 1) and stage (Table 2). The staging system is modified from the TNM classification and is based on the prognostic differences by site and histology that is specific to RMS compared to adult sarcomas (Table 3). A description of a RMS tumor would then include both stage and group. Appropriate staging work-up includes assessment of primary tumor by computed tomography (CT) or magnetic resonance imaging (MRI), and assessment of regional and distant disease. Paratesticular and extremity RMS have a high incidence of lymph node metastases. Therefore, the status of regional lymph nodes (by sentinel node biopsy or node dissection) must be assessed when primary tumors are located at these sites. A bone scan, bilateral bone marrow biopsies and aspirates, and CT scan of the chest are necessary to rule out metastatic disease. At this time, positron emission tomography is not considered a staging tool for RMS but is being evaluated in prospective COG trials.[26]

SITE-SPECIFIC SURGICAL ISSUES

All patients diagnosed with RMS are considered to have micrometastatic disease at diagnosis and therefore all receive chemotherapy. Thus, aggressive resections of apparently marginally resectable or unresectable lesions, is unwarranted. Extremity RMS has a poorer prognosis compared to other sites. In IRS-IV, survival in stage 2

Table 1. IRS clinical grouping classification

Group I: Localized disease, completely resected

Regionalnodes not involved—lymph node biopsy or dissection is required except for head and neck lesions
(A) Confined to muscle or organ of origin
(B) Contiguous involvement—infiltration outside the muscle or organ of origin, as through fascial planes
Notation: This includes both gross inspection and microscopic confirmation of complete resection. Any nodes that may be inadvertently taken with the specimen must be negative. If the latter should be involved microscopically, then the patient is placedin group IIB or group IIC (see below).

Group II: Total gross resection with evidence of regional spread

(A) Grossly resected tumor with microscopic residual disease
Surgeon believes that all the tumor has been removed, but the pathologist finds tumor at the margin of resection, and additional resection to achieve a clean margin is not feasible. No evidence of gross residual tumor; no evidence of regional node involvement; once radiotherapy and/or che motherapy have been started, re-exploration and removal of the area of microscopic residual does not change the patient's group.
(B) Regional disease with involved nodes, completely resected with no microscopic residual
Notation: Complete resection with microscopic confirmation of no residual disease makes this different from group IIA and group IIC. Additionally, in contrast to group IIA, regional nodes (which are completely resected, however) are involved, but the most distal node is histologically negative.
(C) Regional disease with involved nodes, grossly resected, but with evidence of microscopic residual and/or histologic involvement of the most distal regional node (from the primary site) in the dissection
Notation: The presence of microscopic residual disease makes this group different from group IIB, and nodal involvement makes this group different from group IIA.

Group III: Incomplete resection with gross residual disease

(A) After biopsy only
(B) After gross or major resection of the primary (>50%)

Group IV: Distant metastatic disease present at onset

Lung, liver, bones, bone marrow, brain, and distant muscle and nodes
Notation: The above excludes regional nodes and adjacent organ infiltration, which places the patient in a more favorable-grouping (as noted above under group II). The presence of positive cytology in the cerebrospinal fluid, pleural or abdominal fluids, as well as implants on pleural or peritoneal surfaces are regarded as indications for placing the patient in group IV.

and 3 RMS, regardless of group, histology, or amputation, was 55 to 60%.[26] Extremity lesions measured in the longest diameter of 5 cm or greater should be biopsied first in preparation for neoadjuvant chemotherapy. This will allow a more limited resection and avoid the possibility of having positive microscopic margins at the site of primary excision. Unlike adults, postoperative radiation therapy is avoided in extremity lesions in children because of the limb length discrepancy, which will result from radiation therapy at the long-bone growth plates. If the diagnosis of RMS is found to be a surprise to the surgeon who believed he/she was excising a benign lesion, and therefore a marginal or "shelling out" procedure was done and is later found at final pathology to be rhabdomyosarcoma, primary re-excision of the operative site is recommended to avoid the need

Table 2. IRS-modified TNM pretreatment staging classification

Stage	Sites	T	Size	N	M
1	Favorable	T_1 or T_2	a or b	N_0 or N_1 or N_x	M_0
2	Unfavorable	T_1 or T_2	a	N_0 or N_x	M_0
3	Unfavorable	T_1 or T_2	a	N_1	M_0
			b	N_0 or N_1 or N_x	M_0
4	All	T_1 or T_2	a or b	N_0 or N_1	M_1

Favorable sites are the orbit, head and neck (excluding parameningeal sites), genitourinary system (excluding bladder/prostate), and the biliary tract.
Unfavorable sites are the bladder/prostate, extremities, cranial parameningeal sites, and other sites (including the trunk and retroperitoneum, but excluding the biliary tract).
Pretreatment size is determined by external measurement using magnetic resonance imaging or computerized tomography (CT), depending on the anatomic location. For less accessible primary sites, CT is used as a means of lymph node assessment as well. Metastatic sites require some form of imaging (but not histologic confirmation, except for bone marrow examination) confirmation.
Abbreviations: M_0, no distant metastasis; M_1, metastasis present; N_0, regional nodes not clinically involved; N_1, regional nodes clinically involved by neoplasm; N_x, clinical status of regional nodes unknown (especially sites that preclude lymph node evaluation); Size a, $\leq$5 cm in diameter; Size b, >5 cm in diameter; T_1, confined to anatomic site of origin; T_2, extension and/or fixation to surrounding tissue.

Table 3 Rhabdomyosarcoma Risk Stratification Used for Children's Oncology Group

Histology	Clinical Group	Stage	Age	Risk Group
Embryonal, with variants	I, II, III	1	All	Low
Embryonal, with variants	I, II	2, 3	All	Low
Embryonal, with variants	III	2, 3	All	Intermediate
Embryonal, with variants	IV	4	< 10 years	Intermediate
Embryonal, with variants	IV	4	≥ 10 years	High
Alveolar	I, II, III	1, 2, 3	All	Intermediate
Alveolar	IV	4	All	High

for external beam radiation therapy. Mutilating surgery or amputation is to be avoided at the time of initial diagnosis of RMS.

Hays and colleagues found in 1989 that primary re-excision (PRE) after initial marginal resection improved local recurrence and prolonged survival.[27] He reviewed 154 extremity and trunk patients from IRS II (1972 to 1984). Of 154 patients with group IIa, that is node negative with microscopic residual, 41 underwent re-excision of the tumor "bed" with wide margins. PRE down-staged these patients to group 1. The overall survival (OS) of patients with RMS of the trunk or extremity that underwent PRE was 91% compared to 113 patients with stage IIa that were not re-excised in which the 3-year survival rate was 74%. These data have more recently been validated by other studies, including an Italian study in 2001 of patients with localized soft tissue sarcomas. In the Italian cooperative group studies, 126 patients with grade IIa tumors were reviewed. PRE was completed in 53 patients, including 23 with RMS and 30 with NRSTS. Of the 53 patients, 45 had complete histologic excision of the tumor and received chemotherapy without radiation therapy (RT). After PRE, 39 patients remain in their first complete response without RT. In this study, PRE was found to be effective in trunk, extremity, and paratesticular sites, but its role in sarcomas over 5 cm in size is uncertain.[28]

Paratesticular RMS is another site of disease in which the correct surgical approach is critical. When a tumor of the testicle is suspected, the excision should be done through a groin/hernia incision. If a malignant lesion is suspected because of elevation of preoperative serum markers, such as alpha-feto-protein or Beta HCG, the spermatic cord should be mobilized and a high ligation of the cord with orchiectomy should be completed through the groin incision. If there is some question about the malignant nature of the lesion, the spermatic cord should be encircled by a penrose drain or umbilical tape so as to temporarily occlude venous drainage, to avoid extravasation of tumor cells, while an incisional biopsy is completed. Then, when frozen section confirms a malignancy, the spermatic cord should be ligated above

the temporary occlusion. In patients greater than 10 years of age who have no distant organ metastasis, ipsilateral, nerve-sparing retroperitoneal lymph node dissection (INSRLND) should be completed whether or not enlarged nodes are seen on staging CT scan. In patients less than 10 years of age with paratesticular RMS, INSRLND should be reserved for children with enlarged retroperitoneal lymph nodes seen on staging CT scan. A laparascopic or open approach is acceptable. As it stands to date, patients with paratesticular RMS who have pathologically positive retroperitoneal lymph nodes will receive abdominal radiation in addition to adjuvant chemotherapy. On univariate analysis, OS for patients less than 10 years of age with paratesticular RMS is 96% compared to 80% in those patients greater than 10 years of age.[29]

Nonrhabdomyosarcoma Soft Tissue Sarcoma in Children

Approximately 8% of childhood malignancies are soft tissue sarcomas. Half of these are NRSTS. There are over 20 histologic types, and genetic patterns are poorly understood. When surgical resection is feasible, 70% of patients are expected to achieve long-term survival with or without radiation therapy.[30] Patient outcome is largely based on age, the presence of metastasis at diagnosis, and size and depth of the lesion.

Patients less than 1 year of age have an excellent prognosis, whereas the adolescents and young adults have the worse prognosis compared to younger patients or older adults.[31] A review of patients treated at SJCRH between 1962 and 1996 revealed the overall 5-year survival estimate (univariate analysis) for children > 1 year of age was 92% compared to 36% in those 15 to 25 years of age. Patients between 1 and 15 years had an intermediate survival of approximately 60%. Survival after relapse was poor in all age groups except those < 1 year of age. The 5-year estimate of post relapse survival in patients 0 to 1 year of age was 80% compared to the 15 to 25 years in which survival was 21%. Although the type of

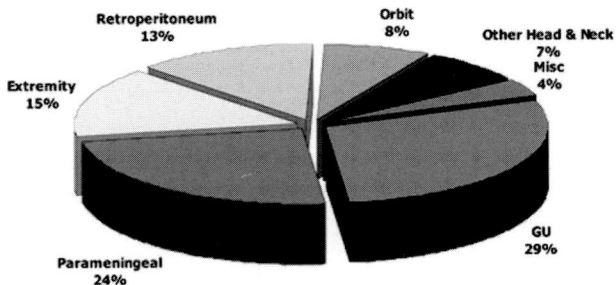

Figure 1 Rhabdomyosarcoma sites.

chemotherapy in these patients was variable, surgical excision was completed for lesions ≥ 5 cm and for most patients, incisional biopsy of lesions > 5 cm was followed by chemotherapy, re-excision, and radiation therapy or amputation.

The treatment for children and adolescents with NRSTS has not previously standardized, nor have there been any pediatric cooperative group trials as in RMS. Because there are over 20 different histologic sites, standardization is difficult. The first risk-based prospective trial of NRSTS in children and adolescents is just beginning and continuing through 2010. In this trial patients with NRSTS will be treated as low, intermediate, or high risk based on criteria previously ascertained in a thorough review of 121 patients by Spunt and colleagues.[32,33] In patients with surgically resected NRSTS, univariate analysis revealed clear risk factors. Positive surgical margins ($p = .004$), tumor size ≥ to 5 cm ($p < .001$), invasiveness ($p = .002$), high grade ($p = .028$), and intra-abdominal primary site ($p = .055$) had a negative impact on event-free survival (EFS). Multivariate analysis verified all of these risk factors except for invasiveness. Local recurrence was predicted by intra-abdominal primary site ($p = .028$), positive surgical margins ($p = .003$), and the omission of radiation therapy (0.043). As expected, the biology of the tumor, that is tumor size ≥ 5 cm, invasiveness, and high grade, predicted distant recurrences.[32] Children and adolescents with initially unresected NRSTS are a subgroup of pediatric NRSTS that are particularly high risk. The 5-year estimated OS and EFS were 56 and 33%, respectively, and post relapse survival was poor—19% despite multimodality therapy.[33]

References

1. Gurney JG, Severson RK, Davis S, et al. Incidence of cancer in children in the United States. Sex-, race-, and 1-year age-specific rates by histologic type. Cancer 1995;75:2186–95.

2. Weber CO. Anatomische untersuchung einer hypertrophische zunge nebst bemerkungen ueber die neubildung quergestreifter muskelfasern, virchow. Arch Pathol Anat 1854;7:115–21.

3. Pappo AS, Shapiro DN, Crist WM, et al. Biology and therapy of pediatric rhabdomyosarcoma. J Clin Oncol 1995;13:2123–39.

4. Maurer HM, Beltangady M, Gehan EA, et al. The Intergroup Rhabdomyosarcoma Study-I. Cancer 1988;61: 209–20.

5. Maurer HM, Gehan EA, Beltangady M, et al. The Intergroup Rhabdomyosarcoma Study-II. Cancer 1993;71: 1904–22.

6. Crist W, Gehan EA, Ragab AH, et al. The Third Intergroup Rhabdomyosarcoma Study. J Clin Oncol 1995;13:610–30.

7. Crist W, Anderson JR, Meza JL, et al. Intergroup Rhabdomyosarcoma Study-IV: results for patients with nonmetastatic disease. J Clin Oncol 2001;19:3091–102.

8. Donaldson SS. The value of adjuvant chemotherapy I the management of sarcomas in children. Cancer 1985;55: 2184–97.

9. Neifeld JP, Maurer HM, Godwin D, et al. Prognostic variables in pediatric rhabdomyosarcoma before and after multi-modal therapy. J Pediatr Surg 1979;14:699–703.

10. Lawrence W, Jegge G, Foote FW. Embryonal rhabdomyosarcoma. Cancer 1964;17:361–76.

11. Flamant F, Hill H. The improvement in survival associated with combined chemotherapy in childhood rhabdomyosarcoma: a historical comparison of 345 patients in the same center. Cancer 1984;53:2417–21.

12. Sutow W, Sullivan MP, Ried HL, et al. Prognosis in childhood rhabdomyosarcoma. Cancer 1970;25:1384–90.

13. Li FP, Fraumeni JF Jr. Rhabdomyosarcoma in children: epidemiologic study and identification of a familial cancer syndrome. J Natl Cancer Inst 1969;43:1365–73.

14. Diller L, Sexsmith E, Gottlieb A, et al. Germline p53 mutations are frequently detected in young children with rhabdomyosarcoma. J Clin Invest 1995;95:1606–11.

15. Matsui I, Tanimura M, Kobayashi N, et al. Neurofibromatosis type 1 and childhood cancer. Cancer 1993; 72:2746–54.

16. Hartley AL, Birch JM, Marsden HB, et al. Neurofibromatosis in children with soft tissue sarcoma. Pediatr Hematol Oncol 1988;5:7–16.

17. Gripp KW, Scott CI Jr, Nicholson L, et al. Five additional Costello syndrome patients with rhabdomyosarcoma: proposal for a tumor screening protocol. Am J Med Genet 2002;108:80–7.

18. Samuel DP, Tsokos M, DeBaun MR. Hemihypertrophy and a poorly differentiated embryonal rhabdomyosarcoma of the pelvis. Med Pediatr Oncol 1999;32:38–43.

19. DeBaun MR, Tucker MA. Risk of cancer during the first four years of life in children from The Beckwith-Wiedemann Syndrome Registry. J Pediatr 1998;132(3 Pt 1):398–400.

20. Horn RC, Enterline HT. Rhabdomyosarcoma: a clinocopathological study and classification of 39 cases. Cancer 1958;11:181–99.

21. Parham DM, Jenkins JJ. Pathology of selected pediatric embryonal neoplasms. Mod Pathol 1994;7:501–19.

22. Agamanolis DP, Dasu S, Krill CE. Tumors of skeletal muscle. Hum Pathol 1986;17:778–95.

23. Shapiro DN, Parham DM, Douglass EC, et al. Relationship of tumor cell ploidy to histologic subtype and treatment outcome in children and adolescents with unresectable rhabdomyosarcoma. J Clin Oncol 1991;9:159–66.

24. Barr FG. Gene fusions involving PAX and FOX family members in alveolar rhabdomyosarcoma. Oncogene 2001;20:5736–46.

25. Barr FG, Qualman SJ, Macris MH, et al. Genetic heterogeneity in the alveolar rhabdomyosarcoma subset without typical gene fusions. Cancer Res 2002;62:4704–10.

26. Breitfeld P, Meyer W. Rhabdomyosarcoma: New windows of opportunity. The Oncologist 2005;10:518–27.

27. Hays DM, Lawerence W, Wharam M, et al. Primary re-excision for patients with microscopic residual tumor following initial excision of sarcomas of trunk and extremity sites. J Ped Surg 1989;24:5–10.

28. Cecchetto G, Gugleilmi M, Inserra A, et al. Primary re-excision: the Italian experience in patients with localized soft tissue sarcomas. Ped Surg Int 2001;17:532–4.

29. Stewart RJ, Martelli H, Oberlin O, et al. Treatment of children with non-metastatic paratesticular rhabdomyosarcoma: results of the Malignant Mesenchymal Tumors studies (MMT 84 and MMT 89) of the international society of pediatric oncology. J Clin Onc 2003;21:793–8.

30. Marcus KC, Grier HE, Shamberger RC, et al. Childhood soft tissue sarcoma: a 20 year experience. J Pediatr 1997;131:603–7.

31. Hayes-Jordan A, Spunt S, Poquette CA, et al. Non-rhabdomyosarcoma soft tissue sarcomas in children: is age at diagnosis an important variable? J Ped Surg 2000;35:948–54.

32. Spunt S, Poquette CA, Hurt YS, et al. Prognostic factors for children and adolescents with surgically resected nonrhabdomyosarcoma soft tissue sarcoma: an analysis of 121 patients treated at St Jude Children's Research Hospital. J Clin Onc 1999;17:3697–705.

33. Spunt S, Hill DA, Motosue AM, et al. Clinical features and outcome of initially unresected non-metastatic pediatric nonrhabdomyosarcoma soft tissue sarcoma. J Clin Onc 2002;20:3225–35.

CHAPTER 82

DIAGNOSTIC BIOPSY, PROGNOSTIC FACTORS, AND STAGING IN MELANOMA

KEITH A. DELMAN, MD

Introduction

The surgical management of melanoma begins with the biopsy. Although the biopsy itself may be a simple procedure, considerable thought is required to appropriately perform one. If a lesion is suspected of being a melanoma, a biopsy should be performed. Careful consideration of the need for subsequent surgical intervention should be made, especially with respect to orientation of closure. Characteristics that are suggestive that a lesion might be a melanoma include asymmetry, border irregularity, color variation, diameter greater than 6 mm, and evolution (the so-called "ABCDEs" of melanoma). In nearly all circumstances, biopsy (and appropriate pathologic analysis), history, and physical examination should provide appropriate information to allow for an initial surgical plan to be determined.

Biopsy Procedures

Although there are multiple methods that can be used to obtain histopathologic information from a suspicious cutaneous lesion, there are limitations to some techniques that make them suboptimal for use in the treatment and diagnosis of melanocytic lesions. It is important to obtain a full-thickness biopsy to provide the clinician definitive information regarding Breslow's depth and other histopathologic features. Current National Comprehensive Cancer Network (NCCN) guidelines recommend the use of excisional biopsy for definitive diagnosis of suspect lesions.[1]

Punch biopsy is an ideal approach for obtaining the information desired to proceed with definitive surgical intervention. This method can be performed safely in the office setting with local anesthesia and minimal morbidity. Surgical punches are available in a multitude of sizes, commonly from 2 to 8 mm. Punch biopsy should be a procedure readily available to the clinician treating patients with melanoma and lesions of the skin. It can be employed in the diagnosis of primary lesions as well as in dermal lesions concerning for recurrence.

In some settings, lesions are too large to be excised in their entirety by punch biopsy. Narrow margin excision should be considered in such scenarios. When performing a narrow margin excision, it is imperative that planning for subsequent wide local excision be considered. Incisions should be oriented in such a fashion as to permit subsequent primary closure of the definitive surgical procedure, if needed. Generally, this means longitudinally in the limbs and along lines of skin tension on the trunk. An alternative approach for lesions too large to undergo complete excision with punch biopsy is to perform a punch biopsy of the area of the greatest suspicion by clinical assessment. The concern with this approach is the potential for sampling error. This method should be utilized sparingly, in situations when other approaches are not feasible.

Frequently, patients are referred to the surgical oncologist by an outside physician, often a dermatologist or family physician, who utilizes a technique other than an excisional, full-thickness biopsy. Shave biopsy is a commonly used alternative method of diagnosis. The concern regarding shave biopsy is the potential failure to obtain a full-thickness assessment of the suspect lesion. As a result of the use of this technique, deep margins are frequently positive, thereby limiting the utility of the histologic information obtained by this approach. If this method is to be used, it should be performed as a deep shave, with the goal of obtaining a full-thickness biopsy being paramount.

Pathologic Analysis

The analysis of a biopsy specimen is as important as the technique used to obtain it. A specimen suspected of being melanoma should be reviewed by an experienced dermatopathologist. It is extremely useful for the surgeon to be familiar with the reporting pathologist, as much of the information obtained from microscopic analysis is not purely objective (ie, rate of tumor infiltrating lymphocytes and extent of regression), and familiarity facilitates an enhanced interpretation of the findings. Definitive surgical intervention can generally be planned with a minimum of reported information. This basic information includes Breslow thickness, presence of histologic ulceration, Clark's level, and margin (deep and lateral) status. These results alone will allow the surgeon to determine margin of excision, and in most circumstances, whether sentinel lymph node biopsy is indicated.

Additional information from pathologic analysis is helpful, and in many centers will guide the surgeon to perform a sentinel lymph node biopsy in lesions that are less than 1.0 mm thick (ie, "high-risk" thin melanomas), but this is a topic covered elsewhere in this book. More significantly, a number of histopathologic characteristics serve as prognostic factors, and therefore help guide the management and follow-up of patients with melanoma. In addition to the basic information listed previously, other useful data that should be reported from pathologic review include the following:

- Anatomic site
- Presence and extent of regression
- Mitotic rate
- Presence and extent of tumor-infiltrating lymphocytes
- Lymphovascular invasion
- Neurotropism
- Presence of vertical growth phase
- Histologic subtype
- Microsatellitosis

The reporting of these additional characteristics is advocated by the NCCN in their 2006 guidelines and the American Academy of Dermatology in their consensus statement from 2001.[1,2]

Prognostic Factors

In preparation for the American Joint Committee on Cancer (AJCC) staging manual's 2002 revision, a multi-

center analysis of 17,600 patients was performed analyzing prognostic factors in melanoma.[3] This undertaking was the largest of its kind ever performed and led to the 2002 version of the AJCC staging system for cutaneous melanoma.[4] Since this analysis, other factors have been identified that are also considered to be useful in assessing prognosis in patients with melanoma. Despite the identification of new prognostic factors, this landmark review provides the foundation for our ability to provide melanoma patients an accurate prognosis for survival and recurrence.

LOCALIZED DISEASE (AJCC STAGE I AND II)

The AJCC analysis included patients from both the era before the routine use of sentinel lymph node (SLN) biopsy and during the era of routine use of SLN biopsy. In the overall review, in patients with clinically localized (stage I and II) melanoma who did not undergo a pathologic assessment of their lymph nodes (ie, SLN biopsy or elective lymphadenectomy), the most significant prognostic factor is the Breslow thickness, followed closely by the presence or absence of primary tumor ulceration. Other factors that significantly affected outcome in patients with clinically localized disease were age, anatomic site, Clark's level of invasion, and gender (Table 1).[3]

In contrast, in patients who did undergo a pathologic assessment of the regional lymph nodes (again, either by SLN biopsy or elective lymphadenectomy), the presence or absence of nodal metastases became the most powerful prognostic indicator, overshadowing both Breslow's depth and tumor ulceration. Additionally, Clark's level and gender were no longer independently significant (Table 2).[3] The impact of nodal status in patients who underwent pathologic analysis of their regional lymphatics in the AJCC review is important in the era of routine SLN biopsy because currently, the vast majority of patients with tumors thicker than 1 mm as well as those with "high-risk" lesions less than 1 mm undergo a routine pathologic assessment of their regional lymphatics. In the era of SLN biopsy, nodal status is therefore the most powerful independent prognostic factor for survival and recurrence in patients with melanoma.

Since the AJCC analysis, several other factors have been reported as useful in assessing survival and recurrence. Recently, two analyses were published, one from the University of Pennsylvania[5] and the other from the Central Malignant Melanoma Registry of the German Dermatological Society.[6] Both groups analyzed melanomas less than 1.0 mm thick. In both reviews, gender was a significant prognostic factor when reviewed under

Table 1 AJCC Melanoma Database Cox Regression Analysis for Patients with Clinically Localized Melanoma

Variable	DF	χ^2 (Wald)	P	Risk Ratio	95% CI
Thickness	1	244.3	< .00001	1.558	1.473–1.647
Ulceration	1	189.5	< .00001	1.901	1.735–2.083
Age	1	45.6	< .00001	1.101	1.071–1.132
Site	1	41	< .00001	1.338	1.224–1.463
Level	1	32.7	< .00001	1.214	1.136–1.297
Sex	1	15.1	0.001	0.836	0.764–0.915

CI = confidence interval; DF = degrees of freedom.
Reprinted with permission from Balch CM et al.[3]

multivariate analysis. Further findings demonstrated that the presence of vertical growth phase as well as the mitotic rate (mitotic figures present vs absent) were also significant prognostic factors. Others have provided evidence for the significance of mitotic rate in predicting survival,[7,8] as well as in predicting the presence of regional metastases.[9] Age has also been shown to be associated with outcome. Sondak and colleagues demonstrated an increased risk of the presence of a positive sentinel lymph node in young patients under the age of 35,[9] whereas advanced age (over age 65) has also been associated with a worse prognosis. The Sunbelt Melanoma Trial noted that advance age was associated with the presence of a greater number of known adverse prognostic indicators such as tumor thickness and ulceration.[10] As many of these reports are single-center, retrospective reviews, these factors will be investigated further at the next AJCC review to try to determine their true significance in predicting survival and recurrence in melanoma.

In addition to these clinical and histopathologic findings, new inroads into our understanding of genetics have generated an interest in the prognosis associated with specific genetic patterns in melanoma. Current interest in this area has focused predominantly on two genes: CDKN2A, which is the locus that encodes the p16 tumor suppressor gene and is commonly mutated in melanoma, and BRAF, which is a component of the mitogen-activated protein kinase pathway. In a study from the John Wayne Cancer Institute, the presence of BRAF mutations was associated with the development of metastatic disease, leading them to the conclusion that BRAF mutations may be a predictor of a metastatic phenotype.[11] Although our understanding of the genetics of melanoma is evolving, mutations in these genes appear prevalent,[12] and it is likely that as our knowledge evolves, we may be able to utilize them to characterize survival and recurrence at the genetic level.

REGIONAL DISEASE

In patients with pathologically confirmed regional nodal metastases, the number of involved lymph nodes as well as whether they are clinically identified (macroscopic) or identified via SLN biopsy (microscopic) have been shown to be prognostic factors.[3,13] Nodal status designations have been separated into groupings with 1 node (N1), 2 or 3 nodes (N2) and 4 or more nodes (N3). The N3 designation also includes patients with matted nodes, or synchronous in-transit and nodal disease. In the substaging of patients with nodal or in-transit disease, the presence of ulceration is the sole primary tumor characteristic that persists as a factor in determining survival and recurrence.[3] Other factors that have been identified as prognostic in this group of patients included the presence or absence of extranodal disease as well as tumor volume.[14–16] A recent study asserts that in patients

Table 2 Cox Regression Analysis for Patients Without Clinical Evidence of Nodal Metastases Whose Regional Lymph Nodes Were Pathologically Staged after Sentinel or Elective Lymphadenectomy

Variable	DF	χ^2 (Wald)	P	Risk Ratio	95% CI
Nodal status	1	100.69	< .00001	2.239	1.913–2.621
Thickness	1	81.85	< .00001	1.583	1.433–1.749
Ulceration	1	78.83	< .00001	1.938	1.674–2.242
Site	1	27.86	< .00001	1.483	1.281–1.716
Age	1	14.25	0.0002	1.095	1.044–1.147
Sex	1	1.88	0.1705	0.9	0.774–1.046
Level	1	0.01	0.9082	1.007	0.896–1.131

CI = confidence interval; DF = degrees of freedom.
Reprinted with permission from Balch CM et al.[3]

with clinically positive nodal disease, the amount of FDG uptake may predict recurrence-free survival.[17] These data are too immature to be clinically useful at the present time, but not surprising given the known predictive value of tumor volume. It may, in fact, portend the future of staging approaches in patients with high-risk disease.

Another factor that, in the age of routine lymphoscintigraphy and SLN biopsy, has been shown to play a potential prognostic role in patients with lymph node metastases is drainage to multiple lymphatic basins. Data from Memorial Sloan-Kettering and The University of Texas M. D. Anderson Cancer Center[18,19] have demonstrated that multibasin drainage for truncal lesions predicts an increased risk of nodal metastases[19] and a lower 5-year overall survival.[18] Unfortunately, these data are contrasted by reports from the Sydney Melanoma Unit that demonstrate that multibasin drainage is not associated with a worse outcome or increased risk of nodal metastases.[20] At present, this requires further analysis before the role of multibasin drainage can be completely characterized.

Interferon remains the sole agent with a demonstrated benefit in patients with nodal metastases. Recently, it has been shown that the presence of autoimmunity in patients receiving interferon is associated with an improved prognosis from treatment.[21] Although interesting, these data are the result of a subanalysis of a larger trial and have not yet been confirmed in a larger investigation, thereby limiting the conclusions that can be drawn from it.

PROGNOSTIC FACTORS IN STAGE IV (DISTANT METASTATIC) MELANOMA

One of the most significant factors in determining outcome in patients with metastatic melanoma is the serum lactate dehydrogenase (LDH). In patients with stage IV disease, 5-year survival can decrease from nearly 20% (in those with distant subcutaneous or nodal metastases) to less than 10% with the presence of an elevated LDH.[4,22,23] Another major factor is the type of distant metastasis. Lesions in visceral organs have a worse prognosis than those present in skin, subcutis, or distant nodes. There has been considerable attention paid to the role of reverse transcriptase-polymerase chain reaction to identify circulating melanoma cells, but this approach has not demonstrated clinical utility as of yet. Furthermore, a number of circulating molecules such as S100 and YKL-40 have also been associated with poorer prognosis in patients with metastatic disease, but these data are limited and have yet to be subjected to rigorous review.

Staging

The American Joint Commission on Cancer staging of melanoma uses a standard tumor-nodes-metastasis (TNM) system. As mentioned previously, the AJCC last revised the staging system in 2002. This revision was the result of an unprecedented analysis of 17,600 patients analyzed from several international centers. As mentioned previously, the analysis included patients from before and after the development of SLN biopsy; therefore, routine pathologic staging of lymph nodes was not performed in all patients analyzed. Despite this, significant revisions from the 1997 staging system did occur. Most significantly were changes in the T stage, which were revised to the following groupings: T1: ≤ 1.00 mm; T2: 1.1 to 2.0 mm; T3: 2.1 to 4.0 mm; and T4: 4.0 mm Breslow's depth. This structure resulted in the best fit for univariate and multivariate Cox regression models.[3] Preparations are currently under way to perform the next revision to the AJCC staging system that is planned for 2009. Currently, the 2002 system is utilized and discussed subsequently.

"T" CLASSIFICATION

The "T" classification has been simplified from previous iterations of the AJCC staging system in that the present system utilizes whole integers rather than fractions for dividing points. As mentioned previously, this is the result of a rigorous analysis by the authors of the current system, during which several different cutoffs were compared and the current system was identified as the best fit in univariate and multivariate analysis. Additional considerations in T stage resulted from Kaplan-Meier survival analyses. The most significant factor to affect prognosis was that the presence of primary tumor ulceration resulted in survival curve that mirrored that of the next highest thickness classification: patients with T1 tumors that were ulcerated had a prognosis similar to patients with T2 nonulcerated tumors, patients with T2 tumors that were ulcerated had a prognosis similar to patients with T3 nonulcerated tumors, and so on (Figure 1). Additionally, Clark's level was noted to be a significant prognostic factor, but only in lesions that were 1.0 mm or less in thickness (T1). Lesions that are this thickness and are Clark's level IV are upstaged in a similar fashion as if they were ulcerated. Clark's level does not play a role in any other setting in the current staging system. This collection of characteristics led to the addition of the subscript "a" or "b" designation in the primary tumor staging system.

Primary tumor thickness (T stage) is currently defined as either not assessable: Tx (as in regressed melanomas or incomplete biopsies); no evidence of the primary tumor:

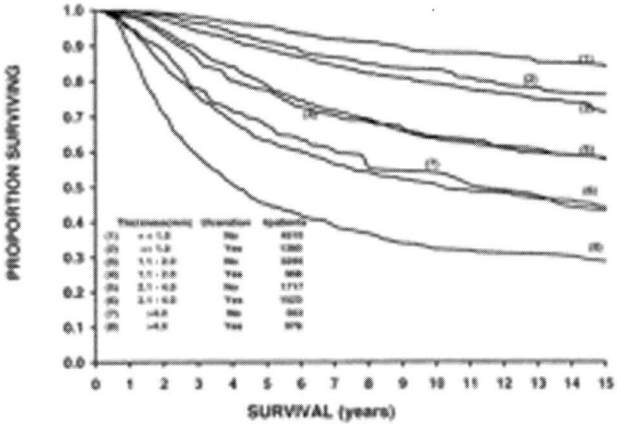

Figure 1 Kaplan-Meier survival curves for patients with localized melanoma stratified by thickness and the presence or absence of ulceration. Note that the presence of ulceration generates a survival curve mirroring that of the next highest T stage. Reprinted with permission from Balch CM et al.[3]

T0 (as in melanomas of unknown primary); tumors less than or equal to 1.0 mm in thickness: T1; tumors 1.01 to 2.00 mm in thickness: T2; tumors 2.01 to 4.0 mm in thickness: T3; or tumors greater than 4.01 mm in thickness: T4 (Table 3).

Patients without nodal metastases are either stage I or stage II as defined by their T stage and the presence or absence of ulceration as mentioned above. Patients who are T1 and nonulcerated (T1a) are the only group in stage IA (patients who are Clark's level IV also get upstaged into T1b/stage IB). These patients have a 5-year survival of approximately 95% based on the AJCC review; however, a recent review of SEER data indicated that this may be a slight underestimation in the patient population in the United States.[24] This may also reflect the fact that the population analyzed in the SEER analysis

Table 3 T Stage by Breslow Thickness. Subgroupings Are Defined by the Presence (Subgroup a) or Absence (Subgroup b) of Ulceration

Primary Tumor Thickness	T Stage Grouping
Primary tumor cannot be accurately assessed (ie, incomplete biopsy)	Tx
No evidence of the primary tumor (ie, melanomas of unknown primary site)	T0
In situ	Tis
≤ 1.0 mm thick	T1
1.01–2.0 mm	T2
2.01–4.0 mm	T3
> 4.0 mm	T4

Adapted from Greene FL et al.[25]

was inclusive only of patients who were treated during the era of routine use of SLN biopsy.

Patients who are T1 and ulcerated (T1b) or T2 and nonulcerated (T2a) are grouped into AJCC stage IB. These individuals have a 5-year survival of approximately 90%. Similarly, patients who are T2 and ulcerated (T2b) or T3 and nonulcerated (T3a) are classified as stage IIA. They carry a 5-year survival of nearly 80%. Patients who are T3 and ulcerated (T3b) or T4 and nonulcerated (T4a) are grouped together into stage IIB. These individuals have a 5-year survival approximating 65%. Patients with lesions thicker than 4 mm and ulcerated (T4b) are the only group in stage IIC. These individuals have a 5-year overall survival of 45%. As with the patients in stage IA, the SEER review revealed that for all stages, prognosis is slightly better in the United States population then that which was reported in the AJCC analysis that included an international population[24] (Table 4).

"N" CLASSIFICATION

Stage III disease is defined as locoregional metastases in the current staging system. Nodal metastases essentially define the stage III classification, as only patients with in-transit lesions or satellite lesions are classified as stage III in the absence of nodal disease. The "N" grouping is defined into 3 major divisions with 5 subdivisions. The N1 classification includes only patients with one involved lymph node. Those identified by sentinel node biopsy or by elective lymphadenectomy, and therefore without clinical evidence of disease, are labeled with a subscript "a" for micrometastases. Those identified by clinical evaluation are subdivided by subscript "b." Patients with 2 or 3 nodes pathologically involved are classified as N2, again with subscripts "a" and "b" designating microscopic disease versus clinically identified or macroscopic disease.

Along with the number of nodes, the primary tumor characteristics play a role in classifying the stage groupings for AJCC stage III patients. Stage IIIA patients are those without ulceration of their primary lesion, and who are not Clark's level IV (T1-4a). Most significantly, however, this grouping is limited to patients with 3 or fewer nodes, with microscopic disease only, that is, N1a or N2a disease.

Patients with ulcerated primary lesions (T1-4b) and microscopic disease limited to 3 nodes (N1-2a) or nonulcerated primary lesions (T1-4a) and macroscopic disease limited to 3 nodes (N1-2b) are collectively grouped into stage IIIB. Also included in this group are patients with in-transit disease or satellite disease *without* metastatic nodes (N2c) regardless of primary tumor characteristics.

Table 4 American Joint Committee on Cancer Staging of Localized Lesions, with Associated 5-Year Survival

AJCC Stage	T Stage Included	5-Yr Survival*
IA	T1a	95%
IB	T1b, T2a	90%
IIA	T2b, T3a	78%
IIB	T3b, T4a	65%
IIC	T4b	45%

*This is a combined figure including both T stage groupings included in AJCC stages that include more than 1 T stage.
Reprinted with permission from Balch CM et al.[4]

Stage IIIC is composed of patients with ulcerated primary lesions (T1-4b) and clinically palpable lymphadenopathy, or patients with N3 disease, which is defined by 4 or more lymph nodes, matted nodes, or nodal disease in conjunction with satellite or in-transit disease. Averaged across all of their subgroupings, 5-year survival for stage IIIA is approximately 67%, IIIB is approximately 52%, and IIIC is 27% (Table 5).

"M" CLASSIFICATION

As with all AJCC staging systems for solid tumors, the "M" classification in melanoma denotes distant metastatic disease. The authors of the 2002 AJCC system developed 3 subgroupings to the M classification, defined by the type of metastasis as well as by the serum lactate dehydrogenase (LDH). Any patient with distant metastases and an elevated serum LDH is classified as M1c. Patients with visceral metastases in organs other than the lungs are also classified as M1c. Patients with lung metastases are classified as M1b, and may have a slightly better prognosis than those in the M1c subgrouping in the short term (despite AJCC data indicating otherwise over 5-years, 1-year survival is noted to be better in patients with lung lesions only). M1a patients are those with distant lesions in the skin or subcutaneous tissue or with distant nodal metastases (nodes in basins other than those identified as primary draining basins at the time of SLN biopsy). Patients with M1a disease have a better 5-year survival than those with M1b or M1c. A pre-

Table 5 American Joint Committee on Cancer Staging of Locoregional Metastases, Including 5-Year Survival

AJCC Stage	T, N Stage Groupings Included	5-Yr Survival*
IIIA	(T1-4a), N1a, N2a	67%
IIIB	(T1-4b), N1a, N2a **or** (T1-4a) N1b, N2b **or** (Any T), N2c	52%
IIIC	(T1-4b), N1b, N2b or (Any T), N3	27%

*This is a combined figure including an average of all subgroupings.
Reprinted with permission from Balch CM et al.[4]

dominance of the role of the M subclassification is for the purposes of stratifying patients for clinical trials. The AJCC groups all patients with M1 disease into stage IV, and these patients have a less than 20% 5-year survival with current treatment regimens.

SUMMARY AND FUTURE DIRECTIONS

The current AJCC system was last revised in 2002 and is scheduled to undergo its next major revision in 2009. The next revision is likely to take a close look at some of the prognostic factors identified in many of the single-center retrospective analyses discussed previously. In the localized disease category, mitotic rate in particular will be specifically addressed for its prognostic value relative to the importance of ulceration. In the regional category, a better understanding concerning the prognosis of patients with microscopic sentinel node disease will have to be analyzed, as an ever increasing percentage of node-positive patients will be diagnosed with early and limited nodal involvement. Furthermore, since ulceration status of the primary is an independent predictor for patients with regional disease, the presence of mitoses in the primary, which like ulceration represents a surrogate for aggressive biology, will have to be analyzed as a potential predictor in the stage III categories.

Currently, the system identifies patients as having either localized (stage I or II), locoregional (stage III), or distant (stage IV) disease. Future systems may include genetic and molecular staging or may utilize predictive algorithms or nomograms to determine individual prognosis.

References

1. National Comprehensive Cancer Network. NCCN clinical practice guidelines in oncology. Jenkintown, PA; 2006. Available at http://www.nccn.org/professionals/physician_gls/f_guidelines.asp. (Accessed October 15, 2006.).

2. Sober AJ, Chuang T-Y, Duvic M, et al. Guidelines of care for primary cutaneous melanoma. J Am Acad Dermatol 2001;45:579–86.

3. Balch CM, Soong SJ, Gershenwald JE, et al. Prognostic factors analysis of 17,600 melanoma patients: validation of the American Joint Committee on Cancer melanoma staging system. J Clin Oncol 2001;19:3622–34.

4. Balch CM, Buzaid AC, Soong SJ, et al. Final Version of the American Joint Committee on Cancer staging system for cutaneous melanoma. J Clin Oncol 2001;19:3635–48.

5. Gimotty PA, Guerry D, Ming ME, et al. Thin primary cutaneous malignant melanoma: a prognostic tree for 10-year metastasis is more accurate than American Joint Committee on Cancer staging. J Clin Oncol 2004;22:3668–76.

6. Leiter U, Buettner PG, Eigentler TK, Garbe C. Prognostic factors of thin cutaneous melanoma: an analysis of the Central Malignant Melanoma Registry of the German Dermatological Society. J Clin Oncol 2004;22:3660–7.

7. Leon P, Daly JM, Synnestvedt M, et al. The prognostic implications of microscopic satellites in patients with clinical stage I melanoma. Arch Surg 1991;126:1461–8.

8. Salman SM, Rogers GS. Prognostic factors in thin cutaneous malignant melanoma. J Dermatolc Surg Oncol 1990;16:413–8.

9. Sondak VK, Taylor JM, Sabel MS, et al. Mitotic rate and younger age are predictors of sentinel lymph node positivity: lessons learned from the generation of a probabilistic model. Ann Surg Oncol 2004;11:247–58.

10. McMasters KM, Noyes RD, Reintgen D, et al. Lessons learned from the Sunbelt Melanoma Trial. J Surg Oncol 2004;86:212–23.

11. Shinozaki M, Fujimoto A, Morton DL, Hoon DSB. Incidence of BRAF oncogene mutation and clinical relevance for primary cutaneous melanomas. Clin Cancer Res 2004;10:1753–7.

12. Haluska FG, Tsao H, Wu H, et al. Genetic Alterations in signaling pathways in melanoma. Clin Cancer Res 2006; 12(7 Pt 2):2301s–7s.

13. Grunhagen DJ, Eggermont AM, van Geel AN, et al. Prognostic factors after cervical lymph node dissection for cutaneous melanoma metastases. Melanoma Res 2005;15: 179–84.

14. Calabro A, Singletary E, Balch C. Patterns of relapse in 1001 consecutive patients with melanoma nodal metastases. Arch Surg 1989;124:1051–5.

15. Gadd MA, Coit DG. Recurrence patterns and outcome in 1019 patients undergoing axillary or inguinal lymphadenectomy for melanoma. Arch Surg 1992;127:1412–6.

16. Gershenwald JE, Berman RS, Porter G, et al. Regional nodal basin control is not compromised by previous sentinel lymph node biopsy in patients with melanoma. Ann Surg Oncol 2000;7:226–31.

17. Bastiaannet E, Hoekstra OS, Oyen WJG, et al. Level of fluorodeoxyglucose uptake predicts risk for recurrence in melanoma patients presenting with lymph node metastases. Ann Surg Oncol 2006;13:1–8.

18. Jimenez RE, Panageas K, Busam KJ, Brady MS. Prognostic implications of multiple lymphatic basin drainage in patients with truncal melanoma. J Clin Oncol 2005;23: 518–24.

19. Porter GA, Ross MI, Berman RS, et al. Significance of multiple nodal basin drainage in truncal melanoma patients undergoing sentinel lymph node biopsy. Ann Surg Oncol 2000;7:256–61.

20. Bonenkamp JJ, Daley C, Colman M, Thompson JF. Drainage to multiple lymphatic fields is not an independent prognostic factor in truncal melanoma. Melanoma Res 2001;11:S78–9.

21. Gogas H, Ioannovich J, Dafni U, et al. Prognostic significance of autoimmunity during treatment of melanoma with interferon. N Engl J Med 2006;354:709–18.

22. Eton O, Legha SS, Moon TE, et al. Prognostic factors for survival of patients treated systemically for disseminated melanoma. J Clin Oncol 1998;16:1103–11.

23. Deichmann M, Benner A, Bock M, et al. S100-Beta, melanoma-inhibiting activity, and lactate dehydrogenase discriminate progressive from nonprogressive American Joint Committee on Cancer stage IV melanoma. J Clin Oncol 1999;17:1891–6.

24. Gimotty PA, Botbyl J, Soong S-j, Guerry D. A population-based validation of the American Joint Committee on cancer melanoma staging system. J Clin Oncol 2005;23: 8065–75.

25. Greene FL, Page DL, Fleming ID, et al, editors. AJCC Cancer Staging Handbook. 6th ed. New York: Springer-Verlag; 2002. p. 243.

Chapter 83

Indications and Techniques of Regional Lymphadenectomy

Keith A. Delman, MD

Paul F. Mansfield, MD

Jeffrey E. Lee, MD

Introduction

The most common site of metastases from melanoma is to the draining lymph nodes. Regional basins that may be involved and can be surgically addressed include axillary, cervical, epitrochlear, inguinal, iliac, and popliteal nodes. Nodal metastases are divided into microscopic (detected at the time of sentinel lymph node biopsy or at the time of elective nodal dissection) or macroscopic (disease identified by clinical evaluation). The current version of the American Joint Committee on Cancer (AJCC) staging system for melanoma includes classification by the number of involved nodes: N1 (1 node positive), N2 (2–3 nodes positive), and N3 (4 or more nodes positive). Standard treatment of melanoma patients found to have occult or clinically evident regional lymph node metastases includes complete dissection of the lymphatic basin. Since patients with regional nodal metastasis from melanoma are at relatively high risk of tumor recurrence, consideration for postoperative systemic adjuvant therapy via high-dose interferon-alpha or, alternatively, a clinical trial is appropriate. This chapter describes the indications for regional lymphadenectomy and the technical approach to each lymphatic basin.

Indications for Regional Lymphadenectomy

The indications for formal lymphadenectomy have become more straightforward. Historically, elective lymphadenectomy was considered in patients without clinical evidence for regional nodal metastasis if they presented with at least an intermediate-risk primary tumor. However, elective lymph node dissection has essentially been supplanted in the modern era by intraoperative lymphatic mapping and sentinel lymph node biopsy. With this technique, patients with clinically localized melanomas without clinical evidence of metastases but with primary tumor characteristics suggesting at least modest risk of harboring occult regional metastatic disease undergo sentinel lymph node (SLN) biopsy. The results of this SLN biopsy dictate the need for subsequent surgical intervention. Unless the SLN biopsy was performed in the setting of a clinical trial with specific proscriptions on completion lymph node dissection, patients with occult metastatic disease identified in their nodal basin by sentinel lymph node should undergo a completion lymphadenectomy of the involved basin. This procedure is commonly termed a "selective lymphadenectomy." Depending on the primary tumor characteristics of the population to which the procedure is applied, approximately 17% of patients who undergo sentinel lymph node biopsy will have a positive sentinel lymph node.[1–4]

Patients with clinical disease involving a regional nodal basin should also undergo lymphadenectomy; this procedure is commonly referred to as a "therapeutic" lymph node dissection. These patients tend to have a higher volume of disease than patients who undergo regional lymphadenectomy for SLN biopsy-detected metastases. In the current AJCC staging system, patients with clinically detected disease are staged separately from those with SLN-detected disease to reflect their relatively poorer prognosis.

Contraindications to Regional Lymphadenectomy

Patients who cannot medically tolerate general anesthesia are generally not considered for regional lymphadenectomy. Although from a technical standpoint some regional lymphadenectomies can be completed under a regional block, the inability to tolerate general anesthesia represents a strong relative contraindication to performing these procedures. Especially with respect to inguinal lymphadenectomy it is often difficult to perform an adequate regional block in these patients. In addition, on occasion there are findings at operation that indicate the need to proceed with extended dissection of the adjacent nodal basin (inguinal to pelvic, for example).

Some patients choose not to pursue completion lymphadenectomy despite counseling and confirmation of the finding of an involved SLN. Approximately 80% of patients with only a single positive SLN will not have any further positive nodes identified at completion lymphadenectomy; this implies that there may be a subset of patients (for example, those with only microscopic disease identified in a single lymph node) in whom such an approach does not result in an elevated risk of melanoma recurrence. However, data from appropriately powered randomized controlled clinical trials are not yet available to assist patients and physicians in deciding when it is safe to forgo completion lymphadenectomy.

Finally, patients with widespread extraregional metastatic disease may be poor candidates for formal lymph node dissection. Surgeons must consider symptoms related to the regional nodal disease, the morbidity of the lymph node dissection, and the potential effectiveness of alternative treatment modalities before proceeding with a regional surgical procedure that does not render the patient disease free. In some patients with distant metastases, however, aggressive surgical intervention to address regional nodal metastasis may be justified, particularly when there is significant morbidity related to the regional disease and distant metastatic disease is limited in extent.

Surgical Technique

GENERAL CONSIDERATIONS

Several issues should be considered when preparing a patient to undergo regional lymphadenectomy. Initial planning should begin at the time of SLN biopsy. The surgeon who performs the SLN biopsy should orient the biopsy incision so as to allow for a subsequent completion lymphadenectomy incision to be performed, including excision of the biopsy scar en bloc with the lymphadenectomy specimen. This planning can be facilitated by first identifying the area of greatest focal gamma activity representing the location of the sentinel lymph node, and then drawing the completion lymphadenectomy incision to include that focus. The incision is then made the appropriate length along the completion lymphadenectomy outline.

Prior to completion lymphadenectomy, patients should undergo a chest x-ray and an age-appropriate preoperative laboratory evaluation. There is no indication for extensive laboratory or radiographic staging of patients who present with clinically localized melanoma. Two recent studies have demonstrated that routine imaging for staging purposes in patients with only a single positive SLN is not indicated.[5,6] In contrast, in patients with multiple positive nodes or in those undergoing therapeutic lymphadenectomy for clinically detected metastases, we routinely perform a formal staging evaluation; though recognize that even in this situation the yield is low. Our standard evaluation for such patients includes a complete blood count; electrolytes; blood urea nitrogen; creatinine; glucose; liver function tests; a chest radiograph; computed tomography of the chest, abdomen, and pelvis; and magnetic resonance imaging of the brain. Patients considered candidates for postoperative adjuvant therapy will require a similar staging evaluation prior to beginning systemic therapy. In order to avoid the need for repeat imaging studies, we will usually delay formal staging of a patient with regional nodal involvement limited to occult disease identified on SLN biopsy until after formal lymphadenectomy and just prior to beginning adjuvant therapy.

At the time of completion lymphadenectomy, patients should receive perioperative prophylactic antibiotics to cover common skin flora. General anesthesia is utilized; we routinely use laryngeal mask airway anesthesia. Sequential compression devices and TED Hose are applied to the lower extremities before induction of anesthesia. If the patient will be undergoing surgery on one of the lower limbs, after induction, the compression device is removed from the operative limb. A Foley catheter is inserted if the patient will have a pelvic or lower extremity dissection, or if the surgical procedure is expected to last more than 3 hours.

AXILLARY LYMPHADENECTOMY

Patient Position

The patient is placed supine on the operating room table with the operative arm extended. A soft roll is placed longitudinally under the upper torso and scapula, elevating the latissimus dorsi muscle. The table is positioned to allow the assistant to stand above the arm and the surgeon to stand inferior to it. It is generally helpful to have a second assistant available for retracting purposes, although this is not mandatory. This person stands on the opposite side from the operative field. We find that using an Iron Intern (or similar retractor system) can be quite helpful, and in teaching situations this allows the student to stand at the end of the arm board on the side of the surgery with a generally excellent view.

Patient Preparation and Draping

We routinely perform an extremely wide prep, from the ipsilateral anterior superior iliac spine, to across the midline, up to the neck, shoulder, and the upper extremity, and down to the midforearm. The forearm is wrapped either in a towel drape clipped with piercing towel clips or with a stockinette. The prep is also carried onto the back, to the lateral edge of the scapula. The body is rolled away from the operative side and elevated slightly. A towel and side drape is placed longitudinally under the patient's side, and the prepped arm is placed on this drape so that it may be moved freely during the procedure. The remainder of the patient is draped to leave the axilla exposed.

Incision and Surgical Technique

We use a "lazy-S" incision for most of our regional lymphadenectomies. The incision should be tailored to remove previous scars, whether from an earlier dissection or from a sentinel lymph node biopsy. The skin ellipse, inclusive of any previous scar, is generally excised en bloc with the lymphadenectomy specimen.

Unlike in breast cancer, the dissection for melanoma is a complete dissection, routinely including levels I, II, and III, the fibrofatty tissue superficial and superior to the axillary vein and sometimes requiring division of the pectoralis minor muscle to gain access to the medial tissue of level III. The incision is carried along the edge of the pectoralis major muscle beginning near its origin for approximately 2 cm, and then is brought down across the axilla and then along the anterior border of the latissimus dorsi muscle for approximately 2 cm (Figure 1). Flaps are then raised medially to the pectoralis border and laterally (or "posteriorly") to the latissimus border. These flaps should be adjusted based on the body habitus of the patient, but generally are approximately 5 mm in thickness. The dissection is carried superiorly to the tendinous portion of the pectoralis major and inferiorly

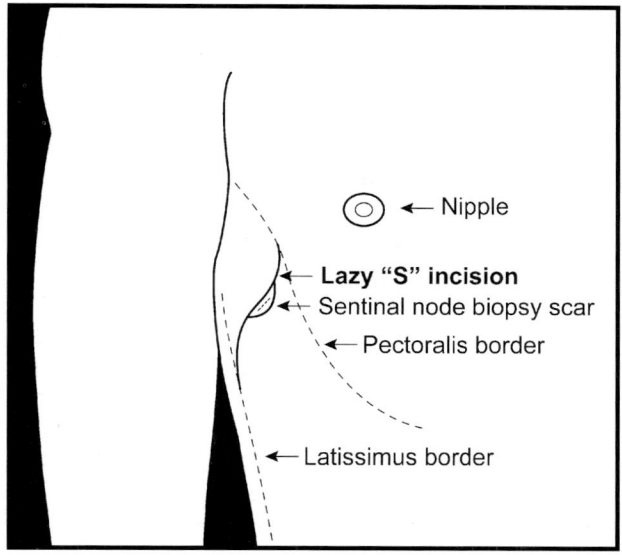

Figure 1 Incision used for complete axillary dissection.

to the junction of the latissimus muscle with the serratus anterior.

Dissection is carried out along the latissimus border, often using a finger or clamp to mobilize the investing fascia along its lateral aspect. This approach offers some protection to the thoracodorsal nerve, as this generally inserts on the medial aspect of the muscle. The dissection is carried up to the tendinous insertion of the muscle, with the surgeon cognizant of the possibility of encountering the thoracodorsal neurovascular bundle approximately midway to one-third of the way inferior to the tendinous insertion. In the course of this dissection, the intercostobrachial is encountered and divided. During the dissection for melanoma, no attempt to salvage this sensory nerve is made. At the apex of the tendinous insertion of the latissimus, the lateral aspect of the axillary vein is encountered. In approximately 5% of patients there may be fibers of the latissimus dorsi that traverse anterior to the axillary vein. There are predictably one or two venous branches in this area that must be clipped or ligated. Once the dissection along the latissimus is carried out, attention is then turned to the pectoralis major. In a fashion similar to the latissimus dissection, the investing fascia of the pectoralis major is mobilized with a clamp, and then dissection is carried out along it and posteriorly to the nodes between the two pectoralis muscles, and then around them ("Rotter's nodes"). The tissue between the pectoralis major and minor muscles is swept into the axilla proper, and the dissection is carried along the pectoralis minor muscle. The medial pectoral nerve is encountered and routinely preserved. Sacrifice of this nerve is rarely necessary and leads to atrophy of the pectoralis minor (which it innervates) and the lateral and superior aspect of pectoralis major (the secondary component of its innervation).

The axillary vein is now skeletonized along its anterior and superior aspects from lateral to medial, with the tissue superficial and superior to it being mobilized down into the wound. Care must be taken in this area as this is on top of the brachial plexus. Flexion of the elbow and shoulder joint bringing the arm up and across the chest often facilitates this dissection at the highest limits of the axilla. At this point we return to the inferior aspect of the axilla and mobilize the inferior tissue from the serratus anterior. Attention is then turned to the medial border of the latissimus dorsi and the thoracodorsal neurovascular bundle is identified and skeletonized up to the axillary vein. A small neurovascular bundle branch from the thoracodorsal courses lateral to medial and inserts adjacent to the long thoracic nerve on the chest wall. We utilize this branch to identify the long thoracic nerve. The axillary contents are dissected free of the serratus anterior and the long thoracic nerve superiorly to the axillary vein. It is important to maintain a knowledge of this nerve as the dissection is carried medially into levels II and III as this nerve can be injured in its proximal extent during this part of the dissection.

A Richardson or Deaver retractor (or deep Iron Intern blade) is then placed behind the pectoralis minor and the musculature of the chest elevated to expose the medial extent of the axillary vein. Small venous branches are clipped or ligated and the tissue is dissected free to the level of Halstead's ligament in a medial to lateral fashion to meet the remainder of the dissection specimen. In some circumstances, the pectoralis minor must be divided to gain access to this area, but we do not perform this routinely. Injury to the axillary vein (or its branches) in this area can be treacherous and extremely difficult to repair, thus great care should be taken during this part of the dissection to avoid any injury to the vessels here. Completion of this part of the dissection should free the specimen from the patient. The wound is then irrigated with saline, and after hemostasis is achieved, a large closed suction drain is placed through a separate stab wound (we use a 19 French (F) round, fluted drain). The drain is brought out, usually within 1 cm of the incision to limit any potential radiation field, should such adjuvant therapy be indicated. The wound is closed using an intradermal stitch and a subcuticular closure.

Postoperative Care

The patient is routinely observed overnight in the hospital with discharge home the next morning. The drain generally remains in place until it is draining less than 30 cc/day for 2 consecutive days. This often may take 2 to 3 weeks; however, we prefer to remove drains within 14 days of surgery and do not regularly leave drains in beyond 3 weeks. The most common complications after axillary lymphadenectomy are seroma and infection. Most patients with low-grade cellulitis can be treated with oral antibiotics, but infected seromas should be evacuated. Approximately 10% of patients undergoing axillary lymphadenectomy for melanoma will develop lymphedema, which despite being a more extensive dissection than that performed for breast cancer, has a lower incidence of swelling.[7–9] The reason for this is not thoroughly understood but may be the result of the disruption of the chest wall lymphatics or, more likely, the regular use of radiation in the management of breast cancer.

INGUINOFEMORAL (SUPERFICIAL GROIN) AND ILIOINGUINAL (DEEP PELVIC) LYMPHADENECTOMY

Patient Position

The patient is placed supine on the operating room table with the hip externally rotated and the knee slightly flexed, exposing the femoral triangle. A small roll may be needed under the knee for support of the joint, although this is not mandatory, and in some patients it is unnecessary. The lateral malleolus should be padded to prevent damage from pressure. In some instances, the scrotum is sutured to the opposite leg to keep it away from the field, particularly if the SLN biopsy scar is very medial on the leg. We generally remove the sequential compression device from the operative limb.

Patient Preparation and Draping

The patient is then prepped widely from just below the knee table to table, into the groin, across the midline to above the umbilicus, and down out onto the flank to the table. Towels are stapled to the patient, leaving most of the thigh exposed, the umbilicus, the pubic bone, and the anterior superior iliac spine, along with the abdominal skin, for a distance approximately 5 cm above the umbilicus. A groin towel is stapled in place in all cases.

Incision and Surgical Technique for Superficial Groin Dissection

We routinely use a longitudinal incision with a "lazy-S" portion across the groin crease, although an alternative linear incision has also been advocated by others. As with all regional lymphadenectomies, if the procedure is being performed after SLN biopsy or other surgical intervention (previous dissection or excisional biopsy), the scar should be excised with the specimen and removed en bloc with the superficial inguinal contents. Our incision generally runs from 5 cm superior and medial to the anterior superior iliac spine, parallel and in the groin crease, and then vertically down the leg in the central portion of the femoral triangle almost to its apex (Figure 2). Once the skin is incised, flaps are raised in medial and lateral directions to the adductor and sartorius muscles, respectively, no further medial than the lateral aspect of the pubic bone and no further lateral than the anterior superior iliac spine at those levels.

Once flaps have been raised, two Adson-Beckman retractors can be utilized for exposure. We begin with the tissue on the external oblique aponeurosis, sweeping the lymph node-bearing tissue approximately 10 cm superior to the inguinal ligament down into the femoral triangle proper. At this point, attention is turned toward the lateral aspect of the dissection and the tissue overlying the sartorius muscle is mobilized, inclusive of the investing fascia. At the medial border of the muscle runs the main trunk of the femoral nerve, which must be

identified and preserved. At the apex of the femoral triangle, where the adductor longus and the sartorius intersect, the tissue is dissected from inferior to superior. There is predictably a small venous branch coursing from the lateral aspect of the leg, which is ligated and divided, as well as a branch of the femoral nerve, which is identified here. This femoral nerve branch is often sacrificed, but can occasionally be salvaged.

The medial aspect of the dissection is carried out over the adductor longus, leaving the fascia on this muscle. The tissue is mobilized toward the femoral vein. The saphenous vein crosses the adductor longus muscle as the vessel enters the femoral triangle and courses toward its junction with the femoral vein. In general, this is identified and ligated during this mobilization. We routinely doubly ligate the distal extent of the retained portion of the vein. In addition, there are frequently extensive lymphatic channels in the tissue surrounding the saphenous vein, which are ligated as well. In some cases (for us, particularly in pediatric patients or in some patients with the primary lesion on the trunk) a saphenous vein-sparing dissection can be carried out. Although technically a bit more challenging, preserving the saphenous vein may result in less lower-extremity edema, as the superficial venous drainage remains intact. If this approach is taken, great care must be taken to be sure to remove all of the lymph node-bearing tissue surrounding the vein, as it is routinely done when the vein is resected.

Attention is turned next toward the femoral artery and its investing fascia, which is incised. The lymph node-bearing tissue is mobilized from the artery in an adventitial plane, taking great care to clip or ligate all small branches, for in this area, even the smallest vessels can bleed substantially. The dissection is carried out over the femoral vein, which lies medial and posterior to the artery, skeletonizing it, with particular attention to its medial aspect, where the preponderance of the remaining lymphatic tissue lies. The tissue from the femoral canal is retracted superiorly and dissected off of the vessels up to the saphenofemoral junction.

At this point, we place a goose-necked vascular clamp on the saphenofemoral junction and complete the resection by dividing the saphenous vein. A 4-0 nonabsorbable monofilament suture is used to oversew the saphenous stump. At this point the sole remaining attachments are the lymphatic channels coursing medial to the vein up to the femoral canal. The lymphatics are divided at the level of the femoral canal and the specimen is removed. Attention is turned to the femoral canal and Cloquet's node. If the patient does not have multiple (4 or more) visibly involved nodes or clinical evidence of disease (even in a single node), we then biopsy Cloquet's

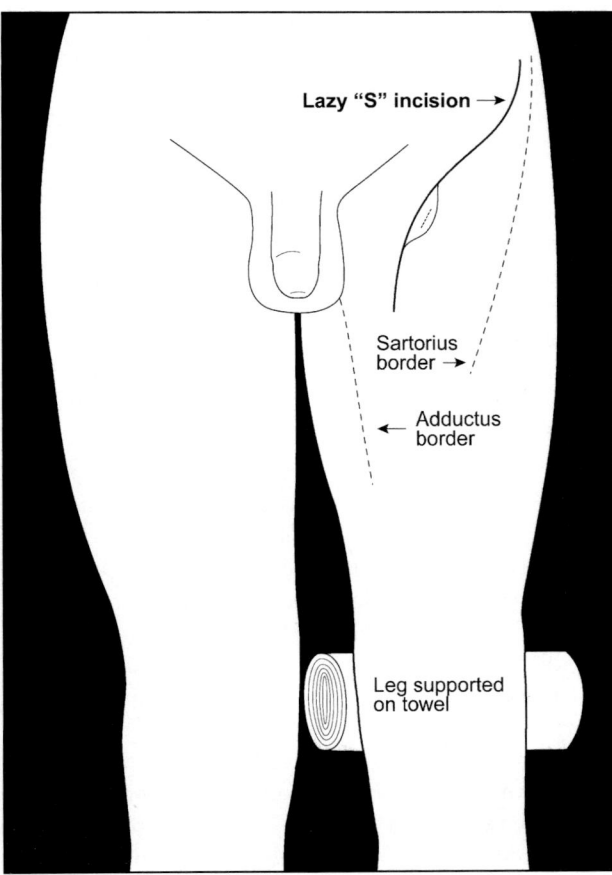

Figure 2 Incision used for superficial and deep groin dissection.

node to indicate the need to pursue a deep groin dissection in patients with only microscopic disease. To gain access to Cloquet's node, the lacunar ligament is incised and a femoral hernia is created. The node lies slightly posterior and medial to the external iliac vein just inside the pelvis. There is, with some reliable frequency, a small vein just inside the pelvis that needs to either be retracted out of the way, or ligated. The node is sent for frozen-section evaluation. The wound is irrigated with saline and packed with a moist gauze until closure.

Incision and Surgical Technique for Deep Pelvic Lymphadenectomy

In patients with evidence of multiple involved nodes, a clinically positive (palpable) node, or a positive Cloquet's node, a deep dissection is carried out. As most patients undergoing a pelvic lymphadenectomy will have a synchronous superficial groin dissection, we simply extend the skin incision vertically a few centimeters up the abdominal wall (the reason for the high prep on the abdomen). Although some authors divide the inguinal ligament routinely, we prefer to use a separate fascial incision for the deep pelvic dissection, using a standard "kidney transplant incision." To achieve this, an 8 to 10 cm incision is made in the external oblique aponeurosis parallel to the inguinal ligament approximately 5 to 6 cm superior to it. The underlying musculature (internal oblique, transversus abdominis) is divided in the direction of their fibers and the peritoneum is then mobilized medially with blunt dissection. A self-retaining retractor is utilized to maintain exposure in this setting (either a Bookwalter or Thompson). The ureter must be identified and protected. The inferior epigastric vessels are identified and either retracted or ligated. All of the lymph node-bearing fatty tissue is dissected free of the external iliac vessels proximally up to the bifurcation of the common iliac into its external and internal branches. The tissue is swept off of the medial aspect of the bladder, visualizing the superior vesicular artery. Great care should be taken not to injure the ureter. Cloquet's node and any tissue not previously removed from the femoral canal are also included with this specimen. It is not unusual in a patient with gross disease to have nodal disease immediately behind the vein as it courses through the inguinal canal. Although gross lymphadenopathy proximal to the iliac bifurcation can and should be resected, patients with disease outside the extent of the standard dissection have a poor prognosis, as this is a sign of biologically aggressive disease. The dissection around the iliac vessels is often aided by the application of vessel loops for retraction and mobilization of these structures.

We send the iliac packet of nodes as a second specimen during superficial and deep groin dissection (the superficial groin nodes being the first specimen). Once resected, attention is turned to the obturator nodes, which lie along the pelvic sidewall and course anterior to the obturator nerve as it travels toward the obturator foramen. This tissue routinely is resected with blunt dissection, although it may be facilitated by the use of a Martin forceps to grasp the packet of nodes. Finger dissection of these nodes is optimal as it allows identification and preservation of the obturator nerve, which is identified as a taut cord beneath the nodal tissue. The obturator vessels course deep to the nerve in this area and can be the source of substantial hemorrhage, which can be difficult to control if disrupted. We do not routinely resect the tissue posterior to the obturator nerve unless it is grossly involved, and then only with great caution.

The obturator packet of lymph nodes is sent as a third specimen in this procedure, allowing the pathologists to characterize the extent of involvement of each compartment of nodal tissue. The pelvis is then irrigated, hemostasis assured and a 19F round, fluted, drain is placed in the pelvis and brought out through a separate skin stab wound within a centimeter of the skin edge. The fascia is closed in layers, and then attention is returned to the femoral compartment again.

If a deep pelvic dissection has been performed simultaneously, the drain for the superficial femoral dissection is brought in from above, through a separate skin stab adjacent to the deep pelvic drain. If the superficial dissection has been performed alone, we routinely bring the drain out below the wound, on the thigh. In all cases, however, we perform a sartorius muscle transposition as a part of the closure of the superficial groin dissection to protect the underlying femoral artery and vein should there be any wound breakdown.

To perform a sartorius muscle transposition, the muscle is divided as close to its insertion on the anterior superior iliac spine as possible. The lateral femoral cutaneous nerve can usually be identified and preserved. The muscle is then mobilized from its lateral attachments. The blood supply to the sartorius is segmental, and the perforating vessels are clipped and divided sequentially until the muscle is free enough to be transposed. Every effort is made to minimize the number of perforating branches that need to be sacrificed in order to preserve as much of the blood supply as possible. The muscle is then either "flipped" over into place or slid laterally, depending on the position in which it lies most effectively. We then use 2-0 nonabsorbable monofilament "U" stitches to anchor the muscle to the inguinal ligament and external oblique fascia. Prior to transposition of the muscle, the femoral canal defect is closed using a single 2-0 monofilament nonabsorbable suture. The lateral and medial aspects of the muscle flap are then anchored, if necessary, using 3-0 absorbable braided suture. The drain is placed superficial to this muscle through the entire femoral triangle. The skin is then closed using 3-0 absorbable deep dermal sutures and skin staples.

Postoperative Care

The patients generally remain in the hospital until the deep drain is removed, which is usually within 3 or 4 days after surgery. We regularly keep patients at bedrest for 24 hours after superficial groin dissection, but then encourage normal ambulation. Patients who undergo superficial groin dissection only are observed overnight and then discharged home. We follow similar patterns of drain management for the superficial drain in these procedures as we do for axillary lymphadenectomy, waiting until less than 30 cc/day of drainage is noted for 2 consecutive days before removing the drain. Again, this often may take 2 to 3 weeks; however, we prefer to remove drains within 14 days of surgery and do not regularly leave drains in beyond 3 weeks. Complications after inguinalfemoral and ilioinguinal dissection occur with greater frequency than in other regional lymphadenectomies. In some reviews, up to 50% of patients will have some type of complication.[10] These complications range from mild, low-cellulitis treatable with oral antibiotics, to deep wound infections requiring opening of the wound. Lymphedema, seroma, and infectious complications are the most common difficulties after surgery in the groin and pelvis, with as many as 20% of patients developing a significant degree of lower extremity swelling.[7,8,10–13]

CERVICAL LYMPHADENECTOMY

Special Considerations

The cervical lymph node basin warrants a brief discussion of issues that pertain specifically to the head and neck. These lymph node basins are at risk of harboring clinical or occult metastasis from primary melanomas of the head and neck region or upper trunk, and are also an occasional site for melanoma metastasis from an unknown primary site. Metastasis to lymph nodes from primary melanomas in the head and neck tend to follow a predictable pattern. Melanomas occurring anterior to the pinna of the ear generally metastasize to the parotid, submandibular, submental, upper jugular, and posterior triangle lymph nodes. Lesions occurring inferior to the

lateral fissure of the lip usually spread to cervical lymph nodes rather than to parotid nodes. Melanomas occurring on the scalp posterior to the pinna of the ear usually spread to occipital, postauricular, posterior triangle, or jugular chain nodes. However, exceptions to these predicted patterns of nodal spread occur, and these exceptions illustrate the benefit of lymphoscintigraphy and SLN biopsy.

Although radical neck dissection was historically recommended as treatment for patients with clinically evident regional melanoma metastasis involving the lateral cervical compartment, modified (also referred to as functional or comprehensive) neck dissection, including levels II, III, IV, and V, but sparing the spinal accessory nerve, the sternocleidomastoid muscle, and the internal jugular vein, has supplanted the more radical operation except in circumstances where there is direct tumor extension to one or more of these important anatomic structures. Since patients with occult disease identified by sentinel lymph node biopsy generally have a lower tumor burden than those with clinically detected disease, it is conceivable that selective neck dissection (including fewer anatomic regions than traditional comprehensive neck dissection) may achieve equivalent regional control and cure rates in selected patients with limited nodal involvement while providing lower morbidity. However, in the absence of more accurate information regarding the anatomic compartments involved in patients undergoing completion lymphadenectomy following excision of an involved sentinel lymph node, we continue to advocate comprehensive neck dissection as standard surgical therapy for patients with occult regional melanoma metastasis identified by sentinel lymph node evaluation.

Patient Position

The patient's shoulders are elevated on a soft shoulder roll; hyperextension of the neck is avoided. For unilateral neck dissection, the patient's face is oriented toward their opposite shoulder. The table is turned 90 degrees. The operating surgeon positions himself at the patient's side, with the surgeon's assistant positioned above the head of the patient.

Patient Preparation and Draping

We prep widely, as with the other regional lymphadenectomies. In the head and neck we alternatively use either a betadine prep or chlorhexadine. The prep is carried across the midline and down onto the chest wall. The ipsilateral face and ear are also prepped along to the shoulder and upper back. A small piece of rolled xeroform gauze is inserted into the ear canal to prevent betadine from drying inside. The corner of the mouth, the inferior aspect of the ear, and the jugular notch should all be visible in the field. We routinely use a split sheet with a bar drape, which is self-adhesive, although if cloth drapes are used they should be sutured to the patient.

Incision and Surgical Technique

Several orientations of skin incisions can be used. Most commonly, we perform a neck dissection for melanoma through an oblique incision along the sternocleidomastoid muscle with an extension in an L-shaped fashion parallel and superior to the clavicle to improve exposure of the eleventh nerve and level V lymph nodes. This chapter does not cover parotidectomy, which would necessitate an incision overlying the preauricular space just anterior to the border of the tragus and extending down over the stylomastoid foramen to meet the sternocleidomastoid incision. An alternative incision for a comprehensive neck dissection includes the oblique incision overlying the sternocleidomastoid with transverse submandibular and supraclavicular extensions forming a letter "I." We prefer to excise gross disease involving skin as well as scars from previous neck operations en bloc as part of the neck dissection when possible (Figure 3). After incision of the skin, subpla-

tysmal flaps are created to the limits of dissection, which include the anterior border of the sternocleidomastoid medially, the trapezius muscle posterolaterally, the submandibular gland superiorly, and the clavicle inferiorly. The great auricular nerve is preserved whenever possible. A rigid retractor is helpful in maintaining exposure; we suture the skin flaps back with 2-0 silk (Figure 4).

The spinal accessory (eleventh) nerve is identified as the trapezius muscle is exposed. The eleventh nerve is usually identified low in the neck and traced cephalad. Care is taken to preserve the more proximal extent of the nerve as it exits from underneath the lateral border of the sternocleidomastoid muscle, and motor branches from the eleventh nerve to the sternocleidomastoid muscle are preserved. To minimize thermal injury, dissection along the eleventh nerve is carried out with sharp dissection and bipolar cautery. The external jugular vein is divided high along the sternocleidomastoid muscle. The anterior border of the sternocleidomastoid muscle is incised. The external jugular vein together with associated lymph nodes and fatty tissue is brought down off the posterolateral aspect of the muscle. The sternocleidomastoid muscle is elevated from its bed, allowing medial and lateral retraction to improve exposure and facilitate complete dissection. We often utilize a ½-inch penrose drain to manipulate this muscle.

The posterior belly of the digastric muscle and the hypoglossal (twelfth) nerve are identified at the superior limit of dissection. Care is taken to preserve the fascia overlying the submandibular gland when possible to avoid injury to the marginal mandibular nerve. Dissection is carried out from cephalad to caudad along the internal jugular vein; fatty and lymphatic tissue is

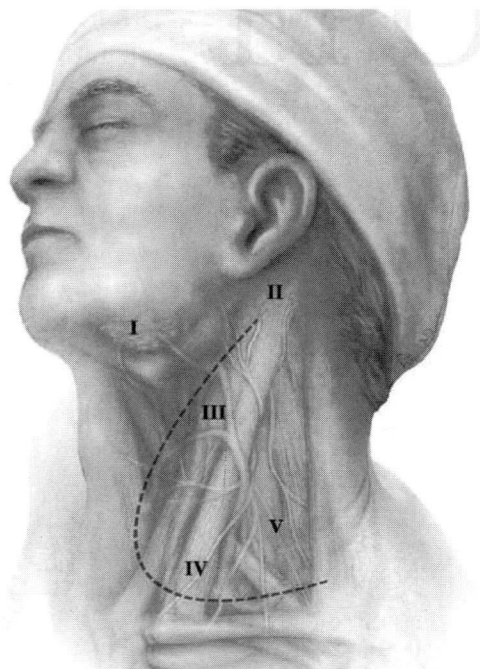

Figure 3 The author's preferred cervical incision, which should be inclusive of any previous biopsy site. The incision extends along the anterior border of the sternocleidomastoid and is carried laterally out over the clavicle.

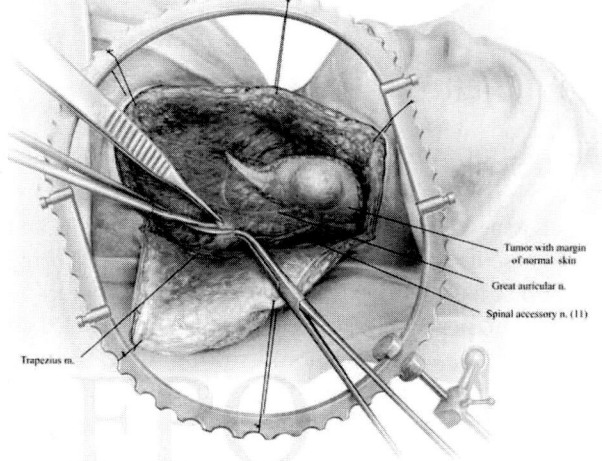

Tumor with margin of normal skin

Great auricular n.

Spinal accessory n. (11)

Trapezius m.

Figure 4 Rigid-ring retractor (Bookwalter) in place to assist with exposure.

reflected off the anterior and lateral borders of the vein and taken with the operative specimen (Figure 5). The vagus nerve is identified within the carotid sheath and preserved. The omohyoid muscle is divided medially as it passes over the internal jugular vein. Occasionally one will encounter gross disease extending into level VI (the central neck), into the upper mediastinum, or below the clavicle. The surgeon should be prepared to extend the operation to include these areas when indicated by preoperative clinical examination or imaging studies, or by intraoperative findings. Dissection is carried down to the base of the neck. During left neck dissection, the thoracic duct is identified as it enters the junction of the internal jugular vein and the subclavian vein at the inferomedial limit of dissection. An accessory thoracic duct may often be identified on the right side. In patients undergoing therapeutic neck dissection for clinically involved lymph nodes, these structures are generally ligated under direct vision. In patients undergoing lymphadenectomy for occult metastatic disease identified by sentinel lymph node biopsy, it may be preferable to leave the thoracic duct or accessory thoracic duct intact.

The specimen is dissected off the posterior aspect of the clavicle. The external jugular vein is divided inferiorly and the omohyoid muscle is divided laterally above the clavicle. The excised portions of the external jugular vein and the omohyoid muscle are resected en bloc with the operative specimen. A deep dissection plane is established just superficial to the deep cervical fascia overlying the scalene muscles. Underneath this fascia lie the brachial plexus, the phrenic nerve, and the transverse cervical vessels. These are preserved. Transverse cervical sensory roots traversing the specimen are divided as they are encountered, and dissection of the specimen is completed in a caudad to cephalad direction over the deep cervical fascia.

After removal of the operative specimen, the patient is placed in Trendelenburg's position and a "Valsalva" insufflation breath is administered by the anesthesia service. Any evidence for venous bleeding or lymphatic leak is identified and controlled by suture ligation at this time. In cases in which there are leaks from multiple lymphatic tributaries (as is sometimes encountered in patients following resection of bulky lymphadenopathy), the sternal head of the sternocleidomastoid muscle can be mobilized to buttress lymphatic closure. A 15F round, closed suction drain is positioned within the wound. The wound is then closed using 3-0 interrupted buried absorbable platysmal sutures and a 4-0 absorbable subcuticular skin suture.

Postoperative Care

Patients generally recover relatively rapidly from neck dissection. Most patients can be discharged the day following surgery. Wound drainage is continued until output is less than 30 cc per day. Drains can usually be removed within 1 week of operation. The overall complication rate for neck dissection is low. Complications include wound seroma, infection, spinal accessory nerve injury, and lymphatic leak. The risk of infection is generally quite low and the incisions almost always heal in a cosmetically satisfactory manner. Patients are routinely given a diet prior to discharge from the hospital, so that the character and volume of drain output can be evaluated for the presence of chyle, which indicates the presence of a lymphatic leak. In patients with low volume lymphatic leaks (< 200 cc per day), a conservative approach via a fat-restricted diet is indicated; the vast majority of these small leaks close spontaneously within a few days. In patients with a high volume lymphatic leak, we favor immediate surgical closure to avoid inflammatory wound problems as well as the inconvenience and anxiety associated with the need for long-term dietary restriction, intravenous hyperalimentation, and octreotide therapy.

EPITROCHLEAR DISSECTION

Patient Position

This type of dissection, as with the popliteal dissection, is relatively rarely performed. The recovery of nodes from these areas is low; however, there appears to have been an increase in the performance of these dissections since the advent of lymphatic mapping and sentinel node biopsy. The patient is positioned supine with the arms extended.

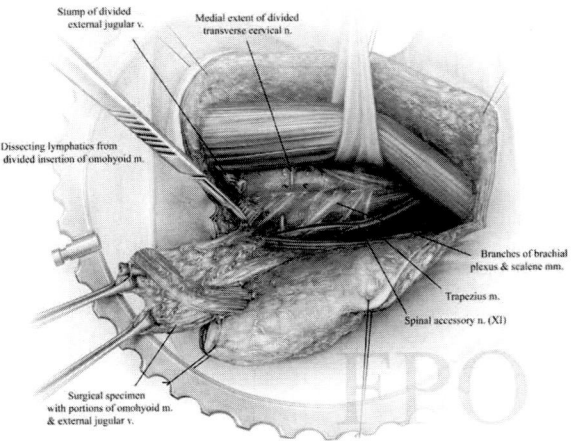

Figure 5 Lymphadenectomy specimen as it is retracted laterally and inferiorly.

If a concurrent axillary dissection is being performed, we plan for this and position the patient appropriately.

Patient Preparation and Draping

If the patient is not having a concurrent axillary lymphadenectomy, an extremity drape is an excellent choice for this procedure. We prep the entire arm up to the axilla and leave the entire distal extremity exposed. Alternatively, a stockinette can be used over the hand and distal forearm. If a concurrent axillary dissection is to be carried out, we generally perform the axillary dissection first, so as to limit interference from the drain in the epitrochlear basin while moving the arm to perform the axillary dissection.

Incision and Surgical Technique

The incision is started 8 cm above and slightly anterior to the medial epichondial and traverses in a slight "hockey stick" fashion across the antecubital fossae for a distance of 4 to 5 cm in the joint crease. The transverse portion of the incision is carried over the tendonous portion of the biceps muscle (Figure 6). Flaps are raised posteriorly to just behind the epichondial and anterolaterally over the biceps muscle. Nodal-bearing tissue is then dissected off the biceps and into the fossa. The fibrofatty, node-bearing tissue between the biceps and triceps muscles is dissected, identifying the brachial artery and vein, and median and ulnar nerves. These structures are all preserved. The nodal-bearing tissue is then swept distally off the vessels and nerves for the remainder of the dissection to the intersection of the biceps muscles and the wrist flexors (Figure 7). A 15F (or in smaller patients, particularly thin women, a 10F) round, fluted drain is placed, usually through an inferior (distal) separate stab wound, and anchored in place.

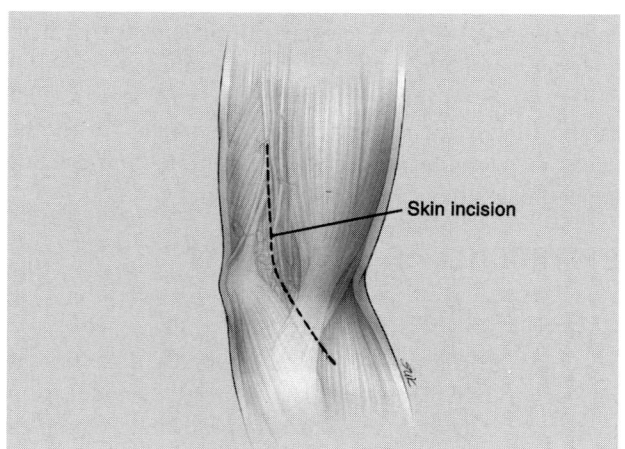

Figure 6 Incision for an epitrochlear dissection, carried medially across the biceps tendon.

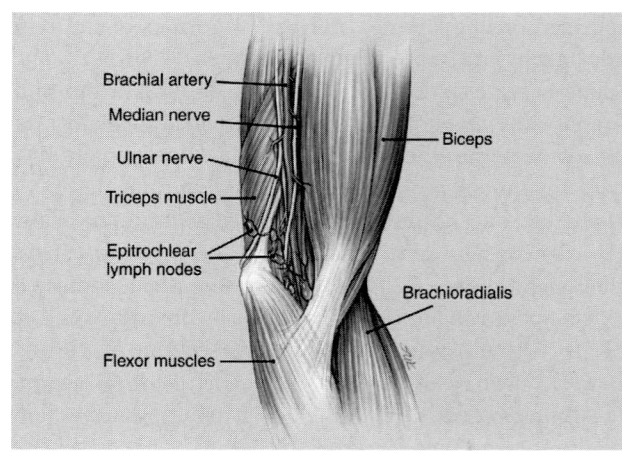

Figure 7 Location of nodal specimen from an epitrochlear lymphadenectomy.

Postoperative Care

Generally the patient remains hospitalized overnight. Drains remain in place until drainage is less than 20 cc/day (since this is generally a smaller space), which is usually a much shorter period than after axillary or inguinal lymphadenectomy, routinely less than a week. As with other regional lymphadenectomies, complications encountered most commonly are seroma or infection; lymphedema is a rare complication after epitrochlear dissection.

POPLITEAL DISSECTION

Patient Position

The patient is positioned prone, with all pressure points padded. The operative leg is slightly flexed at the knee. If a subsequent inguinal lymphadenectomy is being performed, we perform the popliteal dissection first.

Patient Preparation and Draping

The patient is prepped circumferentially from midthigh to the inferior aspect of the belly of the gastrocnemius muscle. A laparotomy sheet or a U-drape are excellent drapes for this procedure. Alternatively, cloth draping may be used as well.

Incision and Surgical Technique

The incision for popliteal dissection can be fashioned in one of two ways. We prefer a "lazy-S" incision from 10 cm above the joint crease on the lateral thigh (overlying the biceps femoris) in a longitudinal fashion, moving transversely across the joint and ending up 10 cm distal to the joint crease longitudinally along the medial aspect of the calf (overlying the gastrocnemius just medial to semimembranosis) (Figure 8). An alternative incision is the mirror image of this incision running from superiomedially to inferiolaterally. The choice of incision may be influenced by the orientation of any previous sentinel node biopsy incision.

Flaps are raised to incorporate a rectangle formed by imaginary extensions of the longitudinal limits of the incision. The goal of these flaps should be to expose the boundaries of the popliteal fossa, which includes the biceps femoris and semitendinosis muscles. Between these muscles, the tibial and common peroneal nerves are identified, exposed, and preserved. The fibrofatty, nodal-bearing tissue is swept from around the nerves and dissected distally while exposing the popliteal artery and vein and removing the nodal-bearing tissue from around them (it is important to address the tissue on the far side of the vessels, as the only nodes in the specimen may be in this area) (Figure 9). The inferior limit of dissection is where the vessels dive behind the gastrocnemius muscle. A round, fluted 15F drain is placed in the wound with the drain generally exiting inferiorly, and the wound is closed using 3-0 absorbable braided sutures in the deep dermis and a running subcuticular 4-0 monofilament suture.

Postoperative Care

Generally the patient remains hospitalized at least overnight. If a concurrent deep pelvic dissection has been performed (as would be the case if dissection was performed in the setting of clinically palpable inguinal adenopathy), the patient may be hospitalized longer, of course. Drains remain in place until drainage is less than 30 cc/day, which is usually a much shorter period than after axillary or inguinal lymphadenectomy. As with other regional lymphadenectomies, complications most commonly are seroma or infection; lymphedema is much

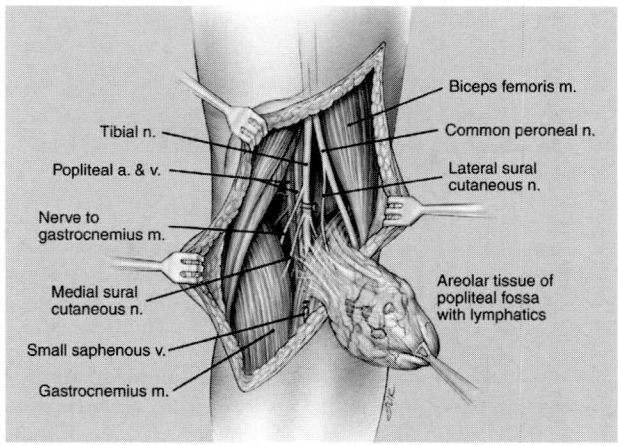

Figure 9 Borders of the dissection for a popliteal dissection along with a depiction of the nodal specimen.

less common after popliteal dissection. Particularly with the popliteal dissection, we find that ambulation is often more difficult, and thus get physical therapy involved shortly after surgery.

Summary

Regional lymphadenectomy is an important component of the comprehensive management of patients with melanoma. Surgical extirpation of all identified disease remains the most useful therapy for this disease. Knowledge of the anatomy of the regional nodal basins is essential to the successful completion of a formal lymph node dissection. As evidence mounts supporting the role of early lymphadenectomy in maximizing the clinical outcome of patients with regional nodal metastasis from melanoma, it is increasingly important that these procedures be performed by individuals knowledgeable about the disease and experienced with indications for surgical intervention, technical details of operative strategy, and appropriate postoperative management.

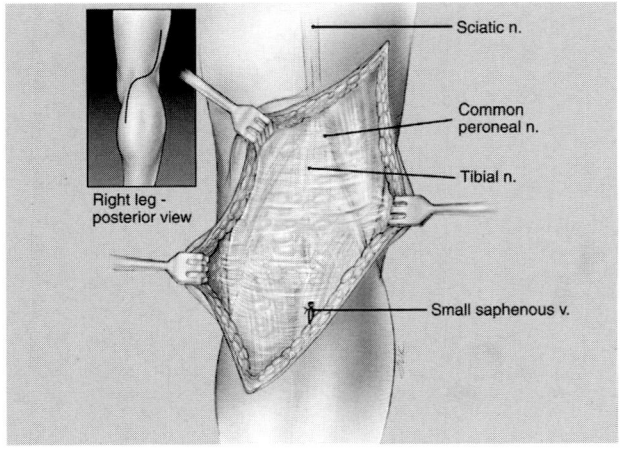

Figure 8 Incision for popliteal lymphadenectomy of the right leg.

References

1. Gershenwald JE, Colome MI, Lee JE, et al. Patterns of recurrence following a negative sentinel lymph node biopsy in 243 patients with stage I or II melanoma. J Clin Oncol 1998;16:2253–60.

2. Wagner JD, Ranieri J, Evdokimow DZ, et al. Patterns of initial recurrence and prognosis after sentinel lymph node biopsy and selective lymphadenectomy for melanoma. Plast Reconstr Surg 2003;112:486–97.

3. Murray DR, Carlson GW, Greenlee R, et al. Surgical management of malignant melanoma using dynamic lymphoscintigraphy and gamma probe-guided sentinel

lymph node biopsy: the Emory experience. Am Surg 2000; 66:763–7.

4. Thompson JF, Stretch JR, Uren RF, Ka VS, Scolyer RA. Sentinel node biopsy for melanoma: where have we been and where are we going? Ann Surg Oncol 2004;11:147S–51S.

5. Aloia TA, Gershenwald JE, Andtbacka RH, et al. Utility of computed tomography and magnetic resonance imaging staging before completion lymphadenectomy in patients with sentinel lymph node-positive melanoma. J Clin Oncol 2006;24:2858–65.

6. Miranda EP, Gertner M, Wall J, et al. Routine imaging of asymptomatic melanoma patients with metastasis to sentinel lymph nodes rarely identifies systemic disease. Arch Surg 2004;139:831–7.

7. Karakousis CP. Surgical procedures and lymphedema of the upper and lower extremity. J Surg Oncol 2006;93:87–91.

8. Serpell JW, Carne PW, Bailey M. Radical lymph node dissection for melanoma. ANZ J Surg 2003;73:294–9.

9. Ballo MT, Strom EA, Zagars GK, et al. Adjuvant irradiation for axillary metastases from malignant melanoma. Int J Radiat Oncol Biol Phys 2002;52:964–72.

10. Beitsch P, Balch C. Operative morbidity and risk factor assessment in melanoma patients undergoing inguinal lymph node dissection. Am J Surg 1992;164:462–6.

11. Hughes TM, Thomas JM. Combined inguinal and pelvic lymph node dissection for stage III melanoma. Br J Surg 1999;86:1493–8.

12. Karakousis CP, Heiser MA, Moore RH. Lymphedema after groin dissection. Am J Surg 1983;145:205–8.

13. Ballo MT, Zagars GK, Gershenwald JE, et al. A critical assessment of adjuvant radiotherapy for inguinal lymph node metastases from melanoma. Ann Surg Oncol 2004;11: 1079–84.

CHAPTER 84

REGIONAL THERAPY FOR INTRANSIT MELANOMA METASTASES

MERRICK I. ROSS, MD

Definitions and Prognosis

The clinical entity of intransit disease is a unique form of regional lymphatic spread of tumor manifesting as nodules in the dermis, subcutaneous tissue, or both. While it may develop in association with a variety of aggressive forms of cutaneous malignancies, either synchronous with the diagnosis of the primary or more frequently in the form of a relapse subsequent to the resection of the primary tumor, it most commonly develops in patients with melanoma.[1,2] Historically, regional cutaneous melanoma metastases had been defined arbitrarily according to their proximity to the primary lesion or wide excision site, as local recurrence, satellites, and intransit disease respectively, for closest to farthest away.[3] These designations are, in reality, just descriptive and have little prognostic relevance, as all three entities, regardless of their distance from the primary, are manifestations of the same biologic events (Figure 1). As a result, the most recent American Joint Commission on Cancer(AJCC) staging criteria includes all three entities in the Regional (N) classifications, as N2c and staged as either IIIb or IIIc depending on the absence or presence of lymph node metastases, respectively.[4] For simplicity purposes, the term intransits, is often used to represent the entire spectrum of regional

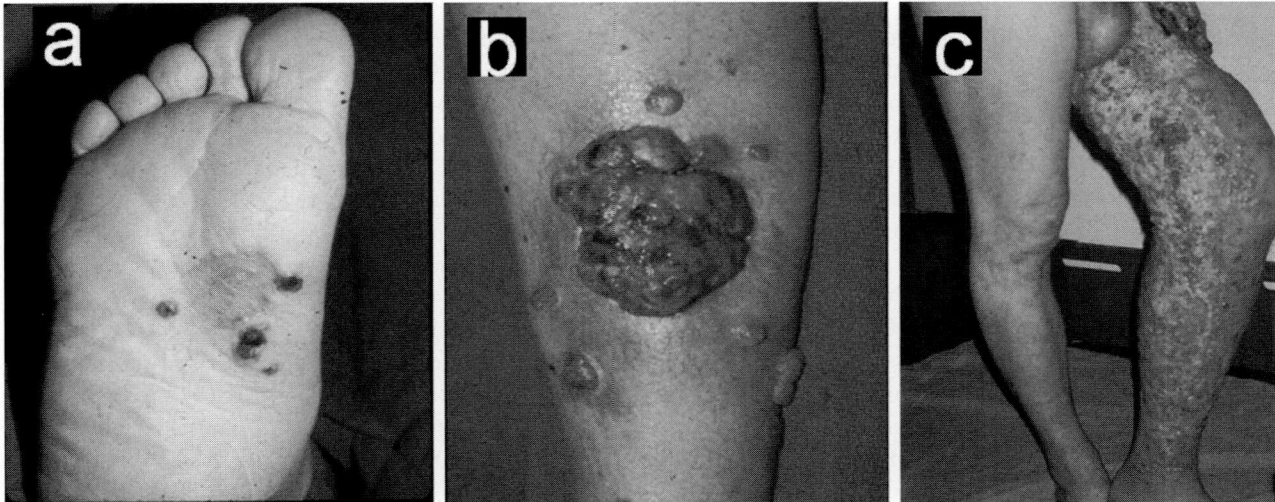

Figure 1 Examples of the clinical spectrum of in-transit disease: (a) local metastases, (b) local metastases and satellites, (c) diffuse in-transit disease; all of which represent manifestations of regional lymphatic spread and classified as AJCC sub-stage N2c.

cutaneous disease. Having said that, it is important to make a distinction between two different biologic entities that are referred to as a "local recurrence". Generally speaking, local recurrence has in the past been defined as any disease relapse that develops in or near the previous primary excision scar or skin graft site. The more common type of local recurrence is really a "local metastasis" and represents dermal lymphatic spread and is therefore part of the above described spectrum of intransit diseases. A "true" local recurrence is not very common and represents re-growth of residual primary disease in the dermis or at the epidermal/dermal interface left behind by an inadequate narrow excision 5 or as a result of a "field effect" of multi-focal atypical melanocytes. Pathologically, his entity may contain a primary junctional component (in-situ disease) with or without an invasive dermal component or a dermal component only. The prognosis is variable and most dependent on the constellation of tumor microstaging findings (thickness or ulceration) and other prognostic factors identified in the recurrent lesion.[5] Therefore, management of "true" local recurrence should be similar to what is recommended for primary melanomas.

Classically, intransit disease is characterized as occurring between the primary site and the ipsilateral regional nodal basin(s),[1] but may also develop solely or in part retrograde to the primary melanoma site, and/or in the soft tissue beyond the proximal basin. While the presentation of multiple tumor nodules is most common, they may occur as a single isolated site. While extremity lesions are clearly more frequent, particularly in the leg,[2] intransit disease may develop in association with or as a consequence of trunk and head and neck melanomas. Regardless of their presentation, such disease is generally a strong predictor of concurrent or subsequent distant metastase.[2-3] A recent study from the MD Anderson group assessed the factors associated with distant failure in patients who developed intransit disease. Based on univariate analysis the clinico-pathologic factors predicting distant relapse were, short disease-free interval (< 12 months) between primary surgery and the development of intransit disease, nodal involvement, subcutaneous location, and large volume of intransit metastases. Based on multivariate analysis the only factor that independently predicted distant relapse was large burden of intransit disease.[2]

While the risk for distant relapse is significant and therefore must be considered when recommending management strategies, treatment of the regional disease is important beacause if left untreated, it can be the source of significant morbidity in the form of bleeding, ulceration, pain, infection, soft tissue swelling, and ambulatory disability.

Incidence and Predictors of Intransit Disease

While intransit disease in general is considered an infrequent event, because among the entire primary invasive melanoma patient population the reported incidence is between 3%–10%,[1] certain high risk subgroups have been identified with higher incidence rates, and in actuality, intransit disease is observed in a significant proportion of the overall relapsing fraction of patients.[1-2]

While little information is available concerning how often newly diagnosed melanoma patients present with intransit metastases, a significant body of literature exists providing accurate incidence rates subsequent to appropriate primary tumor treatment obtained through the long term follow-up of newly diagnosed patients with primary invasive melanomas entered into prospective randomized margins of excision, adjuvant limb perfusion, and elective lymph node dissection trials.[6-10]

The results of 4 margins of excision trials have been published.[6-9] These trials were designed to evaluate the benefit of wider margins of excision in terms of local/regional control and survival within defined prognostic groups, primarily based on tumor thickness and stratified by the appropriate prognostic factors. Therefore, valuable natural history information was obtained. The incidence of intransit disease among the various study populations ranged from a low of 2.5% to a high of 6.3% as summarized in Table 1. These differences can be explained mostly by the differences in mean tumor thickness, ranging from 1.2 mm to 3.1 mm respectively. The adjuvant limb perfusion trial performed as a collaboration of the World Health Organization and the European Organization for the Research and Treatment of Cancer included 900 patients with primary melanomas of at least 1.5mm in thickness to receive wide excision only or wide excision plus adjuvant limb perfusion with Melphalan. The median tumor thickness was 2.8 mm and in the control arm (wide excision only) the intransit recurrence rate was 6.6%.[10]

Collectively, these data confirm that among the stage I and II melanoma population, the subsequent development of intransit disease is not a very common event, but an increased risk for such events is correlated with increasing tumor thickness. As described above, additional primary clinicopathologic factors reported to be associated with intransit recurrence are ulceration, lower extremity site, and nodal metastases.[2]

While these biologic predispositions have been demonstrated, some recent reports have suggested that the type of surgical treatment patients receive may increase the likelihood of developing intransit disease,

Table 1 Incidence of in-transit disease in stage I and II patients enrolled in prospective randomized surgical trials

Study	# Patients	Primary tumor thickness	Incidence
WHO	612	1.0 mm	2.5%
Swedish	989	1.2 mm	3.7%
UK MSG	900	3.1 mm	6.3%
WHO/EORTC	412	2.8 mm	
No ELND			6.6%
ELND			6.4%

In several large series that have reported the incidence of in-transit metastases, the incidence has ranged from 2.5% to 6.6% which clearly depends of the median tumor thickness.

particularly early surgical intervention in the major proximal regional lymph node basin and specifically sentinel lymph node biopsy followed by formal lympha-denectomy.[11–12] These communications suggest the hypothesis that interventions in the proximal nodal basin results in lymphatic stasis which in turn may promote the development of intransit disease. While a relatively high rate of intransit disease has been observed in patients undergoing a node dissection for a positive sentinel node, the authors incorrectly concluded this was a result of the surgical intervention rather than recognizing that these patients represent a high risk subset; thicker primary tumors and a high incidence of ulceration in addition to the fact that these patients manifested lymphatic dissemination as evidenced by the positive nodes.[13] The most contemporary information concerning the incidence and predictors of intransit disease comes from a study including almost 1400 primary melanoma patients all treated initially with wide excision and sentinel node biopsy.[2] The overall incidence of intransit disease was 6% and based on a multivariate analysis, the predictors were sentinel lymph node involvement, thickness, ulceration, lower extremity primary, and age greater than 50. This report also provided valuable information concerning the risk for distant relapse after the diagnosis of intransit disease. With a median follow-up of almost 4 years, slightly

more than 50% of the patients had developed distant disease.

An extension of this report was a result of a collaboration between the M.D. Anderson Cancer Center and the Sydney Melanoma Unit, involving more than 3400 primary melanoma patients treated between 1991 and 2001,[14] (Table 2). The majority of the patients underwent sentinel node biopsy as part of their initial surgical management, but many received wide excision only and more than 200 also received elective node dissection. When comparing the patients who were treated with wide excision only and the group who also were treated with sentinel node biopsy, both exhibited essentially identical primary tumor prognostic factors and an identical incidence of intransit disease.[14] The group of patients who received an elective node dissection as part of their initial surgical management were observed to have a slightly higher incidence of intransit disease. While one may conclude that the greater disruption of lymphatics caused by the full dissection is responsible for the higher intransit event rate, a more likely explanation is that this group had primary tumors that were thicker and had a higher incidence of ulceration than the other groups. Again, multivariate analysis demonstrated that the biologic factors predicted intransit disease rather than the type or extent of surgery in the proximal regional nodal basin.

Table 2 Incidence of in-transit disease according to type of primary surgical treatment MDACC/SMU* Database (N=3,413)

Treatment	# Patients	Thickness	Ulceration	ITM*
WLE	1,035	1.8 mm	24.5%	4.9%
WLE + SLNB	2,149	1.7 mm	22.3%	4.5%
WLE + ELND	229	2.8 mm	40.2%	5.7%

*ITM=in-transit metastases, MDACC/SMU=MD Anderson Cancer Center/Sydney Melanoma Unit
In the current era of lymphatic mapping and SLN bx there has been concern that early surgical intervention in the regional lymph node basins may increase the incidence of IT metastases by leading to disruption of lymphatics. In order to evaluate this further, melanoma patients who underwent surgical intervention at the MDACC or the SMU were combined and the incidence of in-transit metastases in 3 groups of patients was compared, those who underwent WLE alone, those who underwent WLE + SLNB, and those who underwent WLE + ELND. The overall rate of in-transit metastasis was 5.3% and was 4.9% for patients who underwent WLE alone, 4.5% in patients who underwent WLE + SLNB bx, and 5.7% in patients who underwent WLE + ELND. While the incidence of ITM was slightly greater in the WLE + ELND group, this is likely due to thicker primary tumors rather than surgical intervention in the RLN basin. These results suggest that it is tumor biology and not the surgical approach to the regional lymph nodes that determines the risk of IT disease.

Two subsequent reports have similarly not been able to correlate an increase risk of intransit disease with the use of sentinel node biopsy.[15-16]

Further evidence that early surgical intervention in the proximal regional lymph node basin does not promote the clinical appearance of intransit disease can be found in the long term follow-up of primary melanoma patients treated in two additional prospective randomized clinical trials, one addressing the role of adjuvant isolated limb perfusion and the other evaluating margins of excision and simultaneously the role of elective node dissection.[8,10] In the adjuvant perfusion trial the use of elective dissection was not randomized, but in approximately 50% of the patients the surgeon included an elective dissection as part of the initial surgical approach[10] and in the margins of excision trial, the role of elective dissection was the other main study endpoint and therefore, was part of the randomization scheme.[8] In both studies, when comparing the incidence of intransit disease in patients who received elective dissection to those who did not, no differences could be detected. Since an elective node dissection (a formal dissection) represents a more significant disruption of the lymphatics in the regional basin compared to performing a sentinel node biopsy and failed to result in an increased incidence of intransit disease argues strongly against the hypothesis offered by some authors that early mechanical interventions in the regional basin promotes intransit disease.

In summary, the vast majority of the credible available published evidence concerning the predictors of intransit disease in primary melanoma patients argues that it is the biologic events inherent in the primary lesion and the propensity for lymphatic spread of tumor cells that govern such events rather than the lymphatic obstruction that may be associated with performing a sentinel node biopsy.

Management of Intransit Metastases

Historically, the clinical spectrum of intransit disease is one that is feared because it not only represents a form of lymphatic dissemination and an associated risk for synchronous and metachronous distant disease, but it is very difficult to treat and continued regional progression is associated with significant morbidity. Since no clear evidence based standard of care exists, surgical strategies have been logically linked to the extent, the location, and perceived aggressiveness of disease, and therefore run the gamut from simple excision, to regional administration of chemotherapy, and in desperation to amputation. Other approaches have included a variety of systemic therapies (chemotherapy and/or immunother-

apy), intra-lesional injections of biologically active agents (BCG, IL-2, interferon, GMCSF), palliative radiotherapy, laser ablation, electroporation, or combinations of the above either in the context of formal clinical trials or off study in an attempt to find something that may result in a meaningful response and palliation.[17-24] This chapter will focus primarily on the surgical management of extremity intransit disease and discuss some of the guidelines for the use of surgical excision and the available techniques, effectiveness, and morbidity of approaches that utilize regional administration of chemotherapy, i.e. limb perfusion.

Surgical Excision of Intransit Disease

Simple surgical excision can be very effective as the primary modality used in the management of a selected population of patients with intransit disease. In patients with a limited number of nodules where a complete surgical removal with negative margins can be accomplished is a very rational first approach, particularly if the length of disease-free interval prior to the development of intransit disease is long. Such an approach is associated with little morbidity and is relatively inexpensive. Wide margins as recommended for primary melanomas is probably not warranted and may increase the surgical morbidity unnecessarily. While surgical excision is appealing, it should be recognized that these patients have a very high rate of intransit recurrence at other sites in the limb because of the high rate of associated sbuclinical multifocal micrometastatic dissemination. These patients have at least a 50% chance of distant relapse as well, therefore adjuvant systemic therapy such as interferon or participation in clinical trials should be considered. Prognosis of these patients is significantly influenced by the presence of concurrent or previous nodal disease, therefore in those patients who are clinically node negative some have advocated the use of sentinel lymph node staging simultaneous with the surgical excision.[25] In general, the sentinel node localizing agents are injected in proximity to the intransit disease rather than the original site of the primary melanoma.

If the volume of intransit disease is large enough or if multiple nodules are present but still realistically resectable, a clinical trial involving a planned resection to render the patient free of measurable disease, followed by an autologous vaccine made from the resected disease used post-operatively in the adjuvant setting, is an appealing approach as it combines modalities that address the regional disease as well as the systemic microscopic disease that is likely present. To that same end, these patients are also excellent candidates for neoadjuvant clinical trials. Systemic therapies can be administered with intact measurable disease to assess response to therapy and then used post-resection in the adjuvant setting if a pre-resection response is observed.

In patients who develop recurrent intransit disease subsequent to a previous resection, and most will, but manifest an indolent biology (small volume disease after a long disease-free interval) and still have not relapsed at distant sites, additional surgical resections offers a potentially effective treatment strategy that is inexpensive and very well tolerated. However, if multiple sites of intransit recurrences develop rapidly, then complete surgical resection is not only difficult to accomplish, but is doomed to fail. These latter more aggressive subsets represent the majority of patients with intransit disease and should be evaluated for more aggressive approaches such as regional administration of chemotherapy.

Regional Administration of Chemotherapy

While published experience with intra-arterial infusion of chemotherapy with or without the application of a proximal tourniquet,[26-27] most current approaches to the regional administration of chemotherapy as a treatment strategy for intransit disease include isolated limb perfusion (ILP) and the more recently described isolated limb infusion, better referred to as "minimally invasive" limb perfusion (MILP). Both approaches require placement of venous and arterial catheters in establishing a complete perfusion circuit and have the same goal: to delivery high dose chemotherapy to treat most of the limb while at the same time limit the systemic exposure of the drug. The isolation offers the therapeutic advantage of high concentration levels of chemotherapy (approximately a log higher than what would normally be given if that same chemotherapy was to be administered systemically) to increase the cell kill, without systemic toxicity. The rationale for perfusion is that the melanoma cells, which have rapid cell divisions, may be exquisitely sensitive to the high dose of chemotherapy, but the tissues of the limb, except for the skin, have relatively low cell division rates and are therefore relatively resistant to chemotherapy damage. Furthermore, historical experience with amputations as salvage treatment for extensive intransit disease demonstrate that cure rates of 21–33% can be achieved.[28-29] These data suggest that in at least some patients the disease is truly confined to the extremity and control or complete eradication of the regional disease can result in long term survival. Isolated limb perfusion attempts to accomplish such goals, but with limb preservation. Since the available systemic therapies used to treat metastatic melanoma offer only a 10%-15% complete response rate, interest has remained in evaluating regional approaches to this potentially very morbid disease process.[30]

Technical Aspects of Isolated Limb Perfusion

The concept and surgical approach is not new, as it was formally introduced by Creech in the 1950's.[31] As far as the traditional surgical approach is concerned (ILP) some modifications have been adopted, particularly in the sophistication of the monitoring systems used to detect leak of the perfusate from out of the limb to the systemic circulation. Heat was added to the regimen in 1969 with the intent of improving the response rate via the hypothesized mechanism of increasing the uptake of the chemotherapy into the melanoma cells and/or by acting synergistically with the chemotherapy as evidenced in pre-clinical models evaluating the role of heat along with alkylating agents.[32-33] While hyperthermia (39–40 degrees centigrade) is part of the "standard" regimen employed, based on reports claiming improved response rates,[1] no direct comparisons in prospective randomized trials have been carried out to confirm the benefit of adding heat to the perfusion circuit versus performing the perfusion in normothermic conditions. The most common circulation time utilized for drug exposure after the target temperature is reached is one hour. Flow rates are generally 400-600 cc/ min for the leg and 200-400 cc for the arm. A variety of agents have been used, including Melphalan, Nitrogen Mustard, Actinomycin D, and Cisplatin. Most of the experience in terms of response and tolerability has been with Melphalan. Dosing is determined according to the volume of the limb to be treated. The typical dose of Melphalan is 10 mg/liter of leg and 13 mg/liter of arm.

Logistically, the procedure is complicated and requires expertise from nuclear medicine, use of a gamma probe placed over the heart to detect and monitor for leak, and collaboration with a perfusionist to prime and maintain the extracorporeal oxygenated circuit. From a technical perspective, the traditional surgical approach is a demanding procedure with the most important component being the identification and surgical ligation of the collateral arterial and venous side branches along the main vessels to and from the leg or arm in order to accomplish complete isolation of the involved limb. Generally a formal lymph node dissection is performed not only for exposure to the vessels targeted for cannulation and to the collaterals, but also to remove metastatic nodal disease if present. When treating the lower extremity, access to the major vessels can be obtained at the level of the femoral triangle or the iliacs. This decision depends on whether or not nodal disease is present and whether a previous node dissection had been performed. If disease is present in the femoral triangle then a deep dissection is required as well as a superficial inguinal lymphadenectomy, and the perfusion is then easiest to perform at the level of the iliac vessels. If a previous superficial dissection has been performed, then again the iliac basin is the best choice. If a previous superficial and deep dissection has been performed, then the femoral basin is the preferred choice, as redo surgery in the groin is easier and safer at that level compared to redo surgery in the pelvis. If no prior lymph node dissection has taken place and no gross nodal metastases exists, then either approach is acceptable. In treating the arm, an infraclavicular approach to the axillary vessels is generally used.

After the dissection and ligation of the collaterals is accomplished and the cannulas are placed in the vessels (18 or 20 French in the vein and 12-18 French in the artery), an Esmarc or pneumatic tourniquet is placed tight and as proximal as possible around the limb to control the cutaneous collaterals; this completes the isolation. Isolation is critical for two reasons: it avoids systemic toxicity and probably enhances the response rate by keeping the drug concentration in the limb high. A schematic of a completed perfusion set-up is illustrated in Figure 2. Leakage of the perfusate from the limb to the systemic circulation can cause two problems: increase the chance of systemic toxicity and reduce the circulating absolute drug dose in the limb. Such an event is detected by employing a monitoring system that includes the use of red blood cells obtained from the patient that are radio labeled in the Nuclear Medicine department, most commonly with Technitium 99. The radiolablled blood is then delivered to the patient in 2 aliquots, one given systemically and the other in the isolated circuit. A gamma probe is placed over the heart for continuous monitoring for leak, which is detected by a continuous rise in radioactive counts over time. The percent leak is determined by knowing the ratio of radioactivity administered in the circuit to that administered systemically. Generally, a 10 to 1 ratio is easiest to back calculate, as a 10% leak is present when a doubling of the background systemic counts is observed. A leak can occur from the systemic circulation into the circuit as well, which is detected by a gain in volume of the circuit. Avoiding leakage of systemic volume into the perfusion circuit is important so as not to dilute out the concentration of the drug.

The most radical modifications to ILP were developed at the Sydney Melanoma Unit and first reported in 1998 [34-35]. The motivations for change were to make the

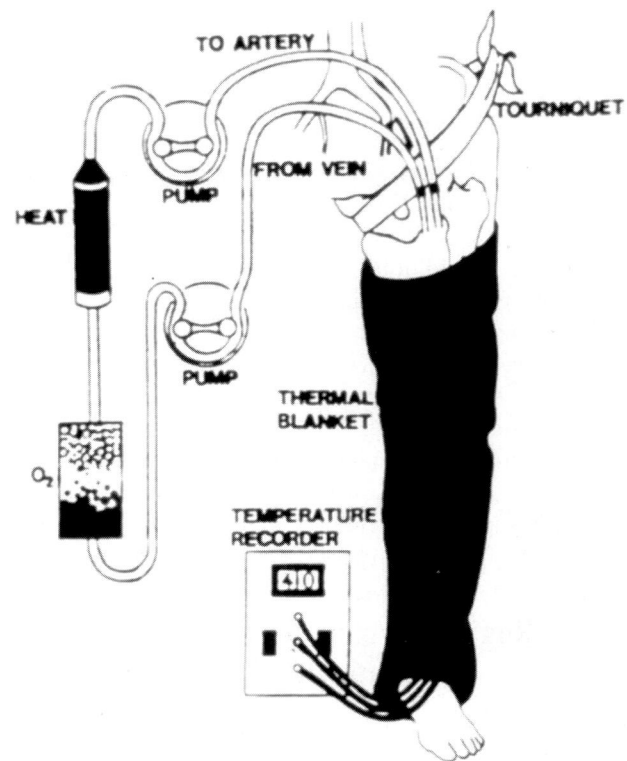

Figure 2 Schematic of perfusion technique. Surgical exposure of the femoral artery and vein is depicted with large bore intra-luminal cannulas secured in place. The cannulas are attached to an extracorpeal pump oxygenator to complete the circuit. A tourniquet is placed around the most proximal aspect of the limb adjacent to the inguinal ligament to complete the isolation. A warming blanket is placed circumferentially around the limb. The chemotherapy is administered through the arterial port and then circulated for one hour at a flow rate of 400-600cc/min.

procedure logistically less complicated, reduce operating room time, reduce costs, and obviate the need for a leak monitoring system. The other motivation for modifying the technique was that preclinical data demonstrated that response rates to melphalan may be enhanced in an anaerobic/acidic environment. As a result, John Thompson studied a minimally invasive approach using small catheters placed percutaneously by interventional radiology and a pneumatic tourniquet that ensures isolation of a low flow non-oxygenated perfusion circuit that is manually circulated with a syringe and stop cocks instead of an extracorporeal pump. The catheters are placed with fluoroscopic guidance through the groin of the uninvolved leg or either groin for an arm perfusion. A schematic and an intra-operative photograph of a completed MILP circuit is depicted in Figures 3 and 4 respectively. The arterial catheter is placed antegrade and the venous catheter retrograde. The low flow (80-120 cc/min) circulation time is 30 minutes, and the ischemia

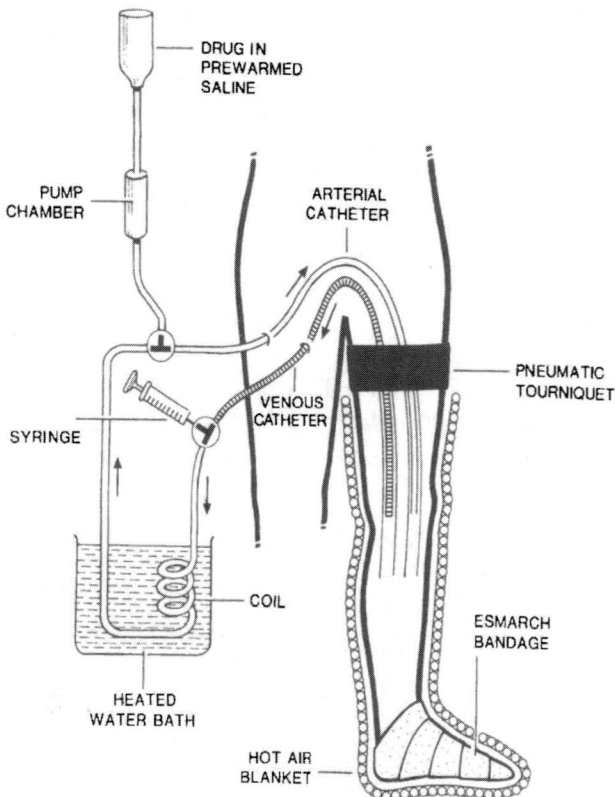

Figure 3 Schematic of MILP set-up. The small bore venous and arterial catheters are placed by interventional radiology through the opposite groin to a level in the limb to be treated below the planned placement of a pneumatic tourniquet. A syringe is attached to the venous port in order to manually circulate the pefusate by drawing from the venous side. The perfusate is heated as it passes through a heating chamber en-route from the venous side to the arterial side. The limb is heated with a warming blanket. The chemotherapy is administered through the arterial port of the circuit.

time ranges from 60-80 minutes, with the resultant PH ranging from 7.0-7.2.

Indications for Limb Perfusion

The use of limb perfusion when measurable intransit disease is present is termed a "therapeutic" perfusion. Appropriate candidates include patients with multiple intransit metastases that realistically are not amenable to surgical resection. A careful staging work-up for distant metastases is mandated to determine if the perfusion is to be carried out with curative intent in addition to an attempt at local regional control and palliaition. Location of the disease within the limb is important. Patients with lesions that are present high and lateral on the extremity will not be included within the perfused area and are therefore not good candidates.

In some patients distant disease may already be present, but the disease in the limb is progressing and causing significant morbidity while the distant disease is limited and asymptomatic. In these palliative situations, establishing a treatment plan that addresses the major symptom complex is rational and furthermore the severe pain, ulceration, bleeding, and infection often associated with extensive intransit disease may limit the ability to administer aggressive forms of systemic therapy. The use of perfusion may effectively control the disease in the limb, at least for a period of time, improve the quality of life, and allow access to a wider range of systemically administered regimens.[36]

Perfusions have also been carried out to prevent recurrence (adjuvantly) in patients identified as having a high risk for developing intransit disease as a major component of or the sole site of first relapse. The goal of adjuvant perfusion is not only to provide durable control of local and regional disease, but also to impact survival by preventing potential sources of future distant failure.

While little formal data is published concerning the effectiveness of perfusion used in the palliative setting, a reasonable body of literature exists concerning the effectiveness of limb perfusion used with curative intent in both the therapeutic and adjuvant settings.

RESULTS OF THERAPEUTIC LIMB PERFUSION

Historically, the reported overall and complete clinical response rates have been 60%–80% and 30%–60%, 1 respectively with ILP using either melphalan as a single agent or in combination with actinomycin and or nitrogen mustard. Some experience with Cisplatin has been reported, but has not been widely used because of higher incidence of severe regional toxicity.[37] As a result, most of the available response data is with melphalan. Initial studies using single agent melphalan at normothermic conditions revealed overall responses ranging from 30%–60% with half of these being complete.[38] In contrast, systemic chemotherapy typically results in less than a 10% complete response rate. It is therefore not surprising that interest persisted in evaluating ILP. The addition of heat to the regimen appeared to increase the overall response rates to approximately 80–90% and CR rates from 25%–60% 1. Various levels of heat, defined as mild hyperthermia (39–40), borderline hyperthermia (40–41), and hyperthermia (41–43) have been utilized. While mild and borderline hyperthermia are reported to result in higher responses than normothermia (37–38), no apparent additional benefit was observed when absolute hyperthermia (42 degrees) was employed, (table 3).[38–41] In contrast, a retrospective study from the

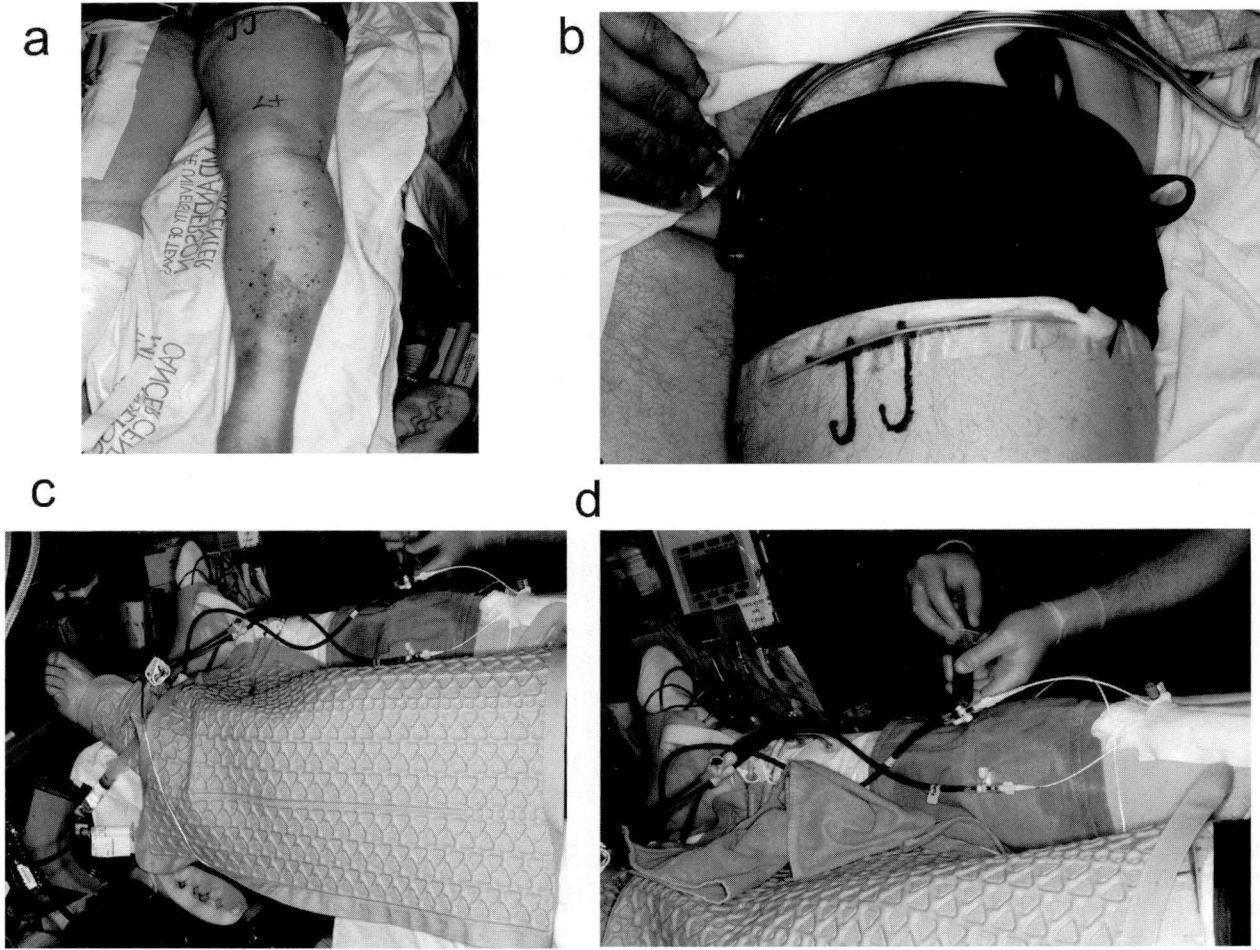

Figure 4 Actual patient undergoing MILP for multiple dermal in-transits below the knee. In (a) the patient has returned from interventional radiology after the catheters have been placed. Panel (b) is a close-up demonstrating the placement of the pneumatic tourniquet and a radio-opaque marker at its inferior extent. This is used as a guide to ensure the tips of the catheters are distal to the tourniquet. The warming blanket around the treated limb is shown in panel (c). In (d) the perfusate is being circulated manually using a syringe attached to the venous port.

Netherlands compared the results of 218 patients treated with mild hyperthermia to 166 patients treated under normothermic conditions failed to reveal any obvious improved responses.[42] An example of a complete response after ILP is shown in figures 5 and 6. Durability of response has not been consistently reported, but common times for relapse in the extremity are between 18–24 months.[38–39] Some investigators have studied a planed double perfusion with some success in terms of feasibility without significantly increasing toxicity.[43] Repeat ILP has also been studied after an initial response and subsequent relapse.[44] A good initial

Table 3 Selected ILP trials with Melphalan: response according to temperature

ILP temperature	Procedure #	CR%	PR%	OR%	Duration of Response (mos)	Author
Normothermia (37–38°C)	58	41	24	65	6	Klaase 1994
Mild hyperthermia (39–40°C)	103	76	23	99	10	Lingam 1996
Borderline hyperthermia (40–41°C)	105	73	13	86	10	Thompson 1997
Hyperthermia (41.5–43°C)	119	46	40	86	ns	Di Filippo 1998
		41–76%		65–99%	6–10 mos	

This table summarizes some of the larger trials of ILP using Melphalan alone. These were performed at varying degrees of hyperthermia, but it has been shown that higher temperatures do lead to an increased risk of Grade IV and V toxicity. Therefore, current ILPs are performed using mild hyperthermia.

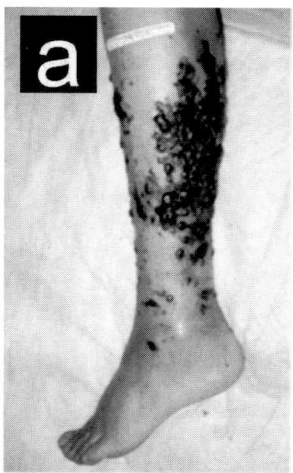
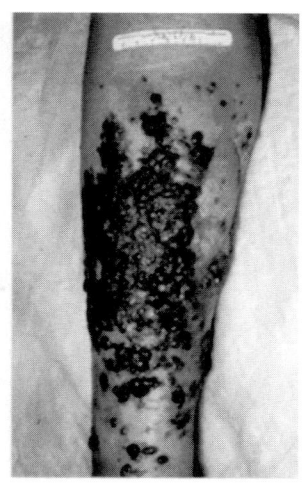
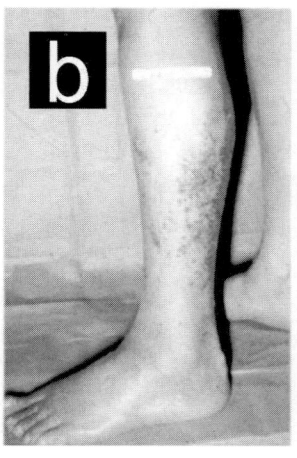
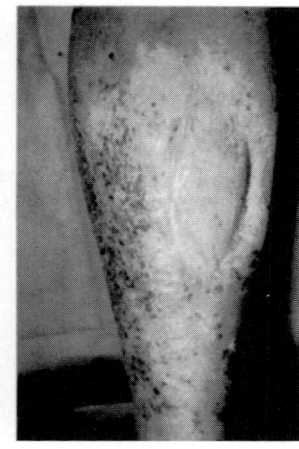

Figure 5 Typical response to hyperthermic limb perfusion with melphalan in this patient with extensive superficially located in-transit disease. Pre-treatment extent of disease is shown in (a) and post-perfusion response in (b) where all that remains is pigmented macrophages in the dermis.

response is generally predictive of another meaningful response.[45]

The most exciting experience was reported in 1992 with the addition of Tumor Necrosis Factor (TNF) to melphalan studied in a relatively small number of patients. In this report, 19 melanoma patients with measurable intact intransit disease were treated with a regimen of preoperative systemically administered gamma interferon and a combination of melphalan and TNF in the perfusion circuit, demonstrating an overall and complete response of 100% and 89%, respectively.[46] This report stimulated a renewed interest in regional therapy followed by a number of clinical trials performed in Europe and in the United States, (Table 4). The 89% CR rate was subsequently confirmed with this regimen in a multi center phase II study in Europe.[47] Figure 7

illustrates the type of response observed with the addition of TNF. In Italy a phase I/II study evaluated various doses of TNF with CR rates ranging from 53%–70%.[48] In the United States, Fraker etal conducted another phase I/II study evaluating two doses of TNF; the regimen previously studied in the Europe and a larger dose, and reported CR rates of 36%–76%[49]. To test the importance of including gamma interferon in the regimen a phase III trial was performed comparing melphalan with TNF versus the triple drug therapy.[50] The results demonstrated a trend for an improved response rate with the addition of gamma interferon, but this difference was not statistically significant. Furthermore, best CR rate in either treatment arm was 78%, essentially identical to that achieved in the US with a similar TNF regimen.

While CR rates were generally higher with TNF containing regimens compared to previously observed CR rates with melphalan alone, regional toxicity appeared to be higher. More regional toxicity could partly be explained by the fact that more meticulous attention was directed to the technical aspects of the procedure in order to avoid the hypotension and potentially lethal events that could be associated with leakage of TNF from the limb to the systemic circulation; which not only ensures high TNF concentration levels in the circuit but also high Melphalan concentration levels. The higher Melphalan levels achieved as a result of more meticulous surgical techniques employed when TNF is added to the perfusion circuit could in part be responsible for the higher response rates observed. To directly address this issue , a phase III randomized trial comparing the triple drug TNF containing regimen (melphalan, TNF and gamma interferon) versus melphalan alone was designed to determine if the TNF results were truly better, and therefore worth the potential for increased regional toxicity, or merely a consequence of more meticulous isolation resulting in a higher chemotherapy concentration in the limb. This trial was stopped early because the supply of TNF utilized for this trial was exhausted, but 103 patients were randomized, and the initial analysis demonstrated a significant improvement in regional complete responses with TNF (56% vs 72%), but similar overall response rates.of 94%.[51] This trial also showed that the higher response rates with TNF compared to Melphalan alone were observed primarily in patients with larger tumor burden. Subsequently, another multi center randomized trial was performed in the United States through the American College of Surgeons Oncology Group ACOS-OG, again to study the impact of adding TNF to the Melphalan regimen, but stratified according to tumor burden (Figure 8). This trial was somewhat different than the previous trial, as interferon gamma was not

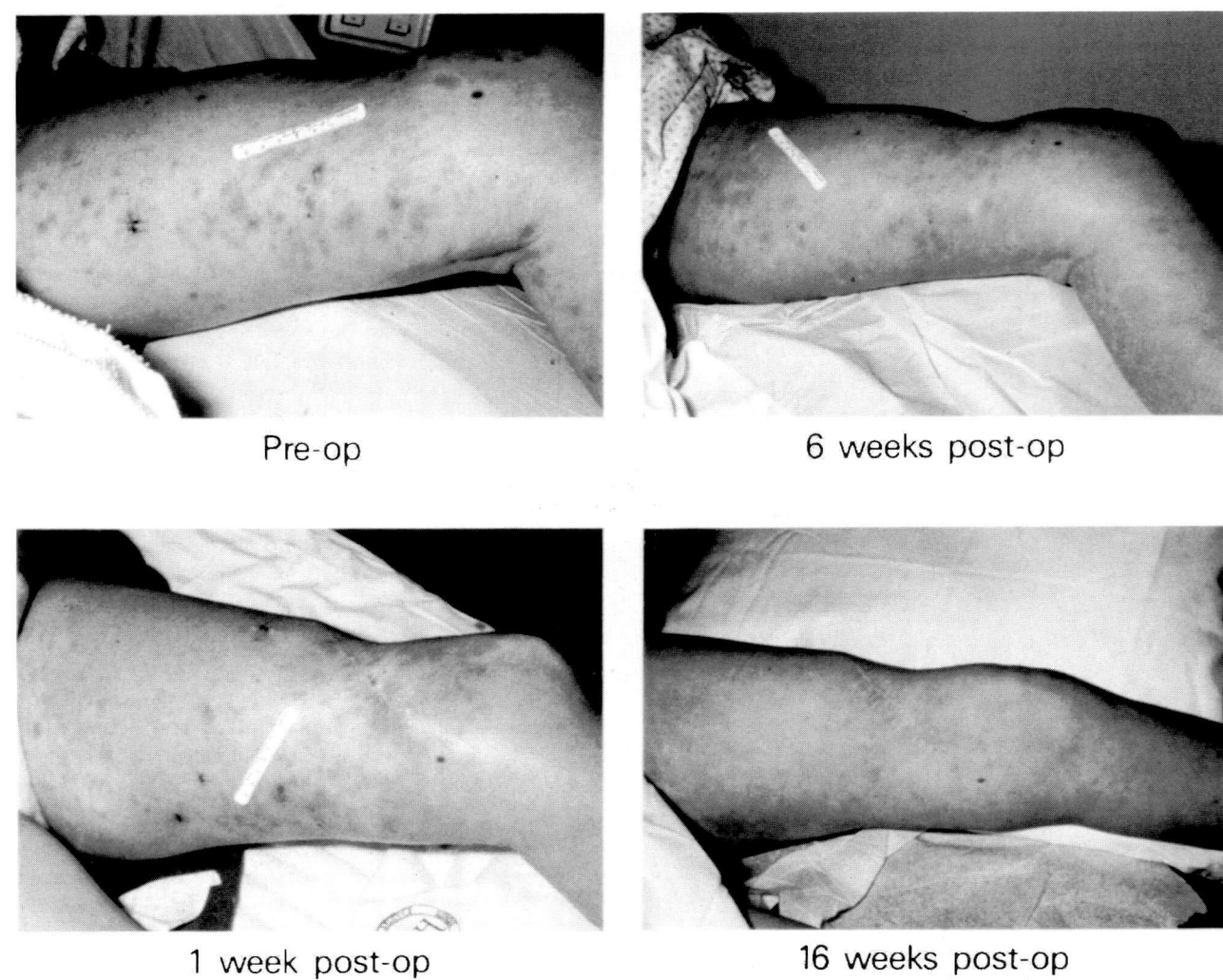

Figure 6 Time course of complete clinical response to melphalan perfusion is illustrated in the four panels above in this patient with extensive sub-dermal in-transit metastases in the medial thigh.

included in the TNF regimen. This modification was based on findings from a randomized trial in Europe that compared the TNF regimen with and without gamma interferon which demonstrated a lack of superiority with interferon gamma, as described above. The overall and complete response at three months were 68% and 25%, respectively.[30] No obvious difference was observed in the TNF containing treatment arm. However, at six months follow-up the durable complete response rate was higher with TNF, but this was not statistically significant, (Table 5). Possible explanations as to why this trial in particular resulted in lower response rates compared to the previous US randomized trial and several of the published European trials with TNF include: patient selection, differences in response criteria, and possibly an under-appreciation for the value of systemically admi-

nistered gamma interferon prior to the perfusion. While the US randomized trial is notably the outlier to date, a more recently published experience from Great Britain reported an overall and complete response rate of 77% and 40%, respectively in 30 patients treated with an ILP regimen of melphalan and TNF.[52] Like the most recent US randomized trial, gamma interferon was not part of the treatment.

Over the past few years, interest in the MILP approach to the regional administration of chemotherapy has increased since the initial publication from the group in Australia.[34] They reported an overall response rate of 85% with more than half being complete responses. Their experience with MILP fared well when compared with their prior experience with ILP (Table 6). Advanced disease stage and extensive limb tumor burden predicted inferior

Table 4 Results of ILP with Melphalan + TNF with and without interferon gamma

Author	Procedure #	CR%	PR%	OR%	Duration of Response (mos)	IFN gamma + or −
Lienard 1992	19	89	11	100	>8	+
Lienrd 1994	58	88	12	100	26	+
Fraker 1996	26	76	16	92	ns	+
Lienard 1999	64	73	22	95	14	+
Fraker 2002	53	72	21	93	ns	+
Corbett 2006	58	26	43	69	ns	−
Hays 2007	30	40	33	77	ns	−

The clinical trials of Melphalan + TNF ILP that followed demonstrated significantly better complete and overall response rates than with Melphalan alone ranging from 59 – 90% for CR and 64 – 100% for OR. In addition, the responses appeared to be more durable.

The Fraker study which was carried out at the NCI was actually a dose escalation study of TNF in which 12 patients were treated with 6mg rather than 4mg of TNF. However, the complete response rate was better in those patients who received 4mg of TNF.

The Lienard study, published in 1999 was a radomized Phase III trial that compare Melphalan + TNF ILP with and without interferon gamma. This study concluded that there was no significant contribution from interferon gamma.

However, none of these studies were randomized to compare Melphalan ILP alone to Melphalan + TNF ILP

responses. One of the theorized advantages of this approach was the opportunity to more easily carry out repeat perfusions. Unfortunately, a report from the same group that summarized the results of patients treated with two planned perfusions several weeks' apart demonstrated slightly increased toxicity without significantly improving responses.[53] Some centers in the US have adopted the minimally invasive approach in place of the traditional ILP, particularly for patients with disease that is more distal in the extremity. Collectively, more than 100 patients from three institutions have been treated with preliminary results similar to those from Australia.[54–55]

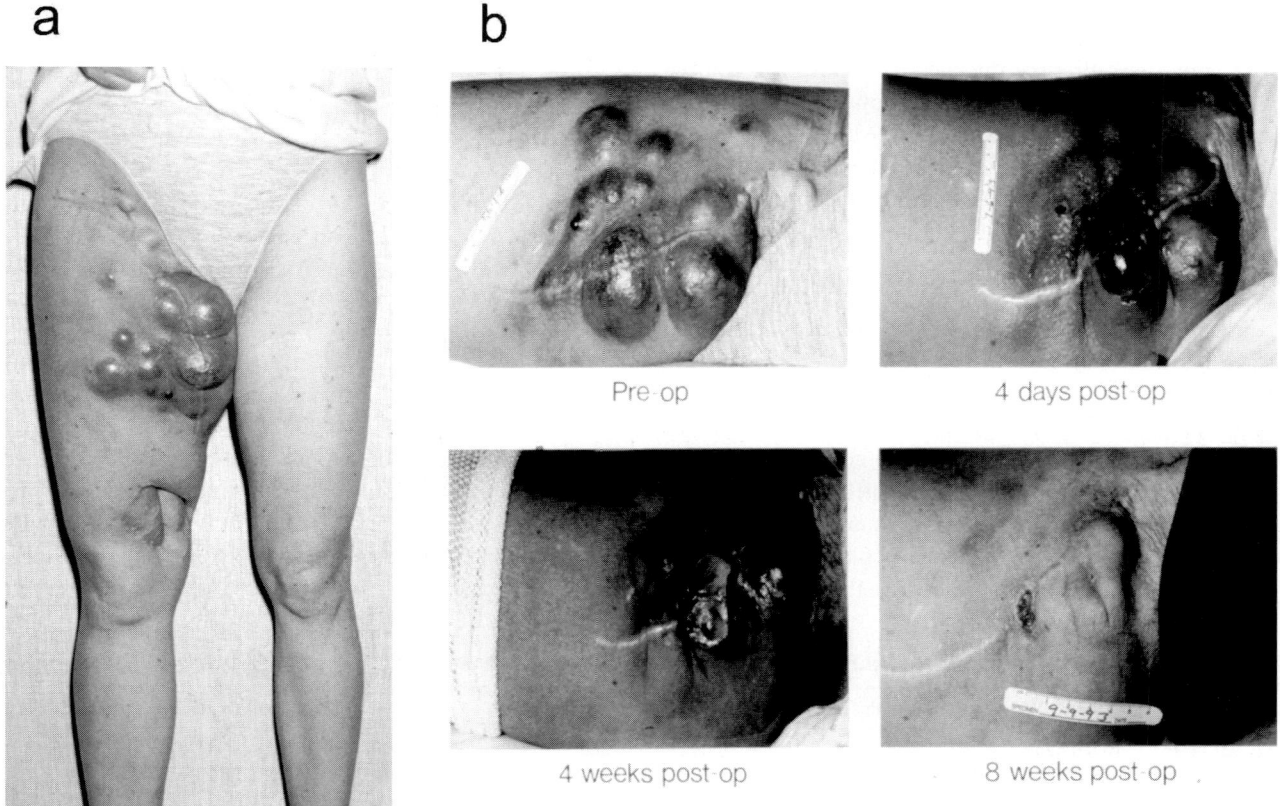

Figure 7 Patient with very bulky in-transit disease in (a) with rapid time to the onset of tumor necrosis shown in the four (b) panels after perfusion, typical of responses observed with TNF containing perfusion regimens.

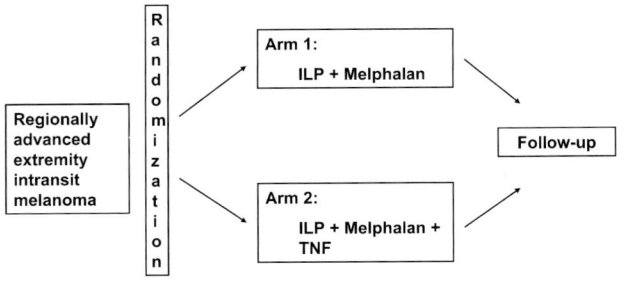

Figure 8 Randomization schema of the ACOS-OG trial comparing the efficacy of ILP with Melphalan alone versus melphalan plus TNF in the treatment of measurable extremity intransit disease.

RESULTS OF ADJUVANT LIMB PERFUSION

The role for adjuvant limb perfusion has been evaluated in only 2 prospective randomized trials. Because of limitations in trial design, the questions of whether or not limb perfusion can prevent intransit disease which in turn may improve survival has not been adequately addressed.

The larger of the two trials, which included almost 900 patients, was carried out through a collaboration between the WHO and the EORTC 10(Figure 9). The phase III design included patients with clinically localized primary melanoma with Breslow thickness >1.5mm, randomized to receive a wide excision of the primary alone or wide excision plus adjuvant limb perfusion with Melphalan. The results revealed a significantly reduced incidence of intransit disease as well as a prolongation in time to intransit failure in the perfusion treatment arm, but no difference in time to or incidence of distant relapse. As a result, the authors appropriately concluded that routine adjuvant perfusion could not be justified in patients with stage II melanoma. In retrospect, the patient population targeted in the study was not high risk for the development of intransit disease. As would have been predicted, the incidence of intransit disease in the control population (median tumor thickness of 2,8 mm) was only 6.6%, hardly a high enough risk to adequately test whether prevention of such intransit events could impact survival. Interestingly, the perfusions did reduce the intransit rate by

Table 6 Single institution results comparing ILP and MILP responses (Sydney Melanoma Unit)

Type of Response	ILP	MILP
CR	58%	41%
PR	27%	44%
OR	85%	85%

50% to 3.3%. While this was statistically different, it was probably not clinically relevant. If one could extrapolate a 50% risk reduction in intransit recurrrence in an identifiable high risk group with at least a 50% incidence of intransit disease, not only may the survival analysis be different, but the routine use of perfusion in this setting may be justified purely on the basis of preventing a potentially morbid and quality of life impacting disease recurrence. Such a high risk group was the focus of interest in the other aforementioned prospective randomized adjuvant perfusion trial. The Swedish Melanoma Study Group enrolled 86 patients with resectable intransit disease to receive excision of the intransit recurrence alone or resection with perfusion. The results demonstrated a significantly improved disease-free survival, but only a trend for improved overall survival,[56] figure 10. Unfortunately the study was small and therefore underpowered. A multi-center experience with limb perfusion utilized after resection of multiple episodes of intransit recurrences resulted in prolonged limb disease-free intervals.[57] While this was not a randomized trial this experience highlights the potential benefit for adjuvant perfusion in high risk patients.

The future for adjuvant perfusion, if any, is currently unknown, but some interest has re-emerged in using the minimally invasive approach described above to study adjuvant perfusion in a cohort of patients predicted to have a high risk for intransit disease as the first site of relapse.

Toxicity of Limb Pefsusion

Acute limb toxicity following perfusions has been graded according to definitions by Wieberdink.[58] Grades 1-V are defined in Table 7 and range from skin erythema to extensive tissue necrosis necessitating amputation respectively. Fortunately, the incidence of the most severe

Table 5 Results of randomized trial of ILP with melphalan alone versus melphalan plus TNF alpha (ACOSOG Z0020 trial)

Response	3-Month Follow-up			6-Month Follow-up		
	Melphalan (N = 58)	Melphalan + TNF (N = 58)	p-value	Melphalan (N = 44)	Melphalan + TNF (N = 45)	p-value
CR	24%	26%	.890	20%	42%	.101
PR	38%	43%		27%	13%	
OR	62%	69%	.435	48%	56%	.460

Trial was halted due to no evidence of clinical efficacy from TNF.

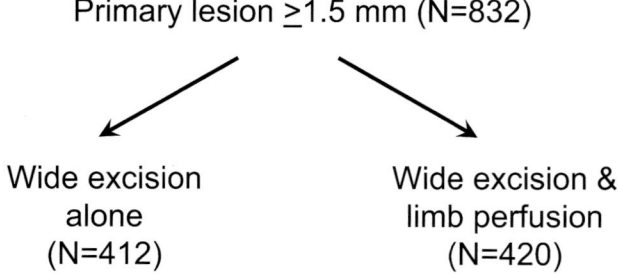

Figure 9 Randomization schema of WHO- EORTC adjuvant ILP protocol in patients with primary melanoma >1.5 mm in thickness.

regional toxicity is generally less than 3%[59] and assuming that complete isolation has been accomplished, systemic toxicity should be non-existent.[60] Creatinine Kinase (CPK) levels and frequent physical examinations in the post-perfusion setting has been the mainstay for the detection of muscle injury and the development of compartment syndrome for the purpose of early intervention with fasciotomies to avoid the devastating

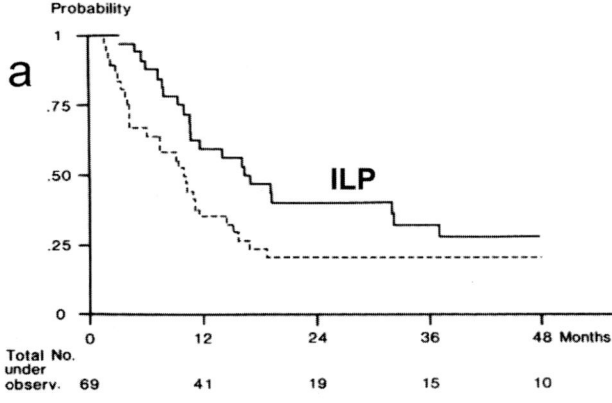

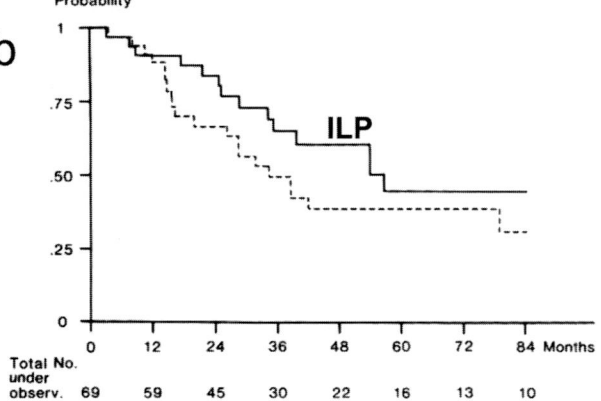

Figure 10 Results of small randomized trial of adjuvant ILP in patients undergoing resection of intransit disease. In (a) a significant improvement in limb-free survival is illustrated with ILP. In (b) a trend for improved survival is observed in the ILP treatment arm.

Table 7 Classification grading of acute tissue reactions after limb perfusion

Grade I	No reaction
Grade II	Slight erythema and/or edema
Grade III	Considerable erythema and/or edema with some blistering; slightly disturbed motility permissible
Grade IV	Extensive epidermolysis and/or obvious damage to the deep tissues, causing definite functional disturbances; threatening or manifest compartmental syndromes
Grade V	Reaction that may necessitate amputation

Adopted from Wieberdink et al., EJCCO 1982, 18:905-910.

In 1982 Wieberdink performed a series of ILPs in x number of patients and developed a toxicity grading system for acute regional tissue reactions after ILP. This grading system is divided into 3 grades with the goal to maintain toxicity at grade 3 or less. This grading system is still used today to describe toxicities from ILP. One of the major drawbacks of this grading system is that it is very subjective and does not take into account more objective information such as CK levels, Limb circumference, and compartment pressures.

In 1982, Wieberdink published a paper that focused on acute regional toxicity following ILP and its relationship to melphalan dosing in an attempt to develop more uniform and standardized melphalan dosing. Wieberdink classified acute regional toxicity into 5 grades which are listed here in this table. The standard dosing of melphalan usually maintains acute regional toxicity in grades I-III. One of the drawbacks of this classification system is that it is subjective. Using this classification system, however, has enabled investigators to refine ILP to maximize tumor response while limiting increases in toxicity.

progression to extensive soft tissue loss and eventual amputation.[61] Relatively high CPK levels may occur in the absence of compartment syndrome but are still reflective of muscle injury and its associated rhabdomyolysis. In order to avoid impairment of kidney function the rate of intravenous fluid administration is increased and alkalinization of the urine may be protective. Some groups institute steroids to limit the muscle inflammation and injury. Based on the SMU experience, MILP is associated with a very low incidence of severe acute reactions, as shown in Table 8. A recent report from the combined MILP experience form MD Anderson and Duke has compared the toxicity and hospital stay after traditional ILP and MILP and summarized in table 9. Surprisingly, hospital stays were significantly longer with MILP at a median of 7 days versus 5 days for those who underwent ILP. The hospital stay for the traditional approach was mainly for recovery from the surgical procedure and after the minimally

Table 8. Acute regional toxicity results after MILP (Sydney Melanoma Unit)

Acute Regional Toxicity	# Patients (N=135)
Grade I	1 (1%)
Grade II	55 (41%)
Grade III	72 (53%)
Grade IV	7 (5%)
Grade V	0

Table 9 Results of combined MDACC-Duke MILP series compared to ILP

Variable	MILP	ILP	
Age	67 (range 32-87)	65 (range 35-83)	
Gender	21 female, 32 male	22 female, 28 male	
Extremity treated	43 lower, 10 upper	47 lower, 3 upper	
CPK peak POD (median)	4 (1.5–7.5d)	1 (0.5 – 1.5d)	P<0.0001
CPK peak value (median, u/L)	1616 (95- 35,194)	545 (151-8409)	P<0.02
Length of stay (median, days)	7 (5 - 10d)	5 (4 - 15d)	P<0.02
WBT grades 1-3	50 (92%)	50 (100%)	
WBT grade 4	3 (6%)	0	
WBT grade 5	0	0	

Zager et al., SSO Mar 2006.

invasive approach it was for monitoring of toxicity because of a later time to develop muscle injury and CPK elevations.[55] Figure 11 demonstrates the differences in CPK elevation time kinetics between the two approaches.

The long term morbidity and health related quality of life after perfusion has been recently studied.[62–63] While long term side effects such as edema, muscle atrophy, decreased range of motion, and limb discomfort, as reported by the patients were not uncommon, they were mild and well tolerated and had little impact on the quality of life assessments.[64]

Future Goals

Perfusion based treatment of intransit melanoma is an excellent model for studying novel anti-neoplastic agents and regimens in both the pre-clinical and patient care settings. Easy access to tumor for biopsies pre and post treatment and the ability to easily monitor response with either physical examination, photography, and/or radiographic imaging makes this model attractive in terms of studying biochemical and molecular markers of response

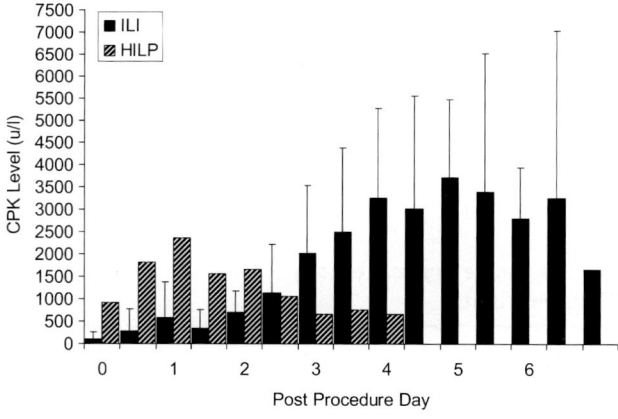

Figure 11 Comparative time course kinetics of CPK elevations post-perfusion with ILP and MILP. The CPK elevations are higher and occur later with MILP.

and toxicity. Excellent preclinical perfusion models are being utilized to identify novel agents and approaches that may be applied to patients. An example of such a strategy is based on a recent preclinical study in mice identified that one of the mechanism in which TNF alpha destroys the integrity of the tumor vasculature is by selectively targeting VE-cadherin.[65] While TNF alpha is not available in the US to be used for perfusions and certainly is too toxic to be administered systemically, plans are ongoing to study other Cadherin inhibitors administered systemically pre perfusion in the hope of increasing the effectiveness of regionally administered Melphalan. Other efforts include identifying genomic signatures for response to melphalan as well as to other agents. Such endeavors will allow the selection of agents to be used for specific patients based on the underlying biology of the tumor. Such rational approaches will not only improve the effectiveness of available therapies but also avoid unnecessary toxicity to those patients determined unlikely to respond.

References

1. Grunhagan DJ, de Wilt JHW, van Geel AN, et al. Isolated limb perfusion for melanoma patients- a review of its indications and the role for tumour necrosis facotr-alpha. Eur J Surg Onco 2006, 32370–381.

2. Pawlik TM, Ross MI, Johnson MM, et al. Predictors and natural history of in-transit melanoma after sentinel lymphadenectomy. Ann Surg Oncol 2005;12(8):587–96.

3. Balch CM, Soong SJ, Gershenwald JE, et al. Prognostic factors analysis of 17,600 melanoma patients: validation of the American Joint Committee on Cancer melanoma staging system. J Clin Oncol 2001;19:3622–3634.

4. Balch CM, Buzaid AC, Soong SJ, et al. Final version of the American Joint Committee on Cancer staging system for cutaneous melanoma. J Clin Oncol 2001;19:3635–48.

5. Brown CD, Zitelli JA. The prognosis and treatment of true local cutaneous recurrent malignant melanoma. Dermatol Surg 1995;21(4):285–90.

6. Veronesi U, Cascinelli N. Narrow excision (1-cm margin). A safe procedure for thin cutaneous melanoma. Arch Surg 1991;126:438–441Alexander HR, Fraker DL, Bartlett DL: Isolated limb perfusion for malignant melanoma. Semin Surg Oncol 1996;12:416–428.

7. Cohn-Cedermark G, Rutqvist LE, Andersson R, et al. Long term results of a randomized study by the Swedish Melanoma Study Group on 2-cm versus 5-cm resection margins for patients with cutaneous melanoma with a tumor thickness of 0.8-2.0 mm. Cancer 2000;89:1495–1501.

8. Balch CM, Urist MM, Karakousis CP, et al. Efficacy of 2-cm surgical margins for intermediate-thickness melanomas (1 to 4 mm). Results of a multi-institutional randomized surgical trial. Ann Surg 1993;218:262–267.

9. Thomas JM, Newton-Bishop J, A'Hern R, et al. Excision margins in high-risk malignant melanoma. N Engl J Med 2004;350:757–766.

10. Koops HS, Vaglini M, Suciu S, et al. Prophylactic isolated limb perfusion for localized, high-risk limb melanoma; results of a multicenter randomized phase III trial. J Clin Oncol 1998;16:2906–2912.

11. Estourgie SH, Nieweg OE, Kroon BB. High incidence of in-transti metastases after sentinel node biopsy in patients with melnoma. Br J Surg 2004;91(10):1370–1.

12. Thomas JM, Clark MA. Selective lymphadenectomy in sentinel node-positive patients may increase the risk of locl/in-transit recurrence in malignant melanoma. Eur J Surg Oncol 2004;30(6):686–91.

13. Pawlik TM, Ross MI, Shaw HM, et al. Re: Selective lymphadenectomy in sentinel node-positive patients may increase the risk of local/in-transit recurrence in malignant melanoma, Thomas and Clark. Eur J Surg Oncol 2005;31(3):323–4.

14. Pawlik TM, Ross MI, Thompson JF, et al. The risk of in-transit metastases depends on tumor biology and not the surgical approach to regional lymph nodes. L Clin Oncol 2005;23(21):4588–90.

15. Cerovac S, Mashadi SA, Williams AM, et al. Is there increased risk of local and in-trnsit recurrence following sentinel lymph node biopsy? J Plast Reconstr Aesthet Surg 2006;59(5):487–93.

16. van Poll D, Thompson JF, Colman MH, et al. A sentinel node biopsy does not increase the incidence of in-transit metastasis in patients with primary cutaneous melanoma. Ann Surg Oncol 2005;12(8):597–608.

17. Hill S, Thomas JM. Use of the carbon dioxide laser to manage cutaneous metastases from malignant melanoma. Br J Surg 1996;83:509–512.

18. Rols MP, Bachaud JM, Giraud P, et al. Electrochemotherapy of cutaneous metasteses in malignant melanoma. Melanoma Res 2000;10:468–474.

19. Heller R, Jaroszeski MJ, Reintgen DS, et al. Treatment of cutaneous and subcutaneous tumors with electroche-motherapy using intralesional bleomycin. Cancer 1998;83:148–157.

20. Hsueh EC, Nathanson L, Foshag LJ, Essner R, et al. Active specific immunotherapy with polyvalent melanoma cell vaccine for patients with in-transit melanoma metastases. Cancer 1999;85:2160–2169.

21. Seegenschmiedt MH, Keiholz L, Altendorf-Hofmann A, et al. Palliative radiotherapy for recurrent and metastatic malignant melanoma: prognostic factors for tumor response and long-term outcome: a 20 year experience. Int J Radiat Oncol Biol Phys 1999;44:607–618.

22. Cohen MH, et al. Intralesional treatment of recurrent cutaneous malignant melanoma: a randomized prospective study of intralesional Bacillus Calmette-Guerin versus intra-lesional dinitrocholorobenzene. Cancer 1978;41:2456–63.

23. Storm FK, Sparks FC, Morton DL. Treatment for melanoma of the lower extremity with intralesional injection of bacilli Calmette Guerin and hyperthermic perfusion. Surg Gynecol Obstet 1979;149:17–21.

24. Von Wussow P, et al. Intralesional interferon-alpha therapy in advanced malignant melanoma. Cancer 1998;61:1071–4.

25. Yao KA, Hsueh EC, Essner R, et al. Is sentinel lymph node mapping indicated for isolated local and in-transit recurrent melanoma? Ann Surg. 2003 Nov, 238(5):743–7.

26. Calabro A, Singletary SE, Carrasco CH, et al. Intraarterial infusion chemotherapy in regionally advanced malignant melanoma. J surg Oncol 1990;43:239–244.

27. Karakousis CP, Kontzoglou K, Driscoll DL. Tourniquet infusion chemotherapy for extremity in-transit lesions in malignant melanoma. Ann Surg Oncol 1997;4:506–510.

28. Jaques DP. Major amputation for advanced malignant melanoma. Surg Gynecol Obstet 1089;169:1–6.

29. Kapma MR, Vrouenraets BC, Nieweg OE, et al. Major amputation for intractable extremity melanoma after failure of isolated limb perfusion. Eur J Sur Oncol 2005;31:95–99.

30. Cornett WR, McCall LM, Petersen RP, et al. Randomized multicenter trial of hyperthermic isolated perfusion with melphalan alone compared with melphalan plus tumor necrosis factor: American College of Surgeons Oncology Group Trial Z0020. L Clin Oncol 2006;24(25):4196–201.

31. Creech O, Krementz ET, Ryan RF, et al. Chemotherapy of cancer: Regional perfusion utilizing an extracorporeal circuit. Ann Surg 1958;148:616–632.

32. Stehlin JS Jr. Hyperthermic perfusion with chemotherapy for cancers of the extremities. Surg Gynecol Obstet 1969;129:305–308.

33. Storm FK, Morton DL. Value of therapeutic hyperthermic limb perfusion in advanced recurrent melanoma of the lower extremity. Am J Surg 1985;150:32–35.

34. Thompson JF, Kam PC, Waugh RC, et al. Isolated limb infusion with cytotoxic agents: a simple alternative to

isolated limb perfusion. Semin Surg Oncol 1998;134:238–247.

35. Thompson JF, Kam PC. Isolated limb infusion for melanoma: a simple but effective alternative to isolated limb perfusion. J Surg Oncol 2004;88:1–3.

36. Takkenberg RB, Vrouenraets AN, Gee V, et al. Palliative isolated limb perfusion for advanced limb disease in stage IV melanoma patients. J Surg Oncol 2005;91:107–111.

37. Thompson JF, Gianoutsos MP. Isolated limb perfusion for melanoma: effectiveness and toxicity of cisplatin compared with that of melphalan and other drugs. World J Surg 1992; 16:227–233.

38. Klaase JM, Kroon BB, Van Geel AN, et al. Limb recurrence-free interval and survival in patients with recurrent melanoma of the extremities treated with normothermic isolated perfusion. J Am Coll Surg 1994;178:564–572.

39. Thompson JF, Hunt JA, Shannon KF, et al. Frequency and duration of remission after isolated limb perfusion for melanoma. Arch Surg 1997;132:903–907.

40. Lingam MK, Byrne DS, Aitchison T, et al. A single centre's experience with isolated limb perfusion in the treatment of recurrent malignant melanoma of the limb. Eur J Cancer 1996;32A(10):1668–73.

41. Di Filippo F, Anza M, Rossi CR, et al. The application of hyperthermia in regional chemotherapy. Sem Surg Oncol 1998;14(3):215–23.

42. Klaase JM, Kroon BB, Eggermont AM, et al. A retrospective comparative study evaluating the results of mild hyperthermia versus controlled normothermic perfusion for recurrent melanoma of the extremities. Eur J Cancer 1995; 31A(1):58–63.

43. Noorda EM, Vrouenraets BC, Nieweg OE, et al. Long-term results of a double perfusion schedule using high dose hyperthemia and melphalan sequentially in extensive melanoma of the lower limb. Melanoma Res 2003;13: 395–399.

44. Klop WM, Vrouenraets BC, Van Geel AN, et al. Repeat isolated limb perfusion with melphalan for recurrent melanoma of the limbs. J Am Coll Surg 1996;192:457–472.

45. Feldman AL, Alexander HR Jr, Bartlett DL, et al. Management of extremity recurrences after complete responses to isolated limb perfusion in patients with melanoma. Ann Surg Oncol 1999;6:562–567.

46. Lienard D, Ewalenko P, Delmotte JJ, et al. High-dose recombinant tumor necrosis factor alpha in combination with interferon gamma and melphalan in isolation perfusion of the limbs for melanoma and sarcoma. J Clin Oncol 1992;10:52–60.

47. Lienard D, Eggermont AM, Schraffordt Koops H, et al. Isolated perfusion of the limb with high-dose tumour necrosis factor-alpha (TNF-alpha), interferon-gamma (IFN-gamma) and melphalan for melanoma stage III:

Results of a multicentre pilot study. Melanoma Res 1994; 4(suppl 1):21–26.

48. Vaglini M, Santinami M, Manzi R, et al. Treatment of in-transit metastases from cutaneous melanoma by isolation perfusion with tumour necrosis factor-alpha (TNF-alpha), melphalan and interferon-gamma (IFN-gamma): Dose-finding experience at the National Cancer Institute of Milan. Melanoma Res 1994;4(suppl 1):35–38.

49. Fraker DL, Alexander HR, Andrich M, et al. Treatment of patients with melanoma of the extremity using hyperthermic isolated limb perfusion with melphalan, tumor necrosis factor, and interferon-gamma: Results of a tumor necrosis factor dose-escalation study. J Clin Oncol 1996;14: 479–489.

50. Lienard D, Eggermont AM, Koops B, et al. Isolated limb perfusion with tumour necrosis factor-alpha and melphalan with or without interferon-gamma for the treatment of in-transit melanoma metastases: A multicentre randomized phase II study. Melanoma Res 1999;9:491–502.

51. Fraker DL, Alexander HR, Ross M, et al. A phase III trial of isolated limb perfusion for extremity melanoma comparing melphalan alone versus melphaln plus tumor necrosis factor (TNF-alpha) plus interferon-gamma (IFN). Ann Surg Onc 2002;9(suppl; abstr 1):S8.

52. Hays AJ, Neuhaus SJ, Clark MA, et al. Isolated limb perfusion with melphalan and tumor necrosis factor alpha for advanced melanoma and soft-tissue sarcoma. Ann Surg Oncol 2007;14(1):230–38.

53. Lindner P, Thompson JF, De Wilt JH, et al. Double isolated limb infusion with cytotoxic agents for recurrent and metastatic limb melanoma. Eur J Surg Oncol 2004;30:433–439.

54. Brady MS, Brown K, Patel A, et al. A phase II trial of isolated limb infusion with melphalan and dactinomycin for reginal melanoma and soft tissue sarcoma of the extremity. Ann Surg Oncol 2002;13:1123–29.

55. Zager JS, Gersehnwald JE, Aldrink J, et al. Isolated limb infiusion for locally recurrent and in-transit extremity melanoma: a combined institutional initial experience. Ann Surg Oncol 2006;13:84, (abstract).

56. Hafstrom L, Rudenstam CM, Blomquist E, et al. Regional hyperthermic perfusion with melphalan after surgery for recurrent malignant melanoma of the extremities. Swedish Melanoma Study Group. J Clin Oncol 1991;9:2091–2094.

57. Noorda EM, Takkenberg B, Vrouenraets BC, et al. Isolated limb perfusion prolongs the limb recurrence-free interval after several episodes of excisional surgery for loco-regional recurrent melanoma. Ann Surg Oncol 2004;11: 491–499.

58. Wieberdink J, Benckhuysen C, Braat RP, et al. Eur J Cancer Clin Oncol 1982;18:905–910.

59. Vrouenraets BC, Kroon BBR, Klaase JM, et al. Severe acute regional toxicity after normothermic or 'mild' hyperther-

mic isolated limb perfusion with melphalan for melanoma. Melanoma Res 1995;5:425–431.

60. Vrouenraets BC, Kroon BB, Ogilvie AC, et al. Absence of severe systemic toxicity after leakage-controlled isolated limb perfusion with tumor necrosis factor-alpha and melphalan. Ann Surg Oncol 1999;6:405–412.

61. Vrouenraets BC, Kroon BB, Klasse JM, et al. Value of laboratory tests in monitoring acue regional toxicity after isolated limb perfusion. Ann Surg Oncol 1997;4(1): 88–94.

62. Vrouenraets BC, Eggermont AM, Klaase JM, et al. Long-term neuropathy after regional isolated perfusion with melphalan for melanoma of the limbs. Eur J Surg Oncol 1994;20:681–85.

63. Vrouenraets BC, In't Veld GJ, Nieweg OE, et al. Long-term functional morbidity after mild hyperthermic isolated limb perfusion with melphalan. Eur J Surg Oncol 1999;25:503–508.

64. Noorda EM, van Kreij RHJ, Vrouenraets BC, et al. The health related quality of life in long-term survivors of melanoma treated with limb perfusion. Eur J Surg Oncol 2007, 1–7.

65. Menon C, Ghartey A, Canter R, et al. Tumor necrosis factor-alpha damages tumor blood vessel integrity by targeting VE-cadherin. Ann Surg 2006;244(4):781–91.

CHAPTER 85

SURGICAL RESECTION OF METASTASES: RATIONALE, INDICATIONS, AND RESULTS

ABIGAIL S. CAUDLE, MD

DAVID W. OLLILA, MD

Introduction

For the majority of patients diagnosed with stage IV melanoma, the only treatment option offered is systemic therapy, either chemotherapy or biologic therapy. However, the results of cytotoxic therapy, dacarbazine or interleukin-2, have been unsatisfactory to date; complete clinical responses are uncommon with 5-year overall survival rates approximately 5%.[1,2] Partial clinical response to either drug improves overall survival by only a few months. Thus, only patients who have a complete clinical response have any reasonable chance to have a durable 5-year survival.[3]

Novel therapeutics are currently being investigated in well-designed phase III clinical trials, and if successful will offer other systemic therapy alternatives. However, until new agents are proven to be efficacious in prospective, randomized clinical trials, the current paradigm for the management of distant metastases in melanoma patients needs to be reevaluated. Conventional teaching has been that surgical resection is not indicated in patients with blood-borne metastases at distant sites, because the cancer is widely disseminated and impractical for a locoregional approach to control. Nevertheless, a number of series show long-term survival following resection of distant metastases in stage IV melanoma patients.[4] In this chapter, we will demonstrate that in properly selected patients with limited sites of stage IV metastatic melanoma, it is time to reposition surgery as the initial treatment option in the treatment paradigm.

Prognosis of Melanoma Patients with Stage IV Disease

As our understanding of the biology of melanoma as a disease process is evolving, so is the staging system. The American Joint Committee on Cancer (AJCC) instated a revised classification system in 2003 that recognized the clinical and pathological features that are distinctive to melanoma and serve as prognostic markers based on the AJCC Melanoma Database.[5] Major revisions to the tumor-nodes-metastasis (TNM) staging system included a designation for tumors with ulceration, a distinction for number of involved lymph nodes as well as microscopically positive versus clinically diagnosed lymph node involvement, and recognition of the variability in metastatic sites. This new classification system was then validated by a prospective database involving 13 institutions and cooperative study groups.[1] This database of 17,600 patients, with all stages of disease and ranges of therapies, included at least 5-year follow-up on 73% of patients and at least 10-year follow-up on 49%.

The fact that site of metastatic disease in melanoma dramatically affects prognosis is reflected in the new AJCC staging system, which divides metastatic disease into M1a for skin, subcutaneous, or distant lymph node metastases; M1b for pulmonary sites; and M1c for other visceral metastases or any other distant site with elevated lactic dehydrogenase. The AJCC validation study analyzed 1,158 stage IV melanoma patients in their database and found that the most significant differences in survival were between visceral and nonvisceral (skin, soft tissue, and distant lymph node) sites. When they further divided the visceral sites, there was a difference in 1-year survival rates of patients with lung metastases versus other visceral organs, but this difference was not significant when looking at 2-year survival.

Skin, soft tissue, and distant lymph nodes metastases represent the most common sites, comprising up to 40% of stage IV melanoma metastases.[6] As discussed previously, multiple studies report that skin, soft tissue, and distant lymph node metastases have better outcomes than other metastatic sites.[1,7,8] Even within this group of M1a patients, certain subsets have been identified with better outcomes. For instance, patients with skin and soft tissue metastasis tend to fare better than those with distant lymph node disease.[9]

The lungs represent the most common site of visceral metastases in melanoma patients, with various series reporting between 12 and 36% of patients having lung metastases.[6,10] Harpole and colleagues[10] looked at 7,564 melanoma patients and estimated the probability of a melanoma patient developing a pulmonary metastasis as 0.13 at 5 years, 0.19 at 10 years, and 0.3 at 20 years. Most pulmonary metastases are asymptomatic, and therefore are detected with screening measures. Routine screening chest radiograph is the most appropriate way to follow melanoma patients. Suspicious nodules found should be further evaluated by CT scan to better characterize the number and character of the lesions. CT-PET is also emerging as a helpful modality to differentiate metastases from benign findings.

Melanoma metastasizes to the gastrointestinal (GI) tract in 2 to 4% of patients in autopsy studies. However, around 50% of patients who die of disseminated melanoma have GI involvement.[11] The small bowel is the most common site involved (75–90%), with colon (20–25%), and stomach (3–16%) following in prevalence.[12] Patients with GI metastases usually are symptomatic with anemia (60%), abdominal pain (29–59%), bleeding (26–40%), obstruction (27%), palpable mass (12%), or weight loss (9%).[13]

Melanoma represents the third most common type of brain metastases in the United States after lung and breast cancers. In patients with stage IV melanoma, 10 to 40% will have intracranial metastases. This is a major source of morbidity and mortality, being identified as the direct cause of death in 95% of these patients.[14] In fact, in autopsy series, up to 75% of patients with disseminated melanoma will have evidence of brain metastases.[15] Unfortunately, the presence of CNS, or intracranial, metastases is a very poor prognostic factor secondary to the fact that it is usually the sign of disseminated disease and the fact that current therapies do not improve the prognosis.

Resection with Curative Intent

RATIONALE

Chemotherapy, biologic therapy, and combined bio-chemotherapy in the treatment of patients with metastatic melanoma has had mixed results. While novel therapeutic agents are continually introduced into clinical trials, the current standard of therapy remains decarbazine, which has a 15 to 20% response rate and unclear affect on overall survival,[16] and interleukin-2 (IL-2), which has a 20 to 25% response rate and 5 to 7% complete response.[17] Only these patients who have a complete response have any chance at a durable result leading to an improved 5-year survival. Given the lack of currently available, efficacious systemic therapies, surgical resection in carefully selected patients with isolated metastasis is gaining popularity.

An important distinction in surgical nomenclature needs to be emphasized. A complete metastasectomy is the surgical removal of all clinically and/or radiographically detected metastases. This is the only operation considered for curative intent in patients with stage IV disease. Incomplete metastesectomy is essentially a palliative operation, aimed at relieving the patient's symptoms and does not improve 5-year survival rates. The following sections will emphasize that only patients who undergo a complete metastasectomy have any chance at substantial 5-year survival.

SKIN, SOFT TISSUE, AND DISTANT LYMPH NODES METASTASES

Even in this subgroup of Stage IV patients with a relatively favorable prognosis, an aggressive surgical approach is warranted provided there is no evidence of other visceral disease. As for all sites, the goal is complete resection when technically feasible. For patients with skin and soft tissue metastases, the median survival after complete resection is 24 months,[9] as compared to 10 to 18 months reported for patients treated with a wide variety of incomplete resections and/or intralesional therapies[7,8] (Table 1). Patients with a solitary metastasis confined to the dermal or subcutaneous tissue that is completely resected have reported 8-year survival rates over 80%.[18] The number of lesions, disease-free interval, and size of lesions have also been noted as prognostic indicators.[19] All efforts should be made to perform complete resection of skin, soft tissue, and lymph node metastases, since these patients have such a favorable prognosis after complete excision.

Table 1 Skin, Soft Tissue, and Lymph Nodes *(Reflects data after complete excision)*

Author	Number of Patients	Median Survival (Months)	5-Year Overall Survival
Markowitz, 1991[9]	72	24	38%
Gadd and Coit, 1992[8]	23	29	22%
Barth, 1995[7]	281	15	14%

PULMONARY METASTASES

Though the prognosis for patients with pulmonary metastases is worse than patients with skin and soft tissue sites, complete resection of isolated metastases still confers a survival advantage. Patient selection plays a critical role in the management of these patients, with a patient's pulmonary reserve and predicted postoperative pulmonary status considered in the decision to pursue complete metastasectomy. Multiple nodules and bilateral disease are not definite contraindications to resection if the patient can be rendered free of disease. The possibility of benign findings as well as other primary tumors must always be considered. However, the presence of multiple lesions is more worrisome for metastatic disease, thus these patients should be fully evaluated for other sites of extrathoracic disease. Identifying patients who can be rendered disease free through pulmonary resection is important since there is no value to putting patients through the risk of operative intervention if this goal cannot be achieved. Though complete resection is the most important prognostic factor, there are other components that have been identified, such as longer disease-free interval, treatment with chemotherapy, negative mediastinal lymph nodes, and presence of a single lesion.[10,20]

The 2 largest studies have reported 5-year overall survival rates of 20 to 27% in patients who were completely resected versus 3 to 4% in those that were not.[10,21] Patients with multiple lesions should be evaluated for surgical options since they may still have a survival advantage after metastasectomy if a complete resection can be performed.[20,21] Given this clear difference in survival, an aggressive surgical approach is justified if there is a reasonable probability to obtain tumor-free margins while insuring a quality postoperative functional status. Though some patients may benefit from palliative resections, only a complete resection offers a survival benefit[22] (Table 2).

ABDOMINAL METASTASES: GASTROINTESTINAL TRACT

As with other sites of stage IV melanoma metastases, the technical ability to perform a complete metastectomy is the best prognostic indicator. Once again, patient selection is important. Because of the close proximity of the organs in the abdominal cavity, a single metastasis may actually involve a portion of multiple organs. For instance, a metastasis on the greater curvature of the stomach may also involve the spleen, colon, and distal pancreas. Given the location of the metastasis and the magnitude of the operation necessary for a complete metastasectomy, the surgeon must assess the predicted postoperative function of the patient after a complete resection. For instance, a patient with multiple small bowel metastases that would require multiple enterectomies for complete resection may result in inadequate enteral absorption. With those things in mind, an aggressive surgical approach is still warranted. Even patients with multiple abdominal sites who can be completely resected fare better with surgical intervention. Multiple studies show improved survival after complete resection with median survival improving from 5 to 8 months to 15 to 28 months after metastectomy (Table 3).[12,23]

ABDOMINAL METASTASES: LIVER

Traditionally, patients with liver metastases, were not considered operative candidates, but there is growing evidence that carefully selected patients may benefit from resection. The largest study looking at this pooled data from the John Wayne Cancer Institute and the Sydney Melanoma Unit, capturing 1,750 patients with liver metastases from melanoma.[24] Of these, 34 patients underwent exploration with intent to resect, of which 24 were resected while 10 were explored without resection. Median survival for patients resected was 28 months as opposed to 4 months for the subgroup that was explored,

Table 2 Pulmonary *(reflects data after complete resection)*

Author	Number of Patients	Median Survival (months)	5-Year Overall Survival
Harpole, 1992[10]	98	20	20%
Tafra, 1995[21]	106	18	27%
Leo, 2000[20]	282	19	22%

Table 3 Gastrointestinal Tract *(Reflects data after complete resection)*

Author	Number of Patients	Median Survival (months)	5-Year Overall Survival
Ricaniadis, 1995[12]	23	28	28%
Ollila, 1996[33]	46	49	41%
Agrawal, 1999[32]	19	15	38%

but not resected. Another small study from England reports disease-free survivals of 76 to 147 months after resection of isolated hepatic metastases.[25]

Some hepatic metastases are not amenable to surgical resection because of location of tumor in relation to bile ducts and vessels, bilobar disease, or preexisting hepatic dysfunction. Another emerging locoregional technology that may be effective in these cases is radiofrequency ablation (RFA), with median survival of 25 months reported after RFA of unresectable lesions. Although patients in this study with more than 3 lesions had lower survival rates than those with 1 or 2 lesions (28.1 m vs 18.5 m), this may prove to confer a survival benefit as opposed to nonoperative management in future studies. Clearly, the results of all of these studies warrant careful consideration for resection in patients with isolated hepatic disease.[26]

OTHER ABDOMINAL SITES

Other abdominal solid organs can be sites of metastatic disease. Patients with isolated splenic metastases completely resected have median survival of 23 months as opposed to 4 to 5 months for patients who had incomplete resections or no operative intervention.[27] The adrenal glands are another site for melanoma metastases with survival rates of 26 to 59 months after complete resections versus 9 to 15 months for patients with nonresectable disease.[13,28] The key in all of these sites seems to be the ability to render the patient disease free.

INTRACRANIAL METASTASES

Intracranial metastases carry a very poor prognosis. Although there are encouraging data with systemic therapy, there is little evidence that current efforts at local control confer any survival benefit. Most studies demonstrate a median survival of 7 to 10 months after resection.[29,30] This does not change even with the addition of whole-brain radiotherapy. The main role of surgery is palliation, with some evidence showing improvement in neurologic symptoms.

Surgery for Palliation

SKIN, SOFT TISSUE, AND LYMPH NODES

Metastases of the skin, soft tissue, and lymph nodes can present with symptoms of pain, functional limitation, and bleeding in patients with disseminated disease but otherwise asymptomatic. These sites are usually amenable to complete excision without associated significant morbidity, and should be pursued as such since complete resection can provide durable palliation and improve quality life.

CHEST

Since most pulmonary metastases are asymptomatic, there is seldom a need for palliative resection. Symptoms such as cough, chest pain, and hemoptysis are usually signs of advanced disease. However, cardiac involvement is becoming increasingly recognized as CT-PET and MRI are used more aggressively. In autopsy studies, almost 50% of patients with disseminated disease have cardiac involvement, although their antemortem symptoms were rarely attributed to cardiac disease. There are scattered reports of palliative or prophylactic cardiac resection to correct electrophysiologic sequelae or to prevent embolic events that are likely to be fatal.[31]

ABDOMINAL

Because of the symptomatic nature of gastrointestinal tract lesions (obstruction and/or bleeding), palliative resection is usually warranted even if complete resection is not possible. These attempts are successful in alleviating symptoms over 90% of the time.[32,33] Symptomatic splenic and adrenal lesions are also effectively treated with palliative resections.[27,28]

INTRACRANIAL

The 2 main treatment options for patients with brain metastases are surgery and stereotactic radiosurgery, although both are usually palliative, as mentioned previously. Stereotactic radiosurgery (SR) uses multiple radiation beams that converge on a single lesion in order to deliver high-dose radiation with minimal effects to the surrounding tissue. This can be administered using a gamma knife that utilizes multiple cobalt sources to deliver a focused high dose, or using a linear accelerator targeted to an area with rapid dose falloff out of the treatment field. Levine and colleagues treated 45 patients in their series, reporting improvement or stabilization of symptoms in 78%.[34] They also noted that 28% of the lesions disappeared radiographically, although their median survival of 8 months points to the fact that this is a palliative procedure.

Stage IV Complete Metastasectomy Trial

Unfortunately, most of the published literature in complete metastasectomy for stage IV melanoma patients is from retrospective, single institutional series. Opponents of this aggressive surgical approach cite the lack of randomized, controlled trial evidence supporting complete metastasectomy in these patients. Furthermore, opponents correctly emphasize the inherent selection bias in any single institution series, with only the candidates most likely to benefit from surgery actually making it to the operating room. Finally, even advocates for complete metastasectomy concede there has been no standardization of the surgical procedures and no surgical quality control.

One of the staunchest advocates of complete metastasectomy in stage IV melanoma patients, Donald L. Morton, MD, recognized these problems and launched a prospective, randomized, international trial for these patients.[35] To be eligible for trial (a phase III randomized, double-blind trial of immunotherapy with a polyvalent melanoma vaccine, Canvaxin plus BCG vs placebo plus BCG as a postsurgical treatment for stage IV melanoma), all patients had to have undergone complete metastasectomy of their stage IV metastases with tumor-free surgical margins. Following surgery, the patients were then randomized to adjuvant Canvaxin immunotherapy and BCG or placebo and BCG. To be clear, the surgical therapy was not randomized, only the postsurgical adjuvant therapy. All patients had to receive a complete metastasectomy as outlined in the protocol, and strict adherence to these guidelines was assured by the surgical monitoring committee for the trial. Although the primary aim of the trial, Canvaxin as a postsurgical adjuvant failed to demonstrate a disease-free or overall survival benefit, several other conclusions can be made from this important trial.

First, uniformity of complete metastasectomies can be accomplished in an international, randomized, controlled trial. Surgeons from across the globe can perform similar complete surgical resections from a variety of anatomic sites and achieve tumor-free surgical margins. This similarity in complete metastasectomies led to a 40% 5-year survival for the entire study cohort. This impressive 5-year overall survival rate has never been achieved in any randomized, controlled stage IV melanoma surgical trial, nor has it has ever been seen in any chemotherapy or biologic therapy trial for stage IV melanoma patients.

These randomized, controlled trial data diffuse several of the arguments against an aggressive surgical approach in patients with stage IV disease. The data strongly support that the best initial option for patients with stage IV disease is not systemic chemotherapy or biologic therapy, but rather, a complete metastasectomy if technically feasible. Thus, the first step for patients with newly diagnosed stage IV disease should be an evaluation of an experienced surgical oncologist to assess resectability.

Conclusion

The limited, currently available systemic therapies for stage IV melanoma patients do not confer the survival advantage of complete metastasectomy. For patients with limited sites of stage IV disease, the time has come to reposition surgery as the first option for patients provided a complete metastasectomy can be performed. Complete metastasectomy, regardless of the anatomic site, confers survival advantages not seen with the currently available cytotoxic agents. This aggressive surgical approach should be tempered with the knowledge that incomplete resections put patients at increased risk without any proven survival benefit and should be reserved only for palliation of symptoms.

The ideal approach to stage IV melanoma patients would be complete metastasectomy followed by a novel adjuvant therapy that is efficacious and can prolong the 5-year survival beyond that of just a surgical resection. Medical oncologists and surgical oncologists need to work together to develop the best therapeutic plan to this group of patients.

References

1. Balch C, Soong S, Gershenwald J, et al. Prognositc factors analysis of 17,600 melanoma patients: validation of the American Joint Committee on Cancer melanoma staging system. J Clin Oncol 2001;19:3622–34.
2. Eton O, Legha S, Moon T, et al. Prognostic factors for survival of patients treated systemically for disseminated melanoma. J Clin Oncol 1998;16:1103–11.
3. Coates A, Segelov E. Long term response to chemotherapy in patients with visceral metastatic melanoma. Ann Oncol 1994;5:249–51.
4. Ollila D, Hsueh E, Stern S, et al. Metastasectomy for recurrent stage IV melanoma. J Surg Oncol 1999;71:209–13.

5. Balch C, Buzaid A, Soong S, et al. Final version of the American Joint Committee on Cancer staging system for cutaneous melanoma. J Clin Oncol 2001;19:3635–48.

6. Balch C, Soong S, Murad T, et al. A multifactorial analysis of melanoma. IV. Prognostic factors in 200 melanoma patients with distant metastases (stage III). J Clin Oncol 1983;1:126–34.

7. Barth A, Wanek L, Morton D. Prognostic factors in 1521 melanoma patients with distant metastases. J Am Coll Surg 1995;181:193–201.

8. Gadd M, Coit D. Recurrence patterns and outcome in 1019 patients undergoing axillary or inguinal lymphadenopathy for melanoma. Arch Surg 1992;127:1412–6.

9. Markowitz J, Cosimi L, Carey R, et al. Prognosis after initial recurrence of cutaneous melanoma. Ann Surg 1991; 214:703–7.

10. Harpole D Jr, Johnson C, Wolfe W, et al. Analysis of 945 cases of pulmonary metastatic melanoma. J Thorac Cardiovasc Surg 1992;103:743–8.

11. Patel J, Didolkar M, Pickren J, et al. Metastatic pattern of malignant melanoma. A study of 216 autopsy studies. Am J Surg 1978;135:807–10.

12. Ricaniadis N, Konstadoulakis M, Walsh D, et al. Gatsrointestinal metastases from malignant melanoma. Surg Oncol 1995;4:105–10.

13. Branum G, Seigler H. Role of surgical intervention in the management of intestinal metastases from malignant melanoma. Am J Surg 1991;162:428–31.

14. Sampson J, Carter J, Friedman A, et al. Demographics, prognosis, and therapy in 702 patients with brain metastases from malignant melanoma. J Neurosurg 1998;88:11–20.

15. Yu C, JCT C, Apuzzo M, et al. Metastatic melanoma to the brain: prognostic factors after gamma knife radiosurgery. Int J Radiat Oncol Biol Phys 2002;52:1277–87.

16. Hill G, Krementz E, Hill H. Dimethyl triazenoimidazole carboxamide and combination therapy for melanoma. IV. Late results after complete response to chemotherapy (Central Oncology Group Protocols 7130, 7131, and 7131A). Cancer 1984;53:1299–305.

17. Rosenberg S, Yang J, Topaliam S, et al. Treatment of 283 consecutive patients with metastatic melanoma or renal cell cancer using high dose bolus interleukin 2. JAMA 1994; 271:907–13.

18. Bowen G, Chang AE, Lowe L, et al. Solitary melanoma confined to the dermal and/or subcutaneous tissue: evidence from revisiting the staging classification. Arch Dermatol 2000;136:1397–9.

19. Wong SL, Coit DG. Role of surgery in patients with stage IV melanoma. Curr Opin Oncol 2004;16:155–60.

20. Leo F, Cagini L, Rocmans P, et al. Lung metastases from melanoma: when is surgical treatment warranted? Br J Cancer 2000;83:569–72.

21. Tafra L, Dale P, Wanek L, et al. Resection and adjuvant immunotherapy from melanoma metastatic to the lung and thorax. J Thorac Cardiovasc Surg 1995;110:119–28.

22. Karp N, Boyd A, DePan H, et al. Thoracoctomy for metastatic malignant melanoma of the lung. Surgery 1990; 107:256–61.

23. Wood T, DiFronzo L, Rose D, et al. Does complete resection of melanoma metastatic to solid intra-abdominal organs improve survival? Ann Surg Oncol 2001;8:658–62.

24. Rose D, Essner R, Hughes T, et al. Surgical resection for metastatic melanoma to the liver: the John Wayne Cancer Institute and Sydney Melanoma Unit experience. Arch Surg 2001;136:950–5.

25. Crook T, Jones O, John T, et al. Hepatic resection for malignant melanoma. Eur J Surg Oncol 2006;32:315–7.

26. Amersi F, McElrath-Garza A, Ahmad A, et al. Long-term survival after radiofrequency ablation of complex unresectable liver tumors. Arch Surg 2006;141:581–8.

27. de Wilt J, McCarthy W, Thompson J. Surgical treatment of splenic metastases in patients with melanoma. J Am Coll Surg 2003;197:38–43.

28. Haigh P, Essner R, Wardlaw J, et al. Long-term survival after complete resection of melanoma metastatic to the adrenal gland. Ann Surg Oncol 1999;6:633–9.

29. Wronski M, Arbit E. Surgical treatment of brain metastases from melanoma: a retrospective study of 91 patients. J Neurosurg 2000;93:9–18.

30. Oredsson S, Ingvar C, Strombald L, et al. Palliative surgery for brain metastases of malignant melanoma. Eur J Surg Oncol 1990;16:451–6.

31. Manner G, Harting M, Russo P, et al. Surgical management of metastatic melanoma to the ventricle. Tex Heart Inst J 2003;30:218–20.

32. Agrawal S, Yao T, Coit D. Surgery for melanoma metastatic to the gastrointestinal tract. Ann Surg Oncol 1999;6:336–44.

33. Ollila D, Essner R, Wanek L, et al. Surgical resection for melanoma metastatic to the gastrointestinal tract. Arch Surg 1996;131:975–9.

34. Levine S, Petrovich Z, Cohen-Gadol A. Gamma knife radiosurgery for metastatic melanoma: an analysis of survival, outcome, and complications. Neurosurgery 1999;44:59–64.

35. Morton D, Mozzilo N, Thompson J, et al. An international, randomized, double-blind, phase 3 study of the specific active immunotherapy agent, onamelatucel-L (Canvaxin™), compared to placebo as a post-surgical adjvuvant in AJCC stage IV melanoma [abstract 12]. Presented at the Society of Surgical Oncology Cancer Symposium, 59th Annual Meeting; 2006 March 23–26; San Diego, CA.

CHAPTER 86

MANAGEMENT OF MELANOMA METASTASES FROM AN UNKNOWN PRIMARY SITE

JANICE N. CORMIER, MD, MPH

YAN XING, MD, MS

Background

Metastatic melanoma arising from an unknown primary site (MUP) was first described in 1952.[1] The diagnostic criteria for MUP were initially proposed in 1963 by Dasgupta and colleagues.[2] Contemporary criteria for diagnosis include (1) metastatic melanoma confirmed clinically, histologically, and immunohistochemically; (2) absence of a previous cutaneous tumor, pigmented or not, that was destroyed or excised without histologic examination; and (3) exclusion of unusual primary sites, including urogenital, otolaryngologic, or ophthamologic sites. MUP has been estimated to account for approximately 1.2 to 8.8% of all melanoma cases (Table 1).[1–23]

Metastatic melanoma should be part of the differential diagnosis of all patients presenting with a metastasis of unknown origin, particularly when lymph nodes are the principal site. Fine-needle aspiration or core biopsy of the metastasis is usually adequate for tissue diagnosis. Immunohistochemical studies have revolutionized the pathologist's ability to identify MUP. For example, melanoma can be positively identified by its immunoreactivity for S-100, vimentin, and HMB-45.[24] In addition, electron microscopy can be performed in the event of equivocal findings to visualize cellular organelles and demonstrate subcellular structures such as melanosomes or premelanosomes, which are diagnostic for melanoma.[24]

Although the true etiology of an MUP is unknown, several suggested explanations were recently summarized by Anbari and colleagues.[17] They include (1) a concurrent, unrecognized melanoma; (2) a previously excised melanoma that was clinically or pathologically misdiagnosed; (3) an antecedent, unrecognized, spontaneously regressed primary melanoma; and (4) the de novo malignant transformation of an aberrant melanocyte. The first two explanations indicate the need for careful history taking, a physical examination, and, when possible, a rereview of all previous biopsies in all patients with a suspected diagnosis of MUP. The validity of explanations 3 and 4 continue to be debated among experts in the field. Clinical and histologic observations favoring the third explanation, namely, the disappearance of a primary lesion as a result of spontaneous regression, date back to 1965 in a study by Smith and Stehlin.[25] In support of the possibility of a regressed primary melanoma resulting in disseminated disease, it has been suggested that the immunologic response that results in primary tumor regression somehow contributes to the more favorable outcomes seen in some series of patients with MUP.[3] In other words, regression may be evidence of a more vigorous host immune response, which may in turn provide a modest survival advantage for patients with MUP compared with patients with known primary tumors. Finally, according to the fourth explanation, MUP is a primary tumor arising from ectopic melanocytes in either a lymph node[26] or a visceral organ that result from aberrant migration of neuroectodermal cells;[27] these melanocytes subsequently undergo primary malignant transformation. Such an explanation is particularly attractive in regards to lymph node disease, as it is not uncommon to find capsular nevus cells in lymph nodes.

Table 1 Summary of Literature Pertaining to Incidence of MUP

First Author, Year	Study Period	Total No. Patients	MUP Patients	Incidence (%)	Stage III No. (%)	Stage IV No. (%)
Pack, 1952[1]	1917–1950	1190	29	2.4	–	–
Dasgupta, 1963[2]	1935–1957	992	37	3.7	24 (65)	13 (35)
Baab, 1975[3]	1944–1969	2446	98	4	54 (55)	44 (45)
Milton, 1977[4]	1950–1977	1854	76	4.1	60 (79)	16 (21)
Giuliano, 1980[5]	1971–1978	980	55	5.6	36 (65)	19 (35)
Lopez, 1982[6]	1955–1976	1593	129	8.1	–	–
Chang, 1982[7]	1948–1975	3805	166	4.4	75 (45)	91 (55)
Panagopoulos, 1983[8]	1940–1975	670	30	4.5	19 (63)	11 (37)
Reintgen, 1983[9]	1972–1982	2612	124	4.7	79 (64)	45 (36)
Klausner, 1983[10]	1973–1981	230	12	5.2	9 (75)	3 (25)
Wong, 1987[11]	1971–1986	4011	188	4.7	188 (100)	0
Jonk, 1990[12]	1961–1986	–	26	–	26 (100)	0
Velez, 1991[13]	1977–1988	1045	64	6.1	34 (53)	30 (47)
Norman, 1992[14]	1986–1989	580	18	3.1	17 (94)	1 (6)
Nasri, 1994[15]	1964–1991	–	46	–	46 (100)	0
Sutherland, 1996[16]	1981–1987	11904	145	1.2	–	–
Anbari, 1997[17]	1978–1996	–	40	–	26 (65)	14 (35)
Schlagenhauff, 1997[18]	1976–1996	3258	75	2.3	67 (89)	8 (11)
Vijuk, 1998[19]	1983–1996	3650	146	4.0	0	146 (100)
Chang, 1998[20]	1985–1994	84836	1893	2.2	814 (43)	1079 (57)
Laveau, 2001[21]	1985–1998	646	19	2.9	8 (42)	11 (58)
Katz, 2005[22]	1986–1996	2485	65	2.6	28 (43)	37 (57)
Cormier, 2006[23]	1990–2001	804	71	8.8	71 (100)	0

MUP = metastatic melanoma of unknown primary site; No. = number.

Clinical Presentation

The usual clinical scenario associated with MUP consists of finding metastatic melanoma in a single lymph node basin, a skin or subcutaneous nodule, or one (or multiple) distant organ sites. It has been estimated that 42 to 79% of patients with MUP present with a metastatic melanoma, which is often described as a "painless mass, in a single nodal basin (see Table 1).[3,7–9,28] The most common region involved in MUP is the axillary nodal basin, which accounts for 50 to 76% of cases. According to several reports, the cervical lymph nodes are the primary nodal basin in 20 to 30% of patients with MUP.[5,8,9,12]

To establish a diagnosis of MUP, one must first perform a clinical evaluation, which includes a total skin examination with biopsy of any suspicious lesions. A knowledge of the regional lymphatic drainage permits a focused examination of the anatomic regions most likely to harbor a previously unrecognized primary or regressed melanoma. Suspicious pigmented lesions or partially depigmented lesions should be excised and subjected to detailed histologic examination. In this regard, it was recently suggested that dermoscopy can play a role in the detection of a previously unknown primary melanoma by narrowing the field of lesions to be removed for histologic examination.[29] By naked-eye examination,

characteristics of a lesion that should be considered suspicious for a regressed primary melanoma include focal areas of white, gray-white, or pink pigmentation of the skin.[30] A Wood's ultraviolet lamp can also be useful in revealing areas of depigmentation or halo nevi. A pathologic review of such lesions often reveals fibroplasia in the papillary dermis with a lymphocytic infiltrate in the acute phase that later disappears, a macrophage infiltrate that consumes melanin, and new blood vessel formation.[31]

The pathologic review of any of prior biopsy specimens, if available, is also mandatory to confirm the absence of a previous or concomitant melanoma. All patients presenting with MUP must be evaluated for the presence and extent of distant metastatic disease. The staging evaluation should include computed tomographic (CT) scans of the chest, abdomen, and pelvis and magnetic resonance imaging (MRI) or CT imaging of the brain. More recently, fluorodeoxyglucose positron emission tomography has been advocated as a more sensitive indicator of metastatic melanoma compared with conventional diagnostic imaging modalities. Additional directed diagnostic evaluation is recommended for some patients with MUP. Such evaluation includes otorhinolaryngologic examinations in patients with metastases to the head and neck region and proctoscopy or gynecologic examination in patients with inguinal lymph node metastases.[18] Ophthalmologic examinations should be reserved for patients with MUP who have visceral metastases, primarily of the liver.

In a recently published study by our group,[23] we compared the characteristics of patients with stage III MUP ($n = 71$) with those of stage III control patients matched for nodal status (N1b, N2b, and N3 only) who had known primary cutaneous tumors ($n = 466$). The median age of the MUP cohort was 51 years (range, 21–71 years) compared with 54 years (range, 15–92 years) for the control group. In general, the cohorts were similar, except for the larger proportion of males (72% vs 58%, $p = 0.024$) and the predominance of axillary nodal disease (76% vs 48%, $p < 0.001$) among patients with MUP. This profile of clinical characteristics is consistent with that observed in several other studies.[2,5,7–9,16,17,22]

Classification

Patients with MUP can be categorized into 2 clinical groups: those with metastatic involvement to lymph nodes and those with nonnodal (eg, visceral involvement or subcutaneous) disease.[24] The involvement of multiple nodal regions is not necessarily an indication of stage IV disseminated disease because midline melanoma of the trunk can metastasize to bilateral or multiple nodal groups. In reports that include both of these groups, the distribution is relatively equal among patients with stage III and stage IV disease (see Table 1).[3–5,7–9,13,14,17,18,20–22] Specifically, in the cohort of 65 patients in the study by Katz and colleagues,[22] 28 (43%) had lymph node metastases, 12 (19%) had cutaneous or subcutaneous metastases, and 25 (39%) had visceral metastases. Of the patients with visceral metastases, 10 (40%) had central nervous system disease.[22] Additionally, Anbari and colleagues[17] reported that of 40 patients with MUP, 65% had lymph node metastasis only, 28% had visceral lesions, and 8% had subcutaneous nodules. In the largest population-based cohort of 1,893 patients with MUP, 43% had nodal disease only (stage III), and 57% had distant metastatic disease.[20]

The sixth edition of the American Joint Committee on Cancer staging system subclassifies stage III disease according to the degree of nodal (N) involvement.[32] In this N classification, the suffix "b" designates macrometastasis, which is empirically defined as clinically detectable disease. Furthermore, because the presence or absence of ulceration of the primary tumor is unknown in patients with MUP, the staging classification IIIB and IIIC cannot be applied to them. Thus, the subclassifications in MUP patients only consist of N1b, implying 1 lymph node with macrometastasis; N2b, implying 2 to 3 nodes with macrometastasis; and N3, implying 4 or more

metastatic regional nodes, matted nodes, or in-transit metastasis(es)/satellite(s) with any metastatic nodes(s). Among the cohort of patients with MUP in our study, 47%, 14%, and 39% presented with N1b, N2b, and N3 disease, respectively.[23]

Outcomes

The fate of patients with MUP has been reported to be highly variable, ranging from apparent cure with years of disease-free survival to rapid progression to distant metastatic disease and death. Dasgupta and colleagues[2] suggested as early as 1963 that survival was similar in patients with known and unknown primary tumors when the studies were controlled for stage of disease. This observation has been supported by several other reports.[5,9,11,13,23,28] However, there continues to be some controversy about the overall prognosis of patients with MUP, with some studies suggesting that these patients have slightly worse prognoses,[4] and others indicating that they have more favorable outcomes.[3,7,11,19,23] Several reasons may account for this discrepancy. First, many of the earliest series were reported in eras prior to contemporary radiologic imaging, so reliable staging with computed tomography was not available. As a result, outcomes were reported for small, heterogeneous groups of patients. Second, many of the studies included only small series of patients from single institutions whose outcomes might not have truly reflected those of larger, population-based cohorts. Third, outcomes were often compared with historical cohorts of patients with known primary cutaneous tumors. In the current era of radiologic imaging and recent modifications to the American Joint Committee on Cancer staging system,[32] more accurate comparisons of survival outcomes for patients with stage III and stage IV MUP can be performed with matched cohorts of patients with known primary cutaneous melanoma.

STAGE III MUP

Lymphadenectomy has been shown to result in 5-year overall survival rates of 29 to 55% in patients with MUP who have involvement of a single regional lymph node basin (Table 2).[2,7,17,22] Whereas several studies[2,11,14,18] have shown that this prognosis is similar to that of patients with stage III melanoma who have known primary tumors, others[6–8,15,17,23] have shown that patients with MUP who present with lymph node involvement may have a better prognosis than their counterparts with known cutaneous primary melanomas. In our MUP study cohort,[23] melanoma recurred in 40 (56%) patients during the follow-up interval: 10 (25%) were regional recurrences (in basins or retrograde in

Table 2 Reported Survival Outcomes Associated with Stage III MUP

First Author, Year	No. Stage III MUP Patients	5-Year DSS (%)	5-Year OS (%)	Median OS (years)
Chang, 1982[7]	75	–	46	–
Panagopoulos, 1983[8]	19	–	29	2.5
Reintgen, 1983[9]	79	–	–	2.6
Wong, 1987[11]	188	–	46	–
Velez, 1991[13]	34	–	45	4.4
Sutherland, 1996[16]	–	19*	–	–
Chang, 1998[20]	814	46	–	–
Katz, 2005[22]	28	–	39	4.0
Cormier, 2006[23]	71	56	55	6.4

DSS = disease-specific survival; MUP = metastatic melanoma of unknown primary site; No. = number; OS = overall survival.
*Includes both stage III and stage IV disease.

transit metastases), 28 (70%) were distant recurrences, and 2 (5%) were synchronous regional and distant recurrences. The types of recurrences were similar in the controls with known primary tumors; of the 282 (61%) patients with recurrence, 82 (29%) had regional recurrence, 175 (62%) had distant recurrence, and 7 (3%) had synchronous regional and distant recurrence. In addition, local disease recurred in 18 (6%) of the patients with known primary tumors. Thirty-five patients (49%) in the MUP group and 267 patients (57%) in the control group died of melanoma. The median disease-specific survival duration was 7.60 years for patients with MUP and 3.56 years for control patients.

The 5-year disease-specific survival rate in patients with MUP was 56% compared with 44% in the control group ($P = 0.04$). Overall, patients with MUP fared better than matched control patients in our study (hazard ratio = 0.73; 95% confidence interval, 0.53–1.01; $p = 0.057$). There were no significant differences in treatment factors (eg, postoperative radiation therapy and systemic therapy) between patients with MUP and control patients. The finding that patients with MUP had more favorable survival outcomes than the control cohort (55% vs 42%, $P = 0.043$) (Figure 1) is consistent with the findings reported in several other studies.[3,7,8,11,15,17] Our finding was also consistent after multivariate analyses, even when an adjustment was made for primary tumor ulceration in the control cohort.

STAGE IV MUP

Not surprisingly, in the studies that included outcomes for patients with both stage III and stage IV MUP, the median and 5-year overall survival rates were significantly shorter for patients with stage IV MUP, ranging from 8 to 14% (Table 3). For example, Katz and colleagues[22] reported that the median survival duration for patients with stage IV MUP was 12 months, with a 5-

year survival rate of 13.9% (95% confidence interval, 4.4–28.6%). Patients with cutaneous or subcutaneous metastases fared better than those with lung or other visceral metastases. Similarly, Chang and colleagues[20] reported that in a large cohort of patients with MUP ($n = 1,893$) from the National Cancer Database, patients with regional disease (stage III) had a 5-year survival rate of 46.3% compared with a rate of only 15.8% for patients with distant (stage IV) disease ($P < 0.0001$). These survival outcomes are similar to the 7- to 9-month median survival duration reported in patients with metastatic melanoma.[33,34]

Treatment Recommendations

In general, a surgical approach has been advocated for isolated nodal or visceral metastatic disease in all

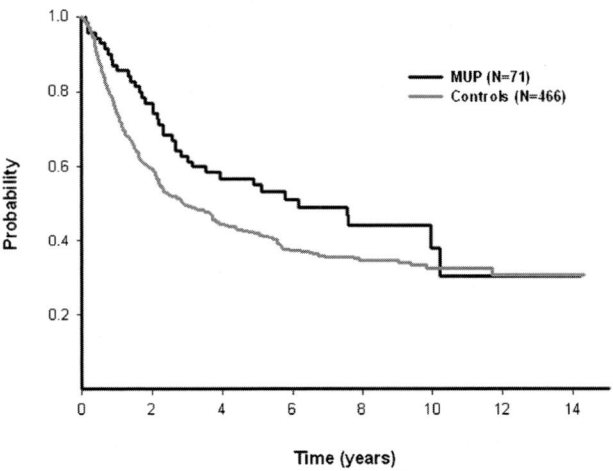

Figure 1 Overall survival duration for patients with stage III MUP compared with that of matched patients (controls) with known primary tumors.

Table 3 Reported Survival Outcomes Associated with Stage IV MUP

First Author, Year	No. Stage IV MUP Patients	5-Year DSS (%)	5-Year OS (%)
Chang, 1982[7]	91	–	8
Velez, 1991[13]	30	–	10
Sutherland, 1996[16]	–	19*	–
Chang, 1998[20]	1079	16	–
Katz, 2005[22]	37	–	14

DSS = disease-specific survival; MUP = metastatic melanoma of unknown primary site; No. = number; OS = overall survival.
*Includes both stage III and stage IV disease.

patients, including those with unknown primary tumors, because subgroups of these patients fare well.[20,35–41] In general, patients with MUP should be fully staged with radiologic imaging prior to treatment decisions being made, and the extent (stage) of disease should be considered.

STAGE III MUP

Therapeutic completion regional nodal dissection is recommended for all patients with stage III MUP. This procedure includes a level I, II, and III axillary node dissection for patients with axillary disease; a superficial inguinofemoral node dissection and (possibly) a deep pelvic node dissection for those with disease in the groin; and a modified neck dissection for patients with cervical disease. In our study of patients with MUP metastatic to nodal basins and a matched control group, all patients underwent completion nodal dissection as their primary treatment; there was no difference between the groups in the median number of regional lymph nodes removed during the procedure.[23] The median number of lymph nodes removed at the time of axillary nodal dissection was 23 for the MUP group versus 22 for the control cohort. The median number of lymph nodes removed at the time of inguinofemoral lymph node dissection was 15 in both groups, and the median number of lymph nodes dissected at the time of cervical lymph node dissection was 18 for the MUP group versus 17 for the control group. In the patients with MUP, additional nodal disease was recovered from the nodal basin 46% of the time with completion node dissection. This information is valuable for determining prognosis in that patients with 1 positive node have a better prognosis than patients with 2 to 3, and the latter patients have a better outcome than patients with 4 or more positive nodes.[23] Patients with stage III MUP should also be considered for adjuvant treatment trials designed for patients with stage III disease and known primary tumors.

Whereas the ultimate goal of completion node dissection is a cure, the benefits of achieving control of bulky regional nodal disease must not be underestimated,

even for patients who are destined to develop distant metastatic disease. To maximize the potential for regional control, we treated 18 (25%) patients with MUP and 90 (19%) control patients in our series with postoperative radiation therapy delivered to the regional nodal basin. Indications for postoperative radiation therapy included (1) extracapsular extension of nodal metastatic disease, (2) lymph node metastasis greater than 3 cm, or (3) more than 3 lymph nodes with disease.

STAGE IV MUP

The prognosis for patients with stage IV melanoma, whether is arises from known or unknown primary tumors, is extremely poor, with a median survival duration ranging from 6 to 12 months, and a 5-year survival rate of less than 10%. More recent trials in selected patients receiving intensive biochemotherapy regimens have resulted in slightly longer median survival durations. However, no chemotherapy or immunotherapy regimen has shown consistent benefit in overall survival for most patients with stage IV melanoma. Similarly, vaccines have shown little clinical activity to date.

Despite the overall poor prognosis, there have been subsets of patients with stage IV disease among whom long-term survival has been reported after aggressive surgical resection of metastatic disease.[35–41] Surgical resection is technically possible in most patients who have only 1 or 2 metastatic sites. In particular, surgical resection with minimal (1 cm) margins is reasonable in patients with MUP who have limited cutaneous or subcutaneous metastases (eg, M1a disease). Additionally, complete metastatectomy, regardless of the anatomic site, should be considered in selected patients whenever possible. Such patients include those in whom surgical resection of metastatic disease can be achieved completely and safely; incomplete resection should be reserved for palliation of symptoms only. Palliative procedures performed in appropriately selected patients have resulted in reliable relief of symptoms and improved quality of life. Furthermore, all patients undergoing resection of metastatic melanoma should be considered for clinical trials with systemic adjuvant therapies, including novel drug therapies and vaccines.

Conclusions

MUP is not a rare entity, accounting for 1.2 to 8.8% of all patients with melanoma. Metastatic melanoma should be considered in the differential diagnosis of all patients who present with a metastasis of unknown origin, particularly when lymph nodes are the principal presenting site. Fine-needle aspiration and immunohistochemical analysis of the metastatic lesion can usually confirm the diagnosis of MUP. Current recommendations for the evaluation of patients with this disease include a review of previous skin biopsy specimens, full skin evaluation, brain imaging (with CT or MRI), and CT imaging of the chest, abdomen, and pelvis to rule out distant metastatic disease. When clinically appropriate, urogenital, otolaryngologic, or ophthamologic examinations should be performed in patients to exclude unusual primary sites. Approximately 50% of patients presenting with MUP have metastatic involvement to lymph nodes only (stage III MUP). The natural history of patients with stage III MUP is similar to that of patients with stage III disease with known primary tumors. Therefore, patients with stage III MUP (and subsets of patients with stage IV MUP) should be treated with an aggressive surgical approach with curative intent and should be considered for adjuvant therapy protocols.

References

1. Pack GT, Gerber DM, Scharnagel IM. End results in the treatment of malignant melanoma; a report of 1190 cases. Ann Surg 1952;136:905–11.

2. Dasgupta T, Bowden L, Berg JW. Malignant melanoma of unknown primary origin. Surg Gynecol Obstet 1963;117: 341–5.

3. Baab GH, McBride CM. Malignant melanoma: the patient with an unknown site of primary origin. Arch Surg 1975; 110:896–900.

4. Milton GW, Shaw HM, McCarthy WH. Occult primary malignant melanoma: factors influencing survival. Br J Surg 1977;64:805–8.

5. Giuliano AE, Moseley HS, Morton DL. Clinical aspects of unknown primary melanoma. Ann Surg 1980;191:98–104.

6. Lopez R, Holyoke ED, Moore RH, Karakousis CP. Malignant melanoma with unknown primary site. J Surg Oncol 1982;19:151–4.

7. Chang P, Knapper WH. Metastatic melanoma of unknown primary. Cancer 1982;49:1106–11.

8. Panagopoulos E, Murray D. Metastatic malignant melanoma of unknown primary origin: a study of 30 cases. J Surg Oncol 1983;23:8–10.

9. Reintgen DS, McCarty KS, Woodard B, et al. Metastatic malignant melanoma with an unknown primary. Surg Gynecol Obstet 1983;156:335–340.

10. Klausner JM, Gutman M, Inbar M, Rozin RR. Unknown primary melanoma. J Surg Oncol 1983;24:129–31.

11. Wong JH, Cagle LA, Morton DL. Surgical treatment of lymph nodes with metastatic melanoma from unknown primary site. Arch Surg 1987;122:1380–3.

12. Jonk A, Kroon BB, Rumke P, et al. Lymph node metastasis from melanoma with an unknown primary site. Br J Surg 1990;77:665–8.

13. Velez A, Walsh DL, Karakousis CP. Treatment of unknown primary melanoma. Cancer 1991;68:2579–81.

14. Norman J, Cruse CW, Wells KE, et al. Metastatic melanoma with an unknown primary. Ann Plast Surg 1992;28:81–4.

15. Nasri S, Namazie A, Dulguerov P, Mickel R. Malignant melanoma of cervical and parotid lymph nodes with an unknown primary site. Laryngoscope 1994;104:1194–8.

16. Sutherland CM, Chmiel JS. Patient characteristics, treatment, and outcome of unknown primary melanoma in the United States for the years 1981 and 1987. Am Surg 1996; 62:400–6.

17. Anbari KK, Schuchter LM, Bucky LP, et al. Melanoma of unknown primary site: presentation, treatment, and prognosis–a single institution study. University of Pennsylvania Pigmented Lesion Study Group. Cancer 1997;79:1816–21.

18. Schlagenhauff B, Stroebel W, Ellwanger U, et al. Metastatic melanoma of unknown primary origin shows prognostic similarities to regional metastatic melanoma: recommendations for initial staging examinations. Cancer 1997;80: 60–5.

19. Vijuk G, Coates AS. Survival of patients with visceral metastatic melanoma from an occult primary lesion: a retrospective matched cohort study. Ann Oncol 1998;9: 419–22.

20. Chang AE, Karnell LH, Menck HR. The National Cancer Data Base report on cutaneous and noncutaneous melanoma: a summary of 84,836 cases from the past decade. The American College of Surgeons Commission on Cancer and the American Cancer Society. Cancer 1998;83: 1664–78.

21. Laveau F, Picot MC, Dereure O, et al. Metastatic melanoma of unknown primary site. Ann Dermatol Venereol 2001; 128:893–8.

22. Katz KA, Jonasch E, Hodi FS, et al. Melanoma of unknown primary: experience at Massachusetts General Hospital and

Dana-Farber Cancer Institute. Melanoma Res 2005;15:77–82.

23. Cormier JN, Xing Y, Feng L, et al. Metastatic melanoma to lymph nodes in patients with unknown primary sites. Cancer 2006;106:2012–20.

24. Chorost MI, Lee MC, Yeoh CB, et al. Unknown primary. J Surg Oncol 2004;87:191–203.

25. Smith JL Jr, Stehlin JS Jr. Spontaneous regression of primary malignant melanomas with regional metastases. Cancer 1965;18:1399–415.

26. Hara K. Melanocytic lesions in lymph nodes associated with congenital naevus. Histopathology 1993;23:445–51.

27. Dasgupta TK, Brasfield RD, Paglia MA. Primary melanomas in unusual sites. Surg Gynecol Obstet 1969;128:841–8.

28. Giuliano AE, Cochran AJ, Morton DL. Melanoma from unknown primary site and amelanotic melanoma. Semin Oncol 1982;9:442–7.

29. Stante M, de Giorgi V, Carli P. Possible role of dermoscopy in the detection of a primary cutaneous melanoma of unknown origin. J Eur Acad Dermatol Venereol 2006;20:299–302.

30. Mihm MC Jr, Fitzpatrick TB, Brown MM, et al. Early detection of primary cutaneous malignant melanoma. A color atlas. N Engl J Med 1973;289:989–96.

31. Patterson J. Regression in primary malignant melanomas. Am J Dermatopathol 1979;1:90.

32. Greene FL, Page DL, Fleming ID, et al, editors. Melanoma of the skin. In: AJCC cancer staging handbook: from the AJCC cancer staging manual, 6th ed. New York: Springer; 2002. p. 239.

33. Balch CM, Buzaid AC, Soong SJ, et al. Final version of the American Joint Committee on Cancer staging system for cutaneous melanoma. J Clin Oncol 2001;19:3635–48.

34. Balch CM, Soong SJ, Gershenwald JE, et al. Prognostic factors analysis of 17,600 melanoma patients: validation of the American Joint Committee on cancer melanoma staging System. J Clin Oncol 2001;19:3622–34.

35. Essner R, Lee JH, Wanek LA, et al. Contemporary surgical treatment of advanced-stage melanoma. Arch Surg 2004;139:961–6.

36. Ollila DW, Caudle AS. Surgical management of distant metastases. Surg Oncol Clin N Am 2006;15:385–98.

37. Rose DM, Essner R, Hughes TM, et al. Surgical resection for metastatic melanoma to the liver: the John Wayne Cancer Institute and Sydney Melanoma Unit experience. Arch Surg 2001;136:950–5.

38. Allen PJ, Coit DG. The surgical management of metastatic melanoma. Ann Surg Oncol 2002;9:762–70.

39. Wood TF, DiFronzo LA, Rose DM, et al. Does complete resection of melanoma metastatic to solid intra-abdominal organs improve survival? Ann Surg Oncol 2001;8:658–62.

40. Meyer T, Merkel S, Goehl J, Hohenberger W. Surgical therapy for distant metastases of malignant melanoma. Cancer 2000;89:1983–91.

41. Leo F, Cagini L, Rocmans P, et al. Lung metastases from melanoma: when is surgical treatment warranted? Br J Cancer 2000;83:569–72.

Chapter 87

Adjuvant Systemic and Adjuvant Radiation Therapy for Melanoma: What the Surgeon Needs to Know

Frank Haluska, MD, PhD

Kevin Kalinsky, MD

Jay Douglas, MD

Introduction

In the United States, cutaneous melanoma is the fifth most common cancer in men. It is the sixth most common in women. Currently, it is estimated that approximately 62,000 people will be diagnosed with melanoma per year, and nearly 7,900 people are expected to die of this disease.[1] The natural history of melanoma typically involves the development of a localized tumor, early involvement of regional lymph nodes, and ultimately the manifestation of disseminated disease. One clinical consequence of this natural history is that patients who ultimately develop advanced disease have identifiable features of high-risk melanoma early in their course. Thus, many of the nearly 8,000 patients who ultimately succumb to melanoma yearly are candidates for early therapy. This therapy is the first focus of this chapter. In particular, we will focus on a variety of therapies that have been tested in the adjuvant setting, and on the use of the sole FDA-approved modality for adjuvant therapy of high-risk melanoma, interferon alpha-2b.

Failure in a regional lymph node basin after a formal lymph node dissection occurs more commonly than many surgeons would like to admit. Such recurrences are difficult to treat and may be the source of significant morbidity in terms of pain, bleeding, and lymphedema. As is the case with distant disease, micrometastatic is in all probability the source of relapse in the regional basin, and predictors for such relapse have been identified. Therapies directed to prevent in-basin relapse in a dissected basin, radiation therapy in particular, is the second focus of this chapter.

It is imperative that surgeons who treat patients with melanoma should not only have a clear understanding of the critical prognostic factors that predict regional and distant relapse and are able to recommend and carry out stage appropriate surgical therapies, but also have at least a basic appreciation for the risks and benefits of the available adjuvant therapies or adjuvant clinical trials. In this way the surgeon plays a central role in the processes of identifying patients eligible for adjuvant therapy and helping patients transition from appropriately aggressive surgery to receive rational regional and systemic strategies.

Adjuvant Systemic Therapy

BACKGROUND

Since metastatic melanoma is known to have a poor prognosis, much research has been conducted in the evaluation for effective adjuvant therapy after primary tumor resection or after dissection of regional lymph node metastases and, more recently, after resection of distant disease in highly selelcted stage IV patients. Although this last subgroup may have the highest risk of subsequent relapse after surgical resection, it is the least-studied subgroup of patients. The concept of adjuvant therapy for melanoma is based on the hypothesis that these therapies may have an effect on residual, micro-metastatic disease that is the source for future relapse. Patients with advanced stages of disease have an increased risk of developing metastases, and ultimately an increased mortality. The goal of adjuvant therapy is to reduce the rate of recurrent melanoma and to increase the overall survival of these patients. Systemic adjuvant treatment of melanoma is considered when a patient is clinically free of disease following surgical excision of a high-risk primary tumor, or once nodal involvement is determined to be present.[2]

A number of adjuvant modalities have been tested in several clinical settings (see Table 1). Until recently, no regimen was shown to provide effective adjuvant therapy, and it is worthwhile to briefly examine the experience with adjuvant therapy to provide context for interferon's utility. Studied agents have included chemotherapy, immunotherapy with a variety of compounds, hormones, and vitamins.

Chemotherapy

In the adjuvant setting, chemotherapy has not been successful.[15] Chemotherapy, however, has limited activity in malignant melanoma. The best single agents include dacarbazine (DTIC), cisplatin, and alkylating agents. For metastastic disease, each has activity (complete response + partial response) in the range of 10%, and in the most recent large randomized trials comparing therapies with

Table 1 Tested Adjuvant Therapies

Chemotherapy (including DTIC, Cisplatin, Alkylating Agents)
BCG
Corynebactium parvum
Levamisole
Megace
Vitamins (including Vitamin A)
Interferon (High, Intermediate, and Low Dose)
Vaccine Therapy
Biochemotherapy

chemotherapy, the activity of DTIC alone is approximately 8% (CITE genasense). Combination chemotherapy, although offering enhanced response rates in single-arm studies, has not been proven to provide significant benefit over single agents in randomized, comparative trials. In the adjuvant setting, dose escalation with autologous transplant has been evaluated as well. Although the number of patients enrolled in this and similar studies is small, this therapeutic approach did not demonstrate a significant overall survival (OS) or disease-free survival (DFS) advantage.[3]

Nonspecific Immunotherapy

Bacillus Calmett-Guérin (BCG), *Corynebacterium*, and levamisole have been studied as adjuvant modalities. These treatments have not demonstrated any statistical impact in the adjuvant setting and are not considered standard therapy.

BCG has been examined as therapy for both the American Joint Committee on Cancer (AJCC) stage II and stage III patients.[4] Six randomized trials evaluated adjuvant BCG for stage II disease; none demonstrated any benefit to treatment. An additional seven trials examined BCG in stage III disease. Only one of these trials, comparing BCG + DTIC with BCG or DTIC, showed a survival benefit to the combined therapy.[5] However, the World Health Organization (WHO) performed a large, randomized trial of adjuvant chemotherapy (DTIC), BCG, or the combination of the two, and did not demonstrate any significant difference in outcomes between the groups.[6]

Randomized trials have also examined the role of *Corynebacterium parvum* as adjuvant immunotherapy, and randomized trials comparing *Corynebactium parvum* with control noted no difference in the groups.[8]

Levamisole, a synthetic imidazothiazole derivative that has been widely used in the treatment of worm infestations, has been used in the adjuvant setting because it has been thought to possess immunostimulatory properties. Four randomized controlled trials have examined the role of levamisole as adjuvant treatment in melanoma. In a review of the available data, the benefit of this medication has been determined to be marginal, and, although the morbidity from levamisole is generally minimal, between 17 and 44% of patients in these trials needed to discontinue this treatment secondary to side effects.[9] Thus, levamisole is not considered a standard therapeutic option for patients with melanoma.

Hormones

Adjuvant hormonal therapy with megace, a synthetic derivative of progesterone, has also been tested in a controlled setting. After a small, randomized trial showed a trend to improvement in survival with megestrol acetate versus placebo treatment, a large prospective phase III study was initiated by the North Central Cancer Treatment Group (NCCTG-897051).[10] However, since this trial was set up, there has been no further interest in this agent for this setting.[10]

Vitamins

Retinoids have also been studied in as adjuvant treatment. Patients with tumors greater than 0.75 mm and clinically negative lymph nodes were randomized oral vitamin A (100,000 IU/d) for 18 months or to observation. At 8-year follow-up, no difference in DFS or OS was identified. Based on this lack of benefit, no further evaluation of vitamin A as adjuvant therapy for melanoma has been warranted.[11]

Interferon

BACKGROUND

Based on the conduct of a randomized trial, interferon alpha-2b is approved by the FDA for the adjuvant therapy of patients with high-risk melanoma. To date, in three large randomized controlled trials carried out by the Easter Cooperative Oncology Group, nearly 1,900 patients with high-risk resected melanoma have been treated. The weight of the evidence suggests that interferon has an important role in the treatment of these patients.

Interferons are a class of natural proteins produced by the cells of the immune system in response to challenges by foreign agents. The term "interferon" was first coined in 1957 by Scottish virologist Alick Isaccs and Swiss researcher Jean Lindenmann, as they noted an interference effect caused by heat-inactivated influenza virus on the growth of live influena virus.[12] In humans, there are three major classes of inteferon (IFN): type I (which includes IFN-alpha, IFN-beta, IFN-omega, and IFN-Tao isoforms), type II (consisting of solely IFN-gamma), and the recently discovered IFN-lambda (with three different isoforms).[13] Type I cells bind to a type I IFN receptor, while type II cells bind to a distinct type II receptor. The IFNs perform a broad spectrum of functions. They generally display antiviral and antitumor activity, activate macrophage and natural killer lymphoctyes, and enhance MCH classes I and II.

While IFN-alpha is secreted by T and B lymphoctyes, INF-beta is secreted by fibroblasts, and INF-gamma by T cells and NK cells. Unlike type I IFNs, IFN-gamma is not directly induced in cells after viral infection. Preparations of INF-alpha, -beta, and -gamma are currently available

and have been mostly produced using (r) DNA technology.

In addition to its use in melanoma, IFN-alpha has been extensively studied in patients with other solid and hematologic tumors, including renal cell, Kaposi's sarcoma, hairy cell leukemia, CML, and follicular lymphoma. Currenlty, IFN-beta 1a is FDA approved for patients with relapsing-remitting multiple sclerosis, and IFN-gamma is FDA approved for use in chronic granulomatous disease.[13]

Interferon in Melanoma

Interferon-alpha was initially evaluated in the setting of metastatic melanoma. As monotherapy, IFN induced response rates of approximately 15%, with complete response rates of approximately 5%.[14] The use of interferon as a single agent in metastatic disease has not been pursued. But as a result of its promising activity, this treatment was pursued in the adjuvant setting. Currently, there are at least twelve randomized phase III trials investigating the role of IFN-alpha for patients with stage II and III melanoma (Table 2). These studies differ by the dose administered, duration of administration, and disease stage of the enrolled patients. Adjuvant trials can be classified into low-dose, intermediate-dose, and high-dose trials, depending on the different dose regimens.[15]

LOW-DOSE INTERFERON

The signficant toxicity that is associated with high-dose interferon (HDI) prompted the study of lower-dose IFN (LDI) in the adjuvant setting. The dose used in these trials is IFN-alpha-3 MU SQ 3 times per week. They differed in the duration of treatment (see Table 2). Six randomized controlled trials have been performed comparing LDI with observation in resected, high-risk patients with melanoma. These trials have inconsistently shown a DFS or OS advantage. The WHO enrolled 444 patients with stage III disease and compared those receiving LDI (IFN-alpha-3 MU SQ 3 times per week for 3 years) versus observation. No significant impact was noted at a median follow-up of 39 months.[16]

In these studies, patients were not required to undergo surgical evaluation of regional lymph nodes with either sentinel lymph node surgery or prophylactic lymph node dissection. The patients were known only to be clinically node negative. Thus, these patients were poorly stratified and do not correspond well to current patients with intermediate-thickness melanomas, as standard of care in the United States is to perform sentinel lymph node biopsy on melanomas > 1 mm or those < 1 mm with negative pathologic features such as Clark's level IV or V

Table 2 Randomized Trials of Adjuvant Interferon for Melanoma

Study	Group (Duration of IFN by # of months)	Overall Survival (±)	Disease Free Survival (±)	Reference
Low-Dose Interferon	Scottish (6)	–	–	(16)
	Austrian (12)	+	–	(17)
	French (18)	+	–	(18)
	EORTC 18871/DKG 80-1 (12)	–	–	(19)
	WHO (36)	–	–	(20)
	UK-AIM High (24)	–	–	(21)
	ECOG 1690 (24)	–	–	(27)
Intermediate-Dose Interferon	EORTC melanoma trial 18952	–	–	(23)
High-Dose Interferon	ECOG 1684 (12)	+	+	(25)
	ECOG 1690 (12)	–	+	(26)
	ECOG 1694 (12)	+	+	(28)
	ECOG 2696 (12)	+	+	(29)

and/or ulceration.[17] Despite the improved toxicity profile with LDI, because of the lack of demonstration of its efficacy, it is not presently FDA approved.

INTERMEDIATE-DOSE INTERFERON

The European Organisation for Research and Treatment of Cancer (EORTC) melanoma trial 18952 is the only study to evaluate the role of intermediate-dose IFN-alpha in the adjuvant setting. There were three arms in this trial. The two treatment arms both received an induction phase of 10 MU/dose subcutaneously (SQ) daily for 1 month followed by either 10 MU SQ 3 times a week for 1 year or 5 MU SQ 3 times a week for 2 years. There were 1,388 patients with stage IIB or III disease recruited prior to closure of the trial. After a median follow-up of approximately 4.5 years, no significant DFS or OS advanatage was noted in either of the treatment groups.

Intermediate-dose interferon was found to not offer significant benefit in the adjuvant setting.[23]

HIGH-DOSE INTERFERON

Background

IFN (HDI) alpha-2b is the only FDA-approved therapy for patients at high risk of recurrence of melanoma. Four randomized phase III US cooperative group trials have examined the use of HDI. In these trials (Table 3) (ECOG 1684, ECOG 1690, ECOG 1694, and ECOG 2696), the year long treatment plan is as follows:

Induction: 20 MU/m^2/d intravenously for 5 days each week for 4 weeks.

Maintenance: 10 MU/m^2 TIW subcutaneously 3 times a week for 48 weeks.

Table 3 High-Dose Melanoma

Study	Patient Number Enrolled (n)	Median Follow-Up	Control OS	HDI OS	P value	Control DFS	HDI DFS	P value	Reference
E1684	287	6.9 years	2.8 years	3.8 years	(P = .0237, one-sided)	1.0 years	1.7 years	(P = .0023, one-sided)	(25)
E1690	642	52 month	Estimated 5 year: 55%	Estimated 5 year: 52%	HR = 1	Estimated 5 year: 35%	Estimated 5 year: 44%	HR = 1.28 (P(2) =.05	(27)
E1694	880	96 weeks	81 (20%)	52 (13%)	HR=1.52 (P$_1$ = .009	151 (39%) of 389	98 (25%) of 385	The HR=1.47 (P$_1$ = .0015)	(28)
E2696	107	Overall Survival Advantage Not seen. Exact numbers not given.	p value for A versus C .303,	p value for B versus C .588.	Not Signficant	Arm C 14.85.	Arm A – not reached. Arm B -30.72 months	Adjusted p value for A vs, C = .016. Adjusted p value for B vs. C = .03.	(29)

Please note, Control OS, HDI OS, Control DFS, and HDI DFS are reported as median numbers.
Please note, the control group in 1694 is not an observation group. This group consists of those patients receiving the vaccination.
Please note, in E2696, the control group is GMK alone (arm C). The HDI is both GMK vaccine plus concurrent HDI (arm A) and GMK vaccine plus sequential HDI (arm B).

The rationale for the initial high-dose intravenous treatment phase is to provide maximal dose intensity while minimizing the induction of anti-IFN antibodies. Because of the substantial relapse rate associated with high-risk melanoma and lack of other effective adjuvant therapies, the results of the first trial listed, ECOG 1684, led to the rapid approval of HDI. The FDA accepted HDI as an adjuvant treatment for stage IIB and stage III disease.[24] However, the results of the above-mentioned trials are inconsistent, ranging from statistically significant improvements in OS and DFS to minimal or no benefit. In addition, this therapy is known to be difficult to tolerate with associated morbidities. Thus, HDI remains a controversial topic in the melanoma literature.

ECOG 1684

The first of these trials is the ECOG 1684 trial, which randomized 287 patients to either observation versus HDI following surgery.[25] The earlier AJCC staging system was used for these patients. Those enrolled were from stage IIB (Breslow depth > 4.00 mm) and stage III (node positive). With a median follow-up of 6.9 years, DFS was improved by IFN therapy (1.7 vs 1.0 years, $p = 0.0023$, one-sided). At 5 years, an 11% absolute increase in RFS was noted (37% vs 26%). OS was also significantly improved (3.8 vs 2.8 years, $p = 0.0237$, one-sided), when analyzed either according to eligible patients or by intention to treat. At 5 years, an absolute increase in survival at 5 years was noted (46% vs 37%).

This improvement in both DFS and OS led to the FDA approval of this treatment for patients with primary lesions thicker than 4 mm or node positive. Of interest, in a follow-up analysis, the overall survival benefit seen in this trial was no longer statistically significant at a median follow-up 12.6 years. DFS was still evident (HR 1.38; P2 = 0.02). It is unclear whether the diminished overall survival is due to cancer-related death or death from competing causes in an aging study population (median age of this population now > 60).[21]

ECOG 1690

Subsequent to ECOG 1684, ECOG designed and implemented the ECOG 1690 trial. The goal of E1690 was in essence to confirm the observation of ECOG 1684. The results, however, did not confirm the findings of ECOG 1684.

Intergroup ECOG 1690 is a 3-armed study, designed to compare HDI, low-dose interferon (LDI-IFN 3MU/d SQ TIW for 2 years), and observation in a similar patient population, T4 or N1.[27] Unlike ECOG 1684, the patients

with clinically negative regional nodes were not required to undergo staging lymph node dissections. Thus, only about one-quarter of the patients with T4 N0 disease were electively dissected.

At 52 months median follow-up, a DFS benefit of HDI versus observation was seen (HR 1.28, $p = .05$) greater than for LDI (HR 1.09, $p = .17$). No overall survival advantage was seen (HR 1.0).

Several reasons have been postulated for the DFS benefit with HDI not translating into an overall survival benefit. First, the observation group in ECOG 1690 had signficant outcome improvement in comparison with the observation group in 1684. This improvement was seen in both disease-free and overall survival. The median overall survival of patients in the ECOG 1690 observation arm was 6 years in ECOG 1684, in comparison with 2.8 years for ECOG 1684. This effect may be due to selection bias. ECOG 1690 had a larger number of patients with T4 N0 (25% vs 11%). Also, a high number of patients in the observation arm received salvage therapy (including 31% who received IFN as their salvage therapy).

Furthering the controversy regarding the effectiveness of HDI, a pooled analysis of 713 patients from ECOG 1684 and ECOG 1690 was published in March 2004.[21] The analysis, a two-sided univariate log-rank comparison of HDI versus observation (median follow-up of 7.2 years) showed that HDI was superior with respect to DFS ($p < 0.006$). However, neither the univariate nor the multivariate analysis of the pooled data demonstrated a statistically significant OS benefit of HDI versus observation. Again, the unusually prolonged postrelapse survival rate of the patients in the ECOG 2690 arm and the crossover use of IFN in these patients are thought be contributing factors to the lack of significant overall survival of HDI.[26]

EGOG 1694

In a third trial, Intergroup ECOG 1694, compared 1 year of HDI versus 2 years of a vaccine called GMK, containing the ganglioside GM2 linked to KLH and given with QS-21 adjuvant.[28] This trial accrued 880 patients with T4 or nodal disease. It closed in October of 1999. The trial was halted in May 2000, with a median of 16 months of follow-up, when interim analysis demonstrated an advantage to interferon. There was no observation-arm group. Both disease-free and overall survival significantly favored HDI.

ECOG 2696

ECOG 2696 is a small, randomized phase II trial, which tested the effect of the combination of HDI plus ganglioside vaccine on the antibody response to GM2 in resected stage IIb, III, and IV.[29] Patients were randomized to GMK vaccine plus concurrent HDI (arm A), GMK vaccine plus sequential HDI (arm B), or GMK alone (arm C). Even though relapse and death were not primary end points of the study, Kaplan-Meier curves of OS and DFS were estimated at a median follow-up of 24 months. A DFS advantage for the two HDI-containing arms, compared with the vaccine-only arm, was noted ($P = 0.016$; $P = 0.03$). There was no benefit in OS.[29]

Toxicities

The side effects of HDI have been well noted. Four major side effect groups typically occur: constitutional, neuropsychiatric, hematologic, and hepatic (Table 4). In ECOG 1684, both treatment delays and dosage reductions were frequently required during therapy, including 50% of treated patients during the induction period and 48% of patients during the maintenance phase. Grade III toxicities were noted in 67% of all treated patients at some point in their therapy. Nine percent had grade IV toxicities. In the course of the trial, 2 patients died of liver toxicity prior to the realization of this toxicity.[25] On subsequent trials there was greater experience with this medication and no lethal toxicity was noted.

The toxicities associated with HDI can be divided into those occurring in the acute setting, which typically diminish over time, and those that develop on a chronic basis. In the acute setting, patients experience fevers, chills, and rigors, usually between 3 and 6 hours after receiving IFN. Patients may also experience constitutional symptoms, such as headaches, myalgias, and malaise. Patients can develop tolerance to these symptoms if the medication is given on a prolonged and uninterrupted basis. However, rigors and chills can recur if a patient's treatment is held for even a few days. Both transaminitis and neutropenia can occur in the acute setting and can be modified by adjusting the IFN dose.[13]

Table 4 Possible Associated Toxicities (25)

Constitutional	Fatigue
	Anorexia
	Weight Loss
	Fever
	Myalgia
Hepatic	Transaminitis
Neuropsychiatric	Depression
	Dizziness/vertigo
	Confusion
Hematologic	Thrombocytopenia
	Anemia
	Leukopenia

The chronic symptoms experienced by patients on IFN include fatigue (70–100% of patients), anorexia (40–70%), and neuropsychiatric symptoms (up to 30%).[30] These symptoms appear to be dose related and cumulative. Much focus has been appropriately been placed on the possible neuropsychiatric side effects of interferon. Patients may experience such central nervous symptoms as somnolence, confusion, lethargy, dizziness, and impaired mental status.[30] Peripheral nervous systems toxicities, such as numbness and tingling, may occur. A significant minority of patients receiving interferon can become depressed and, in some cases, can lead to suicide. These mood disorders can occur in patients without predisposing factors or any prior history of psychiatric problems. The mechanism by which interferon causes psychiatric issue is not well understood; however, some argue that this side effect may be the result of neuroendocrine effects.[13]

Since these side effects can be significant, communication among all members of a treatment team is essential for patients receiving interferon therapy. Although constitutional side effects can be managed with appropriate hydration and acetaminophen, patients receiving HDI should initially be evaluated with at least weekly liver function tests, weekly complete blood counts, and monthly TSH measurements.[13] Also, if a patient is thought to have any risk factors for a mood disorder, it is recommended that the patient be evaluated by a psychiatric expert for evaluation prior to interferon therapy.[13]

Analyzing Toxicity

When considering HDI therapy, the ratio of risks to benefits should be considered. In a review of the ECOG 1684 trial data, patients receiving HDI averaged 5.8 months of severe treatment-related toxicities. When considering the 9 month relapse-free survival advantage, the patients treated with HDI were thought to have an improved quality-of-life survival.[31] Also, based on ECOG 1684, the lifetime cost of HDI per quality adjusted life-year is approximately $15,000 (US). This cost is below the established reference range for cost-effectiveness, $50,000 to $100,000 per quality-adjusted year of life saved.[32] In an attempt to quantify the level of comfort patients possess regarding the toxicity and benefits of interferon, 107 low-risk melanoma patients were evaluated using the standard gamble technique. The researchers found that, on average, patients rated quality of life with melanoma recurrence much lower than even severe interferon toxicity. They concluded that DFS is highly valued by these patients.[33]

Summary of HDI Results

In the above mentioned four randomized trials using HDI (ECOG 1684, ECOG 1690, ECOG 1694, and ECOG 2626), all four studies demonstrate a DFS benefit to HDI, and two demonstrate an OS benefit as well. HDI has assumed a role as standard therapy for patients with stage IIb, IIc, and III disease. HDI should not be considered in patients with serious coexisting illnesses and a life expectancy < 10 years.[34]

From these studies, it is unclear what characteristics would predict response from interferon therapy. Individual studies suggest that the greatest benefit of HDI may be limited to certain patient populations based on the number of lymph nodes involved. But, no consistent pattern has been noted. In the ECOG 1684 trial, only the node-positive patients derived benefit from treatment. However, as already mentioned, only a small number of patients were node negative, 11% of the 280 patients. On the other hand, in the ECOG 1694 trial, the patients with node-negative disease derived the greatest benefit.

Since approximately 15 to 30% of patients who receive interferon treatment develop autoimmune disorder, including thyroiditis and vitiligo, researchers recently examined if there was a prognostic significance to developing autoimmunity after interferon in the adjuvant setting.[35] Two hundred patients with stage IIb, IIC, or III disease were treated with HDI. Patients were observed for signs of autoimmunity, including physical manifestations of vitiligo and serum antithyroid, antinuclear, anti-DNA, and anticardiolipin autoantibodies. With a median duration of 45.6 months, 26% of patients developed autoantibodies and clinical manifestations of autoimmunity. DFS had not been reached among patients with autoimmunity (vs 16 months for patients without signs of autoimmunity) and overall survival was not reached among patients with autoimmunity (vs 37.6 months without autoimmunity). Thus, autoimmunity was an independent prognostic marker for improved DFS and overall survival ($P <$ 0.001). The patients who developed autoimmunity were noted to have an approximate reduction in the risk of recurrence of melanoma by a factor of 50.[36] However, no biomarker is currently available to predict which patients would benefit from this therapy. Although the development of autoimmunity cannot be used as a criterion for selecting patients for the interferon, perhaps those patients with a documented predisposition toward autoimmunity should be a group of patients for whom immunotherapy should be directed. More research is required to further explain this finding, with the eventual goal being to tailor treatment options for specific groups of patients with melanoma.

Ongoing Clinical Trials

HIGH-DOSE INTERFERON

ECOG 1697 is enrolling patients with IB to IIIA melanoma to receive 4 weeks of HDI without a maintenance phase versus observation. The accrual goal is 1,420 patients (Figure 1).

PEGYLATED INTERFERON

EORTC 18991 is a multicenter randomized phase III trial comparing pegylated interferon (once a week for 5 years) with observation alone in patients with stage III melanoma after regional lymph node dissection. The enrollment goal was 900 patients. The trial was activated on 6/00 and closed on August 18, 2003.[2]

BIOCHEMOTHERAPY

Previous attempts have been made to combine the modalities of chemotherapy and biotherapy and develop a treatment that has a better survival outcome in comparison with that achieved with either therapy alone. Small, randomized trials have combined dacarbazine plus BCG as adjuvant treatment. A randomized, controlled trial comparing this combination with observation in patients with high-risk melanoma found no impact on biochemotherapy on survival.[38] In the metastatic setting, a randomized trial of the addition of IFN to DTIC in 271 patients showed no benefit to the combination.[39]

Currently, S0008 is an active trial evaluating high-risk, node-positive patients. This study is a comparison between HDI for 1 year versus 3 cycles of biochemotherapy (including cisplatin, dacarbazine, vinblastine, IL-2, INF, and G-CSF). The enrollment goal is 410 patients (Figure 2).

SENTINEL LYMPH NODE INVOLVEMENT DETECTED BY THE POLYMERASE CHAIN REACTION

The Sunbelt Melanoma Trial is an ongoing, multicenter prospective randomized trial. The study involves 79 centers and over 3,600 patients from across the United States and Canada. Its goal is to determine the effects of lymphadenectomy, with or without adjuvant HDI versus observation alone on DFS and OS with submicroscopic sentinel lymph node metastasis detected only by PCR (ie, these tumors are sentinel lymph node negative by histology and immunohistochemistry).[2]

VACCINE THERAPY

Vaccine therapy, including autologus, allogeneic, and peptide vaccines, have been studied in the management

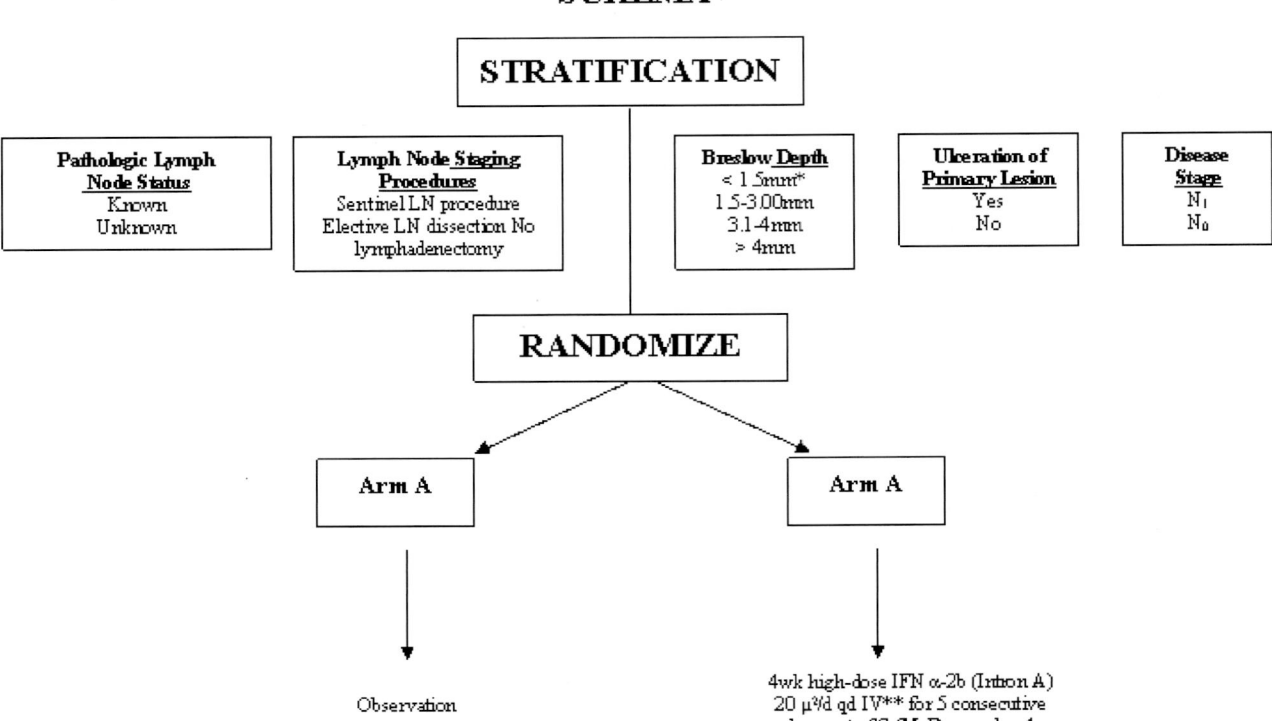

SCHEMA

STRATIFICATION

Pathologic Lymph Node Status	Lymph Node Staging Procedures	Breslow Depth	Ulceration of Primary Lesion	Disease Stage
Known Unknown	Sentinel LN procedure Elective LN dissection No lymphadenectomy	< 1.5mm* 1.5-3.00mm 3.1-4mm > 4mm	Yes No	N₁ N₀

RANDOMIZE

Arm A → Observation

Arm A → 4wk high-dose IFN α-2b (Intron A) 20 μ³/d qd IV** for 5 consecutive days out of 7 (M-F) q week x 4 weeks

* Patients must have one microscopically positive lymph node.
** Please use actual weight when calculating surface area for Arm B. Round dose to nearest 1.0 million unit.

NOTE: Patients must receive their first injection of IFN-2b within 5 business days of randomization
NOTE: Quality of life measures will be administered in Arms A&B at baseline (prior to the administration of T1), at day 22, every 3 months in the period 0-2 years after study entry, and every 6 months in the period.
NOTE: Only Breslow thickness and not Clark level will determine eligibility.

Figure 1 ECOG 1697. From The Don & Sybil Harrington Cancer Center Web site.[37]

of melanoma. None are currently approved as therapy. No phase III trials have shown an overall positive result with this treatment method.[40]

Recently, however, much research has been performed involving melacine, an allogenic melanoma cell line lysate vaccine combined with a potent adjuvant.[41,42] After a response was noted in patients with metastatic disease, SWOG trial 9035 was initiated to compare stage II patients receiving this vaccine versus observation in a randomized, controlled setting. Enrollment criteria for this study included patients with intermediate-thickness (1.5–4.0 mm or Clark's level IV if thickness unknown), clinically or pathologically node-negative melanoma (T3 N0 M0). Even though the overall results of this trial did not display a significant overall improvement in DFS for vaccinated patients, patients with specific HLA types, in this case HLA-A2 and HLA-C3+, showed a highly significant improvement in DFS when vaccinated (5-

year DFS, 77%, compared with 64% for observation ($p = .004$)). No difference was noted between the HLA-C3 + and HLA-C3 patients in the observation group. Also, an overall survival advantage was seen in vaccinated A2C3+ patients versus observation (5-year estimate 89% vs 76%, $p = 0.003$).

Again, this study raises the possibility of future tailored therapy for patients with melanoma, and further studies investigating the role of this melacine in stage II patients are being considered.[41,42]

Another important vaccine study currently enrolling involves MDX-010 (Ipilimumab) ± MDX-1329. MDX-010 is a fully human antibody against human CTLA-4 (cytotoxic T-lymphocyte-associated antigen 4), a molecule on T cells thought to be responsible for suppressing the immune response. The use of an anti–CTLA-4 antibody has also been reported to cause autoimmune disorders in cancer patients and has been associated with

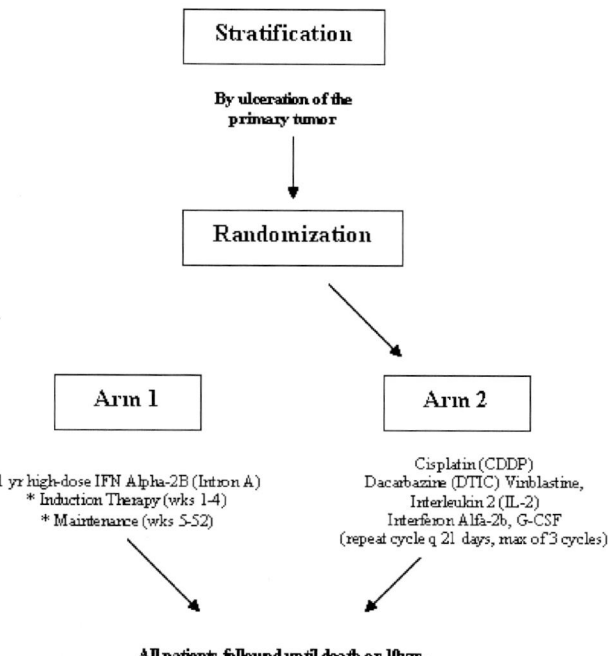

Figure 2 S0008 Schema. From The Don & Sybil Harrington Cancer Center Web site.[37]

tumor regression.[36] MDX-1329 is a vaccine consisting of two gp1000 melanoma peptides. Currently, a phase III trial has been initiated comparing pretreated stage IV or unresectable stage III patients treated with MDX-010 antibody, MDX-1379 melanoma vaccine, or a combination of MDX-010/MDX-1379. If the results of this study are shown to have value in this setting, it is highly likely that these therapies will be used as an adjuvant therapy.

Conclusion

Clinical investigation into new therapies for melanoma is active. Patients with localized disease can be readily categorized into prognostic subsets based on the presence or absence of a number of risk factors. Patients with thick primary lesions, or patients with regional lymph node metastases, are at high risk of the development of metastases and ultimately of dying from their disease. Currently, the only FDA-approved therapy for melanoma is HDI. This medication still remains controversial. The results from randomized controlled trials assessing adjuvant therapy have been mixed. Although the four large trials have shown a DFS advantage, the overall survival benefit has been variable.

Although the FDA has approved HDI for stage IIB-III melanoma, this therapy should not be considered for everyone secondary to its side effect profile. The risks of this treatment for patients with serious comorbidities or

a life expectancy < 10 years outweigh potential benefits. Future research is being directed to tailoring this medication to the subgroup of patients who would derive benefit from this treatment.

Adjuvant Radiotherapy

The use of radiation as adjuvant therapy to prevent regional (in-basin) recurrence in patients who have undergone formal dissection of involved lymph nodes is supported by clinical experience. As discussed below, nodal irradiation appears to improve local control rates, particularly in patients with certain prognostic features.[43] Its impact on survival is less clear. Unfortunately, no large-scale, randomized clinical trials comparing radiotherapy with observation have been completed, so the true impact of radiotherapy remains unclear. A phase III clinical trial currently being conducted by the Trans-Tasman Radiation Oncology Group may rectify this situation.[44] In this trial, patients at high risk of local recurrence following a lymphadenectomy for stage III melanoma are being randomized to surgery alone or surgery plus radiotherapy. The primary end point is locoregional control, with secondary outcome assessments including disease-free survival, overall survival, toxicity, and quality of life.

Evidence supporting the use of adjuvant radiotherapy generally relies on comparisons of local failure in patients receiving adjuvant radiotherapy against rates historically reported for observation-only patients. In retrospective analyses of patients with pathologically involved lymph nodes who did not receive adjuvant therapy, the rates of recurrence in the previously dissected nodal basin ranged from 14 to 30%.[45,46] Certain characteristics increase the likelihood of failure (Table 5),[45] most notably extracapsular extension.[45]

Compared with the nodal recurrence rates reported with observation in these analyses, most studies of adjuvant radiotherapy following complete lymph node dissection have reported lower recurrence rates, ranging from 5 to 20%.[47] Regional recurrence rates remained low in patients with risk factors that predispose to nodal recurrence, including extracapsular extension and multiple positive nodes.[48,49]

An analysis by Ballo and colleagues[50] is of particular value. In this retrospective review of 89 patients with axillary lymph node metastases who had undergone dissection and postoperative radiation, the rate of axillary control was 87% at 5 years. Five-year overall survival was 50%, and 5-year disease-free survival was 46%. Factors associated with reduced axillary control included lymph nodes larger than 6 cm and an unknown location of the primary tumor.[50]

Table 5 Prognostic Factors for Nodal Basin Failure Following Complete Lymph Node Dissection in 338 Patients[45]

Factor	Rate of Recurrence	P Value
Lymph node location		
Cervical	43%	.008
Axillary	28%	
Inguinal	23%	
Extracapsular extension		
Present	63%	< .0001
Absent	23%	
Number of positive lymph nodes		
1 to 3	25%	.0001
4 to 10	46%	
> 10	63%	
Size of largest involved lymph node		
< 3 cm	25%	<.001
3 to 6 cm	42%	
> 6 cm	80%	

Table 6 Five-Year Rates of Lymphedema and Grade 2 (Requiring Medical Intervention) or Grade 3 (Requiring Surgical Intervention) Treatment-Related Complications in Melanoma Patients Managed with Lymphadenectomy Followed by Radiotherapy[49]

Lymph Node Site	Lymphedema (%)	Grade 2/3 Treatment-Related Complications (%)
Epitrochlear ($n = 3$)	0	0
Cervical ($n = 267$)	1	11
Axillary ($n = 154$)	20	30
Inguinal ($n = 42$)	27	39

Whereas most of the studies of radiotherapy in melanoma have not included a control arm, one small study[51] directly compared adjuvant radiotherapy versus no irradiation in patients suffering from melanoma with cervical lymph node involvement. This study was not randomized, and the group receiving radiation ($n = 45$) had more extensive nodal involvement with respect to extracapsular extension and number of involved nodes than the nonirradiated group ($n = 107$). Nevertheless, the group receiving radiotherapy showed a trend toward improved regional control (6.5% recurrence rate compared with 18.7% in the nonirradiated group; $P = .055$), but no significant improvement in survival (40% and 35%, respectively, at 5 years).[51]

Adjuvant radiotherapy is generally well tolerated in patients with melanoma, and some. Lymphedema is the most common complication, affecting approximately 10% of patients.[49] As reported in one study, the mean time to development of edema is approximately 12 months.[50] Lymphedema is also associated with lymph node dissection, so the contribution of radiation to this adverse event is unclear. The rate of treatment-related complications, including lymphedema, depends on the site of lymph node dissection (Table 6), with the highest complication rate associated with inguinal treatment.[49]

On the basis of institutional experience and studies conducted to date, the most appropriate patients with regional melanoma to receive adjuvant nodal basin irradiation are characterized by any the following:[47]

- Extracapsular extension
- ≥ 4 involved lymph nodes
- Lymph node ≥ 3 cm in size
- Cervical lymph node location
- Recurrent nodal disease

ADJUVANT THERAPY WITH CONCURRENT IFN-ALFA-2B AND RADIATION

The combination of IFN-alfa-2b and radiotherapy as adjuvant therapy in patients with melanoma has also been assessed, but mostly from a safety perspective. To date, no randomized clinical trials have examined whether this combination offers an advantage over either therapy alone.

In the experience of the authors, radiation can be given during the maintenance phase of IFN-alfa-2b treatment so as not to add to tolerability concerns during the aggressive induction phase. Even during the maintenance phase, however, combination therapy can result in tolerability problems, perhaps owing to a radiosensitizing effect of IFN. A study of 18 patients with stage III melanoma who received adjuvant radiotherapy during the IFN-alfa-2b maintenance phase found that 7 developed grade III skin reactions and 3 others showed signs of other severe radiation-induced toxicities (pneumonitis, mucositis, and wound dehiscence).[52] Another study of 10 patients with melanoma who had received IFN-alfa-2b treatment during radiation therapy or within 1 month of its completion reported that half experienced severe subacute or late complications of therapy, including peripheral neuropathy, radiation necrosis in the brain, and radiation necrosis in subcutaneous tissue.[53] Close clinical monitoring is therefore required in patients receiving combination treatment with radiation and IFN-alfa-2b. If radiation can be withheld until the full course of IFN-alfa-2b has been given, then this might help to minimize the adverse events.

References

1. American Cancer Society. Cancer facts and figures 2006. Atlanta: American Cancer Society; 2006. p. 1–20.

2. Lens M. Cutaneous melanoma: interferon alpha adjuvant therapy for patients at high risk for recurrent disease. Dermatol Ther 2006;19:9–18.

3. Meisenberg BR, Ross M, Vredenburgh JJ, et al. Randomized trial of high-dose chemotherapy with autologous bone marrow support as adjuvant therapy for high-risk, multi-node-positive malignant melanoma. J Natl Cancer Inst 1993;85:1081–5.

4. Barth A, Morton DL. The role of adjuvant therapy in melanoma management. Cancer 1995;75:726–34.

5. Wood WC, Cosimi AB, Carey RW, Kaufman SD. Randomized trial of adjuvant therapy for "high risk" primary malignant melanoma. Surgery 1978;83:677–81.

6. Veronesi U, Adamus J, Aubert C, et al. A randomized trial of adjuvant chemotherapy and immunotherapy in cutaneous melanoma. N Engl J Med 1982;307:913–6.

7. Haluska FG, Ibrahim N. Therapeutic targets in melanoma: MAPKinase Pathway. Curr Oncol Rep 2006;8:400–5.

8. Thatcher N, Mene A, Banerjee SS, et al. Randomized study of Corynebacterium parvumadjuvant therapy following surgery for (stage II) malignant melanoma. Br J Surg 1986; 73:111–5.

9. Verma S, Quirt I, McCready D, et al. Melanoma Disease Site Group. Systematic review of systemic adjuvant therapy for patients at high risk for recurrent. melanoma. Cancer 2006;106:1431–42.

10. Creagan ET, Ingle N, Schutt AJ, Schaid DJ. A prospective, randomized controlled trial of megestrol acetate among high-risk patients with resected malignant melanoma. Am J Clin Oncol 1989;12:152–5.

11. Meyskens FL Jr, Liu PY, Tuthill RJ, et al. Randomized trial of vitamin A versus observation as adjuvant therapy in high-risk primary malignant melanoma: a Southwest Oncology Group Study. J Clin Oncol 1994;12:2060–5.

12. Isaacs A, Lindenman J. Virus interference I. The interferon. Proc R Soc 1957;147:258–67.

13. Jonasch E, Haluska FG. Interferon in oncological practice: review of interferon biology, clinical applications, and toxicities. Oncologist 2001;6:34–55.

14. Kirkwood JM. Interferon therapy: melanoma. In: DeVita VT, Hellman S, Rosenberg SA, editors. Biologic therapy of cancer. 2nd ed. Philadelphia: J.B. Lippincott; 1995. p. 388–411.

15. Kavanagh D, Hill AD, Djikstra B, et al. Adjuvant therapies in the treatment of stage II and III malignant melanoma. Surgeon 2005;3:245–56.

16. Cameron DA, Cornbleet MC, Mackie RM, et al. Adjuvant interferon alpha-2b in high-risk melanoma: the Scottish study. Br J Cancer 2001;84:1146–9.

17. Pehamberger H, Soyer HP, Steiner A, et al. Adjuvant interferon alpha-2a treatment in resected primary stage II cutaneous melanoma. Austrian malignant melanoma cooperative group. J Clin Oncol 1998;16:1425–9.

18. Grob JJ, Dreno B, de Salmoniere P, et al. Randomised trial of interferon alpha-2a as adjuvant therapy in resected primary melanoma thicker than 1.5 mm without clinically detectable nodal metastases. Lancet 1998;351: 1905–10.

19. Kleeberg UR, Suciu S, Broker EB, et al. Final results of the EORTC 18871/DKG 80-1 randomized phase III trial rIFN-alpha2b versus rIFN-gamma versus ISCADOR M versus observation after surgery in melanoma patients with either high-risk primary (thickness > 3mm) or regional lymph node metastases. Eur J Canc 2004;40:390–402.

20. Cascinelli N, Bufalino R, Morabito A, Mackie R. Results of adjuvant interferon study in WHO melanoma programme. Lancet 1994;343:913–4.

21. Hancock BW, Wheatley K, Harris S, et al. Adjuvant interferon in high-risk melanoma: the AIM HIGH Study—United Kingdom coordinating Committee on Cancer Research (UKCCCR) randomized study of adjuvant low-dose extended duration interferon alpha-2a in high risk resected malignant melanoma. J Clin Oncol 2004;22: 53–61.

22. Balch CM, Buzaid AC, Soong SJ, et al. Final version of the American Joint Committee on Cancer staging system for cutaneous melanoma. J Clin Oncol 2001;19:3635–48.

23. Eggermont AM, Suciu S, MacKie R, et al. EORTC Melanoma Group.Post-surgery adjuvant therapy with intermediate doses of interferon alfa-2b versus observation in patients with stage IIb/III melanoma (EORTC 18952): randomised controlled trial. Lancet 2005;366:1189–96.

24. Sabel MS, Sondak VK. Pros and cons of adjuvant interferon in the treatment of melanoma. Oncologist 2003;8: 451–8.

25. Kirkwood JM, Strawderman MH, Ernstoff MC, et al. Interferon alfa-2b adjuvant therapy of high-risk resected cutaneous melanoma: the Eastern Cooperative Oncology group trial EST 1684. J Clin Oncol 1996;14:7–17.

26. Kirkwood JM, Manola J, Ibrahim J, et al. A pooled analysis of Eastern Cooperative Oncology Group and intergroup trials of adjuvant high-dose interferon for melanoma. Clin Cancer Res 2004;10:1670–7.

27. Kirkwood JM, Ibrahim JG, Sondak VK, et al. High- and low-dose interferon alfa-2b in high-risk melanoma: first analysis of intergroup trial E1690/S9111/C9190. J Clin Oncol 2000;18:2444–58.

28. Kirkwood JM, Ibrahim JG, Sosman JA, et al. High-dose interferon alfa-2b significantly prolongs relapse-free and overall survival compared with the GM2-KLH/QS-21 vaccine in patients with resected stage IIB-III melanoma: results of intergroup trial E1694/S9512/C509801. J Clin Oncol 2001;19:2370–80.

29. Kirkwood JM, Ibrahim J, Lawson DH, et al. High-dose interferon-2b does not diminish antibody response to GM2 vaccination in patients with resected melanoma: results of the Multicenter Eastern Cooperative Oncology Group phase II trial E2696. J Clin Oncol 2001;19:1430–6.

30. Borden EC, Parkinson D. A perspective on the clinical effectiveness and tolerance of interferon-alpha. Semin Oncol 1998;25 suppl 1:3–8.

31. Cole BF, Gelber RD, Kirkwood JM, et al. Quality-of-life-adjusted survival analysis of interferon alfa-2b adjuvant treatment of high-risk resected cutaneous melanoma: an Eastern Cooperative Oncology Group study. J Clin Oncol 1996;14:2666–73.

32. Hillner BE, Kirkwood JM, Atkins MB, et al. Economic analysis of adjuvant interferon alfa-2b in high-risk melanoma based on projections from Eastern Cooperative Oncology Group 1684. J Clin Oncol 1997;15:2351–8.

33. Kilbridge KL, Weeks JC, Sober AJ, et al. Patient preferences for adjuvant interferon alfa-2b treatment., 2001;19:812–23.

34. Dubois RW, Swetter SM, Atkins M, et al. Developing indications for the use of sentinel lymph node biopsy and adjuvant high-dose interferon alfa-2b in melanoma. Arch Dermatol 2001;137:1217–24.

35. Gogas H, Ioannovich J, Dafni U, et al. Prognostic significance of autoimmunity during treatment of melanoma with interferon. N Engl J Med 2006;354:709–18.

36. Koon H, Atkins M. Autoimmunity and immunotherapy for cancer. N Engl J Med 2006;354:758–60.

37. The Don & Sybil Harrington Cancer Center Web site. Available at: https://secure.harringtoncc.org/ (accessed January 13, 2007).

38. Canadian Medical Association. Randomized controlled trial of adjuvant chemoimmunotherapy with DTIC and BCG after complete excision of primary melanoma with a poor prognosis or melanoma metastases. CMAJ 1983;128:929–33.

39. Falkson CI, Ibrahim J, Kirkwood JM, et al. Phase III trial of dacarbazine versus dacarbazine with interferon alpha-2b versus dacarbazine with tamoxifen versus dacarbazine with interferon alpha-2b and tamoxifen in patients with metastatic malignant melanoma: an Eastern Cooperative Oncology Group study. J Clin Oncol 1998;16:1743–51.

40. Atkins MB, Elder DE, Essner R, et al. Innovations and challenges in melanoma: summary statement from the first Cambridge conference. Clin Cancer Res 2006;12:2291s–6s.

41. Sondak VK, Liu P-Y, Tuthill RJ, et al. Adjuvant immunotherapy of resected, intermediate-thickness, node-negative melanoma with an allogeneic tumor vaccine: overall results of a randomized trial of the Southwest Oncology Group. J Clin Oncol 2002;20:2058–66.

42. Sosman JA, Unger JM, Liu P-Y, et al. Adjuvant immunotherapy of resected, intermediate-thickness, node-negative melanoma with an allogeneic tumor vaccine: impact of HLA class I antigen expression on outcome. J Clin Oncol 2002;20:2067–75.

43. Bastiaannet E, Beukema JC, Hoekstra HJ. Radiation therapy following lymph node dissection in melanoma patients: treatment, outcome and complications. Cancer Treat Rev 2005;31:18–26.

44. Immediate radiotherapy or observation after surgery for melanoma involving lymph nodes [study protocol]. National Cancer Institute Web site. Available at: http://clinicaltrials.gov/ (accessed October 20, 2006).

45. Lee RJ, Gibbs JF, Proulx GM, et al. Nodal basin recurrence following lymph node dissection for melanoma: implications for adjuvant radiotherapy. Int J Radiat Oncol Biol Phys 2000;46:467–74.

46. White RR, Stanley WE, Johnson JL, et al. Long-term survival in 2,505 patients with melanoma with regional lymph node metastasis. Ann Surg 2002;235:879–87.

47. Ballo MT, Ang KK. Radiotherapy for cutaneous malignant melanoma: rationale and indications. Oncology (Huntingt) 2004;18:99–107.

48. Ang KK, Peters LJ, Weber RS, et al. Postoperative radiotherapy for cutaneous melanoma of the head and neck region. Int J Radiat Oncol Biol Phys 1994;30:795–8.

49. Ballo MT, Ross MI, Cormier JN, et al. Combined-modality therapy for patients with regional nodal metastases from melanoma. Int J Radiat Oncol Biol Phys 2006;64:106–13.

50. Ballo MT, Strom EA, Zagars GK, et al. Adjuvant irradiation for axillary metastases from malignant melanoma. Int J Radiat Oncol Biol Phys 2002;52:964–72.

51. O'Brien CJ, Petersen-Schaefer K, Stevens GN, et al. Adjuvant radiotherapy following neck dissection and parotidectomy for metastatic malignant melanoma. Head Neck 1997;19:589–94.

52. Gyorki DE, Ainslie J, Joon ML, et al. Concurrent adjuvant radiotherapy and interferon-a2b for resected high risk stage III melanoma—a retrospective single centre study. Melanoma Res 2004;14:223–30.

53. Hazard LJ, Sause WT, Noyes RD. Combined adjuvant radiation and interferon-alpha 2B therapy in high-risk melanoma patients: the potential for increased radiation toxicity. Int J Radiat Oncol Biol Phys 2002;52:796–800.

CHAPTER 88

NONMELANOMA SKIN CANCER

JONATHAN S. ZAGER, MD

MERRICK I. ROSS, MD

Nonmelanoma skin cancers (NMSC) consist mostly of squamous cell carcinoma (SCC) and basal call carcinomas (BCC), which account for greater than 90% of all malignancies of the skin.[6,10,21] Both SCC and BCC are mainly seen in the elderly population (age > 60). Basal cell carcinoma is about 4 to 5 times more frequently diagnosed than SCC, with the relative incidences of SCC and BCC being approximately 38 of 100,000 (SCC) and 147 of 100,000 (BCC) per US population, respectively.[6,10,21] Both SCC and BCC occur with increasing frequency with age, and both tend to occur on sun-exposed areas of the body.[6,10,21]

Another, less frequent NMSC, is Merkel cell carcinoma (MCC). MCC is much less frequent than melanoma and far less frequent than SCC or MCC.[22]

The epidemiology, etiology, and treatment of SCC, BCC, and MCC will be described below.

Squamous Cell Carcinoma

EPIDEMIOLOGY/ETIOLOGY

Squamous cell carcinoma of the skin accounts for approximately 15 to 20% of all skin cancers.[3,4,6,21] It is more common in men than women (approximately 2–3:1) and the incidence increases with age.[6,20] SCC is more common in whites than blacks, and it is most commonly seen on sun-exposed areas of the body such as the lips, ears, scalp, face, and upper body.[6,21]

There are numerous factors that contribute to the etiology of SCC. The most important is solar exposure.[3,4,6,12,21] Mutations of the *TP53* tumor suppressor gene induced by UV light, specifically 280 to 320 nm UV-B, are found in ~50% of SCCs.[3,4,6,12,21] The incidence of SCC also increases with decreased latititud and

proximity to the equator, again directly related to the amount of solar radiation one is exposed to.[3,4,6,12,21]

Immunosuppression is another important risk factor in the development of SCC, with transplant recipients and AIDS patients being at an increased risk of developing a more aggressive course of SCC.[8,12,1,21,24] Both SCC and BCC are reported to occur approximately 65 to 250 times more frequently in transplant recipients and the immunosuppressed than in the general population.[8,12,21] NMSC is the most common malignancy seen in the post-transplant population.[11] Herrero and colleagues report that the relative risk of NMSC in a population of liver transplant recipients was 20.26 (95% confidence interval: 14.66–27.29) as compared with sex- and age-matched population, with a greater incidence of SCC than BCC.[12] The etiology behind this increased incidence in this population appears to be related to total solar exposure pretransplant, increasing age, amount of immunosuppression, and male sex.[12] Often these immunosuppressed patients suffer from a multiple lesions, which appear to be more aggressive. They tend to grow rapidly, show a higher rate of local recurrences, and metastasize in 5 to 8% of the patients.[3,12]

Human papilloma virus (HPV) infection has also been implicated in the development of SCC, especially around the genetalia of males and females. HPV 16 and 18 are the strains most implicated in the etiology of genital SCC. HPV 38 has been shown to be present in up to 50% of NMSC, including its presence in 13% of SCCs and 18% in BCCs. The HPV may also act synergistically with UV-B radiation in inducing SCC.[13]

SCC can also arise from an old scar or burn site, known as a Marjolin's ulcer. These areas of chronic inflammation and chronic healing are known etiologies of SCC. Several other factors have also been implicated in the development of SCC, such as arsenic, tar, and other polycyclic aromatic hydrocarbons.[13,21]

Lastly, a previous diagnosis of any skin malignancy translates into an increased risk of future development of SCC or other NMSC.[16,21,29]

DIAGNOSIS AND STAGING

There are certain skin conditions that mimic SCC. These include benign conditions such as seborrheic keratoses, which are benign proliferations of the epidermis that appear on keratinizing skin. These keratoses usually increase in incidence with age, they are not thought to be directly related to sun exposure, but are common on the head and neck, hands, and trunk. Seborrheic keratoses usually appear as flat to slightly raised brown macules that are plaque-like and have flaky surfaces. These do not give rise to NMSC but can sometimes be confused with melanoma lesions. These can be followed by a dermatologist or surgical oncologist; they also can be treated with liquid nitrogen and numerous other topical pharmaceutical agents.[27]

Keratoacanthomas are well-differentiated squamoproliferative skin lesions that usually grow rapidly and then regress spontaneously. They usually occur on sun-damaged areas of the body, especially on the head and neck. Keratoacanthomas appear as red, or skin colored, round raised nodules with a cratered center. They can be easily confused with SCC and require excision if there are any questions regarding the diagnosis, especially if these lesions are conservatively observed and do not regress over a period 6 to 12 months.[21,27]

Actinic keratoses are premalignant lesions that have potential to develop into SCC. Again these lesions are seen mostly on sun-exposed areas of the body. They appear as scaly, yellow to brown patches of raised skin. Since actinic keratoses have the potential to turn into SCC, they should be treated if they persist through a short period of observation.[21,27] A definitive treatment can be a narrow-margin (0.5 mm) local excision done as an outpatient or in the office. Other treatment options include cryosurgery, curettage, dermabrasion, chemical peels, laser resurfacing, and local pharmacological treatments such as 5-fluorouracil (5-FU), imiquimod, diclofenac, and tretinoin, each with advantages and limitations.[17,21,27]

Any cutaneous lesion suspicious for malignancy should be biopsied. Ideally the biopsy should involve full thickness of the skin to the level of the subcutaneous fat. This type of biopsy can enable the pathologist to determine the depth of the lesion in question. A punch biopsy tool can be used for most lesions. Punch biopsies range from 2 to 8 mm and then the defect can be closed with interrupted 3-0 or 4-0 simple nylon sutures. If the lesion is larger than 1 cm, a punch biopsy can be performed in the office of the most suspicious part of the lesion, or an excisional biopsy with a narrow margin can be performed under local anesthesia. Shave biopsies are not ideal methods of diagnosis since they may or may not involve the entire depth of the lesion. A shave biopsy is usually performed with a No. 15 scalpel after injecting local anesthetic under the skin to raise a wheel. The shave biopsy should be deep enough to involve the deeper layers of the dermis in order to try to get an adequate pathological assessment of the deep margin of the lesion in question.

Bowens disease and Queyrat's erythroplasia of the penis are clinical expressions of SCC in situ. SCC in situ is typically characterized by full-thickness dysplastic involvement of the epidermis without penetration beneath the basement membrane. Bowen's disease is characterized by a persistent, progressive, slightly raised, red, scaly or crusted plaque. The ideal treatment for SCC in situ is local surgical, narrow-margin (0.5 cm) excision. However, other options are topical chemotherapy, cauterization. and liquid nitrogen therapy.[27]

Once the diagnosis of invasive SCC is made, a careful physical examination of the patient, including a full skin survey as well as examination of the major lymph node basins, is performed. Although the metastatic potential is small (2–3% overall), there are certain sites of primary disease, histologic features, and underlying host-related factors that may identify a high risk subset that portend a greater chance of metastatic spread. The regional lymph node basins are the most common site of metastatic spread of SCC, and based on recent prognostic analysis, nodal involvement represents the powerful independent predictor of distant disease.[3,5,15,17,21,27] The immunosuppressed patient is at higher risk of regional and distant metastatic spread of SCC. Thicker tumors > 5 mm, larger tumors > 2 cm in diameter, lesions that arise in scars, the presence of perineural invasion, and poorly differentiated grade are all higher risk features that predict an increased likelihood for metastasis. SCC of the ear and lip both have higher rates of metastases to regional lymph nodes, as do SCC arising from the skin of the genitalia.. All of these higher risk SCCs raise the potential of nodal spread from 2 to 3% to 10 to 30%.[3,5,15,17,21,27]

Some of these primary tumor prognostic factors (tumor size and deep penetration into underlying structures) have been included in the current version of the American Joint Committee on Cancer (AJCC) staging system for NMSC and define the T stages of 1-4[11] (Table 1). Some feel that the current system is antiquated and does not include some of the important prognostic factors. A new system has been proposed

Table 1 Current AJCC Staging System for Cutaneous Squamous Cell Carcinaoma of the Skin

Primary tumor (T)

TX	Primary tumor cannot be assessed
T0	No evidence of primary tumor
Tis	Carcinoma in situ
T1	Tumor 2 cm or less in greatest dimension
T2	Tumor more than 2 cm but not more than 5 cm in greatest dimension
T3	Tumor more than 5 cm in greatest dimension
T4	Tumor invades deep extradermal structures (ie, cartilage, skeletal muscle, or bone)

In the case of multiple simultaneous tumors, the tumor with the highest T category will be classified and the number of separate tumors will be indicated in parentheses, eg, T2 (5)

Regional lymph nodes (N)

NX	Regional lymph nodes cannot be assessed
N0	No regional lymph node metastasis
N1	Regional lymph node metastasis

Distant metastasis (M)

MX	Distant metastasis cannot be assessed
M0	No distant metastasis
M1	Distant metastasis

Stage grouping

Stage 0	Tis	N0	M0
Stage I	T1	N0	M0
Stage II	T2	N0	M0
	T3	N0	M0
Stage III	T4	N0	M0
	Any T	N1	M0
Stage IV	Any T	Any N	M1

Histopathologic grade (G)

GX	Grade cannot be assessed
G1	Well differentiated
G2	Moderately differentiated
G3	Poorly differentiated
G4	Undifferentiated

(Table 2) to establish more relevant prognostic groups, which in turn can help the clinical management decision making in the role for the early diagnosis of nodal disease using sentinel node biopsy and which patients should be considered for adjuvant radiation therapy and/or systemic adjuvant clinical trials. Even though the risk of metastases from SCC overall is low, SCC is very common, which translates into 2,500 deaths per year; therefore, establishing a staging system that is SCC specific and prognostically relevant is a worthwhile endeavor.[11]

TREATMENT

Definitive therapy of SCC can be divided into surgery or nonsurgical treatments. After a definitive diagnosis is made, the ideal and most effective therapy for SCC lesions of the skin is surgical excision. Whether surgical excision can be primarily closed, closed with local rotational flaps or skin grafts, or Mohs' micrographic surgery (discussed below) depends on the anatomic site and size of the SCC, and the quality of the surrounding tissues.[2,14,27] The ideal margin of excision for SCC is not well defined. SCC in situ can be excised with a 0.5 cm margin.[15,21,22,28] This 0.5 cm margin can also be applied to those invasive SCCs smaller than 2 cm without poor pathological features and not invasive into the subcutaneous tissue can also be excised with a 0.5 cm margin.[15,21,22] SCC with high-grade histological features, those with deep invasion into the subcutaneous tissues, or those larger than 2 cm in size should be excised with a 0.5 to 1cm or more margin.[15,21,22] A planned excision along Langer's lines is ideal for the long-term cosmetic results. Mohs' micrographic surgery (discussed below) can be performed for SCCs in sensitive and delicate locations such as the head or neck, or with aggressive histological subtypes where definitive negative margins is ideal to achieve adequate local control.[2,15,28]

Other potential therapies for SCC include curettage in combination with electrocautery, cryotherapy with liquid nitrogen, and laser ablation with a CO_2 laser. These methods are not as good as surgical excision when 5-year disease-free survival rates are concerned; however, they may be used with small or superficial tumors, and the site should be monitored regularly for recurrences.[16,21,29]

Table 2 Proposed Cancer Staging System for Squamous Cell Carcinoma of the Skin

Primary tumor (T)

TX		Primary tumor cannot be assessed
T0		No evidence of primary tumor
Tis		Carcinoma in situ
T1		Invasive tumor up to 1 cm in diameter
	T1a	Less than 2 mm in thickness or contained within the dermis
	T1b	Greater than 2 mm in thickness but less than or equal to 5 mm in thickness or extending into the subcutaneous fat
	T1c	Greater than 5 mm in thickness or invading periosteum, perichondrium, or muscle
	T1d	Tumor demonstrates perineural spread
T2		Invasive more than 1 cm but less than 2 cm in diameter
	T2a	Less than 2 mm in thickness or contained within the dermis
	T2b	Greater than 2 mm in thickness but less than or equal to 5 mm in thickness or extending into the subcutaneous fat
	T2c	Greater than 5 mm in thickness or invading periosteum, perichondrium, or muscle
	T2d	Tumor demonstrates perineural spread
T3		Invasive tumor more than 2 cm but less than 3 cm in diameter
	T3a	Less than 2 mm in thickness or contained within the dermis
	T3b	Greater than 2 mm in thickness but less than or equal to 5 mm in thickness or extending into the subcutaneous fat
	T3c	Greater than 5 mm in thickness or invading periosteum, perichondrium, or muscle
	T4d	Tumor demonstrates perineural spread
T4		Invasive tumor more than 3 cm in diameter
	T4a	Less than 2 mm in thickness or contained within the dermis
	T4b	Greater than 2 mm in thickness but less than or equal to 5 mm in thickness or extending into the subcutaneous fat
	T4c	Greater than 5 mm in thickness or invading periosteum, perichondrium, or muscle
	T4d	Tumor demonstrates perineural spread

Regional lymph nodes (N)

NX	Lymph nodes cannot be assessed
N0	No clinical lymph node disease
N1	Metastasis in a single ipsilateral lymph node less than 3 cm in greatest dimension
N2a	Metastasis in a single ipsilateral lymph node more than 3 cm but less than 6 cm
N2b	Metastasis in multiple ipsilateral lymph nodes, none more than 6 cm in greatest dimension
N2c	Metastasis in bilateral or contralateral lymph nodes, none more than 6 cm in greatest dimension involvement
N2d	Intralymphatic regional metastasis (in-transit or satellite metastasis) without nodal metastasis
N3	Lymph node involvement greater than 6 cm, seventh nerve or skull base involvement

P or p designation

P = parotid disease alone

p = parotid and cervical neck involvement

Examples: N1P, N2p

Metastasis (M)

MX	Metastatic disease cannot be assessed
M0	No clinical metastatic disease
M1	Distant metastasis

Histopathology grade

GX	Tumor grade cannot be assessed
G1	Well differentiated
G2	Moderately differentiated
G3	Poorly differentiated
G4	Desmoplastic

Host (to be captured as a comorbidity)

HX	Immunocompetency of host cannot be determined
H0	Host is not immunocompromised
H1	Immunocompromised host

Clinical stage grouping

Stage 0	Tis	N0	M0
Stage Ia	T1	N0	M0
Stage Ib	T2	N0	M0
Stage Ic	T3	N0	M0
Stage Id	T4	N0	M0
Stage II	Any T	N1	M0
Stage III	Any T	N2	M0
	Any T	N3	M0
Stage IV	Any T	Any N	M1

Topical therapies with 5-FU (5% cream) and imiquimod creams have been shown to be effective against smaller and more superficial invasive SCCs (5-FU) as well as actinic keratoses and SCCs in situ (imiquimod and 5-FU). They are applied 1 to 2 times/day (5-FU) or 3 to 5 days per week (imiquimod) for a period of 2 to 6 weeks (5-FU) or longer (imiquimod). Both treatments can have some side effects seen as local irritation of the skin. Rebiopsy of lesions after a full course of treatment with either 5-FU or imiquimod will confirm adequate therapy. These treatments are usually well tolerated and are best suited for patients who have multiple SCCs or premalignant lesions such as actinic keratoses in a confined area such as the back, chest, or head and neck.[16,17,19,21,29]

The development of regional lymph node disease is not only a predictor for future distant disease, but also represents a difficult clinical scenario as it is often bulky, very difficult to manage, and may be the source of significant morbidity. Therefore, it is rational to identify at diagnosis those patients who are likely to develop regional lymph node disease. In the management of these high-risk patients, a consideration for performing a sentinel lymph node biopsy (SLNB) in addition to wide local excision of the primary site is becoming more commonplace.

Those patients at high risk of nodal metastases from SCC include those with large lesions (> 2cm); poorly differentiated histology; deep lesions (invading into a Breslow depth greater than 5 mm); and those lesions that are recurrent or located on the lip or helix, or immunosuppressed patients (positive HIV status or status postsolid organ transplant).[20,25,30] The regional and distant metastatic potential in these high-risk patients has been reported to be as high as 15 to 45%, when more than one high-risk factor is present in an individual.[20,25,26] These patients may benefit from SLNB, which would enable the clinician to individualize treatment according to nodal status, offering completion nodal dissections and/or radiation to the regional nodal basins as well as systemic chemotherapy or clinical trials to the patient.[25,26] In a retrospective analysis, Mullen and colleagues have identified those patients with SCC who are at high risk of recurrence and death from cutaneous SCC.[20] The authors again identified patients who on univariate analysis had poorly differentiated SCC ($p = 0.016$) (Figure 1), scar SCCs (Marjolin's ulcers) ($p = .008$) (Figure 2), tumor size > 2cm ($p = .006$) (Figure 3), and regional nodal disease at presentation ($p = .0001$) (Figure 4) as factors significantly associated for recurrence or death from disease. On multivariate analysis, these authors identified only regional nodal disease at presentation ($p = .0001$) as significant for recurrence or death.

Weisberg and colleagues have even proposed Mohs' surgery (see below for description of Mohs') in combination with SLNB for high-risk recurrent SCCs.[29] The regional metatstatic rates from recurrent high-risk SCCs have been reported to be as high as 25 to 45%.[30] These authors state in a single case report that patients with large high-risk recurrent lesions can benefit from optimal tumor extirpation via the Mohs' micrographic

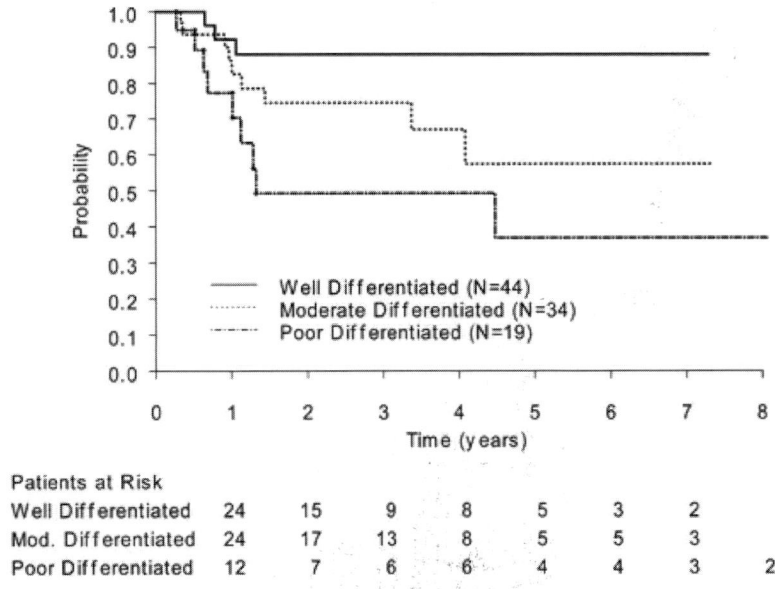

Figure 1 Kaplan-Meyer survival curve according to degree of differentiation.

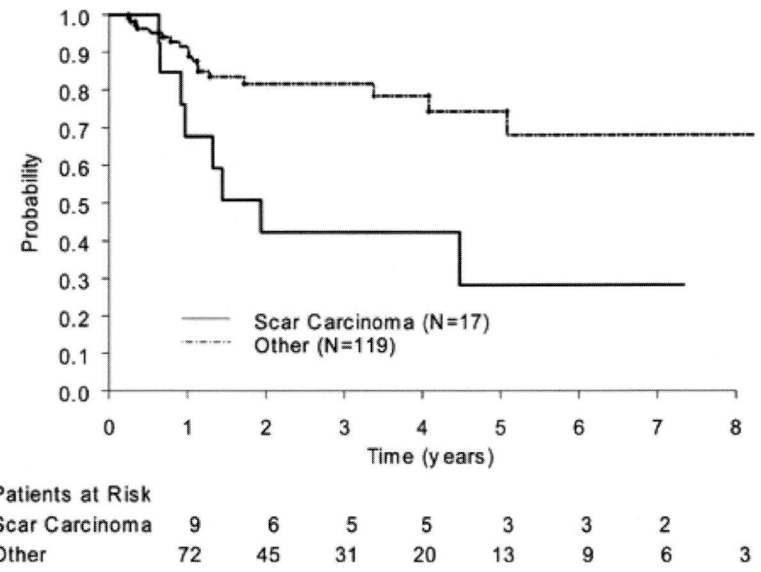

Figure 2 Kaplan-Meyer curve of SCC originating in scar vs all other.

surgical technique, and at the same time have their regional nodal basins evaluated by the SLNB technique. This combination technique of Mohs' and SLNB may be useful in recurrent SCCs in delicate areas of the face, requiring careful pathological margins assessment and evaluation of regional nodal spread.

In the era of widespread use of SLNB for breast cancer and melanoma, this staging procedure can be performed safely, with few false-negative results, and provide valuable prognostic information in patients with high-risk SCC. A recent article reviewed the published experience with SLNB in high-risk primary SCC. Overall, the incidence of a positive SLN is approximately 20%. Most of the series are small, single institutional reports. Further prospective studies should be conducted in order to determine if detection of subclinical microscopic nodal disease in patients with high-risk SCCs would benefit from completion nodal dissection and/or adjuvant therapies.[26] Even in the absence of a survival benefit, the potential for improved regional

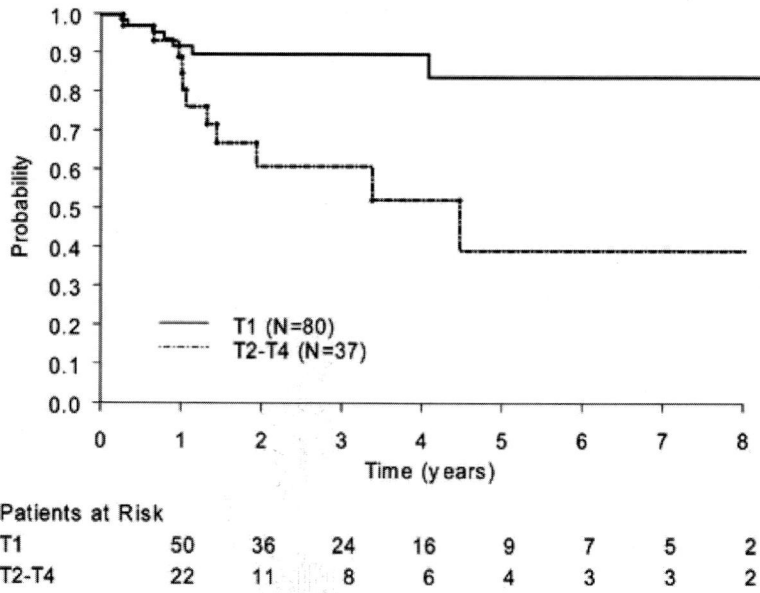

Figure 3 Kaplan-Meyer survival curve according to T stage(T1< 2cm vs T2-T4).

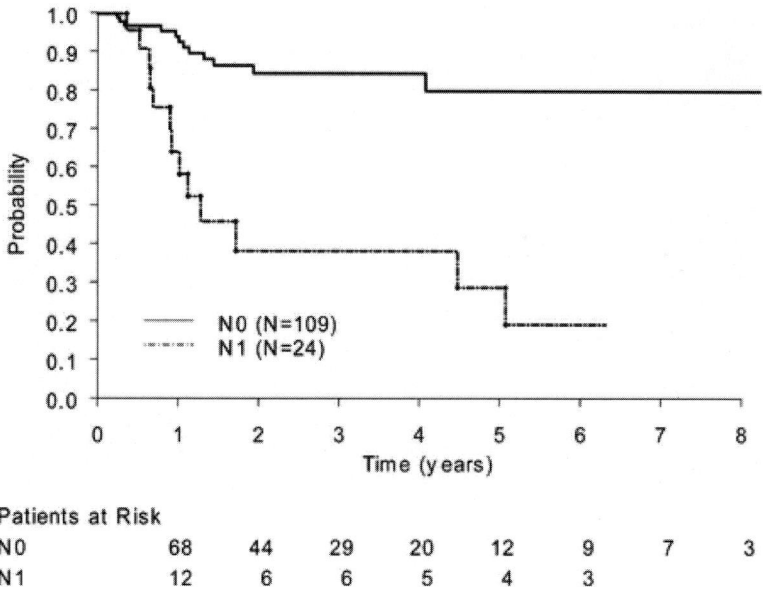

Figure 4 Kaplan-Meyer survival curve according to nodal status.

nodal basin control can be very valuable. Extrapolating from experience with melanoma, management of the regional disease when microscopic is more effective than when clinically apparent. Figure 5 illustrates an example of advanced regional nodal disease that may have been avoided if a sentinel node biopsy would have been performed as part of the initial management of this unfortunate patient who initially presented with a high-risk cutaneous SCC.

Basel Cell Carcinoma

EPIDEMIOLOGY/ETIOLOGY

Basal cell carcinoma (BCC) is the most common malignancy in humans. BCC is 4 to 5 times more common than SCC. BCC typically occurs in areas of chronic sun exposure, is slow growing, and rarely metastasizes. BCC has been referred to as the "rodent ulcer" because of its local destructive capabilities. The overall prognosis approaches 100% 5-year survival with the correct treatment. The estimated annual incidence in the white population is 900,000 people (550,000 male, 350,000 female), whereas the estimated lifetime risk of BCC is 33 to 39% in men and 23 to 28% in women.[7,9,10]

Ultraviolet radiation is the most common cause of BCC.[9] A prior history of sunburns and blistering can oftentimes be elucidated when interviewing patients about sun exposure history.[9] In addition, chronic sun exposure appears to be important in the development of BCC. There usually is a long latency period of greater than 20 years between the sun damage and the clinical onset of BCC. X-ray exposure, arsenic exposure, and immunosuppression have all been implicated as potential causes of BCC.[9,10,21]

A history of previous NMSC (either BCC or SCC) portends an increased risk of developing others (BCC or SCC) in the future. This increased rate of new NMSC can be as high as 35% 5 years after original diagnosis.[9,10,21]

DIAGNOSIS

There are no real premalignant precursor lesions to BCC. However, there are a few inherited syndromes that are associated with an increased incidence of developing BCC.

Nevoid BCC (basal cell nevus syndrome) is an autosomal dominant condition that is associated with an increased incidence of multiple BCCs at an early age as well as other malignancies such as meningiomas and medulloblastomas.[9,10,21]

Bazex's syndrome is another inherited (x-linked dominant) syndrome that is associated with an increased risk of the development of multiple BCCs, much like the nevoid BCC syndrome.[9,10,21]

There are numerous subtypes of BCC. These subtypes vary in level of aggressiveness. BCCs are typically seen on the face, ears, scalp, neck, or upper trunk. Mild trauma in the form of rubbing the lesions or washing or bumping

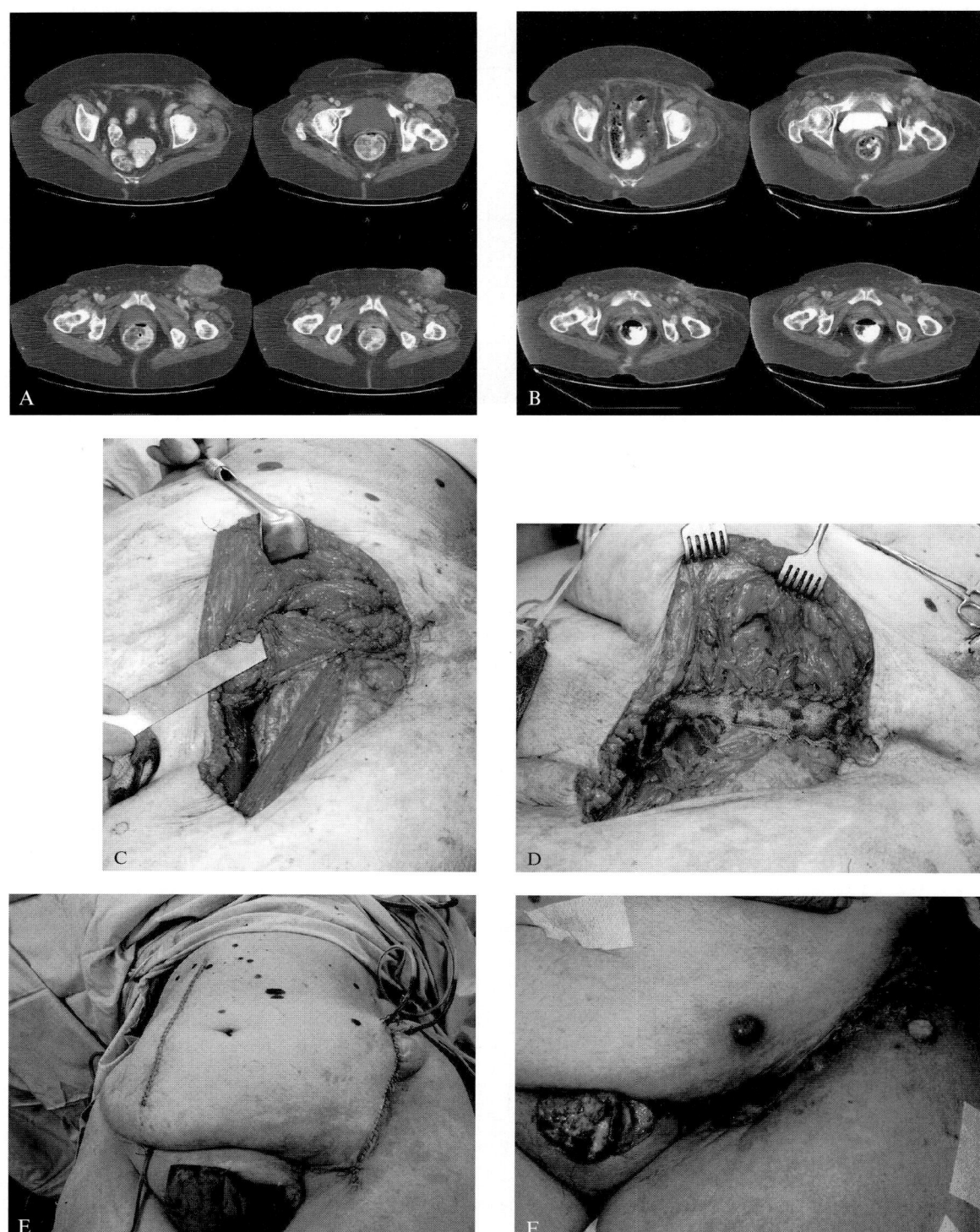

Figure 5 A 56-year-old woman underwent a wide excision of a high-risk SCC on left lower back. Three years later she developed bulky inguinal nodal disease seen on CT scan (A). An excellent partial response was observed with chemoradiation (B). The end result of formal superficial and deep node dissection en bloc with overlying skin and inguinal ligament is pictured (C). The inguinal ligament is reconstructed with mesh (D). The completed surgical procedure after rotation of contralateral rectus muscle flap (E). Unfortunately, massive multifocal regional recurrence developed 7 months later (F).

them into objects may cause some bleeding from the lesion itself. As mentioned above, a sun-exposure history is usually elicited.[9,10,21]

The most common form of BCC is the nodular variant. This variant presents as a waxy, pearly, sometimes umbilicated or ulcerated lesion with rolled or heaped up borders and some spider telengiectasias around the edges. Pigmented, cystic, micronodular, morpheaform, and infiltrating are all descriptive terms for BCC histological variants. The micronodular, morpheaform, and infiltrating subtypes are aggressive in nature. These subtypes should ideally be surgically removed because of tumor extension beyond visible borders. Routine histologic examination of the biopsy specimen can usually differentiate between the various subtypes.[9,10,17,21,22]

TREATMENT

The treatment of BCC is much like that of SCC. Surgical excision with a narrow margin is the most definitive treatment and affords the best potential for cure. In areas where tissue sparing is necessary for best comesis, Mohs' micrographic surgery can be performed (see section below). Mohs' can also be performed with certain subtypes of BCC (ie, infiltrating, micronodular), where extension beyond visible borders may be present and careful histological examination of margins is essential to prevent recurrence.[9,10,17,21,22]

The extent of excision should be to negative margins and, generally, a 4 to 5 mm margin excision can be performed and durable local control and high long-term cure rates achieved ($> 95\%$ 5-year disease-free survival) with all variants of BCC. Local excision can be performed under local anesthesia in an outpatient setting. The specimen should be carefully examined for margin status in pathology.[9,10,18,19,21] For some more aggressive and larger BCCs, plastic and reconstructive surgical techniques may have to be employed to repair large surgical defects. Recurrent tumors are generally more aggressive than primary lesions, and subclinical extension also tends to be greater.[9,10,17,21,22]

Factors to consider in choosing therapy include histologic BCC subtype, location and size of tumors, age of patient, ability of patient to tolerate surgery, and expense. As mentioned above, the morpheaform, micronodular, and infiltrating subtypes are more aggressive as are recurrent BCCs. With these certain clinical scenarios, subclinical extension should be suspected and carefully ruled out in pathology.[9,10,17,21,22]

Curettage, cryotherapy, and topical chemotherapy can also be used in the treatment of BCC as they are used in SCC. The cure rates are less than that with surgical excision, but are still favorable for the most part ($\sim 90\%$).[9,10,17,21,22]

Certain patients with BCC who are likely to be referred for surgical consultation will have very invasive tumors necessitating radical surgical excisions. BCC by nature is a locally destructive ("rodent ulcer") tumor that when left untreated can go on to invade underlying vital structures such as nerves, arteries and veins, skeletal muscle, and bone. These are the type of patients who will require major en bloc resections and likely plastic surgical myocutaneous flap reconstruction.

Mohs' Micrographic Surgery

Mohs' micrographic surgery (MMS) is a surgical technique that employs the removal of all clinically apparent tumor with a narrow margin of normal-appearing tissue. MMS can be performed as an outpatient procedure, or even in the office if a dermatopathologist is available to perform frozen-section analysis on the margins. The margins, including the deep margin, are then marked carefully and oriented for the pathologist to determine immediate intraoperative margin assessment by frozen-section analysis. The frozen sections are oriented in a way that the surgeon and pathologist communicate to determine exactly which specific area or margin of the specimen is involved so that that particular area can be excised again with a narrow rim of normal-appearing tissue, therefore sparing other areas of the excision site further removal of tissue.[2,15,21,28]

There are numerous advantages to MMS. One being the fact that the margins are very carefully assessed and the risk of local recurrence is negligible after the procedure is finished. Secondly, MMS is a good technique for use in areas of the body (ie, head and neck) where tissue sparing is essential for good final cosmesis. Lastly, the reported cure rates using MMS in treating BCC and SCC are very high ($> 98\%$).[2,15,28]

The one main disadvantage of MMS is the time spent in the detailed frozen-section analysis and precision marking of margins to ensure that they are negative.

Merkel Cell Carcinoma

EPIDEMIOLOGY/ETIOLOGY

Merkel cell carcinoma (MCC) is a rare and highly aggressive neoplasm of the skin mechanoreceptors.[1,14,23] It was first described by Toker in 1972 and is characterized by trabecular architecture and the presence of neurosecretory granules within tumor cells.[22] MCC classically presents in the sixth to seventh decade as a painless, rapidly growing, reddish-hued, intradermal nodule.[14,23]

Although no universally accepted staging system exists, commonly utilized classification includes three groups: stage I, clinically localized primary tumors (Ia, ≤ 2 cm diameter; Ib > 2 cm diameter); stage II, regional lymph node involvement; stage III, distant metastatic disease.[1,22] Regional disease and distant metastasis are associated with a worsened prognosis in MCC. Reported 5-year survival rates are as follows: stage I, 60 to 75%; stage II, < 50%; and stage III, < 35%.[1,23]

The overall incidence of this rare skin tumor is approximately 0 to 23 per 100,000 people in the United States. The typical patient is an elderly white male. MCC tends to occur in those over 50 years old and males outnumber females 2 to 3:1. MCC has been reported to be associated with sun exposure, exposure to arsenic, and immunosuppression. There have been reports of an increased incidence of MCC in transplant recipients, patients with chronic lymphocytic leukemia, and those with HIV.[1,23]

DIAGNOSIS

The diagnosis of MCC can be difficult. Although the tumors have the characteristic appearance described above, they sometimes can be mistaken for other small cell tumors (ie, small cell cancer of the lung, lymphoma, neuroblastoma, and melanoma) that have metastasized to the dermis on light microscopy. The differentiation of MCC from these other tumors can be performed with immunohistochemical analysis. Typically, MCC will express neuron-specific enolase and chromogrannin as well as cytokeratin markers and be negative for S100, thyroid transcription factor, and leukocyte common antigens).[1,23]

MCC Merkel cell tumors tend to recur locally and to metastasize early to regional nodes. Local recurrence rates have been reported to be as high as 75%, whereas up to 60 to 75% of patients with clinical stage I disease may develop nodal disease during their disease course.[1,23]

TREATMENT

The recommended treatment of Merkel cell carcinoma has been variable across the literature. This is in part because of the rarity of the disease as well as no specific AJCC staging system exists. For primary tumors, a wide local excision of at least 2 cm is recommended, especially in those tumors that are thicker than 2 cm in diameter. When margins are close or the tumors are in specific areas of the body (head and neck) that preclude wide excision, adjuvant radiation to the primary site has been advocated by most investigators with experience with this disease.[1,13,23]

Those patients with evidence of clinical nodal involvement should have a regional lymphadenectomy, as this will enable better control in the regional nodal basin. Again, adjuvant radiation for those with bulky nodal disease after nodal dissection can be given to decrease the chances for regional failure. For those patients whose disease seems limited to the primary site, intraoperative lymphatic mapping (IOLM) with sentinel lymph node biopsy (SLNB) has been recommended to adequately stage the regional nodal basin. Data presented at the International Sentinel Node Society Meeting in December 2004 from our institution have shown that SLNB is safe and effective in staging the regional nodal basin in MCC.[30] We performed SLNB in a cohort of 32 patients with clinically negative nodes (stage I disease). Twenty-three of the 32 patients had a negative SLNB, none of whom recurred in the regional nodal basin. None of the negative SLNB patients received any further treatment to the mapped nodal basin. There were 2 (10%) recurrences in the negative SLNB group, neither of which was in the regional nodal basin as the first site of recurrence. Of the 9 patients who had a positive SLNB, 6 (66%) had a completion lymphadenectomy and 3 (33%) had definitive external beam radiation therapy (XRT) to the draining nodal basin in lieu of a completion lymphadenectomy. Of the 3 (33%) recurrences in the SLNB-positive group, no patient recurred in the regional nodal basin. Recurrences were mostly distant in nature. In the negative SLNB cohort, 1 patient recurred distantly first, and 1 patient recurred locally followed by distant and regional recurrence. From the SLNB-positive cohort, there were 3 recurrences, 2 of which were distant first, and the third was local followed by distant recurrence. In our study, the disease-free survival at a median follow-up of 21 months was 91% in the SLNB-negative group and 67% in the SLNB-positive group.[31]

The treatment for stage III disease, or distant metastases, is again not well defined. Chemotherapeutic agents such as doxorubicin, cisplatin, 5-FU, and cyclophosphamide have all been used alone and in combination with disappointing results. Overall, the median survival of patients with stage III MCC is approximately 9 months. The overall response rates of chemotherapy usage in MCC are approximately 50 to 68%, with complete response rates being reported as high as 30 to 35%; however, the response rates are not durable with the median response duration being approximately 6 months.[1,14,23]

The optimal management seems to be a wide local excision and SLNB for all patients with stage Ia or Ib disease, with or without external beam radiation for improved local control when margins may be compromised. Nodal dissection and/or XRT to the regional nodal basin seems to be a durable method of controlling regional nodal disease either micro- or macrometastatic disease in the nodal basins. As demonstrated above, there is a propensity for stage II patients to have both local and distant recurrences; therefore, there may be a role in systemic chemotherapy in these high-risk patients. Unfortunately, the current regimens do not provide durable distant control of the disease, and further investigation is warranted in developing a better adjuvant regimen for use in stage III MCC.[23]

References

1. Allen PJ, Bowne WB, Jaques DP, et al. Merkel cell carcinoma: prognosis and treatment of patients from a single institution. J Clin Oncol 2005;23:2300–9.

2. Batra RS, Kelley LC. Predictors of extensive subclinical spread in nonmelanoma skin cancer treated with Mohs micrographic surgery. Arch Dermatol 2002;138:1043–51.

3. Bernstein SC, Lim KK, Brodland DG, Heidelberg KA. The many faces of squamous cell carcinoma. Dermatol Surg 1996;22:243–54.

4. Bogdanov-Berezovsky A, Cohen AD, Glesinger R, et al. Risk factors for incomplete excision of squamous cell carcinomas. J Dermatolog Treat 2005;16:341–4.

5. Brodland DG, Zitelli JA. Surgical margins for excision of primary cutaneous squamous cell carcinoma. J Am Acad Dermatol 1992;27(2 Pt 1):241–8.

6. Chuang TY, Popescu NA, Su WP, Chute CG. Squamous cell carcinoma. A population-based incidence study in Rochester, Minn. Arch Dermatol 1990;126:185–8.

7. Chuang TY, Popescu A, Su WP, Chute CG. Basal cell carcinoma. A population-based incidence study in Rochester, Minnesota. J Am Acad Dermatol 1990;22(3):413–7.

8. Clayton AS, Stasko T. Treatment of nonmelanoma skin cancer in organ transplant recipients: review of responses to a survey. J Am Acad Dermatol 2003;49:413–6.

9. Crowson AN. Basal cell carcinoma: biology, morphology and clinical implications. Mod Pathol 2006;19 Suppl 2:S127–47.

10. De Giorgi V, Massi D, Lotti T. Basal-cell carcinoma [author reply]. N Engl J Med 2006;354:769–71.

11. Dinehart SM, Peterson S. Evaluation of the American Joint Committee on Cancer staging system for cutaneous squamous cell carcinoma and proposal for a new system. Dermatol Surg 2005;31:1379–84.

12. Herrero JI, Espana A, Quiroga J, et al. Nonmelanoma skin cancer after liver transplantation. Study of risk factors. Liver Transpl 2005;11:1100–6.

13. Karagas MR, Nelson HH, Sehr P, et al. Human papillomavirus infection and incidence of squamous cell and basal cell carcinomas of the skin. J Natl Cancer Inst 2006;98:389–95.

14. Koljonen VS. Merkel cell carcinoma. World J Surg Oncol 2006;4:7.

15. Lane JE, Kent DE. Surgical margins in the treatment of nonmelanoma skin cancer and Mohs micrographic surgery. Curr Surg 2005;62:518–26.

16. Limmer BL. Nonmelanoma skin cancer: today's epidemic. Tex Med 2001;97:56–8.

17. Luce EA. Advanced and recurrent nonmelanoma skin cancer. Clin Plast Surg 1997;24:731–45.

18. McCutcheon B, White K, Kotwall C, et al. A preliminary study of imiquimod treatment in variants of basal cell carcinoma. Am Surg 2005;71:662–5.

19. Micali M, Nasca MR, Musumeci ML. Treatment of an extensive superficial basal cell carcinoma of the face with imiquimod 5% cream. Int J Tissue React 2005;27:111–4.

20. Mullen JT, Feng L, Xing Y, et al. Invasive squamous cell carcinoma of the skin: defining a high-risk group. Ann Surg Oncol 2006;13:902–9.

21. Nguyen TH, Ho DQ. Nonmelanoma skin cancer. Curr Treat Options Oncol 2002;3:193–203.

22. Pichardo-Velazquez P, Dominguez-Cherit J, Vega-Memije ME, et al. Surgical option for nonmelanoma skin cancer. Int J Dermatol 2004;43:148–50.

23. Poulsen M. Merkel cell carcinoma of skin: diagnosis and management strategies. Drugs Aging 2005;22:219–29.

24. Purdie KJ, Surentheran T, Sterling JC, et al. Human papillomavirus gene expression in cutaneous squamous cell carcinomas from immunosuppressed and immunocompetent individuals. J Invest Dermatol 2005;125:98–107.

25. Reschly MJ, Messina JL, Zaulyanov LL, et al. Utility of sentinel lymphadenectomy in the management of patients with high-risk cutaneous squamous cell carcinoma. Dermatol Surg 2003;29:135–40.

26. Ross AS, Schmults CD. Sentinel lymph node biopsy in cutaneous squamous cell carcinoma: a systematic review of the english literature. Dermatol Surg 2006;32:1309–21.

27. Smoller BR. Squamous cell carcinoma: from precursor lesions to high-risk variants. Mod Pathol 2006;19 Suppl 2: S88–92.

28. Telfer NR. Mohs micrographic surgery for nonmelanoma skin cancer. Clin Dermatol 1995;13:593–600.

29. Urbach F. Incidence of nonmelanoma skin cancer. Dermatol Clin 1991;9:751–5.

30. Weisberg NK, Bertagnolli MM, Becker DS. Combined sentinel lymphadenectomy and Mohs micrographic surgery for high-risk cutaneous squamous cell carcinoma. J Am Acad Dermatol 2000;43:483–8.

31. Zager JS, Prieto VG, Ballo MT, et al. Clinical significance of positive sentinel nodes in Merkel cell carcinoma. International Sentinel Node Meeting, Los Angeles, CA 2004.

Chapter 89

Surgical Management of Stage I and II Melanoma: Excision Margins, Reconstruction, and Sentinel Node Biopsy

Merrick I. Ross, MD

The vast majority of patients newly diagnosed with melanoma present with disease clinically localized to the primary site (stage I and II). Surgical strategies have included two main components: wide excision of the primary tumor or biopsy site and regional lymph node evaluation. Historically, treatment of melanoma has from a surgical perspective been aggressive, but unfortunately not evidence based. An aggressive surgical approach was based on personal anecdotes suggesting that narrow excisions would lead to local recurrence of disease and not fully dissecting the regional lymph nodes early resulted in patients later developing advanced regional disease that was not only difficult to control but associated with a high rate of incurable distant failure. Because such observations were reported by the surgical leaders of their time, initial surgical management policies were adopted that included wide resection margins of 3 to 5 cm around the primary lesion and frequently an elective lymph node dissection (ELND) of the regional basin. The popularity of the latter procedure was reinforced as a result of retrospective studies claiming that a survival advantage is conferred with ELND[1]. In some centers the wide excision and the elective dissection was carried out in-continuity by an en-bloc removal of the primary site, the anatomically closest regional lymph node group, and the intervening strip of skin, subcutaneous tissue, and underlying fascia. Such an approach was based on the advice offered by Pringle in

1908, who based on his experience with three cases suggested that "All that is removed should be in one continuous strip as far as possible."[2]

Surgery continues to be the single most effective modality for this stage of disease; therefore, establishing rational standards of surgical care, based on relevant biologic and or prognostic information, that would minimize morbidity without sacrificing oncologic goals has been an important challenge. Over the years, as a result of a better understanding of the factors governing or predicting the natural history of melanoma and completed clinical trials designed to study novel techniques or less aggressive surgical approaches, evidence based advances in how surgeons carry out the two main components of primary melanoma management have become a reality. The driving force behind such an evolution in care has been to achieve the fundamental goals of surgical management of the cancer patient: to optimize the chance for cure, establish accurate staging, and provide durable local and regional disease control while at the same time minimizing morbidity. The intent of this chapter is to discuss the relevant evidence supporting the current recommendations for surgical excision of the primary melanoma, offer practical approaches to closing soft tissue defects, provide guidance in managing some of the unusual histologies and difficult anatomic locations, and explore the rationale, utility, technical issues, and controversies of a more selective approach to the clinically node negative regional lymph nodes using sentinel lymph node (SLN) biopsy.

Excision of the Primary Melanoma

Wide surgical resection of the diagnostic biopsy site or residual primary lesion inclusive of a surrounding margin of normal skin en bloc with underlying subcutaneous tissue down to the muscular fascia has been adopted as the surgical standard in the initial management of the primary melanoma. While the goal of an appropriately performed diagnostic biopsy is to establish pathologic microstaging (tumor thickness and ulceration status), the goal of wide local excision is to achieve durable local disease control and to cure those patients who do not already harbor disseminated micrometastases to the regional lymph nodes or distant sites. How wide of an excision margin to employ has been the center of controversy for decades. The vast majority of narrow excision margins (1 cm) followed by primary closure of the resultant surgical defect can be accomplished under local anesthesia with minimal cost and surgical morbidity.[3] On the other hand, wide excision margins ($\geq$ 2 cm) not only are often performed under general anesthesia but depending on the anatomic site may require reconstruction with expensive and sometimes elaborate full thickness advancement or rotation flaps or coverage with cosmetically unappealing skin grafts. Narrow excisions, however, are often thought to result in a higher rate of local/regional failures which in-turn may have survival implications. Because local recurrence (LR) is generally an event associated with a poor prognosis and complicated and potentially morbid treatment strategies may be necessary in the event of LR, prevention of such events is a compelling reason to promote wide excision margins. At the same time,, minimizing treatment related morbidity is another important management goal. Excessive margins without improved outcome can lead to unnecessary treatment morbidities in terms of costs, complications, and cosmetic disfigurement. Therefore, establishing rational standards for the extent of surgical excision margins has been a worthwhile clinical investigation goal.

Historical Perspective and the Emergence of a Contemporary Paradigm

At the beginning of the twentieth century, melanoma was not very common and was usually diagnosed in a locally advanced stage. Based purely on anecdotal experience,

the use of 5 cm radial margins was adopted as the standard approach. The origin of such recommendations is somewhat ambiguous, but is often incorrectly attributed to a report in the late 1800s from Handley who described a wide resection margin including 1 inch (not 5 cm) of surrounding skin and underlying soft tissue[4]. Further supporting the use of 5 cm margins was the pathologic descriptions by Olsen[5] and Wong[6], documenting that atypical melanocytes may extend for 5 cm beyond the primary lesion. Regardless of the origin, the 5 cm excision approach persisted until the 1970s, when a better understanding concerning the natural history of melanoma and the prognostic factors (tumor thickness in particular) that influenced outcome was established[7,8]. Surgeons began to use narrower margins for low-risk lesions with excellent results[9–15]. While several published reports documented a low incidence of LR when narrow margins were used for thin melanomas, other retrospective reports suggested that LR was relatively frequent when such margins were used to treat thicker lesions, suggesting that LR is a function of both inherent biology as well as extent of margin[16]. The paradigm of wider margins being necessary for higher-risk (thicker) lesions emerged and subsequently tested in several prospective randomized surgical trials. If such a paradigm were true, that outcome (the frequency of local and regional events and overall survival [OS]) is impacted by the extent of excision margins, the following assumptions can be made: 1) microscopic satellite disease is more common and exists at a greater distance from the periphery of the primary lesion in association with thicker melanomas, 2) these microsatellites are a source of subsequent clinically apparent local, regional, and distant relapses, and 3) wider margins removes microscopic disease that would be left behind when narrower margins are used, resulting in an improved outcome. The following discussion summarizes the design and results of the completed randomized trials evaluating the role for wide excision in primary melanoma patients. All of these trials were designed and statistically powered according to the hypothesis that the wider margin would be superior to the narrower margin in terms of local-regional control and survival. A concise description of trial randomization schemes and the number of patients included can be found in table 1.

THIN MELANOMA (T1-T2; < 2MM) EXCISION TRIALS

The French Cooperative Group[17], the World Health Organization (WHO)[18–20], and the Swedish Melanoma Study Group (SMSG)[21–22] compared wide and narrow margins of excision in patients with melanomas < 2 mm

TABLE 1 Completed prospective randomized trials addressing surgical excision margins for primary cutaneous melanomas

Surgical trial group	No. of patients	Tumor Thickness (mm)	Randomized Surgical treatment arms
French Cooperative Study	362	≤ 2	2 cm vs. 5 cm
Swedish Melanoma Study Group 1	989	≤ 2	2 cm vs. 5 cm
World Health Organization (WHO) Melanoma Program	612	< 2	1 cm vs 3cm
Intergroup Melanoma Surgical Trial	486	1-4	2 cm vs 4 cm
UK Melanoma Study Group	900	>2	1cm vs. 3 cm
Swedish Melanoma Study Group 2	936	>2	2 cm vs 4cm

thick. While the trials differed somewhat in regards to the number of patients accrued, width of excision margins tested, and threshold of tumor thickness, the result were consistent. Local recurrences were very infrequent (less than 3%), and wider margins had no statistical impact on local or regional events or on long-term survival. As a result, narrow margins (1 cm) were adopted as the standard of care. One centimeter margins were easily embraced by the treating dermatology and surgical communities for melanomas 1 mm or less. Some, however, have been reluctant to adopt a 1 cm margin in their practice for patients with tumors in the range between 1 and 2 mm in thickness.[23] Lingering concerns have been primarily a result of the trend in the WHO study (with progressive follow-up reported in 1988[18], 1991[19], and 1998[20]) toward an increase in the absolute number of LRs in the narrow excision group (Table 2).

TABLE 2 Local recurrence as a first site of recurrent melanoma by tumor thickness range and excision margin in sequential reports of the WHO Study

| Tumor thickness (mm) | Excison Margin | | |
	1 cm	3 cm	Total
Number of patients with lesions ≤1.0 mm	186	173	359
Reported Local Recurrences # (%):			
1988	0 (0)	0 (0)	0 (0)
1991	0 (0)	0 (0)	0 (0)
1998	3 (1.6)	1 (0.6)	4 (1.1)
Number of patients with lesions 1.01– 2.0 mm	119	134	253
Reported Local Recurrences # (%):			
1988	3 (2.5)	0 (0)	3 (1.2)
1991	4 (3.4)	0 (0)	4 (1.1)
1998	5 (4.2)	2 (1.5)	7 (2.8)
Number of patients with all lesions < 2.0 mm	305	307	612
Reported Local Recurrences # (%):			
1988	3 (1.0)	0 (0)	3 (0.5)
1991	4 (1.3)	0 (0)	4 (0.6)
1998	8 (2.6)	3 (1.0)	11 (1.8)

THE INTERGROUP MELANOMA SURGICAL TRIAL (T2-T3 MELANOMAS; 1 TO 4 MM)

The Intergroup Melanoma Surgical Trial was initiated in 1983 and accrued 740 patients with intermediate thickness melanomas (ie, 1.0 to 4.0 mm)[24-26]. Two eligibility groups were established and stratified according to tumor thickness (1 to 2 mm, 2 to 3 mm, and 3 to 4 mm), anatomic site, (trunk, head and neck, and extremity) and primary tumor ulceration. The randomization scheme for Group A (N=468) was a 2cm versus a 4 cm margin for those patients with melanomas located on the trunk or proximal extremity to ensure that the more radical 4 cm margin could be carried out if they were randomly assigned to receive such a treatment. The remaining patients designated as group B (N=272) included those with either head and neck or distal extremity lesions, all of whom underwent a 2 cm excision). Overall, only 28 patients (3.8%) developed an LR, but the survival of these patients was significantly worse compared to the remaining 712 patients who did not, as illustrated in Figure.1.

A multifactorial step-wise regression analysis based on the Cox model was performed for the entire group of 740 patients. The initial report demonstrated that OS was dependent on primary tumor thickness, histologic

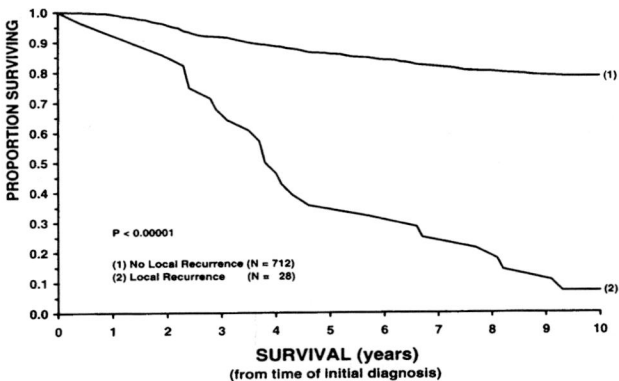

Figure 1 Comparison of survival for patients in Intergroup Trial with and without local recurrence.

Table 3 Multifactorial Analysis of Prognostic Factors in Predicting Survival in Intergroup Trial (Cox Proportional Hazards Model)[24]

Factor	Relative Risk	p-Value
Thickness	1.738	0.0008
Ulceration	2.205	0.0095
Anatomic subsite	1.919	0.0389
Surgical margin	1.526	0.1421

ulceration, and anatomic site, but not influenced by extent of excision margin 3).[24] The updated report in 2001 provides the analyses as it relates to local failure.[26] The only two factors independently predictive of poorer local control were the presence of tumor ulceration ($p <$ .001), and the head and neck site ($p =$ .02), table 4

Among the 468 Group A patients (randomized to 2 cm versus 4 cm margins), no statistical differences in OS, LR incidence rates, or risk for intransit disease was observed between the two treatment arms A summary of the trial results among the randomized treatment arms are shown in Table 5. A trend however, for improved 10-year disease-specific survival was observed in the wider excision cohort, 70% for those who had a 2 cm margin versus 77% for those who had a 4 cm margin ($p =$ .074). Not surprisingly, the incidence of skin grafting was

Table 4 Multivariate Analysis (Cox Model) of Risk for Local Recurrence (Anytime) Among all 740 Patients in Intergroup Trial

Factor	Risk Ratio	p-Value
Tumor ulceration	6.3	0.0001
Anatomic site:		
Head/Neck	9.4	0.01
Extremity	3.5	0.14
Trunk	2.5	0.24
Tumor thickness (<2.0mm vs >2mm)	2.0	0.14
Surgical margin (2cm vs 4cm)	1.0	0.79
Surgical wound closure (skin graft vs primary closure)	0.9	0.75

TABLE 5 Results Summary of Intergroup Melanoma Trail Group A patients. Incidences of events are compared according to randomized extent of excision (4 cm vs 2 cm)

	Excision Margin		
Event	4 cm	2 cm	P value
Local recurrence % (First relapse)	0.9	0.4	NS
Local recurrence (%) (Anytime)	2.6	2.1	NS
In transit metastasis (%) (Anytime)	5.2	5.9	NS
10-Year survival (%)	77	70	.07
Skin graft (%)	46	11	< 0.001
Wound complication (%)	10	10	NS

significantly different among the treatment groups, with higher skin grafting rates (11% versus 46%) experienced by the patients who underwent the wider margin of excision. Postoperative wound complication rates were not however statistically different between the two surgical arms.[25] While almost 90% of the defects created by the 2 cm excisions could be closed primarily in the Group A patients, only in 45% of the Group B patients could this be accomplished as 55% of patients required a skin graft for coverage on these more restrictive anatomic sites.[24]

THICKER MELANOMA (T3-T4, > 2MM) EXCISION TRIALS

Both the United Kingdom Melanoma Study Group (UKMSG) and SMSG have carried out multicentered trials randomizing patients with primary melanomas thicker than 2 mm to receive either a wide or narrow excision margin. While the two trials were very similar in size and in eligibility criteria, the treatment arms studied were different; 2 cm versus 4 cm and 1 cm versus 3 cm for the SMSG and the UKMSG respectively. The results of the UK trial have been published[27] while only preliminary findings are available for the Swedish study, which were presented at the "World Congress on Melanoma" in Vancouver in September 2005.

Interestingly, statistically more locoregional events were observed in patients randomized to the 1 cm treatment arm in the UK trial (37% versus 32%, p < 0.05), table 6. Locoregional relapses were defined collectively as LR, satellite, in-transit, and regional nodal disease. Loco-regional free survival curves according to excision arm is illustrated in figure 2. Additionally, as in the Intergroup Trial, more absolute melanoma-specific deaths occurred in patients who received the narrower excision, but this difference did not reach statistical significance, figure 3. Based on multivariate analyses, width of excision margin was determined to be one of the predictors of locoregional recurrence, but not for OS. Two conclusions may be offered to explain the lack of survival impact: 1) the number of local/regional events that were avoided by wider excision were too small to

Table 6 UK Margins Trial Results (med f/u 5 years)

	1 cm	3 cm	P-value
L/R rec. %	37	32	0.05
local/Intransit %	8.1	5.9	NS
Complications %	7.8	13.9	0.05
General anes. %	32	66	<.001

Multi-variate analysis:
-Predictors of Death: Ulc > thickness > gender > site
-Predictors of L/R: Ulc > thickness > gender > margin
Thomas et al, NEJM, Feb, 2004

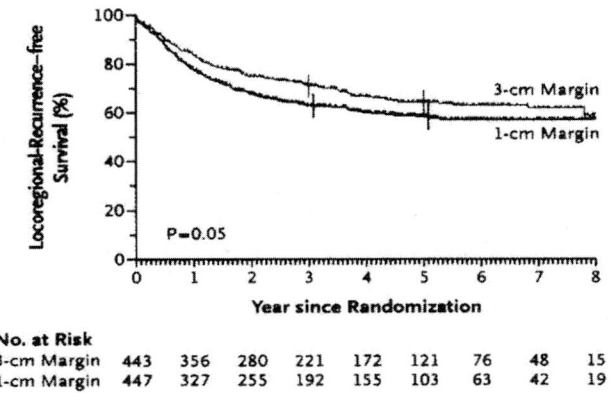

Figure 2 Loco-regional-free survival according to randomized treatment arm in the UKMSG trial. Statistically more events over time were observed in patients wo received the narrow (1cm) excision.

translate into a survival benefit in a study of this size and power, and/or 2) local/regional failures are not consistently a source of distant relapse and therefore more complete removal of clinically occult locally metastatic disease via a wider excision does not significantly alter the natural history of disease. The improved locoregional control observed with wider margins was however associated with an increased use of skin grafts, a greater use of general, anesthesia, and increased surgical morbidity. The study does, however, suggest that at least a percentage of nodal or other local/regional events may be reduced or avoided by wider excisions that presumably remove clinically occult but potentially clinically relevant disease more completely than a narrow excision. These data imply that the clinical appearance of local, intransit, and nodal disease is in part derived from local micrometastases existing at the time of primary diagnosis. In this way the paradigm of wider excisions needed for higher-risk (thicker) melanoma patients is supported.

In contrast, the preliminary results from the Swedish trial revealed that wider margins have no impact on any event, at least within the context of comparing 4 cm to 2cm excisions.

Current Recommendations

Collectively, these trials provide the basis for current recommendations for the extent of surgical margins for melanoma according to tumor thickness (Table 7). In formulating recommendations, the available data must be evaluated in the context of the goals for surgical therapy, optimizing both cure (survival) and local control and minimizing morbidity.

For melanoma in situ, excision of the lesion or biopsy site with a 0.5 to 1 cm border of clinically normal skin and a layer of the subcutaneous tissue is sufficient. Although these lesions are noninvasive, a local recurrence may present as an invasive melanoma with the potential for metastasis. Margin recommendations for melanomas in situ are based on a consensus of the available experience demonstrating excellent local control with the use of such margins.[28] Most in situ melanomas are completely and easily excised with a 0.5 to 1 cm margin and the surgical defect most often closed primarily under local anesthesia. A minority, lentigo maligna type in particular, are insidiously large microscopically and despite the removal of normal appearing skin surrounding the gross extent of the pigmented lesion, histologically positive margins may occasionally be encountered. These particular lesions may require sequential operative excisions to achieve adequate pathologically clear margins and occasionally the use of split thickness skin graft (STSG) or flap closure.

For invasive melanomas ≤ 1 mm thick, an excision with a 1 cm margin of clinically normal skin and

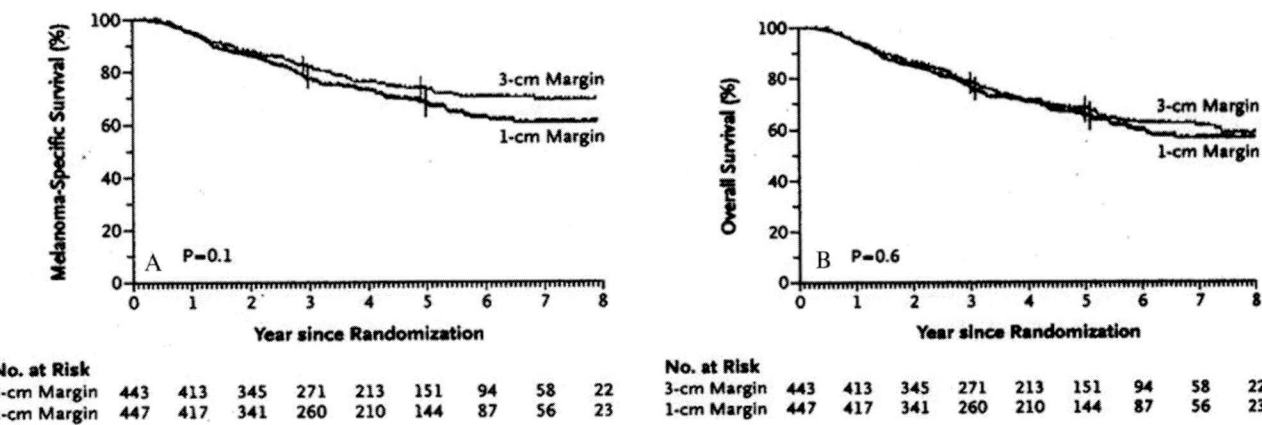

Figure 3 Survival results according to treatment arm in the UKMSG margins of excision trial. A trend for improved melanoma specific survival in the patients who received the wider margin is illustrated in (a), but no difference in overall survival (b) was observed

TABLE 7 Margin of excision recommendations by range of tumor thickness

Tumor thickness (mm)	Excision margin (cm)
In situ	0.5 – 1
0-1	1
1-2	1 or 2*
2-4	2
> 4	2

*A 1 cm margin is appropriate in anatomically restricted areas; otherwise a 2 cm margin is preferable.

underlying subcutaneous tissue appears adequate. The use of this narrow margin for these low-risk patients yields excellent cosmetic and functional results in any anatomic location without compromising therapeutic efficacy. Except for the occasional lesion arising on the distal extremities, scalp, or face in a limited number of patients, essentially all 1 cm excisions can be primarily closed. The data from the WHO randomized trial are the basis for this margin recommendation and a recent report of the excellent results obtained using these surgical guidelines in practice, under local anesthesia in an ambulatory care setting, further supports the recommendation.[3]

The appropriate margin of excision to be used for melanomas between 1 and 2 mm in thickness are derived from both the WHO and Intergroup trials. A trend for an increased incidence of LR in the narrow excision group (1cm margin) was observed in the WHO Trial, however, because of the small number of observed events, this study lacks the statistical power to confirm or refute equivalence in the long-term clinical course between 1 and 3 cm margins. The incidence of LR in the Intergroup Melanoma Trial was lower than in the WHO Trial for the overlapping 1.0 to 2.0 mm thickness patients; 0.6% versus 4.5% respectively, and no apparent advantage in either local control or survival was achieved with 4 cm margins. Since 4cm is not better than 2cm, one must conclude that 3cm is not better than 2cm margins. Furthermore, no study to date has directly compared 1 cm versus 2 cm margins. Therefore, we would recommend a 2 cm surgical margin for these melanomas (1 to 2 mm in thickness) whenever it is anatomically feasible and where the surgical defect can be closed primarily without a skin graft. However, in anatomic locations where a proposed 2 cm margin may compromise adjacent functional or cosmetic structures, or require the use of sophisticated wound reconstruction techniques or a STSG, a 1 cm or some margin < 2 cm and > 1 cm may be preferentially used. Because the OS data from prospective clinical trials reveal no apparent benefit with a wider excision, the use of 1 cm surgical margin either

selectively or exclusively is safe and appropriate for melanomas up to 2.0 mm in thickness.

For melanomas between 2 and 4 mm, a 2 cm surgical margin is currently the recommended standard based on the Intergroup data. The UK Trial, which included a 2 to 4 mm subset that overlapped with the Intergroup Trial, demonstrated improved local/regional control with a 3 cm margin versus a 1 cm margin. While a 3 cm margin may be superior to 1 cm in terms of local control (UK Trial), 4 cm has not been demonstrated to be superior to 2 cm (Intergroup and Swedish trials); logically again,, a 3 cm margin cannot be superior to 2 cms. Therefore, no data exists that supports any surgical approach for this group of patients (2 to 4 mm) that would include margins greater than 2 cm.

Until very recently, recommendations for treating thick (> 4 mm) melanomas have been based on retrospective analyses. Much is known about the natural history of patients with thick melanomas from these studies; these patients are at higher risk for both local recurrence (approximately 10 to 15%) and distant metastases (approximately 60%).[29–32] Prognostic variables and excision margins have been evaluated for patients with thick melanomas in recent years through a collaborative effort of the M. D. Anderson and Moffitt Cancer Centers.[32] Patients were retrospectively analyzed with respect to local recurrence and survival as a function of the extent of the excision margin and other prognostic factors. No decrease in survival (figure 4) or increase in LR rates (figure 5) were observed when margins of 2 cm or less were used, compared to patients with melanomas of similar thickness and constellation of prognostic factors having a wider than 2 cm excision margin. LR appeared to be more a function of primary tumor factors rather than width of excision with the presence of primary tumor ulceration as the only factor influencing local failure identified by univariate analysis (Table 8). Multivariate analysis revealed that OS was impacted by nodal status, tumor ulceration, and thickness > 6 mm, but not by margins width or LR.[32] Despite the retrospective nature of the study, a balance in prognostic factors was observed between the two excision groups. The inference, albeit limited by the retrospective nature of this study of 278 patients treated over a 10-year period, is that 2 cm margins can be safely employed for thicker lesions. Interestingly, while the LR rate was, as anticipated, relatively high (11%), in contrast to findings from the Intergroup Trial, such events did not appear to be associated with a poorer prognosis compared to patients without local failure (Figure 5). Both the UK and Swedish randomized trials included patients in this thickest group (> 4mm). The authors of the UK Trial concluded that 3 cm margins should be used for thicker

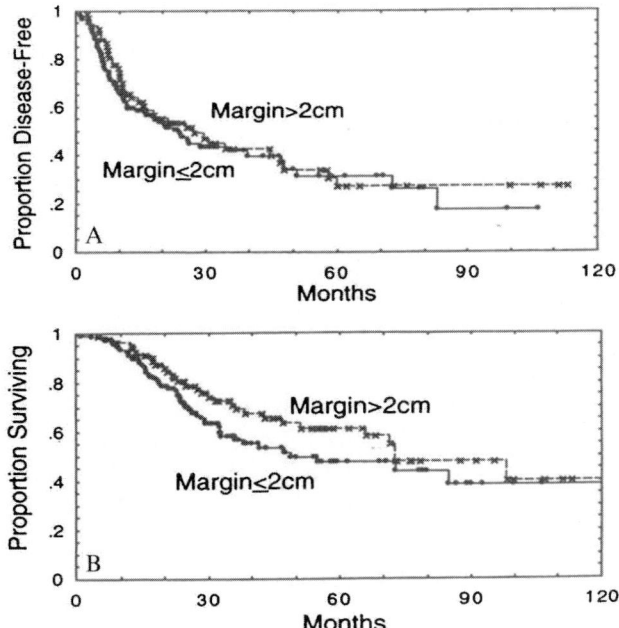

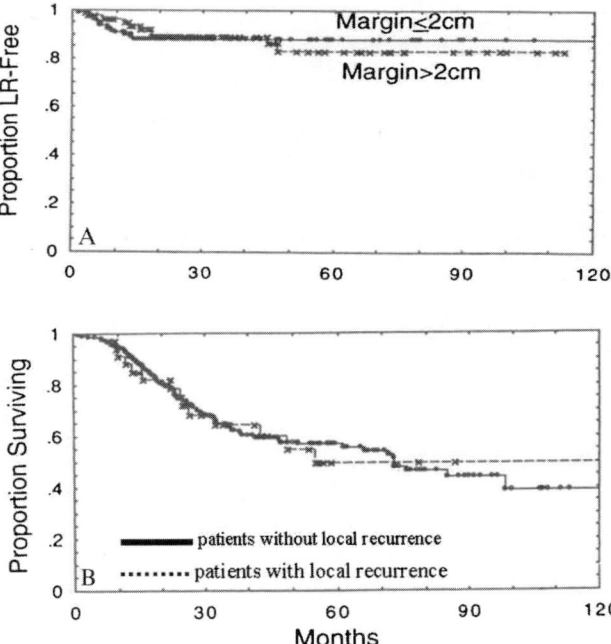

Figure 4 Survival curves for thick melanoma patients according to margins of excision. Disease free and overall survival shown in (a) + (b) respectively. Data points for ≤ 2 cm margins represented as circles and > 2 cm margins as X's.

Figure 5 Local recurrence free survival according to excision margin in thick melanoma patients from MDACC/Moffitt Trial No statistical difference was observed for patients who received a ≤ 2 cm margin (represented by circles) vs. those with a > 2 cm margin (represented by X's) shown in (a). Overall survival was no different whether or not patients with thick melanomas experienced a local recurrence, (b).

melanomas (> 4 mm) because of the improved local/regional control demonstrated with this wider margin. Acceptance of this conclusion has been met with resistance for the following reasons: 1) no survival differences to date has been demonstrated, 2) differences in local/regional events would not be as evident with the routine use of sentinel node biopsy, 3) statistical difference in local events is lost when nodal events are taken out of the analysis, and 4) 3 cm margins are associated with greater surgical morbidity and an increased use of skin grafts. While the UK Trial is currently the only published prospective randomized trial evaluating excision margins in the highest risk group, the preliminary results of the Swedish trial(which includes this group) fails to show any benefit for margins greater than 2 cm.

Based on the currently available evidence it can be simply stated that the appropriate margins of excision for melanomas < 2 mm and > 2 mm are 1 cm and 2 cm, respectively. In this way the vast majority of surgical defects created by the treatment of primary melanoma can be accomplished with primary closure except in the anatomically restricted areas, such as scalp, face, and distal extremities. As time has passed and more data have become available, the paradigm of wider excisions for thicker or worse prognosis lesions is more strongly challenged and the concept that LR and metastatic

TABLE 8 Factors predictive of local recurrence in thick melanoma patients (> 4 cm)

Prognostic Factor	% with Local Recurrence	Univariate P value
Overall	12.2	
Margin		
≤2 cm	11.1	.948
>2 cm	12.2	
Thickness		
4.1-6 mm	11.9	.901
>6 mm	12.7	
Gender		
Male	12.1	.682
Female	12.0	
Nodal status		
Absent	10.3	.057
Present	16.7	
Anatomic Location		.056
Extremity	19.2	
Trunk	6.8	
Head and neck	11.3	
Ulceration		
Absent	10.3	.040
Present	16.7	

dissemination is a function of inherent biology that is not obviously impacted by wide excisions has been promoted. In light of this mounting data that narrower margins may be acceptable, it is not irrational to selectively perform excision margins less than 2 cm for intermediate and thick melanomas that arise in anatomically restrictive areas such as the face, where 2 cm margins may result in significant cosmetic disfigurement or may be impossible to achieve because of proximity to the eyes, ears, nose, or mouth. On then other hand, the data from the UK trial does suggest that very narrow margins (1cm) for higher risk lesions may be too narrow, at least in reference to local and regional events, therefore we should not be cavalier in our approach to excision margins and assume that 1 cm margins is safe for all melanomas. Figure 6 illustrates a potential explanation for the UK data and why 1cm margins may be too narrow in some patients.

Whether it will ultimately be proven that narrower (1 cm) margins is adequate for all melanomas, resulting in reduced morbidity and virtually obviating the need for using skin grafts in the surgical management of primary melanomas as well as dispelling the current paradigm will greatly depend on the long-term results of the UK and the more recent SMSG trials. It should be emphasized, however, that all of the randomized trials to date regarding excision margins for melanoma were designed and powered according to the hypothesis that the wider

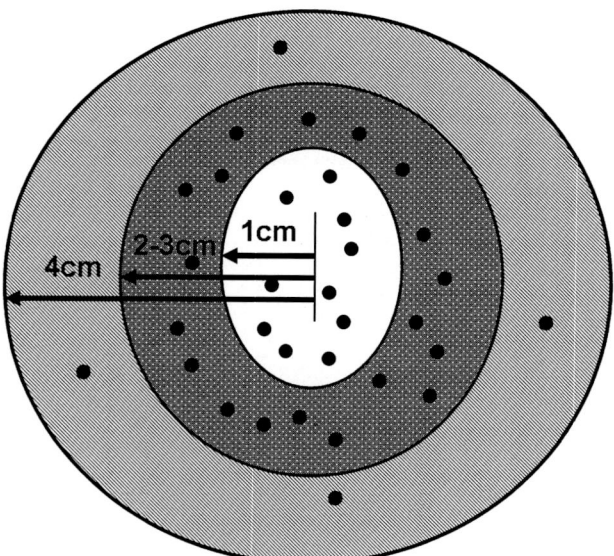

Figure 6 Theoretical diagram illustrating how wider margins removes more microscopic satellites than a narrow 1 cm margin, resulting in a lower incidence of loco-regional failure. Very wide margins (4cm), however, provide little additional benefit as the microscopic satellites, depicted as black circles rarely exist farther than 2cm from the primary site.

excisions would be superior to the more narrow excisions, not that the narrow excision is equivalent—the latter of which would require significantly more patients to accomplish. In response to this critique, discussions are ongoing to initiate an international collaboration to carry out a prospective/randomized margins of excision trial of 1 cm versus 2 cm in the management of melanomas > 2 mm in thickness powered to demonstrate that the narrow margin is equivalent to the wider margin. These patients would also undergo lymphatic mapping and SLN biopsy regardless of randomized excision width. Concerns over trends in survival in favor of wider excision that do not reach statistical significance because of lack of power in trial design as observed in the Intergroup and UK studies will be adequately addressed by this next important clinical trial[33].

EXCISIONS FOR HISTOLOGIC VARIANTS

The Diagnostic Dilemma

The precise histologic diagnosis of a melanocytic skin lesion and its malignant potential can occasionally present a diagnostic dilemma and remain ambiguous, even after tertiary consultation by expert dermatopathologists and the use of specialized histologic staining techniques. For example, it may be difficult to discriminate between a deep penetrating nevus, a Spitz nevus, a malignant Spitz nevus, and a spitzoid melanoma. When confusion exists as to the primary diagnosis, it is best to treat the patient according to the lesion in the differential diagnosis which carries the worst prognosis; a wide excision with 1 or 2 cm margins depending on the measured thickness of the melanocytic proliferation and primary closure is a relatively innocuous surgical procedure relative to the risks of an inadequately excised melanoma. These lesions are currently classified as melanocytic lesions of unknown malignant potential and often manifest spitzoid features and are found more frequently in young adults and children. Interest has emerged in studying the genetics of these lesions using comparative genomic hybridization techniques[34]. This information may provide insights into the expected natural history of these lesions which would be helpful in establishing a more definitive surgical strategy.

Desmoplastic Melanoma

Desmoplastic melanomas are special histological variants of melanoma that are more common in males and tend to exhibit somewhat of a different natural history when compared to other cutaneous lesions of similar Breslow's tumor thickness. Approximately one-third to one-half of patients ultimately diagnosed with a desmoplastic melanoma have undergone a prior biopsy of the index lesion that was incorrectly determined to be benign. As a result, a delay in diagnosis is not uncommon for these lesions and probably explains why the median tumor thickness is greater than other more common histologic subtypes. The fact that many of the lesions do not exhibit the classic signs ("ABCDs") of melanoma, and histologically appear to be very bland, contributes to this delay in diagnosis.

Significant predictors adversely impacting survival are a high mitotic rate and increased tumor thickness. Higher local recurrence rates have been observed, but regional lymph node metastasis are less frequent at initial presentation or as the first site of recurrence. Desmoplastic lesions, particularly those on the head and neck, are often associated with histologic evidence of perineural invasion. When this neurotropism is present there is a greater propensity for local recurrence[35]; therefore, these patients, in particular, may benefit from adjuvant radiation therapy after excision.

Lentigo Maligna (Melanoma)

The terms "Lentigo Maligna" and "Lentigo Maligna Melanoma" are somewhat confusing. Lentigo maligna refers to a specific histologic subtype of melanoma in situ, and a more accurate term is lentigo maligna melanoma in situ. Lentigo maligna melanoma implies that the index process has an invasive component. Regardless of the nomenclature, these lesions can be very large clinically as well as deceivingly extensive microscopically, particularly if they contain a large in situ component. Adding to this problem is that they often develop in chronically sun-exposed areas that are often anatomically restrictive in terms of obtaining margins, such as the face and scalp. Therefore, repair of the surgical defect often requires a skin graft or an elaborate flap closure. To find out after completing the reconstruction that negative margins were not achieved results in a difficult management issue. Making matters worse is that it is very difficult and almost impossible to obtain accurate frozen section margin evaluation at the time of the excision. The following steps are offered in the management of large lentigo maligna lesions in anatomically restrictive and cosmetically sensitive areas: 1) the use of a Wood's Lamp can help more accurately delineate the gross macroscopic peripheral extent, 2) the reconstruction can be delayed after the formal excision for 2 to 3 days to allow time to evaluate the margins with formal permanent histology, 3) a physiologic dressing or duo-derm covering can be placed over the surgical defect at the time of the excision while waiting for the formal pathologic assessment

of margins without compromise to the ultimate reconstruction. Figure 7 shows the resultant surgical defect following the excision of a lentigo maligna melanoma in situ and reconstruction with a rotational flap 2 days later after margin status was established.

Mucosal Primaries

Primary melanomas arising from the mucosal epithelia lining the respiratory, alimentary, and genitourinary tracts have been well documented but are relatively rare. Eighty percent of the non-cutaneous melanomas are ocular in origin with the remaining 20% arising from the mucosae with an annual incidence of only 0.15 per 100,000 persons, representing 3%-4% of all melanomas diagnosed yearly[36,37]; The relative dearth of clinical material and therefore, the absence of large databases, has contributed greatly to the fact that insights into the pathogenesis, natural history, and treatment of mucosal melanoma have not kept pace with the advances made in the understanding and treatment of their cutaneous counterparts. Integral to those advances has to a great extent been the establishment of primary tumor microstaging as one of the critical prognostic indicators for melanoma of the skin. Such information for the mucosal melanomas may not apply or may be difficult to ascertain because of the anatomic sites from which they arise. As a result, determining prognosis by extrapolation from what we know about cutaneous melanoma may not be accurate. As a result, recommendations for treating the primary site in those patients with clinically localized disease is based empirically and offered from those centers with the most experience and long term follow up. Despite the fact that the prognosis for mucosal melanomas is poor, most of the newly diagnosed primary mucosal patients have no evidence of metastatic disease. Therefore treatment of the primary tumor can provide durable local disease control if not cure.

Mucosal melanomas represent a diverse clinical entity. In most published series, lesions of the mucus membranes of the head and neck are the most common followed by those arising in the anorectal region and vulva[37]. Surgical oncologists and general surgeons would more likely be called upon to care for patients with anorectal mucosal primaries.

Ano-rectal Primaries

Primary anorectal mucosal melanoma is an uncommon aggressive malignancy characterized by early systemic dissemination and therefore a poor prognosis. Presenting symptoms are rectal bleeding, rectal pain, or a palpable mass[38-41]. The primary lesions are most often identified at the squamo-columnar junction where most of the melanocytes reside, but can develop purely in rectal (columnar) mucosa or anal (squamous) mucosa.

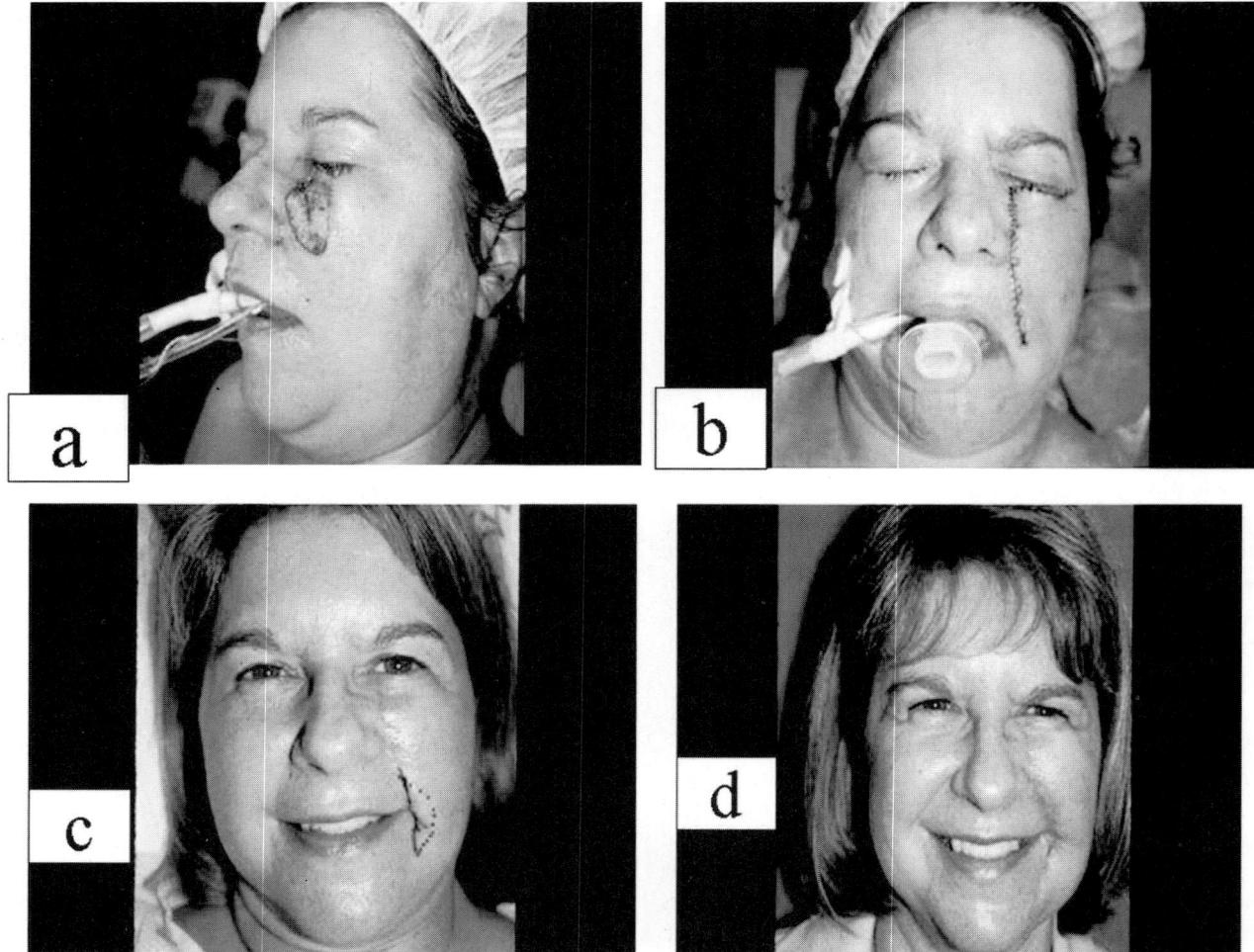

Figure 7 The surgical defect following an excision for a lentigo maligna melanoma in-situ is shown in (A), followed by the rotational flap reconstruction 2 days later, in (b), excision od "dog ear" in (c), and ultimate cosmetic result in ().

Such information may be important when assessing and/or predicting lymphatic drainage patterns and likely sites of regional lymph node failure. Despite the fact that most patients present with clinically localized disease to the primary site (80%) with or without regional lymph node disease but no demonstrable distant disease, the vast majority will succumb to distant dissemination regardless of the extent of local/regional therapy, with a median survival of 25 months[40] The poor overall prognosis is most likely explained by a delay in diagnosis until symptoms develop. The chance for early diagnosis in anorectal melanoma patients, and for almost all mucosal melanomas in general, is limited because these lesions develop in occult anatomic locations. Unlike cutaneous melanoma where early change can readily be visibly detected, mucosal lesions remain asymptomatic until they are locally advanced and ulcerated. While one study demonstrated that lesions less than 2 mm have a more favorable prognosis[36], most lesions present as relatively

large polypoid masses, therefore most of the mucosal primaries are comparable to IIC cutaneous lesions (>4mm in thickness and ulcerated) and are likely to harbor micro-metastatic disease at diagnosis. The only exception is when the diagnosis is made incidentally upon hemorrhoidectomy. Experience with mucosal melanomas further demonstrates the propensity for melanoma in general, to metastasize with relative small primary tumor volumes compared to other solid tumors.

Because of its rarity, standards of care for anorectal have not been well established. Historically, APR with extensive elective pelvic and inguinal lymphadenectomy was promoted[39]. Because survival rates were so poor (<25%), a more conservative and less morbid sphincter preserving approach was selectively employed, with APR reserved for patients with unresectable local recurrences. Local/regional control rates after transanal excision were inferior to those reported after APR as the initial surgical procedure but survival rates unaffected in a negative way[38,41]. Recurrence patterns after local excision include either local tumor relapse and or regional nodal failure (primarily inguinal) in up to 60% of patients[38]. Borrowing the concept of margin negative local excision and adjuvant XRT often used for the common types of rectal cancers combined with what we have learned about adjuvant nodal irradiation and elective nodal basin radiation regimens in the treatment of resected metastatic nodal disease from cutaneous melanoma and control of the regional basin in high risk head and neck cutaneous primaries a rationale treatment strategy has been applied selectively to those patients with resectable anorectal melanoma in the hope of improving local/regional control and still provide sphincter preservation. Transanal excision and adjuvant post-operative XRT delivered in five 30 Gy fractions to the primary surgical site and potential regional nodal basins has been recently evaluated.[42,43] Long-term results, for both local/regional control and overall survival, compare favorably with results achieved with APR but without the associated functional morbidity.[43]

Regional lymph node metastases are a common form of failure in anorectal melanoma patients. Extrapolating from a wealth of experience with lymphatic mapping and SLN biopsy in the management of primary cutaneous melanoma patients such an approach has been applied to anorectal patients who present without clinically or radiographically identifiable nodal disease. While lesions arising at or below the squamo-columnar junction often drain primarily to one or both inguinal basins, lesions above this area are likely to spread through the rectal mesenteric nodes. Using lymphoscintigraphy, individual lymphatic drainage patterns can be defined and SLN biopsy can be performed if drainage to the inguinal nodes is demonstrated. In this way a more selective approach to nodal treatment can be pursued and potentially reducing the morbidity associated with unnecessary lymphadenectomy or nodal irradiation.

TECHNIQUES FOR ROUTINE WOUND CLOSURE

The majority of patients present with early stage cutaneous melanoma and can be effectively treated with a simple elliptical excision of the primary lesion or biopsy site followed by primary closure. Procedures that include excision margins of 2 cm or less can often be accomplished on an outpatient basis with local anesthesia alone or in conjunction with intravenous sedation. From a technical point of view, the long axis of the elliptical excision should be oriented to maximally utilize the available surrounding skin to achieve a dependable and full thickness primary closure and oriented towards the appropriate draining nodal basin where possible. A variety of options for designing the ellipse can be used in order to facilitate closure (Figure 8). The planned excision is influenced by the anatomic site and surgeons' assessment of the elasticity and mobility of the local soft tissues. The elliptical excision may not necessarily be directly linear but may be a "lazy S" type pattern. The width of the oncologically appropriate excision is first circumferentially measured with a ruler from the edge of an intact tumor or previous biopsy site. An elliptical excision, with the long axis of the excision of three to four times the width, is usually the technique of choice to facilitate mobilization of full thickness subcutaneous and skin flaps for primary closure (Figure 9). The excision includes the removal of the skin and underlying subcutaneous tissue down to the muscular fascia (figure 8c); there is no evidence that removal of the muscular fascia provides any improvement or impairment of local control or survival.[44,45]

The specimen should be marked for orientation for accurate histologic margin assessment prior to being severed from the patient. Closure of the defect usually requires the creation of an advancement flap. This is performed by detaching the skin and subcutaneous tissue from the underlying fascial connections in a plane just

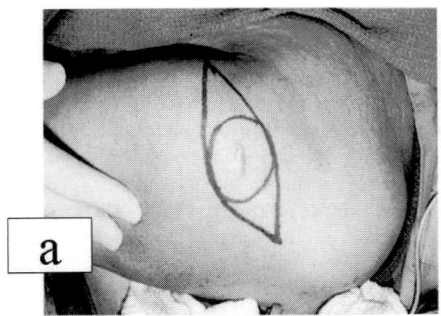 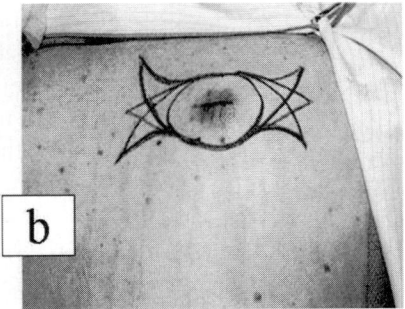 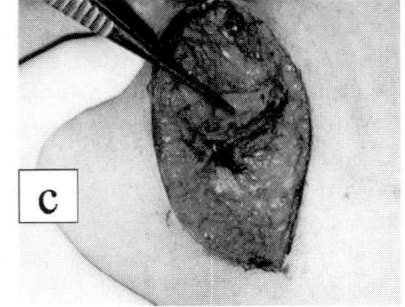

Figure 8 Examples of excision margins. In (a), a 1 cm excision oriented in a linear fashion planned for a proximal extremity lesion and in (b), various options shown for a 2 cm excision on the back to allow primary closure. In (c), the depth of excision extends to, but not including the muscular fascia.

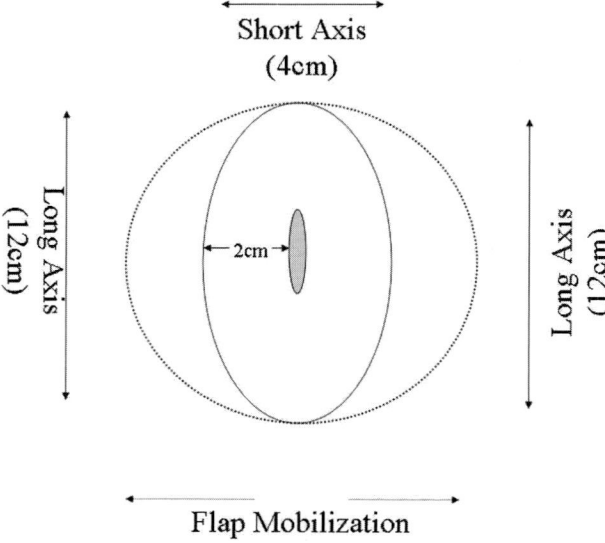

Figure 9 The surgical margin is 2 cm from the biopsy site or the lateral margin of the intact melanoma. The long axis of the incision should be three to four times its width; shematic is depicted in (A) and actual planned excision in (B). After the melanoma is excised, skin flaps are raised in a plane above the deep fascia for a sufficient distance to enable closure of the skin edges without undue tension. The most extensive area of mobilization is near the center of the flaps, and it often is necessary to mobilize the skin flaps for a distance twice that the excised margin. The flaps are usually joined in a two-step procedure; the subcutaneous tissues and deep dermis are joined first, and the skin is approximated by either a standard suture technique or a subcuticular closure.

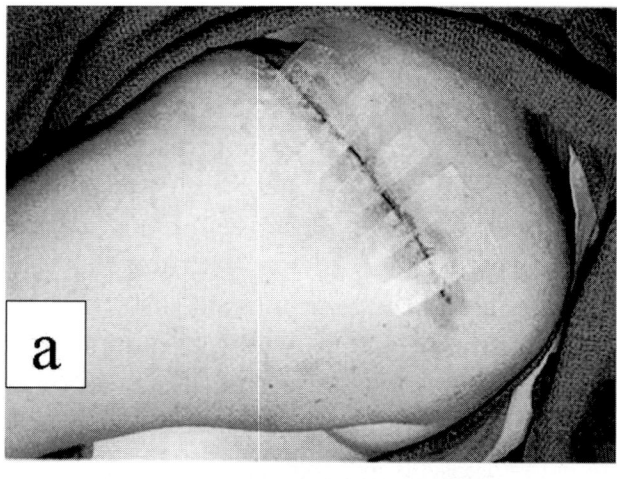

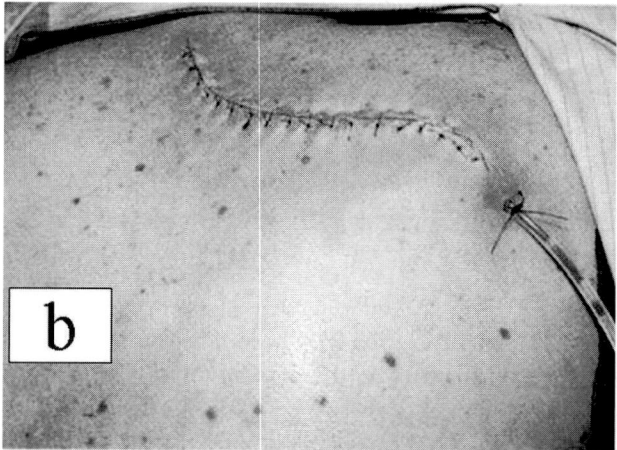

Figure 10 Completed full thickness primary closure is shown without and with a suction drain in (a) and (b) respectively.

deep to the fatty layer of the skin. The flaps should be tailored so that the most central part of the excision is mobilized to the greatest degree because this is the area with greatest tension. The opposing flaps can then be stretched over the defect and the tissues approximated using absorbable interrupted deep intradermal sutures (Figure 10). The skin can then be closed with a running subcuticular closure, with a stapling device, or interrupted nylon sutures depending on the closure tension, the anticipated range of motion and wound-stress predicted for specific anatomic locations. Depending on the size and location of the soft tissue defect, a closed suction drain may be necessary to avoid a seroma (Figure 10b).

The surgical morbidity, cosmetic disfigurement, and financial costs incurred for skin grafts are greater than primary wound closure; primary wound closure with local advancement flaps is almost always preferable. In some anatomic locations, however, primary closure is not possible l, such as the distal extremities or scalp. In such circumstance, closure of the defect is often accomplished with either a split- or full-thickness skin graft or rotation flap closures. In cosmetically sensitive locations, such as on the face rotation flaps offer a cosmetically more satisfying

alternative, (figure) Patient dissatisfaction with the appearance of the healed surgical wound is most often associated with the degree of soft tissue indentation or depression rather than the length of the incision.[46] Avoiding skin grafts when possible, providing the patient with accurate information about the expected postoperative physical appearance, and a candid but empathetic discussion of the potential lethality of inadequately treated melanoma all give the patient an accurate and appropriate perspective to alleviate the negative psychological impact of surgical treatment of the primary.

ANATOMICAL CONSIDERATIONS FOR EXCISION

The preceding surgical techniques can be employed for melanomas in most anatomic sites, such as the trunk, the proximal extremities, and a large percentage of the distal extremities. However, surgical approaches may need to be individualized and modified in other anatomical sites.

Face

Because of the proximity to vital structures and the importance of cosmetic results, excision margins for primary melanomas of the face often need to be limited to avoid injury or deformity to the eyes, nose, ears, or mouth. Figure 11 illustrates the planned excision and steps for reconstruction for a relatively large melanoma of the face adjacent to the right eye. Radiation therapy may be considered to help reduce the risk of local recurrence following the treatment of lesions with very narrow margins and/or when risk of local recurrence is increased.

Ear

Depending on the location of the lesion, primary melanomas of the ear may be best managed with a wedge-type excision or partial amputation (Figure 12). A total auriculectomy is generally reserved for only very locally advanced primary lesions or extensive local recurrences. For patients who wear glasses, special efforts should be made to preserve the upper part of the ear. Excellent prosthetic devices of good functional and cosmetic quality are available for patients who require a more disfiguring excision.

Nose

The shape and contour of the nose is the end result of several aesthetic units. Excisions of primary melanomas involving the nose may therefore need to be individualized according to the location of the planned defect to be reconstructed. While skin grafts can often be used, the cosmetic results are frequently suboptimal. Local rota-tional flaps offer the best option and the type of flap used also depends on which aesthetic unit is being reconstructed. Figures 13 and 14 illustrates the reconstruction of surgical defects resulting from excisions on the tip and sidewall units respectively.

Breast

The skin overlying the breast does not possess qualities that should influence the surgeon to perform more radical excisions (ie, mastectomy) when treating melanomas that arise in this area. In general, mastectomy should not be performed for primary melanomas of the breast skin. Most excisions can be performed in accordance with the above-mentioned guidelines without significant distortion to the contour of the breast. The nipple-areolar complex should be sacrificed only if directly involved by or adjacent to the primary tumor; the nipple areolar complex can be reconstructed in this case.

Digits

Melanomas that arise on the skin or nail bed of the toes are managed with a straightforward amputation at the metatarsal-phalangeal joint. The joint space can usually be covered with adequate soft tissue by raising either a plantar or dorsal soft tissue flap. A significant functional deficit is rarely produced by the total amputation of a single digit from the foot. Because the metatarsal head of the great toe is a critical structure for ambulation, its removal (ie, a ray amputation) should be avoided when performing amputations of the great toe.

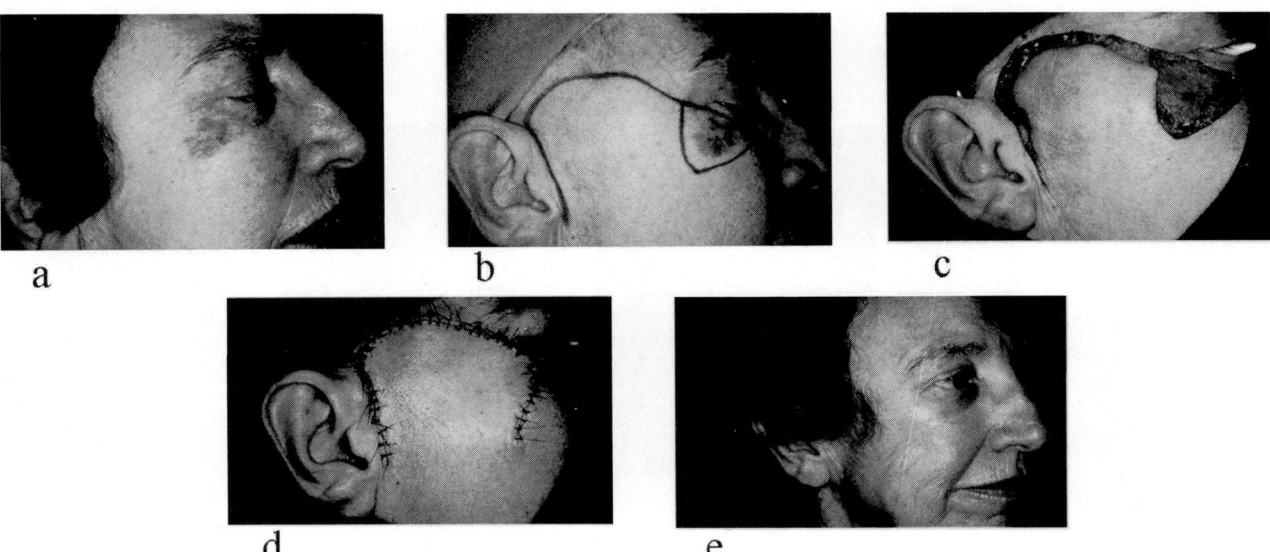

a b c d e

Figure 11 Relatively large lentigo maligna melanoma on the face is shown in (a). The planned excision and rotation flap reconstruction is illustrated in (b). Panels (c-e) shows the resultant surgical defect and raised flap, closure of the defect, and long term cosmetic result, respectively.

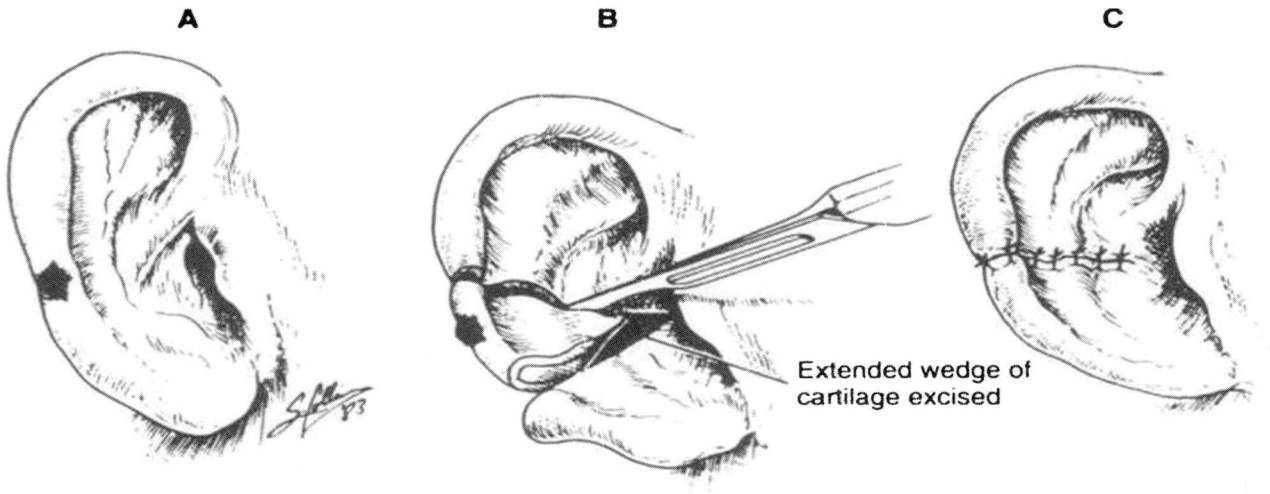

Figure 12 Technique of wedge excision for a melanoma on the outer helix of the ear (A). It is important to carry the incision down to the inner helix of the ear (B), and to include a wedge of the cartilage to the external auditory canal to fully mobilize the ear for closure (C).

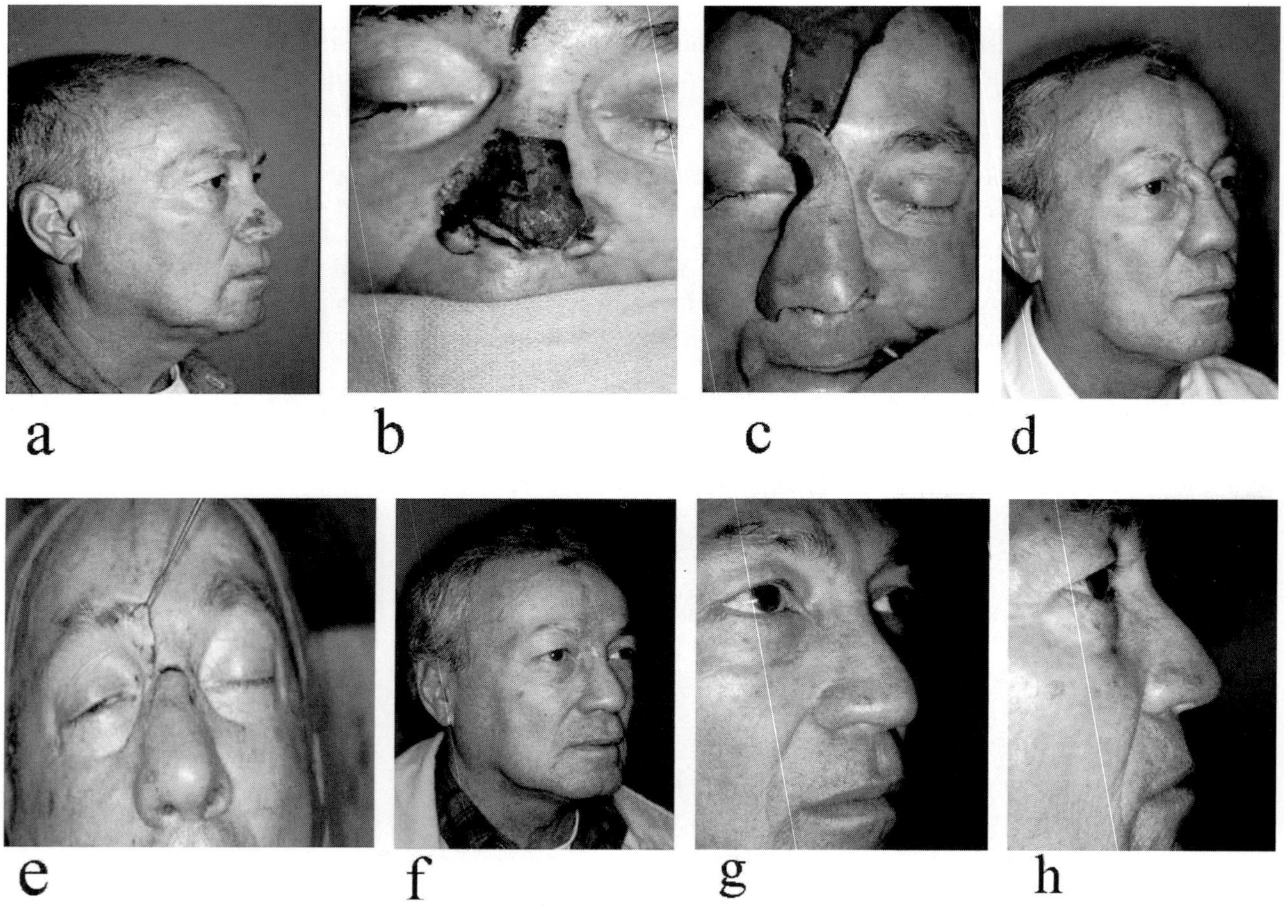

Figure 13 Primary melanoma involving the ala and sidewall aesthetic units of the nose in (a). The surgical defect after an appropriate excision is shown in (b) and inset of forehead pedicle flap in (c). Closure of recipient site in (d), transaction of the pedicle after 3 weeks in(e), and completed reconstruction in (f). Long term result in (g and h).

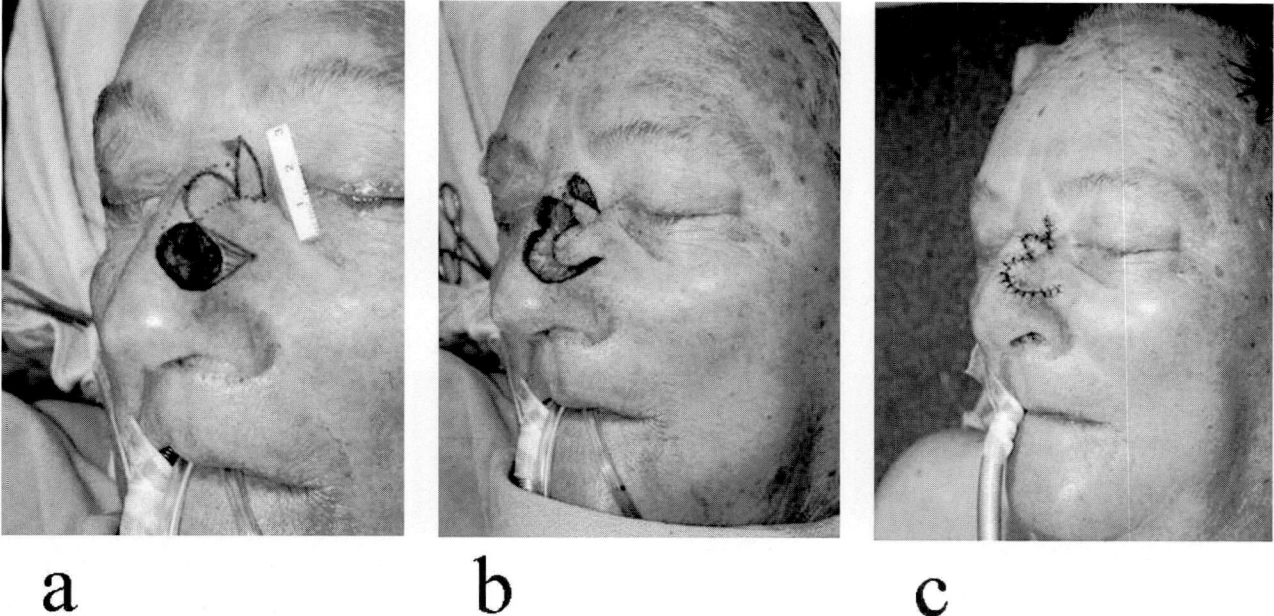

a   b   c

Figure 14 Surgical defect in Lt sidewall subunit of the nose and planned tri-lobe flap reconstruction in (a). Rotation of the lobes in (b) and completed reconstruction in (c). By design, the successive lobes are progressively smaller allowing for primary closure of the smallest defect.

Complete amputations of fingers or thumb give rise to a more significant functional impairment. When excising melanomas on the fingers, amputations should only be used when the distal phalanx, particularly the nail bed, is involved and should be planned in a way to preserve as much length of the digit as possible but without compromising margins. The digit is preferentially amputated proximal to the distal interphalangeal joint of the fingers and the interphalangeal joint of the thumb if the extent of the nail bed or parenchymal involvement and the proximal location of the lesion's border allow (Figure 15). Because the excision of bone offers no oncologic benefit, unless the bone is directly involved, the total amputation of a finger or ray amputation to include the metacarpal bone is not mandated for proximal finger lesions. Adequate soft tissue excisions without amputation can usually be performed for primary lesions located on the proximal portions of the fingers and thumbs. Wound closure may be accomplished by full-thickness skin grafts, local rotational flaps, or full-thickness soft tissue flaps created by the amputation of an adjacent and less functionally important digit or cross finger flap taken from a less functionally important area of an adjacent digit. This latter flap may be selectively used to reconstruct the complete removal of the nail bed and surrounding margin of skin and soft tissue when treating subugual melanomas of the thumb as shown in figure 16, particularly if the functionally important dorsal tendon to the distal phalanx can be spared.

Web Space

Melanomas that occur in the web spaces between the digits may require complicated reconstruction after excision, particularly when the primary lesion is located on the hand or in the web space adjacent to the great toe. En bloc total digital amputation along with removal of the metatarsal or metacarpal head tends to result in significant cosmetic disfigurement and functional defi-

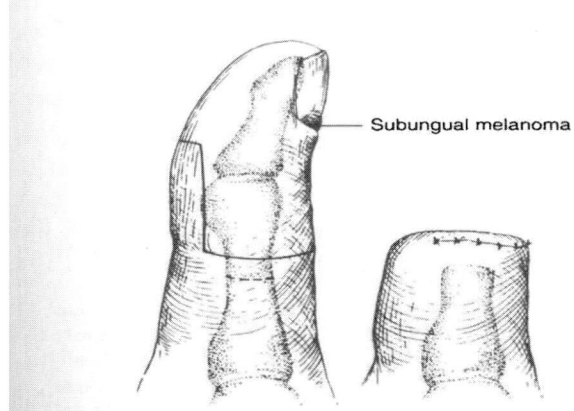

— Subungual melanoma

Figure 15 Schematic amputation of the thumb for removal of a subungual melanoma. The digit is amputated just proximal to the distal interphalangeal joint, with a flap of skin on the volar side to be used as a full-thickness covering over the stump.

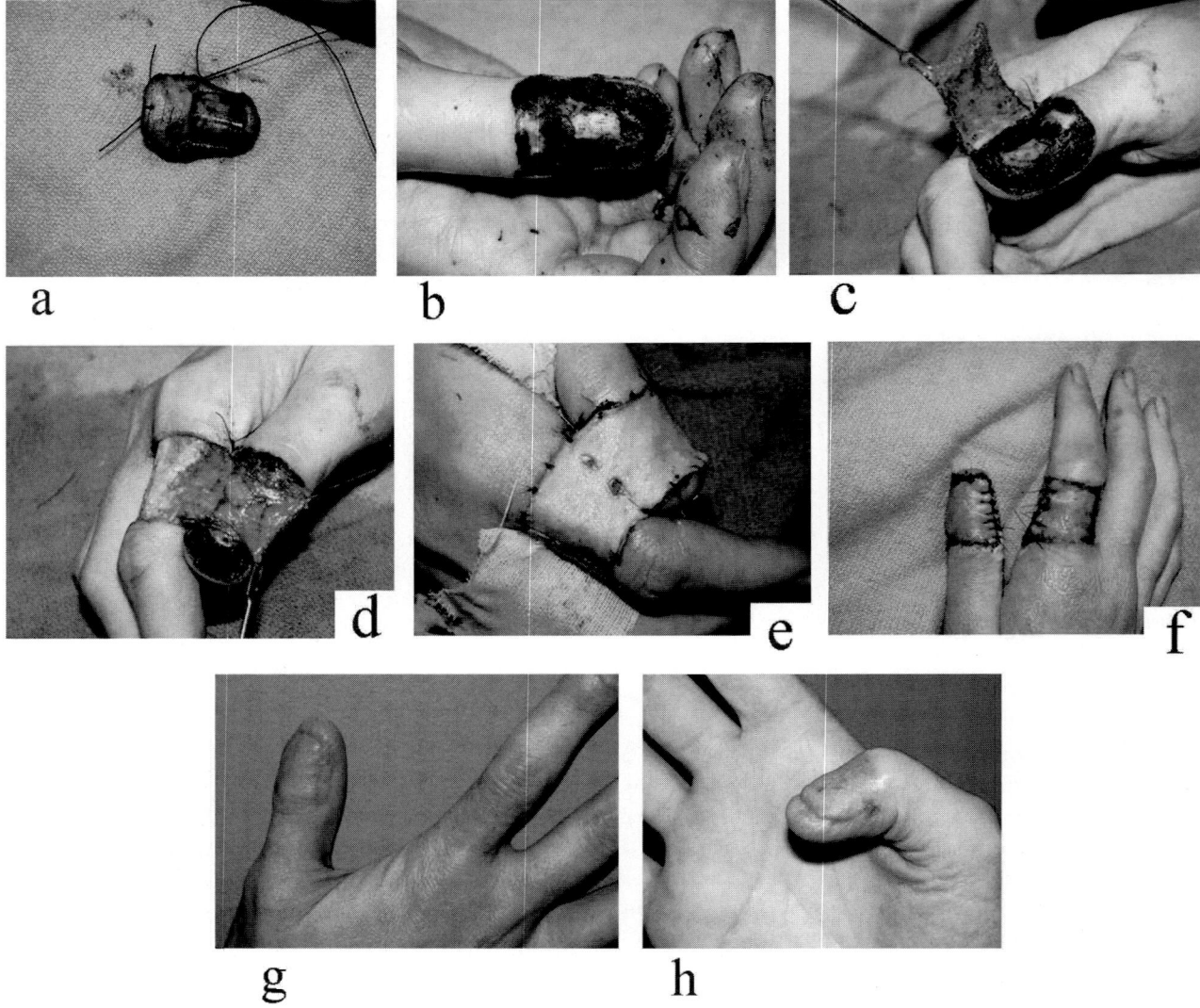

Figure 16 Alternative approach to treat subungual melanoma of the thumb in order to spare the entire length of the thmb. Excision specimen in (a) including the removal of the entire nail bed and matrix with surrounding skin and soft tissue and defect shown in (b). Harvestind of adjact cross finger flap in(c) and inset of flap in the surgical defect in (d) followed by skin grafting in (e). The flap is separated in (f) with long term result shown in (g) and (h).

cits. Soft tissue excisions alone are usually possible in these areas, and the defect can then be covered with either full-thickness skin grafts or local rotational flaps (Figure 17).

Umbilicus

Melanomas can arise in the skin adjacent to, or within, the umbilicus. In these situations adequate surgical margins require removal of the umbilicus and overlying skin. A series of rotational flaps can be used to reconstruct the navel after a circular-type excision if desired (Figure 18).

Foot

Melanomas on the plantar surface of the foot often affect a large surface area. Primary closure after adequate excision is almost invariably impossible. Over non-weight-bearing surfaces such as the arch of the foot, split-thickness skin grafts almost always provide adequate coverage. However, on weight-bearing surfaces, such as over the calcaneus and over the head of the first metatarsal, skin grafts sometimes will not take well and/or do not provide durable soft tissue coverage. Many surgeons have adopted the strategy of first covering the wound with a split or full thickness graft. If it takes well

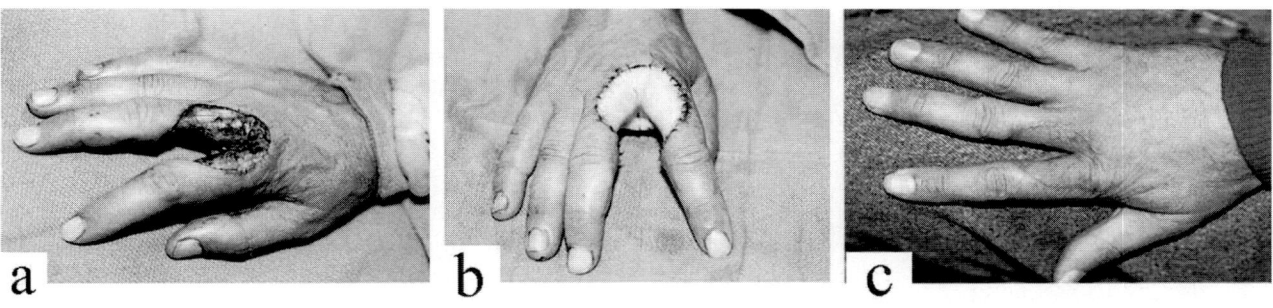

Figure 17 Soft tissue defect following a 2 cm excision of a thick melanoma in the web space in (A). Coverage of the defect with a full-thickness skin graft in (B). Completed result demonstrating preservation of function and cosmesis without compromising surgical margins in (C).

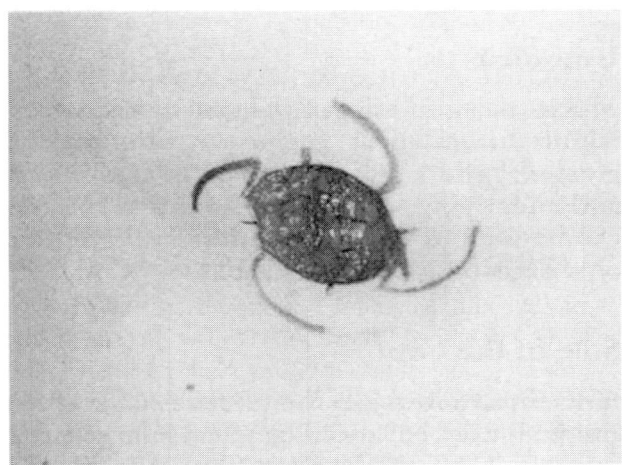

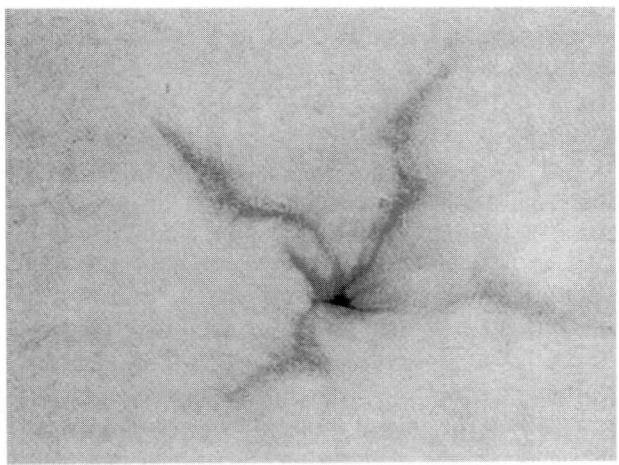

Figure 18 (A), Soft tissue defect following excision of a melanoma in the umbilicus. (B), Closure was accomplished with a series of rotational flaps.

and determined to be acceptably durable for ambulation, then a more complicated plastic surgical reconstruction that may require revisions is avoided. Others prefer to always attempt to reconstruct defects on weight bearing regions with full thickness soft tissue flaps primarily rather than selectively when skin grafts fail. Soft tissue defects created over the ball of the foot can also be covered by amputating the great toe but preserving full-thickness skin and soft tissue on the dorsum of the toe to be used as a rotational flap to cover the defect on the plantar surface of the ball of the foot. Lesions on the heel that require significant soft tissue excisions are more problematic but can often be closed by a rotational flap from the arch of the foot based on the posterior tibial vessels. This full-thickness soft tissue flap can cover the surgical defect on the heel, and the defect created at the nonweight-bearing donor site can be covered with a skin graft (Figure 19). In some situations the defect is too large or positioned too far posterior to allow adequate coverage with this type of flap, and a myocutaneous transfer from a distant site with microvascular recon-struction provides an alternative (Figure 20). These more complicated reconstructions may be especially indicated in situations where a split-thickness skin graft has been attempted and proven inadequate. Another option has recently become popular using a staged approach by placing a wound vac sponge dressing immediately following the excision, followed by placement of a skin graft a few weeks later when a thick and well vascularized bed of granulation tissue has developed. Such a strategy is illustrated in figure 21.

Moh's Surgery

Moh's micrographic surgery uses pathological techniques to map the histologic extent of a particular malignant lesion to allow excision with a minimal surgical margin. The technique is practiced and espoused primarily by dermatologists. The technique originally required in situ

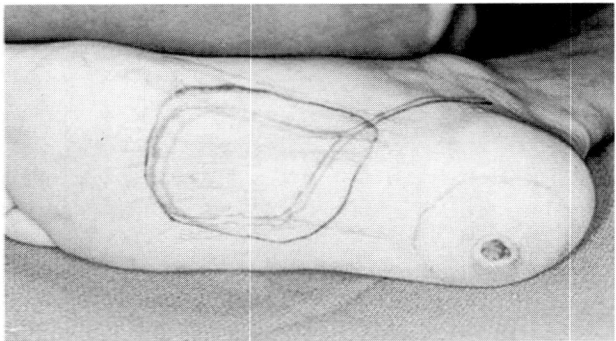

a

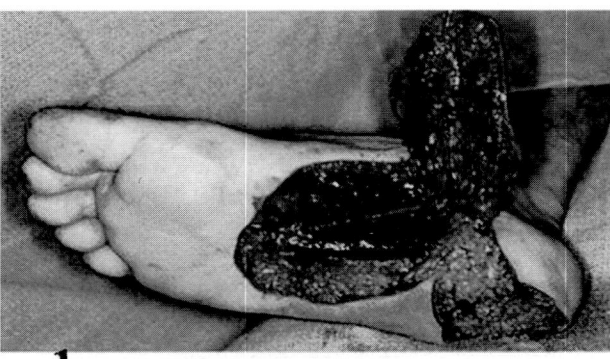

b

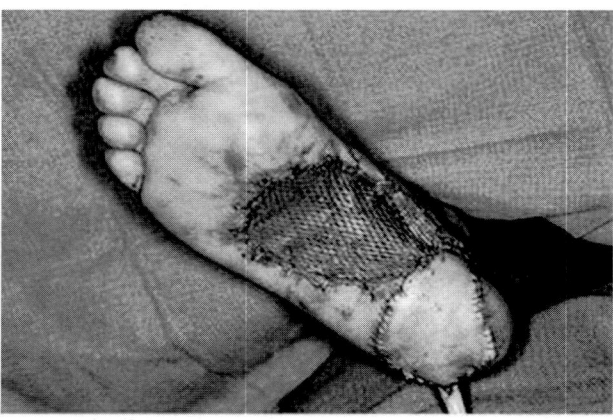

c

Figure 19 (A), Soft tissue defect over weight-bearing area on plantar surface. (B), Creation of full-thickness rotational flaps from non-weight-bearing area. (C), Full-thickness coverage over weight-bearing area and skin graft to non-weight-bearing area completed.

tissue fixation before excision, but most dermatologists now use a fixation technique of excised tissue. Horizontal histologic sections of the excised specimen permit a more complete microscopic examination of the surgical margin than traditional methods. The location of residual tumor at the margins of initial excisions is graphically mapped and malignant extensions are pursued with sequential excisions until the entire tumor is excised. This allows maximum sparing of tumor-free adjacent tissue. In regard to its use as a primary therapy for melanoma, most of the published literature consists of patients with in situ or thin invasive lesions. Local control rates are reported to be excellent for these low-risk lesions and comparable to reported standard surgical approaches but no formal direct comparisons have to this date been pursued.[47,48] Until more data are available, Moh's surgery should be used selectively in special circumstances for melanoma in situ or minimally invasive lesions in anatomically restrictive sites to preserve adjacent vital structures.

Sentinel Node Biopsy: A Rational Strategy in the Management of Stage I and II Melanoma

MANAGEMENT OF THE CLINICALLY UNINVOLVED REGIONAL NODES

While recommendations for the extent of excision margins, described above are widely accepted, the approach to the clinically uninvolved regional lymph nodes has been the source of ongoing controversy. How to best manage the following scenario is illustrative of the dilemma: A 36-year old patient presents following a punch biopsy of a changing pigmented lesion over the left scapula diagnosed as a 1.8 mm melanoma. Physical examination reveals the absence or enlarged lymph nodes in any potential regional lymph node group. The chest X-ray is normal and the patient is otherwise healthy. Traditionally, this patient would have been offered one of two options in addition to excision of the primary tumor: 1) observation of the regional lymph nodes and formal node dissection only if the patient subsequently develops clinically evident (palpable) nodal disease, an approach termed therapeutic lymph node dissection (TLND), 2) formal lymph node as a component of the initial surgical treatment dissection, referred to as elective lymph node dissection (ELND). Both approaches have theoretical as well as very real disadvantages.[1]

A significant percentage of individuals, predicted by increasing tumor thickness or other unfavorable histologic features of the primary tumor[49], harbor clinically undetectable regional lymph node metastases, which in most patients will lead to palpable (macroscopic) nodal disease. Once clinical nodal involvement develops, the ability to achieve long-term survival and durable regional disease control with a (TLND) may be compromised

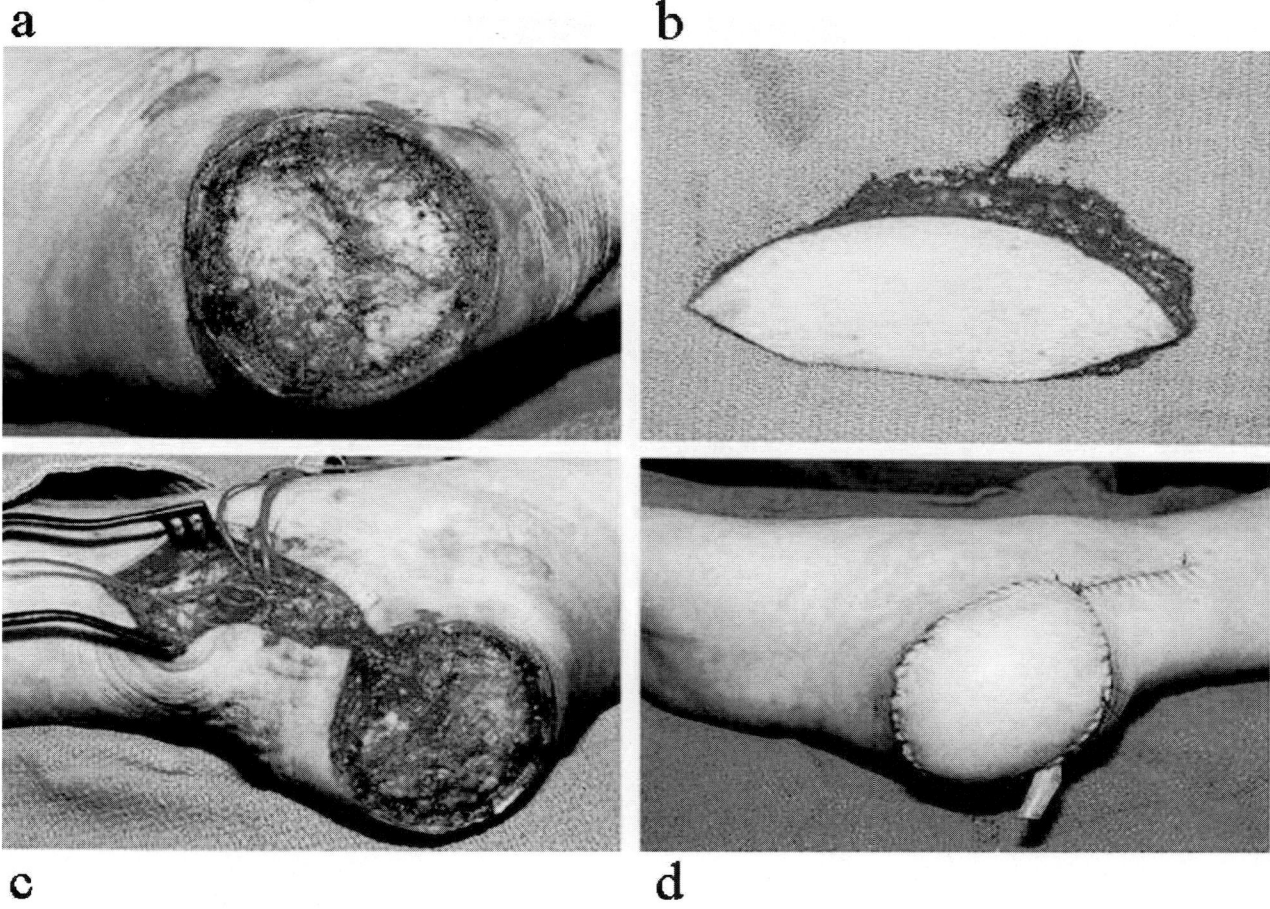

Figure 20 (A), Surgical defect on the heel is too far posterior to be adequately covered by rotational flaps. (B), Distant free myocutaneous flap with vascular pedicle. (C), Exposure of recipient vessels. (D), Complete microvascular anastomosis and free flap reconstruction.

compared to surgical approaches targeted at microscopic nodal burden[49]. In the majority of patients, however, microscopic nodal disease is absent at diagnosis. These patients cannot benefit from an ELND but will be subjected to the cost and morbidity of an unnecessary operation if treated in this manner. Making this controversy even more contentious is the lack of a consistent survival advantage demonstrated in ELND trials[50–53]. A rational compromise emerged when the technique of lymphatic mapping and SLN biopsy was introduced as a minimally invasive method for determining if occult nodal metastases are present[54]. Patients with proven occult nodal disease in the SLN could then undergo an early TLND, and those without disease could be observed, an approach termed *selective lymphadenctomy* [54]

SCIENTIFIC SUPPORT FOR THE SENTINEL NODE CONCEPT

Lymphatic mapping relies on the hypothesis that the dermal lymphatic drainage from cutaneous sites to the regional lymph node basin is an orderly and definable process and that these lymphatic drainage patterns should mimic the metastatic spread of melanoma cells in the lymphatics, figure 22. In this way, the first lymph node(s) receiving lymphatic drainage (the sentinel nodes) are the most likely to contain metastatic disease. The successful identification, surgical removal, and histologic examination of these nodes should provide accurate nodal staging.

To test this hypothesis, clinical studies were performed using intradermal injections of blue lymphatic dyes (isosulfan blue or patent blue V) at the primary tumor site followed by the visual identification of the SLNs in the nodal basin. These studies established the following: 1) SLN identification rates, and 2) the accuracy of the SLN in determining the presence or absence of regional nodal metastases.

The first report published by Don Morton in 1992 evaluated 237 patients and demonstrated an 82% SLN identification rate[54]. Subsequent studies from the M. D. Anderson and Moffitt Cancer Centers[55,56] and the

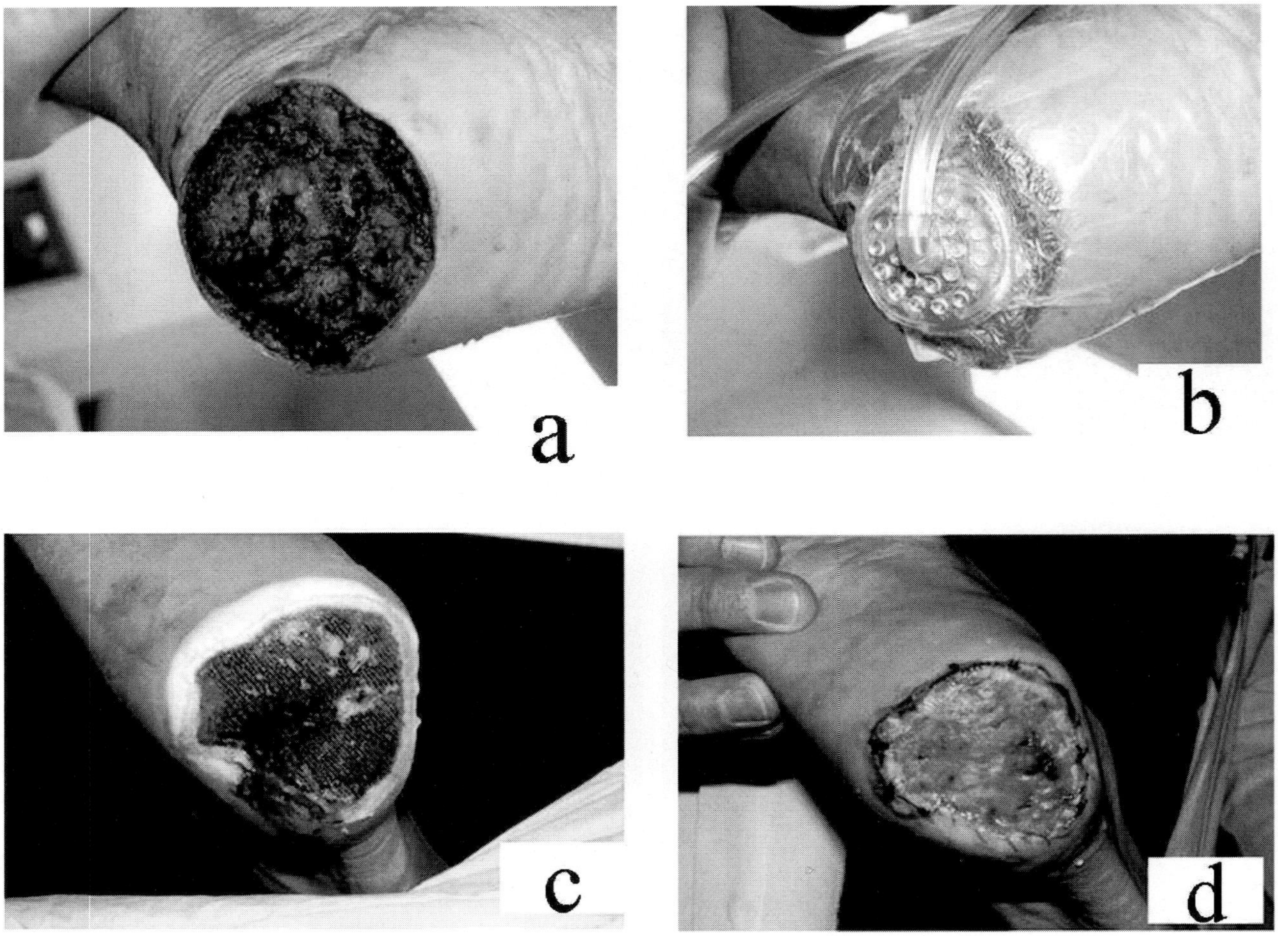

Figure 21 Less complicated alternative to reconstruct a posterior calcaneus defect (a) using a wound vac to promote the growth of a well vascularized thick layer of granulation tissue (b). Bed of vascularized tissue shown in (c) and placement of skin graft in (d).

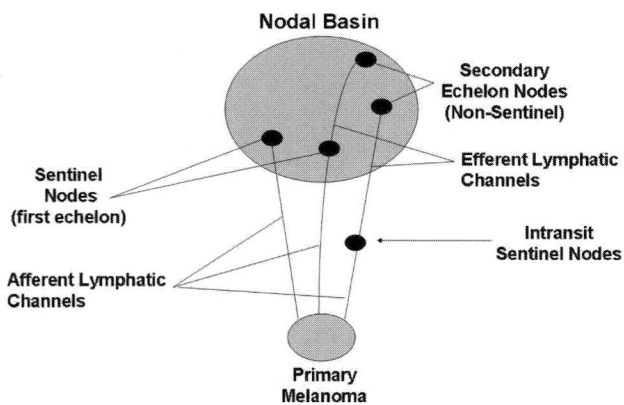

Figure 22 Schematic of potential afferent lymphatic channels draining from a primary cutaneous site to sentinel (first echelon) nodes in the nodal basin. Secondary echelon nodes may be identified by pass through of the intradermally injected blue dye or radio-labeled colloid. Occassionally a sent.inel node is located between the injection site and the formal nodal basin defined here as "intransit" sentinel node, but also referred to as "interval" or "ectopic" sentinel node.

Sydney Melanoma Unit reported similar findings[57]. Accuracy assessment was accomplished through the use of synchronous ELND performed at the time of the SLN biopsy. A false-negative event was defined as the detection of microscopic disease in a non-SLN when the SLN from the same basin was histologically negative. Accordingly, the false-negative rate was then calculated as the number of false-negative events divided by the total number of patients with microscopic nodal disease. Collectively, these initial studies evaluated 402 patients with successful SLN localization, 86 of which were found to have regional node metastases (81 patients with a positive SLN and 5 additional patients with disease only in a non-SLN)[1,55–57]. This low false-negative rate of 5% supported the SLN concept.

Additional evidence that regional node metastasis is an orderly and nonrandom event is provided from the M. D. Anderson Cancer Center reporting on the examination of 105 lymphadenectomy specimens in patients with at least one positive SLN[58]. Investigators found that the SLN was the only node involved in 83 (79%) of the basins, with disease in additional nodes identified in 21% of the lymphadenectomy specimens. Presented in another way, 68% of all the SLNs removed and only 1.8% of all non-SLNs were involved with metastatic disease.[58]

Tremendous interest was generated from these initial studies, and many centers subsequently adopted the selective lymphadenectomy approach for newly diagnosed intermediate and high-risk stage I and II melanoma patients. Improvements in SLN localization techniques, insights into the biologic relevance of the SLN (discussed below), and additional findings supporting the SLN concept emerged. In a report of nearly 250 SLN-negative patients followed for over 3 years, only 10 patients (4%) developed nodal failure within the previously mapped regional basin[59]. Such failures represent a false-negative rate similar to the 5% determined by concomitant ELND. More careful histologic scrutiny of the negative SLNs from these same 10 patients revealed the presence of disease in 8. These data not only further supported the validity of the SLN concept, but also suggested that routine histologic examinations of SLNs may fail to detect clinically relevant disease.

TECHNICAL ADVANCES

Initial SLN identification rates of 80% to 85% using blue dye injections provided a promising beginning. The use of high-resolution cutaneous lymphoscintigraphy[60–62] and an intraoperative hand-held gamma detection device to locate radiolabeled colloids that have accumulated in SLNs after being injected at the primary site have yielded higher SLN identification rates.[58,62–64] The use of a gamma probe was first described by Krag, who reported a 95% SLN identification rate.[64] Studies comparing combined modality techniques (radiocolloid plus blue dye) versus blue dye alone demonstrated a significant increase in SLN identification to 99% with the combined approach.[58,63]

Furthermore, the number of SLNs identified was greater when both modalities were employed compared to blue dye alone (1.74 versus 1.31, respectively[58]). The intraoperative use of the gamma probe provides a method of detection that is independent of and more sensitive than visualization of blue-stained nodes and may locate SLNs that may otherwise be undetected. This more complete removal of SLNs may further reduce the already low false-negative rate. Figure 23 summarizes the components necessary for successful identification and removal of a sentinel node.

These techniques can also aid in the localization of SLNs that may exist outside and/or proximal to the formal nodal basin; referred to as interval, in-transit, or ectopic SLNs[65–69], figure 24. According to published studies, the frequency of such SLN locations is in the range of 5% to 10% of patients, and the frequency of involvement with microscopic disease is the same as that of SLNs harvested from formal basins[69]. The failure to identify these nodes risks under-staging some patients and leaving behind potential sources of clinical recurrences.

BIOLOGIC AND PROGNOSTIC SIGNIFICANCE OF THE SENTINEL NODE

Studies have demonstrated that the incidence of SLN metastases correlates directly with increasing tumor thickness[58,70–73] (Table 9). SLN involvement is also associated with a variety of other known primary tumor factors predictive of OS, including ulceration, lymphatic invasion, mitotic rate, Clark level, anatomic site, and host factors such as age[72–75]. In a multivariate analysis, the two variables that independently predicted SLN involvement were tumor thickness and the presence of ulceration[73] Interestingly, the most recent analysis from the American Joint Commission on Cancer (AJCC) melanoma staging committee demonstrated that the same two factors were also the strongest predictors of survival in stage I and II patients[49,74] This analysis uncovered a unique interaction between tumor thickness and ulceration in that the presence of ulceration within a specific tumor thickness stage worsened the prognosis of patients equivalent to those in the next higher thickness group without ulceration.[74] A similar relationship between thickness and ulceration in terms of predicting the incidence of SLN metastases exists as shown in Table 9[73] These observations support the hypothesis that the prognostic value of tumor thickness and ulceration is largely dependent on the fact that these two same factors predict SLN metastases, and in this way offers convincing evidence that SLN involvement is a biologically important event.

Further supporting this conclusion are findings from survival analyses of large numbers of stage I and II patients managed in prospective selective lymphadenectomy programs. More than one such report revealed that the SLN-negative patients enjoyed a significantly improved survival compared to SLN-positive patients (figure 25), and the histologic status of the SLN was the most powerful independent predictor of OS when compared to previously described primary tumor factors.[77], (table 10). Several similar analyses have since been published from large single institutional as well as multicentered experiences demonstrating that SLN status is the most powerful independent predictor of

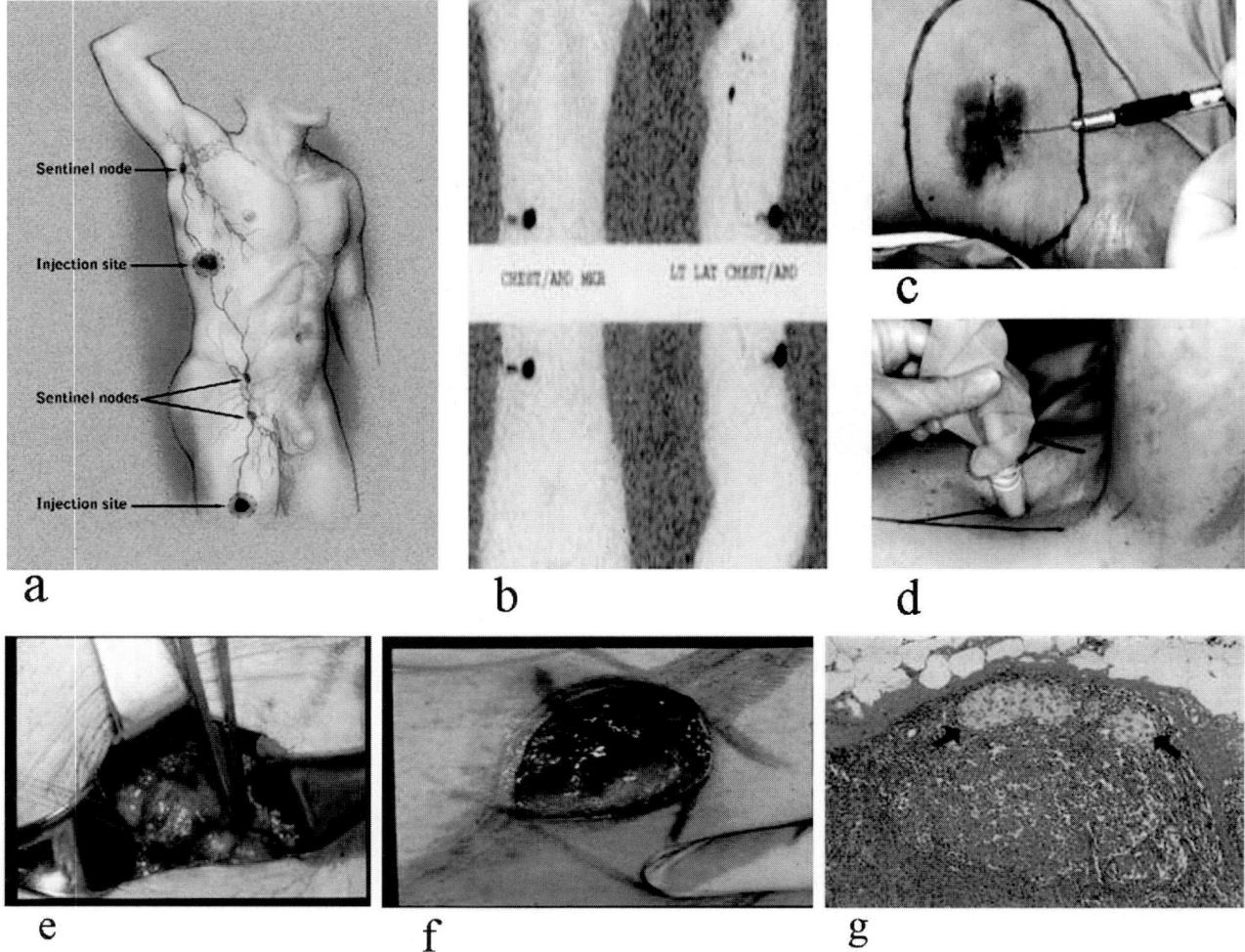

Figure 23 Lymphatic mapping and Sentinel Lymph Node Concept and Technique. The SLN concept is illustrated demonstrating potential afferent drainage patterns from primary tumor sites to the first draining nodes (sentinel node) in the regional basins in (a). Lymphoscintigraphy (b) is an important component of the procedure which identifies nodal basin(s) at risk for primary melanomas arising in ambiguous lymphatic drainage sites and the number sentinel nodes in the basin. In (b) lymphatic drainage from the low back is to the axilla rather thn the closer inguinal basin. Injection of isosulfan blue intradermally around biopsy site in (c), Transcutaneous localizaTion of SLN using gamma detection probe in (d), exploration of nodal basin and visualization of SLN in (e) and (f) and histologic detection of occult metastases in subcapsular sinus in (g)

survival in the clinically node negative primary melanoma patients.[78–80]

Rationale for SLN Biopsy

The original motivation to study SLN biopsy was to resolve the long-standing surgical controversy of how to approach the clinically node-negative regional lymph node basins. Subsequently, results of clinical trials demonstrating survival benefits[52,53] and improved regional disease control afforded by application of node dissection in patients with microscopic nodal involvement and improved survival for the use of adjuvant interferon in node-positive patients[81] provided addi-

tional motivation to incorporate SLN biopsy in the management of stage I and II patients.

Does early node dissection impart a survival benefit?

The potential for improved survival with early node dissection was the goal for the routine application of ELND as part of the initial management of newly diagnosed stage I and II patients. The question of survival impact with the use of ELND relative to nodal observation and therapeutic dissection for those patients who develop clinically detectable nodal disease has been evaluated in four prospective randomized trials. The first

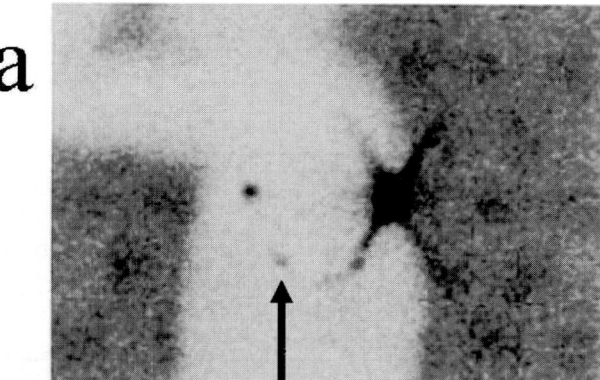

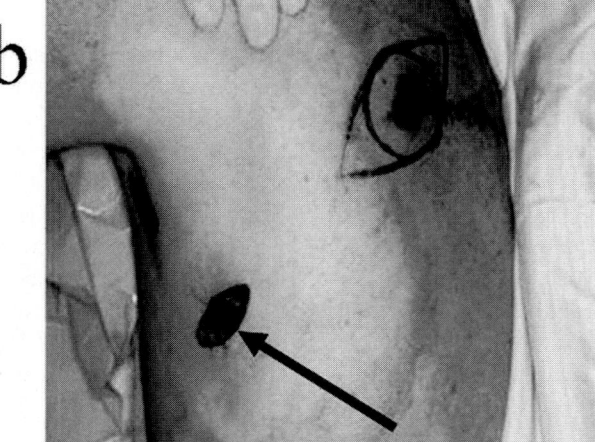

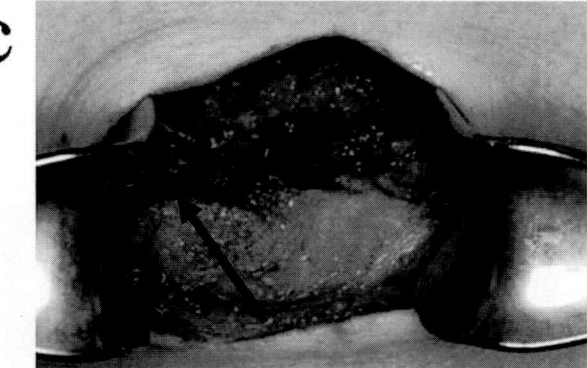

Figure 24 Intransit sentinel node. Lymphoscinitgraphy (a) shows lymphatic drainage pattern from injection site over left upper back to the ipsilateral axilla and an intransit sentinel node (arrow) over the scapular spine. Intra-operative photograph (b)showing the primary site over the upper back and sentinel node biopsy sites in the axilla and intransit region (arrow). Close-up view of exposed intransit node (arrow) with blue afferent channel.

2 trials (one from the World Health Organization and one from the Mayo Clinic[50,51] performed in the 1970s and prior to knowledge concerning primary tumor prognostic factors, demonstrated no survival advantage.

Table 9 Incidence of SLN metastases according to primary tumor factors

Tumor Thickness (mm)	Total No. Patients (N)	Positive SLN		
		All (%)	non-Ulcerated (%)	ulcerated (%)
≤ 1.00	326	4.2	3.9	12.5
1.01–2.00	490	11.4	10.8	21.2
2.01–4.00	310	28.5	23.1	37.0
4.01+	190	45.5	31.2	55.4
Total	1316	17.4	11.9	37.0

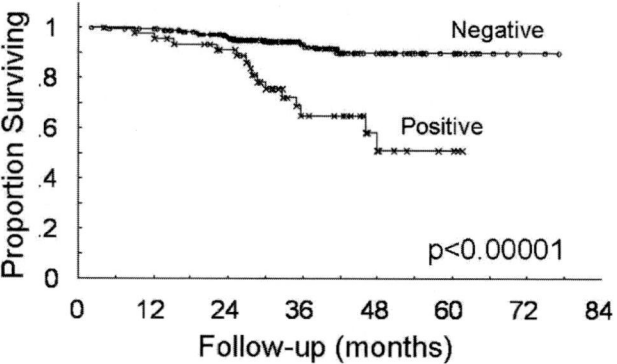

Figure 25 Melanoma specific survival of stage I & II patients according to SLN status.

Accordingly, ELND was strongly contested and largely abandoned. These trials were subsequently criticized because the study populations were at low risk for occult nodal disease and therefore unlikely to benefit from the surgical treatment being tested. Two additional ELND trials were performed targeting the higher-risk clinically node-negative patients.[52,53] Trends for improved survival following ELND were observed in both trials; however, these differences were not statistically significant. While many concluded that early treatment of nodal metastases had little impact on disease progression, others suggested that these trials were underpowered because only the 20% of patients harboring nodal disease could potentially benefit from the procedure.[1] Long-term results published

Table 10 Prognostic Factors Influencing Disease-Specific Survival in Stage I & II Patients Undergoing SLN Biopsy

Prognostic Factor	Multiple covariate		
	Univariate	Hazard Ratio	p-value
Age	NS	-	NS
Sex	NS	-	NS
Axial location	.03	-	NS
Tumor thickness	<.0001	1.1	.04
Clark level > III	.001	2.3	.01
Ulceration	<.0001	3.3	<.0001
SLN status	<.0001	6.5	<.0001

in 1998 from the WHO ELND Trial, which included patients with trunk primaries > 1.5 mm, demonstrated that patients with microscopic nodal disease in the ELND treatment arm experienced improved OS compared to patients who developed clinical adenopathy after randomization to excision alone.[52] Results published in 2000 from the Intergroup ELND Trial in which patients with melanomas 1 to 4 mm in thickness were studied, demonstrated that prospectively stratified subgroups (1 to 2 mm and all non-ulcerated primaries) derived a survival benefit with ELND[53]. While OS rates for the entire study cohorts in both trials were not statistically different, confirming that not all patients can benefit from ELND, these studies do suggest that specific subsets of patients (most notably those with microscopic nodal disease and possibly additional patients with nodal disease undetected by routine histologic techniques) can benefit from earlier dissections. These data offer evidence-based credence to the theoretical concerns of delaying the lymphadenectomy until palpable nodal disease develops and supports the selective lymphadenectomy approach.

The survival impact of the selective lymphadenectomy strategy, using SLN biopsy as an alternative to ELND, was formally studied in a prospective randomized multicentered international trial comparing the outcomes of nodal observation after wide excision to SLN biopsy and completion dissection for patients with microscopic nodal involvement.[79] The design and primary and secondary endpoints of the Multi-center Selective Lymphadenectomy Trial-1 (MSLT-1) are schematized in figure 26. The results of the 3rd interim analysis of the MSLT-1 were recently published in the NEJM[79] Data were available for 1,269 patients. In the biopsy group, the presence of metastases in the SLN was the most important prognostic factor. The 5-year melanoma-specific survival rate was 72.3 ± 4.6% among patients with tumor-positive SLNs and 90.2 ± 1.3% among those with tumor-negative SLNs (P <0.001), confirming the previously reported observations from several other groups. While melanoma-specific death rate at 5 years was similar in the two groups (13.8% in the observation group and 12.5% in the biopsy group), as was melanoma-specific survival rate at 3 years (90.1 ± 1.4% and 93.2 ± 0.9%, respectively) and 5 years (86.6 ± 1.6% and 87.1 ± 1.3%, respectively)While no overall survival advantage was observed when comparing the entire cohort of patients randomized to SLN biopsy compared to those patients who received a wide excision only and nodal observation, a small but statistically different disease-free survival advantage was observed (78.3 ± 1.6% versus 73.1 ± 2.1%, hazard ratio [HR] 0.74, 95% CI 0.59–0.93; P = 0.009). The incidence of SLN micrometastases was 16% while the rate of relapse

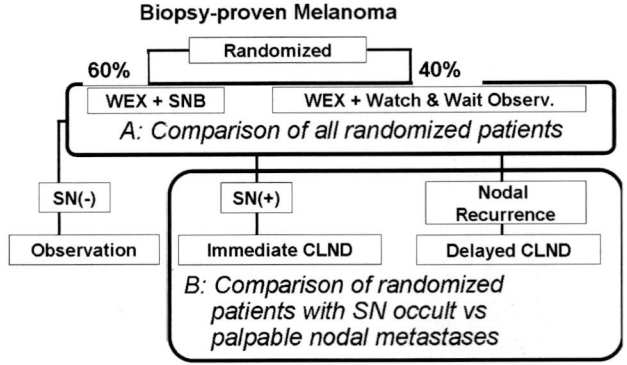

Figure 26 Treatment algorithm for recently completed Multicenter Selective Lymphadenectomy Trial-1

in regional nodes in the observation group was 15.6%. The mean number of tumor-involved nodes at lymphadenectomy was 1.4 in the SNB group and 3.3 in the observation group (P <0.001). A pronounced overall survival advantage was observed when the analysis was performed including only the node positive patients. Compared to the patients who underwent a therapeutic (delayed dissection) for clinical nodal failure after being randomized to nodal observation, the SLN positive patients enjoyed an improved 5-year survival of 20% (72.3 ± 4.6% versus 52.4 ± 5.9%; HR for death 0.51, 95% CI 0.32–0.81; P = 0.004) as shown in figure 27.

The interim results of the MSLT-I Trial provide important insights into the value of selective lymphadenectomy compared with delayed lymphadenectomy. The lack of an overall survival difference between the two treatment arms is not surprising. This trial suffers from the same limitations as the ELND trials: being underpowered because of the low percentage of patients (16%

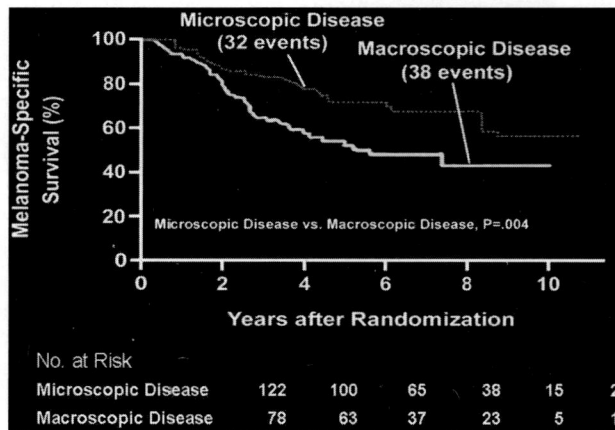

Figure 27 Melanoma-specific survival curves of node positive patients in the MSLT-1 trial. SLN positive patients enjoyed better survival than patients randomized to receive nodal observation and underwent node dssection after developing clinically involved nodes.

in this trial) who could benefit from complete lympha-denectomy. Assuming that early lymphadenectomy for SLN-positive patients is associated with an 20% survival benefit, one would predict an overall survival advantage of no more than 3.2% compared with delayed lympha-denectomy. Nonetheless, survival differences can emerge with longer follow-up, particularly since disease-free survival differences have already been reported. If future events follow the patterns observed in the two ELND trials, more recurrences in the nodal observation arm may develop over time than in the SNB arm.

The results of the secondary survival analysis compar-ing SLN-positive patients with those who developed clinically palpable nodes following nodal observation are particularly noteworthy. The improved survival of the SLN-positive group not only corroborates the results of the WHO trial but also supports the concept that—if left intact—microscopic nodal disease progresses and is associated with a worse prognosis. In some patients, therefore, increasing nodal burden can be a source of systemic dissemination; early treatment of nodal disease can favorably alter the natural history of their disease.

Regional Disease Control

The most common first recurrence in primary melanoma patients initially treated with excision of the primary site alone is palpable lymph node metastases. These patients are generally treated with a TLND for attempts at cure and regional control of disease. Reported in-basin, post-dissection failure rates range from 9 to 50% depending on a variety of factors, including basin site, number and size of involved nodes, and presence of extracapsular extension.[82–86] In-basin recurrences are very difficult to treat surgically and may be the source of significant morbidity in the form of pain, severe lymphedema, venous obstruction, skin ulceration, nerve involvement, and bleeding. In-basin failures in patients treated with ELND and found to harbor microscopic disease, occur in less than 10% of patients and reported to be even lower after completion dissection in SLN-positive patients[87,88]. The potential for improved regional disease control when dissections are performed for microscopic disease further supports the use of SLN biopsy.

HISTOLOGIC EXAMINATION OF SLNS

The fundamental goal of SLN biopsy is to accurately stage the regional basin. This is accomplished first by the accurate identification and complete surgical removal of all the SLNs from the appropriate nodal basins at risk, and then by the careful histologic examination of these nodes. Although the definition of careful histologic examination continues to evolve, it is clear that as

pathologic scrutiny becomes more extensive, it is more feasible to apply novel and sensitive techniques to one or two nodes (SLNs) rather than 20 to 30 nodes submitted following an ELND. Utilizing careful evaluation of the most likely nodes to contain metastatic disease, more accurate nodal staging is possible and is accomplished with little morbidity to the patient.

Historically, the standard approach for evaluating lymph nodes, and therefore initially applied to SLNs as well, was to bivalve a clinically negative node and stain a section from each half with hematoxylin and eosin (H&E). As a result, only a small percent of the lymph node(s) are sampled and likely explains why conven-tional histologic techniques underestimates the incidence of regional nodal disease in stage I and II patients. For example, the incidence of nodal failure following surgical excision alone for primary melanomas 2 to 4 mm is approximately 35%–50%, while the incidence of micro-scopic nodal disease as determined by ELND or SLN biopsy specimens, when applying the routine pathologic technique of bivalving the nodes, is approximately 25 to 40% While subsequent nodal failure may in part result from clinically occult intransit disease, several lines of evidence support the concept that nodal disease is more often present at diagnosis than is demonstrated by conventional histology: 1) step sectioning (ie, better sampling) improves the ability to detect microscopic disease,[59] 2) 80% of patients who develop nodal basin failure after a negative SLN biopsy initially assessed by routine pathology are determined to be node positive following more careful analysis of the paraffin blocks[59,89] and, 3) evaluation of SLNs using the reverse transcrip-tase-polymerase chain reaction (PCR) to detect the presence of messenger-RNA encoding for melanoma-specific proteins (ie, tyrosinase) as potential surrogate markers of nodal disease results in higher SLN-positive rates[90–92] Reports indicate that essentially all H&E positive SLNs and anywhere from 25 to 50% of H&E negative SLNs are PCR positive. While preliminary clinical correlation studies demonstrate that the PCR positive-H&E-negative group exhibit recurrence rates intermediate between the PCR-negative and H&E-positive patients[90–93], long term follow-up failed to demonstrate an overall decreased survival in the PCR+ patients compared to the PCR negative patients in two recently published series.[93,94] As histologic techniques become more sensitive, specificity may be compromised, but the more careful and complete the evaluation of SLNs, the more likely we are to define a true and homogeneous SLN-negative subset.

Current recommendations include multiple H&E sections and immunohistolgy using HMB-45 and MART-1, but established standards are still in evolution[89,95]. Frozen section at the time of SLN biopsy probably reduces the sensitivity and is therefore not recommended,[96] but imprint touch cytology performed on multiple sections of the SLN at the time of the procedure can accurately detect microscopic disease in a significant percentage with occult metastasesand facilitate same day completion dissections without compromising the formal permanent histological examination[97]. PCR evaluation at the present should only be used in the setting of a clinical trial.

Patient Selection for SLN Biopsy

Candidates for SLN biopsy include newly diagnosed primary, clinically node-negative patients predicted to be at intermediate or high-risk of harboring occult nodal disease, based on primary tumor characteristics.[72,73] Specific percent risk thresholds are still in question, but tumor thickness thresholds of 1 mm have gained wide consensus. The routine use of SLN biopsy in patients with thin (<1 mm) is not cost effective because of the overall low risk of nodsal involvement in this group[98]. However, a selective approach in patients with thin melanomas based on the presence of Clark level IV and/ or ulceration, is rational, as these two factors were the most powerful predictors of recurrence in the thin melanoma patients in the recent AJCC analysis[49]. Simply stated, stage IB and higher may be offered SLN biopsy. Other primary tumor prognostic factors commonly used in the decision process in the thin melanoma patients are vertical growth phase. An emerging important primary tumor risk factor for SLN involvement is the presence and number of miitotic figures in the vertical growth phase as a surrogate for aggressive biology.[99,100] In a study from the University of Pennsylvania, those patients with thin melanomas of at least 0.76mm and exhibiting 1 or more mitotic figures per mm^2 the incidence SLN metasteses was 12.5%[100] Increasingly, the presence of mitotic figures is being used to identify the higher risk subset of patients as candidates for SLN biopsy.

It should be emphasized that SLN biopsy is also appropriate for patients with thick melanomas (> 4 mm) even though this group is also at high risk for distant disease, as recently published experiences from more than one center demonstrates that SLN status is the single most important independent predictor of survival.[101–103]

Other clinical scenarios arise where SLN biopsy may be useful: 1) in patients who develop a true local recurrence subsequent to a relatively narrow excision as prior treatment of a primary melanoma; 2) for patients in which the exact tumor thickness cannot be ascertained because of improper placement in the paraffin block, resulting in tangential sectioning when tumor is present at the base secondary to a superficial shave biopsy; when

a manipulation such as cryotherapy or cauterization has been performed on the same lesion prior to the diagnosis of melanoma, 3) when the pathologic diagnosis of an atypical melanocytic lesion is ambiguous but may possibly include a primary melanomas >1 mm in the differential diagnosis[104]; or 4) for patients who have already received a formal wide excision with or without a skin graft and then wish to have accurate assessment of their draining lymph node basins. In this latter situation the accuracy of the technique is in question because the lymphatic drainage of the remaining skin may be different than the skin that existed immediately adjacent to the original primary melanoma. A few small published series compared the incidence of positive SLNs in groups of patients who had already undergone a 1 cm or wider excision to patients who had intact lesions or only an excisional biopsy for diagnosis. The patient groups were matched in terms of primary tumor factors and the incidence of positive SLNs was similar, suggesting that SLN biopsy may still be accurate in these patients.[105]

IS COMPLETION DISSECTION IN PATIENTS WITH A POSITIVE SLN NECESSARY?

This is the next important question that needs to be asked and answered in respect to SLN biopsy. Only 12% – 25% of patients with a positive SLN will be found to have additional microscopic nodal disease within non-sentinel nodes removed by a subsequent therapeutic dissection.[106,107] These data must be viewed with some concern of underestimating disease, as the pathologic techniques used to evaluate additional non-SLN(s) removed through a therapeutic lymphadenectomy procedure has been limited to bisecting lymph nodes rather than multiple step section or special histochemical stains. An international randomized trial (MSLT-2) is currently accruing patents using the basic framework design of a randomization to therapeutic node dissection versus nodal basin observation after a positive SLN biopsy. This trial will answer the following questions: 1) the incidence of nodal failure after removal of a positive SLN in the absence of a completion dissection, 2) the incidence and predictors of additional positive nodes in the same basin, and 3) the survival impact if any, for completion dissection. Some surgeons are already inconsistently omitting the completion dissection in SLN positive patients and others are selectively not recommending completion dissection based on published predictors of non-SLN involvement including patients with primary tumors < 2mm and SLN tumor burden of < 2mm in diameter. Such practices outside of a clinical trial should be discouraged until evidence is available supporting it's safety, and therefore completion dissection should be considered the current standard of care.

CONCLUDING COMMENTS

SLN biopsy is proven to accurately stage the regional lymph node basins in stage I and II melanoma patients with little morbidity and promotes the selective application of formal node dissections. The SLN-positive patients are then treated when the nodal tumor burden is microscopic, optimizing the chance for long-term survival and durable regional control. With the introduction of more sensitive histologic techniques, SLN biopsy offers the opportunity to more accurately stage patients and defines a more pure and homogeneous node-negative population The node-positive patients can then receive standard adjuvant therapy or participate in prospective clinical trials assessing the value of novel adjuvant therapy regimens. The low risk patients can then be safely spared the morbidity of additional surgery and adjuvant therapy. Until molecular studies are readily available and have the ability to accurately determine the metastatic phenotype in primary melanomas, SLN biopsy currently offers the opportunity to accomplish the aforementioned goals in managing stage I and II patients: optimizing the chance for cure, providing durable regional control, accurate staging, and minimizing treatment morbidity.

References

1. Ross MI. Surgical management of stage I and II melanoma patients: Approach to the regional lymph node basin. Seminars in Surgical Oncology 1996;12:394–401.

2. Pringle JA. A method of operation in melanotic tumours of the skin. Edinb Med J 1908;23:496–499.

3. Bono A, et al. Ambulatory narrow excision for thin melanoma (< or = 2 mm): results of a prospective study. Eur J Cancer 1997;33(8):1330–2.

4. Handley WS. The pathology of melanotic growths in relation to their operative treatment. Lancet 1907; i(927):1907.

5. Olsen G. The malignant melanoma of the skin. New theories based on a study of 500 cases. Acta Chir Scand Suppl 1966;365:1–222.

6. Wong CK. A study of melanocytes in the normal skin surrounding malignant melanomata. Dermatologica 1970; 141(3):215–25.

7. Breslow A, Macht SD. Optimal size of resection margin for thin cutaneous melanoma. Surg Gynecol Obstet 1977; 145(5):691–2.

8. Balch CM, et al. Tumor thickness as a guide to surgical management of clinical stage I melanoma patients. Cancer 1979;43(3):883–8.

9. Kelly JW, et al. The frequency of local recurrence and microsatellites as a guide to reexcision margins for cutaneous malignant melanoma. Ann Surg 1984; 200(6):759.

10. Cosimi AB, et al. Conservative surgical management of superficially invasive cutaneous melanoma. Cancer 1984; 53(6):1256–9.

11. Elder DE, et al. Optimal resection margin for cutaneous malignant melanoma. Plast Reconstr Surg 1983;71(1):66–72.

12. Goldman LI, Byrd R. Narrowing resection margins for patients with low-risk melanoma. Am J Surg 1988; 155(2):242–4.

13. Cascinelli N, Van Der Esch EP, Breslow A. The probelm of resection margins. Eur J Cancer 1980;16:1079.

14. Day CL Jr, et al. Narrower margins for clinical stage I malignant melanoma. N Engl J Med 1982;306(8):479–82.

15. O'Rourke MG, Altmann C. R. Melanoma recurrence after excision. Is a wide margin justified? Ann Surg 1993; 217(1):2–5.

16. Milton GW, Shaw HM, McCarthy WH. Resection margins for melanoma. Aust N Z J Surg 1985; 55(3):225–6.

17. Khayat D, Rixe O, Martin G, et al. Surgical margins in cutaneous melanoma (2 cm versus 5 cm for lesions measuring less than 2.1-mm thick). Cancer 2003;97:1941–1946.

18. Veronesi U, et al. Thin stage I primary cutaneous malignant melanoma. Comparison of excision with margins of 1 or 3 cm. N Engl J Med 1988;318(18):1159–62.

19. Veronesi U, Cascinelli N. Narrow excision (1-cm margin). A safe procedure for thin cutaneous melanoma. Arch Surg 1991;126(4):438–41.

20. Cascinelli N. Margin of resection in the management of primary melanoma. Semin Surg Oncol 1998;14(4):272–5.

21. Ringborg U, et al. Resection margins of 2 versus 5 cm for cutaneous malignant melanoma with a tumor thickness of 0.8 to 2.0 mm: randomized study by the Swedish Melanoma Study Group. Cancer 1996;77(9):1809–14.

22. Cohn-Cedermark G, et al. Long term results of a randomized study by the Swedish Melanoma Study Group on 2-cm versus 5-cm resection margins for patients with cutaneous melanoma with a tumor thickness of 0.8–2.0 mm. Cancer 2000;89(7):1495–501.

23. Marsden JR. *Malignant melanoma excision margins. Melanoma Study Group.* Lancet 1993;341(8838):184.

24. Balch CM, et al. Efficacy of 2-cm surgical margins for intermediate-thickness melanomas (1 to 4 mm). Results of a multi-institutional randomized surgical trial. Ann Surg 1993;218(3):262–7; discussion 267–9.

25. Karakousis CP, et al. Local recurrence in malignant melanoma: long-term results of the multiinstitutional randomized surgical trial. Ann Surg Oncol 1996;3(5):446–52.

26. Balch CM, et al. Long-term results of a prospective surgical trial comparing 2 cm vs. 4 cm excision margins for 740 patients with 1-4 mm melanomas. Ann Surg Oncol 2001;8(2):101–8.

27. Thomas JM, Newton-Bishop J, A'Hern R, et al. Excision margins in high-risk malignant melanoma. N Engl J Med 2004;350:757–766.

28. NIH Consensus Conference. Diagnosis and treatment of early melanoma. JAMA 1992;268:1314–1319.

29. Schneebaum S, et al. Cutaneous thick melanoma. Prognosis and treatment. Arch Surg 1987;122(6):707–11.

30. Spellman JE Jr, et al. Thick cutaneous melanoma of the trunk and extremities: an institutional review. Surg Oncol 1994;3(6):335–43.

31. Ball AS, Thomas J. Surgical management of malignant melanoma. Br Med Bull 1995;51(3):584–608.

32. Heaton KM, et al. Surgical margins and prognostic factors in patients with thick (>4mm) primary melanoma. Ann Surg Oncol 1998;5(4):322–8.

33. Johnson TM, Sondak VK. Melanoma margins: the importance and need for more evidence-based trials. Arch Dermatol 2004;140:1148–1150.

34. Bauer J, Bastian BC. Distinguishing melanocytic nevi from melanoma by DNA copy number changes: compartive genmoic hybridization as a reearch and diagnostic tool. Dermatol Ther 2006;19(1):40–9.

35. Quinn MJ, et al. Desmoplastic and desmoplastic neurotropic melanoma: experience with 280 patients. Cancer 1998;83(6):1128–35.

36. Tomicic J, Wanebo HJ. Mucosal melanomas. Surg Clin North Am 2003;83(2):237–52 Review.

37. Patrick RJ, Fenske NA, Messina JL. Primary mucosal melanoma. J Am Acad Dermatol 2007;56(5):828–34.

37a. Goldman S, Glimelium B, Pahlman L. Anorectal malignant melanoma in Sweden: Report of 49 patients. Dis Colon Rectum 1990;33:874–877.

38. Ross M, Pezzi C, Ptzzi T, et al. Patterns of failure in anorectal melanoma. Arch Surg 1990;125:313–316.

39. Brady MS, Kavolius JP, Quan SHQ. Anorectal melanoma: A 64-year experience at Memorial Sloan-Kettering Cancer Center. Dis Colon Rectum 1995;38:146–151.

40. Konstadoulakis MM, Ricaniadis N, Walsh D, et al. Malignant melanoma of the anorectal region. J Surg Oncol 1995;58:118–120.

41. Siegel B, Cohen D, Jacob ET. Surgical treatment of anorectal melanomas. Am J Surg 1983;146:336–338.

42. Bentzen SM, Overgaard J, Thames HD, et al. Clinical radiobiology of malignant melanoma. Radiother Oncol 1989;16:169–182.

43. Ballo MT, Gershenwald JE, Zagars GK, et al. Sphincter – sparing local excision an adjuvant radiation for anal-rectal melanoma. J clin Oncol 2002;20:4555–58.

44. Olsen G. Removal of fascia - Cause of more frequent metastases of malignant melanomas of the skin to regional lymph nodes? Cancer 1964;17:1159.

45. Kenady DE, Brown BW, McBride CM. Excision of under-lying fascia with a primary malignant melanoma: effect on recurrence and survival rates. Surgery 1982;92(4):615–8.

46. Cassileth BR, Lusk EJ, Tenaglia AN. Patients' perceptions of the cosmetic impact of melanoma resection. Plast Reconstr Surg 1983;71(1):73–5.

47. Zitelli JA, Brown C, Hanusa BH. Mohs micrographic surgery for the treatment of primary cutaneous melanoma. J Am Acad Dermatol 1997;37(2 Pt 1):236–45.

48. Zitelli JA, Brown CD, Hanusa BH. Surgical margins for excision of primary cutaneous melanoma. J Am Acad Dermatol 1997;37(3 Pt 1):422–9.

49. Balch CM, Soong SJ, Gershenwald JE, et al. Prognostic factors analysis of 17,600 melanoma patients: validation of the american joint committee on cancer melanoma staging system. J Clin Oncol 2001;19:3622–34.

50. Sim FH, Taylor WF, Pritchard DJ, Soule EH. Lymphadenectomy in the management of stage I malignant melanoma: A prospective randomized study. Mayo Clin Proc 1986;61:697.

51. Veronesi U, Adamus J, Bandiera DC, et al. Inefficacy of immediate node dissection in stage I melanoma of the limbs. N Engl J Med 1977;297:627.

52. Cascinelli N, Morabito A, Santinami M, MaKie RM, Belli F. Immediate or delayed dissection of regional nodes in patients with melanoma of the trunk: A randomised trial. The Lancet 1998;351(9105):793–796.

53. Balch CM, Soong S, Ross MI, Urist MM, Karakousis CP, Temple WJ, Mihm MC, Barnhill RL, Jewell WR, Wanebo HJ, Harrison R. Long-Term Results of a Multi-Institutional Randomized Trial Comparing Prognostic Factors and Surgical Results for Intermediate Thickness Melanomas (1.0 to 4.0 mm). Intergroup Melanoma Surgical Trial. Ann Surg Oncol March 2000;7(2):87–97.

54. Morton D, Wen D, Wong J, et al. Technical details of intraoperative lymphatic mapping for early stage melanoma. Archives Surg 1992;127:392–399.

55. Ross M, Reintgen D, Balch C. Selective lymphadenectomy: Emerging role for lymphatic mapping and sentinel node biopsy in the management of early stage melanoma. Semin Surg Oncol 1993;9:219–223.

56. Thompson J, McCarthy W, Bosch C, et al. Sentinel lymph node status as an indicator of the presence of metastatic

melanoma in regional lymph nodes. Melanoma Res 1995; 5:255–260.

57. Reintgen D, Cruse C, Wells K, et al. The orderly progression of melanoma nodal metastases. Ann Surg 1994;220:759–767.

58. Gerhsenwald JE, Tseng C-h, Thompson W, Mansfield PF, Lee JE, Bouvet M, et al. Improved sentinel lymph node localization in patients with primary melanoma with the use of radiolabeled colloid. Surgery 1998;124(2):203–210.

59. Gershenwald J, Colome M, Lee J, et al. Patterns of recurrence following a negative sentinel lymph node biopsy in 243 patients with stage I or II melanoma. J Clin Oncol 1998;16:2253–2260.

60. Uren R, Howman-Giles R, Thompson J, et al. Lymphoscintigraphy to identify sentinel lymph nodes in patients with melanoma. Melanoma Res 1994;4:395–399.

61. Berger DH, Feig BW, Podoloff D, Norman J, Cruse CW, Reintgen DS, Ross MI. Lymphoscintigraphy as a predictor of lymphatic drainage from cutaneous melanoma. Ann Surg Oncol 1997;4:247–251.

62. Albertini J, Cruse C, Rapaport D, et al. Intraoperative radiolymphoscintigraphy improves sentinel lymph node identification for patients with melanoma. Ann Surg 1996; 223:217–224.

63. Kapteijn BA, Nieweg OE, Liem I, Mooi W, Blam AJ, Muller SH, et al. Localizing the sentinel node in cutaneous melanoma: Gamma probe detection versus blue dye. Annals of Surgical Oncology 1997;4:156–160.

64. Krag D, Meijer S, Weaver D, et al. Minimal-access surgery for staging of malignant melanoma. Arch Surg 1995;130: 654–658.

65. Thompson JF, Uren RF, Shaw HM, McCarthy WH, Quin MJ, O'Brien CJ. Location of sentinel lymph nodes in patients with cutaneous melanoma: new insights into lymphatic anatomy. J Am Coll Surg August 1999; 189(2):195–204.

66. Uren RF, Thompson JF, Howman-Giles R. Sentinel nodes. Interval nodes, lymphatic lakes, and accurate sentinel node identification. Clin Nucl Med. March 2000; 25(3):234–236.

67. Uren RF, Thompson JF, Howman-Giles R, Shaw HM. Melanoma metastases in triangular intermuscular space lymph nodes. Ann Surg Oncol 1999 Dec;6(8):811.

68. Uren RF, Howman-Giles R, Thompson JF, McCarthy WH, Quinn MJ, Roberts JM, Shaw HM. Interval nodes: the forgotten sentinel nodes in patients with melanoma. Arch Surg. 2000 Oct;135(10):1168–72.

69. Sumner WE 3rd, Ross MI, Mansfield PF, Lee JE, Prieto VG, Schacherer CW, Gershenwald JE. Implications of lymphatic drainage to unusual sentinel lymph node sites in patients with primary cutaneous melanoma. Cancer July 2002;95(2):354–360.

70. Thompson JF. The Sydney Melanoma Unit experience of sentinel lymphadenectomy for melanoma. Ann Surg Oncol. 2001 Oct;8(9 Suppl):44S–47S.

71. Cascinelli N, Belli F, Santinami M, Fait V, Testori A, Ruka W, Cavaliere R, Mozzillo N, Rossi CR, MacKie RM, Nieweg O, Pace M, Kirow K. Sentinel lymph node biopsy in cutaneous melanoma: the WHO Melanoma Program experience. Ann Surg Oncol July, 2000;7(6):469–474.

72. McMasters KM, Wong SL, Edwards MJ, Ross MI, Chao C, Noyes RD, Viar V, Cerrito PB, Reintgen DS. Factors that predict the presence of sentinel lymph node metastasis in patients with melanoma. Surgery August 2001; 130(f2):151–156.

73. Rousseau DL Jr, Ross MI, Johnson MM, Prieto VG, Lee JE, Mansfield PF, Gershenwald JE. Revised AJCC staging criteria accurately predict sentinel lymph node positivity in clinically node-negative melanoma patients. Ann Surg Oncol January 2003;10(5):569–574.

74. Sondak VK, Taylor Jm, Sabel MS, et al. Mitotic rate and younger age are predictors of sentinel lymph node positivty: lessons learned from the generation of a probabilistic model. Ann surg oncol 2004;11(3):247–58.

75. Thompson JF, Shaw HM. Should tumor mitotic rate and patient age as well as tumor thickness, be used to select melanoma patients for sentinel node biopsy? Ann surg oncol 2004;11(3):233–35.

76. Balch CM, Buzaid AC, Soong SJ, Atkins MB, Cascinelli N, Coit DG, Fleming ID, Gershenwald JE, Houghton A Jr, Kirkwood JM, McMasters KM, Mihm MF, Morton DL, Reintgen DS, Ross MI, Sober A, Thompson JA, Thompson JF. Final version of the american joint committee on cancer staging system for cutaneous melanoma. J Clin Oncol 2001, Aug 15;19(16):3635–3638.

77. Gershenwald JE, Thompson W, Mansfield PF, Lee JE, Colome MI, Tseng CH, Lee JJ, Balch CM, Reintgen DS, Ross MI. Multi-Institutional Melanoma Lymphatic Mapping Experience: The Prognostic Value of Sentinel Lymph Node Status in 612 Stage I or II Melanoma Patients. Journal of Clinical Oncology March 1999;17(3):976–983.

78. Clary BM, Brady MS, Lewis JJ, Coit DG. Sentinel lymph node biopsy in the management of patients with primary cutaneous melanoma: review of a large single-institutional experience with an emphasis on recurrence. Ann Surg. 2001 Feb;233(2):250–8.

79. Morton DL, et al. Sentnel-node biopsy or nodal observation in melanoma. N Engl J Med 2006 Sep 28; 355(13):1307–17.

80. Cascinelli N, Bombardieri E, Bufalino R, et al. Sentinel and nonsentinel node status in stage IB and II melanoma patients: two-step prognostic indicators of survival. J Clin Oncol 2006;24(27):4464–71.

82. Lee RJ, Gibbs JF, Proulx GM, et al. Nodal basin recurrence following lymph node dissection for melanoma implica-

tions for adjuvant radiotherapy. Int J Radiat Oncol Biol Phys 2000;46:467–474.

84. O'Brien CJ, Coates AS, Petersen-Schaefer K, et al. Experience with 998 cutaneous melanomas of the head and neck over 30 years. Am J Surg 1991;162:310–314.

85. Calabro A, Singletary SE, Balch CM. Patterns of relapse in 1001 consecutive patients with melanoma nodal metastases. Arch Surg 1989;124:1051–5.

86. Ballo MT, Strom EA, Zagars GK, et al. Adjuvant irradiation for axillary metastases from malignant melanoma. Int J Radiat Oncol Biol Phys 2002;52:964–72.

87. Slingluff CL Jr, Stidham KR, Ricci WM, et al. Surgical management of regional lymph nodes in patients with melanoma: experience with 4682 patients (see comments). Ann Surg 1994;219:120–130.

88. Gershenwald JE, Berman RS, Porter G, Mansfield PF, lee JE, Ross MI. Regional Nodal Basin Control is not Compromised by Previous Sentinel Lymph Node Biopsy in Patients with Melanoma. Ann Surg Oncol April 2000; 7(3):226–231.

89. Cook MG, Green MA, Anderson B, et al. The development of optiml pathological assessment of sentinel lymph nodes for Melanoma. J Pathol 2003;200:314–319.

90. Wang X, Heller R, VanVoorhis N, et al. Detection of submicroscopic lymph node metastases with polymerase chain reaction in patients with malignant melanoma. Ann Surg 1994;220(6):768–774.

91. Shivers SC, Wang X, Li W, Joseph E, Messina J, Glass LF, De Conti R, Cruse CW, Berman C, Fenske NA, Lyman GH, Reintgen DS. Molecular staging of malignant melanoma: correlation with clinical outcome. JAMA 1998, Oct. 28;280(16):1410–1415.

92. Reintgen D, Balch C, Kirkwood J, Ross M. Recent advances in the care of the patient with malignant melanoma. Ann Surg 1997;225:1–14.

93. Kammila US, Ghoussein R, Bhattacharya S, Coit DG. Serial follow-up and the prognostic significance of reverse transcriptase-polymerase chain reaction-staged sentinel lymph nodes from melanoma patients. J Clin oncol 2004; 22:3989–96.

94. Scoggins CR, Ross MI, Reintgen DS, et al. Prospective multi-instituional study of reverse transcription polymerase chain reaction for molecular staging of melanoma. J Clin Oncol 2006, Jun 20;24(18).

95. Clark SH, Prieto VG. Processing of sentinel lymph nodes for detection of metastatic melanoma: Proposal for an alternative method to serial sectioning. Lab Invest 2001;14:66A.

96. Stojadinovic A, Allen PJ, Clary BM, Busam KJ, Coit DG. Value of frozen-section analysis of sentinel lymph nodes for primary cutaneous malignant melanoma. Ann Surg. 2002 Jan, 235(1):92–8.

97. Soo V, Shen P, Pichardo R, et al. Intraoperative evaluation of sentinel lymph nodes for metastatic melanoma by imprint cytology. Ann surg oncol 2007;5:1612–7.

98. Agnese DM, Abdessalam SF, Burak WE, et al. Cost-effectivenss of sentinel lymph node biopsy in thin melanomas. Surgery 2003;134:542–8.

99. Thompson JF, Shaw HM. Sentinel node metastasis from thin melanomas with vertical growth phase. Ann Surg Oncol. 2000 May;7(4):251–2.

100. Kesmodel SB, Karakousis GC, Botbyl JD, et al. Mitotic rate as a predictor of sentinel lymph node posistivity in patients with thin melanomas. Ann surg oncol 2005; 12(6):1–10.

101. Gershenwald JE, Mansfield PF, Lee JE, Ross MI. Role for Lymphatic Mapping and Sentinel Lymph Node Biopsy in Patients with Thick (> or = 4 mm) Primary Melanoma. Ann Surg Oncol March 2000;7(2):160–165.

102. Jacobs IA, Chang CK, Salti GI. Role of sentinel lymph node biopsy in patients with thick (>4mm) primary melanoma. Am Surg 2004;70(1):59–62.

103. Carlson GW, Murray DR, Hestly A, et al. Sentinel lymph node mapping for thick (>or=4 mm) melanoma: should we be doing it? Ann Surg Oncol 2003;10(4): 408–15.

104. Lohmann CM, Coit DG, Brady MS, Berwick M, Busam KJ. Sentinel lymph node biopsy in patients with diagnostically controversial spitzoid melanocytic tumors. Am J Surg Pathol. 2002 Jan, 26(1):47–55.

105. Gannon CJ, Rousseau DL, Ross MI, et al. Accuracy of lymphatic mapping and sentinel node biopsy after previous wide local excision in patients with primary melanoma. Cancer 2006;107(11):2647–52.

106. Vylsteke RJCLM, Borgstein PJ, van Leeuwen PAM, et al. Sentinel lymph node tumor load: An independent predictor of additional lymph node involvement and survival in melanoma. Ann Surg Oncol 2005; 12:1–9.

107. Govindarajan A, Ghazarian DM, McCready DR, et al. Histological features of melanoma sentinel lymph node metastases associated with status of the completion lymphadenectomy and rate of subsequent relapse. Ann Surg Oncol 2007;14:906–12.

INDEX